Coders' Desk Reference
for Diagnoses

2007
4th Edition

Notice

Coders' Desk Reference for Diagnoses was conceived to be an accurate and authoritative source of information about coding and reimbursement issues. Every effort has been made to verify accuracy and information is believed reliable at the time of publication. Absolute accuracy cannot be guaranteed, however. This publication is made available with the understanding that the publisher is not engaged in rendering legal or other services requiring a professional license. Please address questions regarding this product to the Ingenix customer service department at:

1.800.INGENIX (464.3649) option 1

or email us at customerservice@ingenix.com.

Acknowledgments

The following staff contributed to the development and/or production of this book:

Anita Hart, RHIA, CCS, CCS-P, *Product Manager*
Mike Desposito, *Product Director and Client Relationships*
Karen Schmidt, BSN, *Technical Director*
Lynn Speirs, *Director, Editorial/Desktop Publishing*
Stacy Perry, *Desktop Publishing Manager*
Lisa Singley, *Project Manager*
Beth Ford, RHIT, CCS, *Clinical/Technical Editor*
Kerrie Hornsby, *Desktop Publishing Specialist*
Kate Holden, *Editor*

Copyright

Copyright 2006 Ingenix

All rights reserved. No part of this publication may be reproduced or transmitted in any form or by any means, electronic or mechanical, including photocopy, recording, or storage in a database or retrieval system, without the prior written permission of the publisher. Printed in the United States of America.

Made in the USA

ISBN 978-1-56337-921-5

About the Technical Editors

Beth Ford, RHIT, CCS

Ms. Ford is a clinical/technical editor for Ingenix. She has extensive background in both the professional and technical components of CPT/HCPCS and ICD-9-CM coding. Ms. Ford has served as a coding supervisor and coding consultant, as well as a health information management director. She is an active member of the American Heath Information Management Association (AHIMA).

Anita C. Hart, RHIA, CCS, CCS-P, *Product Manager*

Ms. Hart's experience includes conducting and publishing research in clinical medicine and human genetics for Yale University, Massachusetts General Hospital, and Massachusetts Institute of Technology. In addition, Ms. Hart has supervised medical records management, health information management, coding and reimbursement, and worker's compensation issues as the office manager for a physical therapy rehabilitation clinic. Ms. Hart is an expert in physician and facility coding, reimbursement systems, and compliance issues. Ms. Hart developed the ICD-9-CM Changes: An Insider's View. She has served as technical consultant for numerous other publications for hospital and physician practices. Currrently, Ms. Hart is the Product Manager for the ICD-9-CM and ICD-10-CM/PCS product lines.

Our Commitment to Accuracy

Ingenix is committed to producing accurate and reliable materials.

To report corrections, please visit www.ingenixonline.com/accuracy or email accuracy@ingenix.com. You can also reach customer service by calling 1.800.INGENIX (464.3649), option 1.

Contents

Introduction 1	070–079 Other Diseases Due to Viruses and Chlamydiae 169
Format 1	
ICD-9-CM Codes and Descriptions 1	080–088 Rickettsioses and Other Arthropod-borne Diseases 176
Additional Descriptors 2	
Narrative 2	090–099 Syphilis and Other Venereal Diseases 178
Coding Clinic References 2	
Documentation Issues 2	100–104 Other Spirochetal Diseases 182
Coding Clarification 2	110–118 Mycoses 183
Coding Scenarios 2	120–129 Helminthiases 186
Illustrations 2	130–136 Other Infectious and Parasitic Diseases 188
ICD-9-CM Conventions 3	
ICD-9-Conventions 3	137–139 Late Effects of Infectious and Parasitic Diseases 191
Three Volume Set 3	
Supplemental Classifications 3	**140–239 Neoplasms** **193**
Approaches to ICD-9-CM Coding 4	140–149 Malignant Neoplasm of Lip, Oral Cavity, and Pharynx 194
Rules of ICD-9-CM Reference 4	
Format 4	150–159 Malignant Neoplasm of Digestive Organs and Peritoneum 198
Typeface 4	
Punctuation 4	160–165 Malignant Neoplasm of Respiratory and Intrathoracic Organs 203
Notes 4	
Instructional Notes 5	170–176 Malignant Neoplasm of Bone, Connective Tissue, Skin, and Breast 207
Modifiers 5	
Abbreviations 5	
Cross-references 5	179–189 Malignant Neoplasm of Genitourinary Organs 211
Official ICD-9-CM Coding Guidelines 7	
Coding Guidelines 7	190–195 Malignant Neoplasm of Other and Unspecified Sites 216
ICD-9-CM Official Guidelines for Coding and Reporting 7	
	196–199 Secondary and Unspecified Malignant Neoplasms 220
Syndromes **53**	
Prefixes and Suffixes **111**	200–208 Malignant Neoplasm of Lymphatic and Hematopoietic Tissue 222
Prefixes 111	
Suffixes 114	210–212 Benign Neoplasms of Digestive and Respiratory System and Intrathoracic Organs 228
Abbreviations, Acronyms, and Symbols **117**	
Anatomy Charts **133**	
001–139 Infectious and Parasitic Diseases .. **143**	213–215 Benign Neoplasms of Bone, Connective, and Soft Tissues ... 229
001–009 Intestinal Infectious Diseases .. 143	
010–018 Tuberculosis 147	216–217 Benign Neoplasms of Integumentary System 230
020–027 Zoonotic Bacterial Diseases 150	
030–041 Other Bacterial Diseases 153	218–222 Benign Neoplasms of Genital Organs 231
042 Human Immunodeficiency Virus (HIV) Infection 160	
	224–225 Benign Neoplasms of Nervous System 232
045–049 Poliomyelitis and Other Non-arthropod-borne Viral Diseases of Central Nervous System 162	
	226–228 Benign Neoplasms of Other and Unspecified Sites 233
050–057 Viral Diseases Accompanied by Exanthem 163	230–234 Carcinoma In Situ 234
	235–238 Neoplasms of Uncertain Behavior 236
060–066 Arthropod-borne Viral Diseases. 167	

239	Neoplasms of Unspecified Nature...................238

240-279 Endocrine, Nutritional and Metabolic Diseases, and Immunity Disorders........241
240-246	Disorders of Thyroid Gland....241
250-259	Diseases of Other Endocrine Glands...................243
260-269	Nutritional Deficiencies.......253
270-279	Other Metabolic and Immunity Disorders..................255

280-289 Diseases of the Blood and Blood-Forming Organs.................265

290-319 Mental Disorders..............279
290-299	Psychoses 279
290-294	Organic Psychotic Conditions...279
295-299	Other Psychoses 283
300-316	Neurotic Disorders, Personality Disorders, and Other Nonpsychotic Mental Disorders............286
317-319	Mental Retardation 297

320-389 Diseases of the Nervous System and Sense Organs.......................299
320-326	Inflammatory Diseases of the Central Nervous System.............299
327	Organic Sleep Disorders.......303
330-337	Hereditary and Degenerative Diseases of the Central Nervous System....................305
338	Pain.....................310
340-349	Other Disorders of the Central Nervous System............311
350-359	Disorders of the Peripheral Nervous System............317
360-379	Disorders of the Eye and Adnexa 321
380-389	Diseases of the Ear and Mastoid Process 343

390-459 Diseases of the Circulatory System 353
390-392	Acute Rheumatic Fever 353
393-398	Chronic Rheumatic Heart Disease 354
401-405	Hypertensive Disease.........356
410-414	Ischemic Heart Disease 362
415-417	Diseases of Pulmonary Circulation.................371
420-429	Other Forms of Heart Disease ..372
430-438	Cerebrovascular Disease 380
440-448	Diseases of Arteries, Arterioles, and Capillaries..............386
451-459	Diseases of Veins and Lymphatics, and Other Diseases of Circulatory System................... 391

460-519 Diseases of the Respiratory System............................397
460-466	Acute Respiratory Infections ...397
470-478	Other Diseases of the Upper Respiratory Tract............400
480-487	Pneumonia and Influenza.....403
490-496	Chronic Obstructive Pulmonary Disease and Allied Conditions..405
500-508	Pneumoconioses and Other Lung Diseases Due to External Agents...................410
510-519	Other Diseases of Respiratory System 412

520-579 Diseases of the Digestive System..419
520-529	Diseases of Oral Cavity, Salivary Glands, and Jaws...........419
530-538	Diseases of Esophagus, Stomach, and Duodenum.............430
540-543	Appendicitis 437
550-553	Hernia of Abdominal Cavity....438
555-558	Noninfectious Enteritis and Colitis....................440
560-569	Other Diseases of Intestines and Peritoneum................442
570-579	Other Diseases of Digestive System 445

580-629 Diseases of the Genitourinary System............................451
580-589	Nephritis, Nephrotic Syndrome, and Nephrosis..............451
590-599	Other Diseases of Urinary System 461
600-608	Diseases of Male Genital Organs 468
610-611	Disorders of Breast 473
614-616	Inflammatory Disease of Female Pelvic Organs 474
617-629	Other Disorders of Female Genital Tract...............475

630-677 Complications of Pregnancy, Childbirth, and the Puerperium 483
630-633	Ectopic and Molar Pregnancy ..483
634-639	Other Pregnancy with Abortive Outcome..................485
640-649	Complications Mainly Related to Pregnancy................488
650-659	Normal Delivery, and Other Indications for Care in Pregnancy, Labor, and Delivery..........498
660-669	Complications Occurring Mainly in the Course of Labor and Delivery..................504

670–677	Complications of the Puerperium 508		905–909	Late Effects of Injuries, Poisonings, Toxic Effects, and Other External Causes 647
680–709 Diseases of the Skin and Subcutaneous Tissue 511			920–924	Contusion with Intact Skin Surface 649
680–686	Infections of Skin and Subcutaneous Tissue 511		925–929	Crushing Injury 650
690–698	Other Inflammatory Conditions of Skin and Subcutaneous Tissue 515		930–939	Effects of Foreign Body Entering Through Orifice............. 651
			940–949	Burns 652
700–709	Other Diseases of Skin and Subcutaneous Tissue 519		950–957	Injury to Nerves and Spinal Cord 655
			953–957	Injury to Nerve Roots, Peripheral, and Superficial Nerves 656
710–739 Diseases of the Musculoskeletal System and Connective Tissue. 525			958–959	Certain Traumatic Complications and Unspecified Injuries 657
710–719	Arthropathies and Related Disorders 525		960–979	Poisoning by Drugs, Medicinal and Biological Substances 658
720–724	Dorsopathies 537			
725–729	Rheumatism, Excluding the Back 542		980–989	Toxic Effects of Substances Chiefly Nonmedicinal as to Source 663
730–739	Osteopathies, Chondropathies, and Acquired Musculoskeletal Deformities 548		990–995	Other and Unspecified Effects of External Causes 666
			996–999	Complications of Surgical and Medical Care, NEC 669
740–759 Congenital Anomalies 555			**V01–V86 Supplementary Classification of Factors Influencing Health Status and Contact with Health Services 677**	
745–747	Congenital Anomalies of the Cardiovascular System 560			
760–779 Certain Conditions Originating in the Perinatal Peroid 579				
			V01–V06	Persons with Potential Health Hazards Related to Communicable Diseases 677
760–763	Maternal Causes of Perinatal Morbidity and Mortality 579			
764–779	Other Conditions Originating in the Perinatal Period 584		V07–V09	Persons with Need for Isolation, Other Potential Health Hazards and Prophylactic Measures 681
780–799 Symptoms, Signs, and Ill-Defined Conditions 597				
			V10–V19	Persons with Potential Health Hazards Related to Personal and Family History 683
780–789	Symptoms 597			
790–796	Nonspecific Abnormal Findings . 614			
797–799	Ill-Defined and Unknown Causes of Morbidity and Mortality 619		V20–V28	Persons Encountering Health Services in Circumstances Related to Reproduction and Development 690
800–999 Injury and Poisoning 621				
800–829	Fractures 621			
805–809	Fracture of Neck and Trunk. ... 624		V30–V39	Liveborn Infants According to Type of Birth 695
810–819	Fracture of Upper Limb 627			
820–829	Fracture of Lower Limb 630		V40–V49	Persons with a Condition Influencing Their Health Status. 697
830–839	Dislocation 632			
840–848	Sprains and Strains of Joints and Adjacent Muscles 634			
			V50–V59	Persons Encountering Health Services for Specific Procedures and Aftercare 703
850–854	Intracranial Injury, Excluding Those with Skull Fracture 635			
860–869	Internal Injury of Thorax, Abdomen, and Pelvis 637		V60–V68	Persons Encountering Health Services in Other Circumstances 708
870–879	Open Wound of Head, Neck, and Trunk 640			
890–897	Open Wound of Lower Limb. ... 644		V70–V82	Persons Without Reported Diagnosis Encountered During Examination and Investigation of Individuals and Populations ... 712
900–904	Injury to Blood Vessels 645			

V72–V82	Screening Exams............714	E878–E879	Surgical and Medical Procedures as the Cause of Abnormal Reaction of Patient or Later Complication, Without Mention of Misadventure at the Time of Procedure....747
V83–V84	Genetics..................721		
V85	Body mass index [BMI]........721		
V86	Estrogen receptor status......722		

E800–E999 Supplementary Classification of External Causes......................723

		E880–E888	Accidental Falls...........749
E800–E807	Railway Accidents..........723	E890–E899	Accidents Caused by Fire and Flames..................751
E810–E819	Motor Vehicle Traffic Accidents................725	E900–E909	Accidents due to Natural and Environmental Factors......753
E820–E825	Motor Vehicle Nontraffic Accidents................727	E910–E915	Accidents Caused by Submersion, Suffocation, and Foreign Bodies..................756
E826–E829	Other Road Vehicle Accidents................729	E916–E928	Other Accidents...........758
E830–E838	Water Transport Accidents...731	E930–E949	Drugs, Medicinal and Biological Substances Causing Adverse Effects in Therapeutic Use...762
E840–E845	Air and Space Transport Accidents................733		
E846–E848	Vehicle Accidents Not Elsewhere Classifiable...............734	E950–E959	Suicide and Self-Inflicted Injury..................768
E850–E858	Accidental Poisoning by Drugs, Medicinal Substances, and Biologicals...............736	E960–E969	Homicide and Injury Purposely Inflicted by Other Persons...770
		E970–E978	Legal Intervention.........772
		E979	Terrorism................773
E860–E869	Accidental Poisoning by Other Solid and Liquid Substances, Gases, and Vapors.........739	E980–E989	Injury Undetermined Whether Accidentally or Purposely Inflicted................774
E870–E876	Misadventures to Patients During Surgical and Medical Care....................744	E990–E999	Injury Resulting fromOperations of War....................777

Introduction

Coders' Desk Reference for Diagnoses is a comprehensive ICD-9-CM coding reference designed for medical offices, hospitals, health insurance companies, educators, and students who seek to expand their understanding of diagnostic coding. The goal is to enrich the user's clinical understanding of ICD-9-CM, so code selection becomes more accurate.

Unlike other ICD-9-CM references, Coders' Desk Reference for Diagnoses includes numeric codes in ICD-9-CM, from 001 to 999, V codes and E codes. In some cases, its narrative discusses clinical issues affecting code selection for comprehensive categories (diabetes, fractures) and in other cases provides code-specific information (sudden infant death syndrome, hydatidiform mole). Because the book does not include the comprehensive index found in the official ICD-9-CM, it does not replace use of an official code book. However, used in conjunction with a code book, Coders' Desk Reference for Diagnoses will provide an unparalleled clinical roadmap to code selection.

Format

Coders' Desk Reference for Diagnoses begins with sections on the history of diagnostic coding; ICD-9-CM conventions, ICD-9-CM coding guidelines; syndromes; common prefixes and suffixes; common abbreviations, acronyms, and symbols; and anatomy charts. It then follows the organization of ICD-9-CM, looking at diseases and their codes beginning with Infectious and Parasitic Diseases (Chapter 1) through Injury and Poisoning (Chapter 17), in numeric order. The V code and E code supplemental classifications are included as well. The basic format of the book is to provide clinical coding support, with illustrations, narrative, definitions, and other resources that will help the user working from the medical record.

ICD-9-CM Codes and Descriptions

The codes in Coders' Desk Reference for Diagnoses are organized in hierarchical context, appearing within an appropriate three-digit rubric. All three-digit rubrics appear in a capitalized format. If the three-digit code is valid, an icon (OK) appears next to the code to indicate it is a valid code for use on a claim form. For example:

129   Intestinal parasitism, unspecified OK

Note that (OK) next to the description with 129 indicates that code 129 represents a valid ICD-9-CM code. There are fewer than 100 valid three-digit codes in ICD-9-CM.

Though all three-digit categories appear in Coders' Desk Reference for Diagnoses, invalid four-digit categories have been eliminated to reduce confusion regarding code choices. With the exception of valid three-digit codes, all other valid codes in Coders' Desk Reference for Diagnoses appear at the same indent, unlike the presentation in ICD-9-CM itself. For example, all valid codes that occur in rubric 088 Other Arthropod-borne diseases, appear as follows:

088.0	Bartonellosis — Bartonella bacilliformis; sandflies; Andes
088.81	Lyme disease — Borrelia burgdorferi; ticks, United States
	AHA: Q2, 1989, 10; Q3, 1990, 14; Q4, 1991, 15
088.82	Babesiosis — Babesia; ticks
	AHA: Q4, 1993, 23
088.89	Other specified arthropod-borne diseases — not elsewhere classified
088.9	Arthropod-borne disease, unspecified — unknown

Note that some valid codes in rubric 088 are four-digit codes and some valid codes in this rubric are five-digit codes. Only valid codes are included.

Should there be information within a four-digit subclassification that applies to all five-digit codes within that subclassification, the invalid four-digit code will appear with a ⌐sth icon, to differentiate it from the valid five-digit codes that follow. For example:

722.8 ⌐sth   Postlaminectomy syndrome

Postlaminectomy syndrome is a complex of symptoms following laminectomy surgery. It includes conditions and syndromes described as postfusion, postmicrosurgery, and postchemonucleolysis.

722.80	Postlaminectomy syndrome, unspecified region — unknown site on spine
722.81	Postlaminectomy syndrome, cervical region — neck, C1-C7

© 2006 Ingenix   ⌐sth Needs fifth digit   OK Valid three-digit code

Coders' Desk Reference for Diagnoses

722.82	Postlaminectomy syndrome, thoracic region — upper back, T1-T12
722.83	Postlaminectomy syndrome, lumbar region — lower back, L1-L5

Because the elimination of invalid four-digit codes could compromise the completeness of the code descriptions as they appear in ICD-9-CM, complete descriptions are used with each code in *Coders' Desk Reference for Diagnoses*. Therefore, while a code would read in an ICD-9-CM book like this:

239	Neoplasms of unspecified nature
239.0	Digestive system

In *Coders' Desk Reference for Diagnoses*, the codes would read like this:

239	Neoplasms of unspecified nature
239.0	Neoplasms of unspecified nature of digestive system

Note that the information from ICD-9-CM's description for 239 has been combined with the information from ICD-9-CM's description for 239.0 to create the description for *Coders' Desk Reference for Diagnoses*.

Additional Descriptors

Following most codes in *Coders' Desk Reference for Diagnoses* are brief descriptors that help differentiate the codes and determine which code is best suited for each clinical situation. For example:

701.9	Unspecified hypertrophic and atrophic condition of skin — skin tag, atrophoderma, pendulous abdomen, redundant skin, or unknown

In this example, the term "atrophoderma" appears as a descriptive term under 701.9 in ICD-9-CM; and the other terms are indexed to 701.9 in the official ICD-9-CM alphabetic index. In other cases, clinical research has provided the synonyms or support information that appears following the dash after a code, as in the case of:

001.0	Cholera due to Vibrio cholerae — Inaba, Ogawa, Hikojima serotypes; classical
001.1	Cholera due to Vibrio cholerae el tor — commonly less severe or asymptomatic
001.9	Cholera, unspecified — unknown whether V. cholerae or V. cholerae el tor

None of the supporting information appears in the official ICD-9-CM code text.

Narrative

Coders' Desk Reference for Diagnoses provides valuable background information on thousands of medical conditions. Information that appears directly after a three-digit category applies to all codes within that rubric. Information that appears following a four-digit subclassification applies to all codes in that subclassification, and information following a five-digit code applies only to that code.

Coding Clinic References

Listed with the ICD-9-CM codes are the AHA (American Hospital Association) Coding Clinic references. These identify diagnostic coding issues and answers on how to code for them properly, based on a patient situation (e.g., inpatient, outpatient). For example:

345	Epilepsy and recurrent seizures
	AHA: Q4, 1992, 23; Q2, 1992, 8; Q1, 1993, 24

Q4 indicates 4th quarter, followed by the year, and 23 is the page number in *AHA Coding Clinic for ICD-9-CM*.

Documentation Issues

This section indicates specific documentation issues that may arise while coding. For example:

> The terms grand mal and tonic-clonic seizures in the documentation do not establish the diagnosis of epilepsy.

Coding Clarification

These assist the user in clarifying coding problems and issues that may come up. For example:

> Recurrent Seizures: Recurrent seizures are not epilepsy, although all seizures in an epileptic patient are recurrent.

Coding Scenarios

The coding scenarios will assist the user in understanding how to code in particular situations. For example:

> A patient with known epilepsy is admitted after having experienced a grand mal seizure.
>
> Code assignment: 345.10, Epilepsy, grand mal status, without mention of intractable epilepsy

Illustrations

Illustrations provide users a better understanding of the anatomical nuances associated with specific codes. The illustrations usually include a labeled anatomical view, and may include narrative that discusses specific conditions or anatomic sites. The illustrations are almost always simplified schematic representations. In many instances, some detail is eliminated in order to make a clear point about the anatomic site that is the focus of the depiction.

ICD-9-CM Conventions

ICD-9-Conventions

The following section summarizes the coding conventions found in ICD-9-CM and the coding conventions that will be found in ICD-10-CM. In ICD-9-CM, the overview compares the following features:

1. Format
2. Typeface
3. Punctuation
4. Notes
5. Instructional notes
6. Modifiers
7. Abbreviations
8. Cross-references

Three Volume Set

1. Volume 1 of ICD-9-CM is a tabular listing of disease and injury divided into 17 sections, generally along anatomic sites. Two supplementary classifications contain alphanumeric codes to report factors influencing health status and other contact with health services (V codes) and causes of injury and poisoning (E codes). Appendixes to Volume 1 provide additional information and references.
2. Volume 2 is an alphabetic index of codes contained in Volume 1 and is important in locating proper diagnoses. An index to external causes of injury (E codes) is included. Three tables are included to assist in the selection of proper codes for hypertension, neoplasms, and drugs and chemicals.
3. A third volume of ICD-9-CM contains codes developed for coding inpatient facility procedures and is not ordinarily consulted for physician or outpatient services. Volume 3 contains both a tabular listing, arranged along anatomic lines, and an alphabetic index. Volume 3 coding issues are outside the framework of this reference manual.

Supplemental Classifications

Volume 1 contains two supplemental code classifications: V codes and E codes. V codes can be used as primary diagnoses when reporting services not related to current medical problems or conditions such as periodic or routine medical exams. E codes are never used as primary diagnoses, providing supplemental information only on the causes of injury and poisoning. See the individual listings for more information.

V codes (V01-V86), describe circumstances that influence a patient's health status and identify reasons for medical encounters resulting from circumstances other than a disease or injury classified in the main part of ICD-9-CM.

V codes are generally used in three instances:

- When a physician identifies a circumstance or problem in a person who is not currently sick but has nonetheless come in contact with health services (to act as an organ donor or to receive a prophylactic vaccination, for example)
- When an ill or injured patient requires specific treatment (such as chemotherapy for malignancy or removal of pins or rods in postoperative orthopedic care)
- When a problem or circumstance that influences the patient's health is not itself a current illness but may affect future medical treatment

The second set of supplemental codes in Volume 1 is the *Supplementary Classification of External Causes of Injury and Poisoning (E800-E999)*, also known as E codes. The E codes are never listed as the primary diagnosis; they are adjunctive. More than one E code may be needed to describe fully the circumstances of an accident. Use them to establish medical necessity to indicate a secondary payer responsible for payment of the service, identify causes of injury and poisoning, and to identify drugs. The index for the E codes is found in Volume 2, following the Table of Drugs and Chemicals.

Approaches to ICD-9-CM Coding

Determining a diagnostic code begins with analysis of the encounter form, operative report, or diagnostic statement for those words or main terms that best identify the patient's current condition or symptoms. Once the current condition or symptom is identified, consult Volume 2, the alphabetic index, to identify the main term associated with the condition or symptom. Next, identify any modifying terms listed below the main term to more specifically describe the condition or symptom. After the most specific main term and modifiers have been identified, look up the corresponding code in Volume 1, the tabular list. Follow any instructions or notes in both the alphabetic index and the tabular list.

Rules of ICD-9-CM Reference

An ironclad rule in diagnostic coding is to never derive a code by consulting only the Volume 2 alphabetic index. It is a reference index to the full tabular listing of Volume 1, which often yields a different code, additional codes, or a more specific code.

The six-step process for assigning diagnostic codes can be summarized as follows:

1. Determine the main terms that describe the patient's condition or symptoms.
2. Look up the main term in Volume 2 where the condition is alphabetized as a noun or adjective.
3. If indicated, follow cross-references such as *see, see also*, and see category to find the correct code.
4. Review subterms and modifying words. Refer to any indented terms under the main term to further clarify the code selection.
5. Verify the code as listed in Volume 2, the alphabetic index, by checking it against Volume 1, the tabular listing.
6. Review all instructions and notes in Volume 1 such as *includes, excludes, code first underlying disease*, or *use additional code* to assure that the correct code has been selected.

In outpatient coding, do not attempt to code "rule out," "probable," "suspect," or "questionable" descriptions in the documentation. While acceptable in a patient's medical record and for inpatient coding, coding rules do not allow their use in outpatient coding. Rather, code the condition, symptoms, signs, test results, or other reasons that can be documented for the medical encounter. (See "Official ICD-9-CM Coding Guidelines" chapter for specifics on inpatient hospital coding.)

Format

ICD-9-CM has an indented format. Subterms are indented two spaces to the right of the term to which they are linked. Continuations of lines too long for columns are indented four spaces.

251.2	Hypoglycemia, unspecified
	Hypoglycemia: Hypoglycemia:
	NOS spontaneous
	reactive

Typeface

Bold type identifies all codes and main terms in the Tabular List (Volume 1), separating them from subordinate information or notes.

Italicized type identifies those categories that cannot be reported as a primary diagnosis and also for all exclusion notes.

Punctuation

- Braces ({ }) enclose a series of terms modified by the statement or terms appearing to the right of the brace.

- Brackets ([ ]) enclose synonyms, alternative wordings, or explanatory phrases. The brackets may be square [ ] or italicized *[ ]*.

- Colon (:) is used in Volume 1 of ICD-9-CM to identify a term that is incomplete without one or more of the descriptors following it. Do not assign the code unless one or more of the descriptors is present in the physician's diagnostic statement.

- Parentheses ( ) enclose supplementary (nonessential) modifiers and do not generally affect code assignment. However, they do serve to confirm for the user that the correct code was selected when the nonessential modifier is present in both ICD-9-CM and the physician's documented diagnosis. Parentheses also enclose many *see also* references.

Notes

Notes are found in Volumes 1 and 2 and have no fixed length. They give general coding instructions. Notes in Volume 1 are indented and printed in plain type, while those in Volume 2 are boxed and italicized. The placement of these notes is as important as their content. Notes at the beginning of a section apply to all categories within the section. Those at the beginning of a subsection apply to all categories within the subsection. Likewise, notes preceding three-digit categories apply to all fourth-digit and fifth-digit codes within that category.

- *Code also* dictates the use of two diagnostic codes. List the etiology (cause) first, followed by the manifestation. The two codes combined represent the primary diagnosis.

- *Code first underlying disease* identifies diagnoses that are not primary and are incomplete when used alone. In such cases the code, its title, and instructions are italicized. This type of instructional note appears only in Volume 1. A code with this instructional note should be recorded second, with the underlying cause recorded first. Italicized brackets identify this situation in Volume 2.

Instructional Notes

To assign diagnostic codes at the highest level of specificity, there are additional notes to follow.

- Excludes indicates terms that are not ordinarily coded under the referenced term. The word "Excludes" is surrounded by a box for easy identification and the corresponding note is italicized. This note does not prevent you from using the excluded code in addition to the code from which it was excluded when both conditions are present.

- Includes appear immediately under a three-digit code title to provide further definition or to give an example of the category contents.

- Use Additional Code in Volume 1 indicates those categories where an additional code is available to provide further information and to give a more complete picture of the diagnosis. The additional code should identify other aspects of the disease, including manifestation, cause, associated condition, and nature of the condition itself.

Modifiers

Essential modifiers are indented two spaces just below the main terms. They are generally presented in alphabetical order, with the exceptions of with and without, which appear before the alphabetized modifiers. Each additional essential modifier clarifies the previous one and is indented two additional spaces to the right. These descriptive terms affect code selection since they describe essential differences in site, etiology, and symptoms. When a main term in the tabular Volume 1 has only one essential modifier, it appears on the same line as the main term, separated by a comma.

Nonessential modifiers are listed immediately to the right of the main term and are enclosed in parentheses. They serve as examples to help translate written terminology into numeric codes and may be present or absent in the diagnostic statement without affecting code assignment.

Abbreviations

NEC (not elsewhere classifiable) indicates that the ICD-9-CM system does not provide a specific code for the condition described in the medical record.

NOS (not otherwise specified) is the equivalent of "unspecified" and is used only when there is a lack of information and documentation to support a specific code selection.

Cross-references

In Volume 2, several types of cross-references are encountered:

- *See* indicates that you should see the condition listed instead of the term you've found in order to assign the correct diagnostic code.

- *See also* indicates that additional information is available. This cross-reference may provide a more specific code or an additional code.

- *See* category directs the user to an additional three-digit category, not just a single code. Again, an appropriate code cannot be assigned unless you follow this instruction.

Official ICD-9-CM Coding Guidelines

Coding Guidelines

ICD-9-CM Official Guidelines for Coding and Reporting

Effective December 1, 2005

Narrative changes appear in bold text.

The guidelines have been updated to include the V Code Table.

The Centers for Medicare and Medicaid Services (CMS) and the National Center for Health Statistics (NCHS), two departments within the U.S. Federal Government's Department of Health and Human Services (DHHS) provide the following guidelines for coding and reporting using the International Classification of Diseases, 9th Revision, Clinical Modification (ICD-9-CM). These guidelines should be used as a companion document to the official version of the ICD-9-CM as published on CD-ROM by the U.S. Government Printing Office (GPO).

These guidelines have been approved by the four organizations that make up the Cooperating Parties for the ICD-9-CM: the American Hospital Association (AHA), the American Health Information Management Association (AHIMA), CMS, and NCHS. These guidelines are included in the official government version of the ICD-9-CM and also appear in *Coding Clinic for ICD-9-CM,* published by the AHA.

These guidelines are a set of rules that have been developed to accompany and complement the official conventions and instructions provided within the ICD-9-CM itself. These guidelines are based on the coding and sequencing instructions in Volumes 1, 2, and 3 of ICD-9-CM, but provide additional instruction. Adherence to these guidelines when assigning ICD-9-CM diagnosis and procedure codes is required under the Health Insurance Portability and Accountability Act (HIPAA). The diagnosis codes (Volumes 1-2) have been adopted under HIPAA for all health care settings. Volume 3 procedure codes have been adopted for inpatient procedures reported by hospitals. A joint effort between the health care provider and the coder is essential to achieve complete and accurate documentation, code assignment, and reporting of diagnoses and procedures. These guidelines have been developed to assist both the health care provider and the coder in identifying those diagnoses and procedures that are to be reported. The importance of consistent, complete documentation in the medical record cannot be overemphasized. Without such documentation accurate coding cannot be achieved. The entire record should be reviewed to determine the specific reason for the encounter and the conditions treated.

The term "encounter" is used for all settings, including hospital admissions. In the context of these guidelines, the term "provider" is used throughout the guidelines to mean physician or any qualified health care practitioner who is legally accountable for establishing the patient's diagnosis. Only this set of guidelines, approved by the cooperating parties, is official.

The guidelines are organized into sections. Section I includes the structure and conventions of the classification and general guidelines that apply to the entire classification, and chapter-specific guidelines that correspond to the chapters as they are arranged in the classification. Section II includes guidelines for selection of principal diagnosis for non-outpatient settings. Section III includes guidelines for reporting additional diagnoses in non-outpatient settings. Section IV is for outpatient coding and reporting.

Section I. Conventions, general coding guidelines and chapter-specific guidelines

A. Conventions for the ICD-9-CM
    1. Format
    2. Abbreviations
        a. Index abbreviations
        b. Tabular abbreviations

3. Punctuation
4. Includes and excludes notes and inclusion terms
5. Other and Unspecified codes
   a. "Other" codes
   b. "Unspecified" codes
6. Etiology/manifestation convention ("code first," "use additional code," and "in diseases classified elsewhere" notes)
7. "And"
8. "With"
9. "See" and "see also"

B. General coding guidelines
   1. Use of both Alphabetic Index and Tabular List
   2. Locate each term in the Alphabetic Index
   3. Level of detail in coding
   4. Code or codes from 001.0 through V86.1
   5. Selection of codes 001.0 through 999.9
   6. Signs and symptoms
   7. Conditions that are an integral part of a disease process
   8. Conditions that are not an integral part of a disease process
   9. Multiple coding for a single condition
   10. Acute and chronic conditions
   11. Combination code
   12. Late effects
   13. Impending or threatened condition

C. Chapter-specific coding guidelines
   1. Chapter 1: Infectious and Parasitic Diseases (001-139)
      a. Human immunodeficiency virus (HIV) infections
      b. Septicemia, systemic inflammatory response syndrome (SIRS), sepsis, severe sepsis, and septic shock
   2. Chapter 2: Neoplasms (140-239)
      a. Treatment directed at the malignancy
      b. Treatment of secondary site
      c. Coding and sequencing of complications
      d. Primary malignancy previously excised
      e. Admissions/encounters involving chemotherapy and radiation therapy
      f. Admission/encounter to determine extent of malignancy
      g. Symptoms, signs, and ill-defined conditions listed in chapter 16
      h. Encounter for prophylactic organ removal
   3. Chapter 3: Endocrine, Nutritional, and Metabolic Diseases and Immunity Disorders (240-279)
      a. Diabetes mellitus
   4. Chapter 4: Diseases of Blood and Blood-Forming Organs (280-289)
      a. Anemia of chronic disease
   5. Chapter 5: Mental Disorders (290-319)
      Reserved for future guideline expansion
   6. Chapter 6: Diseases of Nervous System and Sense Organs (320-389)
      Reserved for future guideline expansion
   7. Chapter 7: Diseases of Circulatory System (390-459)
      a. Hypertension
      b. Cerebral infarction/stroke/cerebrovascular accident (CVA)
      c. Postoperative cerebrovascular accident
      d. Late effects of cerebrovascular disease
      e. Acute myocardial infarction (AMI)
   8. Chapter 8: Diseases of Respiratory System (460-519)
      a. Chronic obstructive pulmonary disease [COPD] and asthma
      b. Chronic obstructive pulmonary disease [COPD] and bronchitis

Official ICD-9-CM Coding Guidelines

9. Chapter 9: Diseases of Digestive System (520-579)

   Reserved for future guideline expansion

10. Chapter 10: Diseases of Genitourinary System (580-629)
    a. **Chronic kidney disease**

11. Chapter 11: Complications of Pregnancy, Childbirth, and the Puerperium (630-677)
    a. General rules for obstetric cases
    b. Selection of OB principal or first-listed diagnosis
    c. Fetal conditions affecting the management of the mother
    d. HIV infection in pregnancy, childbirth and the puerperium
    e. Current conditions complicating pregnancy
    f. Diabetes mellitus in pregnancy
    g. Gestational diabetes
    h. Normal delivery, code 650
    i. The postpartum and peripartum eriods
    j. Code 677 Late effect of complication of pregnancy
    k. Abortions

12. Chapter 12: Diseases Skin and Subcutaneous Tissue (680-709)

    Reserved for future guideline expansion

13. Chapter 13: Diseases of Musculoskeletal and Connective Tissue (710-739)

    Reserved for future guideline expansion

14. Chapter 14: Congenital Anomalies (740-759)
    a. Codes in categories 740-759, Congenital anomalies

15. Chapter 15: Newborn (Perinatal) Guidelines (760-779)
    a. General perinatal rules
    b. Use of codes V30-V39
    c. Newborn transfers
    d. Use of category V29
    e. Use of other V codes on perinatal records
    f. Maternal causes of perinatal morbidity
    g. Congenital anomalies in newborns
    h. Coding additional perinatal diagnoses
    i. Prematurity and fetal growth retardation
    j. Newborn sepsis

16. Chapter 16: Signs, Symptoms and Ill-Defined Conditions (780-799)

17. Chapter 17: Injury and Poisoning (800-999)
    a. Coding of injuries
    b. Coding of fractures
    c. Coding of burns
    d. Coding of debridement of wound, infection, or burn
    e. Adverse effects, poisoning and toxic effects
    f. **Complications of care**

18. Classification of Factors Influencing Health Status and Contact with Health Service (Supplemental V01-V86)
    a. **Introduction**
    b. V codes use in any health care setting
    c. V codes indicate a reason for an encounter
    d. Categories of V codes
    e. **V Code Table**

19. Supplemental Classification of External Causes of Injury and Poisoning (E codes, E800-E999)
    a. General E code coding guideline
    b. Place of occurrence guideline
    c. Adverse effects of drugs, medicinal and biological substances guidelines
    d. Multiple cause E code coding guidelines
    e. Child and adult abuse guideline

f. Unknown or suspected intent guideline
   g. Undetermined cause
   h. Late effects of external cause guidelines
   i. Misadventures and complications of care guidelines
   j. Terrorism guidelines

Section II. Selection of Principal Diagnosis
A. Codes for symptoms, signs, and ill-defined conditions
B. Two or more interrelated conditions, each potentially meeting the definition for principal diagnosis
C. Two or more diagnoses that equally meet the definition for principal diagnosis
D. Two or more comparative or contrasting conditions
E. A symptom(s) followed by contrasting/comparative diagnoses
F. Original treatment plan not carried out
G. Complications of surgery and other medical care
H. Uncertain diagnosis
I. **Admission from observation unit**
   1. **Admission following medical observation**
   2. **Admission following post-operative observation**
J. **Admission from outpatient surgery**

Section III. Reporting Additional Diagnoses
A. Previous conditions
B. Abnormal findings
C. Uncertain diagnosis

Section IV. Diagnostic Coding and Reporting Guidelines for Outpatient Services
A. Selection of first-listed condition
B. Codes from 001.0 through V86.1
C. Accurate reporting of ICD-9-CM diagnosis codes
D. Selection of codes 001.0 through 999.9
E. Codes that describe symptoms and signs

F. Encounters for circumstances other than a disease or injury
G. Level of detail in coding
   1. ICD-9-CM codes with three, four, or five digits
   2. Use of full number of digits required for a code
H. ICD-9-CM code for the diagnosis, condition, problem, or other reason for encounter/visit
I. "Probable," "suspected," "questionable," "rule out," or "working diagnosis"
J. Chronic diseases
K. Code all documented conditions that coexist
L. Patients receiving diagnostic services only
M. Patients receiving therapeutic services only
N. Patients receiving preoperative evaluations only
O. Ambulatory surgery
P. Routine outpatient prenatal visits

Section I. Conventions, general coding guidelines and chapter-specific guidelines
The conventions, general guidelines, and chapter-specific guidelines are applicable to all health care settings unless otherwise indicated.

A. Conventions for the ICD-9-CM
The conventions for the ICD-9-CM are the general rules for use of the classification independent of the guidelines. These conventions are incorporated within the index and tabular of the ICD-9-CM as instructional notes. The conventions are as follows:

1. **Format:**

    The ICD-9-CM uses an indented format for ease in reference

2. **Abbreviations**

    a. **Index abbreviations**

        NEC "Not elsewhere classifiable"-This abbreviation in the index represents "other specified." When a specific code is not available for a condition, the index directs the coder to the "other specified" code in the tabular.

    b. **Tabular abbreviations**

        NEC "Not elsewhere classifiable"-This abbreviation in the tabular represents "other specified." When a specific code is not available for a condition, the tabular includes an NEC entry under a code to identify the code as the "other specified" code (See section I.A.5.a.,"Other" codes).

NOS "Not otherwise specified"-This abbreviation is the equivalent of unspecified. (See section I.A.5.b., "Unspecified" codes)

3. **Punctuation**

[ ]   Brackets are used in the Tabular List to enclose synonyms, alternative wording, or explanatory phrases. Brackets are used in the index to identify manifestation codes. (See section I.A.6., Etiology/manifestations)

( )   Parentheses are used in both the index and tabular to enclose supplementary words that may be present or absent in the statement of a disease or procedure without affecting the code number to which it is assigned. The terms within the parentheses are referred to as nonessential modifiers.

:   Colons are used in the Tabular List after an incomplete term needs one or more of the modifiers following the colon to make it assignable to a given category.

4. **Includes and excludes notes and inclusion terms**

Includes: This note appears immediately under a three-digit code title to further define, or give examples of, the content of the category.

Excludes: An excludes note under a code indicates that the terms excluded from the code are to be coded elsewhere. In some cases the codes for the excluded terms should not be used in conjunction with the code from which they are excluded. An example of this is a congenital condition excluded from an acquired form of the same condition. The congenital and acquired codes should not be used together. In other cases, the excluded terms may be used together with an excluded code. An example of this is when fractures of different bones are coded to different codes. Both codes may be used together if both types of fractures are present.

Inclusion terms: List of terms included under certain four- and five- digit codes. These terms are the conditions for which that code number is to be used. The terms may be synonyms of the code title, or, in the case of "other specified" codes, the terms are a list of the various conditions assigned to that code. The inclusion terms are not necessarily exhaustive. Additional terms found only in the index may also be assigned to a code.

5. **Other and unspecified codes**

   a. **"Other" codes**—Codes titled "other" or "other specified" (usually a code with a fourth digit of 8 or fifth digit of 9 for diagnosis codes) are for use when the information in the medical record provides detail for which a specific code does not exist. Index entries with NEC in the line designate "other" codes in the tabular. These index entries represent specific disease entities for which no specific code exists so the term is included within an "other" code.

   b. **"Unspecified" codes**—Codes (usually a code with a fourth digit of 9 or fifth of 0 for diagnosis codes) titled "unspecified" are for use when the information in the medical record is insufficient to assign a more specific code.

6. **Etiology/manifestation convention ("code first," "use additional code," and "in diseases classified elsewhere" notes)**—Certain conditions have both an underlying etiology and multiple body system manifestations due to the underlying etiology. For such conditions, the ICD-9-CM has a coding convention that requires the underlying condition to be sequenced first followed by the manifestation. Wherever such a combination exists, there is a "use additional code" note at the etiology code, and a "code first" note at the manifestation code. These instructional notes indicate the proper sequencing order of the codes, etiology followed by manifestation.

In most cases the manifestation codes will have in the code title, "in diseases classified elsewhere." Codes with this title are a component of the etiology/manifestation convention. The code title indicates that it is a manifestation code. "In diseases classified elsewhere," codes are never permitted to be used as first listed or principal diagnosis codes. They must be used in conjunction with an underlying condition code, and they must be listed following the underlying condition.

There are manifestation codes that do not have "in diseases classified elsewhere" in the title. For such codes a "use additional code" note will still be present and the rules for sequencing apply.

In addition to the notes in the tabular, these conditions also have a specific index entry structure. In the index both conditions are listed together with the etiology code first followed by the manifestation codes in brackets. The code in brackets is always to be sequenced second.

The most commonly used etiology/manifestation combinations are the codes for diabetes mellitus, category 250. For each code under category 250 there is a use additional code note for the manifestation that is specific for that particular diabetic manifestation. Should a patient have more than one manifestation of diabetes, more than one code from category 250 may be used with as many manifestation codes as are needed to fully describe the patient's complete diabetic condition. The category 250 diabetes codes should be sequenced first, followed by the manifestation codes.

"Code first" and "use additional code" notes are also used as sequencing rules in the classification for certain codes that are not part of an etiology/manifestation combination. See section I.B.9., "Multiple coding for a single condition."

7. **"And"**

The word "and" should be interpreted to mean either "and" or "or" when it appears in a title.

8. **"With"**

The word "with" in the Alphabetic Index is sequenced immediately following the main term, not in alphabetical order.

9. **"See" and "see also"**

The "see" instruction following a main term in the index indicates that another term should be referenced. It is necessary to go to the main term referenced with the "see" note to locate the correct code.

A "see also" instruction following a main term in the index instructs that there is another main term that may also be referenced that may provide additional index entries that may be useful. It is not necessary to follow the "see also" note when the original main term provides the necessary code.

B. **General coding guidelines**
1. **Use of both Alphabetic Index and Tabular List** — Use both the Alphabetic Index and the Tabular List when locating and assigning a code. Reliance on only the Alphabetic Index or the Tabular List leads to errors in code assignments and less specificity in code selection.

2. **Locate each term in the alphabetic index** — Locate each term in the Alphabetic Index and verify the code selected in the Tabular List. Read and be guided by instructional notations that appear in both the Alphabetic Index and the Tabular List.

3. **Level of detail in coding** — Diagnosis and procedure codes are to be used at their highest number of digits available.

ICD-9-CM diagnosis codes are composed of codes with either three, four, or five digits. Codes with three digits are included in ICD-9-CM as the heading of a category of codes that may be further subdivided by the use of four and/or fifth digits, which provide greater detail.

A three-digit code is to be used only if it is not further subdivided. Where fourth-digit subcategories and/or fifth-digit subclassifications are provided, they must be assigned. A code is invalid if it has not been coded to the full number of digits required for that code. For example, acute myocardial infarction, code 410, has fourth digits that describe the location of the infarction (e.g., 410.2 Of inferolateral wall), and fifth digits that identify the episode of care. It would be incorrect to report a code in category 410 without a fourth and fifth digit.

ICD-9-CM Volume 3 procedure codes are composed of codes with either three or four digits. Codes with two digits are included in ICD-9-CM as the heading of a category of codes that may be further subdivided by the use of third and/or fourth digits, which provide greater detail.

4. **Code or codes from 001.0 through V86.1** — The appropriate code or codes from 001.0

through V86.1 must be used to identify diagnoses, symptoms, conditions, problems, complaints, or other reason(s) for the encounter/visit.

5. **Selection of codes 001.0 through 999.9** — The selection of codes 001.0 through 999.9 will frequently be used to describe the reason for the admission/encounter. These codes are from the section of ICD-9-CM for the classification of diseases and injuries (e.g., infectious and parasitic diseases; neoplasms; symptoms, signs, and ill-defined conditions, etc.).

6. **Signs and symptoms** — Codes that describe symptoms and signs, as opposed to diagnoses, are acceptable for reporting purposes when a related definitive diagnosis has not been established (confirmed) by the provider. Chapter 16 of ICD-9-CM, "Symptoms, Signs, and Ill-defined Conditions" (codes 780.0-799.9) contain many, but not all, codes for symptoms.

7. **Conditions that are an integral part of a disease process** — Signs and symptoms that are integral to the disease process should not be assigned as additional codes.

8. **Conditions that are not an integral part of a disease process** — Additional signs and symptoms that may not be associated routinely with a disease process should be coded when present.

9. **Multiple coding for a single condition** — In addition to the etiology/manifestation convention that requires two codes to fully describe a single condition that affects multiple body systems, there are other single conditions that also require more than one code. "Use additional code" notes are found in the tabular at codes that are not part of an etiology/manifestation pair where a secondary code is useful to fully describe a condition. The sequencing rule is the same as the etiology/manifestation pair where a secondary code is useful to fully describe a condition. The sequencing rule is the same; "use additional code" indicates that a secondary code should be added.

    For example, for infections that are not included in chapter 1, a secondary code from category 041 Bacterial infection in conditions classified elsewhere and of unspecified site, may be required to identify the bacterial organism causing the infection. A "use additional code" note will normally be found at the infectious disease code, indicating a need for the organism code to be added as a secondary code.

    "Code first" notes are also under certain codes that are not specifically manifestation codes but may be due to an underlying cause. When a "code first" note is present and an underlying condition is present, the underlying condition should be sequenced first.

    "Code, if applicable, any causal condition first" notes indicate that this code may be assigned as a principal diagnosis when the causal condition is unknown or not applicable. If a causal condition is known, then the code for that condition should be sequenced as the principal or first-listed diagnosis.

    Multiple codes may be needed for late effects, complication codes, and obstetric codes to more fully describe a condition. See the specific guidelines for these conditions for further instruction.

10. **Acute and chronic conditions** — If the same condition is described as both acute (subacute) and chronic, and separate subentries exist in the Alphabetic Index at the same indentation level, code both and sequence the acute (subacute) code first.

11. **Combination code** — A combination code is a single code used to classify:

    - Two diagnoses
    - A diagnosis with an associated secondary process (manifestation)
    - A diagnosis with an associated complication

    Combination codes are identified by referring to subterm entries in the Alphabetic Index and by reading the inclusion and exclusion notes in the Tabular List.

    Assign only the combination code when that code fully identifies the diagnostic conditions involved or when the Alphabetic Index so directs. Multiple coding should not be used when the classification provides a combination code that clearly identifies all of the elements documented in the diagnosis. When the combination code lacks necessary specificity in describing the manifestation or complication, an additional code should be used as a secondary code.

12. **Late effects** — A late effect is the residual effect (condition produced) after the acute phase of an illness or injury has terminated. There is no time limit on when a late effect code can be used. The residual may be apparent early, such as in cerebrovascular accident cases, or it may occur months or years later, such as that due to a previous injury. Coding of late effects generally requires two codes sequenced in the following order: The condition or nature of the late effect is sequenced first... The late effect code is sequenced second.

    An exception to the above guidelines are those instances where the code for late effect is followed by a manifestation code identified in the Tabular List and title, or the late effect code has been expanded (at the fourth- and fifth-digit levels) to include the manifestation(s). The code for the acute phase of an illness or injury that led to the late effect is never used with a code for the late effect.

13. **Impending or threatened condition** — Code any condition described at the time of discharge as "impending" or "threatened" as follows:

    If it did occur, code as confirmed diagnosis. If it did not occur, reference the Alphabetic Index to determine if the condition has a subentry term for "impending" or "threatened" and also reference main term entries for "Impending" and for "Threatened." If the subterms are listed, assign the given code. If the subterms are not listed, code the existing underlying condition(s) and not the condition described as impending or threatened.

C. Chapter-specific coding guidelines

In addition to general coding guidelines, there are guidelines for specific diagnoses and/or conditions in the classification. Unless otherwise indicated, these guidelines apply to all health care settings. Please refer to section II for guidelines on the selection of principal diagnosis.

1. **Chapter 1: Infectious and Parasitic Diseases (001-139)**
    a. **Human immunodeficiency virus (HIV) infections**
       1) **Code only confirmed cases** — Code only confirmed cases of HIV infection/illness. This is an exception to the hospital inpatient guideline section II, H. In this context, "confirmation" does not require documentation of positive serology or culture for HIV; the provider's diagnostic statement that the patient is HIV positive or has an HIV-related illness is sufficient.

       2) **Selection and sequencing of HIV codes**
          (a) **Patient admitted for HIV-related condition** — If a patient is admitted for an HIV-related condition, the principal diagnosis should be 042, followed by additional diagnosis codes for all reported HIV-related conditions.

          (b) **Patient with HIV disease admitted for unrelated condition** — If a patient with HIV disease is admitted for an unrelated condition (such as a traumatic injury), the code for the unrelated condition (e.g., the nature of injury code) should be the principal diagnosis. Other diagnoses would be 042 followed by additional diagnosis codes for all reported HIV-related conditions.

          (c) **Whether the patient is newly diagnosed** — Whether the patient is newly diagnosed or has had previous admissions/encounters for HIV conditions is irrelevant to the sequencing decision.

          (d) **Asymptomatic human immunodeficiency virus** — V08 Asymptomatic human immunodeficiency virus [HIV]infection, is to be applied when the patient without any documentation of symptoms is listed as being "HIV positive," "known HIV," "HIV test positive," or similar terminology. Do not use this code if the term "AIDS" is used or if the patient is treated for any HIV-related illness or is described as having any condition(s) resulting from his/her HIV positive status; use 042 in these cases.

(e) **Patients with inconclusive HIV serology** — Patients with inconclusive HIV serology, but no definitive diagnosis or manifestations of the illness, may be assigned code 795.71 Inconclusive serologic test for human immunodeficiency virus [HIV].

(f) **Previously diagnosed HIV-related illness** — Patients with any known prior diagnosis of an HIV-related illness should be coded to 042. Once a patient has developed an HIV-related illness, the patient should always be assigned code 042 on every subsequent admission/encounter. Patients previously diagnosed with any HIV illness (042) should never be assigned to 795.71 or V08.

(g) **HIV infection in pregnancy, childbirth and the puerperium** — During pregnancy, childbirth, or the puerperium, a patient admitted (or presenting for a health care encounter) because of an HIV-related illness should receive a principal diagnosis code of 647.6x Other specified infectious and parasitic diseases in the mother classifiable elsewhere but complicating the pregnancy, childbirth or the puerperium, followed by 042 and the code(s) for the HIV-related illness(es). Codes from chapter 15 always take sequencing priority.

Patients with asymptomatic HIV infection status admitted (or presenting for a health care encounter) during pregnancy, child-birth, or the puerperium should receive codes of 647.6x and V08.

(h) **Encounters for testing for HIV** — If a patient is being seen to determine his/her HIV status, use code V73.89 Screening for other specified viral disease. Use code V69.8 Other problems related to lifestyle, as a secondary code if an asymptomatic patient is in a known high risk group for HIV. Should a patient with signs or symptoms or illness, or a confirmed HIV related diagnosis be tested for HIV, code the signs and symptoms or the diagnosis. An additional counseling code V65.44 may be used if counseling is provided during the encounter for the test.

When a patient returns to be informed of his/her HIV test results, use code V65.44 HIV counseling, if the results of the test are negative.

If the results are positive but the patient is asymptomatic, use code V08 Asymptomatic HIV infection. If the results are positive and the patient is symptomatic, use code 042 HIV infection, with codes for the HIV-related symptoms or diagnosis. The HIV counseling code may also be used if counseling is provided for patients with positive test results.

b. **Septicemia, systemic inflammatory response**

syndrome (SIRS), sepsis, severe sepsis, and septic shock

1) **Sepsis as principal diagnosis or secondary diagnosis**

    (a) Sepsis as principal diagnosis-If sepsis is present on admission and meets the definition of principal diagnosis, the underlying systemic infection code (e.g., 038.xx, 112.5, etc.) should be assigned as the principal diagnosis, followed by code 995.91 Systemic inflammatory response syndrome due to infectious process without organ dysfunction, as required by the sequencing rules in the Tabular List. Codes from subcategory 995.9 can never be assigned as a principal diagnosis.

    (b) Sepsis as secondary diagnoses-When sepsis develops during the encounter (it was not present on admission), the sepsis codes may be assigned as secondary diagnoses, following the sequencing rules provided in the Tabular List.

    (c) Documentation unclear as to whether sepsis present on admission-If the documentation is not clear whether the sepsis was present on admission, the provider should be queried. After provider query, if sepsis is determined at that point to have met the definition of principal diagnosis, the underlying systemic infection (038.xx, 112.5, etc.) may be used as the principal diagnosis along with code 995.91 Systemic inflammatory response syndrome due to infectious process without organ dysfunction.

2) **Septicemia/sepsis** — In most cases, it will be a code from category 038 Septicemia, that will be used in conjunction with a code from subcategory 995.9 such as the following:

    (a) **Streptococcal sepsis** — If the documentation in the record states streptococcal sepsis, codes 038.0 and code 995.91 should be used, in that sequence.

    (b) **Streptococcal septicemia** — If the documentation states streptococcal septicemia, only code 038.0 should be assigned; however, the provider should be queried whether the patient has sepsis, an infection with SIRS.

    (c) **Sepsis or SIRS must be documented** — Either the term sepsis or SIRS must be documented to assign a code from subcategory 995.9.

3) **Terms "sepsis," " severe sepsis," or "SIRS"** — If the terms sepsis, severe sepsis, or SIRS are used with an underlying infection other than septicemia, such as pneumonia, cellulitis, or a

nonspecified urinary tract infection, a code from category 038 should be assigned first, then code 995.91, followed by the code for the initial infection. The use of the terms sepsis or SIRS indicates that the patient's infection has advanced to the point of a systemic infection so the systemic infection should be sequenced before the localized infection. The instructional note under subcategory 995.9 instructs to assign the underlying systemic infection first.

Note: The term "urosepsis" is a nonspecific term. If that is the only term documented then only code 599.0 should be assigned based on the default for the term in the ICD-9-CM index, in addition to the code for the causal organism if known.

4) **Severe sepsis** — For patients with severe sepsis, the code for the systemic infection (e.g., 038.xx, 112.5, etc) or trauma should be sequenced first, followed by either code 995.92 Systemic inflammatory response syndrome due to infectious process with organ dysfunction, or code 995.94 Systemic inflammatory response syndrome due to noninfectious process with organ dysfunction. Codes for the specific organ dysfunctions should also be assigned.

5) **Septic shock**

   (a) Sequencing of septic shock-Septic shock is a form of organ dysfunction associated with severe sepsis. A code for the initiating underlying systemic infection followed by a code for SIRS (code 995.92) must be assigned before the code for septic shock. As noted in the sequencing instructions in the Tabular List, the code for septic shock cannot be assigned as a principal diagnosis.

   (b) Septic shock without documentation of severe sepsis-Septic shock cannot occur in the absence of severe sepsis. A code from subcategory 995.9 must be sequenced before the code for septic shock. The use additional code notes and the code first note provide sequencing instructions.

6) **Sepsis and septic shock associated with abortion** — Sepsis and septic shock associated with abortion, ectopic pregnancy, and molar pregnancy are classified to category codes in chapter 11 (630-639).

7) **Negative or inconclusive blood cultures** — Negative or inconclusive blood cultures do not preclude a diagnosis of septicemia or sepsis in patients with clinical evidence of the condition; however, the provider should be queried.

8) **Newborn sepsis** — See section I.C.15.j for information on the coding of newborn sepsis.

9) **Sepsis due to a postprocedural infection** — Sepsis resulting from a

postprocedural infection is a complication of care. For such cases code 998.59 Other postoperative infections, should be coded first followed by the appropriate codes for the sepsis. The other guidelines for coding sepsis should then be followed for the assignment of additional codes.

10) External cause of injury codes with SIRS — An external cause code is not needed with codes 995.91 Systemic inflammatory response syndrome due to infectious process without organ dysfunction, or 995.92 Systemic inflammatory response syndrome due to infectious process with organ dysfunction

Refer to section I.C.19.a.7 for instruction on the use of external cause of injury codes with codes for SIRS resulting from trauma.

2. Chapter 2: Neoplasms (140-239)
General guidelines

Chapter 2 of the ICD-9-CM contains the codes for most benign and all malignant neoplasms. Certain benign neoplasms, such as prostatic adenomas, may be found in the specific body system chapters. To properly code a neoplasm it is necessary to determine from the record if the neoplasm is benign, in situ, malignant, or of uncertain histologic behavior. If malignant, any secondary (metastatic) sites should also be determined.

The neoplasm table in the Alphabetic Index should be referenced first. However, if the histological term is documented, that term should be referenced first, rather than going immediately to the neoplasm table, in order to determine which column in the neoplasm table is appropriate. For example, if the documentation indicates "adenoma," refer to the term in the Alphabetic Index to review the entries under this term and the instructional note to "see also neoplasm, by site, benign." The table provides the proper code based on the type of neoplasm and the site. It is important to select the proper column in the table that corresponds to the type of neoplasm. The tabular should then be referenced to verify that the correct code has been selected from the table and that a more specific site code does not exist.

See section I. C. 18.d.4. for information regarding V codes for genetic susceptibility to cancer.

a. **Treatment directed at the malignancy** — If the treatment is directed at the malignancy, designate the malignancy as the principal diagnosis.

b. **Treatment of secondary site** — When a patient is admitted because of a primary neoplasm with metastasis and treatment is directed toward the secondary site only, the secondary neoplasm is designated as the principal diagnosis even though the primary malignancy is still present.

c. **Coding and sequencing of complications** — Coding and sequencing of complications associated with the malignancies or with the therapy thereof are subject to the following guidelines:

1) **Anemia associated with malignancy** — When admission/encounter is for management of an anemia associated with the malignancy, and the treatment is only for anemia, **the appropriate anemia code (such as code 285.22 Anemia in neoplastic disease)** is designated as the principal diagnosis and is followed by the appropriate code(s) for the malignancy.

Code 285.22 may also be used as a secondary code if the patient suffers from anemia and is being treated for the malignancy.

2) **Anemia associated with chemotherapy, immunotherapy and radiation therapy** — When the admission/encounter is for management of an anemia associated with chemotherapy, **immunotherapy,** or radiotherapy and the only treatment is for the anemia, the anemia is sequenced first followed by **code E933.1. The appropriate neoplasm code should be assigned as an additional code.**

3) **Management of dehydration due to the malignancy** — When the admission/encounter is for management of dehydration due to the malignancy or the therapy, or a combination of both, and only the dehydration is being treated (intravenous rehydration), the dehydration is sequenced first, followed by the code(s) for the malignancy.

4) **Treatment of a complication resulting from a surgical procedure** — When the admission/encounter is for treatment of a complication resulting from a surgical procedure, designate the complication as the principal or first-listed diagnosis if treatment is directed at resolving the complication.

d. **Primary malignancy previously excised** — When a primary malignancy has been previously excised or eradicated from its site and there is no further treatment directed to that site and there is no evidence of any existing primary malignancy, a code from category V10 Personal history of malignant neoplasm, should be used to indicate the former site of the malignancy. Any mention of extension, invasion, or metastasis to another site is coded as a secondary malignant neoplasm to that site. The secondary site may be the principal or first-listed with the V10 code used as a secondary code.

e. **Admissions/encounters involving chemotherapy, immunotherapy, and radiation therapy**

1) **Episode of care involves surgical removal of neoplasm** — When an episode of care involves the surgical removal of a neoplasm, primary or secondary site, followed by adjunct chemotherapy or radiation treatment **during the same episode of care**, the neoplasm code should be assigned as principal or first-listed diagnosis, using codes in the 140-198 series or where appropriate in the 200-203 series.

2) **Patient admission/encounter solely for administration of chemotherapy, immunotherapy, and radiation therapy** — If a patient admission/encounter is solely for the administration of chemotherapy, **immunotherapy** or radiation therapy, assign code V58.0 Encounter for radiation therapy, **V58.11 Encounter for antineoplastic chemotherapy, or V58.12 Encounter for antineoplastic immunotherapy** as the first-listed or principal diagnosis. If a patient receives **more than one of these therapies during the same admission, more than one of these codes may be assigned, in any sequence.**

3) **Patient admitted for radiotherapy/chemotherapy and immunotherapy and develops complications** — When a patient is admitted for the purpose of radiotherapy, **immunotherapy,** or chemotherapy and develops complications such as uncontrolled nausea and vomiting or dehydration, the principal or first-listed diagnosis is V58.0 Encounter for radiotherapy, **V58.11 Encounter for antineoplastic chemotherapy, or V58.12 Encounter for antineoplastic immunotherapy** followed by any codes for the complications.

See section I.C.18.d.8. for additional information regarding aftercare V codes.

f. **Admission/encounter to determine extent of malignancy** — When the reason for admission/encounter is to determine the extent of the malignancy, or for a procedure such as paracentesis or thoracentesis, the primary malignancy or appropriate metastatic site is designated as the principal or first-listed diagnosis, even though chemotherapy or radiotherapy is administered.

g. **Symptoms, signs, and ill-defined conditions listed in chapter 16** — Symptoms, signs, and ill-defined conditions listed in chapter 16 characteristic of, or associated with, an existing primary or secondary site malignancy cannot be used to replace the malignancy as principal or first-listed diagnosis, regardless of the number of admissions or encounters for treatment and care of the neoplasm.

h. See section I.C.18.d.14, Encounter for prophylactic organ removal

3. **Chapter 3: Endocrine, Nutritional, and Metabolic Diseases and Immunity Disorders (240-279)**

   a. **Diabetes mellitus** — Codes under category 250 Diabetes mellitus, identify complications/manifestations associated with diabetes mellitus. A fifth-digit is required for all category 250 codes to identify the type of diabetes mellitus and whether the diabetes is controlled or uncontrolled.

   1) Fifth digits for category 250: The following are the fifth digits for the codes under category 250:

      0   type II or unspecified type, not stated as uncontrolled

      1   type I, [juvenile type], not stated as uncontrolled

      2   type II or unspecified type, uncontrolled

      3   type I, [juvenile type], uncontrolled

      The age of a patient is not the sole determining factor, though most type I diabetics develop the condition before reaching puberty. For this reason type I diabetes mellitus is also referred to as juvenile diabetes.

   2) **Type of diabetes mellitus not documented** — If the type of diabetes mellitus is not documented in the medical record the default is type II.

   3) **Diabetes mellitus and the use of insulin** — All type I diabetics must use insulin to replace what their bodies do not produce. However, the use of insulin does not mean that a patient is a type I diabetic. Some patients with type II diabetes mellitus are unable to control their blood sugar through diet and oral medication alone and do require insulin. If the documentation in a medical record does not indicate the type of diabetes but does indicate that the patient uses insulin, the appropriate fifth digit for type II must be used. For type II patients who routinely use insulin, code V58.67 Long-term (current) use of insulin, should also be assigned to indicate that the patient uses insulin. Code V58.67 should not be assigned if insulin is given temporarily to bring a type II patient's blood sugar under control during an encounter.

   4) **Assigning and sequencing diabetes codes and associated conditions** — When assigning codes for diabetes and its associated conditions, the code(s) from category 250 must be sequenced before the codes for the associated conditions. The diabetes codes and the secondary codes that correspond to them are paired codes that follow the etiology/manifestation convention of the classification (See section I.A.6., Etiology/manifestation convention). Assign as many codes from category 250 as needed to identify all of the associated conditions that the patient has. The corresponding secondary codes are listed under each of the diabetes codes.

      (a) **Diabetic retinopathy/diabetic macular edema-Diabetic macular edema, code 362.07, is only present with diabetic retinopathy. Another code from subcategory 362.0 Diabetic retinopathy, must be used with code 362.07. Codes under subcategory 362.0 are diabetes manifestation codes, so they must be used following the appropriate diabetes code.**

   5) **Diabetes mellitus in pregnancy and gestational diabetes**

      (a) For diabetes mellitus complicating pregnancy, see aection I.C.11.f., Diabetes mellitus in pregnancy.

      (b) For gestational diabetes, see section I.C.11, g., Gestational diabetes.

   6) **Insulin pump malfunction**

      (a) Underdose of insulin due to insulin pump failure-An underdose of insulin due to an insulin pump failure should be assigned 996.57 Mechanical complication due to insulin pump, as the principal or first listed code, followed by the appropriate diabetes mellitus code based on documentation.

(b) Overdose of insulin due to insulin pump failure-The principal or first-listed code for an encounter due to an insulin pump malfunction resulting in an overdose of insulin should also be 996.57 Mechanical complication due to insulin pump, followed by code 962.3 Poisoning by insulins and antidiabetic agents, and the appropriate diabetes mellitus code based on documentation.

4. **Chapter 4: Diseases of Blood and Blood Forming Organs (280-289)**

a. **Anemia of chronic disease-**Subcategory 285.2 Anemia in chronic illness, has codes for anemia in chronic kidney disease, code 285.21; anemia in neoplastic disease, code 285.22; and anemia in other chronic illness, code 285.29. These codes can be used as the principal/first-listed code if the reason for the encounter is to treat the anemia. They may also be used as secondary codes if treatment of the anemia is a component of an encounter but not the primary reason for the encounter. When using a code from subcategory 285 it is also necessary to use the code for the chronic condition causing the anemia.

1) **Anemia in chronic kidney disease-**When assigning code 285.21 Anemia in chronic kidney disease. It is also necessary to assign a code from category 585 Chronic kidney disease to indicate the stage of chronic kidney disease. See I.C.10.a., Chronic kidney disease (CKD). 6

2) **Anemia in neoplastic disease-**When assigning code 285.22 Anemia in neoplastic disease, it is also necessary to assign the neoplasm code that is responsible for the anemia. Code 285.22 is for use for anemia that is due to the malignancy, not for anemia due to antineoplastic chemotherapy drugs, which is an adverse effect.

See I.C.2.c.1., Anemia associated with malignancy.

See I.C.2.c.2., Anemia associated with chemotherapy, immunotherapy and radiation therapy.

See I.C.17.e.1., **Adverse effects.**

5. **Chapter 5: Mental Disorders (290-319)**
Reserved for future guideline expansion

6. **Chapter 6: Diseases of Nervous System and Sense Organs (320-389)**
Reserved for future guideline expansion

7. **Chapter 7: Diseases of Circulatory System (390-459)**

a. **Hypertension**

Hypertension Table

The hypertension table, found under the main term, "Hypertension," in the Alphabetic Index, contains a complete listing of all conditions due to or associated with hypertension and classifies them according to malignant, benign, and unspecified.

1) **Hypertension, essential, or NOS** — Assign hypertension (arterial) (essential) (primary) (systemic) (NOS) to category code 401 with the appropriate fourth digit to indicate malignant (.0), benign (.1), or unspecified (.9). Do not use either .0 malignant or .1 benign unless medical record documentation supports such a designation.

2) **Hypertension with heart disease** — Heart conditions (425.8, 429.0-429.3, 429.8, 429.9) are assigned to a code from category 402 when a causal relationship is stated (due to hypertension) or implied (hypertensive). Use an additional code from category 428 to identify the type of heart failure in those patients with heart failure. More than one code from category 428 may be assigned if the patient has systolic or diastolic failure and congestive heart failure.

The same heart conditions (425.8, 429.0-429.3, 429.8, 429.9) with hypertension, but without a stated casual relationship, are coded separately. Sequence according to the circumstances of the admission/encounter.

3) **Hypertensive kidney disease with chronic renal failure** — Assign codes from category 403, Hypertensive kidney disease, when conditions classified to categories 585-587 are present. Unlike hypertension with heart disease, ICD-9-

CM presumes a cause-and-effect relationship and classifies renal failure with hypertension as hypertensive renal disease.

4) **Hypertensive heart and kidney disease** — Assign codes from combination category 404, Hypertensive heart and **kidney** disease, when both hypertensive **kidney** disease and hypertensive heart disease are stated in the diagnosis. Assume a relationship between the hypertension and the **kidney** disease, whether or not the condition is so designated. Assign an additional code from category 428 to identify the type of heart failure. More than one code from category 428 may be assigned if the patient has systolic or diastolic failure and congestive heart failure.

5) **Hypertensive cerebrovascular disease** — First assign codes from 430-438 Cerebrovascular disease, then the appropriate hypertension code from categories 401-405.

6) **Hypertensive retinopathy** — Two codes are necessary to identify the condition. First assign the code from subcategory 362.11 Hypertensive retinopathy, then the appropriate code from categories 401-405 to indicate the type of hypertension.

7) **Hypertension, secondary** — Two codes are required: one to identify the underlying etiology and one from category 405 to identify the hypertension. Sequencing of codes is determined by the reason for admission/encounter.

8) **Hypertension, transient** — Assign code 796.2 Elevated blood pressure reading without diagnosis of hypertension, unless patient has an established diagnosis of hypertension. Assign code 642.3x for transient hypertension of pregnancy.

9) **Hypertension, controlled** — Assign appropriate code from categories 401-405. This diagnostic statement usually refers to an existing state of hypertension under control by therapy.

10) **Hypertension, uncontrolled** — Uncontrolled hypertension may refer to untreated hypertension or hypertension not responding to current therapeutic regimen. In either case, assign the appropriate code from categories 401-405 to designate the stage and type of hypertension. Code to the type of hypertension.

11) **Elevated blood pressure** — For a statement of elevated blood pressure without further specificity, assign code 796.2, Elevated blood pressure reading without diagnosis of hypertension, rather than a code from category 401.

b. **Cerebral infarction/stroke/cerebrovascular accident (CVA)** — The terms stroke and CVA are often used interchangeably to refer to a cerebral infarction. The terms stroke, CVA, and cerebral infarction NOS are all indexed to the default code 434.91, Cerebral artery occlusion, unspecified, with infarction. Code 436, Acute, but ill-defined, cerebrovascular disease, should not be used when the documentation states stroke or CVA.

c. **Postoperative cerebrovascular accident** — A cerebrovascular hemorrhage or infarction that occurs as a result of medical intervention is coded to 997.02, Iatrogenic cerebrovascular infarction or hemorrhage. Medical record documentation should clearly specify the cause- and-effect relationship between the medical intervention and the cerebrovascular accident in order to assign this code. A secondary code from the code range 430-432 or from a code from subcategories 433 or 434 with a fifth digit of "1" should also be used to identify the type of hemorrhage or infarct.

This guideline conforms to the use additional code note instruction at category 997. Code 436, Acute, but ill-defined, cerebrovascular disease, should not be used as a secondary code with code 997.02.

d. **Late effects of cerebrovascular disease**

1) **Category 438, late effects of cerebrovascular disease** — Category 438 is used to indicate conditions classifiable to categories 430-437 as the causes of late effects (neurologic deficits), themselves classified elsewhere. These "late effects" include neurologic deficits

that persist after initial onset of conditions classifiable to 430-437. The neurologic deficits caused by cerebrovascular disease may be present from the onset or may arise at any time after the onset of the condition classifiable to 430-437.

2) **Codes from category 438 with codes from 430-437** — Codes from category 438 may be assigned on a health care record with codes from 430-437, if the patient has a current cerebrovascular accident (CVA) and deficits from an old CVA.

3) **Code V12.59** — Assign code V12.59 (and not a code from category 438) as an additional code for history of cerebrovascular disease when no neurologic deficits are present.

e. **Acute myocardial infarction (AMI)**

1) **ST elevation myocardial infarction (STEMI) and non-ST elevation myocardial infarction (NSTEMI)**-The ICD-9-CM codes for acute myocardial infarction (AMI) identify the site, such as anterolateral wall or true posterior wall. Subcategories 410.0-410.6 and 410.8 are used for ST elevation myocardial infarction (STEMI). Subcategory 410.7 Subendocardial infarction, is used for non-ST elevation myocardial infarction (NSTEMI) and nontransmural MIs.

2) **Acute myocardial infarction, unspecified**-Subcategory 410.9 is the default for the unspecified term acute myocardial infarction. If only STEMI or transmural MI without the site is documented, query the provider as to the site or assign a code from subcategory 410.9.

3) **AMI documented as nontransmural or subendocardial, but site provided**-If an AMI is documented as nontransmural or subendocardial but the site is provided, it is still coded as a subendocardial AMI. If NSTEMI evolves to STEMI, assign the STEMI code. If STEMI converts to NSTEMI due to thrombolytic therapy, it is still coded as STEMI.

8. **Chapter 8: Diseases of Respiratory System (460-519)**

a. **Chronic obstructive pulmonary disease [COPD] and asthma**

1) **Conditions that comprise COPD and asthma** — The conditions that comprise COPD are obstructive chronic bronchitis, subcategory 491.2, and emphysema, category 492. All asthma codes are under category 493 Asthma. Code 496 Chronic airway obstruction, not elsewhere classified, is a nonspecific code that should be used only when the documentation in a medical record does not specify the type of COPD being treated.

2) **Acute exacerbation of chronic obstructive bronchitis and asthma** — The codes for chronic obstructive bronchitis and asthma distinguish between uncomplicated cases and those in acute exacerbation. An acute exacerbation is a worsening or a decompensation of a chronic condition. An acute exacerbation is not equivalent to an infection superimposed on a chronic condition, though an exacerbation may be triggered by an infection.

3) **Overlapping nature of the conditions that comprise COPD and asthma** — Due to the overlapping nature of the conditions that make up COPD and asthma, there are many variations in the way these conditions are documented. Code selection must be based on the terms as documented. When selecting the correct code for the documented type of COPD and asthma, it is essential to first review the index and then verify the code in the Tabular List. There are many instructional notes under the different COPD subcategories and codes. It is important that all such notes be reviewed to ensure correct code assignment.

4) **Acute exacerbation of asthma and status asthmaticus** — An acute exacerbation of asthma is an increased severity of the asthma symptoms, such as wheezing and shortness of breath. Status asthmaticus refers to a patient's

failure to respond to therapy administered during an asthmatic episode and is a life-threatening complication that requires emergency care. If status asthmaticus is documented by the provider with any type of COPD or with acute bronchitis, the status asthmaticus should be sequenced first. It supersedes any type of COPD, including that with acute exacerbation or acute bronchitis. It is inappropriate to assign an asthma code with fifth-digit 2, with acute exacerbation, together with an asthma code with fifth-digit 1, with status asthmaticus. Only the fifth-digit 1 should be assigned.

b. **Chronic obstructive pulmonary disease [COPD] and bronchitis**

　1) Acute bronchitis with COPD — Acute bronchitis, code 466.0, is due to an infectious organism. When acute bronchitis is documented with COPD, code 491.22 Obstructive chronic bronchitis with acute bronchitis, should be assigned. It is not necessary to also assign code 466.0. If a medical record documents acute bronchitis with COPD with acute exacerbation, only code 491.22 should be assigned. The acute bronchitis included in code 491.22 supersedes the acute exacerbation. If a medical record documents COPD with acute exacerbation without mention of acute bronchitis, only code 491.21 should be assigned.

9. **Chapter 9: Diseases of Digestive System (520-579)**

Reserved for future guideline expansion

10. **Chapter 10: Diseases of Genitourinary System (580-629)**

a. **Chronic kidney disease**

　1) Stages of chronic kidney disease (CKD)-The ICD-9-CM classifies CKD based on severity. The severity of CKD is designated by stages I-V. Stage II, code 585.2, equates to mild CKD; stage III, code 585.3, equates to moderate CKD; and stage IV, code 585.4, equates to severe CKD. Code 585.6 End-stage renal disease (ESRD), is assigned when the provider has documented end-stage renal disease (ESRD). If both a stage of CKD and ESRD are documented, assign code 585.6 only.

　2) Chronic kidney disease and kidney transplant status-Patients who have undergone kidney transplant may still have some form of CKD because the kidney transplant may not fully restore kidney function. Code V42.0 may be assigned with the appropriate CKD code for patients who are status post kidney transplant, based on the patient's post-transplant stage. The use additional code note under category 585 provides this instruction.

Use of a 585 code with V42.0 does not necessarily indicate transplant rejection or failure. Patients with mild or moderate CKD following a transplant should not be coded as having transplant failure unless it is documented in the medical record. For patients with severe CKD or ESRD it is appropriate to assign code 996.81 Complications of transplanted organ, kidney transplant, when kidney transplant failure is documented. If a post kidney transplant patient has CKD and it is unclear from the documentation whether there is transplant failure or rejection, it is necessary to query the provider.

　3) Chronic kidney disease with other conditions-Patients with CKD may also suffer from other serious conditions, most commonly diabetes mellitus and hypertension. The sequencing of the CKD code in relationship to codes for other contributing conditions is based on the conventions in the tabular list. See I.C.3.a.4. for sequencing instructions for diabetes.

See I.C.4.a.1. for anemia in CKD.

See I.C.7.a.3. for hypertensive kidney disease.

See I.C.17.f.1.b. Transplant complications, for instructions on coding of documented rejection or failure.

11. **Chapter 11: Complications of Pregnancy, Childbirth, and thePuerperium (630-677)**
   a. **General rules for obstetric cases**
      1) **Codes from chapter 11 and sequencing priority** — Obstetric cases require codes from chapter 11, codes in the range 630-677 Complications of pregnancy, childbirth, and the puerperium. Chapter 11 codes have sequencing priority over codes from other chapters. Additional codes from other chapters may be used in conjunction with chapter 11 codes to further specify conditions. Should the provider document that the pregnancy is incidental to the encounter, then code V22.2 should be used in place of any chapter 11 codes. It is the provider's responsibility to state that the condition being treated is not affecting the pregnancy.
      2) **Chapter 11 codes used only on the maternal record** — Chapter 11 codes are to be used only on the maternal record, never on the record of the newborn.
      3) **Chapter 11 fifth digits** — Categories 640-648, 651-676 have required fifth-digits, which indicate whether the encounter is antepartum, postpartum and whether a delivery has also occurred.
      4) **Fifth digits, appropriate for each code** — The fifth digits, which are appropriate for each code number, are listed in brackets under each code. The fifth digits on each code should all be consistent with each other. That is, should a delivery occur all of the fifth digits should indicate the delivery.
   b. **Selection of OB principal or first-listed diagnosis**
      1) **Routine outpatient prenatal visits** — For routine outpatient prenatal visits when no complications are present, codes V22.0 Supervision of normal first pregnancy, and V22.1 Supervision of other normal pregnancy, should be used as the first-listed diagnoses. These codes should not be used in conjunction with chapter 11 codes.
      2) **Prenatal outpatient visits for high-risk patients** — For prenatal outpatient visits for patients with high-risk pregnancies, a code from category V23 Supervision of high-risk pregnancy, should be used as the principal or first-listed diagnosis. Secondary chapter 11 codes may be used in conjunction with these codes if appropriate.
      3) **Episodes when no delivery occurs** — In episodes when no delivery occurs, the principal diagnosis should correspond to the principal complication of the pregnancy, which necessitated the encounter. Should more than one complication exist, all of which are treated or monitored, any of the complication codes may be sequenced first.
      4) **When a delivery occurs** — When a delivery occurs, the principal diagnosis should correspond to the main circumstances or complication of the delivery. In cases of cesarean delivery, the selection of the principal diagnosis should correspond to the reason the cesarean delivery was performed unless the reason for admission/encounter was unrelated to the condition resulting in the cesarean delivery.
      5) **Outcome of delivery** — An outcome of delivery code, V27.0-V27.9, should be included on every maternal record when a delivery has occurred. These codes are not to be used on subsequent records or on the newborn record.
   c. **Fetal conditions affecting the management of the mother**
      1) **Fetal condition responsible for modifying the management of the mother** — Codes from category 655 Known or suspected fetal abnormality affecting management of the mother, and category 656 Other fetal and placental problems affecting the management of the mother, are assigned only when the fetal condition is actually responsible for

modifying the management of the mother, i.e., by requiring diagnostic studies, additional observation, special care, or termination of pregnancy. The fact that the fetal condition exists does not justify assigning a code from this series to the mother's record.

2) **In utero surgery** — In cases when surgery is performed on the fetus, a diagnosis code from category 655 Known or suspected fetal abnormalities affecting management of the mother, should be assigned identifying the fetal condition. Procedure code 75.36 Correction of fetal defect, should be assigned on the hospital inpatient record.

No code from chapter 15, the perinatal codes, should be used on the mother's record to identify fetal conditions. Surgery performed in utero on a fetus is still to be coded as an obstetric encounter.

d. **HIV infection in pregnancy, childbirth and the puerperium** — During pregnancy, childbirth, or the puerperium, a patient admitted because of an HIV-related illness should receive a principal diagnosis of 647.6X Other specified infectious and parasitic diseases in the mother classifiable elsewhere, but complicating the pregnancy, childbirth, or the puerperium, followed by 042 and the code(s) for the HIV-related illness(es).

Patients with asymptomatic HIV infection status admitted during pregnancy, childbirth, or the puerperium should receive codes of 647.6X and V08.

e. **Current conditions complicating pregnancy** — Assign a code from subcategory 648.x for patients that have current conditions when the condition affects the management of the pregnancy, childbirth, or the puerperium. Use additional secondary codes from other chapters to identify the conditions, as appropriate.

f. **Diabetes mellitus in pregnancy** — Diabetes mellitus is a significant complicating factor in pregnancy. Pregnant women who are diabetic should be assigned code 648.0x Diabetes mellitus complicating pregnancy, and a secondary code from category 250 Diabetes mellitus, to identify the type of diabetes.

Code V58.67 Long-term (current) use of insulin, should also be assigned if the diabetes mellitus is being treated with insulin.

g. **Gestational diabetes** — Gestational diabetes can occur during the second and third trimester of pregnancy in women who were not diabetic prior to pregnancy. Gestational diabetes can cause complications in the pregnancy similar to those of pre-existing diabetes mellitus. It also puts the woman at greater risk of developing diabetes after the pregnancy. Gestational diabetes is coded to 648.8x Abnormal glucose tolerance. Codes 648.0x and 648.8x should never be used together on the same record.

Code V58.67 Long-term (current) use of insulin, should also be assigned if the gestational diabetes is being treated with insulin.

h. **Normal delivery, code 650**

1) **Normal delivery** — Code 650 is for use in cases when a woman is admitted for a full-term normal delivery and delivers a single, healthy infant without any complications antepartum, during the delivery, or postpartum during the delivery episode. Code 650 is always a principal diagnosis. It is not to be used if any other code from chapter 11 is needed to describe a current complication of the antenatal, delivery, or perinatal period. Additional codes from other chapters may be used with code 650 if they are not related to or are in any way complicating the pregnancy.

2) **Normal delivery with resolved antepartum complication** — Code 650 may be used if the patient had a complication at some point during her pregnancy, but the complication is not present at the time of the admission for delivery.

3) **V27.0 Single liveborn, outcome of delivery** — V27.0 Single liveborn, is the only outcome of the delivery code appropriate for use with 650.

i. **The postpartum and peripartum periods**

1) **Postpartum and peripartum periods** — The postpartum period begins immediately after delivery and continues for six weeks following delivery. The peripartum period is defined as the last

Official ICD-9-CM Coding Guidelines

month of pregnancy to five months postpartum.

2) **Postpartum complication** — A postpartum complication is any complication occurring within the six-week period.

3) **Pregnancy-related complications after six-week period** — Chapter 11 codes may also be used to describe pregnancy-related complications after the six-week period should the provider document that a condition is pregnancy related.

4) **Postpartum complications occurring during the same admission as delivery** — Postpartum complications that occur during the same admission as the delivery are identified with a fifth digit of 2. Subsequent admissions/encounters for postpartum complications should be identified with a fifth digit of 4.

5) **Admission for routine postpartum care following delivery outside hospital** — When the mother delivers outside the hospital prior to admission and is admitted for routine postpartum care and no complications are noted, code V24.0 Postpartum care and examination immediately after delivery, should be assigned as the principal diagnosis.

6) **Admission following delivery outside hospital with postpartum conditions** — A delivery diagnosis code should not be used for a woman who has delivered prior to admission to the hospital. Any postpartum conditions and/or postpartum procedures should be coded.

j. **Code 677 Late effect of complication of pregnancy**

1) **Code 677** — Code 677 Late effect of complication of pregnancy, childbirth, and the puerperium is for use in those cases when an initial complication of a pregnancy develops a sequelae requiring care or treatment at a future date.

2) **After the initial postpartum period** — This code may be used at any time after the initial postpartum period.

3) **Sequencing of code 677** — This code, like all late effect codes, is to be sequenced following the code describing the sequelae of the complication.

k. **Abortions**

1) **Fifth digits required for abortion categories** — Fifth digits are required for abortion categories 634-637. Fifth-digit 1, incomplete, indicates that all of the products of conception have not been expelled from the uterus. Fifth-digit 2, complete, indicates that all products of conception have been expelled from the uterus prior to the episode of care.

2) **Code from categories 640-648 and 651-659** — A code from categories 640-648 and 651-659 may be used as additional codes with an abortion code to indicate the complication leading to the abortion.

Fifth-digit 3 is assigned with codes from these categories when used with an abortion code because the other fifth digits will not apply. Codes from the 660-669 series are not to be used for complications of abortion.

3) **Code 639 for complications** — Code 639 is to be used for all complications following abortion. Code 639 cannot be assigned with codes from categories 634-638.

4) **Abortion with liveborn fetus** — When an attempted termination of pregnancy results in a liveborn fetus assign code 644.21 Early onset of delivery, with an appropriate code from category V27 Outcome of delivery. The procedure code for the attempted termination of pregnancy should also be assigned.

5) **Retained products of conception following an abortion** — Subsequent admissions for retained products of conception following a spontaneous or legally induced abortion are assigned the appropriate code from category 634 Spontaneous abortion, or 635 Legally induced abortion, with a fifth digit of 1 (incomplete). This advice is appropriate even when the patient was discharged previously with a discharge diagnosis of complete abortion.

© 2006 Ingenix ✓5th Needs fifth digit ⬛OK Valid three-digit code

12. **Chapter 12: Diseases of Skin and Subcutaneous Tissue (680-709)**
Reserved for future guideline expansion

13. **Chapter 13: Diseases of Musculoskeletal and Connective Tissue (710-739)**
Reserved for future guideline expansion

14. **Chapter 14: Congenital Anomalies (740-759)**

   a. **Codes in categories 740-759 Congenital anomalies** — Assign an appropriate code(s) from categories 740-759, Congenital anomalies, when an anomaly is documented. A congenital anomaly may be the principal/first-listed diagnosis on a record or a secondary diagnosis. **When a congenital anomaly does not have a unique code assignment, assign additional code(s) for any manifestations that may be present.**

   When the code assignment specifically identifies the congenital anomaly, manifestations that are an inherent component of the anomaly should not be coded separately. Additional codes should be assigned for manifestations that are not an inherent component.

   Codes from Chapter 14 may be used throughout the life of the patient. If a congenital anomaly has been corrected, a personal history code should be used to identify the history of the anomaly. **Although present at birth, a congenital anomaly may not be identified until later in life. Whenever the condition is diagnosed by the physician, it is appropriate to assign a code from codes 740-759.**

   For the birth admission, the appropriate code from category V30 Liveborn infants, according to type of birth should be sequenced as the principal diagnosis, followed by any congenital anomaly codes, 740-759.

15. **Chapter 15: Newborn (Perinatal) Guidelines (760-779)**
For coding and reporting purposes the perinatal period is defined as birth through the 28th day following birth. The following guidelines are provided for reporting purposes. Hospitals may record other diagnoses as needed for internal data use.

   a. **General perinatal rules**

   1) **Chapter 15 codes** — They are never for use on the maternal record. Codes from chapter 11, the obstetric chapter, are never permitted on the newborn record. Chapter 15 code may be used throughout the life of the patient if the condition is still present.

   2) **Sequencing of perinatal codes** — Generally, codes from chapter 15 should be sequenced as the principal/first-listed diagnosis on the newborn record, with the exception of the appropriate V30 code for the birth episode, followed by codes from any other chapter that provide additional detail. The "use additional code" note at the beginning of the chapter supports this guideline. If the index does not provide a specific code for a perinatal condition, assign code 779.89 Other specified conditions originating in the perinatal period, followed by the code from another chapter that specifies the condition. Codes for signs and symptoms may be assigned when a definitive diagnosis has not been established.

   3) **Birth process or community acquired conditions** — If a newborn has a condition that may be either due to the birth process or community acquired and the documentation does not indicate which it is, the default is due to the birth process and the code from chapter 15 should be used. If the condition is community acquired, a code from chapter 15 should not be assigned.

   4) **Code all clinically significant conditions** — All clinically significant conditions noted on routine newborn examination should be coded. A condition is clinically significant if it requires:

   - Clinical evaluation; or
   - Therapeutic treatment; or
   - Diagnostic procedures; or
   - Extended length of hospital stay; or
   - Increased nursing care and/or monitoring; or
   - Has implications for future health care needs

   Note: The perinatal guidelines listed above are the same as the general coding guidelines for "additional diagnoses," except for the final point regarding implications for future health care needs. Codes should be assigned for conditions that have been specified by the provider as having implications for future health care needs. Codes from the perinatal chapter should not be assigned unless the provider has established a definitive diagnosis.

b. Use of codes V30-V39 — When coding the birth of an infant, assign a code from categories V30-V39, according to the type of birth. A code from this series is assigned as a principal diagnosis and assigned only once to a newborn at the time of birth.

c. Newborn transfers — If the newborn is transferred to another institution, the V30 series is not used at the receiving hospital.

d. Use of category V29

1) **Assigning a code from category V29** — Assign a code from category V29 Observation and evaluation of newborns and infants for suspected conditions not found, to identify those instances when a healthy newborn is evaluated for a suspected condition that is determined after study not to be present. Do not use a code from category V29 when the patient has identified signs or symptoms of a suspected problem; in such cases, code the sign or symptom.

    A code from category V29 may also be assigned as a principal diagnosis for readmissions or encounters when the V30 code no longer applies. Codes from category V29 are for use only for healthy newborns and infants for which no condition after study is found to be present.

2) **V29 code on a birth record** — A V29 code is to be used as a secondary code after the V30 Outcome of delivery, code.

e. Use of other V codes on perinatal records — V codes other than V30 and V29 may be assigned on a perinatal or newborn record code. The codes may be used as a principal or first-listed diagnosis for specific types of encounters or for readmissions or encounters when the V30 code no longer applies.

See section I.C.18 for information regarding the assignment of V codes.

f. Maternal causes of perinatal morbidity — Codes from categories 760-763 Maternal causes of perinatal morbidity and mortality, are assigned only when the maternal condition has actually affected the fetus or newborn. The fact that the mother has an associated medical condition or experiences some complication of pregnancy, labor, or delivery does not justify the routine assignment of codes from these categories to the newborn record.

g. Congenital anomalies in newborns — For the birth admission, the appropriate code from category V30 Liveborn infants according to type of birth, should be used, followed by any congenital anomaly codes, categories 740-759. Use additional secondary codes from other chapters to specify conditions associated with the anomaly, if applicable.

Also, see section I.C.14 for information on the coding of congenital anomalies.

h. Coding additional perinatal diagnoses

1) **Assigning codes for conditions that require treatment** — Assign codes for conditions that require treatment or further investigation, prolong the length of stay, or require resource utilization.

2) **Codes for conditions specified as having implications for future health care needs** — Assign codes for conditions that have been specified by the provider as having implications for future health care needs.

    Note: This guideline should not be used for adult patients.

3) **Codes for newborn conditions originating in the perinatal period** — Assign a code for newborn conditions originating in the perinatal period (categories 760-779), as well as complications arising during the current episode of care classified in other chapters, only if the diagnoses have been documented by the responsible provider at the time of transfer or discharge as having affected the fetus or newborn.

i. Prematurity and fetal growth retardation — Providers utilize different criteria in determining prematurity. A code for prematurity should not be assigned unless it is documented. The fift-digit assignment for codes from category 764 and subcategories 765.0 and 765.1 should be based on the recorded birth weight and estimated gestational age.

A code from subcategory 765.2 Weeks of gestation, should be assigned as an additional code with category 764 and codes from 765.0 and 765.1 to specify weeks of gestation as documented by the provider in the record.

j. **Newborn sepsis** — Code 771.81 Septicemia [sepsis]of newborn, should be assigned with a secondary code from category 041 Bacterial infections in conditions classified elsewhere and of unspecified site, to identify the organism. It is not necessary to use a code from subcategory 995.9 Systemic inflammatory response syndrome (SIRS), on a newborn record. A code from category 038 Septicemia, should not be used on a newborn record. Code 771.81 describes the sepsis.

16. *Chapter 16: Signs, Symptoms and Ill-Defined Conditions (780-799)*
Reserved for future guideline expansion

17. *Chapter 17: Injury and Poisoning (800-999)*
a. **Coding of injuries** — When coding injuries, assign separate codes for each injury unless a combination code is provided, in which case the combination code is assigned. Multiple injury codes are provided in ICD-9-CM but should not be assigned unless information for a more specific code is not available. These codes are not to be used for normal, healing surgical wounds or to identify complications of surgical wounds.

The code for the most serious injury, as determined by the provider and the focus of treatment, is sequenced first.

  1) **Superficial injuries** — Superficial injuries such as abrasions or contusions are not coded when associated with more severe injuries of the same site.

  2) **Primary injury with damage to nerves/blood vessels** — When a primary injury results in minor damage to peripheral nerves or blood vessels, the primary injury is sequenced first with additional code(s) from categories 950-957 Injury to nerves and spinal cord, and/or 900-904 Injury to blood vessels. When the primary injury is to the blood vessels or nerves, that injury should be sequenced first.

b. **Coding of fractures** — The principles of multiple coding of injuries should be followed in coding fractures. Fractures of specified sites are coded individually by site in accordance with both the provisions within categories 800-829 and the level of detail furnished by medical record content. Combination categories for multiple fractures are provided for use when there is insufficient detail in the medical record (such as trauma cases transferred to another hospital), when the reporting form limits the number of codes that can be used in reporting pertinent clinical data, or when there is insufficient specificity at the fourth-digit or fifth-digit level. More specific guidelines are as follows:

  1) **Multiple fractures of same limb** — Multiple fractures of same limb classifiable to the same three-digit or four-digit category are coded to that category.

  2) **Multiple unilateral or bilateral fractures of same bone** — Multiple unilateral or bilateral fractures of same bone(s) but classified to different fourth-digit subdivisions (bone part) within the same three-digit category are coded individually by site.

  3) **Multiple fracture categories 819 and 828** — Multiple fracture categories 819 and 828 classify bilateral fractures of both upper limbs (819) and both lower limbs (828), but without any detail at the fourth-digit level other than open and closed type of fractures.

  4) **Multiple fractures sequencing** — Multiple fractures are sequenced in accordance with the severity of the fracture. The provider should be asked to list the fracture diagnoses in the order of severity.

c. **Coding of burns** — Current burns (940-948) are classified by depth, extent, and by agent (E code). Burns are classified by depth as first degree (erythema), second degree (blistering), and third degree (full-thickness involvement).

  1) **Sequencing of burn codes and related condition** — Sequence first the code that

reflects the highest degree of burn when more than one burn is present.

(a) **When the reason for the admission or encounter is for treatment of external multiple burns, sequence first the code that reflects the burn of the highest degree.**

(b) **When a patient has both internal and external burns, the circumstances of admission govern the selection of the principal diagnosis or first-listed diagnosis.**

(c) **When a patient is admitted for burn injuries and other related conditions such as smoke inhalation and/or respiratory failure, the circumstances of admission govern the selection of the principal or first-listed diagnosis.**

2) **Burns of the same local site** — Classify burns of the same local site (three-digit category level, 940-947) but of different degrees to the subcategory identifying the highest degree recorded in the diagnosis.

3) **Non-healing burns** — Non-healing burns are coded as acute burns. Necrosis of burned skin should be coded as a non-healed burn.

4) **Code 958.3 Posttraumatic wound infection** — Assign code 958.3 Posttraumatic wound infection, not elsewhere classified, as an additional code for any documented infected burn site.

5) **Assign separate codes for each burn site** — When coding burns, assign separate codes for each burn site. Category 946 Burns of multiple specified sites, should only be used if the locations of the burns are not documented. Category 949 Burn, unspecified, is extremely vague and should rarely be used.

6) **Burns classified according to extent of body surface involved** — Assign codes from category 948 Burns, when the site of the burn is not specified or when there is a need for additional data. It is advisable to use category 948 as additional coding when needed to provide data for evaluating burn mortality, such as that needed by burn units. It is also advisable to use category 948 as an additional code for reporting purposes when there is mention of a third-degree burn involving 20 percent or more of the body surface.

In assigning a code from category 948:

- Fourth-digit codes are used to identify the percentage of total body surface involved in a burn (all degree).

- Fifth digits are assigned to identify the percentage of body surface involved in third-degree burn.

- Fifth-digit zero (0) is assigned when less than 10 percent or when no body surface is involved in a third-degree burn.

- Category 948 is based on the classic "rule of nines" in estimating body surface involved: head and neck are assigned 9 percent, each arm 9 percent, each leg 18 percent, the anterior trunk 18 percent, posterior trunk 18 percent, and genitalia 1 percent. Providers may change these percentage assignments where necessary to accommodate infants and children who have proportionately larger heads than adults and patients who have large buttocks, thighs, or abdomen that involve burns.

7) **Encounters for treatment of late effects of burns** — Encounters for the treatment of the late effects of burns (i.e., scars or joint contractures) should be coded to the residual condition (sequelae) followed by the appropriate late effect code (906.5-906.9). A late effect E code may also be used, if desired.

8) **Sequelae with a late effect code and current burn** — When appropriate, both a sequelae with a late effect code, and a current burn code may be assigned on

the same record (when both a current burn and sequelae of an old burn exist).

d. **Coding of debridement of wound, infection, or burn** — Excisional debridement involves an excisional debridement (surgical removal or cutting away), as opposed to a mechanical (brushing, scrubbing, washing) debridement.

For coding purposes, excisional debridement is assigned to code 86.22.

Nonexcisional debridement is assigned to code 86.28.

e. **Adverse effects, poisoning and toxic effects** — The properties of certain drugs, medicinal and biological substances, or combinations of such substances, may cause toxic reactions. The occurrence of drug toxicity is classified in ICD-9-CM as follows:

1) **Adverse effect** — When the drug was correctly prescribed and properly administered, code the reaction plus the appropriate code from the E930-E949 series. Codes from the E930-E949 series must be used to identify the causative substance for an adverse effect of drug, medicinal and biological substances, correctly prescribed and properly administered. The effect, such as tachycardia, delirium, gastrointestinal hemorrhaging, vomiting, hypokalemia, hepatitis, renal failure, or respiratory failure, is coded and followed by the appropriate code from the E930-E949 series.

Adverse effects of therapeutic substances correctly prescribed and properly administered (toxicity, synergistic reaction, side effect, and idiosyncratic reaction) may be due to (1) differences among patients, such as age, sex, disease, and genetic factors, and (2) drug-related factors, such as type of drug, route of administration, duration of therapy, dosage, and bioavailability.

2) **Poisoning**

(a) **Error was made in drug prescription** — Errors made in drug prescription or in the administration of the drug by provider, nurse, patient, or other person, use the appropriate poisoning code from the 960-979 series.

(b) **Overdose of a drug intentionally taken** — If an overdose of a drug was intentionally taken or administered and resulted in drug toxicity, it would be coded as a poisoning (960-979 series).

(c) **Nonprescribed drug taken with correctly prescribed and properly administered drug** — If a nonprescribed drug or medicinal agent was taken in combination with a correctly prescribed and properly administered drug, any drug toxicity or other reaction resulting from the interaction of the two drugs would be classified as a poisoning.

(d) **Sequencing of poisoning** — When coding a poisoning or reaction to the improper use of a medication (e.g., wrong dose, wrong substance, wrong route of administration) the poisoning code is sequenced first, followed by a code for the manifestation. If there is also a diagnosis of drug abuse or dependence to the substance, the abuse or dependence is coded as an additional code.

See section I.C.3.a.6.b. if poisoning is the result of insulin pump malfunctions and section I.C.19 for general use of E codes.

3) **Toxic effects**

(a) **Toxic effect codes** — When a harmful substance is ingested or comes in contact with a person, this is classified as a toxic effect. The toxic effect codes are in categories 980-989.

(b) **Sequencing toxic effect codes** — A toxic effect code should be sequenced first, followed by the codes that identify the result of the toxic effect.

(c) **External cause codes for toxic effects** — An external cause code from categories E860-E869 for accidental exposure, code E950.6 or E950.7 for intentional self-harm, category E962 for assault, or categories E980-E982 for undetermined, should also be assigned to indicate intent.

f. **Complications of care**

   1) **Transplant complications**

      (a) **Transplant complications other than kidney**-Codes under subcategory 996.8 Complications of transplanted organ, are for use for both complications and rejection of transplanted organs. A transplant complication code is only assigned if the complication affects the function of the transplanted organ. Two codes are required to fully describe a transplant complication, the appropriate code from subcategory 996.8 and a secondary code that identifies the complication.

      Pre-existing conditions or conditions that develop after the transplant are not coded as complications unless they affect the function of the transplanted organs.

      Post-transplant surgical complications that do not relate to the function of the transplanted organ are classified to the specific complication. For example, a surgical wound dehiscence would be coded as a wound dehiscence, not as a transplant complication.

      Post-transplant patients who are seen for treatment unrelated to the transplanted organ should be assigned a code from category V42 Organ or tissue replaced by transplant, to identify the transplant status of the patient. A code from category V42 should never be used with a code from subcategory 996.8.

      (b) **Kidney transplant and chronic kidney disease**-Patients with chronic kidney disease (CKD) following a transplant should not be assumed to have transplant failure or rejection unless it is documented by the provider. If documentation supports the presence of failure or rejection, then it is appropriate to assign code 996.81 Complications of transplanted organs, kidney, followed by the appropriate CKD code.

18. *Classification of Factors Influencing Health Status and Contact with Health Service (Supplemental V01-V86)*

    Note: The chapter-specific guidelines provide additional information about the use of V codes for specified encounters.

    a. **Introduction** — ICD-9-CM provides codes to deal with encounters for circumstances other than a disease or injury. The Supplementary Classification of Factors Influencing Health Status and Contact with Health Services (V01-V86) is provided to deal with occasions when circumstances other than a disease or injury (codes 001-999) are recorded as a diagnosis or problem.

    There are four primary circumstances for the use of V codes:

    1) A person who is not currently sick encounters the health services for some specific reason, such as to act as an organ donor, to receive prophylactic care, such as inoculations or health screenings, or to receive counseling on health related issues.

    2) A person with a resolving disease or injury, or a chronic, long-term condition requiring continuous care, encounters the health care system for specific aftercare of that disease or injury (e.g., dialysis for renal disease; chemotherapy for malignancy; cast change). A diagnosis/symptom code should be used whenever a current, acute diagnosis is being treated or a sign or symptom is being studied.

Coders' Desk Reference for Diagnoses

3) Circumstances or problems influence a person's health status but are not in themselves a current illness or injury.

4) Newborns, to indicate birth status

b. **V codes use in any health care setting** — V codes are for use in any healthcare setting. V codes may be used as either a first-listed (principal diagnosis code in the inpatient setting) or secondary code, depending on the circumstances of the encounter. Certain V codes may only be used as first listed, others only as secondary codes. See section I.C.18.e, V code table.

c. **V codes indicate a reason for an encounter** — They are not procedure codes. A corresponding procedure code must accompany a V code to describe the procedure performed.

d. **Categories of V codes**

1) **Contact/exposure** — Category V01 indicates contact with or exposure to communicable diseases. These codes are for patients who do not show any sign or symptom of a disease but have been exposed to it by close personal contact with an infected individual or are in an area where a disease is epidemic. These codes may be used as a first-listed code to explain an encounter for testing, or, more commonly, as a secondary code to identify a potential risk.

2) **Inoculations and vaccinations** — Categories V03-V06 are for encounters for inoculations and vaccinations. They indicate that a patient is being seen to receive a prophylactic inoculation against a disease. The injection itself must be represented by the appropriate procedure code. A code from V03-V06 may be used as a secondary code if the inoculation is given as a routine part of preventive health care, such as a well-baby visit.

3) **Status** — Status codes indicate that a patient is either a carrier of a disease or has the sequelae or residual of a past disease or condition. This includes such things as the presence of prosthetic or mechanical devices resulting from past treatment.

A status code is informative, because the status may affect the course of treatment and its outcome. A status code is distinct from a history code. The history code indicates that the patient no longer has the condition.

A status code should not be used with a diagnosis code from one of the body system chapters, if the diagnosis code includes the information provided by the status code. For example, code V42.1 Heart transplant status, should not be used with code 996.83 Complications of transplanted heart. The status code does not provide additional information. The complication code indicates that the patient is a heart transplant patient.

The status V codes/categories are:

V02 — Carrier or suspected carrier of infectious diseases-Carrier status indicates that a person harbors the specific organisms of a disease without manifest symptoms and is capable of transmitting the infection.

V08 — Asymptomatic HIV infection status-This code indicates that a patient has tested positive for HIV but has manifested no signs or symptoms of the disease.

V09 — Infection with drug-resistant microorganisms-This category indicates that a patient has an infection that is resistant to drug treatment. Sequence the infection code first.

V21 — Constitutional states in development

V22.2 — Pregnant state, incidental-This code is a secondary code only for use when the pregnancy is in no way complicating the reason for visit. Otherwise, a code from

Official ICD-9-CM Coding Guidelines

	the obstetric chapter is required.
V26.5x	Sterilization status
V42	Organ or tissue replaced by transplant
V43	Organ or tissue replaced by other means
V44	Artificial opening status
V45	Other postsurgical states
V46	Other dependence on machines
V49.6	Upper limb amputation status
V49.7	Lower limb amputation status
V49.81	Postmenopausal status
V49.82	Dental sealant status
V49.83	Awaiting organ transplant status
V58.6	Long-term (current) drug use-This subcategory indicates a patient's continuous use of a prescribed drug (including such things as aspirin therapy) for the long-term treatment of a condition or for prophylactic use. It is not for use for patients who have addictions to drugs.

Assign a code from subcategory V58.6 Long-term (current) drug use, if the patient is receiving a medication for an extended period as a prophylactic measure (such as for the prevention of deep vein thrombosis) or as treatment of a chronic condition (such as arthritis) or a disease requiring a lengthy course of treatment (such as cancer). Do not assign a code from subcategory V58.6 for medication being administered for a brief period of time to treat an acute illness or injury (such as a course of antibiotics to treat acute bronchitis).

V83	Genetic carrier status- Genetic carrier status indicates that a person carries a gene, associated with a particular disease, which may be passed to offspring who may develop that disease. The person does not have the disease and is not at risk of developing the disease.
V84	Genetic susceptibility status- Genetic susceptibility indicates that a person has a gene that increases the risk of that person developing the disease.

Codes from category V84 Genetic susceptibility to disease, should not be used as principal or first-listed codes. If the patient has the condition to which he/she is susceptible and that condition is the reason for the encounter, the code for the current condition should be sequenced first. If the patient is being seen for follow-up after completed treatment for this condition and the condition no longer exists, a follow-up code should be sequenced first, followed by the appropriate personal history and genetic susceptibility codes. If the purpose of the encounter is genetic counseling associated with procreative management, a code from subcategory V26.3 Genetic counseling and testing, should be assigned as the first-listed code, followed by a code from category V84.

Additional codes should be assigned for any applicable family or personal history. See Section I.C.18.d.14. for information on prophylactic organ removal due to a genetic susceptibility.

Note: Categories V42-V46, and subcategories V49.6, V49.7 are for use only if there are no complications or malfunctions of the organ or tissue replaced, the amputation site, or the equipment on which the patient is dependent.

4) **History (of)** — There are two types of history V codes, personal and family. Personal history codes explain a patient's past medical condition that no longer exists and is not receiving any treatment but that has the potential for recurrence, and therefore may require continued monitoring. The exceptions to this general rule are category V14 Personal history of allergy to medicinal agents, and subcategory V15.0 Allergy, other than to medicinal agents. A person who has had an allergic episode to a substance or food in the past should always be considered allergic to the substance.

Family history codes are for use when a patient has a family member(s) who has had a particular disease that causes the patient to be at higher risk of also contracting the disease.

Personal history codes may be used in conjunction with follow-up codes and family history codes may be used in conjunction with screening codes to explain the need for a test or procedure. History codes are also acceptable on any medical record regardless of the reason for visit. A history of an illness, even if no longer present, is important information that may alter the type of treatment ordered.

The history V code categories are:

V10	Personal history of malignant neoplasm
V12	Personal history of certain other diseases
V13	Personal history of other diseases

Except: V13.4 Personal history of arthritis, and V13.6 Personal history of congenital malformations. These conditions are life-long so are not true history codes.

V14	Personal history of allergy to medicinal agents
V15	Other personal history presenting hazards to health

Except: V15.7 Personal history of contraception

V16	Family history of malignant neoplasm
V17	Family history of certain chronic disabling diseases
V18	Family history of certain other specific diseases
V19	Family history of other conditions

5) **Screening** — Screening is the testing for disease or disease precursors in seemingly well individuals so that early detection and treatment can be provided for those who test positive for the disease. Screenings that are recommended for many subgroups in a population include routine mammograms for women over 40, a fecal occult blood test for everyone over 50, an amniocentesis to rule out a fetal anomaly for pregnant women over 35, because the incidence of breast cancer and colon cancer in these subgroups is higher than in the general population, as is the incidence of Down's syndrome in older mothers.

The testing of a person to rule out or confirm a suspected diagnosis because the patient has some sign or symptom is a diagnostic examination, not a screening. In these cases, the sign or symptom is used to explain the reason for the test.

A screening code may be a first-listed code if the reason for the visit is specifically the screening exam. It may also be used as an additional code if the screening is done during an office visit for other health problems. A screening code is not necessary if the screening is inherent to a routine examination, such as a Pap smear done during a routine pelvic examination. | Should a condition be discovered during the screening then the code for the condition may be assigned as an additional diagnos

The V code indicates that a screening exam is planned. A procedure code is required to confirm that the screening was performed.

The screening V code categories:

V28	Antenatal screening
V73-V82	Special screening examinations

6) **Observation** — There are two observation V code categories. They are for use in very limited circumstances when a person is being observed for a suspected condition that is ruled out. The observation codes are not for use if an injury or illness or any signs or symptoms related to the suspected condition are present. In such cases the diagnosis/symptom code is used with the corresponding E code to identify any external cause.

The observation codes are to be used as principal diagnosis only. The only exception to this is when the principal diagnosis is required to be a code from the V30 Live born infant, category. Then the V29 observation code is sequenced after the V30 code. Additional codes may be used in addition to the observation code but only if they are unrelated to the suspected condition being observed.

The observation V code categories:

V29	Observation and evaluation of newborns for suspected condition not found

For the birth encounter, a code from category V30 should be sequenced before the V29 code.

V71	Observation and evaluation for suspected condition not found

7) **Aftercare** — Aftercare visit codes cover situations when the initial treatment of a disease or injury has been performed and the patient requires continued care during the healing or recovery phase, or for the long-term consequences of the disease. The aftercare V code should not be used if treatment is directed at a current, acute disease or injury, the diagnosis code is to be used in these cases. Exceptions to this rule are codes V58.0 Radiotherapy, and **codes from subcategory V58.1 Encounter for chemotherapy and immunotherapy for neoplastic conditions.** These codes are to be first listed, followed by the diagnosis code when a patient's encounter is solely to receive radiation therapy or chemotherapy for the treatment of a neoplasm. Should a patient receive both chemotherapy and radiation therapy during the same encounter, codes V58.0 and V58.1 may be used together on a record with either one being sequenced first.

The aftercare codes are generally first listed to explain the specific reason for the encounter. An aftercare code may be used as an additional code when some type of aftercare is provided in addition to the reason for admission and no diagnosis code is applicable. An example of this would be the closure of a colostomy during an encounter for treatment of another condition.

Certain aftercare V code categories need a secondary diagnosis code to describe the resolving condition or sequelae, for others, the condition is inherent in the code title.

Additional V code aftercare category terms include fitting and adjustment, and attention to artificial openings.

Status V codes may be used with aftercare V codes to indicate the nature of the aftercare. For example code V45.81 Aortocoronary bypass status, may be used with code V58.73 Aftercare following surgery of the circulatory system, NEC, to indicate the surgery for which the aftercare is being performed. Also, a transplant status code may be used following code V58.44 Aftercare following organ transplant, to identify the organ transplanted. A status code should not be used when the aftercare code indicates the type of status, such as using V55.0 Attention to tracheostomy with V44.0 Tracheostomy status.

The aftercare V category/codes:

Code	Description
V52	Fitting and adjustment of prosthetic device and implant
V53	Fitting and adjustment of other device
V54	Other orthopedic aftercare
V55	Attention to artificial openings
V56	Encounter for dialysis and dialysis catheter care
V57	Care involving the use of rehabilitation procedures
V58.0	Radiotherapy
V58.11	**Encounter for antineoplastic chemotherapy**
V58.12	**Encounter for antineoplastic immunotherapy**
V58.3	Attention to surgical dressings and sutures
V58.41	Encounter for planned post-operative wound closure
V58.42	Aftercare, surgery, neoplasm
V58.43	Aftercare, surgery, trauma
V58.44	Aftercare involving organ transplant
V58.49	Other specified aftercare following surgery
V58.7x	Aftercare following surgery
V58.81	Fitting and adjustment of vascular catheter
V58.82	Fitting and adjustment of non-vascular catheter
V58.83	Monitoring therapeutic drug
V58.89	Other specified aftercare

8) **Follow-up** — The follow-up codes are used to explain continuing surveillance following completed treatment of a disease, condition, or injury. They imply that the condition has been fully treated and no longer exists. They should not be confused with aftercare codes that explain current treatment for a healing condition or its sequelae. Follow-up codes may be used in conjunction with history codes to provide the full picture of the healed condition and its treatment. The follow-up code is sequenced first, followed by the history code.

A follow-up code may be used to explain repeated visits. Should a condition be found to have recurred on the follow-up visit, then the diagnosis code should be used in place of the follow-up code.

The follow-up V code categories:

V24	Postpartum care and evaluation
V67	Follow-up examination

9) **Donor** — Category V59 is the donor codes. They are used for living individuals who are donating blood or other body tissue. These codes are only for individuals donating for others, not for self-donations. They are not for use to identify cadaveric donations.

10) **Counseling** — Counseling V codes are used when a patient or family member receives assistance in the aftermath of an illness or injury, or when support is required in coping with family or social problems. They are not necessary for use in conjunction with a diagnosis code when the counseling component of care

is considered integral to standard treatment.

The counseling V categories/codes:

V25.0	General counseling and advice for contraceptive management
V26.3	Genetic counseling
V26.4	General counseling and advice for procreative management
V61	Other family circumstances
V65.1	Person consulted on behalf of another person
V65.3	Dietary surveillance and counseling
V65.4	Other counseling, not elsewhere classified

11) **Obstetrics and related conditions** — See section I.C.11., the obstetrics guidelines for further instruction on the use of these codes.

V codes for pregnancy are for use in those circumstances when none of the problems or complications included in the codes from the obstetrics chapter exist (a routine prenatal visit or postpartum care). Codes V22.0 Supervision of normal first pregnancy, and V22.1 Supervision of other normal pregnancy, are always first listed and are not to be used with any other code from the OB chapter.

The outcome of delivery, category V27, should be included on all maternal delivery records. It is always a secondary code.

V codes for family planning (contraceptive) or procreative management and counseling should be included on an obstetric record either during the pregnancy or the postpartum stage, if applicable.

Obstetrics and related conditions V code categories:

V22	Normal pregnancy
V23	Supervision of high-risk pregnancy

Except: V23.2 Pregnancy with history of abortion. Code 646.3 Habitual aborter, from the OB chapter is required to indicate a history of abortion during a pregnancy.

V24	Postpartum care and evaluation
V25	Encounter for contraceptive management

Except V25.0x (See section I.C.18.d.11, Counseling)

V26	Procreative management

Except V26.5x Sterilization status, V26.3 and V26.4 (See section I.C.18.d.11., Counseling)

V27	Outcome of delivery
V28	Antenatal screening (See section I.C.18.d.6., Screening)

12) **Newborn, infant and child** — See section I.C.15, the newborn guidelines, for further instruction on the use of these codes.

Newborn V code categories:

V20	Health supervision of infant or child
V29	Observation and evaluation of newborns for suspected condition not found (See section I.C.18.d.7, Observation).
V30-V39	Liveborn infant according to type of birth

13) **Routine and administrative examinations** — The V codes allow for the description of encounters for routine examinations, such as a general check-up or, examinations for administrative purposes, such as a pre-employment

physical. The codes are for use as first-listed codes only, and are not to be used if the examination is for diagnosis of a suspected condition or for treatment purposes. In such cases the diagnosis code is used. During a routine exam, should a diagnosis or condition be discovered, it should be coded as an additional code. Pre-existing and chronic conditions and history codes may also be included as additional codes as long as the examination is for administrative purposes and not focused on any particular condition.

Preoperative examination V codes are for use only in those situations when a patient is being cleared for surgery and no treatment is given.

The V code categories/code for routine and administrative examinations:

V20.2	Routine infant or child health check Any injections given should have a corresponding procedure code.
V70	General medical examination
V72	Special investigations and examinations

Except V72.5 and V72.6

14) **Miscellaneous V codes** — The miscellaneous V codes capture a number of other health care encounters that do not fall into one of the other categories. Certain of these codes identify the reason for the encounter, others are for use as additional codes that provide useful information on circumstances that may affect a patient's care and treatment.

Prophylactic Organ Removal

For encounters specifically for prophylactic removal of breasts, ovaries, or another organ due to a genetic susceptibility to cancer or a family history of cancer, the principal or first-listed code should be a code from subcategory V50.4 Prophylactic organ removal, followed by the appropriate genetic susceptibility code and the appropriate family history code.

If the patient has a malignancy of one site and is having prophylactic removal at another site to prevent either a new primary malignancy or metastatic disease, a code for the malignancy should also be assigned in addition to a code from subcategory V50.4. A V50.4 code should not be assigned if the patient is having organ removal for treatment of a malignancy, such as the removal of the testes for the treatment of prostate cancer.

Miscellaneous V code categories/codes:

V07	Need for isolation and other prophylactic measures
V50	Elective surgery for purposes other than remedying health states
V58.5	Orthodontics
V60	Housing, household, and economic circumstances
V62	Other psychosocial circumstances
V63	Unavailability of other medical facilities for care
V64	Persons encountering health services for specific procedures, not carried out
V66	Convalescence and palliative care
V68	Encounters for administrative purposes
V69	Problems related to lifestyle

15) **Nonspecific V codes** — Certain V codes are so nonspecific, or potentially redundant with other codes in the classification, that there can be little justification for their use in the inpatient setting. Their use in the outpatient setting should be limited to those

Official ICD-9-CM Coding Guidelines

instances when there is no further documentation to permit more precise coding. Otherwise, any sign or symptom or any other reason for a visit that is captured in another code should be used.

Nonspecific V code categories/codes:

V11	Personal history of mental disorder-A code from the mental disorders chapter, with an in remission fifth digit, should be used.
V13.4	Personal history of arthritis
V13.6	Personal history of congenital malformations
V15.7	Personal history of contraception
V23.2	Pregnancy with history of abortion
V40	Mental and behavioral problems
V41	Problems with special senses and other special functions
V47	Other problems with internal organs
V48	Problems with head, neck, and trunk
V49	Problems with limbs and other problems

Exceptions:

V49.6	Upper limb amputation status
V49.7	Lower limb amputation status
V49.81	Postmenopausal status
V49.82	Dental sealant status
V49.83	Awaiting organ transplant status
V51	Aftercare involving the use of plastic surgery
V58.2	Blood transfusion, without reported diagnosis
V58.9	Unspecified aftercare
V72.5	Radiological examination, NEC
V72.6	Laboratory examination

Codes V72.5 and V72.6 are not to be used if any sign or symptoms, or reason for a test is documented. See section IV.K. and section IV.L. of the outpatient guidelines.

V Code Table

Items in bold indicate a change from the April 2005 table. Items underlined have been moved within the table since April 2005.

FIRST LISTED: V codes/categories/subcategories which are only acceptable as principal/first listed.

Codes:

V22.0	Supervision of normal first pregnancy
V22.1	Supervision of other normal pregnancy
V46.12	Encounter for respirator dependence during power failure
V46.13	**Encounter for weaning from respirator [ventilator]**
V56.0	Extracorporeal dialysis
V58.0	Radiotherapy

V58.0 and **V58.1** may be used together on a record with either one being sequenced first, when a patient receives both chemotherapy and radiation therapy during the same encounter.

V58.11	**Encounter for antineoplastic chemotherapy**

V58.0 and V58.11 may be used together on a record, with either one being sequenced first, when a patient

receives both chemotherapy and radiation therapy during the same encounter.

V58.12   Encounter for antineoplastic immunotherapy

Categories/Subcategories:

V20	Health supervision of infant or child
V24	Postpartum care and examination
V29	Observation and evaluation of newborns for suspected condition not found

Exception: A code from the V30-V39 may be sequenced before the V29 if it is the newborn record.

V30-V39	Liveborn infants according to type of birth
V57	**Care involving use of rehabilitation procedures**
V59	Donors
V66	Convalescence and palliative care

Exception: V66.7 Palliative care

V68	Encounters for administrative purposes
V70	General medical examination

Exception: V70.7 Examination of participant in clinical trial

V71	Observation and evaluation for suspected conditions not found
V72	Special investigations and examinations

Exceptions:

V72.4	**Pregnancy examination or test**	
V72.5	Radiological examination, NEC	
V72.6	Laboratory examination	
V72.86	**Encounter for blood typing**	

FIRST OR ADDITIONAL: V code categories/subcategories which may be either principal/first-listed, or additional codes.

Codes:

V15.88	History of fall
V43.22	Fully implantable artificial heart status
V46.14	**Mechanical complication of respirator [ventilator]**
V49.81	Asymptomatic postmenopausal status (age-related) (natural)
V49.84	Bed confinement status
V49.89	**Other specified conditions influencing health status**
V70.7	Examination of participant in clinical trial
V72.5	**Radiological examination, NEC**
V72.6	**Laboratory examination**
V72.86	**Encounter for blood typing**

Categories/Subcategories:

V01	Contact with or exposure to communicable diseases
V02	Carrier or suspected carrier of infectious diseases
V03-V06	Need for prophylactic vaccination and inoculations
V07	Need for isolation and other prophylactic measures
V08	Asymptomatic HIV infection status
V10	Personal history of malignant neoplasm
V12	Personal history of certain other diseases
V13	Personal history of other diseases

Exception:

V13.4	Personal history of arthritis
V13.69	Personal history of other congenital malformations

Official ICD-9-CM Coding Guidelines

V16-V19	Family history of disease	V67	Follow-up examination
V23	Supervision of high-risk pregnancy	V69	Problems related to lifestyle
V25	Encounter for contraceptive management	**V72.4**	**Pregnancy examination or test**
		V73-V82	Special screening examinations
V26	Procreative management	V83	Genetic carrier status

Exception:

V26.5   Sterilization status

ADDITIONAL ONLY: V code categories/subcategories which may only be used as additional codes, not principal/first listed.

Codes:

V28	Antenatal screening	V13.61	Personal history of hypospadias
V45.7	Acquired absence of organ	V22.2	Pregnancy state, incidental
V49.6x	**Upper limb amputation status**	**V46.11**	**Dependence on respirator, status**
V49.7x	**Lower limb amputation status**	V49.82	Dental sealant status
V50	Elective surgery for purposes other than remedying health states	V49.83	Awaiting organ transplant status
V52	Fitting and adjustment of prosthetic device and implant	V66.7	Palliative care
V53	Fitting and adjustment of other device	V85	Body mass index

Categories/Subcategories:

V54	Other orthopedic aftercare	V09	Infection with drug-resistant microorganisms
V55	Attention to artificial openings	V14	Personal history of allergy to medicinal agents
V56	Encounter for dialysis and dialysis catheter care	V15	Other personal history presenting hazards to health

Exception:

V56.0 Extracorporeal dialysis

Exception:

V15.7   Personal history of contraception

V58.3	Attention to surgical dressings and sutures	**V15.88**	**History of fall**
V58.4	Other aftercare following surgery	V21	Constitutional states in development
V58.7	Aftercare following surgery to specified body systems, not elsewhere classified	V26.5	Sterilization status
V58.8	Other specified procedures and aftercare	V27	Outcome of delivery
V61	Other family circumstances	V42	Organ or tissue replaced by transplant
V63	Unavailability of other medical facilities for care	V43	Organ or tissue replaced by other means
V65	Other persons seeking consultation without complaint or sickness		

	Exception:	V49.0	Deficiencies of limbs
	V43.22 Fully implantable artificial heart status	V49.1	Mechanical problems with limbs
		V49.2	Motor problems with limbs
V44	Artificial opening status	V49.3	Sensory problems with limbs
V45	Other postsurgical states	V49.4	Disfigurements in limbs
	Exception: Subcategory V45.7 Acquired absence of organ	V49.5	Other problems with limbs
V46	Other dependence on machines	V49.9	Unspecified condition influencing health status
	Exception: V46.12 Encounter for respirator dependence during power failure	V51	Aftercare involving the use of plastic surgery
V46.13	**Encounter for weaning from respirator [ventilator]**	V58.2	Blood transfusion, without reported diagnosis
~~V49.6x~~	~~Upper limb amputation status~~	V58.5	Orthodontics
~~V49.7x~~	~~Lower limb amputation status~~	V58.9	Unspecified aftercare
V58.6	**Long-term current drug use**	V72.5	Radiological examination, NEC
V60	Housing, household, and economic circumstances	V72.6	Laboratory examination

19. Supplemental Classification of External Causes of Injury and Poisoning (E-codes, E800-E999)

V62	Other psychosocial circumstances
V64	Persons encountering health services for specified procedure, not carried out
V84	Genetic susceptibility to disease
V85	**Body Mass Index**

NONSPECIFIC CODES AND CATEGORIES:

V11	Personal history of mental disorder
V13.4	Personal history of arthritis
V13.69	Personal history of congenital malformations
V15.7	Personal history of contraception
V40	Mental and behavioral problems
V41	Problems with special senses and other special functions
V47	Other problems with internal organs
V48	Problems with head, neck, and trunk

Introduction: These guidelines are provided for those who are currently collecting E codes in order that there will be standardization in the process. If your institution plans to begin collecting E codes, these guidelines are to be applied. The use of E codes is supplemental to the application of ICD-9-CM diagnosis codes. E codes are never to be recorded as principal diagnoses (first-listed in non-inpatient setting) and are not required for reporting to CMS.

External causes of injury and poisoning codes (E codes) are intended to provide data for injury research and evaluation of injury prevention strategies. E codes capture how the injury or poisoning happened (cause), the intent (unintentional or accidental; or intentional, such as suicide or assault), and the place where the event occurred.

Some major categories of E codes include:
- Transport accidents
- Poisoning and adverse effects of drugs, medicinal substances and biologicals
- Accidental falls
- Accidents caused by fire and flames

- Accidents due to natural and environmental factors
- Late effects of accidents, assaults or self injury
- Assaults or purposely inflicted injury
- Suicide or self inflicted injury

These guidelines apply to the coding and collection of E codes from records in hospitals, outpatient clinics, emergency departments, other ambulatory care settings and provider offices, and nonacute care settings, except when other specific guidelines apply.

a. **General E code coding guidelines**

1) **Used with any code in the range of 001-V86.1** — An E code may be used with any code in the range of 001-V86.1, which indicates an injury, poisoning, or adverse effect due to an external cause.

2) **Assign the appropriate E code for all initial treatments** — Assign the appropriate E code for the initial encounter of an injury, poisoning, or adverse effect of drugs, not for subsequent treatment.

3) **Use the full range of E codes** — Use the full range of E codes to completely describe the cause, the intent and the place of occurrence, if applicable, for all injuries, poisonings, and adverse effects of drugs.

4) **Assign as many E codes as necessary** — Assign as many E codes as necessary to fully explain each cause. If only one E code can be recorded, assign the E code most related to the principal diagnosis.

5) **The selection of the appropriate E code** — The selection of the appropriate E code is guided by the Index to External Causes, which is located after the Alphabetical Index to Diseases and by inclusion and exclusion notes in the Tabular List.

6) **E code can never be a principal diagnosis** — An E code can never be a principal (first-listed) diagnosis.

7) **External cause code(s) with systemic inflammatory response syndrome (SIRS)** — An external cause code(s) may be used with codes 995.93 Systemic inflammatory response syndrome due to noninfectious process without organ dysfunction, and 995.94 Systemic inflammatory response syndrome due to noninfectious process with organ dysfunction, if trauma was the initiating insult that precipitated the SIRS. The external cause(s) code should correspond to the most serious injury resulting from the trauma. The external cause code(s) should only be assigned if the trauma necessitated the admission in which the patient also developed SIRS. If a patient is admitted with SIRS but the trauma has been treated previously, the external cause codes should not be used.

b. **Place of occurrence guideline** — Use an additional code from category E849 to indicate the place of occurrence for injuries and poisonings. The place of occurrence describes the place where the event occurred and not the patient's activity at the time of the event.

Do not use E849.9 if the place of occurrence is not stated.

c. **Adverse effects of drugs, medicinal and biological substances guidelines**

1) **Do not code directly from the Table of Drugs** — Do not code directly from the Table of Drugs and Chemicals. Always refer back to the Tabular List.

2) **Use as many codes as necessary to describe** — Use as many codes as necessary to describe completely all drugs, medicinal or biological substances.

3) **If the same E code would describe the causative agent** — If the same E code would describe the causative agent for more than one adverse reaction, assign the code only once.

4) **If two or more drugs, medicinal or biological substances** — If two or more drugs, medicinal or biological substances are reported, code each individually unless the combination code is listed in the Table of Drugs and Chemicals. In that case, assign the E code for the combination.

5) **When a reaction results from the interaction of a drug(s)** — When a reaction results from the interaction of a drug(s) and alcohol, use poisoning codes and E codes for both.

6) **If the reporting format limits the number of E codes** — If the reporting format limits the number of E codes that can be used in reporting clinical data, code the one most related to the principal diagnosis. Include at least one from each category (cause, intent, place) if possible.

If there are different fourth-digit codes in the same three-digit category, use the code for "other specified" of that category. If there is no "other specified" code in that category, use the appropriate "unspecified" code in that category.

If the codes are in different three-digit categories, assign the appropriate E code for other multiple drugs and medicinal substances.

7) **Codes from the E930-E949 series** — Codes from the E930-E949 series must be used to identify the causative substance for an adverse effect of drug, medicinal and biological substances, correctly prescribed and properly administered. The effect, such as tachycardia, delirium, gastrointestinal hemorrhaging, vomiting, hypokalemia, hepatitis, renal failure, or respiratory failure, is coded and followed by the appropriate code from the E930-E949 series.

d. **Multiple cause E code coding guidelines** — If two or more events cause separate injuries, an E code should be assigned for each cause. The first listed E code will be selected in the following order:

E codes for child and adult abuse take priority over all other E codes. See section I.C.19.e., Child and adult abuse guidelines.
E codes for terrorism events take priority over all other E codes except child and adult abuse.
E codes for cataclysmic events take priority over all other E codes except child and adult abuse and terrorism.
E codes for transport accidents take priority over all other E codes except cataclysmic events and child and adult abuse and terrorism.
The first-listed E code should correspond to the cause of the most serious diagnosis due to an assault, accident, or self-harm, following the order of hierarchy listed above.

e. **Child and adult abuse guideline**

1) **Intentional injury** — When the cause of an injury or neglect is intentional child or adult abuse, the first-listed E code should be assigned from categories E960-E968 Homicide and injury purposely inflicted by other persons, (except category E967). An E code from category E967 Child and adult battering and other maltreatment, should be added as an additional code to identify the perpetrator, if known.

2) **Accidental intent** — In cases of neglect when the intent is determined to be accidental E code E904.0 Abandonment or neglect of infant and helpless person, should be the first-listed E code.

f. **Unknown or suspected intent guideline**

1) **If the intent (accident, self-harm, assault) of the cause of an injury or poisoning is unknown** — If the intent (accident, self-harm, assault) of the cause of an injury or poisoning is unknown or unspecified, code the intent as undetermined, E980-E989.

2) **If the intent (accident, self-harm, assault) of the cause of an injury or poisoning is questionable** — If the intent (accident, self-harm, assault) of the cause of an injury or poisoning is questionable, probable or suspected, code the intent as undetermined, E980-E989.

g. **Undetermined cause** — When the intent of an injury or poisoning is known, but the cause is unknown, use codes E928.9 Unspecified accident, E958.9 Suicide and self-inflicted injury by unspecified means, and E968.9 Assault by unspecified means.

These E codes should rarely be used, as the documentation in the medical record, in both the inpatient outpatient and other settings, should normally provide sufficient detail to determine the cause of the injury.

h. **Late effects of external cause guidelines**

1) **Late effect E codes** — Late effect E codes exist for injuries and poisonings but not for adverse effects of drugs, misadventures, and surgical complications.

Official ICD-9-CM Coding Guidelines

2) **Late effect E codes (E929, E959, E969, E977, E989, or E999.1)** — A late effect E code (E929, E959, E969, E977, E989, or E999.1) should be used with any report of a late effect or sequela resulting from a previous injury or poisoning (905-909).

3) **Late effect E code with a related current injury** — A late effect E code should never be used with a related current nature of injury code.

4) **Use of late effect E codes for subsequent visits** — Use a late effect E code for subsequent visits when a late effect of the initial injury or poisoning is being treated. There is no late effect E code for adverse effects of drugs. Do not use a late effect E code for subsequent visits for follow-up care (e.g., to assess healing, to receive rehabilitative therapy) of the injury or poisoning when no late effect of the injury has been documented.

i. **Misadventures and complications of care guidelines**

1) **Code range E870-E876** — Assign a code in the range of E870-E876 if misadventures are stated by the provider.

2) **Code range E878-E879** — Assign a code in the range of E878-E879 if the provider attributes an abnormal reaction or later complication to a surgical or medical procedure, but does not mention misadventure at the time of the procedure as the cause of the reaction.

j. **Terrorism guidelines**

1) **Cause of injury identified by the federal government (FBI) as terrorism** — When the cause of an injury is identified by the federal government (FBI) as terrorism, the first-listed E code should be a code from category E979 Terrorism. The definition of terrorism employed by the FBI is found at the inclusion note at E979. The terrorism E code is the only E code that should be assigned. Additional E codes from the assault categories should not be assigned.

2) **Cause of an injury is suspected to be the result of terrorism** — When the cause of an injury is suspected to be the result of terrorism a code from category E979 should not be assigned. Assign a code in the range of E codes based on the documentation of intent and mechanism.

3) **Code E979.9 Terrorism, secondary effects** — Assign code E979.9 Terrorism, secondary effects, for conditions occurring subsequent to the terrorist event. This code should not be assigned for conditions that are due to the initial terrorist act.

4) **Statistical tabulation of terrorism codes** — For statistical purposes these codes will be tabulated within the category for assault, expanding the current category from E960-E969 to include E979 and E999.1.

Section II. Selection of Principal Diagnosis

The circumstances of inpatient admission always govern the selection of principal diagnosis. The principal diagnosis is defined in the Uniform Hospital Discharge Data Set (UHDDS) as "that condition established after study to be chiefly responsible for occasioning the admission of the patient to the hospital for care."

The UHDDS definitions are used by hospitals to report inpatient data elements in a standardized manner. These data elements and their definitions can be found in the July 31, 1985, *Federal Register* (vol. 50, no. 147), pp. 31038-40.

Since that time the application of the UHDDS definitions has been expanded to include all non-outpatient settings (acute care, short-term, long-term care and psychiatric hospitals; home health agencies; rehab facilities; nursing homes, etc.).

In determining principal diagnosis the coding conventions in the ICD-9-CM, Volumes 1 and 2 take precedence over these official coding guidelines. (See section I.A., Conventions, for the ICD-9-CM).

The importance of consistent, complete documentation in the medical record cannot be overemphasized. Without such documentation the application of all coding guidelines is a difficult, if not impossible, task.

A. **Codes for symptoms, signs, and ill-defined conditions**

Codes for symptoms, signs, and ill-defined conditions from chapter 16 are not to be used as principal diagnosis when a related definitive diagnosis has been established.

B. Two or more interrelated conditions, each potentially meeting the definition for principal diagnosis

When there are two or more interrelated conditions (such as diseases in the same ICD-9-CM chapter or manifestations characteristically associated with a certain disease) potentially meeting the definition of principal diagnosis, either condition may be sequenced first, unless the circumstances of the admission, the therapy provided, the Tabular List, or the Alphabetic Index indicate otherwise.

C. Two or more diagnoses that equally meet the definition for principal diagnosis

In the unusual instance when two or more diagnoses equally meet the criteria for principal diagnosis as determined by the circumstances of admission, diagnostic workup and/or therapy provided, and the Alphabetic Index, Tabular List, or another coding guidelines do not provide sequencing direction, any one of the diagnoses may be sequenced first.

D. Two or more comparative or contrasting conditions

In those rare instances when two or more contrasting or comparative diagnoses are documented as "either/or" (or similar terminology), they are coded as if the diagnoses were confirmed and the diagnoses are sequenced according to the circumstances of the admission. If no further determination can be made as to which diagnosis should be principal, either diagnosis may be sequenced first.

E. A symptom(s) followed by contrasting/comparative diagnoses

When a symptom(s) is followed by contrasting/comparative diagnoses, the symptom code is sequenced first. All the contrasting/comparative diagnoses should be coded as additional diagnoses.

F. Original treatment plan not carried out

Sequence as the principal diagnosis the condition, which after study occasioned the admission to the hospital, even though treatment may not have been carried out due to unforeseen circumstances.

G. Complications of surgery and other medical care

When the admission is for treatment of a complication resulting from surgery or other medical care, the complication code is sequenced as the principal diagnosis. If the complication is classified to the 996-999 series and the code lacks the necessary specificity in describing the complication, an additional code for the specific complication should be assigned.

H. Uncertain diagnosis

If the diagnosis documented at the time of discharge is qualified as "probable," "suspected," "likely," "questionable," "possible," or "still to be ruled out," code the condition as if it existed or was established. The bases for these guidelines are the diagnostic workup, arrangements for further workup or observation, and initial therapeutic approach that correspond most closely with the established diagnosis.

Note: This guideline is applicable only to short-term, acute, long-term care and psychiatric hospitals.

I. Admission from observation unit

1. Admission following medical observation-When a patient is admitted to an observation unit for a medical condition that either worsens or does not improve, and is subsequently admitted as an inpatient of the same hospital for this same medical condition, the principal diagnosis would be the medical condition that led to the hospital admission.

2. Admission following post-operative observation-When a patient is admitted to an observation unit to monitor a condition (or complication) that develops following outpatient surgery and then is subsequently admitted as an inpatient of the same hospital, hospitals should apply the Uniform Hospital Discharge Data Set (UHDDS) definition of principal diagnosis as "that condition established after study to be chiefly responsible for occasioning the admission of the patient to the hospital for care."

J. Admission from outpatient surgery

When a patient receives surgery in the hospital's outpatient surgery department and is subsequently admitted for continuing inpatient care at the same hospital, the following guidelines should be followed in selecting the principal diagnosis for the inpatient admission:

- If the reason for the inpatient admission is a complication, assign the complication as the principal diagnosis.

- If no complication, or other condition, is documented as the reason for the inpatient admission, assign the reason for the outpatient surgery as the principal diagnosis.

- If the reason for the inpatient admission is another condition unrelated to the surgery, assign the unrelated condition as the principal diagnosis.

Section III. Reporting Additional Diagnoses
GENERAL RULES FOR OTHER (ADDITIONAL) DIAGNOSES

For reporting purposes the definition for "other diagnoses" is interpreted as additional conditions that affect patient care in terms of requiring:

- Clinical evaluation; or
- Therapeutic treatment; or
- Diagnostic procedures; or
- Extended length of hospital stay; or
- Increased nursing care and/or monitoring.

The UHDDS item #11-b defines other diagnoses as "all conditions that coexist at the time of admission, that develop subsequently, or that affect the treatment received and/or the length of stay. Diagnoses that relate to an earlier episode which have no bearing on the current hospital stay are to be excluded." UHDDS definitions apply to inpatients in acute care, short-term, long-term care and psychiatric hospital settings. The UHDDS definitions are used by acute care short-term hospitals to report inpatient data elements in a standardized manner. These data elements and their definitions can be found in the July 31, 1985, *Federal Register* (vol. 50, no. 147), pp. 31038-40.

Since that time the application of the UHDDS definitions has been expanded to include all non-outpatient settings (acute care, short-term, long-term care and psychiatric hospitals; home health agencies; rehab facilities; nursing homes, etc.).

The following guidelines are to be applied in designating other diagnoses when neither the Alphabetic Index nor the Tabular List in ICD-9-CM provides direction. The listing of the diagnoses in the patient record is the responsibility of the attending provider.

A. Previous conditions

If the provider has included a diagnosis in the final diagnostic statement, such as the discharge summary or the face sheet, it should ordinarily be coded. Some providers include in the diagnostic statement resolved conditions or diagnoses and status-post procedures from previous admission that have no bearing on the current stay. Such conditions are not to be reported and are coded only if required by hospital policy.

However, history codes (V10-V19) may be used as secondary codes if the historical condition or family history has an impact on current care or influences treatment.

B. Abnormal findings

Abnormal findings (laboratory, x-ray, pathologic, and other diagnostic results) are not coded and reported unless the provider indicates their clinical significance. If the findings are outside the normal range and the attending provider has ordered other tests to evaluate the condition or prescribed treatment, it is appropriate to ask the provider whether the abnormal finding should be added.

Please note: This differs from the coding practices in the outpatient setting for coding encounters for diagnostic tests that have been interpreted by a provider.

C. Uncertain Diagnosis

If the diagnosis documented at the time of discharge is qualified as "probable," "suspected," "likely," "questionable," "possible," or "still to be ruled out," code the condition as if it existed or was established. The bases for these guidelines are the diagnostic workup, arrangements for further workup or observation, and initial therapeutic approach that correspond most closely with the established diagnosis.

Note: This guideline is applicable only to short-term, acute, long-term care and psychiatric hospitals.

Section IV. Diagnostic Coding and Reporting Guidelines for Outpatient Services

These coding guidelines for outpatient diagnoses have been approved for use by hospitals/providers in coding and reporting hospital-based outpatient services and provider-based office visits.

Information about the use of certain abbreviations, punctuation, symbols, and other conventions used in the ICD-9-CM Tabular List (code numbers and titles), can be found in section IA of these guidelines, under "Conventions for the ICD-9-CM." Information about the correct sequence to use in finding a code is also described in section I.

The terms "encounter" and "visit" are often used interchangeably in describing outpatient service contacts and, therefore, appear together in these guidelines without distinguishing one from the other.

Though the conventions and general guidelines apply to all settings, coding guidelines for outpatient and provider reporting of diagnoses will vary in a number of instances from those for inpatient diagnoses, recognizing that:

- The Uniform Hospital Discharge Data Set (UHDDS) definition of principal diagnosis applies only to inpatients in acute, short-term, long-term care and psychiatric hospitals.
- Coding guidelines for inconclusive diagnoses (probable, suspected, rule out, etc.) were developed for inpatient reporting and do not apply to outpatients.

A. Selection of first-listed condition

In the outpatient setting, the term "first-listed diagnosis" is used in lieu of principal diagnosis.

In determining the first-listed diagnosis the coding conventions of ICD-9-CM, as well as the general and disease-specific guidelines take precedence over the outpatient guidelines.

Diagnoses often are not established at the time of the initial encounter/visit. It may take two or more visits before the diagnosis is confirmed.

The most critical rule involves beginning the search for the correct code assignment through the Alphabetic Index. Never begin searching initially in the Tabular List as this will lead to coding errors.

1. **Outpatient surgery**-When a patient presents for outpatient surgery, code the reason for the surgery as the first-listed diagnosis (reason for the encounter), even if the surgery is not performed due to a contraindication.

2. **Observation stay**-When a patient is admitted for observation for a medical condition, assign a code for the medical condition as the first-listed diagnosis. When a patient presents for outpatient surgery and develops complications requiring admission to observation, code the reason for the surgery as the first reported diagnosis (reason for the encounter), followed by codes for the complications as secondary diagnoses.

B. Codes from 001.0 through V86.1

The appropriate code or codes from 001.0 through V86.1 must be used to identify diagnoses, symptoms, conditions, problems, complaints, or other reason(s) for the encounter/visit.

C. Accurate reporting of ICD-9-CM diagnosis codes

For accurate reporting of ICD-9-CM diagnosis codes, the documentation should describe the patient's condition, using terminology which includes specific diagnoses as well as symptoms, problems, or reasons for the encounter. There are ICD-9-CM codes to describe all of these.

D. Selection of codes 001.0 through 999.9

The selection of codes 001.0 through 999.9 will frequently be used to describe the reason for the encounter. These codes are from the section of ICD-9-CM for the classification of diseases and injuries (e.g. infectious and parasitic diseases; neoplasms; symptoms, signs, and ill-defined conditions, etc.).

E. Codes that describe symptoms and signs

Codes that describe symptoms and signs, as opposed to diagnoses, are acceptable for reporting purposes when a diagnosis has not been established (confirmed) by the provider. Chapter 16 of ICD-9-CM, Symptoms, Signs, and Ill-defined Conditions (codes 780.0-799.9) contain many, but not all, codes for symptoms.

F. Encounters for circumstances other than a disease or injury

ICD-9-CM provides codes to deal with encounters for circumstances other than a disease or injury. The Supplementary Classification of Factors Influencing Health Status and Contact with Health Services (V01.0-V86.1) is provided to deal with occasions when circumstances other than a disease or injury are recorded as diagnosis or problems.

G. Level of Detail in Coding

1. **ICD-9-CM codes with three, four, or five digits** — ICD-9-CM is composed of codes with either three, four, or five digits. Codes with

three digits are included in ICD-9-CM as the heading of a category of codes that may be further subdivided by the use of fourth and/or fifth digits, which provide greater specificity.

2. **Use of full number of digits required for a code** — A three-digit code is to be used only if it is not further subdivided. Where fourth-digit subcategories and/or fifth-digit subclassifications are provided, they must be assigned. A code is invalid if it has not been coded to the full number of digits required for that code. See also discussion under section I.b.3., General coding guidelines, Level of detail in coding.

H. **ICD-9-CM code for the diagnosis, condition, problem, or other reason for encounter/visit**

List first the ICD-9-CM code for the diagnosis, condition, problem, or other reason for encounter/visit shown in the medical record to be chiefly responsible for the services provided. List additional codes that describe any coexisting conditions. In some cases the first-listed diagnosis may be a symptom when a diagnosis has not been established (confirmed) by the physician.

I. **"Probable," "suspected," "questionable," "rule out," or "working diagnosis"**

Do not code diagnoses documented as "probable," "suspected," "questionable," "rule out," or "working diagnosis." Rather, code the condition(s) to the highest degree of certainty for that encounter/visit, such as symptoms, signs, abnormal test results, or other reason for the visit. **Please note:** This differs from the coding practices used by short-term, acute care, long-term care, and psychiatric hospitals.

J. **Chronic diseases**

Chronic diseases treated on an ongoing basis may be coded and reported as many times as the patient receives treatment and care for the condition(s).

K. **Code all documented conditions that coexist**

Code all documented conditions that coexist at the time of the encounter/visit, and require or affect patient care treatment or management. Do not code conditions that were previously treated and no longer exist. However, history codes (V10-V19) may be used as secondary codes if the historical condition or family history has an impact on current care or influences treatment.

L. **Patients receiving diagnostic services only**

For patients receiving diagnostic services only during an encounter/visit, sequence first the diagnosis, condition, problem, or other reason for encounter/visit shown in the medical record to be chiefly responsible for the outpatient services provided during the encounter/visit. Codes for other diag-noses (e.g., chronic conditions) may be sequenced as additional diagnoses.

For outpatient encounters for diagnostic tests that have been interpreted by a physician and the final report is available at the time of coding, code any confirmed or definitive diagnosis(es) documented in the interpretation. Do not code related signs and symptoms as additional diagnoses.

Please note: This differs from the coding practice in the hospital inpatient setting regarding abnormal findings on test results.

M. **Patients receiving therapeutic services only**

For patients receiving therapeutic services only during an encounter/visit, sequence first the diagnosis, condition, problem, or other reason for encounter/visit shown in the medical record to be chiefly responsible for the outpatient services provided during the encounter/visit. Codes for other diag-noses (e.g., chronic conditions) may be sequenced as additional diagnoses.

The only exception to this rule is that when the primary reason for the admission/encounter is chemotherapy, radiation therapy, or rehabilitation, the appropriate V code for the service is listed first, and the diagnosis or problem for which the service is being performed is listed second.

N. **Patients receiving preoperative evaluations only**

For patients receiving preoperative evaluations only, sequence first a code from category V72.8 Other specified examinations, to describe the pre-op consultations. Assign a code for the condition to describe the reason for the surgery as an additional diagnosis. Code also any findings related to the pre-op evaluation.

O. **Ambulatory surgery**

For ambulatory surgery, code the diagnosis for which the surgery was performed. If the postoperative diagnosis is known to be different from the preoperative diagnosis at the time the diagnosis is confirmed, select the postoperative diagnosis for coding, since it is the most definitive.

P. Routine outpatient prenatal visits

For routine outpatient prenatal visits when no complications are present, code V22.0 Supervision of normal first pregnancy, or V22.1 Supervision of other normal pregnancy, should be used as the principal diagnosis. These codes should not be used in conjunction with chapter 11 codes.

Syndromes

The term syndrome is commonly misused by the lay public to embrace a very broad spectrum of diseases and illnesses, many of which are not accepted by the traditional western medical fraternity. A syndrome is the composite of signs and symptoms that give a picture of the disease process. In genetics, a syndrome constitutes a pattern of related abnormalities that may be genetically related.

Syndromes may be eponymic — named for an individual, or several individuals (e.g., Tourette's, Ostrum-Furst). Others may be simply descriptive (e.g., cat-cry, acquired immune deficiency); some names are associated with several unrelated syndromes (see Weber). Other syndromes may be referenced by either description or eponym (e.g., bruising syndrome, or Diamond-Gardner syndrome).

The symptoms that comprise a syndrome may be singular or plural, specific, or broadly outlined. Syndromes may be physical or behavioral, congenital, or found later in life; and while syndromes are not diseases, they are used to describe diseases seen daily by health care givers. Commonly known diseases may be known by their accompanying syndromes, which complicates proper coding of ICD-9-CM codes.

ICD-9-CM contains a list of nearly 1,500 syndromes cross-referenced under its numeric system. The following list contains most of those syndromes, explained and cross-referenced by number and name. Many syndromes carry a number of names, which are noted within parenthesis in each entry. Similar syndromes with negligible differences are also grouped together to ease use.

5q minus
(238.74) The most commonly observed structural chromosome abnormality in patients with myeloid disorders, in which a portion of the long arm of chromosome 5 is missing.

13
(758.1) (Patau's, trisomy D, D1) Variable symptoms of newborns with an extra chromosome in group D. Condition is usually fatal within two years and includes mental retardation and malformed ears, cardiac defects, convulsions, and others.

16-18 or E
(758.2) (Edward's, trisomy E, E3) Congenital malformations in which extra chromosome is group E. Includes mental retardation, abnormal skull shape, malformed ears, small mandible, cardiac defects, short sternum, and other symptoms.

21 or 22
(758.0) (Down, G, mongolism) Retardation with numerous markers varying from one person to another. Symptoms include retarded growth, flat face with short nose, epicanthic skin folds, protruding lower lip, rounded ears, thickened tongue, pelvic dysplasia, broad hands and feet, stubby fingers, and absence of Moro reflex.

Abercrombie's
(277.39) One of a group of syndromes characterized by accumulation of insoluble fibrillar proteins (amyloid) in various organs and tissues of the body, compromising vital functions.

Achard-Thiers
(255.2) Aranodactyly with small, receding mandible, broad skull, and laxity of joints in hands and feet.

Acid pulmonary aspiration
(997.3) (Mendelson's) Pulmonary disorder resulting from aspirating the contents of stomach following vomiting or regurgitation.

Acquired immune deficiency
(042) (AIDS) A contagious retroviral disease resulting from infection with human immunodeficiency virus (HIV) that can, in severe cases, suppress vital immunity. Several opportunistic infections, such as Kaposi's sarcoma and pneumocystitis pneumonia, are associated with this syndrome.

Acrocephalosyndactylism
(755.55) (Apert's) A chromosomal condition with webbing of digits and a pointed head and variety of defects. Often associated with other chromosomal abnormalities.

Acute brain syndrome with transient delirium
(293.0) Metabolic encephalopathy with altered state of consciousness or acute confusional state due to an underlying disease or condition.

Acute chest
(282.62) Sickle cell anemia complication with acute bony and soft tissue chest pain with pulmonary infiltrates present on x-ray, due to impaired breathing secondary to pain.

Acute coronary
(411.1) (intermediate coronary) Unstable angina pectoris that has not yet developed into an acute myocardial infarction but requires immediate treatment.

Acute promyelocytic leukemia differentiation
(205.00, 205.01) A subtype of acute myeloid leukemia caused by translocation fusion between chromosomes 15 and 17, associated with abnormal bleeding.

Acute psycho-organic
(293.0) Describes a mental health condition in which delirium and confusion interfere with day-to-day activities or therapy as a result of emotional, organic, chemical, endocrine, or metabolic disorders or causes.

Acute respiratory distress
(518.82, 518.5, 769) (ARDS) An acute state characterized by severe dyspnea, pulmonary infiltrates, and hypoxemia (deficient oxygenation of blood) occurring in certain clinical situations. Adult ARDS following trauma or surgery is coded to 518.5. Newborn ARDS is coded to 769.

Adair-Dighton
(756.51) (van der Hoeve's) Hereditary condition with symptoms including blue sclera, little growth, brittle bones, and deafness.

Adams-Stokes (-Morgagni)
(426.9) (Stokes-Adams, Morgagni's disease, and Spens) Heart block often causing slow or absent pulse, vertigo, syncope, convulsions, and sometimes Cheyne-Stokes respiration.

Addisonian
(255.4) (Bernard-Sergent) Acute adrenal insufficiency caused by illness, trauma, or large amounts of hormones used as therapy. Symptoms include hypotension, hyperthermia, hyponatremia, hyperkalemia, hypoglycemia, nausea, and vomiting.

Adie (-Holmes)
(379.46) Paralysis of conjugate movement of eyes without paralysis of convergence. Caused by lesions of midbrain.

Adiposogenital
(253.8) (Babinski-Fröhlich, Fröhlich) Obesity and hypogonadism in adolescent boys. Rare accompanying dwarfism is thought to indicate hypothyroidism.

Adrenogenital
(255.2) A generalized type of syndrome, inappropriately virilizing or feminizing, caused by inborn enzyme defects in gonadal hormone synthesis, due to adrenal function disorders associated with congenital adrenal hyperplasia and adrenal cortex tumors.

Adult maltreatment
(995.8x) Abuse of an adult with emotional or physical violence, or neglect. Most often committed against spouses and elders.

Adult respiratory distress
(518.5) Pulmonary insufficiency following surgery, shock, or trauma.

Adult sleep apnea
(780.53) Episodes of inadequate or irregular breathing during sleep manifesting with snoring, periods of arrested or irregular breathing, and disruption of sleep.

Affective NEC
(293.83) (affective organic NEC) Organic disorder in which the patient exhibits a number of changes in personality such as amotivation, depression, outbursts, and poor social judgment.

Afferent loop NEC
(537.89) (Gastrojejunal loop obstruction) Distended afferent loop with illness and pain caused by acute or chronic obstruction of the duodenum and jejunum proximal to a gastrojejunostomy.

African macroglobulinemia
(273.3) (Waldenström's) Earmarked by an increase in macroglobulins in the blood with symptoms of hyperviscosity such as weakness, fatigue, bleeding disorders, and visual disturbances.

Ahumada-Del Castillo
(253.1) (Argonz-Del Castillo) Lactation and amenorrhea not following pregnancy characterized by hyperprolactinemia and pituitary adenoma.

Alagille
(759.89) (Watson-Miller) Congenital familial syndrome marked by intrahepatic cholestasis due to hypoplasia of the interlobular biliary duct, neonatal

jaundice, and hepatomegaly. Symptoms include dysmorphic (flat) facies, with prominent forehead, mongoloid slant, mild hypertelorism, straight or bulbous nose, and skeletal anomalies; occasionally diffuse xanthomas (palms, extensor areas, creases), pruritus, mesosystolic murmur, growth and mental retardation, and in males, hypogonadism.

Albright (-Martin)
(275.49) (Martin-Albright, Seabright-Bantam) Similar to hypoparathyroidism and caused by a failure to respond to parathyroid hormone. Short stature, obesity, short metacarpals, and ectopic calcification.

Albright-McCune-Sternberg
(756.59) (McCune-Albright, Albright's hereditary osteodystrophy) Patchy skin pigmentation, endocrine dysfunctions, and polyostotic fibrous dysplasia.

Alcohol abstinence
(291.81) Alcohol withdrawal characterized by symptoms that develop after the discontinuation or reduction in heavy and prolonged alcohol use including tremor, insomnia, nausea or vomiting, transient hallucinations, psychomotor agitation, anxiety, and seizures.

Alcohol withdrawal
(291.81) (alcohol) Absence of alcohol in an alcohol-dependent individual with physiological and psychological symptoms. Severity may result in death.

Alcoholic amnestic
(291.1) Physical and emotional symptoms resulting from profound ingestion of alcohol.

Alder's
(288.2) Polymorphonuclear leukocyte, or white blood cell granulation anomaly.

Aldrich (-Wiskott)
(279.12) (Wiskott-Aldrich) Inherited immunodeficiency with eczema, thrombocytopenia, recurrent pyogenic infection, and increased susceptibility to infection with encapsulated bacteria.

Alibert-Bazin
(202.1x) Malignant neoplasm resembling a fungus and growing outside of the body.

Alice in Wonderland
(293.89) Organic disorder with patient presenting an illusion of dreams, feelings of levitation, and alteration of passage of time. Associated with epilepsy, migraines, and other problems of the parietal part of brain.

Allen-Masters
(620.6) Pelvic pain resulting from old laceration of broad ligament received during delivery.

Alport's
(759.89) Progressive sensorineural hearing loss, ocular defects, and glomerulonephritis, or pyelonephritis. Cause is inherited.

Alveolar capillary block
(516.3) (Hamman-Rich) Chronic inflammation and progressive fibrosis of pulmonary alveolar walls, with progressive dyspnea leading to death by oxygen deprivation or right heart failure.

Amnestic
(294.0) Amnestic dementia in which the patient has no short-term or long-term memories but is not delirious.

Amotivational
(292.89) Patient who chooses not to participate in day-to-day activities or therapy as a result of emotional, organic, or chemical causes.

Amyostatic
(275.1) Accumulation of copper in the brain, cornea, kidney, liver, and other tissues causing cirrhosis of the liver and deterioration in the basal ganglia of the brain.

Androgen insensitivity
(259.5) (Goldberg (-Maxwell) (-Morris) hairless women, male pseudohemaphroditism, nonvirilizing, testicular feminization) Genetic condition affecting the development of reproductive organs marked by female external genitalia or a degree of both male and female genitalia. Amenorrhea noticed in teen years, with short, incompletely developed vagina and rudimentary or absent uterus and fallopian tubes, scanty or absent axillary/public hair, and testicles that may require removal.

Angelman
(759.89) Emergence in early childhood of a pattern of interrupted development, stiff, jerky gait, absence or impairment of speech, excessive laughter, and seizures.

Angina
(413.9) Acute, choking pain most notable in the pectoral region of the chest and implying the onset of a heart attack.

Angina cruris
(443.9) (Charcot's) Number of symptoms in a moving limb including pain, tension, and weakness but absent at rest. Caused by occlusive arterial diseases of the limbs.

Antimongolism
(758.39) Mental and growth retardation, hypertonia, high-arched palate, micrognathia, microcephaly and an anti-mongoloid obliquity of the palpebral fissures.

Antley-Bixler
(759.89) Congenital condition characterized by multiple skeletal fusions with renal and cardiac anomalies. Prognosis for survival is poor.

Antiphospholipid-antibody
(795.79) (Anticardiolipid) An inflammatory disorder that affects many body systems manifested by circulating antiphospholipid antibodies with thrombosis and vascular occlusion, thrombocytopenia, and heart valve disease. Spontaneous abortion also occurs with this syndrome. When anticardiolipid antibody is associated with a definitive clinical diagnosis, assign the code for the specific clinical diagnosis.

Anton (-Babinski)
(307.9) A form of cortical blindness caused by damage to the occipital lobe and where the patient denies the visual impairment.

Apert's
(755.55) Chromosomal condition with webbing of digits, a pointed head, and varieties of defects. Often associated with other chromosomal abnormalities.

Apert-Gallais
(255.2) Type I acrocephalosyndactyly with a peaked head, fusion of digits (specifically the second through fifth digits), and severe acne vulgaris of forearms.

Aphasia-apraxia-alexia
(784.69) (Bianchi's) Sensory aphasic condition with alexia and apraxia associated with lesions in the left parietal lobe.

Apical ballooning
(429.83) (broken heart, Takotsubo) A reversible left ventricular dysfunction in patients without coronary disease, precipitated by emotional or physiological stress.

Arc-welders'
(370.24) Temporary or permanent spot blindness resulting from observing bright light unprotected.

Arch
(446.7) (Martorell-Fabre, Raed-Harbitz, Takayasu-Onishi) Progressive obliteration of brachiocephalic trunk and left subclavian and left common carotid arteries above their source in the aortic arch. Symptoms include ischemia, transient blindness, facial atrophy, and many others.

Arcuate ligament
(447.4) Compression of the celiac artery by the median arcuate ligament in the diaphragm.

Argentaffin, argentaffinoma
(259.2) (Bjorck-Thorson, Cassidy-Scholte, Hedinger's) Carcinoid tumors causing severe attacks of cyanotic flushing of the skin, diarrhea watery stools, bronchoconstrictive attacks, hypotension, edema, and ascites.

Argonz-Del Castillo
(253.1) (Ahumada-Del Castillo) Lactation and amenorrhea not following pregnancy and characterized by hyperprolactinemia and pituitary adenoma.

Argyll Robertson
(094.89) (syphilitic), 379.49 (nonsyphilitic) A condition where the pupil of the eye is small and unresponsive to changes in light intensity.

Arm-shoulder
(337.9) (Claude Bernard-Homer, Reilly's, Steinbrocker's) Disorder following a heart attack with pain and stiffness in the shoulder and swelling and pain in the hand.

Armenian
(277.31) Syndrome characterized by attacks of recurrent high fevers accompanied by pain and inflammation in the lining of the chest and abdominal cavities, skin or joints, and blood vessels.

Arnold-Chiari
(741.0) Cerebellomedullary malformation syndrome. Displacement of the caudal spinal cord due to tethering with or without spina bifida and other problems such as meningomyelocele.

Syndromes

Arnold-Chiari with spina bifida
(741.0x) (Arnold-Chiari) Displacement of the caudal spinal cord due to tethering with or without spina bifida and other problems such as meningomyelocele.

Arrillaga-Ayerza
(416.0) (arteriosclerosis) Cyanosis and hypertension resulting from sclerosis of the pulmonary arteries.

Arteriomesenteric duodenum occlusion
(537.89) (Gastrojejunal loop obstruction) Distended afferent loop with illness and pain caused by acute or chronic obstruction of the duodenum and jejunum proximal to a gastrojejunostomy.

Arteriosclerosis depressive
(293.83) Organic disorder in which the patient exhibits changes in personality such as amotivation, depression, outbursts, poor social judgment, etc., caused by constriction of the arteries to the brain.

Arteriovenous steal
(996.73) A complication of arteriovenous fistula placed for dialysis. Blood can be "stolen" or diverted between vessels resulting in ischemic pain, tingling, numbness, temperature changes, or skin breakdown.

Artery compression
(447.4) Compression of the celiac artery by the median arcuate ligament in the diaphragm.

Artery entrapment
(447.8) Malignant atrophic papulosis.

Artery, superior
(557.1) (Wilkie's) Complete or partial block of the superior mesenteric artery with vomiting, pain, blood in the stool, distended abdomen, and resulting in bowel infarction.

Asherman's
(621.5) Adhesions in the endometrial cavity causing amenorrhea and infertility.

Aspiration
(770.1x) Intrauterine fetal aspiration of amniotic fluid contaminated by meconium.

Ataxia-telangiectasia
(334.8) (Boder-Sedgwick, Louis-Bar) Gonadal hypoplasia, insulin resistance and hyperglycemia, liver function problems, increased sensitivity to ionizing radiation, ataxia, and nystagmus.

Audry's
(757.39) Increased thickening of the skin on extremities and face with clubbing of fingers and deformities in bone of the limb.

Auriculotemporal
(350.8) (Frey's) Localized sweating and flushing of the cheek and ear in response to chewing.

Automatism
(348.8) Infarction of the postero-inferior thalamus causing transient hemiparesis, severe loss of sensation with crude pain in the limbs, or vasomotor or trophic disturbances.

Autosomal deletion
(758.3x) Chromosomal disorder due to the absence of certain portions of a chromosome resulting in congenital abnormalities and/or mental retardation, and developmental delays.

Avellis'
(344.89) (Babinski-Nageotte, Benedikt's, Brown-Sequard, Cestan's, Cestan-Chenais, Foville's, Gubler-Millard, Jackson's, Weber-Leyden) Paraplegia and anesthesia over part of the body caused by lesions in the brain or spinal cord.

Axenfeld's
(743.44) A dysgenesis of the eye marked through widened trabecular meshwork, large iridial bands, and glaucoma.

Ayerza (-Arrillaga)
(416.0) Cyanosis and hypertension, resulting from sclerosis of the pulmonary arteries.

Baader's
(695.1) Necrolysis of the skin caused by toxins.

Baastrup's
(721.5) Kissing spine. Malformation of the spine in which kyphosis becomes so great nonadjacent vertebrae touch.

Babinski-Fröhlich
(253.8) (Frölich) Obesity and hypogonadism in adolescent boys with rare accompanying dwarfism, thought to indicate hypothyroidism.

Babinski-Nageotte
(344.89) (Avellis, Benedikt's, Brown-Sequard, Cestan's, Cestan-Chenais, Foville's, Gubler-Millard, Jackson's, Weber-Leyden) Paraplegia and anesthesia over part of the body caused by lesions in the brain or spinal cord.

Baby or child maltreatment
(995.5x) Child abuse through physical violence, emotional violence, starvation, or neglect.

Bagratuni's
(446.5) (Horton's, giant cell arteritis) Temporal arteritis.

Balint's
(368.16) (Balint's, Holmes', Riddoch's) Cortical paralysis of visual fixation, optic ataxia, and disturbance of visual attention with normal eye movements.

Ballantyne (-Runge)
(766.22) Placental dysfunction occurring in postmature fetuses.

Ballooning posterior leaflet
(424.0) (Barlow's) "Mid-late" systolic click of the heart due to massive protrusion of the mitral valvular leaflet in the left atrial cavity.

Barlow's
(424.0) "Mid-late" systolic click of the heart due to massive protrusion of the mitral valvular leaflet in the left atrial cavity.

Baron Munchausen
(301.51) (see Munchausen)

Barraquer (-Simon)
(272.6) Progressive lipodystrophy, a progressive atrophy of the subcutaneous fat of the face.

Barré-Guillain
(357.0) (Guillain-Barré, Landry, Fisher's, Strohl, Miller) Disorder of the immune system with paraplegia of limbs, flaccid paralysis, ophthalmoplegia, ataxia, and areflexia.

Barré-Liéou
(723.2) Irritation of the nerve roots emanating from the posterior cervical spinal cord.

Barrett's
(530.85) Metiplastic disorder associated with gastrointestinal reflux in the esophagus caused by stricture constructed of epithelium.

Bársony-Polgár
(530.5) (Barsony-Teschendorf) Strong, uncoordinated contraction of the esophagus evoked by deglutition in the elderly. Appears as a series of concentric narrows or as spiral on an x-ray.

Bartter's
(255.13) Found in children with hypokalemic alkalosis, elevated renin or angiotensin levels, low or normal blood pressure, no edema, and retarded growth.

Basedow's
(242.0x) (Basedow, Parry's, Grave's disease) Fatigue, nervousness, emotional lability and irritability, heat intolerance and increased sweating, weight loss, palpitation, and tremor of hands and tongue. May be autoimmune in etiology.

Basilar artery
(435.0) (Raymond-Cestan) Quadriplegia, anesthesia, and nystagmus. Due to obstruction of twigs of the basilar artery, causing lesions in the pontine region.

Basofrontal
(377.04) (Foster-Kennedy, Gowers-Paton-Kennedy) Meningioma of the optic nerve, marked by central scotoma and contralateral choked disk.

Bassen-Kornzweig
(272.5) Retinal pigmentary degeneration, malabsorption, engorgement of upper intestinal cells with triglycerides, neuromuscular abnormalities, and an absence from plasma of low density lipoproteins.

Batten-Steinert
(359.2) Condition in which the peritoneal cover of the liver converts to a white mass resembling cake icing.

Battered child (baby)
(995.54) Injuries sustained by a baby or child from physical abuse, usually inflicted by a caregiver; also known as shaken baby syndrome.

Baumgarten-Cruveilhier
(571.5) Cirrhosis of the liver with patent paraumbilical, varicose periumbilical, or umbilical veins.

Bean's
(228.0x) (Blue rubber bleb) A cavernous hemangioma of the skin or internal organs.

Bearn-Kunkel (-Slater)
(571.49) Chronic hepatitis with autoimmune manifestations.

Beau's
(429.1) Cardiac arrest.

Bechterew-Strümpell-Marie
(720.0) Rheumatoid inflammation of the vertebrae.

Syndromes

Beck's
(433.8x) Occlusion of the spinal artery as result of injury, disk damage, or cardiovascular disease.

Beckwith (-Wiedemann)
(759.89) Congenital disorder with macroglossia, gigantism, dysplasia of the renal medulla, visceromegaly, adrenocortical cytomegaly, and exomphalos.

Behçet's
(136.1) A chronic condition linked to disturbances in the immune system where small blood vessels become locally inflamed, causing ulcerations of the oral and pharyngeal mucous membranes, skin lesions, and Inflammation of joints.

Bekhterev-Strümpell-Marie
(720.0) Rheumatoid inflammation of the vertebrae.

Benedikt's
(344.89) (Avellis, Babinski-Nageotte, Benedikt's, Brown-Sequard, Cestan's, Cestan-Chenais, Foville's, Gubler-Millard, Jackson's, Weber-Leyden) Paraplegia and anesthesia over part of the body caused by lesions in the brain or spinal cord.

Bernard-Horner
(337.9) (Horner's syndrome) Enophthalmos (backward displacement of the eyeball in the orbit), constricted pupil, drooping eyelid (ptosis), and facial dryness caused by brain stem lesion to the ipsolateral side interrupting the sympathetic nerves of the face.

Bernard-Sergent
(255.4) Acute adrenal insufficiency caused by illness or trauma or by large amounts of hormones used as therapy. Symptoms include hypotension, hyperthermia, hyponatremia, hyperkalemia, hypoglycemia, nausea, and vomiting.

Bernhardt-Roth
(355.1) Tingling, formication, itching, and other symptoms on the outer side of the lower part of the thigh. Caused by lateral femoral cutaneous nerve.

Bernheim's
(428.0) Right heart failure accompanied by enlarged liver, distended neck veins, and edema without pulmonary congestion, caused by hypertrophied septum.

Bertolotti
(756.15) Fusion of the bottom lumbar vertebra to the top sacral vertebra, making a sixth sacral vertebra accompanied by sciatica and scoliosis.

Bianchi's
(784.69) Sensory aphasic condition with alexia and apraxia and lesions in the left parietal lobe.

Biedl-Bardet
(759.89) (Biemond's) Mental retardation, pigmentary retinopathy, obesity, polydactyly, and hypogonadism.

Biemond's
(759.89) Mental retardation, pigmentary retinopathy, obesity, polydactyly, and hypogonadism.

Bifurcation
(444.0) (Leriche's) Obstruction of the terminal aorta causing fatigue in the hips, thighs, or calves and pallor of lower extremities and impotence in exercising males.

Big Spleen
(289.4) (hypersplenism) Enlarged spleen caused by cirrhosis of liver or portal or splenic vein thrombosis causing anemia, hyperplasia of marrow precursors of deficient cell type.

Bilateral polycystic ovarian
(256.4) Acute adrenal insufficiency caused by illness, trauma, or by large amounts of hormones used as therapy with hypotension, hyperthermia, hyponatremia, hyperkalemia, hypoglycemia, nausea, and vomiting.

Bing-Horton's (cluster headache)
(346.2x) Idiopathic unilateral headaches that reoccur in brief, sudden attacks that may disappear entirely over time.

Biörck (-Thorson)
(259.2) (Cassidy-Scholte, Hedinger's) Carcinoid tumors that cause cyanotic flushing of the skin, diarrhea watery stools, bronchoconstrictive attacks, hypotension, edema, and ascites.

Blackfan-Diamond
(284.01) (Diamond-Blackfan, Kaznelson's) Congenital anemia that manifests during infancy and requires a number of blood transfusions to maintain life.

Black lung
(500) (coal miner's pneumoconiosis, anthracosis) Blockage of bronchioles by "coal macules" brought about by aspiration of coal dust.

Blind loop
(579.2) Loop of small intestine detached surgically or detaching itself and, in the former case, becomes bacterial, and, in the latter case, accepts feces but cannot discharge it, becoming infected.

Bloch-Siemens
(757.33) (Block-Sulzberger) Pigmented lesions appear in linear, zebra stripe, and other configurations and preceded by vesicles and bullae and followed by verruca lesions.

Bloch-Sulzberger
(757.33) (Block-Siemens) Pigmented lesions appear in linear, zebra stripe, and other configurations and preceded by vesicles and bullae and followed by verruca lesions.

Bloom (-Machacek) (-Torre)
(757.39) Butterfly-shaped lesions on the face and hands, dolichocephalic skull and narrow face, and dwarfism with normal body proportions.

Blount-Barber
(732.4) Bow-legs in children.

Blue toe
(445.02) A complication of pancreatitis characterized by tissue ischemia secondary to cholesterol crystal or atherothrombotic embolization, which leads to occlusion of small vessels that may present as cyanosis of digits, such as the toes.

Boder-Sedgwick
(334.8) (Boder-Sedgwick, Louis-Bar) Gonadal hypoplasia, insulin resistance and hyperglycemia, liver function problems, increased sensitivity to ionizing radiation, ataxia, and nystagmus.

Body or sinus, carotid
(337.0) (Charcot-Weiss-Baker, Sluder's) Stimulation of an overactive carotid sinus, causing a marked drop in blood pressure, which, in turn, may stop the heart.

Bonnevie-Ullrich
(758.6) Short stature, webbed neck, congenital heart disease, and mental retardation.

Bonnier's
(386.19) Ocular disturbances, deafness, nausea, thirst, anorexia, and symptoms resulting from a lesion of Deiters' nucleus and its connections.

Borjeson-Forssman-Lehmann
(759.89) Rare syndrome manifested by severe mental defects, epilepsy, obesity, microcephaly, uneven facial features, enlarged ears, hypogonadism, short stature, and anomaly of digits.

Bouveret (-Hoffmann)
(427.2) Rapid action of the heart with sudden onset and cessation.

Bowel
(579.3) Hypoglycemia and malabsorption following surgery.

Bowel distress
(564.1) Abdominal pain, watery stools, and gas.

Brachial plexus
(353.0) (Naffziger's) Anesthesias and vascular contraction in extremities caused by pressure of brachial plexus and subclavian artery against first thoracic rib.

Brachio-oto-renal
(759.89) (Brachio-optic, Melnick-Fraser) A genetic autosomal dominant disorder that includes anomalies of the ear, cysts in the neck, hearing loss, and malformations of the kidney.

Bradycardia-tachycardia
(427.81) Rapid action of the heart followed by protracted or transient stopping of the heart.

Brailsford-Morquio
(277.5) Accumulation of mucopolysaccharide sulfates affecting the eye, ear, skin, teeth, skeleton, joints, liver, spleen, cardiovascular system, respiratory system, and central nervous system.

Brandt's
(686.8) (Danbolt) Zinc metabolism defect in young children with blisters, crusting, oozing eruptions, loss of hair, and diarrhea.

Brennemann
(289.2) Lymphadenitis in the mesentery and retroperitoneal area as a sequel of throat infection.

Briquet's (Brissaud-Marie)
(300.81) Personality disorder more prevalent among women involving concurrent alcoholism and

somatization whereby the patient reports physical complaints absent of medical indication.

Brissaud-Meige
(244.9) Hypothyroidism resulting from acquired injury of thyroid gland or presence of cretinism.

Brock's
(518.0) Incomplete expansion of the right middle lobe of a lung with chronic pneumonitis.

Broken heart
(429.83) (apical ballooning, Takotsubo) A reversible left ventricular dysfunction in patients without coronary disease, precipitated by emotional or physiological stress.

Brown spot
(756.59) (McCune-Albright, Albright's hereditary osteodystrophy) Patchy skin pigmentation, endocrine dysfunctions, and polyostotic fibrous dysplasia.

Brown's tendon sheath
(378.61) Limited elevation of eye, marked by paresis of inferior oblique muscle.

Brown-Séquard
(344.89) (Avellis, Babinski-Nageotte, Benedikt's, Cestan's, Cestan-Chenais, Foville's, Gubler-Millard, Jackson's, Weber-Leyden) Paraplegia and anesthesia over part of the body caused by lesions in the brain or spinal cord.

Bruck-de Lange
(759.89) Congenital cerebral condition involving dwarfism, mental deficiency, and brachycephaly.

Brugada
(746.89) A congenital heart anomaly in which the hypertrophy (enlargement) is localized to the left ventricle.

Brugsch's
(757.39) Increased thickening of the skin on extremities and face with clubbing of fingers and deformities in bone of the limb.

Bruising
(287.2) (Diamond-Gardner, Gardner-Diamond) Bruising occurring easily and large in women, involving surrounding tissues, resulting in pain, and spawning others.

Buchem's
(733.3) Multiple fractures and bowing of all extremities, thickening of skull bones, and osteoporosis beginning in childhood.

Budd-Chiari
(453.0) Thrombosis of the hepatic vein with enlargement of the liver and severe hypertension.

Büdinger-Ludloff-Läwen
(717.89) An old disruption of ligaments in the knee.

Bulbar
(335.22) (Duchenne's) Paralysis-based symptoms from defects in the medulla oblongata.

Bundle of Kent
(426.7) Muscular bundle forming a direct connection between the ventricle and atrial walls.

Bürger-Grütz
(272.3) Abdominal pain, hepatosplenomegaly, pancreatitis, and eruptive xanthomas in a genetic condition.

Burke's
(577.8) Pancreatic insufficiency and chronic neutropenia.

Burnett's
(275.42) Disorder of the kidneys induced by ingestion of large amounts of alkali and calcium in the therapy of a peptic ulcer. Reversible in the early stages, but can lead to renal failure.

Burnier's
(253.3) (Levi, Lorain-Levi) Dwarfism resulting from malfunction of the pituitary gland.

Burning feet
(266.2) (Gopalan's) Severe discomfort of the feet and other extremities with excessive sweating and elevated skin temperature, and believed to be caused by a riboflavin deficiency.

Bywaters'
(958.5) Traumatic anuria following crushing, especially of kidneys.

Caffey's
(756.59) Soft tissue swelling over the affected bones, irritability, and fever, and running periods of exacerbation and remission.

Calvé-Legg-Perthes
(732.1) Disease of the growth centers, especially the top of the femur, in which the epiphyses is replaced by new calcification.

Capillary leak
(518.82) (ARDS) An acute state characterized by severe dyspnea, pulmonary infiltrates, and hypoxemia (deficient oxygenation of blood) occurring in certain clinical situations.

Carcinogenic thrombophlebitis
(453.1) Spontaneous development of thromboses in the upper and lower limbs because of visceral neoplasm.

Carcinoid
(259.2) (Bjorck-Thorson, Cassidy-Scholte, Hedinger's) Carcinoid tumors causing cyanotic flushing of the skin, diarrhea watery stools, bronchoconstrictive attacks, hypotension, edema, and ascites.

Cardiacus negros
(416.0) (Arrilaga-Ayerza) Cyanosis and hypertension resulting from sclerosis of the pulmonary arteries.

Cardiopulmonary obesity
(278.8) (Pickwick) Obesity, hypoventilation, somnolence, and erythrocytosis.

Cardiorespiratory distress (idiopathic), newborn
(769) (Hyaline membrane) Respiratory distress resulting from reduced amounts of lung surfactant in premature infants. Frequently fatal.

Cardiovasorenal
(272.7) Abnormal accumulations of neutral glycolipids in histiocytes in blood vessel walls, cornea verticillata, paresthesia in extremities, cataracts, and angiokeratomas on the thighs, buttocks, and genitalia.

Carini's
(757.1) Scaling of skin accompanying other congenital syndromes.

Carpal tunnel
(354.0) Pain and tingling, numbness, or burning in the hand resulting from compression of the median nerve by tendons. Often called a repetitive motion injury.

Carpenter's
(759.89) Small head with mental retardation as result of genetic disorder.

Cassidy (-Scholte)
(259.2) (Bjorck-Thorson, Hedinger's) Carcinoid tumors that cause cyanotic flushing of the skin, diarrheal watery stools, bronchoconstrictive attacks, hypotension, edema, and ascites.

Cat-cry
(758.31) (Cri-du-chat) Microcephaly, antimongoloid palpebral fissures, epicanthal folds, micrognathia, strabismus, mental and physical retardation, and a cat-like whine.

Cauda equina
(344.60) Aching pain of the perineum, bladder, and sacrum, radiating in a sciatic fashion, due to compression of spinal nerve roots.

Cauda equina with neurogenic bladder
(344.61) Aching pain of the perineum, bladder, and sacrum, radiating in a sciatic fashion, due to compression of spinal nerve roots. Symptoms include paralysis of organs and limbs served by those roots, including the bladder.

Central pain
(338.0) Neurological condition caused by injury to or dysfunction of the central nervous system.

Cerebellomedullary malformation
(741.0x) (Arnold-Chiari) Displacement of the caudal spinal cord due to tethering with or without spina bifida and meningomyelocele.

Cerebrohepatorenal
(759.89) Craniofacial abnormalities, hypotonia, hepatomegaly, polycystic kidneys, jaundice, and death in infancy.

Cervical compression
(721.1) Cervical spondylosis.

Cervical paralysis
(337.0) (Charcot-Weiss-Baker, Sluder's) Overactive carotid sinus, causing a marked drop in blood pressure stopping or blocking the heart.

Cervical (root) (spine) NEC
(723.8) Symptoms originating form the cervical spine.

Cervical sympathetic
(723.2) (cervicocranial) Irritation of nerve roots emanating from posterior cervical spinal cord.

Cervicodorsal outlet
(353.2) Pain or anesthesias affecting the neck and the upper back.

Céstan (-Raymond)
(433.8x) Quadriplegia, anesthesia, and nystagmus caused by obstruction of twigs of the basilar artery and lesions in the pontine region.

Céstan's
(344.89) (Avellis, Babinski-Nageotte, Benedikt's, Brown-Sequard, Cestan-Chenais, Foville's, Gubler-Millard, Jackson's, Weber-Leyden) Paraplegia and anesthesia over part of the body caused by lesions in the brain or spinal cord.

Céstan-Chenais
(344.89) (Avellis, Babinski-Nageotte, Benedikt's, Brown-Sequard, Cestan's, Foville's, Gubler-Millard, Jackson's, Weber-Leyden) Paraplegia and anesthesia over part of the body caused by lesions in the brain or spinal cord.

Chancriform
(114.1) Symptoms resembling a chancre.

Charcot's
(443.9) Pain, tension, and weakness in a moving limb but absent at rest and caused by occlusive arterial diseases of the limbs.

Charcot-Marie-Tooth
(356.1) Pain across the shoulder and upper arm.

Charcot-Weiss-Baker
(337.0) (Sluder's) Overactive carotid sinus, causing a marked drop in blood pressure stopping or blocking the heart.

CHARGE association
(759.89) CHARGE is an acronym for a recognizable pattern of birth defects which include Coloboma (a cleft or failure to close the eyeball), Heart defects, Atresia of the choanae (blockage of the back of the nasal passage), Retardation (referring to various degrees of physical and or developmental delay), Genital and urinary difficulties (including underdevelopment of reproductive organs) and Ear abnormalities (deformed pinna and or hearing loss). The specific combination of features may vary widely among patients. The underlying cause is unknown.

Cheadle (-Möller) (-Barlow)
(267) Anemia, spongy gums, weakness, induration of leg muscles, and mucocutaneous hemorrhages.

Chédiak-Higashi (-Steinbrinck)
(288.2) (Chediak-Higashi, Dohle body, Hegglin, Jordan's, May) Hepatosplenomegaly, lymphadenopathy, anemia, thrombocytopenia and changes in the bones, cardiopulmonary system, skin, psychomotor skills, abnormalities of granulation, and nuclear structure of white cells open the patient to infection.

Chiari's
(453.0) Thrombosis of the hepatic vein with enlargement of the liver and severe hypertension.

Chiari-Frommel
(676.6x) Unphysiological lactation and amenorrhea following pregnancy caused by hyperprolactinemia and a pituitary adenoma.

Chiasmatic
(368.41) Impairment of vision, limitations of the field of vision, scotoma, headache, syncope, and vertigo.

Chilaiditi's
(751.4) Interposition of the colon between the liver and diaphragm.

Child maltreatment
(995.5x) Child abuse through physical violence, emotional violence, starvation, or neglect.

Chondroectodermal dysplasia
(756.55) (Ellis-van Creveld) Congenital dwarfism with defective development of the cardiac septum, skin, hair, and teeth.

Chorea-athetosis-agitans
(275.1) Accumulation of copper in the brain, cornea, kidney, liver, and other tissues causing cirrhosis of the liver and deterioration in the basal ganglia of the brain.

Christian's
(277.89) (Hand-Schüller-Christian) Multiple-system defects of the membranous bones, exophthalmos, diabetes insipidus, soft tissues, and bone involvement.

Chromosome 4 short arm deletion
(758.39) (Cri-du-chat) Microcephaly, antimongoloid palpebral fissures, epicanthal folds, micrognathia, strabismus, mental and physical retardation, and a cat-like whine.

Chronic alcoholic
(291.2) Numerous symptoms caused by constant, long-time ingestion of alcohol affecting the nervous and gastrointestinal systems.

Chronic fatigue
(780.71) Persistent fatigue that significantly reduces daily activity with chronic sore throat, mild fever,

muscle weakness, myalgia, headaches, and neurological problems.

Chronic mesenteric
(557.1) (Wilkie's) Complete or partial block of the superior mesenteric artery with symptoms of vomiting, pain, blood in the stool, and distended abdomen resulting in bowel infarction.

Chronic pain
(338.4) Persistent condition, often occurring as a result of past injuries, infections, or surgical interventions, in which the nervous system generates pain signals that may be ongoing for weeks to years. Chronic pain may also be due to ongoing disease processes, such as arthritis, cancer, or recurrent infections. Some patients suffer chronic pain in the absence of past injury or physical damage.

Churg-Strauss
(446.4) Form of systemic inflammation and cell death of vessels with prominent lung involvement, manifested by severe asthma, among other respiratory disorders.

Clarke-Hadfield
(577.8) Pancreatic infantilisim with enlarged liver, fatty stools, and pancreatic atrophy in an under-developed child.

Claude Bernard-Horner
(337.9) (Horner's syndrome) Enophthalmos (backward displacement of the eyeball in the orbit), constricted pupil, drooping eyelid (ptosis), and facial dryness caused by brain stem lesion to the ipsolateral side interrupting the sympathetic nerves of the face.

Clerambault
(297.8) The delusional belief that someone, often a person of high social status, is in love with the patient.

Clifford's
(766.22) Placental dysfunction occurring in postmature fetuses.

Climacteric
(627.2) Chills, depression, hot flashes, headache, and irritability in menopausal women.

Clouston
(757.31) Congenital thickened nails and sparse or absent scalp hair, often accompanied by keratoderma of the palms and soles.

Coagulation-fibrinolysis (ICF)
(286.6) (coagulopathy) Decrease of elements needed for coagulation of blood causing profuse bleeding.

Cockayne's
(759.89) Dwarfism with deafness, retinal atrophy, mental retardation, and photo sensitivity.

Cockayne-Weber
(757.39) Dwarfism with a precociously senile appearance, pigmentary degeneration of the retina, optic atrophy, deafness, sensitivity to sunlight, and mental retardation.

Coffin-Lowry
(759.89) A genetic disorder characterized by craniofacial and skeletal abnormalities, mental retardation, short stature, and hypotonia (skeletal muscle weakness).

Cogan's
(370.52) Abrupt onset of interstitial keratitis, tinnitus, and vertigo followed by deafness.

Cold injury (newborn)
(778.2) Birth injury resulting from hypothermia.

Collet (-Sicard)
(352.6) Unilateral lesions of the ninth, tenth, eleventh, and twelfth cranial nerves producing paralysis of the vagal, glossal, and other nerves and the tongue on the same side.

Compartment(al) (anterior) (deep) (posterior)
(729.7x) (Nontraumatic) Swelling within the fascial layers that results in increased pressure, causing constriction of muscles, blood vessels, and nerves. Underlying causes include seizures, nephrotic syndrome, or everyday exercise activities.

(958.9x) (Traumatic or NOS) Early complication of trauma resulting from the compression of nerves and tendons.

Compression
(958.5) Traumatic anuria following crushing.

Concussion
(310.2) Persistent personality disturbance following a blow to the head featuring affective instability, bursts of aggression, apathy and indifference, impaired social judgment, and suspiciousness or paranoid ideation.

Condemned mucosa
(146.x-149.x) A malignant neoplasm involving multiple primary sites including the tonsils, and

other areas such as the floor of the mouth, tongue, and/or hypopharyngeal wall. Code each site as documented.

Congenital muscle hypoplasia
(756.89) Dysplasia of the fingernails and toenails, hypoplasia of the patella, iliac horns, thickening of the glomerular lamina densa, and a flask-shaped femur.

Congenital oculofacial paralysis
(352.6) (Collet-Sicard) Unilateral lesions of the ninth, tenth, eleventh, and twelfth cranial nerves producing paralysis of the vagal, glossal, and other nerves and the tongue on the same side.

Congenital Q-T
(426.82) (long QT, prolonged QT interval, Romano-Ward) Potentially fatal condition precipitated by vigorous exertion, emotional upset, or startling moments due to an imbalance in the electrical timing controlling the pumping action of the heart's ventricles. Patient is susceptible to recurrent episodes of syncope and rapid arrhythmias that can become malignant, leading to sudden death.

Conjunctivourethrosynovial
(099.3) A symptom of Reiter's disease.

Conn (-Louis)
(255.12) Headaches, nocturia, polyuria, fatigue, hypertension, hypokalemic alkalosis, potassium depletion, hypervolemia, and decreased renin activity, caused by a benign pituitary tumor; primary aldosteronism.

Conradi (-Hünermann)
(756.59) Asymmetric shortening of the limbs and scoliosis. Caused by both genetic and maternal medication sources.

Conus medullaris
(336.8) (Froin's) Cerebral spinal fluid of a yellowish hue signaling neoplastic or inflammatory obstruction.

Cooke-Apert-Gallais
(255.2) Type I acrocephalosyndactyly with peak head and fusion of digits (specifically the second through fifth digits) and severe acne vulgaris of forearms.

Cornelia de Lange's
(759.8x) Mental retardation, eyebrows across bridge of nose, hairline well down on forehead, uptilted tip of nose with depressed bridge of nose, and small head with low-set ears.

Corticosexual
(255.2) A generalized type of syndrome, inappropriately virilizing or feminizing, caused by inborn enzyme defects in gonadal hormone synthesis, due to adrenal function disorders associated with congenital adrenal hyperplasia and adrenal cortex tumors.

Costello
(759.89) (Fasciocutaneoskeletal) (FCS) An extremely rare disorder characterized by growth delay after birth leading to short stature, distinct craniofacial features, mental retardation, and multiple anomalous physical characteristics.

Costochondral junction
(733.6) (Tietze's) Painful swelling of costal cartilages, especially of the second rib and interpreted as coronary artery disease.

Costovertebral
(253.0) Arthritis of spine accompanying acromegaly, resembling rheumatoid arthritis and progressing to bony ankylosis with lipping of vertebral margins.

Cotard's
(297.1) Paranoia marked by sensory disturbances, delusions of negation, and suicidal ideations.

Cowden
(759.6) (multiple hamartoma) inherited disorder characterized by hamartomas of stomach and gastrointestinal tract, breast, thyroid carcinoma, and brain. An increased incidence of malignant tumors of the breast, endometrial tissues, and thyroid gland is also described.

Craniovertebral
(723.2) Nerve root irritation emanating from posterior cervical spinal cord.

Creutzfeldt-Jakob
(046.1) Progressive destruction of the pyramidal and extrapyramidal systems with progressive dementia, wasting of muscles, tremor, and other symptoms leading to death.

Cri-du-chat
(758.31) (Cat-cry) Microcephaly, antimongoloid palpebral fissures, epicanthal folds, micrognathia, strabismus, mental and physical retardation, and a cat-like whine.

Crib death
(798.0) (Sudden infant death) Unexpected death of healthy infant under 12 months old.

Crocodile tears
(351.8) (Melkersson-Rosenthal) Facial paralysis with dramatic lacrimation during eating prompted by lesion on the seventh cranial nerve, causing impulses to be misdirected from salivary glands to lacrimal glands.

Croup
(464.4) Obstruction of the larynx caused by allergy, foreign body, infection, or new growth in infants and children.

CRST
(710.1) (cutaneous systemic sclerosis) Induration and thickening of the skin with circulatory and organ changes in the face and hands. The name is an acronym for calcinosis, usually of the fingers, Raynaud's, sclerodactyly (hardened skin and bone deformity of the fingers), and telangiectasia (microvascular red spotting of the skin). Esophageal involvement is termed CREST syndrome.

Cruveilhier-Baumgarten
(571.5) Cirrhosis of the liver with patent paraumbilical, varicose periumbilical, or umbilical veins.

Cubital tunnel
(354.2) Lesion of the ulnar nerve, affecting movement and feeling of hand.

Cuiffini-Pancoast
(162.3) (Hare's) Neoplasm of upper lobe of lung.

Curschmann (-Batten) (-Steinert)
(359.2) Condition in which the peritoneal cover of the liver converts into a white mass resembling cake icing.

Cushing's
(255.0) Abdominal striae, acne, hypertension decreased carbohydrate tolerance, moon face, obesity, protein catabolism, and psychiatric disturbances resulting from increased adrenocortical secretion of cortisol caused by ACTH-dependent adrenocortical hyperplasia or tumor, or by effects of steroids.

Cutaneocerebral angioma
(759.6) (Kalischer's) Formation of multiple angiomas in skin of head and scalp.

Cutaneous nerve of thigh
(355.1) Tingling, formication, itching, and other symptoms on lower part of the thigh. Caused by lateral femoral cutaneous nerve.

Cystic duct stump
(576.0) Recurrence of gall bladder pain following removal of the organ.

D_1
(758.1) (Patau's, trisomy D) Extra chromosome in group D. Condition is usually fatal within two years and includes mental retardation, malformed ears, cardiac defects, convulsions, and other symptoms.

Dameshek
(282.49) One of hemolytic anemias that share a common decreased rate of synthesis of hemoglobin polypeptide chains and classified according to chain involved; erythroblastic anemia.

Dana-Putnam
(281.0) [336.2] Numbness, tingling, weakness, a sore tongue, dyspnea, faintness, pallor of the skin and mucous membranes, anorexia, diarrhea, loss of weight, and fever. Strikes in the fifth decade.

Danbolt (-Closs)
(686.8) (Brandt's) Zinc metabolism defect in young children with blisters, crusting, oozing eruptions, loss of hair, and diarrhea.

Dandy-Walker
(742.3) Hydrocephalus with atresia of the foramina of Luschka and Magendie.

Danlos'
(756.83) (Meekeren, Ehlers) Group of congenital connective tissue diseases with overly elastic skin, hyperextensive joints, and fragility of blood vessels and arteries.

Davies-Colley
(733.99) (Cyriax) Arthritis with degeneration of cartilage leading to collapse of the ears, nose, and tracheobronchial tree. Death may occur as the respiratory system is affected.

De Lange's
(759.89) Inherited deformity with impaired development, mental retardation, eyebrows growing across bridge of nose, hairline well down on forehead, uptilted tip of nose with depressed bridge of nose, and small head with low-set ears.

De Toni-Fanconi (-Debré)
(270.0) (Harts) Renal tubular malfunction, including cystinosis and osteomalacia and caused by inherited disorders or resulting from multiple myeloma or proximal epithelial growth.

Dead fetus
(641.3x) Loss of non-clotting blood and lengthy retention of dead fetus following tachycardia and related symptoms.

Debré
(270.0) (Harts) Renal tubular malfunction, including cystinosis and osteomalacia and caused by inherited disorders or resulting from multiple myeloma or proximal epithelial growth.

Defeminization
(255.2) Mature masculine somatic characteristics by prepubescent male, girl, or woman showing at birth or developing later as result of adrenocortical dysfunction.

Defibrination
(286.6) Dilution of fibrin by enzyme action.

Deficiency
(260) Any syndrome resulting from deficiencies in proteins, hormones, calories, trace minerals, vitamins, and other chemicals necessary for function or growth.

Degos'
(447.8) Malignant atrophic papulosis.

Deiters' nucleus
(386.19) (Bonnier) Ocular disturbances, deafness, nausea, thirst, anorexia, and symptoms traced to vagus centers resulting from lesion of Deiters' nucleus and its connections.

Déjérine-Roussy
(338.0) Infarction of the postero-inferior thalamus causing transient hemiparesis, severe loss of superficial and deep sensation with crude pain in the limbs, and vasomotor or trophic disturbances.

Déjérine-Thomas
(333.0) (Hallervorden-Spatz) Nerves between the striatum and pallidum are completely demyelinated.

Del Castillo's
(606.0) Cessation of menses not associated with pregnancy.

Deletion chromosomes
(758.39) General description of syndromes such as antimongolism and cat-cry in which chromosomes are missing rather than duplicated.

Delusional
(293.81) Organic disorder including hallucinations, beliefs about being followed, being poisoned, etc., and not meeting criteria for schizophrenia.

Dementia-aphonia, of childhood
(299.1x) Dementia in which child becomes mute.

Depersonalization
(300.6) Patient feels detached from his or her body and experiences the feeling of being an automaton or in a dream-like state. Depersonalization must be a primary symptom and not part of schizophrenia or another disorder.

Dercum's
(272.8) (Ander's) Deposits of painful symmetrical nodular or pendulous masses of fat in various body regions.

Diabetes-dwarfism-obesity
(258.1) Endocrine dysfunction causing diabetes and affecting growth and weight.

Diabetes mellitus-hypertension-nephrosis
(250.4x) [581.81] High blood pressure and kidney failure resulting from diabetes in which carbohydrate utilization is reduced and lipid and protein use is enhanced.

Diabetes mellitus in newborn infant
(775.1) Diabetes mellitus

Diabetes-nephrosis
(250.4x) [581.81] High blood pressure and kidney failure resulting from diabetes in which carbohydrate utilization is reduced and lipid and protein use is enhanced.

Diabetic amyotrophy
(250.6x) [358.1] Muscular atrophy resulting from diabetes.

Diamond-Blackfan
(284.01) (Blackfan-Diamond, Kaznelson's) Congenital anemia of infancy requiring a number of blood transfusions to maintain life.

Diamond-Gardener
(287.2) Bruising occurring easily and large, involving surrounding tissues, resulting in pain, and spawning others. Assumed to be a form of autoimmune problem.

Diaper
(270.0) Infantile form of Fanconi's syndrome with cystinosis.

Dialysis dysequilibrium
(276.9) A set of complications arising from dialysis that includes nausea, vomiting, hypertension, and convulsions that result in rapid removal of urea from the extracellular fluid compartments, with movement of water into the vessels and resultant cerebral edema. Code also the underlying disease, such as chronic renal failure, hypertensive renal disease, or diabetes mellitus, and the kidney dialysis status, V45.1.

DIC
(286.6) Decrease of elements needed for coagulation of blood causing profuse bleeding.

Diencephalohypophysial
(253.8) Problem with the thalamus or pituitary gland not otherwise specified.

DiGeorge's
(279.11) Hypoplasia or aphasia of the thymus and parathyroid gland with congenital heart defects, anomalies of the great vessels, esophageal atresia, seizures, and facial deformities.

Dighton's
(756.51) (van der Hoeve's) Blue sclera, little growth, brittle bones, and deafness.

Di Guglielmo's
(207.0x) Condition characterized by large numbers of nucleated red cells appearing in the bone marrow and blood.

Disseminated platelet thrombosis
(446.6) Fatal disease with central nervous system involvement due to formation of fibrin or platelet thrombi in arterioles and capillaries in many organs.

Doan-Wiseman
(289.53) Primary splenic neurtropenia. Syndrome characterized by profound neutropenia and leukopenia, splenomegaly, susceptibility to infection, and hypercellular bone marrow.

Döhle body
(288.2) (Chediak-Higashi, Hegglin, Jordan's, May) Hepatosplenomegaly, lymphadenopathy, anemia, thrombocytopenia, changes in the bones, cardiopulmonary system, skin, and psychomotor skills. Granulation and nuclear structure of white cells opens patient to infection and results in death.

Donohue's
(259.8) Slow physical and mental development, elfin facial features such as wide-set eyes and low-set ears, and severe endocrine disorders indicated by enlarged sexual organs. Rare and fatal.

Double athetosis
(333.71) A form of acquired torsion dystonia manifested by abnormal, uncontrolled, slow, and writhing movements of the extremities, tongue, or face.

Double whammy
(360.81) Dislocation of eye ball.

Down
(758.0) (Trisomy 21, mongolism) Retardation with numerous markers varying from one person to another. Symptoms include retarded growth, flat face with short nose, epicanthic skin folds, protruding lower lip, rounded ears, thickened tongue, pelvic dysplasia, broad hands and feet, stubby fingers, and absence of Moro reflex.

Dressler's
(411.0) Fever, leukocytosis, chest pain, evidence of pericarditis, pleurisy, and pneumonia occurring days or weeks after a myocardial infarction. Postcardiotomy Dressler's is reported with ICD-9-CM code 429.4.

Drug withdrawal
(292.0) A number of physical symptoms resulting from long-time ingestion of, and dependence on, therapeutic and illicit drugs.

Drug withdrawal, infant, of dependent mother
(779.5) A number of physical symptoms suffered by newborns whose drug-dependent mothers allowed drugs to cross the placenta.

Drug-induced
(292.84) Description of symptoms, physiological and psychological, produced by drug abuse or dependence.

Drum
(381.02) Symptom of a number of syndromes affecting the ear.

Dry eye
(375.15) Lacrimal glands are unable to provide enough moisture to cover the eye.

Dry skin
(701.1) Keratosis producing lesions appearing as dry skin.

DSAP
(692.75) (Disseminated Superficial Actinic Porokeratosis) Skin disorder occurring on sun-exposed skin and characterized by numerous superficial, keratotic, brownish-red macules.

Duane's
(378.71) (Still-Turk-Duane, Duane-Stilling-Turk) Simultaneous retraction of eye muscles causing an inability to abduct the affected eye with retraction of the globe.

Dubin-Johnson
(277.4) (Dubin-Sprinz) Nonhemolytic jaundice thought as a defect in concentrated bilirubin and other organs causing a brown granular pigment in the hepatic duct.

Duchenne's
(335.22) Paralysis symptoms caused by medulla oblongata.

Due to mesenteric artery insufficiency
(557.1) (Wilkie's) Blocked superior mesenteric artery with vomiting, pain, blood in the stool, distended abdomen, and bowel infarction.

Dumping
(564.2) Emptying of contents of jejunum with nausea, sweating, weakness, palpitation, syncope, warmth, and diarrhea. Occurs after eating in patients who have had partial gastrectomy and gastrojejunostomy.

Duplay's
(726.2) Inflammation of subacromial or subdeltoid bursa.

Dupré's
(781.6) Irritation of spinal cord and brain mimicking meningitis, but in which there is no swelling of membranes.

During labor
(668.0x) (Mendelson's) Disorders of lung following vomiting and regurgitation by obstetric patients.

Dyke-Young
(283.9) (Hayem-Widal) Anemia caused by exposure to trauma, poisons, and other causes.

Dysmyelopoietic
(298.8) A variety of closely related disorders with various etiological factors characterized by chronic (pain) cytopenias. The code assignment is based on the pathologic diagnosis from bone marrow biopsy, i.e. leukemia (208.xx), preleukemia (288.8).

Dyspraxia
(315.4) Organic disorder affecting patient's ability to perform coordinated acts and not due to psychotic diagnosis.

Dyssynergia cerebellaris myoclonica
(334.2) (Hunt's) Disorder marked by myoclonus epilepsy and muscular tremors associated with disturbance of muscle tone and coordination.

E_3
(758.2) (Edward's, trisomy E) Congenital malformations in which extra chromosome is group E. Includes mental retardation, abnormal skull shape, malformed ears, small mandible, cardiac defects, short sternum, and other symptoms.

Eagle-Barrett
(756.71) (Prune belly) Congenital absence of muscles of abdomen and genitourinary anomalies.

Eagle's
(733.99) Pain resulting from an elongated styloid process of the temporal bone. Code also any associated condition, such as glossopharyngeal neuralgia (352.1) or impingement of the carotid artery (447.1).

Eale's
(362.18) Retinal vasculitis marked by phlebitis, arteritis, and endarteritis.

Eaton-Lambert
(199.1) [358.1] (Lambert-Eaton) Progressive proximal muscle weakness resulting from antibodies directed against motor-nerve axon terminals.

Ebstein's
(746.7) (Hypoplastic left heart) Hypoplasia or atresia of the left ventricle and aorta or mitral valve with respiratory distress and extreme cyanosis. Cardiac failure and death often result in early infancy.

Ectopic ACTH secretion
(255.0) (Cushing) Abdominal striae, acne, hypertension decreased carbohydrate tolerance, moon face, obesity, protein catabolism, and psychiatric disturbances resulting from increased adrenocortical secretion of cortisol caused by ACTH-dependent adrenocortical hyperplasia or tumor, or administration of steroids.

Eczema-thrombocytopenia
(279.12) (Aldrich, Wiskott-Aldrich) Immunodeficiency shown by eczema, thrombocytopenia, and recurrent pyogenic infection with increased susceptibility to infection from encapsulated bacteria.

Eddowes'
(756.51) (Ekman's, Spurway's) Blue sclera, little growth, brittle and malformed bones, and malformed teeth.

Edwards'
(758.2) (E, trisomy E) Congenital malformations in which extra chromosome is group E. Includes mental retardation, abnormal skull shape, malformed ears, small mandible, cardiac defects, short sternum, and other symptoms.

Efferent loop
(537.89) (Gastrojejunal loop obstruction) Distended efferent loop with illness and pain caused by acute or chronic obstruction of the duodenum and jejunum proximal to a gastrojejunostomy.

Ehlers-Danlos
(756.83) (Meekeren, Ehlers, Danlos) Congenital connective tissue diseases with overly elastic skin, hyperextensive joints, and fragility of blood vessels and arteries.

Eisenmenger's
(745.4) Pulmonary hypertension with congenital communication between two circulations so that a right to left shunt results.

Ekbom's
(333.94) (restless legs) Indescribable uneasiness, restlessness, or twitching in the legs after going to bed. Often caused by poor circulation or antipsychotic medications, it can lead to insomnia.

Ekman's
(756.51) (Eddowes', Spurway's) Blue sclera, little growth, brittle and malformed bones, and malformed teeth.

Electric feet
(266.2) (Gopalan's) Discomfort of feet and other extremities, excessive sweating, elevated skin temperature, and riboflavin deficiency.

Ellis-van Creveld
(756.55) Dwarfism with defective development of cardiac septum, skin, hair, and teeth.

Ellison-Zollinger
(251.5) (Zollinger-Ellison) Peptic ulceration with gastric hypersecretion, tumor of the pancreatic islets, and hypoglycemia.

Embryonic fixation
(270.2) (Mendes, van der Hoeve-Halbertsma-Waardenburg, Waardenburg-Klein) Eyebrow or upper or lower eyelid sags.

Empty sella
(253.8) Sella turcica containing no pituitary gland caused by herniating arachnoid, radiotherapy, or surgery.

Endocrine-hypertensive
(255.3) (Schroeder's, Slocumb's) Disorder of adrenal medullary tissue with hypertension, attacks of palpitation, headache, nausea, dyspnea, anxiety, pallor, and profuse sweating.

Engel-von Recklinghausen
(252.01) (Jaffe-Lichtenstein-Uehlinger) Osteitis with fibrous degeneration and formation of cysts with fibrous nodules on affected bones.

Enteroarticular
(099.3) (Fiessinger-Leroy-Reiter) Association of arthritis, iridocyclitis, urethritis, and diarrhea.

Eosinophilia myalgia
(710.5) Painful muscles resulting from accumulation of a large number of granular leukocytes.

Epidemic vomiting
(078.82) (Winter's disease) Nausea and vomiting attacking a group of people suddenly without prior illness or malaise. Headache, vomiting, abdominal pain, and giddiness end quickly.

Erb (-Oppenheim) - Goldflam
(358.00) (Goldflam, Erb, Hoppe) Myoneural conduction-caused progressive muscular weakness beginning in face and throat.

Erdheim's
(253.0) Arthritis of spine accompanying acromegaly, resembling rheumatoid arthritis and progressing to bony ankylosis with lipping of vertebral margins.

Erlacher-Blount
(732.4) Disease causing bow-legs in children; tibia vara.

Erythrocyte fragmentation
(283.19) (Lederer-Brill) Fragmentation of red blood cells.

Euthyroid sick
(790.94) A transient alteration in thyroid hormone metabolism secondary to other illness, surgery, trauma, infectious disease, or stress. Lab values present are not indicative of hypothyroidism.

Evan's
(287.32) An autoimmune hemolytic anemia with immune thrombocytopenia, and sometimes combined with neutropenia, having no known underlying etiology, and varying in their onset, course, and duration. Spontaneous remission and exacerbation occur with autoantibodies acting against specific antigens to different blood components: red blood cells, platelets, and neutrophils.

Exhaustion
(300.5) Hypersomatic disorder.

Eye retraction
(378.71) (Duane, Still-Turk-Duane) Retraction of eye muscles with inability to abduct the affected eye with retraction of the globe.

Eyelid-malar-mandible
(756.0) (Franceschetti's) Malformations of derivatives of the first branchial arch, with palpebral fissures sloping outward and downward with notches in the outer third of the lower lids, defects of malar bones and zygoma, hypoplasia of the jawbone, high or cleft palate, low-set ears, unusual hair growth, and pits between mouth and ear.

Faber's
(280.9) (Hayem-Faber) Central pallor in the red blood cells caused by lack of red cell hemoglobin in blood; achlorhydric anemia.

Fabry (-Anderson)
(272.7) Neutral glycolipids in histiocytes in blood vessel walls, cornea verticillata, paresthesia in extremities, cataracts and angiokeratomas on the thighs, buttocks, and genitalia. Death comes from cardiac, cerebrovascular, and renal complications.

Facial diplegia
(352.6) (Collet-Sicard) Unilateral lesions of the ninth, tenth, eleventh, and twelfth cranial nerves producing paralysis of the vagal, glossal, other nerves, and the tongue on the same side. Most usually result of injury.

Fallot's
(745.2) Also called tetralogy of Fallot. Congenital cardiac defects with pulmonary stenosis, interventricular septal defect, dextroposeptum and venous as well as arterial blood, and right ventricular hypertrophy.

Familial acanthosis nigricans
(701.2) Velvety acanthosis with gray, black, or brown pigmentation on axillae and other body folds. In adults, it results from internal carcinoma. In children, it results from obesity-producing endocrine disturbance.

Familial eczema-thrombocytopenia
(279.12) (Aldrich, Wiskott-Aldrich) Eczema, thrombocytopenia, and recurrent pyogenic infection with increased susceptibility to infection from encapsulated bacteria.

Fanconi's
(284.09) Constitutional aplastic anemia; congenital pancytopeniain which the bone marrow fails to produce the normal amount of blood components.

Fanconi (-de Toni) (-Debré)
(270.0) (Harts) Renal tubular malfunction, including cystinosis and osteomalacia caused by inherited disorders, the result of multiple myeloma, or proximal epithelial growth.

Farber (-Uzman)
(272.8) Swollen joints, lymphadenopathy, subcutaneous nodules, and accumulation in lysosomes of affected cells of PAS-positive lipid consisting of ceramide. Begins soon after birth and caused by deficiency of ceramidase.

Fasciocutaneoskeletal (FCS)
(759.89) (Costello) An extremely rare disorder characterized by growth delay after birth leading to short stature, distinct craniofacial features, mental retardation, and multiple anomalous physical characteristics.

Fatigue NEC
(300.5) Hypersomatic disorder with no identifiable pathology.

FDH
(757.39) (Focal dermal hypoplasia) Linear areas of dermal hyperplasia with soft yellow nodules of fat. Areas are widely distributed and resemble striae distensae.

Feil-Klippel
(756.16) Shorter than average neck and a low hairline. Caused by fewer than average cervical

vertebrae or fusion of hemivertebrae into one bony mass.

Felty's
(714.1) Splenomegaly, leukopenia, arthritis, hypersplenism, anemia and other symptoms.

Feminizing
(255.2) A generalized type of syndrome, inappropriately feminizing, caused by inborn enzyme defects in gonadal hormone synthesis, due to adrenal function disorders associated with congenital adrenal hyperplasia and adrenal cortex tumors.

Fertile eunuch
(257.2) Hypogonadism with gynecomastia, hypospadias, and postpubertal testicular atrophy. Caused by an inherited defect of androgen receptors and insensitivity to testosterone.

Fetal alcohol
(760.71) Growth deficiency, craniofacial anomalies, and limb defects among offspring of mothers who are chronic alcoholics.

Fiedler's
(422.91) Acute, isolated infection of heart muscle.

Fiessinger-Leroy (-Reiter)
(099.3) (Fiessinger-Leroy-Reiter) An association of arthritis, iidocyclitis, and urethritis, sometimes with diarrhea. While symptoms may recur, the arthritis is constant.

Fiessinger-Rendu
(695.1) Necrolysis of the skin caused by toxins.

First arch
(756.0) (Franceschetti's) Malformations of the first branchial arch with palpebral fissures sloping outward and downward with notches in the outer third of the lower lids, defects of malar bones and zygoma, hypoplasia of the jawbone, high or cleft palate, low-set ears, unusual hair growth, and pits between mouth and ear.

Fish odor
(270.8) Rare disorder, also known as trimethylaminuria, in which the body's normal metabolic processes fail, causing the chemical trimethylamine to accumulate in the body. An unpleasant, rotten fish odor is emitted through the sweat, urine, and breath. This disorder may be genetic, or may be a secondary side-effect of treatment with large doses of levocarnitine.

Fisher's
(357.0) (Guillain-Barré, Landry, Strohl, Miller) Paraplegia of limbs, flaccid paralysis, ophthalmoplegia, ataxia, and areflexia caused by disorder of immune system.

Fitz-Hugh and Curtis
(098.86) Peritonitis of the upper abdominal region in persons with a history of gonorrheal or other infections.

Fitz's
(577.0) Acute infection of the pancreas with the formation of necrotic areas, bleeding in the gland, fever, leukocytosis, nausea, and pain.

Flajani (-Basedow)
(242.0x) (Basedow, Parry's, Grave's disease) Fatigue, nervousness, emotional lability and irritability, heat intolerance and increased sweating, weight loss, palpitation, and tremor of hands and tongue caused by excess thyroidal hormones.

Flush
(259.2) (Bjorck-Thorson, Cassidy-Scholte, Hedinger's) Carcinoid tumors causing severe attacks of cyanotic flushing of the skin, diarrheal watery stools, bronchoconstrictive attacks, hypotension, edema, and ascites.

Foix-Alajouanine
(336.1) Ophthalmoplegia, paresis of the sympathetic nerves, and neuroparalytic keratitis from compression of lateral wall of the cavernous sinus.

Fong's
(756.89) Dysplasia of the fingernails and toenails, hypoplasia of patella, iliac horns, thickening of the glomerular lamina densa, and a flask-shaped femur.

Foramen magnum
(348.4) Compression of brain from the space above.

Forbes-Albright
(253.1) Persistent nonpuerperal lactation and amenorrhea caused by pituitary tumor, marked by secretion of excessive amounts of prolactin.

Fossa compression
(348.4) Compression of brain from the fossa underneath.

Foster-Kennedy
(377.04) (Gowers-Paton-Kennedy) Meningioma of optic nerve with central scotoma and contralateral choked disk.

Foville's
(344.89) (Avellis, Babinski-Nageotte, Benedikt's, Brown-Sequard, Cestan's, Cestan-Chenais, Gubler-Millard, Jackson's, Weber-Leyden) Paraplegia and anesthesia over part of the body caused by lesions in the brain or spinal cord.

Fragile X
(759.83) Mental retardation, enlarged testes, big jaw, high forehead, and long ears in males. In females, fragile X presents mild retardation and heterozygous sexual structures. In some families, males have shown no symptoms but carry the gene.

Franceschetti's
(756.0) Malformations of derivatives of the first branchial arch, marked by palpebral fissures sloping outward and downward with notches in the outer third of the lower lids, defects of malar bones and zygome, hypoplasia of the jawbone, high or cleft palate, low-set ears, unusual hair growth, and pits between mouth and ear.

Fraser's
(759.89) Cryptophthalmus with ear malformations, cleft palate, laryngeal deformity, displacement of umbilicus and nipples, digital malformation, separation of symphysis pubis, maldeveloped kidneys, and masculine female genitals.

Freeman-Sheldon
(759.89) (Whistling face syndrome) Deviation of hands and face with protrusion of lips as in whistling, sunken eyes, and small nose.

Frey's
(705.22) Localized sweating and flushing of cheek and ear in response to chewing.

Friderichsen-Waterhouse
(036.3) Fulminating meningococcal septicemia in children below 10 years of age with vomiting, cyanosis, diarrhea, purpura, convulsions, circulatory collapse, meningitis, and hemorrhaging into the adrenal glands.

Friedrich-Erb-Arnold
(757.39) Thickening of skin on extremities and face with clubbing of fingers and deformities in bone of the limb.

Fröhlich's
(253.8) (Babinski-Fröhlich, Launois-Cléret, Renon-Delille) Obesity and hypogonadism in adolescent boys. Dwarfism indicates hypothyroidism.

Froin's
(336.8) Alteration in the cerebral spinal fluid resulting in a yellowish hue and indicative of neoplastic or inflammatory obstruction.

Frommel-Chiari
(676.6x) Hyperprolactinemia and a pituitary adenoma causing unphysiological lactation and amenorrhea following pregnancy.

Frontal lobe
(310.0) Changes in behavior following damage to the frontal areas of the brain including reduction in self-control, foresight, creativity, spontaneity, emotional vivaciousness, and empathy.

Fuller Albright's
(756.59) (McCune-Albright; Albright's hereditary osteodystrophy) Patchy skin pigmentation, endocrine dysfunctions, and polyostotic fibrous dysplasia.

Functional hyperinsulinism
(251.1) (Harris', organic hyperinsulinism) Hyperinsulinism due to organic endogenous factors with hypoglycemia, weakness, perspiration, jitteriness, tachycardia, mental confusion, and vision disturbances.

Gaisböck's
(289.0) Associated with hypertension, but without hyposplenomegaly.

Ganser's, hysterical
(300.16) Psychotic-like condition (but without symptoms and signs of a traditional psychosis) occurring in prisoners who feign insanity or who suffer head injury.

Gardner-Diamond
(287.2) Bruising occurring easily and large, involving surrounding tissues, resulting in pain, and spawning others. Assumed to be a form of autoimmune deficiency.

Gastrojejunal loop obstruction
(537.89) A distended afferent loop marked by illness and pain. Caused by acute or chronic obstruction of the duodenum and jejunum proximal to a gastrojejunostomy.

Gay bowel
Abdominal pain, cramps, bloating, flatulence, nausea, vomiting, or diarrhea caused by enteric bacteria, viruses, fungi, parasites, or trauma as experienced by homosexual males. Assign codes for the specific symptoms and their underlying etiologies (if known).

Gayet-Wernicke's
(265.1) Thiamine deficiency, disturbances in ocular motility, pupillary alterations, nystagmus, ataxia with tremors, and co-existing organic toxic psychosis. Most often due to alcoholism.

Gee-Herter-Heubner
(579.0) Catarrhal dysentery. Malabsorption syndrome of all ages precipitated by gluten-containing foods. Wasting and fatigue in both adults and children. Children suffer growth retardation and irritability. Adults suffer difficulty in breathing and clubbing of fingers.

Gélineau's
(347.00) Narcolepsy, a form of epilepsy where the patient abruptly falls asleep rather than suffering grand or petite mals.

Geniculate ganglion
(053.11) (Hunt's) Facial paralysis, otalgia, and herpes zoster caused by viral infection in seventh cranial nerve and geniculate ganglion.

Gerhardt's
(478.30) Paralysis of vocal cords causing inspiratory dyspnea.

Gerstmann
(784.69) Right-left disorientation, finger agnosia, agraphia, and constructional apraxia, due to lesion in the angular gyrus of the dominant hemisphere of the brain.

Gilbert's
(277.4) Benign elevation of unconjugated bilirubin with no liver damage or other deformities.

Gilford (-Hutchinson)
(259.8) (Hutchinson-Gilford) Precocious senility with death from coronary artery disease occurring before 10 years of age.

Gilles de la Tourette's
(307.23) Motor and vocal tics occurring many times a day beginning before age 21 and in which the type of tic changes over time.

Gillespie's
(759.89) Congenital dysplasia of the eyes, teeth, and extremities.

Glénard's
(569.89) Bloating, gas, pain, and fullness experienced in left upper abdominal quadrant with pain sometimes radiating up into left chest. Downward displacement of viscera may cause bulging of abdomen and other symptoms.

Glinski-Simmonds
(253.2) Wasting of pituitary gland as result of some other condition or affliction.

Glucuronyl transferase
(277.4) Benign elevation of unconjugated bilirubin with no liver damage or other deformities.

Glue ear
(381.20) Painless secretion of mucoid fluid in the middle ear, stopping up the eustachian tube and causing hearing loss.

Goldberg (-Maxwell) (-Morris)
(259.5) (Androgen insensitivity, hairless women, male pseudohemaphroditism, nonvirilizing, testicular feminization) Genetic condition affecting the development of reproductive organs marked by female external genitalia or a degree of both male and female genitalia. Amenorrhea noticed in teen years, with short, incompletely developed vagina and rudimentary or absent uterus and fallopian tubes, scanty or absent axillary/public hair, and testicles that may require removal.

Goldenhar's
(756.0) Epibulbar dermoid cysts, preauricular appendages, micrognathia, and vertebral anomalies.

Goldflam-Erb
(348.00) (Hoppe) Progressive muscular weakness beginning in face and throat caused by a defect in myoneural conduction.

Goltz-Gorlin
(757.39) Irregular linear streaks of skin atrophy, skeletal malformations, papillomas of the lips and labia, and occasional alopecia.

Goodpasture's
(446.21) Renal condition where nephritis progresses rapidly to death, leaving lungs showing extensive hemosiderosis or bleeding.

Gopalan's
(266.2) (burning feet) Severe discomfort of the feet and other extremities associated with excessive sweating and elevated skin temperature; believed to be caused by a riboflavin deficiency.

Gorlin-Chaudhry-Moss
(759.89) Congenital lesion of the basal cells.

Gougerot (-Houwer) - Sjögren
(710.2) (Sicca) Complex of symptoms of unknown source in middle aged women in which following triad exists: keratoconjunctivitis sicca, xerostomia, and connective tissue disease (usually rheumatoid arthritis but sometimes systemic lupus erythematosus). Cause may be abnormal immune response.

Gougerot-Blum
(709.1) Purpuric skin eruption seen on the legs, thighs, and lower trunk of men 40 to 60 years of age and characterized by minute rust-colored papules that fuse into plaques.

Gougerot-Carteaud
(701.8) Benign neoplasm producing finger-like projections from epithelial surface in girls nearing puberty. Papillas begin on back and between breasts, eventually spreading over the torso and throughout the body.

Gouley's
(423.2) Restrictive pericarditis.

Gowers'
(780.2) (vasovagal attack) Fall in blood pressure, slow pulse, and convulsions. Believed to be sudden stimulation of vagal nerve by receptors in heart, carotid sinus, or aortic arch.

Gowers-Paton-Kennedy
(377.04) (Foster-Kennedy, Gowers-Paton-Kennedy) Meningioma of optic nerve with central scotoma and contralateral choked disk.

Gradenigo's
(383.02) Localized meningitis in fifth and sixth cranial nerves, causing paralysis and pain in the temporal region.

Gray or grey
(779.4) Effects of chloramphenicol taken by mother during gestation on the newborn.

Greig's
(756.0) Abnormal increase in the interorbital distance with cleidocranial or craniofacial malformations, along with occasional mental deficiencies.

Gubler-Millard
(344.89) (Avellis, Babinski-Nageotte, Benedikt's, Brown-Sequard, Cestan's, Cestan-Chenais, Foville's, Jackson's, Weber-Leyden) Paraplegia and anesthesia over half or part of the body caused by lesions in the brain or spinal cord.

Guérin-Stern
(754.89) Congenital immobility of most joints, fixed in various postures, with little muscle development and growth.

Gulf war
Various factors, either individual or combined, such as exposure to smoke from burning oil wells, pesticides, infectious diseases, vaccines, cocktails given to soldiers, or toxic chemicals. External factors result in symptoms such as fatigue, joint pain, headache, abdominal pain, diarrhea, irregular temperatures, tumors, memory loss, motor neuron disease, and leukemia. Assign codes for the specific manifestations, with the appropriate external cause (E code) as identified.

Guillain-Barré (-Strohl)
(357.0) (Landry, Fisher's, Strohl, Miller) Often follows viral infections and may be a disorder of immune system with paraplegia of limbs, flaccid paralysis, ophthalmoplegia, ataxia, and areflexia.

Gunn's
(742.8) (jaw-winking) Eyelids widen during chewing, sometimes with an elevation of the upper lid when the mouth is open and closing of the lid when the mouth is closed.

Günther's
(277.1) Cutaneous photosensitivity leading to mutilating skin lesions, homolytic anemia and splenomegaly, and greatly increased urinary excretion of uroporphyrin.

Gustatory sweating
(350.8) (Frey's) Localized sweating and flushing of cheek and ear in response to chewing.

H_3O
(759.81) Rounded face, almond-shaped eyes, strabismus, low forehead, hypogonadism,

hyposomia, mental retardation, and an insatiable appetite.

Hadfield-Clarke
(577.8) Pancreatic infantilism with enlarged liver, fatty stools, and pancreatic atrophy in an underdeveloped child.

Haglund-Läwen-Fründ
(717.89) Traumatic separation of the cartilage of the patella with fissures.

Hairless women
(259.5) (Androgen insensitivity, Goldberg (-Maxwell) (-Morris), male pseudohemaphroditism, nonvirilizing, testicular feminization) Genetic condition affecting the development of reproductive organs marked by female external genitalia or a degree of both male and female genitalia. Amenorrhea noticed in teen years, with short, incompletely developed vagina and rudimentary or absent uterus and fallopian tubes, scanty or absent axillary/public hair, and testicles that may require removal.

Hallervorden-Spatz
(333.0) (Dejerine-Thomas) Nerves between the striatum and pallidum are completely demyelated.

Hamman's
(518.1) Pneumothorax or pneumopericardium resulting from presence of air or gas in the mediastinum beginning spontaneously or from trauma or disease. Sometimes induced to aid in diagnosis.

Hamman-Rich
(516.3) Chronic inflammation, progressive fibrosis of the pulmonary alveolar walls, and progressive dyspnea leading to death by oxygen deprivation or right heart failure.

Hand-foot
(282.61) (Herrick's) Sickle cell anemia.

Hand-Schüller-Christian
(277.89) (Christian) Histiocytosis with an occasional accumulation of cholesterol, defects of the membranous bones, exophthalmos, diabetes insipidus, and multiple-system, soft tissue, and bone involvement.

Hanot-Chauffard (-Troisier)
(275.0) Hypertrophic cirrhosis with pigmentation and diabetes mellitus.

Hare's
(162.3) (Cuiffini-Pancoast) Neoplasm of upper lobe of lung.

Harkavy
(446.0) (MCLS) Fever, conjunctival injection reddening of the oral cavity, ulcerative gingivitis, cervical lymph nodes, and skin eruptions that cover the hands and feet. Skin becomes puffy and sloughs off.

Harris'
(251.1) Hyperinsulinism due to organic endogenous factors, hypoglycemia, weakness, perspiration, jitteriness, tachycardia, mental confusion, and vision disturbances.

Hart's
(270.0) Renal tubular malfunction, cystinosis, and osteomalacia caused by inherited disorders or the result of multiple myeloma or proximal epithelial growth.

Hayem-Faber
(280.9) (Faber) Central pallor in red blood cells caused by lack of red cell hemoglobin in blood; achlorhydric anemia.

Hayem-Widal
(283.9) (Dyke-Young, Widal) One of a group of anemic syndromes caused by exposures to trauma, poisons, and other causes that decreases the number of red blood cells; acquired hemolytic jaundice.

Heat prostration
(992.4) Salt and water depletion following exposure to sunlight and heat, causing heat exhaustion.

Heberden's
(413.9) (angina pectoris) Severe pain in the chest caused by ischemia of the heart prompted by coronary artery disease.

Hedinger's
(259.2) (Bjorck-Thorson, Cassidy-Scholte) Malignant carcinoid tumors causing severe attacks of cyanotic flushing of skin, diarrheal watery stools, bronchoconstrictive attacks, hypotension, edema, and ascites.

Hegglin's
(288.2) (Chediak-Higashi, Dohle body, Jordan's, May) Hepatosplenomegaly, lymphadenopathy, anemia, thrombocytopenia, and changes in the bones, cardiopulmonary system, skin, and

psychomotor skills. Abnormalities of granulation and nuclear structure of white cells open patients to infection and result in death.

Heller's
(299.1x) Dementia in which a child becomes mute with irritability, tantrums, and other behavioral disorders.

HELLP
(642.5x) A group of symptoms occurring with preeclampsia or eclampsia: H=hemolysis, EL=elevated liver function tests, and LP=low platelet counts.

Hemolytic-uremic
(283.11) Nonautoimmune hemolytic anemia with severe thrombocytopenia and purpura, accompanied by acute renal failure, usually seen in children, but can be present at any age.

Hemophagocytic lymphohistiocytosis
(288.4) (HLH) A rare disorder in which an overly abundant amount of histocytes, as well as lymphocytes, begin to penetrate and accumulate in normal tissue and cause damage to a variety of organs. Primary (genetic) HLH is inherited; secondary HLH develops as a response to an abnormal or diseased immune system.

Hench-Rosenberg
(719.3x) Repeated episodes of arthritis and periarthritis without fever or changes in joints.

Henoch-Schönlein
(287.0) Eruption of purpuric lesions with joint pain and swelling, colic, passage of bloody stools, and glomerulonephritis in young children.

Hepatorenal
(572.4) (Heyd's, hepatourologic) Acute renal failure in patients with disease of the biliary or liver tract. Caused by decreased renal blood flow, damaging both organs.

Hercules
(255.2) (Apert-Gallais, Cooke) Type I acrocephalosyndactyly with peaked head, fusion of digits (specifically the second through fifth digits), and severe acne vulgaris of forearms.

Herpetic geniculate ganglionitis
(053.11) (Hunt's) Facial paralysis, otalgia, and herpes zoster caused by viral infection in seventh cranial nerve and geniculate ganglion.

Herrick's
(282.61) Sickle cell anemia.

Herter (-Gee)
(579.0) (Heubner-Herter) Catarrhal dysentery. Inherited malabsorption syndrome of all ages precipitated by gluten-containing foods with wasting and fatigue. Children suffer growth retardation and irritability. Adults suffer difficulty in breathing and clubbing of fingers.

Heyd's
(572.4) Acute renal failure with disease of the biliary or liver tract. Cause is decreased renal blood flow, damaging both organs.

HHHO
(759.81) (H_3O) Rounded face, almond-shaped eyes, strabismus, low forehead, hypogonadism, hyposomia, mental retardation, and an insatiable appetite.

Hoffa (-Kastert)
(272.8) Traumatic proliferation of fatty tissue on knee joint.

Hoffmann's
(244.9) [359.5] Hypothyroidism beginning during infancy as result of acquired injury of thyroid gland or presence of cretinism.

Hoffmann-Bouveret
(427.2) Rapid action of the heart having sudden onset and cessation.

Holiday heart
(427.xx) Usually transient cardiac arrhythmias, sometimes due to excessive alcohol ingestion, following a vacation or weekend away from work. Code both the cardiac arrhythmia and the acute ingestion of alcohol. Code also any alcohol dependence or associated cardiomyopathy.

Holländer-Simons
(272.6) Loss of subcutaneous fat of the upper torso, the arms, the neck, and face but with an increase in fat on and below the pelvis.

Holmes'
(368.16) (Balint's, Riddoch's) Cortical paralysis of visual fixation, optic ataxia, and disturbance of visual attention. Eye movements are normal.

Holmes-Adie
(379.46) (Adie, Holmes, Markus, Saenger's) Pathological reaction in which the pupil does not

react to changes in light and changes if focus is changed. Cause is certain tendon deficiency.

Hoppe-Goldflam
(358.0) (Goldflam, Erb, Hoppe) Progressive muscular weakness beginning in face and throat caused by a defect in myoneural conduction.

Horner's
(337.9) (Claude Bernard-Horner) Enophthalmos (backward displacement of the eyeball in the orbit), constricted pupil, drooping eyelid (ptosis), and facial dryness caused by brain stem lesion to the ipsolateral side interrupting the sympathetic nerves of the face.

Hospital addiction
(301.51) (Multiple operations, Münchhausen) Description of psychosomatic behavior with physical symptoms exhibited by some patients with histrionic personality disorder.

Hunt's
(053.11) (Ramsey-Hunt) Facial paralysis, otalgia, and herpes zoster caused by viral infection in seventh cranial nerve and geniculate ganglion.

Hunter (-Hurler)
(277.5) Mucopolysaccharide sulfates affecting the eye, ear, skin, teeth, skeleton, joints, liver, spleen, cardiovascular system, respiratory system, and central nervous system.

Hutchinson-Boeck
(135) (Lofgren, Schaumann's, Besnier-Boeck-Schaumann) Disorder with fibrosis, lymph nodes, skin, enlarged liver, eyes, enlarged spleen, phalangeal bones, parotid glands, and systemic granulomas composed of epithelioid and multinucleated giant cells.

Hutchinson-Gilford
(259.8) (Gilford) Precocious senility with death from coronary artery disease occurring before 16 years of age.

Hyperabduction
(447.8) Malignant atrophic papulosis.

Hyperactive bowel
(564.9) Abdominal pain, watery stools, and gas.

Hyperaldosteronism with hypokalemic alkalosis
(255.13) (Bartter's) Low or normal blood pressure, no edema, retarded growth, hypokalemic alkalosis, and elevated renin or angiotensin levels.

Hypercalcemic
(275.42) (Albright-Martin, Seabright-Bantam) Similar to hypoparathyroidism, Failure to respond to parathyroid hormone causing short stature, obesity, short metacarpals, and ectopic calcification.

Hypersomnia-bulimia
(349.89) (Kleine-Levin, Parry-Romberg) Hypersomnia associated with bulimia and occurring in males between 10 to 25 years of age. Ravenous appetite is followed by prolonged sleep, along with behavioral disturbances, impaired thought processes, and hallucinations.

Hypersympathetic
(337.9) (Claude Bernard-Homer, Reilly's, Steinbrocker's) Pain and stiffness in the shoulder and swelling and pain in the hand following heart attack.

Hypertransfusion, newborn
(776.4) Polycythemia of newborn resulting from blood flow from mother.

Hyperviscosity
(273.3) Increase in macroglobulins in the blood, hyperviscosity, weakness, fatigue, bleeding disorders, and visual disturbances.

Hypoglycemic
(251.2) (idiopathic familial hypoglycemia) Hypoglycemia described as unspecified

Hypoperfusion
(769) (Hyaline membrane) Respiratory distress in premature neonates associated with reduced amounts of lung surfactant. Frequently fatal.

Hypopituitarism
(253.2) Decreasing production of pituitary hormones caused by lessening activity of the anterior lobe of the hypophysis.

Hypoplastic left heart
(746.7) Hypoplasia or atresia of the left ventricle and aorta or mitral valve with respiratory distress and extreme cyanosis. Cardiac failure and death often result in early infancy.

Hypotension, maternal
(669.2x) Significantly reduced blood pressure during pregnancy.

Hypotonia-hypomentia-hypogonadism-obesity
(759.81) (Prader-Willi) Rounded face, almond-shaped eyes, strabismus, low forehead, hypogonadism,

hyposomia, mental retardation, and an insatiable appetite.

ICF (intravascular coagulation fibrinolysis)
(286.6) Decrease of elements needed for coagulation of blood and profuse bleeding.

Idiopathic cardiorespiratory distress, newborn
(769) (Hyaline membrane, respiratory distress) Respiratory distress in premature neonates associated with reduced amounts of lung surfactant. Frequently fatal.

Idiopathic nephrotic
(581.9) Affects the kidneys of a child with unknown cause.

Iliotibial band friction
(728.89) An overuse injury caused by repetitive friction of the iliotibial band across the lateral femoral epicondyle. Also known as "runners knee," injury to the iliotibial band extending from the thigh over the knee and attaching to the tibia may result in lateral hip, thigh, or knee pain.

Immobility
(728.3) Paralysis of legs and lower part of body.

Immunologic deficiency
(279.00) (Antibody deficiency) Inherited immune deficiencies characterized by insufficient antibodies.

Inappropriate secretion of antidiuretic hormone
(253.6) (Schwartz-Bartter) Low or normal blood pressure, no edema, and retarded growth found in children with hypokalemic alkalosis and elevated renin or angiotensin levels.

Infant of diabetic mother
(775.0) Babies born to diabetic mothers that are larger than average and may experience endocrine disturbances, hypoglycemia, transient tachypnea, or polycythemia. They may be at increased risk for congenital defects, heart failure, or other diseases.

Infantilism
(253.3) Profound retardation of mental and physical development

Inferior vena cava
(459.2) Obstruction of the vena cava.

Inspissated bile, newborn
(774.4) Biliary obstruction in newborn resulting from plugging of outflow tract.

IRDS (idiopathic respiratory distress)
(769) (Hyaline membrane) Respiratory distress in premature neonates associated with reduced amounts of lung surfactant. Frequently fatal.

Itsenko-Cushing
(255.0) (Cushing) Increased adrenocortical secretion of cortisol caused by ACTH-dependent adrenocortical hyperplasia or tumor with abdominal striae, acne, hypertension decreased carbohydrate tolerance, moon face, obesity, protein catabolism, and psychiatric disturbances.

IVC (intravascular coagulopathy)
(286.6) Decrease of elements needed for coagulation of blood. Later stages are marked by profuse bleeding.

Ivemark's
(759.0) Organs of left side of the body are a mirror image of organs on right side. Splenic agenesis and cardiac malformation are associated.

Jaccoud's
(714.4) Post rheumatic fever arthritis with fibrous changes in the joint capsules and tendons. Malformation of the joints resembles rheumatoid arthritis.

Jackson's
(344.89) (Avellis, Babinski-Nageotte, Benedikt's, Brown-Sequard, Cestan's, Cestan-Chenais, Foville's, Gubler-Millard, Weber-Leyden) Paraplegia and anesthesia over part of the body. Caused by lesions in the brain or spinal cord.

Jadassohn-Lewandowski
(757.5) Abnormal thickness and elevation of nail plates with palmar and plantar hyperkeratosis. The tongue is whitish.

Jaffe-Lichtenstein (-Uehlinger)
(252.01) (Engel-von Recklinghausen) Osteitis with fibrous degeneration and formation of cysts, along with fibrous nodules on affected bones due to malfunctioning parathyroid gland.

Jahnke's
(759.6) Angioma in trigeminal nerve, homolateral meningeal angioma with intracranial calcification, and/or angioma of choroid.

Jakob-Creutzfeldt
(046.1) Progressive dementia, wasting of muscles, tremor, and other symptoms. Communicable, rare spongiform encephalopathy occurring in middle life

with progressive destruction of the pyramidal and extrapyramidal systems to death.

Jaksch (-Hayem-Luzet)
(285.8) An anemic disorder among children under age three characterized by acute hemolytic anemia, infections, and gastrointestinal disorders.

Jaw-winking
(742.8) Eyelids widen during chewing, sometimes with an elevation of upper lid when mouth is open and closing of the lid when mouth is closed.

Jejunal
(564.2) (dumping) Emptying of contents of jejunum with nausea, sweating, weakness, palpitation, syncope, warmth, and diarrhea occurring after eating in patients who have had partial gastrectomy and gastrojejunostomy.

Jet lag
(327.35) Imbalance of the normal circadian rhythm resulting from airplane travel through a number of time zones. Leads to fatigue, irritability, and other constitutional disturbances.

Jeune's
(756.4) (ATD–asphyxiating thoracic dystrophy) Pelvis and phalanges are malformed, and cartilage of rib cage is unable to support breath action, leading to asphyxia.

Job's
(288.1) Autosomal disorder of neutrophils with abnormal or absent chemotactic responses, eczema, and staphylococcal abscesses on the skin. Patients tend to be females with fair skin and red hair.

Jordan's
(288.2) (Chediak-Higashi, Dohle body, Hegglin, May) Hepatosplenomegaly, lymphadenopathy, anemia, and thrombocytopenia with changes in the bones, cardiopulmonary system, skin, and psychomotor skills. Abnormalities of granulation and nuclear structure of white cells opens patient to infection and results in death.

Joseph-Diamond-Blackfan
(284.01) (Blackfan-Diamond, Kaznelson's) Congenital anemia of infancy requiring a number of blood transfusions to maintain life.

Jugular foramen
(352.6) (Collet-Sicard) Unilateral lesions of the ninth, tenth, eleventh, and twelfth cranial nerves producing paralysis of the vagal, glossal, and other nerves and the tongue on the same side resulting from injury.

Kahler's
(203.0x) Malignant neoplasm associated with anemia, hemorrhages, recurrent infections, and weakness that originates in bone marrow.

Kalischer's
(759.6) Multiple angiomas in skin of head and scalp.

Kallmann's
(253.4) Failure of sexual development resulting from inadequate secretion of pituitary gonadotropins. Associated with anosmia due to agenesis of the olfactory lobes in the brain, a product of X-linked inheritance.

Kartagener's
(759.3) Reversal of the position or location of organs or viscera.

Kasabach-Merritt
(287.39) Small number of platelets in circulating blood, causing bruising.

Kast's
(756.4) (Maffucci's) Benign cartilaginous growths in bones with bleeding in viscera and skin.

Kaznelson's
(284.01) (Diamond-Blackfan, Joseph) Congenital anemia of infancy and requiring a number of blood transfusions to maintain life.

Kearns-Sayre
(277.87) (Occulocraniosomatic) A mitochondrial defect associated with chronic progressive paralysis of the external eye muscles, cardiac conduction defects, short stature, pigmentary degeneration of the retina, deafness, and intellectual and hearing loss.

Kelly's
(280.8) (Paterson-Brown-Kelly, Plummer-Vinson) Condition in middle-aged women with hypochromic anemia, cracks or fissures at the corners of the mouth, painful tongue, and dysphagia due to esophageal stenosis or webs.

Kinsbourne
(333.2) (infantile myoclonic encephalopathy) (Opsoclonus myoclonus) A rare neurological disorder characterized by an unsteady gait, myoclonus (muscle spasms), and opsoclonus (irregular, rapid eye movements). Other symptoms may include

speech difficulties, decreased muscle tone, irritability, and fatigue. It is often manifested in children with tumors.

Kimmelstiel-Wilson
(250.4x) [581.81] High blood pressure and kidney failure resulting from a form of diabetes in which carbohydrate utilization is reduced and lipid and protein enhanced.

Klauder's
(695.1) Necrolysis of skin caused by toxins.

Klein-Waardenburg
(270.2) (Mendes, van der Hoeve-Halbertsma-Waardenburg, Waardenburg-Klein) Eyebrow or upper or lower eyelid sags.

Kleine-Levin
(327.13) (Parry-Romberg) Hypersomnia with bulimia occurring in males between 10 to 25 years of age. Ravenous appetite is followed by prolonged sleep, along with behavioral disturbances, impaired thought processes, and hallucinations.

Klinefelter's
(758.7) (XXY) Male in development, but with seminal tube dysgenesis, gynecomastia, and urinary gonadotropins.

Klippel-Feil
(756.16) Shorter than average neck and a low hairline caused by fewer than average cervical vertebrae or fusion of hemivertebrae into one bony mass.

Klippel-Trenaunay
(759.89) One extremity with hypertrophy of bone and soft tissues, hemangiomas on the skin, and port-wine stain over the bone.

Klumpke (-Déjérine)
(767.6) Atrophic paralysis of forearm and hand as result of birth trauma to brachial plexus.

Klüver-Bucy (-Terzian)
(310.0) Bilateral temporal lobe ablation with psychic hyperreactivity to visual stimuli or blindness, increased oral and sexual activity, and depressed drive and emotional reactions.

Köhler-Pellegrini-Stieda
(726.62) Calcification of medial collateral ligament of the knee.

König's
(564.89) Alternating constipation and diarrhea with pain meteorism and gurgling sounds in the right iliac fossa.

Korsakoff (-Wernicke)
(294.0) Amnestic dementia in which the patient cannot remember short-term or long-term memories but is not delirious.

Kostmann's
(288.01) Infantile genetic agranulocytosis characterized by recurrent bacterial infections, most commonly infection of the mouth and perirectum.

Kunkel
(571.49) (lipid hepatitis) Chronic hepatitis with autoimmune manifestations.

Langdon Down
(758.0) (mongolism) Congenital retardation with retarded growth, flat face with short nose, epicanthic skin folds, protruding lower lip, rounded ears, thickened tongue, pelvic dysplasia, broad hands and feet, stubby fingers, and absence of Moro reflex.

Larsen's
(755.8) Numerous congenital dislocations with anomalies of the bones and flattened facial features.

Launois'
(253.0) Pituitary secretions causing gigantism beginning before puberty with eosinophilic cell hyperplasia, eosinophilic adenoma, or chromophobe adenoma.

Launois-Cléret
(253.8) (Babinski-Frölich, Renon-Delille) Marked by obesity and hypogonadism in adolescent boys with dwarfism indicating hypothyroidism.

Laurence-Moon (-Bardet) - Biedl
(759.89) Retardation, pigmentary retinopathy, obesity, polydactyly, and hypogonadism.

Lawford's
(759.6) (Kalischer's) Formation of multiple angiomas in skin of head and scalp.

Lederer-Brill
(283.19) Anemic syndrome noted for fragmentation of red blood cells.

Legg-Calvé-Perthes
(732.1) Disease of children in growth centers, especially at top of femur, in which the epiphyses is replaced by new calcification.

Lennox-Gastaut with and without toxic seizures
(345.0x) Severe epilepsy with usual onset in early childhood. Seizures are difficult to treat, varying in type and occurring frequently, causing falls and injuries.

Lennox's
(345.0x) Childhood epilepsy with slow brain waves.

Lenticular
(275.1) Accumulation of copper in the brain, cornea, kidney, liver, and other tissues causing cirrhosis of the liver and deterioration in the basal ganglia of the brain.

Lepore hemoglobin
(282.49) Cardiac defects, coarse facial features, multiple lentigines, pulmonary stenosis, abnormalities of the genitalia, sensorineural deafness, and skeletal changes.

Léri-Weill
(756.59) Dorsal dislocation of the distal ulna and carpal bones, bowing of the radius, and mesomelic dwarfism.

Leriche's
(444.0) Obstruction of the terminal aorta causing fatigue in the hips, thighs, and calves; pallor of lower extremities; and impotence of exercising males.

Lermoyez
(386.00) Vertigo, nausea, vomiting, tinnitus, and progressive deafness caused by endolymphatic hydrops.

Lesch-Nyhan
(277.2) Physical and mental retardation, compulsive self-mutilation of the lips and fingers through biting, impaired renal function, choreoathetosis, spastic cerebral palsy, and purine synthesis and consequent hyperuricemia and uricaciduria.

Leukocyte
(288.09) A severe neutropenia with associated abnormal neutrophil motility. The etiology is unknown. Characterized by infections, most commonly of the mucous membranes and skin.

Lev's
(426.0) (Rytand-Lipstitch) Bundle branch block in patient with normal coronary arteries and myocardium resulting from calcification of the conducting system.

Levi's
(253.3) (Burier, Lorain-Levi) (pituitary dwarfism) Dwarfism resulting from the absence of functional anterior pituitary gland.

Li-Fraumeni cancer
(V84.01) A rare inherited cancer syndrome produced by mutations of gene p53, characterized by increased susceptibility to breast cancer, soft tissue sarcomas, and several other malignancies, all occurring at unusually early ages.

Lichtheim's
(281.0) [336.2] Numbness and tingling, weakness, a sore tongue, dyspnea, faintness, pallor of the skin and mucous membranes, anorexia, diarrhea, loss of weight, and fever. Most often strikes in the fifth decade.

Lightwood's
(588.89) Variety of syndromes resulting from metabolic acidosis springing from renal malfunction.

Lignac (-Fanconi)
(270.0) Metabolic disorder of kidney, involving failure to reabsorb water, minerals, and other substances as well as failure to transport.

Likoff's
(413.9) Severe pain in the chest caused by ischemia of heart prompted by coronary artery disease in menopausal women.

Liver-kidney
(572.4) (Heyd's) Acute renal failure in patients with disease of biliary or liver tract. Cause seems to be decreased renal blood flow, damaging both organs.

Lloyd's
(258.1) Endocrine dysfunction causing diabetes and affecting growth and weight.

Lobe (lung) (right)
(518.0) (Brock) Incomplete expansion of right middle lobe of lung with chronic pneumonitis.

Lobectomy behavior
(310.0) Symptomatic description of Klüver-Bucy syndrome.

Löffler's
(518.3) Transient infiltrations of lungs by eosinophilia resulting in coughing, fever, and dyspnea.

Löfgren's
(135) (Hutchinson-Boeck, Schaumann's, Besnier-Boeck-Schaumann) Involves fibrosis in lungs, lymph nodes, skin, liver, eyes, spleen, phalangeal bones, and parotid glands. Identified by systemic granulomas composed of epithelioid and multinucleated giant cells.

Long arm 18 or 21 deletion
(758.39) Autosomal deletion causing a variety of symptoms.

Long QT syndrome
(426.82) (congenital QT, prolonged QT interval, Romano-Ward) Potentially fatal condition precipitated by vigorous exertion, emotional upset, or startling moments due to an imbalance in the electrical timing controlling the pumping action of the heart's ventricles. Patient is susceptible to recurrent episodes of syncope and rapid arrhythmias that can become malignant, leading to sudden death.

Looser (-Debray) - Milkman
(268.2) (Milkman) Osteoporosis with frequent fractures striking middle-aged women.

Lorain-Levi
(253.3) (Burier, Levi) Dwarfism resulting from absence of functional anterior pituitary gland.

Louis-Bar
(334.8) (Boder-Sedgwick) Gonadal hypoplasia, insulin resistance and hyperglycemia, liver function problems, ataxia, nystagmus, and increased sensitivity to ionizing radiation.

Lowe's
(270.8) (Lowe-Terrey-MacLachlan) Aminoaciduria, cataracts, mental retardation, hydrophthalmia, rickets, and reduced ammonia production by the kidney.

Lower radicular, newborn
(767.4) Damage of nerve root during birth.

Lown (-Ganong)-Levine
(426.81) Electrocardiographic disorder indicated by a short P-R interval with normal duration of the QRS complex.

Lucey-Driscoll
(774.30) Retention jaundice in newborn infants resulting from defective bilirubin conjugation, a product of a steroid in mother's blood being transferred to the infant.

Lutembacher's
(745.5) Atrial septal defect associated with mitral stenosis.

Lyell's
(695.1) Necrolysis of skin caused by toxins.

MacLeod's
(492.8) (Swyer-James) Acquired unilateral hyperlucent lung with severe airway obstruction during expiration.

Macrogenitosomia praecox
(259.8) 1) Excessive bodily development with unusual growth of sexual organs; 2) a description of symptoms indicating Donohue's and other syndromes.

Macroglobulinemia
(273.3) (Waldenström's) Earmarked by increase in macroglobulins in the blood. Has symptoms of hyperviscosity such as weakness, fatigue, bleeding disorders, and visual disturbances.

Macrophage activation syndrome
(288.4) A hemophagocytic syndrome caused by excessive creation and production of T cells and macrophages, often a life-threatening complication of systemic-onset juvenile rheumatoid arthritis.

Maffucci's
(756.4) (Maffucci's) Benign cartilaginous growths in bones with bleeding in viscera and skin.

Magnesium-deficiency
(781.7) Tetany. Any number of syndromes affecting newborns and others. Hyperexcitability of nerve and muscles due to decrease in concentration of extracellular ionized calcium, resulting in calcium and magnesium deficiency.

Malabsorption
(579.9) A number of syndromes in which the body does not adequately absorb dietary constituents and loses nonabsorbed substances in the stool. Due to muscle, digestive, or lymphatic defect.

Malignant carcinoid
(259.2) (Bjorck-Thorson, Cassidy-Scholte, Hedinger's) Carcinoid tumors causing cyanotic flushing of skin, diarrheal watery stools, bronchoconstrictive attacks, hypotension, edema, and ascites.

Mallory-Weiss
(530.7) A tear in esophagus following several hours or days of vomiting, marked by vomiting of blood.

Mandibulofacial
(756.0) (Franceschetti's, mandibulofacial dysostosis) Malformations of derivatives of the first branchial arch, marked by palpebral fissures sloping outward and downward with notches in the outer third of the lower lids, defects of malar bones and zygome, hypoplasia of the jawbone, high or cleft palate, low-set ears, unusual hair growth, and pits between mouth and ear.

Manic depression
(296.80) (bipolar) Alternating major depressive and manic periods.

Mankowsky's
(731.2) (Pierre Marie-Bamberger) Symmetrical osteitis of limbs localized to phalanges and terminal epiphyses of the long bones of forearm and leg. Symptoms include kyphosis of spine and affection of joints.

Maple syrup
(270.3) Anomaly in amino acid metabolism marked by urine and perspiration odor, hypertonicity, convulsions, coma, and death.

Marable's
(447.4) Compression of celiac artery by median arcuate ligament in diaphragm.

Marchesani (-Weill)
(759.89) Short stature, heavy musculature, reduced joint mobility, myopic, glaucoma, and many other symptoms.

Marchiafava-Micheli
(283.2) Paroxysmal nocturnal hemoglobinuria.

Marcus Gunn's
(742.8) (jaw-winking) Eyelids widen during chewing, sometimes with elevation of upper lid when the mouth is open and closing of lid when mouth is closed.

Marfan's
(759.82) Unusually long extremities, subluxation of the lens, dilation of the aorta, and other symptoms.

Marie-Bamberger
(731.2) (Hagner's) A condition characterized by clubbed fingers and toes, vasomotor disturbances of the hands and feet; it occurs in association with pulmonary diseases. Also known as hypertrophic pulmonary osteoarthropathy.

Marie's
(253.0) Secondary to chronic conditions in lung and heart, localized to phalanges and terminal epiphyses of long bones of arm and leg, and accompanied by kyphosis. Caused by pituitary disorder.

Marinesco-Sjögren
(334.2) (Marinesco-Garland, Torsten-Sjögren's, or cataract-oligophrenia) A rare, inherited neurologic disorder characterized by cerebellum and intraocular lens degeneration (cataracts) with mental retardation. Code also the associated cataract, if it is the focus of treatment.

Markus-Adie
(379.46) Paralysis of conjugate movement of eyes without paralysis of convergence. Caused by lesions of midbrain.

Maroteaux-Lamy
(277.5) Accumulation of mucopolysaccharide sulfates affecting eye, ear, skin, teeth, skeleton, joints, liver, spleen, cardiovascular system, respiratory system, and central nervous system.

Martin-Albright
(275.49) (Albright-Martin, Seabright-Bantam) Short stature, obesity, short metacarpals, and ectopic calcification. Similar to hypoparathyroidism and caused by failure to repond to parathyroid hormone.

Martorell-Fabré
(446.7) (Martorell-Fabré, Raed-Harbitz, Takayasu-Onishi) Ischemia, transient blindness, facial atrophy, and many others. Progressive obliteration of the brachiocephalic trunk and the left subclavian and common carotid arteries above their source in the aortic arch.

Massive aspiration of newborn
(770.18) Newborn aspiration pneumonia or pneumonitis caused by inhalation of uterine or birth canal contents, causing significant and serious newborn respiratory compromise, not specifically identified as aspiration pneumonia or pneumonitis from blood, meconium, or clear amniotic fluid.

Masters-Allen
(620.6) Pelvic pain resulting from old laceration of broad ligament received during delivery.

Mastocytosis
(757.33) Inherited disorder of skin (and sometimes other structures) in which pigmented lesions appear in linear, zebra stripe, and other configurations and are preceded by vesicles and bullae and followed by verrucal lesions.

Maternal hypotension
(669.2x) Significantly reduced blood pressure during pregnancy.

Maternal obesity
(646.1x) Edema or excessive weight gain in pregnancy with no hypertension.

May (-Hegglin)
(288.2) (Chediak-Higashi, Dohle body, Hegglin, Jordan's, May) Hepatosplenomegaly, lymphadenopathy, anemia, thrombocytopenia, along with changes in the bones, cardiopulmonary system, skin, and psychomotor skills. Abnormalities of granulation and nuclear structure of white cells open child to infection and result in death.

McArdle (-Schmid) (-Pearson)
(271.0) Glucose-6-phosphatase deficiency due to inherited defects of glycogen metabolism resulting in excess accumulation of glycogen in muscle, characterized by myopathies and hepatorenal effects.

McCune-Albright
(756.59) (Albright's hereditary osteodystrophy) Patchy skin pigmentation, endocrine dysfunctions, and polyostotic fibrous dysplasia.

McQuarrie
(251.2) Hypoglycemia described as primary and unspecified, reactive, or spontaneous.

Meconium aspiration
(770.12) (MAS) Newborn inhalation of meconium while still in utero or with the first breath, generally defined as the presence of meconium beyond the vocal cords, often blocking the lungs, initiating an inflammatory response, and causing significant and serious respiratory compromise.

Median arcuate ligament
(447.4) Compression of celiac artery by median arcuate ligament in diaphragm.

Meekeren-Ehlers-Danlos
(756.83) (Meekeren, Ehlers, Danlos) Group of congenital connective tissue diseases with overly elastic skin, hyperextensive joints, and fragility of blood vessels and arteries.

Meige-Milroy
(757.0) (Nonne-Milroy-Meige) Lymphatic edema of the legs (and face and arms in severe cases) caused by obstruction of lymphatic ducts.

Melkersson (-Rosenthal)
(351.8) (crocodile tears) Facial paralysis with dramatic lacrimation during eating. Caused by lesion on seventh cranial nerve, prompting impulses to be misdirected from salivary glands to lacrimal glands.

Melnick-Fraser
(759.89) (Brachio-oto-renal) A genetic autosomal dominant disorder that includes anomalies of the ear, cysts in the neck, hearing loss, and malformations of the kidney.

Mende's (ptosis-epicanthus)
(270.2) (Mendes, van der Hoeve-Halbertsma-Waardenburg, Waardenburg-Klein) Eyebrow or upper or lower eyelid sags.

Mendelson's
(997.3) Pulmonary disorders caused by aspirating of lung following vomiting or regurgitation during medical procedure.

Ménétrier's
(535.2x) Giant hypertrophy of gastric mucosa.

Ménière's
(386.00) Vertigo, nausea, vomiting, tinnitus, and progressive deafness caused by endolymphatic hydrops.

Meningo-eruptive
(047.1) Enteric cytopathogenic human orphan (ECHO) virus. Common form of virus (which has many variations) is meningo-eruptive, with fever and aseptic meningitis.

Meningococcic
(036.3) (Friderichsen-Waterhouse, Waterhouse,) Acute fulminating meningococcal septicemia occurring in children below 10 years of age with vomiting, cyanosis, diarrhea, purpura, convulsions, circulatory collapse, meningitis, and hemorrhaging into adrenal glands.

Menkes'
(759.89) Congenital abnormality in copper absorption characterized by severe cerebral

degeneration and arterial changes resulting in death in infancy.

Menopause
(627.2) Chills, depression, hot flashes, headache, and irritability.

Menstruation
(625.4) (Premenstrual, PMS) Monthly physiological and emotional distress during the several days preceding menses with symptoms of nervousness, fluid retention, weight gain, and depression.

Mesenteric artery
(557.1) (Wilkie's) Complete or partial block of the superior mesenteric artery with symptoms of vomiting, pain, blood in the stool, and distended abdomen. Results in bowel infarction.

Metastatic carcinoid
(259.2) (Bjorck-Thorson, Cassidy-Scholte, Hedinger's) Carcinoid tumors that causes cyanotic flushing of skin, diarrheal watery stools, bronchoconstrictive attacks, hypotension, edema, and ascites.

Meyenburg-Altherr-Uehlinger
(733.99) Arthritis with degeneration of cartilage leading to collapse of ears, nose, and tracheobronchial tree. Death may occur as respiratory system is affected.

Meyer-Schwickerath and Weyers
(759.89) Abnormally small nose with anteverted nostrils, dental anomalies, and missing phalanges of toes.

Micheli-Rietti
(282.49) Hemolytic anemias that share a common decreased rate of synthesis of one or more hemoglobin polypeptide chains and are classified according to the chain involved.

Michotte
(721.5) Kissing spine. Malformation of spine in which kyphosis becomes so great nonadjacent vertebrae touch.

Micrognathia-glossoptosis
(756.0) Description of anomalies of face and skull.

Microphthalmos
(759.89) Reduction in the size of the eye, opacities of the cornea and lens, and scarring of the retina.

Midbrain
(348.8) Infarction of postero-inferior thalamus causing transient hemiparesis, severe loss of superficial and deep sensation with crude pain in the hypalgic limbs, vasomotor, or trophic disturbances.

Mieten's
(759.89) Congenital malformations affecting multiple systems.

Mikity-Wilson
(770.7) Symptoms include hypercapnia and cyanosis of rapid onset during first month of life and frequently result in death. Rare pulmonary insufficiency in newborn babies, especially those with low birth weight.

Mikulicz's
(527.1) Complex of lacrimal and salivary gland swelling, which may include enlargement associated with other syndromes, such as Sjögren's.

Milk alkali
(275.42) (Burnett's) (milk drinkers) Disorder of kidneys induced by ingestion of large amounts of alkali and calcium in therapy of a peptic ulcer. While reversible in the early stages, it can lead to renal failure.

Milkman (-Looser-Debray)
(268.2) Osteoporosis striking middle-aged women with frequent fractures.

Millard-Gubler
(344.89) (Avellis, Babinski-Nageotte, Benedikt's, Brown-Sequard, Cestan's, Cestan-Chenais, Foville's, Gubler-Millard, Jackson's, Weber-Leyden) Paraplegia and anesthesia over half or part of the body. Caused by lesions in brain or spinal cord.

Miller-Dieker
(758.33) A chromosomal microdeletion with microcephaly, small mandible, growth retardation, failure to thrive, and developmental delays.

Miller Fisher's
(357.0) (Guillain-Barré, Landry, Fisher's, Strohl, Miller) Often follows viral infections and may be a disorder of the immune system with symptoms of paraplegia of limbs, flaccid paralysis, ophthalmoplegia, ataxia, and areflexia.

Milles'
(759.6) (Kalischer's) Formation of multiple angiomas in skin of head and scalp.

Milroy
(757.0) (Nonne-Milroy-Meige) Lymphatic edema of the legs (and face and arms in severe cases) caused by obstruction of lymphatic ducts.

Minkowski-Chauffard
(282.0) Hemolytic anemia with spherocytosis, fragility of erythrocytes, splenomegaly, and jaundice.

Mirizzi's
(576.2) Stone in cystic duct and chronic cystitis leading to spasms and scarring of connective tissue and obstruction of hepatic ducts.

Mohr's
(759.89) (Oral-Fascial-Digital) Cranial, facial, lingual, mandibular, digital, and palatal abnormalities.

Monofixation
(378.34) Strabismus of slight degree.

Moore's
(345.5x) Epilepsy with unilateral clonic movements starting in one group of muscles and spreading to adjacent groups, following the movement of the epilepsy through the contralateral motor cortex.

Morel-Moore
(733.3) (Morel-Morgagni, -Stewart-Morel) Thickening of the inner table of the frontal bone related to obesity in women nearing menopause.

Morgagni-Adams-Stokes
(426.9) (Stokes-Adams; Morgagni's disease; and Spens) Heart block causing slow or absent pulse, vertigo, syncope, convulsions, and Cheyne-Stokes respiration.

Morquio (-Brailsford) (-Ullrich)
(277.5) Accumulation of mucopolysaccharide sulfates affecting the eye, ear, skin, teeth, skeleton, joints, liver, spleen, cardiovascular system, respiratory system, and central nervous system.

Morris
(259.5) (Androgen insensitivity, hairless women, male pseudohemaphroditism, nonvirilizing, testicular feminization) Genetic condition affecting the development of reproductive organs marked by female external genitalia or a degree of both male and female genitalia. Amenorrhea noticed in teen years, with short, incompletely developed vagina and rudimentary or absent uterus and fallopian tubes, scanty or absent axillary/public hair, and testicles that may require removal.

Morton's
(355.6) Pain in the forefoot caused by a lesion of the plantar nerve.

Moschcowitz (-Singer-Symmers)
(446.6) Central nervous system involvement due to formation of fibrin or platelet thrombi in arterioles and capillaries in many organs.

Mounier-Kuhn
(748.3) Tracheobronchomegaly. Acquired Mounier-Kuhn is reported with ICD-9-CM code 519.19.

Mucha-Habermann
(696.2) Chronic dermatosis of unknown origin with scaling lesions that produce small pox-like scars. Recurrence of attacks are common, but disease is self-limiting.

Mucocutaneous lymph node
(446.1) (Harkavy) Fever, conjunctival injection reddening of the oral cavity, ulcerative gingivitis, cervical lymph nodes, skin eruptions that cover the hands and feet, and skin becoming puffy and sloughs off.

Multiple pterygium
(759.89) A rare syndrome characterized by short stature, facial anomalies, multiple webbing anomalies, joint contractures, vertebral fusion defects, rocker-bottom feet, hydrops, and lung hypoplasia.

Münchhausen
(301.51) (Hospital addiction, Multiple operations) Emotional condition in which patient exhibits physical, but psychosomatic, symptoms.

Münchmeyer's
(728.11) Diffuse progressive ossifying polymyositis.

Muscle deficiency
(756.71) (Prune Belly, Eagle-Barrett) Absence of muscles of abdomen and genitourinary anomalies. Intestinal outlines are visible on patient's skin.

Myelodysplastic
(238.7x) Neoplasm of lymphatic and hematopoietic tissues, affecting the spinal cord.

Myeloproliferative
(238.79) Unusual proliferation of myelopoietic tissue.

Naffziger's
(353.0) Raynaud-like symptoms of vascular contractions caused by pressure of brachial plexus and subclavian artery against first thoracic rib.

Nager-de Raynier
(756.0) Franceschetti's syndrome with limb deformities consisting of absence of the radius, radioulnar synostosis, and hypoplasia or absence of thumbs.

Nail-patella
(756.89) Dysplasia of the fingernails and toenails, hypoplasia of the patella, iliac horns, thickening of the glomerular lamina densa, and a flask-shaped femur.

Nebécourt's
(253.3) (Burier, Lorain-Levi) Dwarfism resulting from absence of functional anterior pituitary gland.

Neill-Dingwall
(759.89) Small head and dwarfism. One of many syndromes affecting several body systems, but not elsewhere specified.

Nerve compression
(354.8) Pain in upper and posterior part of the shoulder radiating into neck and occiput, down the arm, and around the chest. Caused by abnormal positioning between the scapula and thorax, pain includes tingling in the fingers.

Netherton's
(757.1) Scaling of skin showing a peripheral double margin in and around the vagina.

Neurocutaneous
(759.6) Occurrence of nevi and skeletal deformities as result of gliosis and abiotrophy of central nervous system.

Neuroleptic malignant
(333.92) Description of the effects of antipsychotic drugs on behavior and cognition.

Newborn of diabetic mother
(775.0) Maternal diabetes mellitus affecting fetus or newborn with hypoglycemia.

Niemann-Pick
(272.7) Accumulation of phospholipid in histiocytes in the bone marrow, liver, lymph nodes, and spleen, cerebral involvement, and red macular spots similar to Tay-Sachs disease. Most commonly found in Jewish infants.

Nonne-Milroy-Meige
(757.0) (Milroy) Lymphatic edema of the legs (and face and arms in severe cases) caused by obstruction of lymphatic ducts.

Nonpsychotic posttraumatic brain
(310.2) Persistent personality disturbance of nonpsychotic origin following blow to the head with affective instability, bursts of aggression, apathy and indifference, impaired social judgment, and suspiciousness or paranoid ideation.

Noonan's
(759.89) (Ulrich-Turner) Ptosis, hypogonadism webbed, neck, congenital heart disease, short stature; once diagnosed as Turner's syndrome until this female component was identified.

Nucleus ambiguous-hypoglossal
(352.6) (Collet-Sicard) Unilateral lesions of the ninth, tenth, eleventh, and twelfth cranial nerves producing paralysis of vagal, glossal, other nerves, and tongue on the same side. Most usually result of injury.

OAV (oculoauriculovertebral dysplasia)
(756.0) (Goldenhar's) Number of anomalies, including epibulbar dermoids, preauricular appendages, micrognathia, and vertebral.

Oculocraniosomatic
(277.87) (Kearn-Sayre) A mitochondrial defect associated with chronic progressive paralysis of the external eye muscles, cardiac conduction defects, short stature, pigmentary degeneration of the retina, deafness, and intellectual and hearing loss.

Oculocutaneous
(364.24) (Vogt-Koyanagi) Uveomeningitis with patchy depigmentation of hair, eyebrows, and lashes; retinal detachment, deafness, and tinnitus may also result.

Oculoglandular
(372.02) Syndrome of the eyes and glands.

Oculomotor
(378.81) (Parinaud's) Paralysis of conjugate movement of the eyes without paralysis of convergence. Caused by lesions of the midbrain.

Ogilvie
(560.89) Colonic obstruction with symptoms of persistent contraction of intestinal musculature. Caused by defect in sympathetic nerve supply.

Ophthalmica, postherpetic
(053.19) Any symptoms of herpes arising in eye.

Syndromes

Ophthalmoplegia-cerebellar ataxia
(378.52) Paralysis of one or more optic muscles or failure to control muscles.

Oppenheim-Urbach
(250.8x) [709.3] Diabetes with skin disorder.

Oral-facial-digital
(759.89) (Papillon-Leage and Psaume) Defects of the oral cavity, face, and hands including bifid tongue, cleft palate, missing teeth, pug-nose, depressed nasal bridge, mental retardation, and others. Syndrome is lethal in males.

Organic affective
(293.83) Patient may exhibit a number of changes in personality such as amotivation, depression, outbursts, poor social judgment, and others.

Organic anxiety
(293.84) Anxiety secondary to the direct physiological effects of a general medical condition. Symptoms may include persistent anxious state, panic attacks, obsessions, or compulsions.

Organic personality
(310.1) Persistent personality disturbance of nonpsychotic origin featuring affective instability, bursts of aggression, apathy and indifference, impaired social judgment, and suspiciousness or paranoid ideation.

Ormond's
(593.4) (Ormond's) Retroperitoneal structures involving and often obstructing ureters sometimes following certain types of chemical treatment; there is no identified cause.

Orthostatic hypotensive-dysautonomic dyskinetic
(333.0) (Hallervorden-Spatz, Dejerine-Thomas) Nerves between the striatum and pallidum are completely demyelated.

Osler-Weber-Rendu
(448.0) A post-pubescent disorder with small telangiectasia and dilated venules developing slowly on the skin and mucus membranes of the lips, nasopharynx, and tongue.

Osteodermopathic hyperostosis
(757.39) Irregular linear streaks of skin atrophy, skeletal malformations, and papillomas of lips.

Osteoporosis-osteomalacia
(268.2) (Milkman, Looser, Debray) Osteoporosis striking middle-aged women with frequently-suffered fractures.

Österreicher-Turner
(756.89) Dysplasia of the fingernails and toenails, hypoplasia of the patella, iliac horns, thickening of the glomerular lamina densa, and a flask-shaped femur.

Ostrum-Furst
(756.59) Deformities of neck, platybasia, and Sprengel's neck.

Otolith
(386.19) (Bonnier) Ocular disturbances, deafness, nausea, thirst, anorexia, and symptoms traced to vagus centers as result of a lesion of Deiters nucleus and its connections.

Otopalatodigital
(759.89) Defects of ear, oral cavity, face, and hands.

Outlet
(353.0) (Naffziger's) Vascular contractions of the digits similar to Raynaud's, caused by pressure of brachial plexus and subclavian artery against first thoracic rib.

Ovarian remnant
(620.8) Pelvic pain typically occurring several weeks or several months following surgical removal of the ovaries, often due to the survival of an ovarian fragment after the operation.

Ovarian vein
(593.4) (Ormond's) Retroperitoneal structures involving and often obstructing the ureters following certain types of chemical treatment; there is no identified cause.

Overuse
(Repetitive Motion) Injuries such as tendinitis, carpal tunnel syndrome, and bursitis related to sustained repetitive motions or to "overuse," usually from performing a certain specific task that taxes one anatomical area and impairs function. Code to the specific injury or condition.

Owren's
(286.3) (Stewart-Prower) Deficiencies of clotting factors noticeable from birth.

P-R interval
(426.81) (Lown-Ganong) Electrocardiographic disorder indicated by a short P-R interval with normal duration of the QRS complex.

Pacemaker
(429.4) Functional deficiency following heart surgery in which the triggering mechanism of the heart may be irregular.

Paget-Schroetter
(453.8) Stress thrombosis of subclavian or axillary vein.

Pancoast's
(162.3) (Hare's, Cuiffini) Neoplasm of upper lobe of the lung.

Panhypopituitary
(253.2) Secretion of all anterior pituitary hormones is inadequate or absent after childbirth.

Parabiotic (transfusion) donor (twin)
(772.0) Transfusion of blood from one fetus to another.

Parabiotic (transfusion) recipient (twin)
(776.4) Polycythemia of newborn as result of blood flow from mother.

Paranoid type
(293.81) Organic disorder with hallucinations, beliefs about being followed, being poisoned, etc.; and not meeting criteria for schizophrenia.

Parinaud's
(378.81) Paralysis of conjugate movement of eyes without paralysis of convergence caused by lesions of the midbrain.

Parkes Weber and Dimitri
(759.6) (Kalischer's) Formation of multiple angiomas in skin of head and scalp.

Parry's
(242.0x) (Basedow, Grave's disease) Fatigue, nervousness, emotional lability and irritability, heat intolerance and increased sweating, weight loss, palpitation, and tremor of hands and tongue. Autoimmune in etiology and caused by excess thyroidal hormones.

Parry-Romberg
(349.89) (Kleine-Levin) Hypersomnia associated with bulimia and occurring in males between 10 to 25 years of age with ravenous appetite followed by prolonged sleep, along with behavioral disturbances, impaired thought processes, and hallucinations.

Parsonage-Aldren-Turner
(353.5) Paroxysmal pain extending length of one of many nerves.

Patau's
(758.1) (Patau's, trisomy D) Variety of symptoms in newborns with extra chromosome in group D and number of symptoms, including mental retardation and malformed ears, cardiac defects, convulsions, and others.

Patellofemoral
(719.46) Anterior knee pain commonly occurring in athletes, caused by irritation on the undersurface of the patella and leading to softening and erosion of the cartilage lining the joint.

Paterson (-Brown) (-Kelly)
(280.8) (Kelly, Plummer-Vinson) Condition in middle-aged women with hypochronic anemia of cracks or fissures at the corners of the mouth, painful tongue, and dysphagia due to esophageal stenosis or webs.

Payr's
(569.89) Bloating, gas, pain, and fullness experienced left upper abdominal quadrant with pain sometimes radiating up into left chest.

Pectoral girdle
(447.8) Malignant atrophic papulosis.

Pelger-Huët
(288.2) (Chediak-Higashi, Dohle body, Hegglin, Jordan's, May) Patients present with hepatosplenomegaly, lymphadenopathy, anemia, thrombocytopenia, along with changes in bones, cardiopulmonary system, skin, and psychomotor skills. Abnormalities of granulation and nuclear structure of white cells open child to infection and result in death.

Pellagra-cerebellar ataxia-renal aminoaciduria
(270.0) (Harts, Toni, Fanconi, Debre) Renal tubular malfunction, including cystinosis and osteomalacia, caused by inherited disorders or the result of multiple myeloma or proximal epithelial growth.

Pellagroid
(265.2) Resembling pellagra or a description of pellagra.

Syndromes

Pellegrini-Stieda
(726.62) (Köhler-Pellegrini-Stieda) Calcification of medial collateral ligament of knee.

Pellizzi's
(259.8) Precocious development of external sexual organs, precocious development of long bones, and hydrocephalus indicating lesion of pineal body.

Pendred's
(243) Familial goiter paired with congenital nerve deafness due to defective organic binding of iodine in the thyroid.

Penfield's
(345.5x) Epilepsy with unilateral clonic movements starting in one group of muscles and spreading to adjacent groups, following the movement of the epilepsy through the contralateral motor cortex.

Penta X
(758.81) Pentasomy. Presence of three additional chromosomes of one type.

Perabduction
(447.8) Malignant atrophic papulosis.

Periurethral fibrosis
(593.4) (Ormond's) Retroperitoneal structures involving and often obstructing the ureters.

Petges-Cléjat
(710.3) (Unverricht-Wagner) Polymyositis occurring with characteristic skin changes including rash on upper eyelids with edema, a rash on the forehead, neck, shoulders, trunk, and arms, and papules on knuckles.

Peutz-Jeghers
(759.6) Formation of multiple hematomas.

Phantom limb
(353.6) Itching, dull ache, or sharp, shooting pains mimicking the nerves of amputated limb.

Pharyngeal pouch
(279.11) (DiGeorge's) Hypoplasia or aphasia of the thymus and parathyroid gland with congenital heart defects, anomalies of the great vessels, esophageal atresia, and facial deformities result from aphasia or hypoplasia of thymus and parathyroid glands. Seizures may accompany most severe cases.

Pick-Herxheimer
(701.8) Atrophy of skin throughout body and of unknown cause.

Pickwickian
(278.8) Obesity, hypoventilation, somnolence, and erythrocytosis. After Pickwick, Dicken's character.

PIE
(518.3) (Löffler's) Transient infiltrations of lungs by eosinophilia, resulting in coughing, fever, and dyspnea.

Pierre Marie-Bamberger
(731.2) (Mankowsky's) Symmetrical osteitis of limbs localized to phalanges, terminal epiphyses of long bones of forearm and leg, kyphosis of the spine, and affection of the joints.

Pierre Mauriac's
(258.1) Endocrine dysfunction causing diabetes and affecting growth and weight.

Pigment dispersion, iris
(364.53) Lack of pigment in iris.

Pineal
(259.8) (Pellizzi's) Precocious development of external sexual organs, precocious development of long bones, and hydrocephalus indicating lesion of pineal body.

Pink puffer
(492.8) (Swyer-James) Acquired unilateral hyperlucent lung with severe airway obstruction during expiration, oligemia, and a small hilum.

Pituitary
(253.0) Excessive pituitary secretions causing gigantism and beginning before puberty.

Placental dysfunction
(762.2) (placental insufficiency) Fetal hypoxia and malnutrition resulting from lack of nutrition and oxygen transferred from mother. Due to degeneration of placenta and identified by yellow vernix.

Placental transfusion
(762.3) Birth of one anemic twin and one plethoric twin due to forcing of blood of one twin into other.

Plantar fascia
(728.71) Disorder of the fascia at the bottom of the foot.

Plica
(727.83) (Synovial plica) Bands of remnant synovial tissue in the knee that become irritated as a result of inflammation or injury. Symptoms include pain, swelling, "clicking" sensation, joint weakness, and

locking of the knee from fibrosis and calcification of the synovial plica.

Plug (newborn) NEC
(777.1) Meconium obstruction of newborn's intestines, resulting from unusually thick or hard meconium.

Plummer-Vinson
(280.8) (Kelly, Paterson-Brown-Vinson) Condition in middle-aged women with hypochronic anemia, marked by cracks or fissures at the corners of mouth, painful tongue, and dysphagia due to esophageal stenosis or webs.

Pneumorenal
(446.21) (Goodpasture's) Renal condition in which nephritis progresses rapidly to death, with lungs showing extensive hemosiderosis or bleeding.

POEMS
(273.8) A condition combining polyneuropathy, organomegaly, endocrinopathy, M-protein, and skin changes. The syndrome is characterized by a wide range of symptoms affecting multiple systems, including peripheral neuropathy, papilledema, hepatosplenomegaly, gynecomastia, hypogonadism, impotence, amenorrhea, glucose intolerance, adrenal insufficiency, hypothyroidism, hyperpigmentation, pachyderma, hirsutism, anasarca, angiomas, and hyperhidrosis. Code also any manifestations.

Polycythemic
(289.0) Gaisböck's syndrome.

Polysplenia
(759.0) Organs of left side of body are mirror image of organs on right side. Splenic agenesis and cardiac malformation are associated.

Pontine
(433.8x) Quadriplegia, anesthesia, and nystagmus due to the obstruction of twigs of the basilar artery, causing lesions in pontine region.

Post-gastric surgery
(564.2) (Dumping) Emptying of contents of jejunum with nausea, sweating, weakness, palpitation, syncope, warmth, and diarrhea. Occurs after eating in patients who have had partial gastrectomy and gastrojejunostomy.

Post-tubal ligation
Symptoms of excessive or frequent menstruation, dysmenorrheal, and pelvic pain in patients who are status post tubal ligation sterilization procedure. Code to specific symptom with V26.51.

Postartificial
(627.4) Menopausal symptoms suffered by some women following destruction of their ovaries, including chills, depression, hot flashes, headache, and irritability.

Postcholecystectomy
(576.0) Recurrence of gall bladder pain following removal of organ.

Postconcussional
(310.2) (postcontusional, postencephalitic) Persistent personality disturbance of nonpsychotic origin following blow to head and featuring affective instability, bursts of aggression, apathy and indifference, impaired social judgment, and suspiciousness or paranoid ideation.

Posterior interosseous nerve
(354.3) Entrapment of the posterior interosseous nerve at various anatomical sites along its course in the upper forearm resulting in pain and/or palsy.

Posterior reversible encephalopathy
(348.39) Syndrome distinguished by headaches, seizures, confusion, loss of vision, and radiological findings of cortical and subcortical edema bilaterally.

Posthepatitis
(780.79) Chronic Fatigue Syndrome. Marked by persistent or relapsing fatigue not resolved by bed rest that significantly reduces daily activity. Other symptoms include chronic sore throat, mild fever, muscle weakness, myalgia, headaches, and neurological problems. Patients are primarily women. The syndrome arises sporadically with no confirmed etiology but is known to occur in clusters.

Postherpetic
(053.19) Description of any symptoms of herpes arising in parts of body.

Postinfarction
(411.0) (Dressler) Fever, leukocytosis, chest pain, evidence of pericarditis, pleurisy and pneumonia occurring days or weeks after a myocardial infarction.

Postlaminectomy
(722.8x) Spinal disorder and pain resulting from a buildup of scar tissue after a laminectomy has been performed.

Postleukotomy
(310.0) Klüver-Bucy or postlobotomy syndrome.

Postmastectomy lymphedema
(457.0) Edema of arms and hands following a mastectomy requiring removal of adjacent lymph nodes.

Postmature (of newborn)
(766.22) Placental dysfunction occurring in postmature fetuses.

Postmyocardial infarction
(411.0) (Dressler) Fever, leukocytosis, chest pain, evidence of pericarditis, pleurisy, and pneumonia occurring days or weeks after myocardial infarction.

Postpartum panhypopituitary
(253.2) Secretion of all anterior pituitary hormones is inadequate or absent after childbirth.

Postphlebitic
(459.1x) Deep vein thrombosis with edema, pain, purpura, and increased cutaneous pigmentation, eczema dermatitis, pruritus, ulceration, and cellulitis.

Postpolio
(138) Inflammation of spinal cord following polio. Symptoms vary.

Postsurgical nonabsorption
(579.3) Hypoglycemia and malnutrition following surgery.

Posttraumatic
(294.0) Amnestic dementia in which patient cannot remember short-term or long-term memories but is not delirious.

Postural orthostatic tachycardia
(427.89, 458.0) Excessive tachycardia in the upright position, without evidence of cardiac disease, in combination with orthostatic symptoms such as dizziness, lightheadedness, or syncope.

Postvagotomy
(564.2) (dumping) Emptying of contents of jejunum with nausea, sweating, weakness, palpitation, syncope, warmth, and diarrhea. Occurs after eating in patients who have had partial gastrectomy and vagotomy.

Potain's
(536.1) Dilation of stomach with indigestion.

Potassium intoxication
(276.7) (potassium overload) Excessive potassium, causing a number of symptoms.

Potter's
(753.0) Renal agenesis with hypoplastic lungs and associated neonatal respiratory distress, hemodynamic instability, acidosis, cyanosis, edema, and characteristic facial features. Death usually occurs from lack of oxygen.

Premenstrual tension
(625.4) (Premenstrual, PMS) Monthly physiological and emotional distress during the days preceding menses with symptoms of nervousness, fluid retention, weight gain, and depression.

Pre-infarction
(411.1) Sudden onset of angina pectoris; often a precursor to myocardial infarction.

Pre-ulcer
(536.9) (Reichmann) Excessive secretion of gastric juice either constantly or during digestion only.

Prinzmetal
(786.52) Chest pain secondary to large vessel spasm that may interfere with breathing.

Profichet's
(729.9) Calcareous nodules in the subcutaneous tissues primarily around larger joints. The nodules ulcerate and exhibit nervous symptoms.

Progeria
(259.8) (Hutchinson-Gilford) Precocious senility with death from coronary artery disease occurring before 10 years of age.

Progressive pallidal degeneration
(333.0) (Hallervorden-Spatz, Dejerine-Thomas) Condition in which the nerves between the striatum and pallidum are completely demyelated.

Prolonged gestation
(766.22) Gestation beyond 42 completed weeks.

Prolonged Q-T interval
(426.82) (congenital QT, long QT, Romano-Ward) Potentially fatal condition precipitated by vigorous exertion, emotional upset, or startling moments due to an imbalance in the electrical timing controlling the pumping action of the heart's ventricles. Patient is susceptible to recurrent episodes of syncope and rapid arrhythmias that can become malignant, leading to sudden death.

Prune belly
(756.71) (Eagle-Barrett) Congenital absence of muscles of abdomen and genitourinary anomalies. Intestinal outlines are visible on skin.

Prurigo-asthma
(691.8) Several itchy skin eruptions of unknown cause accompanying asthma.

Pseudocarpal tunnel
(354.0) Pain and tingling, numbness, or burning in the hand as result of compression of median nerve by tendons.

Pseudohermaphroditism-virilism-hirsutism
(255.2) Possession of mature masculine somatic characteristics by a prepubescent male, girl, or woman. This syndrome may show at birth or develop later as result of adrenocortical dysfunction.

Pseudoparalytica
(358.00) (Goldflam, Erb, Hoppe) Progressive muscular weakness beginning in face and throat and caused by a defect in myoneural conduction.

Pseudo-Turner's
(759.89) (Bonnevie-Ullrich) Congenital disorder with short stature, mental retardation, and a webbed neck but, unlike Turner's, patients can be of either sex and have normal chromosomes and no renal abnormalities.

Pterygolymphangiectasia
(758.6) (XO) Congenital disorder characterized by short stature and webbed neck. Patients of either sex suffer congenital heart disease, mental retardation, and other symptoms.

Ptosis-epicanthus
(270.2) (Mendes, van der Hoeve-Halbertsma-Waardenburg, Waardenburg-Klein) Eyebrow or upper or lower eyelid sags.

Pulmonary sulcus
(162.3) (Cuiffini-Pancoast, Hare's) Neoplasm of upper lobe of lung.

Putnam-Dana
(281.0) [336.2] Numbness and tingling, weakness, a sore tongue, dyspnea, faintness, pallor of the skin and mucous membranes, anorexia, diarrhea, loss of weight, and fever. Strikes in fifth decade.

Pyloroduodenal
(537.89) (Gastrojejunal loop obstruction) Distended efferent loop causing illness and pain with acute or chronic obstruction of the duodenum and jejunum proximal to a gastrojejunostomy.

Pyriformis
(355.0) Lesion on the sciatica nerve causing a pear shaped area of pain and paresthesia.

Radicular
(353.0) (Naffziger's) A disorder presenting symptoms similar to Raynaud's, caused by pressure of brachial plexus and subclavian artery against first thoracic rib.

Raeder-Harbitz
(446.7) (Martorell-Fabre, Takayasu-Onishi) Progressive obliteration of brachiocephalic trunk and left subclavian and left common carotid arteries above their source in the aortic arch. Symptoms include ischemia, transient blindness, facial atrophy, and many others.

Rapid time-zone change
(307.35) (jet lag) Imbalance of normal circadian rhythm resulting from airplane travel through a number of time zones. Leads to fatigue, irritability, and other constitutional disturbances.

Raymond (-Céstan)
(433.8x) Identified through symptoms of quadriplegia, anesthesia, and nystagmus due to the obstruction of twigs of the basilar artery, causing lesions in the pontine region.

Raynaud's
(443.0) (Patriots disease) Constriction of the arteries of the digits caused by cold or emotion. Temperature drops in extremities as much as 30 degrees Fahrenheit, and skin turns white with red and blue mottling. Caused by nerve or arterial damage and can be prompted by stress.

RDS
(769) (Hyaline membrane) Reduced amounts of lung surfactant in premature neonates with respiratory distress. Frequently fatal.

Recipient twin
(776.4) Polycythemia of newborn due to donor twin transfusion.

Refsum's
(356.3) Deafness, retinitis pigmentosa, polyneuritis, nystagmus, and cerebellar signs.

Reichmann
(536.8) Excessive secretion of gastric juice either constantly or during digestion only.

Reifenstein's
(259.5) Hypogonadism with gynecomastia, hypospadias, and postpubertal testicular atrophy. Caused by inherited defect of androgen receptors and insensitivity to testosterone.

Reilly's
(337.9) (Claude Bernard-Homer, Steinbrocker's) Pain and stiffness in the shoulder, with puffy swelling and pain in the hand following a heart attack.

Reiter's
(099.3) (Fiessinger-Leroy-Reiter) Arthritis, iridocyclitis, and urethritis, sometimes with diarrhea. While symptoms may recur, arthritis is constant.

Renal glomerulohyalinosis-diabetic
(250.4x) [581.81] High blood pressure and kidney failure resulting from a form of diabetes in which carbohydrate utilization is reduced and that of lipid and protein enhanced.

Rendu-Osler-Weber
(448.0) Post-pubescent disorder with small telangiectases and dilated venules developing slowly on skin and mucus membranes of lips, tongue, nasopharynx, tongue, and face.

Renofacial
(753.0) Renal agenesis with hypoplastic lungs and associated neonatal respiratory distress, hemodynamic instability, acidosis, cyanosis, edema, and characteristic facial features. Death usually occurs from lack of oxygen.

Rénon-Delille
(253.8) (Babinski-Frölich, Launois-Cléret) Obesity and hypogonadism in adolescent boys. Rare accompanying dwarfism is thought to indicate hypothyroidism.

Respiratory distress
(769) (Hyaline membrane) Premature neonates with respiratory distress and associated with reduced amounts of lung surfactant. Frequently fatal.

Restless legs
(333.94) (Ekbom's) Indescribable uneasiness, restlessness, or twitching in the legs after going to bed. Often caused by poor circulation or antipsychotic medications, it can lead to insomnia.

Retraction
(378.71) (Still-Turk-Duane) Simultaneous retraction of eye muscles causing an inability to abduct the affected eye with retraction of the globe.

Retroperitoneal fibrosis
(593.4) (Ormond's) Retroperitoneal structures obstructing ureters following certain types of chemical treatment; there is no identified cause.

Retroviral seroconversion (acute)
(V08) Syndrome seen in 50 percent to -90 percent of adults recently infected with HIV in which detectable antibodies develop in the blood as a result of the infection. Symptoms often develop within two to six weeks following exposure and are similar to the flu, with sore throat, myalgia, fever, facial and trunk rash, headache, diarrhea, and enlarged glands.

Rett's
(330.8) Progressive disease affecting grey matter of the brain, where infant females present ataxia, autism, dementia, seizures, loss of purposeful use of the hands, and cerebral atrophy.

Reye's
(331.81) Condition of childhood spawned by a spirochetic or viral disease of the upper respiratory system. Symptoms include recurrent vomiting, brain swelling, disturbances of consciousness, and seizures. Often fatal. Can be prompted by use of aspirin.

Reye-Sheehan's
(253.2) (Sheehan's) Secretion of all anterior pituitary hormones is inadequate or absent presenting after childbirth.

Riddoch's
(368.16) (Balint's, Holmes', Riddoch's) Cortical paralysis of visual fixation, optic ataxia, and disturbance of visual attention. Eye movements are normal.

Ridley's
(428.1) Left heart failure marked by acute edema of lung.

Rieger's
(743.44) Dysgenesis of eye marked through widened trabecular meshwork, large iridial bands, and glaucoma.

Rietti-Greppi-Micheli
(282.49) One of a group of hemolytic anemias sharing a common decreased rate of synthesis of one

or more hemoglobin polypeptide chains and are classified according to chain involved.

Riley-Day
(742.8) Eyelids widen during chewing, sometimes with an elevation of the upper lid when mouth is open and closing of lid when mouth is closed.

Robin's
(756.0) (Pierre Robin's) Brachygnathia and cleft palate, upward displacement of the larynx, and angulation of the manubrium sterni. May be paired with others or the sole hyperplasia.

Rokitansky-Kuster-Hauser
(752.49) Absence of vagina and uterus with normal karyotype and ovaries. Amenorrhea.

Romano-Ward
(426.82) (congenital QT, long QT, prolonged QT interval) Potentially fatal condition precipitated by vigorous exertion, emotional upset, or startling moments due to an imbalance in the electrical timing controlling the pumping action of the heart's ventricles. Patient is susceptible to recurrent episodes of syncope and rapid arrhythmias that can become malignant, leading to sudden death.

Romberg's
(349.89) (Kleine-Levin, Parry-Romberg) Hypersomnia associated with bulimia and occurring in males between 10 to 25 years of age. Ravenous appetite following prolonged sleep, along with behavioral disturbances, impaired thought processes, and hallucinations.

Rosai-Dorfman
(277.8x) A rare disorder characterized by proliferation of histiocytes in the lymph nodes, skin, central nervous system, kidney, or digestive tract. Symptoms and physical findings vary depending upon the specific anatomy affected.

Rosen-Castleman-Liebow
(516.0) Chronic disease of lungs marked by chest pain, weakness, hemoptysis, dyspnea, and productive cough. Ventilation of affected areas is prevented by a proteinaceous material.

Roth's
(355.1) Feeling of tingling, formication, itching, and other symptoms on the outer side of the lower part of the thigh caused by lateral femoral cutaneous nerve.

Rothmund's
(757.33) Pigmentation and atrophy of the skin, along with cataracts, saddle nose, bone defects, disturbance of hair growth, and hypogonadism.

Rotor's
(277.4) Nonhemolytic jaundice differing from Dubin-Johnson syndrome in that it does not produce liver pigmentation.

Rubella
(771.0) Developmental abnormalities of newborn baby as resulting from transplacental transference of rubella during the first trimester of pregnancy. Symptoms include ocular and cardiac lesions, deafness, microcephaly, mental retardation, hepatitis, encephalitis, and others.

Rubinstein-Taybi's
(759.89) Congenital defects including broad thumb and great toe, antimongoloid slant to the eyes, beaked nose, prominent forehead, low set ears, high arched palate, mental retardation, and cardiac defects.

Rud's
(759.89) Dwarfism, hypogonadism, and epilepsy with scaly skin as result of inherited disorder.

Ruiter-Pompen (-Wyers)
(272.7) (Fabry's) Corneal opacities; burning pain in palms, soles, and abdomen; chronic paresthesia on hands and feet; cardiopulmonary involvement; edema of the legs; osteoporosis; retarded growth; and delayed puberty. Patients die of renal, cardiac, or cerebrovascular failure.

Runge's
(766.22) (Ballantyne) Placental dysfunction occurring in postmature fetuses.

Russell (-Silver)
(759.89) Suprasellar lesions in anterior third ventricle, hampering a child's ability to thrive. Despite elevated growth hormones, child is emaciated and looses body fat.

Rytand-Lipsitch
(426.0) (Lev's) Bundle branch block in a patient with normal coronary arteries and myocardium resulting from calcification of conducting system.

Sacralization-scoliosis-sciatica
(756.15) (Bertolotti) Fusion of bottom lumbar vertebra to top sacral vertebra, making a sixth sacral

vertebra. Other symptoms include sciatica and scoliosis.

Saenger's
(379.46) Paralysis of conjugate movement of eyes without paralysis of convergence. Caused by lesions of midbrain.

Sandifer
(530.81, 723.5) Syndrome seen in infants who are affected with symptoms of head tilt (torticollis) and prominent spitting from reflux. Symptoms tend to cease and disappear as the child matures.

Sanfilippo's
(277.5) Results from accumulation of mucopolysaccharide sulfates affecting the eye, ear, skin, teeth, skeleton, joints, liver, spleen, cardiovascular system, respiratory system, and central nervous system.

Scaglietti-Dagnini
(253.0) Arthritis of spine accompanying acromegaly, resembling rheumatoid arthritis, and progressing to bony ankylosis with lipping of vertebral margins.

Scalded skin
(695.1) Necrolysis of skin caused by toxins.

Scalenus anticus
(353.0) (Naffziger's) A disorder presenting symptoms similar to Raynaud's, caused by pressure of brachial plexus and subclavian artery against first thoracic rib.

Scapulocostal
(354.8) Pain in upper and posterior part of the shoulder radiating into neck and occiput, down the arm, and around the chest. Caused by abnormal positioning between scapula and thorax, pain can include tingling in the fingers.

Scapuloperoneal
(359.1) A position of fetus in which the scapula rests closest to the perineal area.

Schaumann'
(135) (Hutchinson-Boeck, Lofgren, Besnier-Boeck-Schaumann) Involves the lungs with resulting fibrosis, lymph nodes, skin, liver, eyes, spleen, phalangeal bones, and parotid glands. Identified by systemic granulomas composed of epithelioid and multinucleated giant cells.

Scheie's
(277.5) Accumulation of mucopolysaccharide sulfates affecting the eye, ear, skin, teeth, skeleton, joints, liver, spleen, cardiovascular system, respiratory system, and central nervous system.

Scheuthauer-Marie-Sainton
(755.59) Defective bone formation in skull, often associated with other symptoms.

Schirmer's
(759.6) (Kalischer's) Formation of multiple angiomas in skin of the head and scalp.

Schizophrenic, of childhood
(299.9x) Description of schizophrenia occurring in childhood.

Schmidt's
(258.1) Hypofunction of endocrine glands involving Hashimoto's thyroiditis, hypoparathyroidism, adrenal insufficiency, and underfunctioning gonads.

Schneider's
(047.9) Viral meningitis that is unspecified.

Scholte's
(259.2) (Bjorck-Thorson, Cassidy-Scholte, Hedinger's) Carcinoid tumors causing cyanotic flushing of skin, diarrheal watery stools, bronchoconstrictive attacks, hypotension, edema, and ascites.

Scholz (-Bielschowsky-Henneberg)
(330.0) Metachromatic leukodystrophy, a disturbance of white substance of brain.

Schroeder's
(255.3) (Slocumb's) Disorder of adrenal medullary tissue resulting in hypertension accompanied with attacks of palpitation, headache, nausea, dyspnea, anxiety, pallor, and profuse sweating.

Schüller-Christian
(277.89) (Hand-Schüller-Christian) Histiocytosis with occasional accumulation of cholesterol. Symptoms include defects of the membranous bones, exophthalmos and diabetes insipidus. There is often also a multiple-system, soft tissue, and skeletal involvement.

Schwartz (-Jampel)
(756.89) Dysplasia of fingernails and toenails, hypoplasia of patella, iliac horns, thickening of glomerular lamina densa, and flask-shaped femur.

Schwartz-Bartter
(253.6) Found in children with hypokalemic alkalosis and elevated renin or angiotensin levels with low or normal blood pressure, no edema, and retarded growth.

Scimitar
(747.49) Venous drainage of right lung into the inferior vena cava with hypoplasia of the right lung. Name comes from the convex shadow of the anomalous vein to the right of the lower border of the heart in an x-ray.

Sclera
(756.51) (van der Hoeve's) Blue sclera, little growth, brittle bones, and deafness.

Sclerocystic ovary
(256.4) (Stein, Stein-Leventhal) Oligomenorrhea or amenorrhea, anovulation and infertility, and hirsutism. Most often caused by bilateral polycystic ovaries.

Sea-blue histiocyte
(272.7) (Ruiter-Pompen-Wyers, Fabry's) Corneal opacities; burning pain in palms, soles, and abdomen; chronic paresthesia of hands and feet; cardiopulmonary involvement; edema of the legs; osteoporosis; retarded growth; and delayed puberty. Patients die of renal, cardiac, or cerebrovascular failure.

Seabright-Bantam
(275.49) (Albright-Martin, Martin-Albright) Similar to hypoparathyroidism, caused by failure to respond to parathyroid hormone with short stature, obesity, short metacarpals, and ectopic calcification.

Seckel's
(759.89) Dwarfism with low birth weight, microcephaly, large eyes, beaked nose, receding mandible, and moderate mental retardation.

Secrétan's
(782.3) Traumatic, recurrent edema or hemorrhage of the back of the hand.

Secretoinhibitor
(710.2) (Gougerot-Houwer, Sjögren) Complex of symptoms of unknown source in middle aged women in which the following triad exists: keratoconjunctivitis sicca, xerostomia, and connective tissue disease (usually rheumatoid arthritis but sometimes systemic lupus erythematosus. Cause may be an abnormal immune response.

Senear-Usher
(694.4) Eruption of the skin on the face, scalp, and trunk with lesions scaling erythematosus.

Senilism
(259.8) Progeria syndrome which includes marked senility by 10 years of age.

Serotonin
(333.99) A potentially fatal side effect from a combination of two or more drugs, one of which is often a selective serotonergic enhancing drug. Multiple psychiatric and non-psychiatric manifestations occur: euphoria, intoxication, drowsiness, sustained rapid eye movement, overreactive reflexes, rapid muscle contraction and relaxation, sweating, rigidity, high body temperature, hypomania, confusion, diarrhea, loss of consciousness, and death. Code according to guidelines for adverse effects and/or poisoning.

Serous meningitis
(348.2) Meningitis with serious inflammation in subarachnoid and ventricle spaces and little change in cerebrospinal fluid.

Sertoli cell
(606.0) Congenital germinal epithelium absence of the testes.

Severe acute respiratory
(079.82) (SARS) A life-threatening respiratory disease caused by a strain of coronavirus that presents with a range of flu-like conditions, such as fever, chills, cough, headache, and myalgia. Diagnosis is based upon clinical, laboratory, and etiological findings.

Shaken baby
(995.55) A range of severe injuries sustained by forceful, excessive, violent shaking of a baby, including subdural hematoma, skull fractures, and internal bleeding. Shaken baby may result in death or disability. Code also any associated injuries.

Shaver's
(503) Condition resulting from the ingestion of bauxite fumes and fine particles of alumina and silica in the aluminum mining and manufacturing process. Symptoms include pulmonary emphysema and pneumothorax.

Sheehan's
(253.2) (Reye-Sheehan) Secretion of all anterior pituitary hormones is inadequate or absent; presenting after childbirth.

Shock lung
(518.5) Respiratory distress following surgery, shock, or trauma.

Shoulder-arm
(337.9) (Claude Bernard-Homer, Reilly's, Steinbrocker's, shoulder-hand) Clinical disorder following a heart attack, marked by pain and stiffness in the shoulder, with puffy swelling and pain in the hand.

Shwachman
(288.02) (Shwachman-Diamond) Moderate to severe neutropenia that presents in infancy, with infections, diarrhea, difficulties in feeding, dwarfism, chondrodysplasia, and pancreatic exocrine insufficiency.

Shy-Drager
(333.0) (Hallervorden-Spatz, Dejerine-Thomas) Condition in which the nerves between the striatum and pallidum are completely demyelated.

Sicard's
(352.6) (Collet-Sicard) Unilateral lesions of ninth, tenth, eleventh, and twelfth cranial nerves producing paralysis of the vagal, glossal, and other nerves and tongue on same side. Usually result of injury.

Sicca
(710.2) (Gougerot-Houwer, Sjögren) Complex of symptoms of unknown source in middle-aged women in which the following triad exists: keratoconjunctivitis sicca, xerostomia, and connective tissue disease (usually rheumatoid arthritis but sometimes systemic lupus erythematosus). Cause may be an abnormal immune response.

Sick sinus
(427.81) Dysfunction of cardiac conduction nodes that produces a wide variety of arrhythmias. Symptoms include palpitations and syncope.

Sideropenic
(280.8) Eczema, thrombocytopenia, and recurrent pyogenic infection. Patients suffer an increased susceptibility to infection with encapsulated bacteria.

Siemens' ectodermal dysplasia
(757.31) Congenitally absent sweat glands, smooth finely wrinkled skin, sunken nose, malformed teeth, sparse hair, and deformed nails. Sometimes absent breast tissue, mental retardation, or syndactyly.

Siemens' keratosis follicularis spinulosa
(757.39) Inherited condition in which the hair follicles are replaced by keratosis.

Silfverskiöld's
(756.50) A dominant inherited disease with skeletal changes in extremities.

Silver's
(759.89) Dwarfism marked by late closure of anterior fontanel, bilateral body asymmetry, low birth weight, clinodactyly of the fifth fingers, triangular facial shape, and carp mouth.

Silvestroni-Bianco
(282.49) One of a group of hemolytic anemias that shares common decreased rate of synthesis of one or more hemoglobin polypeptide chains and are classified according to chain involved.

Simons'
(272.6) (Hollander-Simons) Characterized by loss of subcutaneous fat of upper torso, the arms, the neck, and the face but with an increase in fat on and below the pelvis.

Sinus tarsi
(726.79) Caused by posterior tibial nerve at ankle, syndrome can produce significant neuropathy.

Sinusitis-bronchiectasis-situs inversus
(759.3) (Kartagener's) Transposition or misplacement of organs or viscera.

Sipple's
(193) Familial endocrine adenomatosis

Sjögren (-Gougerot)
(710.2) (Gougerot-Houwer) Complex of symptoms of unknown source in middle aged women in which the following triad exists: keratoconjunctivitis sicca, xerostomia, and connective tissue disease (usually rheumatoid arthritis but sometimes systemic lupus erythematosus). Cause may be an abnormal immune response.

Sjögren-Larsson
(757.1) Congenital malformation of the skin with scaling and spastic paraplegia.

Slocumb's
(255.3) (Schroeder's) Disorder of adrenal medullary tissue resulting in hypertension accompanied with attacks of palpitation, headache, nausea, dyspnea, anxiety, pallor, and profuse sweating.

Sluder's
(337.0) (Charcot-Weiss-Baker) Stimulation of an overactive carotid sinus, causing a marked drop in blood pressure, which, in turn, may stop or block the heart.

Smith-Lemli-Opitz
(759.89) Mental retardation, small stature, ptosis, male genital anomalies, anteverted nostrils, and syndactyly of the second and third toes.

Smith-Magenis
(758.33) A chromosomal microdeletion resulting in brachycephaly, incomplete development of facial bones, speech delay, vocal abnormalities, growth retardation, and developmental delays.

Sneddon-Wilkinson
(694.1) Non-inflammatory intimal hyperplasia of medium-sized vessels.

Sotos'
(253.0) Increased birth weight and length, accelerated growth rate for the first four or five years with no elevation of serum growth hormone levels, followed by revision to normal growth rate, antimongoloid slant, prognathism, hypertelorism, dolichocephalic skull, impaired coordination, and moderate mental retardation may be present.

Specified focal (partial)
(310.8) Persistent personality disturbance of nonpsychotic origin with one of the following symptoms: affective instability, bursts of aggression, apathy and indifference, impaired social judgment, and suspiciousness or paranoid ideation.

Spens'
(426.9) (Stokes-Adams; Morgagni's disease) Heart block often causing slow or absent pulse, vertigo, syncope, convulsions, and Cheyne-Stokes respiration.

Sphallo-pharyngo-laryngeal hemiplegia
(352.6) (Collet-Sicard) Unilateral lesions of the ninth, tenth, eleventh, and twelfth cranial nerves producing paralysis of the vagal, glossal, and other nerves and the tongue on the same side. Most usually result of injury.

Spherophakia-brachymorphia
(759.89) (Weill-Marchesani) Abnormally round and small lens of the eyes, short stature, and brachydactyly.

Spinal artery
(433.8x) (Beck's) Occlusion of spinal artery as result of injury, disk damage, or cardiovascular disease.

Splenic agenesis
(759.0) Congenital disorder in which organs of left side of body are a mirror image of the organs on the right side. Splenic agenesis and cardiac malformation are associated.

Splenic flexure
(569.89) Bloating, gas, pain, and fullness experienced in left upper abdominal quadrant with pain sometimes radiating up into left chest.

Splenic neutropenia
(289.53) Inherited disorder with bronchiectasis and pancreatic insufficiency, resulting in malnutrition, sinusitis, short stature, and bone abnormalities.

Spousal abuse
(995.8x) Maltreatment (abuse) of spouses with emotional or physical violence.

Spurway's
(756.51) (Ekman's, Eddowes') Blue sclera, little growth, brittle and malformed bones, and malformed teeth.

Staphylococcal scalded skin
(695.1) Necrolysis of skin caused by toxins.

STARTLE
(759.89) (333.99) (Startle disease) (hyperexplexia) (familial startle disease) (Kok disease) Congenital, autosomal dominant, neurological disorder in which persistent, excessive "startle" reactions occur due to an unexpected noise, movement, or touch. This disorder is frequently misdiagnosed as a form of epilepsy. Code also any other manifestations.

Steal
(435.1) A number of symptoms in a moving limb including pain, tension, and weakness but absent at rest. Caused by occlusive arterial diseases of limbs.

Stein's
(256.4) (Stein-Leventhal) Oligomenorrhea or amenorrhea, anovulation and infertility, and hirsutism. Most often caused by bilateral polycystic ovaries.

Steinbrocker's
(337.9) (Claude-Bernard-Horner, Reilly's) Pain and stiffness in the shoulder with puffy swelling and pain in the hand following a heart attack.

Syndromes

Stevens-Johnson
(695.1) Necrolysis of skin caused by toxins.

Stewart-Morel
(733.3) Thickening of inner table of the frontal bone associated with obesity in women nearing menopause.

Stickler's
(759.89) (hereditary progressive arthro-ophthalmopathy) An autosomal dominant connective tissue disease characterized by an increased occurrence of retinal detachments, joint disorders, cataracts, and facial and dental anomalies. It is usually diagnosed in childhood, but varying degrees of presentation may delay the diagnosis. Code additional manifestations.

Stiff-man
(333.91) Increasing but fluctuating rigidity of upper limb and axial muscles and increasing cerebral and spinal disease but with increased electrical activity.

Still-Felty
(714.1) Splenomegaly, leukopenia, arthritis, hypersplenism, anemia and other symptoms.

Stilling-Türk-Duane
(378.71) (Duane) Simultaneous retraction of eye muscles causing an inability to abduct affected eye with retraction of globe.

Stokes (-Adams)
(426.9) (Morgagni's disease, and Spens) Heart block often causing slow or absent pulse, vertigo, syncope, convulsions, and Cheyne-Stokes respiration.

Straight-back
(756.19) Loss of the anterior concavity in the upper thoracic vertebrae causing spine to move forward and compress the heart between sternum and vertebral body.

Sturge-Kalischer-Weber
(759.6) Subclavian steal

Subclavian-carotid obstruction
(446.7) (Martorell-Fabre, Raed-Harbitz, Takayasu-Onishi) Occurs in the brachiocephalic trunk and the left subclavian and left common carotid arteries above their source in the aortic arch. Symptoms include ischemia, transient blindness, facial atrophy, and many others.

Subcoracoid-pectoralis minor
(447.8) Malignant atrophic papulosis.

Subperiosteal hematoma
(267) (Barlow, Moller, Cheadle) Anemia, spongy gums, weakness, induration of leg muscles, and mucocutaneous hemorrhages.

Subphrenic interposition
(751.4) Interposition of colon between liver and diaphragm.

Sudden infant death
(798.0) (crib death) Unexpected death of healthy infant typically under 12 months old.

Sudeck's
(733.7) (Sudeck-Leriche) Post-traumatic osteoporosis associated with vasospasm.

Sump
(997.4) A surgical complication in which a sump (pit or well) develops in the distal, nonfunctioning part of the common bile duct. Accumulation of GI debris and calculi results in obstruction of the stoma, which produces cholangitis and/or cholestasis.

Sundown
A phenomenon by which a person with dementia resulting from another underlying disease, such as Alzheimer's, may experience hallucinations or changes in behavior and orientation, especially at night. Code the underlying condition.

Suprarenal cortical
(255.3) (Schroeder's, Slocumb's) Disorder of adrenal medullary tissue resulting in hypertension with attacks of palpitation, headache, nausea, dyspnea, anxiety, pallor, and profuse sweating.

Supraspinatus
(726.10) Pain on abduction of shoulder and tenderness upon deep pressure of supraspinatus tendon.

Swallowed blood
(777.3) Swallowed blood syndrome in the newborn, causing hematemesis and melena.

Sweet's
(695.89) Disease of women marked by plaque-like lesions on face, neck, and upper extremities and conjunctivitis, mucosal lesion, malaise, fever, and arthralgia.

Swyer-James
(492.8) (MacLeod's) Acquired unilateral hyperlucent lung with severe airway obstruction during expiration, oligemia, and a small hilum.

Symonds'
(348.2) (Symonds') Meningitis with serious inflammation in subarachnoid and ventricle spaces and little change in the cerebrospinal fluid.

Sympathetic paralysis
(337.0) (Charcot-Weiss-Baker, Sluder's) Stimulation of overactive carotid sinus, causing a marked drop in blood pressure, which, in turn, may stop or block the heart.

Syndactylic oxycephaly
(755.55) (Apert's) Chromosomal condition with primary symptoms including webbing of digits and a pointed head with variations of defects. Often associated with other chromosomal abnormalities.

Systemic fibrosclerosing
(710.8) Widespread formation of fibrous tissue.

Systemic inflammatory response
(995.9x) An acute inflammatory response to systemic infection or trauma that progresses to coagulopathy and organ failure. SIRS is manifested by two or more of the following symptoms: fever, tachycardia, tachypnea, leukocytosis, or leukopenia. The underlying systemic infection must be coded first.

Tachycardia-bradycardia
(427.81) Rapid action of heart followed by protracted or transient stopping of heart.

Takayasu (-Onishi)
(446.7) (Martorell-Fabre, Raed-Harbitz) Brachiocephalic trunk and the left subclavian and left common carotid arteries above their source in the aortic arch. Symptoms include ischemia, transient blindness, facial atrophy, and many others.

Takotsubo
(429.83) (apical ballooning, broken heart) A reversible left ventricular dysfunction in patients without coronary disease, precipitated by emotional or physiological stress.

Tapia's
(352.6) (Collet-Sicard) Unilateral lesions of ninth, tenth, eleventh, and twelfth cranial nerves producing paralysis of vagal, glossal, and other nerves and tongue on the same side. Usually a result of injury.

Tarsal tunnel
(355.5) Caused by posterior tibial nerve at the ankle, syndrome can produce significant neuropathy.

Taussig-Bing
(745.11) Complete transposition of aorta, with major vessels transposed, high septal ventricular defect, and other symptoms.

Taybi's
(759.89) Condition affecting ears, palate, mouth, and fingers.

Teething
(520.7) Eruption of teeth in small child.

Tegmental
(344.89) (Avellis, Babinski-Nageotte, Benedikt's, Brown-Sequard, Cestan's, Cestan-Chenais, Foville's, Gubler-Millard, Jackson's, Weber-Leyden) Paraplegia and anesthesia over part of the body. Caused by lesions in the brain or spinal cord.

Telangiectasis-pigmentation-cataract
(757.33) (Rothmund's) An inherited disorder marked by pigmentation and atrophy of skin, along with cataracts, saddle nose, bone defects, disturbance of hair growth, and hypogonadism.

Temporal
(383.02) (Gradenigo's) Localized meningitis in fifth and sixth cranial nerves, causing paralysis and pain in temporal region.

Temporomandibular joint-pain-dysfunction [TMJ]
(524.60) Headache, dizziness, tinnitus, and other symptoms resulting from dysfunction of the mandibular joint.

Terry's
(362.21) Retinopathy occurring in premature infants treated with high amounts of oxygen. Retina converts into a fibrous mass stunting growth of eye, resulting in blindness.

Terson's
Vitreous and retinal hemorrhages that occur as a result of sudden increase in intracranial pressure due to a subarachnoid hemorrhage. Code the specified types of hemorrhaging present.

Testicular feminization
(259.5) (Androgen insensitivity, hairless women, Goldberg (-Maxwell) (-Morris), male pseudohemaphroditism, nonvirilizing) Genetic condition affecting the development of reproductive organs marked by female external genitalia or a degree of both male and female genitalia. Amenorrhea noticed in teen years, with short,

incompletely developed vagina and rudimentary or absent uterus and fallopian tubes, scanty or absent axillary/public hair, and testicles that may require removal.

Tethered (spinal) cord
(742.59) Adhesions distorting spinal cord in the caudal area and associated with Arnold-Chiari syndrome and spina bifida.

Thalamic
(338.0) Infarction of postero-inferior thalamus causing transient hemiparesis and severe loss of superficial and deep sensation with crude pain in the limbs. Limbs frequently have vasomotor or trophic disturbances.

Thibierge-Weissenbach
(710.1) Systemic disorder of connective tissue marked by induration and thickening of the skin, with circulatory and organ changes. May reside in the face and hands for some time. Also includes Raynaud's phenomenon and, in some cases, esophageal problems.

Thoracic outlet
(353.0) (Naffziger's) Disorder presenting symptoms similar to Raynaud's, caused by pressure of brachial plexus and subclavian artery against first thoracic rib.

Thoracogenous rheumatic
(731.2) (Mankowsky's, Pierre Marie-Bamberger) Symmetrical osteitis of the limbs localized to the phalanges and terminal epiphyses of the long bones of the forearm and leg. Symptoms include kyphosis of the spine and affection of the joints.

Thorson-Biörck
(259.2) (Cassidy-Scholte, Hedinger's) Carcinoid tumors causing cyanotic flushing of skin, diarrheal watery stools, bronchoconstrictive attacks, hypotension, edema, and ascites.

Thrombocytopenia with absent radii
(287.33) (TAR) Congenital abnormality that affects both blood and bone structure, specifically presenting with low platelet counts through childhood and the absence of the radius in both arms. The thumb is present without the radius.

Thrombopenia-hemangioma
(287.39) Small number of platelets in circulating blood, causing bruising.

Thyroid-adrenocortical insufficiency
(258.1) Insufficient production of hormones by the pituitary and thyroid glands.

Tibial
(958.8) Early complication of trauma.

Tietze's
(733.6) Painful swelling of unknown origin of one or more costal cartilages, especially of second rib. Patients may interpret chest pain as coronary artery disease.

Time-zone
(327.35) (jet lag) Imbalance of the normal circadian rhythm resulting from airplane travel through a number of time zones. Leads to fatigue, irritability, and other constitutional disturbances.

Tobias'
(162.3) (Cuiffini-Pancoast, Hare's) Neoplasm of the upper lobe of the lung.

Tolosa-Hunt
(378.55) Cavernous sinus syndrome produced by idiopathic granuloma.

Toni-Fanconi
(270.0) (Harts) Renal tubular malfunction, including cystinosis and osteomalacia that may be caused by inherited disorders or may be the result of multiple myeloma or proximal epithelial growth.

TORCH
(771.2) An acronym for toxoplasmosis, other parasitic, rubella virus, cytomegalovirus, and herpes simplex virus. A parasitic or viral infection of the fetus or newborn by one of the TORCH agents that can result in motor problems or mental, neurological, visual, or auditory deficiencies. Code specified infection/organism and also any associated anomalies.

Torsades de Pointes
(427.1) A distinctive pattern of paroxysmal ventricular tachycardia with a waxing and waning effect of the QRS complexes on ECG. It may be self limiting, or can progress to ventricular fibrillation.

Touraine's
(756.89) Dysplasia of the fingernails and toenails, hypoplasia of the patella, iliac horns, thickening of the glomerular lamina densa, and a flask-shaped femur.

Touraine-Solente-Golé
(757.39) Thickening of the skin on extremities and face with clubbing of fingers and deformities in bone of limb.

Toxic oil
(710.5) Pain in muscles as a result of accumulation of a large number of granular leukocytes.

Toxic shock
(040.82) Staphylococci producing an endotoxin, presenting a high fever, vomiting and diarrhea, decreasing blood pressure, a skin rash, and shock. Hyperemia of several mucous membranes also occurs.

Transfusion donor
(772.0) Transfusion of fetus's blood across the placenta to mother's blood supply.

Transfusion recipient
(776.4) Polycythemia of newborn as result of blood flow from mother.

Traumatic shock
(958.4) Particularly dangerous state of shock following a traumatic injury.

Treacher Collins'
(756.0) (Franceschetti's) Malformations of derivatives of the first branchial arch, marked by palpebral fissures sloping outward and downward with notches in the outer third of the lower lids, defects of malar bones and zygome, hypoplasia of the jawbone, high or cleft palate, low-set ears, unusual hair growth, and pits between mouth and ear.

Trigeminal plate
(259.8) Progeria, which includes marked senility by 10 years of age.

Triple X female
(758.81) Three X chromosomes where the only confirmed symptom is the occurrence of twin Barr bodies in a typical cell.

Troisier-Hanot-Chauffard
(275.0) Hypertrophic cirrhosis with pigmentation and diabetes mellitus.

Trousseau's
(453.1) Spontaneous development of thromboses in upper and lower limbs as a result of visceral neoplasm.

Tumor lysis
(584.8) A side effect of massive doses of chemotherapy on the bloodstream resulting in higher than normal concentrations of phosphates, potassium, and uric acid, with a decrease in calcium. The metabolic abnormalities are secondary to the release of intracellular products after cell lysis. Hyperuricemia occurs secondary to toxicity, which leads to kidney failure. Report also the appropriate external cause code.

Türk's
(378.71) (Duane, Still-Turk-Duane) Simultaneous retraction of eye muscles causing an inability to abduct affected eye with retraction of the globe.

Turner's
(758.6) (XO, Turner-Varney) Congenital disorder characterized by short stature, webbed neck, congenital heart disease, mental retardation, and other symptoms.

Twin-to-twin transfusion
(762.3) The birth of one anemic twin and one plethoric twin due to the forcing of blood of one twin into the other.

Type I
(348.4) Brain damage as result of compression.

Uehlinger's
(757.39) Thickening of skin on extremities and face with clubbing of fingers and deformities in bone of limb.

Ullrich (-Bonnevie) (-Turner)
(758.6) (XO, Turner-Varney) Congenital disorder characterized by short stature, webbed neck, congenital heart disease, mental retardation, and other symptoms.

Ullrich-Feichtiger
(759.89) Congenital abnormalities, depressed nose, small eyes, hypertelorism, and protuberant ears.

Universal joint, cervix
(620.6) (Allen-Masters, Masters-Allen) Pelvic pain resulting from old laceration of broad ligament received during delivery.

Unverricht-Wagner
(710.3) (Petges-Clejat) Polymyositis occurring with characteristic skin changes that include a rash on upper eyelids with edema, a rash on the forehead, neck, shoulders, trunk, and arms, and papules on the knuckles.

Upward gaze
(378.81) (Parinaud's) Paralysis of conjugate movement of eyes without paralysis of convergence. Caused by lesions of the midbrain.

Urbach-Oppenheim
(250.8x) [709.3] Diabetes with skin disorder.

Urbach-Wiethe
(272.8) Deposition of hyaline material in the skin and mucosa of mouth, pharynx, hypopharynx, and larynx. Skin lesions as pustules on faces and exposed surfaces of arms and legs, which heal and form scars.

Urethro-oculoarticular
(099.3) (Fiessinger-Leroy-Reiter, urethro-oculosynovial) Association of arthritis, iridocyclitis, and urethritis, sometimes with diarrhea. While symptoms may recur, the arthritis is constant.

Urohepatic
(572.4) (Heyd's) Acute renal failure in patients with disease of biliary or liver tract. Cause seems to be decreased renal blood flow, damaging both organs.

Uveocutaneous
(364.24) (Vogt-Koyanagi) Uveomeningitis marked by patchy depigmentation of hair, eyebrows, and lashes. Retinal detachment, deafness, and tinnitus may also result.

Vagoaccessory
(352.6) (Collet-Sicard, vagohypoglossal) Unilateral lesions of the ninth, tenth, eleventh, and twelfth cranial nerves producing paralysis of the vagal, glossal, and other nerves and the tongue on the same side. Most usually result of injury.

Valve prolapse
(424.0) (Barlow's) "Mid-late" systolic click due to massive protrusion of mitral valvular leaflet in left atrial cavity.

Van Buchem's
(733.3) Multiple fractures and bowing of all extremities, thickening of skull bones, and osteoporosis.

Van der Hoeve's
(756.51) Blue sclera, little growth, brittle bones, and deafness.

Van der Hoeve-Halbertsma-Waardenburg
(270.2) (Mendes, Waardenburg-Kleinvan, der Hoeve-Waardenburg-Gualdi, ptosis-epicanthus) Eyebrow or upper or lower eyelid sags.

Van Neck-Odelberg
(732.1) Disease of growth centers, especially at the top of the femur, in which the epiphyses is replaced by new calcification.

Vascular insufficiency
(557.1) (Wilkie's) Complete or partial block of the superior mesenteric artery with symptoms of vomiting, pain, blood in the stool, and distended abdomen. Results in bowel infarction.

Vascular loop
(388.5) Compression of the eighth cranial nerve, interfering with inner ear circulation and resulting in deafness, vertigo, and tinnitus.

Vascular splanchnic
(557.0) Visceral circulation syndrome.

Vasomotor
(443.9) (Charcot's) Symptoms in a moving limb including pain tension, and weakness but absent at rest. Caused by occlusive arterial diseases of the limbs.

Vasomotor acroparesthesia
(443.89) (Nothangel's Type) Paresthesia of the tips of the extremities or attacks of tingling resulting from nerve compression at several levels, and cyanosis. May result in gangrene of the affected areas.

Vasovagal
(780.2) (Gower's) Fall in blood pressure, slow pulse, and convulsions. Believed to be sudden stimulation of the vagal nerve by receptors in the heart, carotid sinus, or aortic arch.

VATER
(759.89) Vertebral defects, anal atresia, tracheoesophageal fistula with esophageal atresia, and radial and renal anomalies.

Velo-cardio-facial
(758.32) A chromosomal abnormality causing varying degrees of immune deficiency, cardiac or ventricular septal defects, mild mental retardation, dysmorphic facial features, and cleft palate.

Vena cava
(459.2) Obstruction of the vena cava.

Verbiest's
(435.1) (Charcot's) Symptoms in a moving limb including pain, tension, and weakness but absent at rest. Caused by occlusive arterial diseases of the limbs.

Verner-Morrison
(259.3) Severe diarrhea occurring as an affect of a vasoactive intestinal peptide secreted by functional islet cell tumors of the pancreas; which also results in metabolic abnormalities such as hypokalemia and achlorhydria. Code also tumor of the pancreas.

Vernet's
(352.6) (Collet-Sicard) Unilateral lesions of the ninth, tenth, eleventh, and twelfth cranial nerves producing paralysis of the vagal, glossal, and other nerves and the tongue on the same side. Most usually result of injury.

Video display tube
(723.8) (VDT) Chronic neck and back pain developing from sitting at a computer.

Villaret's
(352.6) (Collet-Sicard) Unilateral lesions of the ninth, tenth, eleventh, and twelfth cranial nerves producing paralysis of the vagal, glossal, and other nerves and the tongue on the same side. Most usually result of injury.

Vinson-Plummer
(280.8) (Kelly, Plummer-Vinson, Paterson-Brown-Vinson) Condition in middle-aged women with hypochromic anemia, marked by cracks or fissures at the corners of the mouth, painful tongue, and dysphagia due to esophageal stenosis or webs.

Viral
(079.99) An unspecified viral infection with symptoms such as swollen glands, extreme fatigue, fever, and upper respiratory symptoms, with nonexudative pharyngitis or palpable, tender lymph nodes.

Virilism
(255.2) (virilizing adrenocortical hyperplasia, congenital) Mature masculine somatic characteristics by a prepubescent male, girl, or woman. This syndrome may show at birth or develop later as result of adrenocortical dysfunction.

Visceral larval migrans
(128.0) Prolonged migration of nematode larvae in the viscera, which can cause hypereosinophilia, hepatomegaly, and pneumonitis.

Visual disorientation
(368.16) (Balint's, Holmes', Riddoch's) Cortical paralysis of visual fixation, optic ataxia, and disturbance of visual attention. Eye movements are normal.

Vitamin B6 deficiency
(266.1) Pellagra, a deficiency-caused syndrome exhibiting gastrointestinal disturbance, erythema, nervous disorders, and mental disturbances.

Vogt's
(333.71) Spastic diplegia with athetosis and pseudobulbar paralysis found with a lesion of the caudate nucleus and putamen.

Vogt-Koyanagi (-Harada)
(364.24) Uveomeningitis marked by patchy depigmentation of hair, eyebrows, and lashes. Retinal detachment, deafness, and tinnitus may also result.

Von Bechterew-Strümpell
(720.0) Rheumatoid inflammation of vertebrae.

Von Graefe's
(378.72) Progressive external ophthalmoplegia, a slowly progressive bilateral myopathy only affecting the muscles around the eye, including lids. Paralysis of the muscles around the eye results.

Von Hippel-Lindau
(759.6) Formation of multiple angiomas on the retina.

Von Schroetter
(453.8) Stress thrombosis of the subclavian or axillary vein.

Waardenburg-Klein
(270.2) (Mendes, van der Hoeve-Halbertsma-Waardenburg) Eyebrow or upper or lower eyelid sags.

Wagner (-Unverricht)
(710.3) (Petges-Clegat, Unverricht-Wagner) Polymyositis occurring with characteristic skin changes that include a rash on the upper eyelids with edema, a rash on the forehead, neck, shoulders, trunk, and arms, and papules on the knuckles.

Waldenström's
(273.3) Increase in macroglobulins in the blood. Has symptoms of hyperviscosity such as weakness, fatigue, bleeding disorders, and visual disturbances.

Waldenström-Kjellberg
(280.8) (Kelly, Plummer-Vinson, Paterson-Brown-Vinson) Condition in middle-aged women with hypochronic anemia, marked by cracks or fissures at the corners of the mouth, painful tongue, and dysphagia due to esophageal stenosis or webs.

Water retention
(276.6) Fluid overload caused by electrolyte and acid-base imbalance.

Waterhouse (-Friderichsen)
(036.3) Acute fulminating meningococcal septicemia occurring in children below 10 years of age. Symptoms include vomiting, cyanosis, diarrhea, purpura, convulsions, and circulatory collapse. The patient will often display meningitis and hemorrhaging into the adrenal glands.

Weakness
(300.5) (neurasthenia) Hypersomatic disorder with no identifiable pathology.

Web
(756.89) Dysplasia of the fingernails and toenails, hypoplasia of the patella, iliac horns, thickening of the glomerular lamina densa, and a flask-shaped femur.

Weber's
(344.89) (Avellis, Babinski-Nageotte, Benedikt's, Brown-Sequard, Cestan's, Cestan-Chenais, Foville's, Gubler-Millard, Jackson's, Weber-Leyden) Paraplegia and anesthesia over half or part of the body. Caused by lesions in the brain or spinal cord.

Weber-Christian
(729.30) Relapsing febrile nodular nonsuppurative panniculitis with development of nodules that spread centrifugally with erythematous borders and clearing centrally to form pigmented plaques.

Weber-Cockayne
(757.39) Dwarfism with a precociously senile appearance, pigmentary degeneration of the retina, optic atrophy, deafness, sensitivity to sunlight, and mental retardation.

Weber-Dimitri
(759.6) (Kalischer's) Formation of multiple angiomas in the skin of the head and scalp.

Weber-Gubler
(344.89) (Avellis, Babinski-Nageotte, Benedikt's, Brown-Sequard, Cestan's, Cestan-Chenais, Foville's, Gubler-Millard, Jackson's, Weber-Leyden) Paraplegia over half or part of the body. Caused by lesions in the brain or spinal cord.

Weber-Osler (-Rendu)
(448.0) Small telangiectasias and dilated venules that develop slowly on the skin and mucus membranes of the lips, tongue, nasopharynx, tongue, and the face.

Wegener's
(446.4) Necrotizing granulomatous vasculitis involving the upper and lower respiratory tracts, which is thought to be a hypersensitivity to unknown antigens.

Weill-Marchesani
(759.89) Abnormally round and small lens, short stature, and brachydactyly.

Weingarten
(518.3) Transient infiltrations of lungs by eosinophilia, resulting in night coughing, fever, and dyspnea.

Weiss-Baker
(337.0) (Charcot-Weiss-Baker, Sluder's) Stimulation of an overactive carotid sinus, causing a marked drop in blood pressure, which, in turn, may stop or block the heart.

Weissenbach-Thibierge
(710.1) Systemic disorder of the connective tissue marked by induration and thickening of the skin, with circulatory and organ changes. May reside in the face and hands for some time. Also includes Raynaud's phenomenon and, in some cases, esophageal problems.

Werlhof-Wichmann
(287.39) Small number of platelets in circulating blood, causing bruising.

Wermer's
(258.0) Tumors in more than one endocrine gland, including the pancreatic islets and parathyroid glands. Syndrome is inherited.

Werner's
(259.8) Premature aging in the adult as result of genetic trait and characterized by sclerodermal skin changes, cataracts, muscular atrophy, diabetes mellitus, baldness, and high incidence of neoplasm.

Wernicke's
(265.1) (Gayet-Wernicke) Thiamine deficiency, disturbances in ocular motility, pupillary

alterations, nystagmus, and ataxia with tremors. Organic toxic psychosis often coexists. Most often due to alcoholism.

Wernicke-Korsakoff
(294.0) Nonalchoholic amnestic dementia where the patient cannot remember short-term or long-term memories but is not delirious.

Westphal-Strümpell
(275.1) (Wilson) Defect in the metabolism of copper. Marked by accumulation of copper in the brain, cornea, kidney, liver, and other tissues causing cirrhosis of the liver and deterioration in the basal ganglia of the brain.

Wet brain
(303.9x) Description of chronic alcoholism.

Wet feet
(991.4) (immersion foot, trench foot) Blotchy cyanosis, increased sweating, paresthesia, and edema. Caused by hypothermia.

Whiplash
(847.0) Acute cervical sprain caused by hyperextension of the neck (C4-C5) during an accident, usually in an automobile.

Whipple's
(040.2) Radical removal of the head of the pancreas, duodenum, and distal third of the stomach. Jejunum is connected to the stomach, pancreas, and bile duct.

"Whistling face"
(759.89) (Freeman-Sheldon) Deviation of hands and face, with protrusion of lips as in whistling, sunken eyes, and small nose.

Widal (-Abrami)
(283.9) (Dyke-Young, Hayem-Widal) One of anemic syndromes caused by exposures to trauma, poisons, and other causes that decreases the number of red blood cells.

Wilkie's
(557.1) Complete or partial block of the superior mesenteric artery with symptoms of vomiting, pain, blood in the stool, and distended abdomen. Results in bowel infarction.

Wilkinson-Sneddon
(694.1) Non-inflammatory intimal hyperplasia of medium sized vessels.

Willan-Plumbe
(696.1) Eruption of circumscribed, discrete, reddish, silvery-scaled maculopapules on the knees, elbows, scalp, and trunk.

Willi-Prader
(759.81) Rounded face, almond-shaped eyes, strabismus, low forehead, hypogonadism, hyposomia, mental retardation, and an insatiable appetite.

Williams
(759.89) A congenital disorder with onset at birth or early infancy and manifests with feeding problems, developmental delays, hypotonia, facial "elfin" anomalies, cataracts, and aortic stenosis. Code also any associated manifestations.

Wilson's
(275.1) (Westphal-Strümpell) Defect in the metabolism of copper with accumulation of copper in the brain, cornea, kidney, liver, and other tissues causing cirrhosis of the liver and deterioration in the basal ganglia of the brain.

Wilson-Mikity
(770.7) Pulmonary insufficiency in newborn babies, especially those with low birth weight with hypercapnia and cyanosis of rapid onset during the first month of life and resulting frequently in death.

Winking
(307.20) Tic motor disorder not otherwise specified.

Wiskott-Aldrich
(279.12) Immunodeficiency shown by eczema, thrombocytopenia, and recurrent pyogenic infection. Patients suffer an increased susceptibility to infection with encapsulated bacteria.

Woake's
(471.1) (polypoid sinus degeneration) Polyp-like growths that hamper sinus function.

XO
(758.6) (Turner's) Short stature, webbed neck, congenital heart disease, mental retardation, and other symptoms.

Yellow vernix
(762.2) (placental dysfunction) Marked by placental dysfunction, infarction, and insufficiency.

Zahorsky
(074.0) (herpangina) Vesicular pharyngitis caused by Coxsackie virus.

Zellweger

(277.86) (cerebrohepatorenal) A rare congenital autosomal recessive disorder associated with a lack of peroxisomal enzymes in the liver and kidneys and characterized by polycystic kidneys, hepatomegaly, jaundice, hypotonia, and craniofacial abnormalities, causing death in infancy.

Zieve's

(571.1) Acute hepatitis or cirrhosis of the liver associated with alcoholism.

Zollinger-Ellison

(251.5) (Ellison-Zollinger) Peptic ulceration with gastric hypersecretion, tumor of the pancreatic islets, and hypoglycemia.

Zuelzer-Ogden

(281.2) Folate-deficiency anemia caused by a drug, congenital, dietary, or other reason.

Prefixes and Suffixes

The uniquely efficient language of medicine is possible thanks to the prefixes and suffixes attached to roots. Changing prefixes and suffixes allows subtle and overt changes in meaning of the terms. The following prefixes and suffixes are paired with their meanings.

Prefixes

Prefixes are one half of the medical language equation and are attached to the beginning of words. For example, the prefix "eu-," meaning good or well, combined with the Greek word for death, "thanatos," produces euthanasia — a good death.

a-, an-	without, away from, not
ab-	from, away from, absent
acro-	extremity, top, highest point
ad-	indicates toward, adherence to, or increase
adeno-	relating to a gland
adip-	relating to fat (also adipo-)
aero-	relating to gas or air
all-	meaning another, other, or different
allo-	indicates difference or divergence from the norm
ambi-	both sides; about or around (also amphi-)
an-	without
angi-	relating to a vessel
aniso-	dissimilar, unequal, or asymmetrical
ankylo-	bent, crooked, or two parts growing together
ante-	in front of, before
antero-	before, front, anterior
anti-	in opposition to, against
antro-	relating to a chamber or cavity
arch-	beginning, first, principal (also arche-, archi-)
archo-	relating to the rectum or anus
arterio-	relating to an artery
arthro-	relating to a joint
astro-	star-like or shaped
atelo-	incomplete or imperfect
auto-	relating to the self
axio-	relating to an axis (also axo-)
balano-	relating to the glans penis or glans clitoridis
baro-	relating to weight or heaviness
basi-	relating to the base or foundation (also basio-)
bi-	double, twice, two
blasto-	relating to germs
blenn-	relating to mucus (also blenno-)
blepharo-	relating to the eyelid
brachi-	relating to the arm (also brachio-)
brachy-	short
brady-	meaning slow or prolonged
broncho-	relating to the trachea
cac-	meaning diseased or bad (also caci-, caco-)
cardio-	relating to the heart
carpo-	relating to the wrist
cata-	down from, down, according to
celo-	indicating a tumor or hernia; cavity
cervico-	relating to the neck or neck of an organ
chilo-	relating to the lip (also cheilo-)
chole-	relating to the gallbladder
cleido-	relating to the clavicle

cyst-	relating to the urinary bladder or a cyst (also cysto-)	idio-	distinct or individual characteristics
cyto-	in relation to cell	ileo-	relating to the ileum (part of the small intestine)
dacry-	pertaining to the lacrimal glands	ilio-	relating to the pelvis
dactyl-	relating to the fingers or toes	infra-	meaning inferior to, beneath, under
demi-	half the amount		
desmo-	relating to ligaments	irid-	relating to the iris
deuter-	secondary or second	ischio-	relating to the hip
dextro-	meaning on or to the right	iso-	equal
dorsi-	relating to the back (also dorso-)	jejuno-	relating to the jejunum (part of the small intestine)
dys-	painful, bad, disordered, difficult	juxta-	next to, near
echo-	reverberating sound	karyo-	relating to the nucleus of a cell
ecto-	external, outside	kerato-	relating to the cornea or horny tissue
ectro-	congenital absence of something	laparo-	flank, loins; operations through the abdominal wall
endo-	within, internal		
entero-	relating to the intestines	laryngo-	relating to the larynx
epi-	on, upon, in addition to	lien-	relating to the spleen
eu-	well, healthy, good, normal	lip-	relating to fat (also lipo-)
exo-	outside of, without	lith-	relating to a hard or calcified substance (also litho-)
fibro-	relating to fibers or fibrous tissue	lumbo-	relating to the loin region
galacto-	relating to milk	macro-	meaning oversized, large
gastro-	relating to the stomach and abdominal region	mal-	bad, poor, ill
		melano-	dark or black in color
genito-	relating to reproduction	meningo-	relating to membranes covering the brain and spine
gono-	relating to the genitals, offspring, origination	mesio-	toward the middle; secondary (also meso-)
gyn-	relating to the female gender		
hema-	relating to blood (also hemato-)	meta-	indicates a change
		mis-	bad, improper
hemi-	half	my-	relating to muscle (also myo-)
hepato-	relating to the liver	myc-	relating to fungus (also myco-)
histo-	relating to tissue	myelo-	relating to bone marrow or the spinal cord
homeo-	indicates resemblance or likeness (also homo-)	narco-	indicates insensate condition or numbness
hydro-	relating to fluid, water, or hydrogen	necro-	indicates death or dead tissue
		nephr-	relating to the kidney
hyper-	excessive, above, exaggerated	noci-	relating to injury or pain
hypo-	below, less than, under	nycto-	relating to darkness or night
hyster-	relating to either the womb or hysteria (also hystero-)	odont-	relating to the teeth
		oligo-	indicates few or small

Prefix	Meaning	Prefix	Meaning
omo-	relating to the shoulder	proso-	indicates toward the front, anterior, forward
omphalo-	relating to the navel		
onco-	relating to a mass, tumor, or swelling	pseudo-	indicates false or imagined
		pulmo-	relating to the lungs and respiration
onycho-	relating to the finger- or toenails	pyelo-	relating to the pelvis
oophor-	relating to the ovaries	pygo-	relating to the buttocks or rump
opistho-	indicates behind or backwards		
		pyle-	relating to an opening/orifice of the portal vein
orchi-	relating to the testicles (also orchido-)	pyloro-	relating to the pylorus, the stomach opening into the duodenum
oscheo-	relating to the scrotum		
osteo-	having to do with bone		
oto-	relating to the ear	pyo-	relating to pus
pachy-	indicates heavy, large, or thick	pyreto-	indicates a fever, heat
		rachi-	relating to the spine (also rachio-)
pali-	repetition, back again, recurring (also palin-)	recto-	meaning straight or relating to the rectum
panto-	indicates the whole or all	retro-	indicates behind, backward, in a reverse direction
para-	indicates near, similar, beside, or past	rheo-	indicates a flow or stream of fluid
patho-	indicates sensitivity, feeling, or suffering	rhino-	relating to the nose
ped-	relating to the foot (also pedi-)	sacro-	relating to the sacrum, the base of the vertebral column
peri-	about, around, or in the vicinity	salpingo-	relating to the fallopian or eustachian tubes
pero-	indicates being maimed or deformed	sarco-	relating to flesh
phaco-	relating to the lens of the eye	scapho-	indicates deformed condition, shaped like a boat
phago-	relating to eating and ingestion	scapulo-	relating to the shoulder
pharyngo-	relating to the pharynx	schisto-	indicates cleft or split; a fissure
phlebo-	relating to the vein		
phreno-	relating to the diaphragm; head or mind	scoto-	relating to darkness; visual field gap
pimel-	relating to fat	sial-	relating to saliva
platy-	indicates wide or broad	sinistro-	meaning on or to the left
pleio-	more, additional	somato-	relating to the body
pleur-	relating to the side or ribs	spheno-	relating to the sphenoid bone at the base of the skull
pneum-	relating to respiration, air, the lungs	sphygmo-	relating to the pulse
pod-	relating to the feet (also podo-)	splanch-	relating to the intestines; viscera
poly-	indicates much or many	steato-	relating to fat
procto-	relating to the rectum and/or anus	stetho-	relating to the chest
		stomato-	relating to the mouth

Prefix	Meaning
sym-	indicates together with, along with, beside
syn-	indicates being joined together
tachy-	indicates swift or fast
tarso-	relating to the foot; margin of the eyelid
teleo-	indicates complete or perfectly formed
teno-	relating to tendons
terato-	indicates being seriously deformed, esp. a fetus
thalamo-	relating to the thalamus, origin of nerves in the brain
thanato-	relating to death
thoraco-	relating to the chest
thrombo-	relating to blood clots
thymo-	relating to the thymus
toco-	relating to birth
trachelo-	relating to the neck
trichi-	relating to hair; hair-like shape (also tricho-)
tympano-	relating to the eardrum
typhlo-	relating to the cecum; relating to blindness
vaso-	relating to blood vessels
ventro-	relating to the abdomen; anterior surface of the body
vesico-	relating to the bladder
viscero-	relating to the abdominal organs
xeno-	relating to a foreign substance
xero-	indicates a dry condition

Suffixes

Suffixes are the other half of the equation. These are attached to the ends of words.

Suffix	Meaning
-agra	indicating severe pain
-algia	pain
-ase	denoting an enzyme
-blast	incomplete cellular development
-centesis	puncture
-cephal	having to do with the head
-cle	meaning small or little (also -cule)
-cyte	having to do with cells
-dactyl	having to do with fingers
-desis	binding or fusion
-ectomy	excision, removal
-ferous	produces, causes, or brings about
-fuge	drive out or expel
-genic	indicates production, causation, generation
-gram	drawn, written, and recorded
-graphic	written or drawn
-ia	state of being, condition (abnormal)
-iasis	condition
-itis	inflammation
-lysis	release, free, reduction of
-metry	scientific measurement
-odynia	indicates pain or discomfort
-oid	indicates likeness or resemblance
-ology	study of
-oma	tumor
-orraphy	suturing
-oscopy	to examine
-osis	condition, process
-ostomy	indicates a surgically created artificial opening
-otomy	indicates a cutting
-pagus	indicates fixed or joined together
-pathic	indicates a feeling, diseased condition, or therapy
-penia	indicates a deficiency; less than normal
-pexy	fixation
-philia	inordinate love of or craving for something
-phobia	abnormal fear of or aversion to something
-plasty	indicates surgically formed or molded
-plegia	indicates a stroke or paralysis
-poietic	indicates producing or making
-praxis	indicates activity, action, condition, or use

-rhage	indicates bleeding or other fluid discharge (also -rhagia)
-rhaphy	indicates a suture or seam joining two structures
-rrhagia	indicates an abnormal or excessive fluid discharge
-rrhexis	splitting or breaking
-spasm	contraction
-taxy	arrangement, grouping (also -taxis)
-tomy	indicates a cutting
-trophy	relating to food or nutrition
-tropic	indicates an affinity for or turning toward
-tropism	responding to an external stimulus

Abbreviations, Acronyms, and Symbols

The acronyms, abbreviations, and symbols used by health care providers speed communications. The following list includes the most often seen acronyms, abbreviations, and symbols. In some cases, abbreviations have more than one meaning. Multiple interpretations are separated by a slash (/). Abbreviations of Latin phrases are punctuated.

<	less than
>	greater than
@	at
A	assessment/blood type
a (ante)	before
a fib	atrial fibrillation
a flutter	atrial flutter
A2	aortic second sound
a.a.	of each
AA	Alcoholics Anonymous
AAHP	American Association of Health Plans
AAL	anterior axillary line
AAMT	American Association for Medical Transcription
AAPCC	adjusted average per capita cost
AAPPO	American Association of Preferred Provider Organizations
AAROM	active assistive range of motion
ATT	alpha-1 antitrypsin
ab	abortion
AB	blood type
abd	abdomen
ABE	acute bacterial endocarditis
ABG	arterial blood gas
abn.	abnormal
ABO	referring to ABO incompatibility
abs. fev.	without fever
a.c.	before eating
ACD	absolute cardiac dullness
ACE	angiotensin converting enzyme/ adrenal cortical extract
ACL	anterior cruciate ligament
ACLS	advanced cardiac life support
ACP	acid phosphatase
acq.	acquired
ACTH	adrenocorticotropic hormone
ACVD	acute cardiovascular disease
ad lib	as desired, at pleasure
ad part. dolent.	to the aching parts
a.d.	right ear/to, up to
ad. us. ext.	for external use
ADA	American Dental Association, or Americans with Disabilities Act
ADEM	acute disseminated encephalomyelitis
ADH	antidiuretic hormone
ad. hib.	to be administered
ADL	activities of daily living
ad. lib.	as desired
adm	admission, admit
ADM	alcohol, drug or mental disorder
ADP	adenosine diphosphate
ADS	alternative delivery system
adst. feb.	when fever is present
AE	above the elbow
AF	atrial fibrillation

AFB	acid fast bacilli	ANSI/HISB	ANSI Health Information Standards Board
A/G	albumin-globulin ratio		
AGA	appropriate (average) for gestational age	ant	anterior
		AOD	arterial occlusive disease
AgNO3	silver nitrate	AODM	adult onset diabetes mellitus
AHA	American Hospital Association	A&P	auscultation and percussion
AHC	alternative health care	A-P	anterior posterior
AHIMA	American Health Information Management Association	Ap	apical
		AP	antepartum/anterior-posterior
AI	aortic insufficiency	APC	Ambulatory Payment Classification
AICD	automatic implant cardioverter defibrillator		
		APM	arterial pressure monitoring
AID	artificial insemination donor/ acute infectious disease	approx	approximately
		appy.	appendectomy
AIDS	acquired immunodeficiency syndrome	aq.	water (aqua)
		ARC	AIDS-related complex
AIH	artificial insemination by husband	ARD	acute respiratory disease
AK	above the knee	ARDS	adult respiratory distress syndrome
AKA	above knee amputation		
ALA	aminolevulinic acid	ARF	acute respiratory/renal failure
alb. (albus)	white	AROM	active range of motion/artificial rupture of membranes
alk. phos.	alkaline phosphatase		
ALL	acute lymphocytic leukemia	art.	artery, arterial
ALP	alkaline phosphatase	AS	aortic stenosis/ arteriosclerosis
ALS	advanced life support	a.s.	left ear
ALT	alanine aminotransferase	ASAP	as soon as possible
alt. dieb.	every other day	ASC	ambulatory surgery center
alt. hor.	every other hour	ASC-H	atypical squamous cell cannot exclude high grade squamous intraepithelial lesion
alt. noc.	every other night		
a.m.	morning		
ama	against medical advice		
AMA	American Medical Association	ASC-US	atypical squamous cell of undetermined significance
amb	ambulate		
AMGA	American Medical Group Association	ASCVD	arteriosclerotic cardiovascular disease
		ASCX12N	American Standard Committee standard for claims and reimbursement
AMI	acute myocardial infarction		
AML	acute myelogenous leukemia		
AMML	acute myelomonocytic leukemia	ASD	atrial septal defect
AMP	adenosine monophosphate/ ampule	ASHD	arteriosclerotic heart disease
		ASO	administrative services only
ANA	American Nursing Association, or antinuclear antibodies	ASR	age/sex rate
		Asst	assistance (min= minimal; mod= moderate)
ANS	autonomic nervous system		
ANSI	American National Standards Institute	AST	aspartate aminotransferase
		ATP	adenosine triphosphate
ANC	Absolute neutrophil count	a.u.	each ear, both ears

AUR	ambulatory utilization review	C&S	culture and sensitivity
A-V	arterioveneous	C	centigrade/complements/cervical vertebrae
AV	atrioventricular		
AVF	arteriovenous fistula	c	with
ax	auxiliary	C-collar	cervical collar
AZT	azidothymidine	CA	cancer
Ba	barium	CA 125	cancer antigen 125
bal.	bath	Ca	calcium/cancer
B&B	bowel and bladder	CABG	coronary artery bypass graft
BB	blow bottles	CAD	coronary artery disease
BBA	Balanced Budget Act of 1997	CAPD	continuous ambulatory peritoneal dialysis
BBB	bundle branch block		
BCC	basal cell carcinoma	caps.(capsula)	capsule
BCP	birth control pill	CAT	computerized axial tomography
BE	barium enema/below the elbow	cath	catheterize
BI	biopsy	CBC	complete blood count
bib.	drink	CBR	complete bed rest
b.i.d.	two times a day	cc	chief complaint
b.i.n.	twice a night	CCPD	continuous cycling peritoneal dialysis
b.i.s.	twice		
BK	below the knee	CCU	coronary care unit
BKA	below knee amputation	CDC	Centers for Disease Control
BLS	basic life support	CDG	congenital disorder of glycosylation
BM	bowel movement		
BMI	body mass index	CDGS	carbohydrate-deficient glycoprotein syndrome
BMR	basal metabolic rate		
BMT	bone marrow transplant	CDH	congenital dislocation of hip
BO	body order	CE	cardiac enlargement
BOW	bag of water	CEA	carcinoembryonic antigen
BP	blood pressure	CF	cystic fibrosis
BPD	bronchopulmonary displasia	CGF	congenital generalized fibromatosis
BPH	benign prostatic hypertrophy		
Br	breastfeeding	CH,Chol	cholesterol
BRBPR	bright red blood per rectum	CHD	congenital heart disease/congestive heart disease
BrC	breast care		
BS	bachelor of surgery/breath sounds/bowel sounds	CHF	congestive heart failure
		CI	confidence interval/chloride
BSA	body surface area	CIN	cervical intraepithelial neoplasia
BSC	bedside commode	CIS	carcinoma in situ
BSD	bedside drainage	CKD	chronic kidney disease
BUN	blood urea nitrogen	cl liqs	clear liquids
BUR	back-up rate (ventilator)	CLD	chronic lung disease/chronic liver disease
BUS	Bartholin urethra skenes		
bx	biopsy	CLL	chronic lymphatic leukemia
		c.m.	tomorrow morning
		cm	centimeter

cm2	square centimeters	CQI	Continuous Quality Improvement
CMC	carpometacarpal	CR	creatine
CMG	cystometrogram	CRC	community rating by class
CMHC	community mental health center	CRF	chronic renal failure
CML	chronic myelogenous leukemia	CRH	corticotropic releasing hormone
CMP	competitive medical plan	crit.	hematocrit
CMRI	cardiac magnetic resonance imaging	CROS	contralateral routing of signals
		CRP	C-reactive protein
CMS	circulation motion sensation	C/S	cesarean section
CMS	Centers for Medicare and Medicaid Services	CS	central service
		CSF	cerebrospinal fluid
CMS-1500	a universal billing form developed by CMS	CT	computerized tomography/corneal thickness/ carpal tunnel syndrome
CMV	cytomegalovirus		
cn	cranial nerves	CTLSO	cervical-thoracic-lumbar-sacral-orthosis
c.n.	tomorrow night		
CNM	certified nurse midwife	CTZ	chemoreceptor trigger zone
CNP	continuous negative airway pressure	cu	cubic
		CV	cardiovascular
CNS	central nervous system	CVA	cerebral vascular accident/ cerebrovascular accident/ costovertebral angle
co	cardiac output		
c/o	complaints of		
CO2	carbon dioxide	CVD	cardiovascular disease, cerebrovascular disease
COB	coordination of benefits		
COBRA	Consolidated Omnibus Budget Reconciliation Act	CVI	chronic venous insufficiency
		CVL	central venous line
COC	certificate of coverage	CVMS	clean voided midstream urine
COLD	chronic obstructive lung disease	CVP	central venous pressure
CON	certificate of need	CVU	cerebrovascular unit
conc.	concentration	CW	closed ward
cont.	continue	CXR	chest x-ray
COPD	chronic obstructive pulmonary disease	cysto	cystoscopy
		D	day/diopter
CP	cerebral palsy	DAW	dispense as written
CPAP	continuous positive airway pressure	D&C	dilation and curettage
		D/C	discharge/discontinue
CPB	cardiopulmonary bypass	dc	discontinue
CPD	cephalopelvic disproportion	DC	dual choice
CPK	creatine phosphokinase	DC'd	discharged/discontinued
CPM	continuous passive motion	DCA	deferred compensation administrator
CPR	cardiopulmonary resuscitation, or computer-based patient record		
		DCI	duplicate coverage inquiry
CPT	chest physical therapy	DCR	dacrocytstorhinostomy
CPT	Physicians' Current Procedural Terminology	DDST	Denver Developmental Screening Test
CPT 1, CPT 2	carnitine palmityltransferase	DE	dose equivalent

decem	ten	DUE	drug use evaluation
decub.	decubitus ulcer/lying down	duo	two
def.	deficient, deficiency	DVT	deep vein thrombosis
del	delivery	D/W	dextrose in water
dep.	dependent	dx	diagnosis
det.	let it be given	DX	diagnosis code
DEXA	dual energy x-ray absorptiometry	dz	disease
dexter, dextra	the right	ead.	the same
DHEA	dehydroepiandrosterone	EBL	estimated blood loss
DHHS	Department of Health and Human Services	EBV	Epstein-Barr virus
		ECCE	extracapsular cataract extraction
DHT	dihydrotestosterone	ECF	extended care facility, extracellular fluid
DIC	disseminated intravascular coagulopathy	ECG	electrocardiogram
DIF	direct immunofluorescence	ECHO	enterocytopathogenic human orphan virus/echocardiogram
disp	disposition		
DJD	degenerative joint disease	ECMO	extracorporeal membrane oxygenation
DKA	diabetic ketoacidosis		
DM	diabetes mellitus	ECT	electro-convulsive therapy/ emission computerized tomography
DMD	Duchenne muscular dystrophy		
DME	durable medical equipment		
DNA	deoxyribonucleic acid	ectopic	ectopic pregnancy (OB)
DNP	do not publish	ED	emergency department/effective dose
DNR	do not resuscitate		
DO	Doctor of Osteopathy	EDC	estimated date of confinement/ expected date of confinement
DOA	dead on arrival		
DOB	date of birth	EDI	electronic data interchange
DOE	dyspnea on exertion	EEG	electroencephalogram
DOH	Department of Health	EENT	eye, ear, nose, and throat
DOS	date of service	EGA	estimated gestational age
DPR	drug price review	EGD	esophagus, stomach and duodenum
DPT	days per thousand		
DPT	diphtheria - pertussis - tetanus	EKG	electrocardiogram
D/R	dayroom	E/M	evaluation and management
DR	delivery room	EMG	electromyograme.m.p.
Dr	doctor	as directed	
DRG	diagnosis related group	en	an enema, a clyster
Dsg	dressing	en bloc	in total
DSM-IV	Diagnostic and Statistical Manual of the American Psychiatric Association's Task Force on Terminology, Fourth Edition	eng.	engorged
		ENG	electronystagmogram
		ENT	ear, nose, and throat
		EO	elbow orthosis
		EOB	explanation of benefits
DSS	dioctyl sulfosoccinate	EOG	electrooculography
DTs	delirium tremens	EOM	end of month
DTRs	deep tendon reflexes	EOM	extraocular motion

EOMB	explanation of Medicare benefits	FI	firm one finger down from umbilicus
EOMI	extraocular motion intact		
EOP	external occipital protuberance	fl	fluid
Epis.	episiotomy	fluro	fluoroscopy
EPO	epoetin alfa	FM	face mask
EPS	electrophysiologic stimulation	FNP	family nurse practitioner
EPSDT	early periodic screening, diagnosis and treatment	FP	family planning/family practitioner
ER	emergency room	FR	family relationship
ER-	estrogen receptor negative status	FSA	flexible spending account
ER+	estrogen receptor positive status	FSE	fetal scalp electrode
ERC	endoscopic retrograde cholangiography	FSH	follicle stimulating hormone
		FTND	full term normal delivery
ERCP	endoscopic retrograde cholangiopancreatography	FTSG	full thickness skin graft
		FTT	failure to thrive
ERG	electroretinogram	F/U	follow-up
ERISA	Employee Retirement Income Security Act of 1974	FUO	fever of unknown origin
		fx	fracture
ESR	erythrocyte sedimentation rate	G	gram
ESRD	end stage renal disease	GA	gastric analysis
EST	electroshock therapy	gav.	gavage
ESWL	extracorporeal shockwave lithotripsy	GB	gallbladder
		GDM	gestational diabetes mellitus
et	and	GFR	glomerular filtration rate
ET	endotracheal	GH	growth hormone
ETOH	alcohol	GI	gastrointestinal
Ex	examination	GIFT	gamete intrafallopian transfer
ext.	extremity	GISA	glycopeptide intermediate staphylococcus aureus
F (on OB)	firm		
F	Fahrenheit/female	GLC	gas liquid chromatography
FAS	fetal alcohol syndrome	GMP	guanosine monophosphate
FB (fb)	fingerbreadth	GnRH	gonadotropin-releasing hormone
FB	foreign body	GP	general practitioner
FBR	foreign body removal	gr.	grain
FBS	fasting blood sugar	grav	number of pregnancies
FDP	fibrin degradation products	GS	general surgeon
Fe	female/iron	GSRA	glycopeptide resistant staphylococcus aureus
FEV	forced expiratory volume		
FFP	fresh frozen plasma	gsw	gunshot wound
FFS	fee for service equivalency	gt./gtt.	drop/drops
FFS	fee for service reimbursement	GU	genitourinary
FH	family history	Gu	guiac
FHR	fetal heart rate	GxT	graded exercise test
FHT	fetal heart tone	gyn	gynecology
		h (hora)	hour

H2O	water	HIE	hypoxic-ischemic encephalopathy
H2O2	hydrogen peroxide	HIPAA	Health Insurance Portability and Accountability Act of 1996
HA	headache/hearing aide		
HAA	hepatitis antigen B	HIV	human immunodeficiency virus
HAAb	hepatitis antibody A	HLV	herpes-like virus
HaAg	hepatitis antigen A	HMD	hyaline membrane disease
HAI	hemaglutination test	HMO	health maintenance organization
HAV	hepatitis A virus	HMS	hepatosplenomegaly
HB	headbox/hepatitis B	H.O.	house officer
HBsAb	hepatitis surface antibody B	HORF	high output renal failure
HBcAg	hepatitis antigen B	H&P	history and physical
HBD	hydroxybutyril dehydrogenase	HPs	hot packs
Hbg	hemoglobin	HPF	high power field
HBO	hyperbaric oxygen	HPG	human pituitary gonadotropin
HbO2	oxyhemoglobin	HPI	history of present illness
HBP	high blood pressure	HPV	human papilloma virus
HBsAg	hepatitis antigen B	HR	Harrington rod/heart rate/hour
HBV	hepatitis B vaccine	HRT	hormone replacement therapy
HCFA	Health Care Financing Administration. See CMS	HS	heelstick/hour of sleep
		HSBG	heelstick blood gas
HCFA-1500	see CMS-1500	HSG	hysterosalpingogram
HCG	human chorionic gonadotropin	HSP	health service plan
HCl	hydrochloric acid	HSV	herpes simplex virus
HCPCS	Healthcare Common Procedural Coding System	ht.	height
		HTLV/III	human T-cell lymphotropic virus / three
Hct	hematocrit		
Hctz	hydrochlorothiazide	HTN	hypertension
HCVD	hypertensive cardiovascular disease	HVA	homovanillic acid
		Hx	history
HD	hip disarticulation	hypo	hypodermic injection
h.d.	at bedtime	IA	intra-arterial
HDL	high-density lipoproteins	IAB	intra-aortic balloon
HEDIS	Health Plan Employer Data and Information Set	IABC	intra-aortic balloon counterpulsation
HEENT	head, eyes, ears, nose, and throat	IABP	intra-aortic balloon pump
HGH	human growth hormone	IBS	irritable bowel syndrome
Hg/Hgb	hemoglobin	IBW	ideal body weight
HGSIL	high grade squamous intraepithelial lesion	ICCE	intracapsular cataract extraction
		ICD-9-CM	International Classification of Diseases, Ninth Revision, Clinical Modification
HH	hard of hearing		
HHA	home health agency		
HHS	Department of Health and Human Services	ICD-10	International Classification of Diseases, Tenth Revision
HIAA	hydroxyindolacetic acid	ICD-10-PCS	International Classification of Diseases, Tenth Revision, Procedural Coding System
Hib	Hemophilus influenzae vaccine		

ICF	intermediate care facility	IV	intravenous
ICH	intracranial/cerebral hemorrhage	IVC	inferior vena cava, intravenous cholangiogram
ICP	intracranial pressure		
ICS	intercostal space	IVF	in vitro fertilization
ICSH	interstitial cell stimulating hormone	IVH	intraventricular hemorrhage
		IVP	intravenous pyelogram
ICU	intensive care unit	JCAHO	Joint Commission on Accreditation of Healthcare Organizations
ID	infective dose		
I&D	incision and drainage		
Id31	radioactive iodine	JODM	juvenile onset diabetes mellitus
IDDM	insulin dependent diabetis mellitus	JVP	jugular venous pressure
IDH	isocitric dehydrogenase	K	potassium
IDM	infant of diabetic mother	Kcal	kilocalorie
Ig	immunoglobulin, gamma	KCL	potassium chloride
IH	infectious hepatitis	kg	kilogram
IM	internal medicine/intramuscular/ infectious mononucleosis	KO	keep open/knee orthosis
		KUB	kidneys, ureters, bladder
IMC	intermediate care	KVO	keep vein open
IME	independent medical evaluation	L	left/lumbar vertebrae
IMO	integrated multiple option	L&A	light and accommodation
IMV	intermittent mandatory ventilation	LA	left atrium
		LAD	left anterior descending
inc.	incision	LAP	leucine aminopeptidase
indep	independent	LAT	lateral
INF	inferior, infusion	LAV	lymphadenopathy associated virus
INH	inhalation solution		
INJ	injection	LAVH	laparascopic assisted vaginal hysterectomy
instill	instillation		
I&O	intake and output	LB	legbag
IOL	intraocular lens	LBB	left bundle branch
IOP	intraocular pressure	LBBB	left bundle branch block
IP	intraperitoneal/interphalangeal	LBP	lower back pain
IPA	individual practice association	LCAD	long chain acyl CoA dehydrogenase deficiency
IPD	intermittent peritoneal dialysis		
IPPB	intermittent positive pressure breathing	LCHAD	long chain 3-hydroxyacyl CoA dehydrogenase deficiency
IQ	intelligence quotient	LCP	licensed clinical psychologist
ISC	infant servo-control	LCSW	licensed clinical social worker
ISG	immune serum globulin	LD	lethal dose
ISN	integrated service network	LDH	lactate dehydrogenase
IT	intrathecal administration	LDL	low-density lipoproteins
ITP	idiopathic thrombocytopenia purpura	LE	lower extremity/lupus erythematosis
IU	international units	LEEP	loop electrocautery excision procedure
IUD	intrauterine device		
		LFT	liver function test

LGA	large for gestational age	MAP	mean arterial pressure
LGSIL	low grade squamous intraepithelial lesion	MASER	microwave amplification by stimulated emission of radiation
LH	luteinizing hormone	MBC	minimum bactericidal concentration/maximum breathing capacity
LHF	left heart failure		
LHR	leukocyte histamine release		
Li	lithium	MBD	minimal brain dysfunction
lido	lidocaine	mcg	microgram
liq.	solution (liquor)	MCAD	medium chain acyl CoA dehydrogenase deficiency
LKS	liver, kidneys, spleen		
LLL	left lower lobe	MCH	mean corpuscular hemoglobin
LLQ	left lower quadrant	MCI	Mild cognitive impairment
LMD	local medical doctor	MCL	midclavicular line
LML	left medio lateral position	MCP	metacarpophalangeal
LMP	last menstrual period	MCR	modified community rating
LMS	left mentum anterior position (chin)	MCT	mediastinal chest tube
		MCV	mean corpuscular volume
LMT	left mentum transverse position	MD	medical doctor
LOA	leave of absence	MD	muscular dystrophy/myocardial disease/manic depression
LOC	level of consciousness/loss of consciousness	MDC	major diagnostic category
		MDD	manic-depressive disorder
LOM	limitation of motion	MDS	Myelodysplastic syndrome
LOP	left occiput posterior position	Mec	meconium
LOT	left occiput transverse position	MED	minimal effective dose
LP	lumbar puncture	med/surg	Medical, surgical
LPM	liters per minute	Medigap	Medicare supplemental insurance
LR	lactated Ringer's/log roll	meds	medications
LS fusion	lumbar sacral fusion	Medsupp	Medicare supplemental insurance
LSA	left sacrum anterior position	MELAS	mitochondrial encephalopathy, lactic acidosis and stroke-like episodes
LSB	left sternal border		
LSO	lumbar sacral orthosis		
LT	left	mEq	milliequivalent
LTC	long term care	mEq/1	milliequivalent per liter
lul	left upper lobe	MERRF	myoclonus with epilepsy and with ragged red fibers
luq	left upper quadrant		
LUTS	lower urinary tract symptoms	MFD	minimum fatal dose
LV	left ventricle	MFT	muscle function test
lymphs	lymphocytes	mg	milligram
lytes	electrolytes	Mg	magnesium
M	manifest refraction/male	MHC	mental health clinic
M1	mitral first sound	MH/CD	mental health/chemical dependency
M2	mitral second sound		
MA1	volume respirator	MH/SA	mental health/substance abuse
MAC	maximum allowable cost	MI	myocardial infarction
MAD	monoamine oxidase (inhibitor)	min	minimum/minimal/minute

misce.	miscellaneous	NCQA	National Committee on Quality Assurance
ML	midline		
ml	milliliter	NCR	no cardiac resuscitation
MLC	midline catheter	NCV	nerve conduction velocity
mm	millimeter	NCVHS	National Committee on Vital Health Statistics
mmHg	millimeters of mercury		
MMPI	Minnesota Multiphasic Personality Inventory	NDC	national drug code
		NEC	necrotizing enterocolitis/not elsewhere classified
MMRV	measles, mumps, rubella vaccine		
MOD	multiple organ dysfunction	neg.	negative
MOM	milk of magnesia	NF	National Formulary
mono	monocyte/mononucleosis	NG	nasogastric
MPD	maximum permissible dose	NGU	nongonococcal urethritis
MR	mitral regurgitation	NIDDM	non-insulin dependent diabetes mellitus
MRA	magnetic resonance angiography		
MRI	magnetic resonance imaging	NJ	nasojejunal
MS	morphine sulfate/multiple sclerosis	NKA	no known allergies
		NKMA	no known medical allergies
MSLT	multiple sleep latency testing	NNR	new and nonofficial remedies
MSO	management service organization	NOS	not otherwise specified
MSRA	methicillin-resistant staphylococcus aureus	novem.	nine
		NP	neuropsychiatry/nurse practitioner
MSS	medical social services		
MSW	master's in social work	NP-CPAP	nasopharyngeal continuous positive airway pressure
MTD	right eardrum		
MTM	metamucil	NPN	Non-par Not Approved/nonprotein nitrogen
MTP	metatarsophalangeal		
MTS	left eardrum	n.p.o.	nothing by mouth
multip.	multipara - pregnant woman who has more than one child	npt	normal pressure and temperature
		NS	normal saline/not significant
		NSAID	nonsteroidal anti-inflammatory drug
MVP	mitral valve prolapse		
MWS	Mickety-Wilson syndrome	NSD	nominal standard dose
N	nitrogen	NSR	normal sinus rhythm
N2O	nitrous oxide	NST	nonstress test
Na	sodium	NSTEMI	non-ST elevation myocardial infarction
NaCl	sodium chloride (salt)		
NAD	no appreciable disease	NSVB	normal spontaneous vaginal bleeding
NAT	nonaccidental trauma		
NB	newborn	NSVD	normal spontaneous vaginal delivery
NBICU	newborn intensive care unit		
NBT	nitroblue tetrazolium	NT	nasotracheal/nontender
NCA	neurocirculatory asthenia	NTE	neutral thermal environment
NCHS	National Center for Health Statistics	NTP	normal temperature and pressure
		N&V	nausea and vomiting
NCPR	no cardiopulmonary resuscitation	o	no information

Abbreviations, Acronyms, and Symbols

O	blood type/oxygen	PAB	premature atrial beats
O2	oxygen	PAC	pre-admission certification
OA	open access	PAC	premature atrial contraction
OA	osteoarthritis	PACU	post anesthesia care unit
OAG	open angle glaucoma	PAD	pulmonary artery diastolic
OB	obstetrics	PAP	Papanicolaou test or smear/pulmonary artery pressure
OB-GYN	obstetrics and gynecology		
OC	open crib/oral contraceptive/office call	Par	participating provider
		PAR	post anesthesia recovery/parenteral
OCT	ornithine carbamyl transterase/oxytocin challenge test		
		para	along side of/number of pregnancies, as para 1, 2, 3, etc
octo.	eight		
o.d.	right eye	PARR	post anesthesia recovery room
OFC	occipitofrontal circumference	part. vic.	in divided doses
oint	ointment	PAT	paroxysmal atrial tachycardia
OJ	orange juice	path	pathology
o.m.	every morning/otitis media	PBA	pseudobulbar affect
OMS	oralmaxillary surgery	PBI	protein-bound iodine
OMT	osteopathic manipulation therapy	PC	packed cells
o.n.	every night	p.c.	after eating
ONH	optic nerve head	PCA	patient controlled analgesia
O&P	ova and parasites	PCD	polycystic disease
OPD	outpatient department	PCG	phonocardiogram
OPG	oculoplethysmography	PCN	penicillin
ophth	ophthalmology	PCN	primary care network
OPV	oral polio vaccine	PCP	primary care physician
OR	operating room	PCPM	per contract per month
ORIF	open reduction internal fixation	PCTA	percutaneous transluminal angioplasty
ortho.	orthopedics		
o.s.	left eye	PCV	packed cell volume
os, oris	mouth	PCW	pulmonary capillary wedge
OSA	obstructive sleep apnea	PD	postural drainage/Parkinson's disease
OST	oxytocin stress test		
OT	occupational therapy	PDA	patent ductus arteriosus
OTC	over-the-counter	PE	physical examination/pulmonary embolism/pulmonary edema
OTD	organ tolerance dose		
OTH	other routes of administration	PEC	pre-existing condition
o.u.	each eye, both eyes	Peds	pediatrics
ov.	ovum/office visit	PEG	pneumoencephalogram
OW	open ward	PEN	parenteral and enteral nutrition
oz.	ounce	PENS	percutaneous electrical nerve stimulation
P	plan/after/pulse, phosphorus		
P2	pulmonic 2nd sound	PERRLA	pupils equal, regular, reactive to light and accommodation
PA	physician assistant/posteroanterior/pulmonary artery		
		PET	positron emission tomography
		PFC	persistent fetal circulation

PFT	pulmonary function test	PREs	progressive resistive exercises
PG	prostaglandin	preg	pregnant
PH	past history	previa	placenta previa
PharmD	Doctor of Pharmacy	primip	primipara - a woman having her first child
pH	potential of hydrogen		
PI	present illness	p.r.n.	as needed for
PICC	peripherally inserted central catheter	PRO	professional (or peer) review organization
PID	pelvic inflammatory disease	PROM	premature rupture of membranes
PKU	phenylketonuria	PSA	prostate specific antigen
PMG	primary medical group	PSP	phenolsulfonphthalein
PMHx	past medical history	PsyD	Doctor of Psychology
PMI	point of maximum intensity	PT	physical therapy/prothrombin time
PMPM	per member per month		
PMPY	per member per year	Pt	patient/prothrombin time
PMN	polymorphonuclear neutrophil leukocytes	PTA	prior to admission/percutaneous transluminal angioplasty
PMS	premenstrual syndrome	PTB	patellar tendon bearing (cast)
PNC	premature nodal contraction	PTCA	percutaneous transluminal coronary angioplasty
PND	paroxysmal nocturnal dyspnea/ post nasal drip	PTH	parathyroid hormone
PNS	peripheral nervous system	PTSD	post-traumatic stress disorder
p/o	by mouth	PTT	partial thromboplastin time
PO	(per os) by mouth/post operative	PUD	peptic ulcer discase
POD	post operative day	pulv.	powder
polys	polymorphonuclear neutrophil leukocytes	PVC	premature ventricular contraction
		PVD	premature ventricular depolarization
POR	problem oriented record		
POS	place of service/point of service/ point of sale	PVL	paraventricular leukomalasia
		Px	prognosis
pos.	positive	Q.	every
post or PM	postmortem exam or autopsy	q.2h	every two hours
PP	postprandial	q.a.m.	every morning
p.p.	near point of visual accommodation	q.d.	every day
		q.h.	every hour
PPD	percussion and postural drainage	q.h.s.	every night
PPH	post partum hemorrhage	q.i.d.	four times daily
PPO	preferred provider organization	q.n.	every night
PPP	protamine paracoagulation	q.o.d.	every other day
p.r.	far point of visual accommodation/through the rectum	q.q.h.	every four hours
		QA	quality assurance
		QM	quality management
pr	per return	qns	quantity not sufficient
PRBC	packed red blood cells	qs	quantity sufficient
PRES	posterior reversible encephalopathy syndrome	quotid	daily

Abbreviations, Acronyms, and Symbols

R	respiration/right atrium	ROM	range of motion
r	roentgen units (x-rays)	ROP	right occiput posterior position
R&C	reasonable and customary	ROS	review of systems
R,R,& E	round, regular, and equal	RPG	retrograde pyelogram
R/O	rule out	RR	recovery room
RA	rheumatoid arthritis/refractory anemia	RRA	registered record administrator
		RRR	regular rate and rhythm
RAEB-1	refractory anemia w/excess blasts-1	RS	reducing substances
		RSV	respiratory syncytial virus
RAEB-2	refractory anemia w/excess blasts-2	RT	recreational therapist/respiratory therapist/resting tracing/right
RARS	refractory anemia w/ringed sideroblasts	RUL	right upper lobe
		ruq	right upper quadrant
RBB	right bundle branch	RV	right ventricle
RBBB	right bundle branch block	Rx	take (prescription; treatment)
RBC	red blood cell	RxN	reaction
RBOW	ruptured bag of water	s	without
RBRVS	resource based relative value scale	s.c.	subcutaneous
RCD	relative cardiac dullness	s.l.	under the tongue, sublingual
RCMD	refractory cytopenia w/ multilineage dysplasia	S.O.S.	if necessary (si opus sit)
		S/P	status post
RCMD-RS	refractory cytopenia w/ multilineage dysplasia and ringed sideroblasts	SAH	subarachnoid hemorrhage
		SALT	serum alanine aminotransferase
		SAST	serum aspartate aminotransferase
RDS	respiratory distress syndrome	SB	sinus bradycardia
REM	rapid eye movement	SBFT	small bowel follow through
RESA	radial cryosurgical ablation	S-C disease	sickle cell hemoglobin-c disease
resp	respiration, respiratory	SCAD	short chain acyl CoA dehydrogenase deficiency
Retro	retrospective rate derivation		
rev.	revise, revision	SCI	spinal cord injury
Rh neg	Rhesus factor negative	SCID	severe combined immunodeficiency
Rh	Rhesus		
RHD	rheumatic heart disease	SCR	standard class rate
RHF	right heart failure	sed rate	sedimentation rate of erythrocytes
RIA	radioimmunoassay	SEM	systolic ejection murmur
RL	Ringer's lactate	sex	six
RLE	right lower extremity	SG	Swan-Ganz
RLF	rentrolental fibroplasia	SGA	small for gestational age
RLL	right lower lobe	SGOT	serum glutamic oxaloacetic acid
rlq	right lower quadrant	SH	social history
RLS	restless legs syndrome	SHBG	sex hormone binding globulin
RML	right middle lobe	SIADH	syndrome of inappropriate antidiuretic hormone
RN	registered nurse		
RNA	ribonucleic acid	SIDS	sudden infant death syndrome
ROA	right occiput anterior position	sine	without

SISI	short increment sensitivity index	TB	tuberculosis
SLE	systemic lupus erythematosus	TBA	to be arranged
SMI	supplementary medical insurance program	TBG	thyroxine/thyroid binding globulin
SNF	skilled nursing facility	TBI	total body irradiation
SNS	sympathetic nervous system	TBSA	total body surface area
SOAP	subjective objective assessment plan	TC&DB	turn, cough, and deep breathe
		Td	tetanus
SOB	shortness of breath	TEFRA	Tax Equity and Fiscal Responsibility Act
sol.	solution		
SOP	standard operation procedure	temp	temperature
SPD	summary plan description	TENS	transcutaneous electrical nerve stimulation
SQ	status quo/subcutaneous		
SROM	spontaneous rupture of membranes	TFT	transfer factor test
		THA	total hip arthroplasty
ss	half	Thal	Thalassemia
ST	sinus tachycardia	THC	tetrahydrocannabinol
staph	staphylococcus	TI	tricuspid insufficiency
stat	immediately	TIA	transient ischemic attack
STD	sexually transmitted disease	TKA	total knee arthroplasty
STEMI	ST elevation myocardial infarction	TM	tympanic membrane
STH	somatotrophic hormone	TMJ	temporomandibular joint
strep	streptococcus	TNS	transcutaneous nerve stimulator/stimulation
STS	serology test for syphilis		
STSG	split thickness skin graft	TO	telephone order
STU	skin test unit	TOA	tubo-ovarian abscess
subcu	subcutaneous	TORCH	Toxoplasmosis, Other (includes syphilis), Rubella, Cytomegalo virus, and Herpes virus
supp	suppository		
Sv	scalp vein		
SVC	service	TP	total protein
SVCS	superior vena cava syndrome	TPN	total parenteral nutrition
Sx	sign/symptom	TPR	temperature, pulse, respiration
T	temperature/tender/thoracic vertebrae	Tr	tinctura, tincture/trace
		TRALI	transfusion-related acute lung injury
T&A	tonsils and adenoids		
t.i.d.	three times daily	TRAM	transverse rectus abdominos musculocutaneous
T3	triiodothyronine		
T4	thyroxine	trans	transverse
TAA	tumor-associated antigen	TRF	thyrotropin releasing factor
TAH	total abdominal hysterectomy	TRH	thyrotropin releasing hormone
TAR	thrombocytopenia with absent radii syndrome	Ts	tension by Schiotz
		TSA	tumor specific antigen
TAT	tetanus antitoxin/turnaround time	TSD	Tay-Sachs disease
		TSE	testicular self-exam
Tb	tubercule bacillus	TSH	thyroid stimulating hormone
		TSS	toxic shock syndrome

Abbreviations, Acronyms, and Symbols

TTN	transient tachypnea of newborn	VIP	vasoactive intestinal peptide
TULIP	transurethral ultrasound guided laser induced prostate	Vit	vitamin (followed by specific letter)
		VLCAD	very long chain acyl CoA dehydrogenase deficiency
TUR	transurethral resection		
TURP	transurethral resection of prostate	VO	verbal order
Tx	treatment	VO2	maximum oxygen consumption
U	unit	VP	vasopressin/voiding pressure
U&C	usual and customary	VPC	ventricular premature contraction
U/A	urinalysis	VPRC	volume of packed red cells
UAC	umbilical artery catheter/ catheterization	VS	vital signs/vesicular sound
		VSD	ventricular septal defect
UB-92	Uniform Billing Code of 1992	vv	veins
UC	unit clerk	w/HSBH	warmed heelstick blood gas
UCHD	usual childhood diseases	WB	whole blood
UCR	usual, customary and reasonable	WBC	white blood count
UE	upper extremity	WC	wheelchair
UFR	uroflowmetry	WCC	well child care
UGI	upper gastrointestinal	WD	well developed
UMN	upper motor neuron	W-D	wet to dry (dressings)
UPIN	universal physician identification number	WHO	World Health Organization
		WLS	wet lung syndrome
UPP	urethra pressure profile	WN	well nourished
UR	utilization review	WNL	within normal limits
ur.	Urine	Wt	weight
UR/QA	utilization review/quality assurance	x	except
		YTD	year-to-date
URI	upper respiratory infection	ZIFT	zygote intrafallopian transfer
URN	utilization review nurse		
US	unstable spine/ultrasound		
UTI	urinary tract infection		
UV	ultraviolet light		
UVC	umbilical vein catheter		
V Fib	ventricular fibrillation		
V tach	ventricular tachycardia		
VA	Veterans Administration		
Va	visual acuity		
VBAC	vaginal birth after cesarean		
VC	vena cava		
VCG	vectorcardiogram		
VD	venereal disease		
VDH	valvular disease of the heart		
VDRL	venereal disease report		
VEP	visual evoked potential		
VF	visual field/ventricular fibrillation		
VIN	vulvar intraepithelial neoplasia		

Anatomy Charts

Skeletal System

Lymphatic System

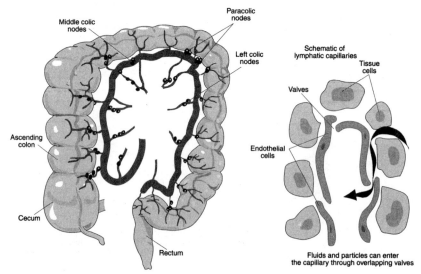

Lymphatic drainage of the colon follows blood supply

Fluids and particles can enter the capillary through overlapping valves

Endocrine System

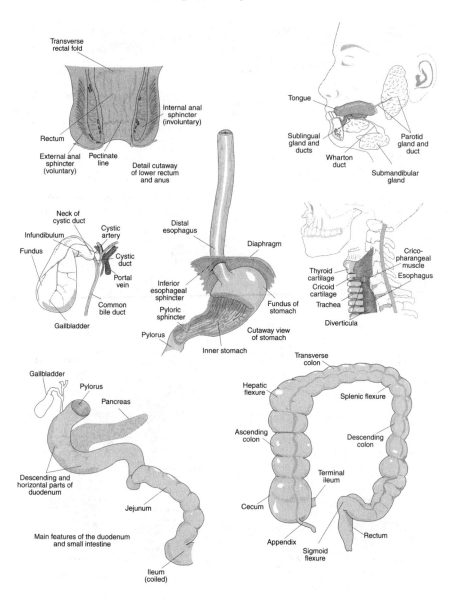

Digestive System

Nervous System

Circulatory System: Arterial

Circulatory System: Venous

Urogenital Tracts

Respiratory System

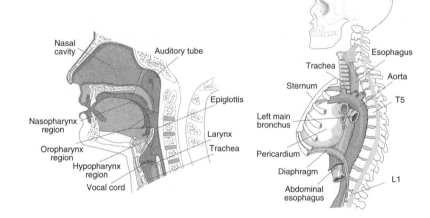

001–139

Infectious and Parasitic Diseases

This section of ICD-9-CM includes communicable diseases, as well as diseases of unknown origin but possibly due to infectious organisms. Infective organisms classified to this chapter include bacteria, chlamydia, fungi, helminths, mycoplasmas, protozoans, rickettsias, and viruses. The diseases may be further divided in ICD-9-CM by anatomic site.

Infectious and parasitic agents live in soil, water, and in the air — virtually everywhere. When these agents infect a host, there are three possible outcomes. The host's immune system can successfully defeat the infective agent. In this outcome, the host may test positive for exposure to the infective agent, but show no symptoms of active disease. In the second outcome, the host can lose ground against the agent, and an equalized state in which the host cannot eradicate the low-grade infection stabilizes. This is generally considered a chronic condition. In its acute form of infection, the infective agent can prevail, causing a multiplication of organisms and an overwhelming infection in the patient. Care must be taken to determine the status of the host before assigning codes. A patient testing positive for tuberculosis, for instance, but exhibiting no symptoms of active disease, would be classified to 795.5 *Nonspecific reaction to tuberculin skin test without active tuberculosis*, rather than to an active TB infection in the 010-018 (active tuberculosis) codes.

In some cases, infectious and parasitic diseases are classified by anatomical site rather than source of infection and found in other chapters of ICD-9-CM. Examples of this include pneumonia and other respiratory infections (460-466), influenza (487), and certain other localized infections. Also, codes reporting contact with infectious diseases, suspected carriers of infectious diseases, and prophylactic vaccination against infectious disease can be found in the supplementary classification of factors influencing health status (V01-V06).

001–009   Intestinal Infectious Diseases

001   Cholera

Cholera is an infection of the entire bowel due to *Vibrio cholerae* and presents with profuse diarrhea, cramps, and vomiting. It is spread through the ingestion of food or water contaminated with feces of an infected person. Cholera is endemic to parts of Asia, Africa, the Middle East, and also portions of the Gulf Coast of the United States. In endemic areas, outbreaks are usually limited to warm seasons. If the infection is imported to other locales, an outbreak can occur in any season.

Symptoms of cholera can be mild or life-threatening. Hypovolemia poses the greatest risk, as it can lead to severe metabolic acidosis and possibly renal tubular necrosis. Cholera responds to antibiotics, and with treatment, the mortality rate from cholera is less than one percent.

A toxic effect of antimony is called "antimonial cholera," but has no relation to a *V. cholerae* infection.

001.0	Cholera due to Vibrio cholerae — *Inaba, Ogawa, Hikojima serotypes; classical*
001.0	Cholera due to Vibrio cholerae — *Inaba, Ogawa, Hikojima serotypes; classical*
001.1	Cholera due to Vibrio cholerae el tor — *commonly less severe or asymptomatic*
001.9	Unspecified cholera — *unknown whether V. cholerae or V. cholerae el tor*

Coding Clarification

Antimonial cholera is reported with 985.4. Report carrier or suspected carrier of cholera with V02.0, and exposure to cholera with V01.0. Vaccination against cholera is reported with V03.0.

002 Typhoid and paratyphoid fevers

Typhoid fever is a systemic bacterial disease caused by the unique human strain of salmonella, *Salmonella typhi*. Outbreaks of typhoid are rare, because most of the cases are acquired during foreign travel to underdeveloped countries. Paratyphoid is similar in presentation to typhoid, though usually milder, caused by any of several organisms: *S. paratyphi* (paratyphoid A), *S. schottmulleri* (paratyphoid B), or *S. hirschfeldii* (paratyphoid C). The means of infection, clinical course, pathology, and treatment are similar to those for typhoid.

Typhoid and paratyphoid cause high fever, abdominal pain, and rash. Intestinal hemorrhage may occur in severe cases of typhoid. The bacilli are generally transmitted by the ingestion of food or water that is contaminated with feces from an infected person. While typhoid and paratyphoid A are strictly human diseases, paratyphoid B and C have been found in other animals and fowl. Contamination of food and water by infected animals or fowl can spread paratyphoid B and C. In either case, the organism moves through the gastrointestinal tract and enters the bloodstream through the lymphatic system.

002.0	Typhoid fever — *Widal negative*
002.1	Paratyphoid fever A — *serotype paratyphi A*
002.2	Paratyphoid fever B — *serotype schottmulleri*
002.3	Paratyphoid fever C — *serotype hirschfeldii*
002.9	Unspecified paratyphoid fever — *unknown paratyphoid serotype*

Coding Clarification

Report a carrier or suspected carrier of typhoid with V02.1 and vaccination against typhoid with V03.1. When typhoid presents with specific manifestations, report those manifestations secondary to the typhoid infection (endocarditis, 421.1; pneumonia, 484.8; perichondritis, 478.71; osteomyelitis, 730.8x; spinal inflammation, 720.81).

003 Other salmonella infections

This classification is called "other" salmonella infections because typhoid and paratyphoid infections are caused by strains of salmonella. This classification includes all other salmonellas — more than 1,500 serotypes — except congenital salmonella. Salmonella remains a significant health problem in the United States. About 85 percent of salmonella infections present as gastroenteritis. The other 15 percent present as septicemia or as another infectious disease.

Salmonella gastroenteritis, also known as enteritis, is caused by the ingestion of contaminated foods. Meat, poultry, raw milk, and eggs are the most common sources. Other reported sources include infected pet turtles or lizards, infected dyes, or contaminated marijuana. Immunosuppressed patients are most susceptible to localized salmonella infection.

003.0	Salmonella gastroenteritis — *gastrointestinal infection*
003.1	Salmonella septicemia — *bloodstream infection*
003.20	Unspecified localized salmonella infection — *unknown localized site*
003.21	Salmonella meningitis — *infection of membranes of brain/spinal cord*
003.22	Salmonella pneumonia — *infection of lungs*
003.23	Salmonella arthritis — *infection of joint*
003.24	Salmonella osteomyelitis — *infection of bone*
003.29	Other localized salmonella infections — *other localized site*
003.8	Other specified salmonella infections — *other salmonella infection*
003.9	Unspecified salmonella infection

Coding Clarification

A carrier or suspected carrier of salmonella (other than typhoid or paratyphoid infections) is reported with V02.3.

004 Shigellosis

Shigellosis is a bacterium that causes an acute infection of the bowel with fever, irritability, drowsiness, anorexia, nausea, vomiting, diarrhea, abdominal pain, and distension. Blood, pus, and mucus are found in the stool. Ingestion of food contaminated by feces of infected individuals is the most common source of infection. Incubation period is one to four days.

There are four species in the *Shigella* genus and they differ according to their biochemical reactions. All cause dysentery in humans and some primates.

004.0	Shigella dysenteriae — *subgroup A, severe dysenteria; type 1 can be fatal in children; Schmitz bacillus, Bacillus dysenteriae or Bacterium dysenteriae*
004.1	Shigella flexneri — *subgroup B; Shigella paradysenteriae and Flexner's bacillus*
004.2	Shigella boydii — *subgroup C; tropical locales, causing severe diarrhea*
004.3	Shigella sonnei — *subgroup D, milder dysentery; Sonne-Duval bacillus or Bacterium sonnei.*
004.8	Other specified shigella infections — *other than A,B,C,D*
004.9	Unspecified shigellosis — *unknown shigella infection*

Coding Clarification
Carrier or suspected *Shigella* carrier is reported with V02.3.

005 Other food poisoning (bacterial)
Food poisoning as reported with a code from category 005 reports the ingestion of bacteria that leads to gastrointestinal infection.

Staphylococcal enterotoxin is a common cause of food poisoning that can occur when an infected food handler introduces the staph into egg, milk, or meat products. The infection multiplies in the protein-rich media. An acute bout of diarrhea and vomiting usually occurs within a few hours of ingestion, and resolves within several hours. Hypovolemia poses the greatest risk to the elderly, the young, and the immunosuppressed, but this form of food poisoning rarely is fatal.

Clostridium botulinum is a neurotoxic bacterium and ingestion of contaminated food leads to optic neurology symptoms including diplopia, loss of accommodation, or blepharoptosis. Gastrointestinal symptoms including vomiting and diarrhea may precede neurological symptoms. No fever is present. Improperly canned food is the most common source of botulism. With treatment, the mortality rate of botulism is still significant although at less than 10 percent.

Food poisoning by *V. vulnificus* is the result of eating raw seafood. Resulting gastroenteritis can be severe and may be fatal to persons with liver disease.

Bacillus cereus (005.89) is commonly found in soil, milk, and dried food such as cereals, herbs, and spices. Meat pies, fried rice, and puddings are frequently implicated in outbreaks.

Botulism is a muscle-paralyzing disease caused by a toxin made by the bacterium *Clostridium botulinum*.

There are three main types of botulism:

- Food-borne botulism occurs when a person ingests pre-formed toxin that leads to illness within a few hours to days. Food-borne botulism is a public health emergency because the contaminated food may still be available to persons other than the patient. Food-borne botulism can occur in all age groups. With food-borne botulism, symptoms begin within six hours to two weeks (most commonly between 12 and 36 hours) after eating toxin-containing food. Symptoms of botulism include double vision, blurred vision, drooping eyelids, slurred speech, difficulty swallowing, dry mouth, muscle weakness that always descends through the body: shoulders are affected, then upper arms, lower arms, thighs, calves, etc. Paralysis of breathing muscles can cause a person to stop breathing and die, unless assistance with breathing (mechanical ventilation) is provided.
- Infant botulism occurs in a small number of susceptible infants each year who harbor *C. botulinum* in their intestinal tract.
- Wound botulism occurs when wounds are infected with *C. botulinum*, which secretes the toxin.

The Centers for Disease Control (CDC) maintains a supply of antitoxin against botulism. The antitoxin is effective in reducing the severity of symptoms if administered early in the course of the disease. Most patients eventually recover after weeks to months of supportive care.

005.0	Staphylococcal food poisoning — Staphylococcal toxemia due to food
005.1	Botulism — *Clostridium botulinum*
005.2	Food poisoning due to Clostridium perfringens (C. welchii) — *enteritis necroticans*
005.3	Food poisoning due to other Clostridia — *other or unknown*
005.4	Food poisoning due to Vibrio parahaemolyticus — *from fish; common to Japan*
005.81	Food poisoning due to Vibrio vulnificus — *severe enteritis from seafood; may progress to septicemia*
005.89	Other bacterial food poisoning — *Bacillus cereus*
005.9	Unspecified food poisoning

Coding Clarification
C. perfringens is commonly found in soil, air, and water. When the bacterium contaminates meat, it forms spores that cause mild gastroenteritis in type A or severe, life-threatening gastroenteritis in type C. Both are reported with 005.2.

C. perfringens is commonly found in soil, air, and water. When the bacterium contaminates meat, it forms spores that cause mild gastroenteritis in type A or severe, life-threatening gastroenteritis in type C. Both are reported with 005.2.

Report 005.1 *Botulism* for food poisoning by *C. botulinum* if botulism was contracted as a result of terrorist acts. E997.1 *Injury due to biological warfare* may be reported in addition to code rubric 005.1. If there is only a suspicion that the patient has been exposed, report V74.8 *Special screening for other specified bacterial and spirochetal diseases* to report the medical necessity of botulism testing.

006 Amebiasis
There are 50 million annual cases of amebiasis worldwide, with 40,000 to 50,000 deaths attributed to amebiasis annually.

Amebiasis is most common in tropical areas where crowded living conditions and poor sanitation exist. Africa, Latin America, Southeast Asia, and India have significant health problems associated with amebiasis. In amebiasis, protozoa can live in the large intestine without causing symptoms or it can invade the colon wall causing colitis, acute dysentery, or chronic diarrhea. The infection may spread through the blood to the liver, and, rarely, to the lungs, brain, or other organs.

Transmission occurs through ingestion of feces in contaminated food or water, use of human feces as fertilizer, or person-to-person contact. Malnutrition and alcoholism predispose a person to more severe disease, as does immunosuppression. Recent travel to a tropical region is a risk factor. In the United States, immunosuppressed populations, people living in institutions, people with disabilities, and male homosexuals are considered higher risk groups, although the infection rate in the United States is low at less than 1 percent.

006.0	Acute amebic dysentery without mention of abscess — *sudden, severe dysentery*
006.1	Chronic intestinal amebiasis without mention of abscess — *persistent dysentery*
006.2	Amebic nondysenteric colitis — *inflamed colon but no dysentery*
006.3	Amebic liver abscess — *liver infection*
006.4	Amebic lung abscess — *lung with or without liver infection*
006.5	Amebic brain abscess — *brain with or without lung and/or liver*
006.6	Amebic skin ulceration — *cutaneous amebiasis*
006.8	Amebic infection of other sites — *including seminal vesicle, bladder, appendix or other site infection, ameboma*
006.9	Unspecified amebiasis — *unknown or unspecified*

Coding Clarification
Codes in the rubric 006 are used to report infection or ulceration due to *Entamoeba histolytica*. If the ameba is other than *E. histolytica,* report 007.8 instead. Meningoencephalitis due to *Naegleria gruber* is reported with 136.2. Carrier or suspected carrier of amebic disease is reported with V02.2.

007 Other protozoal intestinal diseases
Giardia lamblia is the most common intestinal parasite in the United States and is classified to this rubric. Giardiasis is an infection of the lumen of the small intestine, spread by contaminated food and water or by direct contact. Commonly, contaminated water from lakes or streams is a source of the disease. Most cases are asymptomatic, but those with symptoms experience diarrhea, nausea, lassitude, anorexia, and weight loss.

Cryptosporidiosis is usually transmitted person-to-person and the symptoms are mild and self-limited in a healthy population. However, cryptosporidiosis is frequently seen as an opportunistic infection in the acquired immune deficiency syndrome (AIDS), causing profound dehydration and electrolyte imbalances. There is no specific antibiotic therapy for cryptosporidiosis. Treatment consists of rehydration and electrolyte management.

007.0	Balantidiasis — *Balantidium coli infection*
007.1	Giardiasis — *Giardia lamblia, lambliasis infection*
007.2	Coccidiosis — *Isospora belli, Isospora hominis infection*
007.3	Intestinal trichomoniasis — *Trichomonas infection*
007.4	Cryptosporidiosis — *Cryptosporidium infection is self-limiting in immunocompetent cattle workers, debilitating in immunosuppressed patients* AHA: Q4, 1997, 30
007.5	Cyclosporiasis — *dysentery from Cyclospora infection* AHA: Q4, 2000, 38
007.8	Other specified protozoal intestinal diseases — *including chilomastigiasis, craigiasis*
007.9	Unspecified protozoal intestinal disease — *unknown*

Coding Clarification
In the case of an AIDS patient with cryptosporidiosis and volume depletion, report the AIDS first (042), followed by cryptosporidiosis (007.4) and volume depletion (276.50-276.52).

008 Intestinal infections due to other organisms
Intestinal infections caused by *Escherichia* coli are covered in the 008 rubric. The infections are classified by the degree of penetration into intestinal tissue.

008.00	Intestinal infection due to unspecified E. coli — *not otherwise specified* AHA: Q4, 1992, 17
008.01	Intestinal infection due to enteropathogenic E. coli — *inflammation of intestines* AHA: Q4, 1992, 17
008.02	Intestinal infection due to enterotoxigenic E. coli — *toxic reaction in intestinal mucosa, causing voluminous watery secretions* AHA: Q4, 1992, 17
008.03	Intestinal infection due to enteroinvasive E. coli — *infection penetrates intestinal mucosa* AHA: Q4, 1992, 17

Infectious and Parasitic Diseases

008.04	Intestinal infection due to enterohemorrhagic E. coli — *infection penetrates intestinal mucosa, causing ulceration and bleeding* **AHA:** Q4, 1992, 17		
008.09	Intestinal infection due to other intestinal E. coli infections **AHA:** Q4, 1992, 17		
008.1	Intestinal infection due to Arizona group of paracolon bacilli — *Arizona (bacillus)*		
008.2	Intestinal infection due to aerobacter aerogenes — *Enterobacter aerogenes*		
008.3	Intestinal infections due to proteus (mirabilis) (morganii) — *Morganella morganii, Salmonella morganii*		
008.41	Intestinal infections due to staphylococcus		
008.42	Intestinal infections due to pseudomonas **AHA:** Q2, 1989, 10		
008.43	Intestinal infections due to campylobacter		
008.44	Intestinal infections due to yersinia enterocolitica		
008.45	Intestinal infections due to clostridium difficile		
008.46	Intestinal infections due to other anerobes		
008.47	Intestinal infections due to other gram-negative bacteria		
008.49	Intestinal infection due to other organisms **AHA:** Q1, 1988, 6; Q2, 1989, 10		
008.5	Intestinal infection due to unspecified bacterial enteritis		
008.61	Intestinal infection, enteritis due to rotavirus		
008.62	Intestinal infection, enteritis due to adenovirus		
008.63	Intestinal infection, enteritis due to Norwalk virus		
008.64	Intestinal infection, enteritis due to other small round viruses (SRVs)		
008.65	Intestinal infection, enteritis due to calcivirus		
008.66	Intestinal infection, enteritis due to astrovirus		
008.67	Intestinal infection, enteritis due to enterovirus not elsewhere classified		
008.69	Intestinal infection, enteritis due to other viral enteritis **AHA:** Q1, 2003, 10		
008.8	Intestinal infection due to other organism, NEC		

Coding Clarification
Infections or food poisoning caused by other agents are reported with codes in the 005 rubric.

Gastroenteritis and enteritis due to a specified virus is coded to 008.61-008.69.

Use 008.69 to report a specified virus when it is not elsewhere classified or 008.8 to report the infection when it is not elsewhere classified or otherwise specified.

009 Ill-defined intestinal infections
Colitis is the inflammation of the colon, while enteritis is the inflammation of the intestine, especially small intestine. Gastroenteritis is inflammation of the mucous membranes of the stomach and intestines. Diarrhea describes copious, loose bowels without evidence of infection or inflammation of the gastrointestinal tract.

009.0	Infectious colitis, enteritis, and gastroenteritis — *known to be infectious* **AHA:** Q2, 1988, 10; Q3, 1999, 4
009.1	Colitis, enteritis, and gastroenteritis of presumed infectious origin — *presumed to be infectious* **AHA:** Q3, 1999, 6
009.2	Infectious diarrhea — *known to be infectious*
009.3	Diarrhea of presumed infectious origin — *presumed to be infectious* **AHA:** Nov-Dec, 1987, 7

Coding Clarification
Use this series of codes only when more specific information in not available. If the source of infection is known, use an infective enteritis code from the 001-008 series. Noninfective colitis, enteritis, or gastroenteritis is reported with codes in the 555-558 series, and diarrhea due to noninfectious causes is reported with 787.91. Allergic diarrhea is reported with 558.3; nervous diarrhea with 306.4.

Coding Scenario
An acute lymphoblastic leukemia patient presents with extreme abdominal pain, having finished his course of chemotherapy the previous week. His laboratory findings are as follows: profound neutropenia- white count of.2, absolute neutrophil count of 20. The hematologist has diagnosed acute neutropenic enterocolitis due to chemotherapy. Abdominal surgery is not required.

Code assignment: The physician must be queried as to the nature of the enterocolitis- infectious vs. noninfectious.

If the enteritis is infectious, the codes are as follows: 288.03 *Drug induced neutropenia;* 009.1 *Colitis, enteritis, and gastroenteritis, of presumed infectious origin;* E933.1 *Adverse effect of antineoplastic drugs;* and 204.00 *Lymphoid leukemia, acute, without mention of remission.*

010–018 Tuberculosis
Tuberculosis (TB) is a bacterial infection that usually attacks the lungs, but which may also affect other organs. The disease is caused by *Mycobacterium tuberculosis*. TB is transmitted by inhaling air droplets exhaled by an infected person, or sometimes the infection is absorbed through the skin. Medical technicians handling TB specimens may contract the disease through skin wounds. TB

has also been reported in people who have received tattoos or circumcisions in nonsterile conditions.

Symptoms of TB include coughing, chest pain, shortness of breath, loss of appetite, weight loss, fever, chills, and fatigue. Children and people with weakened immune systems are the most susceptible to TB.

A person may become infected with TB bacteria and not develop the disease. The immune system may destroy the bacteria completely. Only 5 to 10 percent of people infected with TB actually become sick.

010 Primary tuberculous infection

Primary TB is the stage of the disease absent of any noticeable symptoms. The disease is not contagious in the early stage. Macrophages, immune cells that detect and destroy foreign matter, ingest the TB bacteria and transport them to the lymph nodes where they may be inhibited, destroyed, or may multiply.

The following fifth-digit subclassification is for use with categories 010-018:

0   unspecified
1   bacteriological or histological examination not done
2   bacteriological or histological examination unknown (at present)
3   tubercle bacilli found (in sputum) by microscopy
4   tubercle bacilli not found (in sputum) by microscopy, but found by bacterial culture
5   tubercle bacilli not found by bacteriological examination, but tuberculosis confirmed histologically
6   tubercle bacilli not found by bacteriological or histological examination but tuberculosis confirmed by other methods (inoculation of animals)

010.0 [sth]   Primary tuberculous complex — *first infection, lung*
010.1 [sth]   Tuberculous pleurisy in primary progressive tuberculosis — *first infection, lung and lung lining*
010.8 [sth]   Other primary progressive tuberculosis infection — *primary site other than pulmonary*
010.9 [sth]   Primary tuberculous infection, unspecified — *unknown primary tuberculosis*

011 Pulmonary tuberculosis

If the bacteria multiply, active primary tuberculosis will develop along with typical symptoms of TB: coughing, night sweats, weight loss, and fever. A chest x-ray typically shows shadows or fluid collection between the lung and its lining.

If the bacteria are suppressed but not destroyed, they will be contained in a mass known as a granuloma or tubercle: a wall of immune cells around inactive bacteria to protect the body from infection. As long as the immune system remains strong, the TB bacteria remain walled off and inactive. The tubercle gradually collects calcium deposits to form a Ghon focus.

Initial tubercles in the lung usually heal, leaving permanent scars that appear as shadows in chest x-rays. At this primary stage of TB, the disease does not progress, but bacteria may remain dormant in the body for many years. If the immune system becomes weakened, the tubercle opens, releases the bacteria, and the infection may develop into secondary TB.

011.0 [sth]   Tuberculosis of lung, infiltrative — (Use additional code to identify any associated silicosis, 502) — *clusters of TB bacilli in lung*
011.1 [sth]   Tuberculosis of lung, nodular — (Use additional code to identify any associated silicosis, 502) — *infiltration of TB leads to formation of nodules*
011.2 [sth]   Tuberculosis of lung with cavitation — (Use additional code to identify any associated silicosis, 502) — *further infiltration of TB leads to cavities*

AHA: For code 011.20: Q4, 1994, 36

011.3 [sth]   Tuberculosis of bronchus — (Use additional code to identify any associated silicosis, 502) — *clusters of TB bacilli in bronchial tissue*
011.4 [sth]   Tuberculous fibrosis of lung — (Use additional code to identify any associated silicosis, 502) — *TB cells in lungs surrounded by fibrous tissue*
011.5 [sth]   Tuberculous bronchiectasis — (Use additional code to identify any associated silicosis, 502) — *TB causes bronchial dilation and cough*
011.6 [sth]   Tuberculous pneumonia (any form) — (Use additional code to identify any associated silicosis, 502) — *TB causes inflammatory reaction of lung*
011.7 [sth]   Tuberculous pneumothorax — (Use additional code to identify any associated silicosis, 502) — *TB causes spontaneous rupture of lung tissue*
011.8 [sth]   Other specified pulmonary tuberculosis — (Use additional code to identify any associated silicosis, 502) — *not elsewhere classified*
011.9 [sth]   Unspecified pulmonary tuberculosis — (Use additional code to identify any associated silicosis, 502) — *unknown type*

012 Other respiratory tuberculosis

Rubric 012 is used to report tuberculosis of respiratory sites other than the lung without lung involvement, such as the pleura; intrathoracic lymph nodes; trachea or bronchus alone; larynx (including the glottis); and the mediastinum, nasopharynx, nose, or sinus.

Tuberculosis of other respiratory sites, such as the nose, can be due to a primary or secondary infection with *Mycobacterium tuberculosis*.

A pleural effusion occurs after the initial infection. The result of a release of a small amount of tuberculoprotein within the lung into the plural space causing an inflammatory response and a resulting accumulation of fluid.

At the time of the initial infection, hilar and mediastinal lymph nodes become seeded with bacilli, and other lymph nodes may also become involved. The infection may progress to clinical significance, may become active at a late date, or may never become active.

012.0 ⌐sth Tuberculous pleurisy — *inflammation of lung lining*
012.1 ⌐sth Tuberculosis of intrathoracic lymph nodes — *hilar, mediastinal, tracheobronchial lymph infection*
012.2 ⌐sth Isolated tracheal or bronchial tuberculosis — *without lung involvement*
012.3 ⌐sth Tuberculous laryngitis — *infection of glottis*
012.8 ⌐sth Other specified respiratory tuberculosis — *mediastinum, nasopharynx, nose, or sinus infection, other*

013 Tuberculosis of meninges and central nervous system

Nearly all TB in the United States originates as a pulmonary disease, though before pasteurization, infection commonly occurred at other anatomical sites with the ingestion of contaminated milk or milk products. Today in the United States, sites other than the lung are considered secondary to pulmonary infection.

013.0 ⌐sth Tuberculous meningitis — *infection of cerebral or spinal meninges*
013.1 ⌐sth Tuberculoma of meninges — *enlarged tubercle in lining or brain or spinal cord*
013.2 ⌐sth Tuberculoma of brain — *enlarged tubercle in brain*
013.3 ⌐sth Tuberculous abscess of brain — *abscess of brain*
013.4 ⌐sth Tuberculoma of spinal cord — *enlarged tubercle in spinal cord*
013.5 ⌐sth Tuberculous abscess of spinal cord — *abscess of spinal cord*
013.6 ⌐sth Tuberculous encephalitis or myelitis — *inflammation of brain or spinal cord*
013.8 ⌐sth Other specified tuberculosis of central nervous system — *other CNS site*
013.9 ⌐sth Unspecified tuberculosis of central nervous system — *unknown CNS site*

014 Tuberculosis of intestines, peritoneum, and mesenteric glands

Infection of the intestinal tract by the tuberculin bacillus can occur through the blood, through swallowing the organisms from the pulmonary tract, or through penetration of the intestinal layers from granuloma or from other infected sites.

Wide-spread, intra-abdominal infection may result in peritonitis, which may present in an exudative form with ascites, or a fibrotic form with slight to no ascites but with intraperitoneal adhesions. Peritoneal tuberculosis is often associated with a concomitant pleural effusion.

014.0 ⌐sth Tuberculous peritonitis — *inflammation of the lining of the abdomen*
014.8 ⌐sth Tuberculosis of intestines, peritoneum, and mesenteric glands, other

015 Tuberculosis of bones and joints

Tuberculosis of the bone or joints is usually limited to cases in which the primary TB occurs during childhood. Sometimes, the symptoms do not present themselves for years. In joint disease, arthritis is present. In bone infection, bone may be destroyed. In Pott's disease, the patient may be asymptomatic until deformity occurs or vertebrae collapse.

015.0 ⌐sth Tuberculosis of vertebral column — (Use additional code to identify manifestation: 711.4, 720.81, 727.01, 730.8, 737.4) — *Pott's disease, sacrum, spine, vertebra, lordosis, scoliosis, intervertebral*
015.1 ⌐sth Tuberculosis of hip — (Use additional code to identify manifestation: 711.4, 727.01, 730.8) — *joint or bone infection*
015.2 ⌐sth Tuberculosis of knee — (Use additional code to identify manifestation: 711.4, 727.01, 730.8) — *joint or bone infection*
015.5 ⌐sth Tuberculosis of limb bones — (Use additional code to identify manifestation: 711.4, 727.01, 730.8) — *long bones, hands, feet, wrist, ankle, dactylitis*
015.6 ⌐sth Tuberculosis of mastoid — (Use additional code to identify manifestation: 711.4, 727.01, 730.8) — *mastoiditis*
015.7 ⌐sth Tuberculosis of other specified bone — (Use additional code to identify manifestation: 711.4, 727.01, 730.8) — *jaw, bony pelvis, shoulder blade, other bone*
015.8 ⌐sth Tuberculosis of other specified joint — (Use additional code to identify manifestation: 711.4, 727.01, 730.8) — *wrist, ankle, sacroiliac, shoulder, other joint*
015.9 ⌐sth Tuberculosis of unspecified bones and joints — (Use additional code to identify manifestation: 711.4, 727.01, 730.8) — *cartilage, ganglion, rheumatism, other synovitis or tenosynovitis*

016 Tuberculosis of genitourinary system

Code tuberculosis of the genitourinary system with the appropriate code from the following range, based on the specific organ affected.

016.0 ⌐sth Tuberculosis of kidney — (Use additional code to identify manifestation: 583.81, 590.81) — *renal, perinephritic*
016.1 ⌐sth Tuberculosis of bladder — *cystitis*
016.2 ⌐sth Tuberculosis of ureter — *ureter only*
016.3 ⌐sth Tuberculosis of other urinary organs — *urethra*

016.4 ⌐sth Tuberculosis of epididymis
016.5 ⌐sth Tuberculosis of other male genital organs —
(Use additional code to identify manifestation:
601.4, 608.81) — *bulbourethral gland, Cowper's
gland, penis, prepuce, prostate, scrotum,
spermatic cord, testis*
016.6 ⌐sth Tuberculous oophoritis and salpingitis —
fallopian tube, ovary
016.7 ⌐sth Tuberculosis of other female genital organs —
*broad ligament, cervix, endometrium, placenta,
uterus*
016.9 ⌐sth Genitourinary tuberculosis, unspecified —
unknown genitourinary site

017 Tuberculosis of other organs

Code tuberculosis of other organs with the appropriate code from the following range, based on the specific organ affected.

017.0 ⌐sth Tuberculosis of skin and subcutaneous cellular
tissue — *cellulitis, colliquativa, cutis,
scrofuloderma*
017.1 ⌐sth Erythema nodosum with hypersensitivity
reaction in tuberculosis — *Bazin's disease,
erythema induratum, tuberculosis indurativa*
017.2 ⌐sth Tuberculosis of peripheral lymph nodes —
axilla, cervical, neck
017.3 ⌐sth Tuberculosis of eye — (Use additional code to
identify manifestation: 363.13, 364.11, 370.31,
370.59, 379.09) — *conjunctiva, globe, iris,
lacrimal apparatus, retina*
017.4 ⌐sth Tuberculosis of ear — *inner ear, middle ear;
excludes mastoid*
017.5 ⌐sth Tuberculosis of thyroid gland — *thyroid*
017.6 ⌐sth Tuberculosis of adrenal glands — *bronze
(Addison's) disease*
017.7 ⌐sth Tuberculosis of spleen — *spleen*
017.8 ⌐sth Tuberculosis of esophagus — *esophagus*
017.9 ⌐sth Tuberculosis of other specified organs — (Use
additional code to identify manifestation: 420.0,
422.0, 424.91) — *artery, breast, buccal cavity,
endocardium, muscle, palate, parotid,
parathyroid, pericardium, perineum, pituitary,
thymus, stomach, vein*

018 Miliary tuberculosis

Tuberculosis bacilli may be seeded to distant organs through the lymphatic or vascular system. Miliary tuberculosis is named for the pale, disseminated lesions that resemble millet seeds. Miliary tuberculosis is most commonly seen in bone marrow, eye, lymph nodes, liver, spleen, kidney, adrenal gland, prostate, seminal vesicle, fallopian tube, endometrium, or meninges. Affected organs may eventually develop progressive, isolated organ infection.

018.0 ⌐sth Acute miliary tuberculosis — *sudden, severe
onset*
018.8 ⌐sth Other specified miliary tuberculosis — *other*
018.9 ⌐sth Unspecified miliary tuberculosis — *unknown*

Coding Clarification

Some tuberculosis codes are found in other sections of ICD-9-CM. Congenital tuberculosis is reported with 771.2, and the late effects of tuberculosis are reported with codes in the 137 series. If an asymptomatic person tests positive for TB, report 795.5. Report exposure to TB without further information on tests or infection status with V01.1, and report the need for a BCG inoculation against TB with V03.2. Do not report personal history of tuberculosis (V12.01) in patients with active disease.

When coding tuberculosis of bones or joints, report the TB code first (015.xx), followed by codes that best describe the manifestation, such as arthropathy (subclassification 711.4), necrosis or osteitis (730.8x), or synovitis/tenosynovitis (727.01). In Pott's disease, also report any curvature of spine (737.43) or spondylitis (720.81).

When coding tuberculosis of the genitourinary system, report the TB code first (016.xx), followed by codes that best describe the manifestation, such as nephropathy (583.81), prostatitis (601.4), or pyelitis (590.81).

When coding tuberculosis of other organs, report the TB code first (017.xx), followed by codes that best describe the manifestation, such as episcleritis (379.09), myocarditis (422.0), or interstitial keratitis (370.59).

020–027 Zoonotic Bacterial Diseases

020 Plague

Plague, an acute infection caused by the bacillus *Yersinia pestis*, occurs in three forms among people: bubonic plague, pneumonic plague, and septicemic plague. All three varieties have been called "black death" because in untreated cases, respiratory failure precedes death by several hours, and during this time, the hypoxic victim's skin may turn deep purple. Plague responds well to modern antibiotics. In the United States, sporadic infections are seen primarily in the Southwest.

Bubonic plague is transmitted by the bite of insects that are normally rodent parasites. The most important of these insects is the rat flea *Xenopsylla cheopis*. Bubonic plague is characterized by buboes: enlarged, inflamed lymph nodes in the groin, armpit, or neck. Other symptoms include headache, fever, nausea, vomiting, and aching joints. Untreated, bubonic plague's fatality rate is 30 to 75 percent.

Infectious and Parasitic Diseases

Septicemic plague may be initiated by direct contact of contaminated hands, food, or objects with the mucous membranes of the nose or throat. Untreated, pneumonic plague's fatality rate is 95 percent; septicemic, nearly 100. In treated cases, the fatality drops to 10 percent or less.

Pneumonic plague is characterized by lung infection and, as a primary infection, is often transmitted by inhaling bacteria-carrying air droplets exhaled by an infected person. Secondary pneumonic plague begins as another form of plague before infecting the lungs.

Pneumonic plague occurs when *Y. pestis* infects the lungs. The first signs of illness in pneumonic plague are fever, headache, weakness, and cough productive of bloody or watery sputum. The pneumonia progresses over two days to five days and may cause septic shock and, without early treatment, death.

Person-to-person transmission of pneumonic plague occurs through respiratory droplets, which can only infect those who have face-to-face contact with the ill patient.

Early treatment of pneumonic plague is essential. Several antibiotics are effective, including streptomycin, tetracycline, and chloramphenicol.

There is no vaccine against plague. Prophylactic antibiotic treatment for seven days will protect persons who have had face-to-face contact with infected patients.

Complications of antibiotics may include nausea, diarrhea, CNS disturbance, local IV site reactions, and abnormalities of hepatic enzymes, eosinophilia, headache, rash, restlessness, vomiting, abdominal pain/discomfort, headache, rash, and restlessness. Code first the symptom of the adverse effect and then the E code for Adverse Effects of a Drug in Therapeutic Use.

020.0	Bubonic plague — *most common, with swollen lymph glands*
020.1	Cellulocutaneous plague — *inflammation and necrosis of the skin*
020.2	Septicemic plague — *infection in bloodstream*
020.3	Primary pneumonic plague — *plague infects lung first*
020.4	Secondary pneumonic plague — *infection spreads to lung*
020.5	Pneumonic plague, unspecified
020.8	Other specified types of plague
020.9	Unspecified plague

Coding Clarification

Rubric 020 is only used for patients with plague. If exposure to plague has been substantiated, report V01.89 *Contact with or exposure to other communicable diseases.* If there is only a suspicion that the patient has been exposed, report V74.8 *Special screening for other specified bacterial and spirochetal diseases* to report the medical necessity of plague testing.

Another code that may become appropriate is V03.3 *Prophylactic inoculation against plague.*

If plague was contracted as a result of terrorist acts, E997.1 *Injury due to biological warfare* may be reported in addition to the appropriate code from rubric 020.

If the patient is isolated for contact with plague, report V07.0 Isolation of individual after contact with infectious diseases.

Other coding issues may include reactions to vaccination, such as anaphylactic shock due to serum 999.4, and other serum reaction 999.5. See Complications, vaccination.

021 Tularemia

A sudden fever, chill, headache, myalgia, and fatigue characterize tularemia.

It is a fairly uncommon disease, seen in the United States mostly in Oklahoma, Missouri, and Alaska. The infective agent, *Francisella tularensis,* enters the body through a tick bite or by direct contact with the skin. The bacillus can penetrate unbroken skin, and can therefore be transmitted by handling tainted meat or cleaning wild game, usually rodents such as squirrels or rabbits.

Tularemia responds well to antibiotic treatment and, with treatment, death is rare. Without treatment, mortality of tularemia is about 5 percent. Once infected, the patient develops immunity.

021.0	Ulceroglandular tularemia — *lesion at cutaneous site of bacillus penetration*
021.1	Enteric tularemia — *intestinal infection*
021.2	Pulmonary tularemia — *infection of lung and/or bronchus*
021.3	Oculoglandular tularemia — *conjunctival infection with possible spread to cornea, lacrimal systems*
021.8	Other specified tularemia — *glandular or other*
021.9	Unspecified tularemia — *site unknown*

Coding Clarification

Tularemia codes are selected on the basis of site of initial infection: skin, lung, gastrointestinal system, eye, or other site.

To report prophylactic vaccination against tularemia, see V03.4.

022 Anthrax
AHA: Q4, 2002, 70

Anthrax infection can occur in three forms: cutaneous (skin), inhalation, and gastrointestinal. Symptoms vary according to the form of infection, but usually occur within seven days.

In most cases, the anthrax bacterium enters a cut or abrasion on the skin. This is called cutaneous anthrax. Skin infection begins as a raised itchy bump that resembles an insect bite. The bump develops into a vesicle and, from there, a painless ulcer, usually 1.0 centimeter to 3.0 centimeters in diameter, within 48 hours. Lymph glands in the adjacent area may swell. Not long afterward, the lesions turn black, a hallmark of skin anthrax, as tissue begins to die. About 20 percent of untreated cases of cutaneous anthrax will result in death. However, death is rare with drug therapy.

Pulmonary anthrax is caused by inhalation of the anthrax bacterium. It generally takes two to five days for symptoms to appear, though in some cases, spores lodged in the lungs may take up to 60 days to germinate. Initially, symptoms mimic those of the flu — fever, nausea, muscle aches, and cough — and after several days, as the immune system fails to rid the body of the bacteria, more severe signs appear, including difficulty breathing, high fever, and shock. Fatality is 90 percent if left untreated.

The intestinal form of anthrax is rare, and may follow the consumption of contaminated meat. Intestinal anthrax is characterized by an acute gastroenteritis progressing into septicemia.

Anthrax is caused by the bacterium *B. anthracis*, which once inside the body emerges from the dormant spore phase, begins to reproduce, and in the process of reproduction, produces toxins that can lead to organ failure. DNA analysis can determine the strain of anthrax in an outbreak and whether the strain has been genetically manipulated.

Pulmonary and cutaneous anthrax are the types of anthrax contracted in recent bioterrorism in the United States, with the pulmonary form most likely to result in death because the germs burrow into lung tissue, where they come in close contact with lymph vessels.

There are several types of lab tests that can detect the presence of anthrax, although no single screen can provide a definitive diagnosis. Culturing a sample taken from the mucous membranes, in the case of pulmonary anthrax, is the most conclusive way to confirm anthrax. An antibody-antigen test is another way to confirm anthrax and this test takes less time than the several days for confirmation through culture.

Antibiotics administered early are effective against the disease and, at the time of the bioterrorism, Cipro was the only medication available in the United States approved as an effective drug against anthrax due to the testing (on animals) the Food and Drug Administration (FDA) requires for labeling a product. The FDA has since fast-tracked approval for penicillin and doxycycline. A company manufacturing an anthrax vaccine for the U.S. military stopped its production in 1998, due to quality control standards cited by the FDA. In the wake of the attacks, the company has reapplied for approval, but in the interim, the federal government has been pushing two newer vaccines into clinical trials.

Complications of antibiotics may include nausea, diarrhea, CNS disturbance, local IV site reactions, and abnormalities of hepatic enzymes, eosinophilia, headache, rash, restlessness, vomiting, abdominal pain/discomfort, headache, rash, and restlessness.

022.0	Cutaneous anthrax — *infection through superficial wound*
022.1	Pulmonary anthrax — *infection in lungs*
022.2	Gastrointestinal anthrax — *acute gastrointestinal infection*
022.3	Anthrax septicemia — *infection in bloodstream*
022.8	Other specified manifestations of anthrax — *other site of infection*
022.9	Unspecified anthrax — *unknown site of infection*

Coding Clarification
Rubric 022 is used only in patients who have contracted anthrax. Do not use these codes for false positive tests or for negative tests in cases of exposure. If an asymptomatic person tests positive for anthrax by nasal swab, report with code 795.31.

If septicemia is due to anthrax, report 022.3; do not report a code from rubric 038.

In the case of pulmonary anthrax with pneumonia, also report the pneumonia, 484.5, in addition to code 022.1.

Report code V01.81, *Contact with or exposure to anthrax*, in cases of persons who have been in the proximity of anthrax spores or who have been linked to persons with a known exposure, even in cases in which the patient tests negative for anthrax if there is documentation of exposure. If there is only a suspicion that the patient has been exposed, report V71.82, *Observation and evaluation for suspected exposure to anthrax.*

Another code that may become appropriate as a result of bioterrorism includes V03.89 *Need for prophylactic vaccination and inoculation against other single bacterial disease.*

If anthrax was contracted as a result of terrorist acts, E997.1 *Injury due to biological warfare* may be reported in addition to the appropriate code from rubric 022.

Other coding issues may include reactions to vaccination, such as anaphylactic shock due to serum 999.4, and other serum reaction 999.5. See Complications, vaccination.

023 Brucellosis

Brucellosis is also known as "undulant fever" or "Bangs disease" and is a systemic infection caused by exposure to any of several *Brucella* species. The species are specific to the type of animal usually infected: sheep/goats, cattle, swine, or dogs.

The infection enters the body through a break in the skin. Onset of symptoms can be within three days to 30 days. Symptoms of brucellosis infection in humans include fever, night sweats, fatigue, anorexia, weight loss, headache, and arthralgia. In animals, the primary sign of infection is abortion in females and epididymitis in males.

Worldwide, brucellosis remains a major source of disease in humans and domesticated animals. *B. abortus* is the most common form in the United States.

023.0	Brucella melitensis — *contact infected sheep/goats*
023.1	Brucella abortus — *contact infected cattle*
023.2	Brucella suis — *contact infected swine*
023.3	Brucella canis — *contact infected dogs*
023.8	Other brucellosis — *more than one source*
023.9	Burcellosis, unspecified — *unknown animal contact*

024 Glanders

Glanders is an equine disease communicable to man and caused by *Burkholderia mallei* (formerly *Pseudomonas mallei*). Nearly all cases of glanders in the United States occur among people who are professionally or recreationally exposed to horses, although glanders can be transmitted from human to human and in the laboratory. Glanders cases have been extremely rare in the United States since the 1940s. Outbreaks do occur in South America,

Asia, Africa, and the Middle East. Symptoms of glanders include headache, chills, fever, and vomiting.

025 Melioidosis

Also known as Whitmore's disease or pseudoglanders, melioidosis is a rare infection caused by *Pseudomonas pseudomallei*. Most cases are limited to Asia. The disease is acquired through exposure to contaminated soil or water to a break in the skin. Symptoms range from a skin lesion at the site of infection, to pneumonia or septicemia. Patients with melioidosis may suffer relapses years after the initial infection has resolved.

026 Rat-bite fever

Rat-bite fever begins with a rat bite, scratch, or ingestion of contaminated food or water. While the initial wound may heal promptly, it usually becomes swollen and painful again within a few weeks of the bite. At that time, regional lymph nodes may swell and there may be chills, fever, and a skin rash. Periods of relapse may subside and recur. Code selection is based on the type of infection: *Spirillum minus* or *Streptobacillus moniliformis*.

026.0	Spirillary fever — *Spirillum minus infection, Sodoku*
026.1	Streptobacillary fever — *Streptobacillus moniliformis infection, Haverhill fever*
026.9	Unspecified rat-bite fever — *unknown*

027 Other zoonotic bacterial diseases

Use this rubric to report zoonotic bacterial disease not described earlier in the chapter.

027.0	Listeriosis — (Use additional code to identify manifestation, 320.7) — *infection by Listeria monocytogenes*
027.1	Erysipelothrix infection
027.2	Pasteurellosis — *infection by Pasteurella multocida (P. septica)*
027.8	Other specified zoonotic bacterial diseases — *Yersinia septica, others*
027.9	Unspecified zoonotic bacterial disease — *unknown*

Coding Clarification

In all cases, code the zoonotic bacterial disease first, followed by manifestations of the infection, as in the case of listeriosis with meningitis (320.7). Report congenital listeriosis infection with 771.2.

030–041 Other Bacterial Diseases

030 Leprosy

Mycobacterium leprae causes leprosy. Leprosy, also known as Hansen's disease, can be treated effectively with several drugs. If left untreated, the disease can result in severe disfigurement, especially of the feet, hands, and face. It is rarely fatal.

Ninety percent of the 900,000 leprosy cases worldwide occur in just 16 nations, with India and Brazil having the highest numbers of cases. Only 7,000 registered cases of leprosy currently exist in the United States. Most of these patients are immigrants who acquired the disease in their home countries.

Leprosy has two main forms: tuberculoid and lepromatous. In tuberculoid leprosy, skin lesions are few and small, with few bacteria present. Lepromatous leprosy, is a more severe disease, with symptomatic widespread lesions and significant bacteria.

Leprosy is not easily transmitted, but likely is transmitted person-to-person through nasal droplets released from an infected person. Less than 5 percent of people who are infected with *M. leprae* actually develop leprosy. For most, the immune system fights off infection. Immunosuppressed patients are no more likely to develop leprosy and research has not discovered what, if anything, predisposes a person to the disease.

Treating leprosy using multidrug therapy can halt the progression of the disease, though there are side effects. Inflammation develops in patients when leprosy bacteria are killed and erythema nodosum leprosum (ENL) is a risk in patients during drug therapy. The painful skin sores characteristic of ENL are thought to be a result of abnormal immune reactions to the killed bacteria.

030.0	Lepromatous leprosy (type L) — *widespread lesions and bacteria*
030.1	Tuberculoid leprosy (type T) — *small lesions, few bacteria*
030.2	Indeterminate leprosy (group I) — *uncharacteristic, early manifestation*
030.3	Borderline leprosy (group B) — *transitional; neither tuberculoid or lepromatous; dimorphous*
030.8	Other specified leprosy — *not elsewhere classified*
030.9	Unspecified leprosy — *unknown type*

Coding Clarification
When coding leprosy, report the leprosy code, and identify any manifestations in addition to the leprosy, such as arthropathy (711.4x), infective and deformity-creating dermatitis of the eyelid (373.4) or corneal lesion (371.89).

031 Diseases due to other mycobacteria
Mycobacteria cause leprosy and tuberculosis. In this rubric, other mycobacterial diseases are classified by site of infection.

Mycobacterium avium-intracellulare (MAC) affects up to 40 percent of human immunodeficiency virus (HIV)-infected people in the United States, while the disseminated form of the disease (DMAC) affects 15 to 24 percent of AIDS patients and other people with severely impaired immune systems. Severe anemia, fever, night sweats, anorexia, and diarrhea characterize DMAC. It is a significant cause of AIDS morbidity.

031.0	Pulmonary diseases due to other mycobacteria — *lung infection; Battey disease, M. avium, M. intracellulare, M. kansasii, M. fortuitum, M. xenopi*
031.1	Cutaneous diseases due to other mycobacteria — *skin infection; Buruli ulcer; M. marinum (M. balnei)*
031.2	Disseminated diseases due to other mycobacteria — *more than one site; DMAC, MAC* **AHA:** Q4, 1997, 31
031.8	Other specified diseases due to other mycobacteria — *not elsewhere classified; kasongo, kakerifu*
031.9	Unspecified diseases due to mycobacteria — *unknown or atypical*

Coding Clarification
When coding AIDS-related cases, sequence the code for AIDS (042) first, followed by the code for MAC or DMAC (031.2).

032 Diphtheria
An acute, contagious disease, diphtheria is one of the childhood diseases that common immunizations protect against. (The D in DPT is for the diphtheria vaccine). The infective agent is *Corynebacterium diphtheriae*.

Diphtheria usually presents with sore throat, with its hallmark fibrous membrane most commonly seen on the tonsil or nasopharynx. This membrane can combine with pharyngeal edema to obstruct breathing. However, diphtheria can attack other organs rather than presenting as a sore throat, and the codes in this rubric are therefore classified by site of infection.

032.0	Faucial diphtheria — *tonsillar*
032.1	Nasopharyngeal diphtheria — *deep, soft tissue of nose and pharynx*
032.2	Anterior nasal diphtheria — *superficial, soft tissue of the nose*
032.3	Laryngeal diphtheria — *larynx*
032.81	Conjunctival diphtheria — *conjunctiva*

Infectious and Parasitic Diseases

032.82	Diphtheritic myocarditis — *wall of the heart*
032.83	Diphtheritic peritonitis — *abdominal membrane lining*
032.84	Diphtheritic cystitis — *bladder*
032.85	Cutaneous diphtheria — *skin*
032.89	Other specified diphtheria — *neurological or other complication*
032.9	Unspecified diphtheria

Coding Clarification
Report carrier or suspected carrier of diphtheria with V02.4 and report prophylactic vaccination against diphtheria with V03.5 (diphtheria alone).

Vaccinations for diphtheria in combination with other diseases are in the V06 series of codes.

033 Whooping cough
An acute, contagious disease, whooping cough is one of the childhood diseases that common immunizations protect against. The P in DPT is for the pertussis (whooping cough) vaccine.

The infective agent in whooping cough is *Bordetella pertussis*. A milder disease clinically indistinguishable from *B. pertussis* is caused by *B. parapertussis*. *B. bronchiseptica* also creates symptoms of whooping cough.

The course of whooping cough is approximately six weeks and has three stages: catarrhal (nocturnal cough, sneezing, and lacrimation); paroxysmal (thick mucus, choking spells); and convalescence, when the severity of the symptoms diminishes. Mortality for the most severe form of whooping cough, pertussis, is about 2 percent in children younger than 1.

033.0	Whooping cough due to Bordetella pertussis (P. pertussis) — (Use additional code to identify any associated pneumonia, 484.3) — *B. pertussis*
033.1	Whooping cough due to Bordetella parapertussis (B. parapertussis) — (Use additional code to identify any associated pneumonia, 484.3) — *B. parapertussis*
033.8	Whooping cough due to other specified organism — (Use additional code to identify any associated pneumonia, 484.3) — *B. bronchiseptica*
033.9	Whooping cough, unspecified organism — (Use additional code to identify any associated pneumonia, 484.3) — *unknown organism*

Coding Clarification
Report any pneumonia concurrent to whooping cough separately with 484.3. The pneumonia should be coded as a secondary diagnosis.

Prophylactic vaccination is reported with V03.6 (pertussis alone) or with a code from the V06 series for pertussis vaccination in combination with other prophylactic vaccinations.

034 Streptococcal sore throat and scarlet fever
Strep throat is a common pharyngeal infection presenting with a red, sore throat and fever. Strep throat responds readily to antibiotic treatment. Without antibiotics, strep throat can progress into scarlet fever, typified by a red blush to the skin of the chest and abdomen, that blanches under pressure. Streptococcal infections can progress to endocarditis, pneumonias, and septicemias.

| 034.0 | Streptococcal sore throat — *simple strep throat* |
| 034.1 | Scarlet fever — *red rash spreading from trunk* |

Coding Clarification
Carrier or suspected carrier of streptococcus is reported with V02.51 for Group B and V02.52 for other strains of streptococcus.

For streptococcal angina, use code 034.0.

035 Erysipelas OK
Formerly called St. Anthony's fire, erysipelas is a hot, bright red, superficial cellulitis, involving dermal lymphatics that is usually caused by a streptococcal infection.

Coding Clarification
If the erysipelas infection is of the external ear, report the erysipelas first, and the site of infection with 380.13. For erysipelas as a maternal complication of childbirth, see rubric 670.

036 Meningococcal infection
Neisseria meningitidis is a common cause of meningitis. Also called meningococcus, the bacteria may invade the spinal cord, brain, heart, joints, optic nerve, or bloodstream. A pink or petechial rash may accompany the disease. Although the bacterium is found in the nasopharynx of 5 percent of the population, only a fraction of carriers ever develop the disease. It is seen most commonly in infants or in epidemics among persons who live in close quarters (barracks, schools).

036.0	Meningococcal meningitis — *infection of membranes lining brain or spinal cord*
036.1	Meningococcal encephalitis — *infection of brain*
036.2	Meningococcemia — *invasion of bloodstream*
036.3	Waterhouse-Friderichsen syndrome, meningococcal — *vascular collapse and shock*
036.40	Meningococcal carditis, unspecified — *site of heart infection unknown*
036.41	Meningococcal pericarditis — *infection of lining of heart*
036.42	Meningococcal endocarditis — *infection within heart cavities*

036.43	Meningococcal myocarditis — *infection of muscle of heart*
036.81	Meningococcal optic neuritis — *infection of optic nerve*
036.82	Meningococcal arthropathy — *infection of joint*
036.89	Other specified meningococcal infections — *other specific site of infection*
036.9	Unspecified meningococcal infection — *unknown site of infection*

Coding Clarification
Prophylactic meningococcal vaccination is administered during epidemics and is reported with V03.89.

Carrier or suspected carrier of meningitis is reported with V02.59.

037 Tetanus 🆗

Tetanus is an infection by *Clostridium tetani,* and is commonly called "lockjaw" because of the tonic spasms that occur in voluntary muscles. *C. tetani* is found in soil and animal feces, and infection may result from insignificant or deep wounds. The infected patient may have difficulty swallowing, speaking, or respiration as a result of the tonic spasms caused by the infection.

In the United States, the highest number of tetanus cases is seen among intravenous drug abusers and in burn victims or as a complication of abortion or pregnancy. See the index of ICD-9-CM for entries relating to tetanus occurring as a result of abortion or childbirth.

Tetanus has a high mortality rate and is one of the diseases that common childhood immunizations protect against. (The T in DPT is for tetanus vaccine.)

Coding Clarification
Report prophylactic vaccination for tetanus with V03.7. If tetanus immunization occurs in conjunction with other immunizations, see the V06 series of immunization codes.

038 Septicemia
AHA: Q3, 1988, 12; Q4, 1988, 10; Q2, 2004, 16

Septicemia is the invasion of the bloodstream that results in multisystemic infection. Codes in this series are classified according to the infective bacterial agent.

Septicemia, also called septic syndrome or sepsis, occurs when a localized infection (a urinary tract infection, operative wound infection, or infected tooth) metastasizes and the bacterium is spread throughout the body. The disease is acute, and symptoms may include shaking chills, fever, abdominal pain, vomiting, and diarrhea. Septicemia treatments include antibiotic therapy, drainage of any abscess, or reoperation.

The incidence of septicemia in staphylococcal infection is related to the organism identified. As many as 90 percent of *Staphylococcus aureus* infection cases are true sepsis, while less than 50 percent of non-aureus *Staphylococcus* cases are true sepsis.

Use additional code for systemic inflammatory response syndrome (SIRS), 995.91-995.92.

038.0	Streptococcal septicemia — *other than Streptococcus pneumoniae* AHA: Q3, 1988, 12; Q4, 1988, 10; Q2, 1996, 5; Q4, 2003, 79
038.10	Unspecified staphylococcal septicemia — *unknown staphylococcus* AHA: Q3, 1988, 12; Q4, 1988, 10; Q4, 1997, 32
038.11	Staphylococcus aureus septicemia — *also called Staphylococcus pyogenes* AHA: Q3, 1988, 12; Q4, 1988, 10; Q4, 1997, 32; Q4, 1998, 42; Q2, 2000, 5; Q1, 2005, 7
038.19	Other staphylococcal septicemia
038.2	Pneumococcal septicemia — *septicemia from bacteria common to pneumonia* AHA: Q3, 1988, 12; Q4, 1988, 10; Q1, 1991, 13; Q2, 1996, 5
038.3	Septicemia due to anaerobes — *due to bacteroides* AHA: Q3, 1988, 12; Q4, 1988, 10
038.40	Septicemia due to unspecified gram-negative organism — *not otherwise specified* AHA: Q3, 1988, 12; Q4, 1988, 10
038.41	Septicemia due to hemophilus influenzae (H. influenzae) — *also called Pfeiffer's bacillus* AHA: Q3, 1988, 12; Q4, 1988, 10
038.42	Septicemia due to Escherichia coli (E. coli) — *also called colon bacillus and Escherich's bacillus* AHA: Q3, 1988, 12; Q4, 1988, 10; Q3, 2003, 73
038.43	Septicemia due to pseudomonas — *family Pseudomonadaceae* AHA: Q3, 1988, 12; Q4, 1988, 10
038.44	Septicemia due to serratia — *family Enterobacteriaceae* AHA: Q3, 1988, 12; Q4, 1988, 10
038.49	Other septicemia due to gram-negative organism — *including Proteus vulgaris* AHA: Q3, 1988, 12; Q4, 1988, 10
038.8	Other specified septicemia — *not elsewhere classified* AHA: Q3, 1988, 12; Q4, 1988, 10

Infectious and Parasitic Diseases

038.9 Unspecified septicemia — *disseminated, unknown cause*
AHA: Q3, 1988, 12; Q4, 1988, 10; Q2, 1996, 6; Q3, 1996, 16; Q1, 1998, 5; Q3, 1999, 5,9; Q2, 2000, 3; Q4, 2003, 79; Q2, 2004, 16; Q2, 2005, 18, 19

Documentation Issues

"Sepsis" may be an ambiguous term in the medical record and coding should differentiate generalized sepsis represented in this code rubric from other bacterial infections.

Current official coding guidelines assume the terms "sepsis" and "severe sepsis" are associated with SIRS. Code the underlying condition first, then assign the code for sepsis (995.91) or severe sepsis (995.92). By contrast, the term "septicemia" prompts physician query regarding whether "sepsis" and therefore "SIRS" are also present. Sequencing for sepsis and septicemia due to underlying infections are determined by the circumstances of admission and instructional terms within the text.

When the documentation states the diagnosis of septicemia with shock or general sepsis with septic shock, code and list the septicemia first and use an additional code for SIRS, followed by a code for the septic shock.

If the documentation has an unclear diagnostic statement as to the site or organ-specific sepsis (e.g., urosepsis), it may require clarification from the physician for accurate code selection.

If the physician has documented urosepsis, verify which of the following the diagnosis is intended to mean:

- Generalized sepsis caused by leakage of urine or toxic urine by-products into the general vascular circulation, code 038.x
- Urine contaminated by bacteria, bacterial by-products, or other toxic material but without other findings, code 599.0

When the physician documents that the sepsis is secondary to a urinary tract infection (UTI) and the blood and urine cultures reveal the presence of the infection, it would be appropriate to code both the septicemia and the UTI.

If the medical record documentation identifies that the septicemia is due to *Candida albicans*, a code would not be selected from the bacterial disease series, categories 030-041. *C. albicans* is one of the mycotic infections and is classified as such. The correct code would be 112.5 *Disseminated candidiasis*.

If the physician documents both pneumococcal pneumonia (481) and pneumococcal septicemia (038.2), both conditions should be coded.

Coding Clarification

Complication of Care: When septicemia is caused by a complication of care (e.g., indwelling urinary catheter, vascular access device), the complication code should be listed as principal/primary diagnosis. Additional codes should be assigned for the septicemia from category 038, and the organism responsible for the sepsis should also be coded if it is not included in the category 038 code descriptor.

Infection Originating in the Perinatal Period: Sepsis of newborn should be coded to 771.81 *Septicemia [sepsis] of newborn*. Do not assign codes from the 038 or 995.9 categories for perinatal infections. A secondary code from category 041 may be assigned to identify the organism, if known.

Negative Blood Cultures: Septicemia is defined as evidence of infection with fever or hypothermia, tachypnea, tachycardia, and impaired organ system perfusion, such as altered mental status, oliguria, and relative hypotension. Metabolic acidosis may also be present secondary to impaired organ perfusion, as evidenced by either an increased lactate level, increased anion gap, or reduced blood pH. So, although the blood culture may be negative, it may still be appropriate to code the septicemia in view of the clinical findings.

Neutropenic/Nadir Sepsis: This is a true sepsis; even though the white cell counts and temperature are at low points, bacteria is still present in the condition. Two codes need to be assigned for this condition: code 038.9 *Unspecified septicemia* and 288.00 *Neutropenia, unspecified* for the neutropenia.

Noncardiogenic Acute Pulmonary Edema: When acute pulmonary edema is secondary to septicemia it should be coded as an additional code to the septicemia. Use codes 038.9 *Septicemia* and 518.4 *Acute edema of lung, unspecified*.

Sepsis Secondary to Urinary Tract Infection: If a localized urinary infection has entered into the patients blood stream and has developed into a generalized sepsis, use only a code from category 038. Code 599.0 *Urinary tract infection, site not specified* would not be reported as an additional code. If the code from category 038 identifies the causative organism (e.g., pseudomonas septicemia 038.43) it would not be necessary to report a code from category 041. Code also the presence of SIRS if documented.

Coders' Desk Reference for Diagnoses

Septicemia with Pneumonia: Septicemia occurring with pneumonia is a true septic infection and should be coded in addition to the pneumonia. Hospital code sequencing is dependent upon the circumstances of the admission.

Streptococcus Pneumoniae: *Streptococcus pneumoniae* is the microbiological term for the germ that causes pneumococcal disease, so only one code is necessary, code 038.2 *Pneumococcal septicemia*.

The following types of septicemia should be coded as follows: Shigella septicemia, 004.9; Salmonella septicemia, 003.1; gonococcal septicemia, 098.89; herpetic septicemia, 054.5; postoperative septicemia, 998.59; septicemia from anthrax, 022.3.

Coding Scenario
A patient is admitted with an infection of the gastrostomy site. Physician documentation confirms the blood culture result that gastrostomy site growth of *Staphylococcal aureus* has invaded the bloodstream.

Code assignment: 536.41 *Infection of gastrostomy* and 038.11 *Staphylococcus aureus septicemia*

A patient with chronic renal failure is seen with an infection of his vascular access device. Physician documentation indicates that the patient has septicemia due to the vascular access device.

Code assignment: 996.62 *Infection and inflammatory reaction due to vascular device, implant and graft*, 038.9 *Unspecified septicemia*, and 585.9 *Chronic kidney disease, unspecified*

A 2-day-old infant is readmitted to the hospital with neonatal staphylococcal septicemia.

Code assignment: 771.81 *Septicemia [sepsis] of newborn* and 041.10 *Staphylococcus, unspecified*

A patient is diagnosed with generalized sepsis and septic shock following an abortion performed two days ago.

Code assignment: 639.0 *Genital and pelvic infection following abortion* and 639.5 *Shock following abortion*

A 3-year-old is admitted via the emergency department with sores on the mouth and a fever. The physician documents Nadir sepsis and neutropenia as the discharge diagnosis.

Code assignment: 038.9 *Unspecified septicemia* and 288.00 *Neutropenia, unspecified*

A patient is diagnosed with severe pneumococcal sepsis due to pneumococcal pneumonia. Evidence of SIRS, with organ dysfunction and resultant septic shock, is documented in the medical record.

Code assignment: 038.2 *Pneumococcal septicemia*, 481 *Pneumococcal pneumonia*, 995.92 *Severe sepsis*, and 785.52 *Septic shock*.

039 Actinomycotic infections
Infections by *Actinomyces israelii* are classified in this rubric according to site, at which multiple, communicating abscesses often form granulated tissue. The disease is most commonly seen in adult males and is slowly progressive, although it is sometimes seen as a local complication of intrauterine device (IUD) placement in women.

Code	Description
039.0	Cutaneous actinomycotic infection — *superficial skin infection*
039.1	Pulmonary actinomycotic infection — *lung involvement with chest pain, fever, cough*
039.2	Abdominal actinomycotic infection — *intestinal involvement with anorexia, pain, fever, vomiting and irregular bowels*
039.3	Cervicofacial actinomycotic infection — *"lumpy jaw" in oral mucosa or neck*
039.4	Madura foot — *deep foot infection following penetrating injury*
039.8	Actinomycotic infection of other specified sites — *site not elsewhere classified, multiple sites, or generalized*
039.9	Actinomycotic infection of unspecified site — *unknown site*

040 Other bacterial diseases
Gas gangrene is the result of infection by the *Clostridium* bacteria, usually at the site of injury or a recent surgical wound. It is an acute condition, with red, extremely painful tissue swelling in quick progression to surrounding areas. Involved tissue is destroyed. Gas gangrene has a high mortality rate. *Clostridia* species of bacteria produce many toxins that cause tissue death and systemic symptoms, including sweating, fever, and shock. Untreated, gas gangrene can lead to renal failure, coma, and death. Treatments include wound debridement, amputation, antibiotics, and hyperbaric oxygen treatment.

Whipple's disease primarily effects middle-aged men and presents as chronic diarrhea, anemia, arthralgia, and abdominal pain.

040.0	Gas gangrene — *clostridial myonecrosis, malignant edema* **AHA:** Q1, 1995, 11
040.1	Rhinoscleroma — *Klebsiella rhinoscleromatis infection of nose, nasopharynx*
040.2	Whipple's disease — *intestinal lipodystrophy*

Infectious and Parasitic Diseases

040.3	Necrobacillosis — *Fusobacterium necrophorum* abscess or necrosis	041.04	Streptococcus infection in conditions classified elsewhere and of unspecified site, group D [Enterococcus] — (Note: This code is to be used as an additional code to identify the bacterial agent in diseases classified elsewhere and bacterial infections of unspecified nature or site)
040.81	Tropical pyomyositis — *including Bungpagga*		
040.82	Toxic shock syndrome — (Use additional code to identify the organism) — *Use additional code to identify the organism*		
	AHA: Q4, 2002, 44	041.05	Streptococcus infection in conditions classified elsewhere and of unspecified site, group G — (Note: This code is to be used as an additional code to identify the bacterial agent in diseases classified elsewhere and bacterial infections of unspecified nature or site)
040.89	Other specified bacterial diseases — *not elsewhere classified, including toxic shock syndrome*		
	AHA: Nov-Dec, 1986, 7		

Coding Clarification

Gas gangrene associated with abortion, pregnancy, or labor and delivery should be reported with codes from that section of ICD-9-CM. Check the ICD-9-CM index for more information. Also check the ICD-9-CM index for a complex list of gangrene diagnoses other than gas gangrene.

Arteriosclerosis with gas gangrene is reported with two codes: 440.29 *Other atherosclerosis of native arteries of extremities* and 040.0 *Gas gangrene*. It is inappropriate to use code 440.24 as this code only includes ischemic gangrene.

041	**Bacterial infection in conditions classified elsewhere and of unspecified site**	041.09	Other streptococcus infection in conditions classified elsewhere and of unspecified site — (Note: This code is to be used as an additional code to identify the bacterial agent in diseases classified elsewhere and bacterial infections of unspecified nature or site)
	AHA: July-Aug, 1984, 19; Q2, 2001, 12		

This rubric of ICD-9-CM provides supplemental codes to identify bacterial agents in diseases classified elsewhere. They usually are sequenced after the disease manifestation. Codes in this rubric can also be used to classify bacterial infections of unspecified nature or site.

041.00	Unspecified streptococcus infection in conditions classified elsewhere and of unspecified site — (Note: This code is to be used as an additional code to identify the bacterial agent in diseases classified elsewhere and bacterial infections of unspecified nature or site)	041.10	Unspecified staphylococcus infection in conditions classified elsewhere and of unspecified site — (Note: This code is to be used as an additional code to identify the bacterial agent in diseases classified elsewhere and bacterial infections of unspecified nature or site)
			AHA: Q2, 2006, 15
		041.11	Staphylococcus aureus infection in conditions classified elsewhere and of unspecified site — (Note: This code is to be used as an additional code to identify the bacterial agent in diseases classified elsewhere and bacterial infections of unspecified nature or site)
			AHA: Q2, 2006, 16
041.01	Streptococcus infection in conditions classified elsewhere and of unspecified site, group A — (Note: This code is to be used as an additional code to identify the bacterial agent in diseases classified elsewhere and bacterial infections of unspecified nature or site)	041.19	Other staphylococcus infection in conditions classified elsewhere and of unspecified site — (Note: This code is to be used as an additional code to identify the bacterial agent in diseases classified elsewhere and bacterial infections of unspecified nature or site)
041.02	Streptococcus infection in conditions classified elsewhere and of unspecified site, group B — (Note: This code is to be used as an additional code to identify the bacterial agent in diseases classified elsewhere and bacterial infections of unspecified nature or site)	041.2	Pneumococcus infection in conditions classified elsewhere and of unspecified site — (Note: This code is to be used as an additional code to identify the bacterial agent in diseases classified elsewhere and bacterial infections of unspecified nature or site)
		041.3	Friedländer's bacillus infection in conditions classified elsewhere and of unspecified site — (Note: This code is to be used as an additional code to identify the bacterial agent in diseases classified elsewhere and bacterial infections of unspecified nature or site) — *Klebsiella pneumoniae infection*
			AHA: July-Aug, 1984, 19; Q2, 2001, 12
041.03	Streptococcus infection in conditions classified elsewhere and of unspecified site, group C — (Note: This code is to be used as an additional code to identify the bacterial agent in diseases classified elsewhere and bacterial infections of unspecified nature or site)	041.4	Escherichia coli (E. coli) infection in conditions classified elsewhere and of unspecified site — (Note: This code is to be used as an additional code to identify the bacterial agent in diseases classified elsewhere and bacterial infections of unspecified nature or site)
		041.5	Hemophilus influenzae (H. influenzae) infection in conditions classified elsewhere and of unspecified site — (Note: This code is to be used as an additional code to identify the

	bacterial agent in diseases classified elsewhere and bacterial infections of unspecified nature or site)
041.6	Proteus (mirabilis) (morganii) infection in conditions classified elsewhere and of unspecified site — (Note: This code is to be used as an additional code to identify the bacterial agent in diseases classified elsewhere and bacterial infections of unspecified nature or site)
041.7	Pseudomonas infection in conditions classified elsewhere and of unspecified site — (Note: This code is to be used as an additional code to identify the bacterial agent in diseases classified elsewhere and bacterial infections of unspecified nature or site)
041.81	Mycoplasma infection in conditions classified elsewhere and of unspecified site — (Note: This code is to be used as an additional code to identify the bacterial agent in diseases classified elsewhere and bac-terial infections of unspecified nature or site)
041.82	Bacterial infection in conditions classified elsewhere, Bacteroides fragilis — (Note: This code is to be used as an additional code to identify the bacterial agent in diseases classified elsewhere and bacterial infections of unspecified nature or site)
041.83	Clostridium perfringens infection in conditions classified elsewhere and of unspecified site — (Note: This code is to be used as an additional code to identify the bacterial agent in diseases classified elsewhere and bacterial infections of unspecified nature or site)
041.84	Infection due to other anaerobes in conditions classified elsewhere and of unspecified site — (Note: This code is to be used as an additional code to identify the bacterial agent in diseases classified elsewhere and bacterial infections of unspecified nature or site) — *gram negative anaerobes, Bacteroides (fragilis)* AHA: July-Aug, 1984, 19; Q2, 2001, 12
041.85	Infection due to other gram-negative organisms in conditions classified elsewhere and of unspecified site — (Note: This code is to be used as an additional code to identify the bacterial agent in diseases classified elsewhere and bacterial infections of unspecified nature or site) — *Aerobacter aerogenes, Mima polymorpha, Serratia* AHA: July-Aug, 1984, 19; Q1, 1995, 18; Q2, 2001, 12
041.86	Helicobacter pylori (H. pylori) infection — (Note: This code is to be used as an additional code to identify the bacterial agent in diseases classified elsewhere and bacterial infections of unspecified nature or site) — *associated with peptic ulcers* AHA: July-Aug, 1984, 19; Q4, 1995, 60; Q2, 2001, 12
041.89	Infection due to other specified bacteria in conditions classified elsewhere and of unspecified site — (Note: This code is to be used as an additional code to identify the bacterial agent in diseases classified elsewhere and bacterial infections of unspecified nature or site) — *not elsewhere classified* AHA: July-Aug, 1984, 19; Q2, 2001, 12; Q2, 2003, 7; Q2, 2006, 7
041.9	Bacterial infection, unspecified, in conditions classified elsewhere and of unspecified site — (Note: This code is to be used as an additional code to identify the bacterial agent in diseases classified elsewhere and bacterial infections of unspecified nature or site)

Coding Clarification

Helicobacter pylori with chronic gastritis is reported with two codes: 535.10 *Atrophic gastritis* and 041.86 *Helicobacter pylori (H. pylori)*.

When coding a disease caused by an infectious organism, report the disease first, followed by the code that identifies the infectious agent. For example, urinary tract infection due to *E. coli* is sequenced as 599.0, then 041.4.

Coding Scenario

A patient is seen in the clinic for painful urination and fever. A urine culture shows the bacterial agent *Pseudomonas*. The physician's diagnostic statement confirms a urinary tract infection due to *Pseudomonas*.

Code assignment: 599.0 *Urinary tract infection, site not specified* and 041.7 *Pseudomonas*

042 Human Immunodeficiency Virus (HIV) Infection

HIV is divided into two categories: HIV-1 and HIV-2. HIV-1 is seen worldwide; HIV-2 is limited to Africa and other countries and is seldom seen in the United States. HIV-1 has far-ranging health effects and manifestations. This code is reserved for patients with active HIV-1 infections, or AIDS. HIV-2 cases are reported with 079.53.

HIV-1 is a blood-borne virus in that it is transmitted through body fluids containing blood or plasma. Transmission of HIV-1 can occur sexually or non-sexually through the exchange of body fluids infected with a high concentration of the virus, mainly blood, semen, or vaginal/cervical secretions.

In HIV-1, the body's immune system is attacked, reducing its ability to protect itself against a variety of illnesses. Over time, the infected person becomes more susceptible to opportunistic infections or cancers that attack the body and can cause death. AIDS related complex (ARC) includes general lymphadenopathy, anorexia, fever, malaise, diarrhea, anemia, oral hairy leukoplakia, and oral candidiasis.

042 Human immunodeficiency virus [HIV] OK
AHA: July-Aug, 1987, 8; Q3, 1990, 17; Q2, 1992, 11; Q1, 1993, 21; Q4, 1997, 30,31; Q1, 1999, 14; Q1, 2003, 15; Q1, 2004, 5; Q2, 2004, 11; Q1, 2005, 7

Documentation Issues
In cases where the medical record documentation indicates "possible," "probable," or "questionable" AIDS, not confirmed, without manifestations, that record should be returned to the physician for further clarification. Physicians also need to be aware that unacceptable terminology and abbreviations in the medical record should not be used. These terms only cause confusion in code selection.

Do not use 042 in cases of "rule-out" or "suspected" AIDS; this diagnosis can create a flag in the patient's data files that could interfere with their ability to obtain life or health insurance.

Coding Clarification
If the patient is being treated for AIDS or an AIDS-related illness, the code for HIV-1 infection (042) should be sequenced first, followed by codes for manifestations of HIV-1 infection. If the patient is being treated for an illness unrelated to AIDS, for example, an injury, AIDS would be reported secondarily to the injury.

Patients with an HIV-related illness should be coded to category 042, located in Chapter 1 of the tabular list, Infectious and Parasitic Diseases. Notes in the tabular section advise the coder to use additional codes to identify all manifestations of HIV-1 and to use an additional code (079.53) to identify HIV-2 infection, if present.

Patients with physician-documented asymptomatic HIV infections who have never had an HIV-related illness should be coded to category V08, located in Chapter 18 of the tabular list, which are V Codes. A note is provided under this category that specifically indicates that this code is only to be used when no HIV infection symptoms or conditions are present. If any HIV infection symptoms or conditions are present, the coder is referred to code 042.

Patients (including infants) with inconclusive HIV test results should be classified with code 795.71, located under the Other nonspecific immunological findings subcategory (795.7) in Chapter 16 of the tabular list, Symptoms, Signs and Ill-Defined Conditions. A note is provided that clearly identifies that this code is only to be used when a test finding is reported as nonspecific. Negative findings are not coded.

HIV During Pregnancy: The obstetric code, 647.6x, should be used followed by the appropriate HIV code.

HIV Testing: For asymptomatic patients that solely want testing to identify their HIV status, use code V73.89 *Screening for other specified viral disease.* In addition, use code V69.8 *Other problems related to lifestyle,* if the patient is known to be a high risk individual.

If the patient returns for the results that are negative, use code V65.44 *Human immunodeficiency virus (HIV) counseling.* If the results were positive and the patient is asymptomatic, use code V08 *Asymptomatic HIV infection.* If the results were positive and they are symptomatic, use code 042 *Human Immunodeficiency virus (HIV) disease* with additional codes to identify the HIV-related symptoms or diagnosis. In addition, if counseling is performed, an additional code V65.44 *Human immunodeficiency virus (HIV) counseling* may be used.

AIDS Wasting Syndrome: Assign 042 *Human immunodeficiency virus (HIV) disease* and use the additional code 799.4 *Cachexia.* Also code any associated conditions that are documented.

Positive Newborn Testing: If a newborn has a positive ELISA or Western Blot test for HIV the correct code is 795.71 *Nonspecific serologic evidence of human immunodeficiency virus [HIV].* These tests may reflect the antibodies of the mother and not the baby. If the mother is positive for HIV, the antibody may cross the placenta to the newborn. The antibodies may be carried up to 18 months producing a false-positive result. These false-positive results during the newborns' first 18 months are due to the mother's antibodies that the newborn carries. The newborn may later lose those antibodies, indicating that he or she was actually never infected.

Pediatric HIV: Patients with any prior diagnosis of HIV-related illness should be assigned 042 for every subsequent admission, regardless of age or CDC classification.

Coding Scenario
A patient is admitted to the hospital with acute bronchitis. Three months ago, the patient tested positive for HIV but has not yet shown any symptoms of HIV disease.

Code assignment: 466.0 *Acute bronchitis* and V08 *Asymptomatic HIV infection*

A patient that is six months' pregnant is being treated for pneumocystosis secondary to HIV.

Code assignment: 647.63 *Pregnancy complicated by other viral diseases, antepartum condition or complication*, 042 *Human immunodeficiency virus (HIV) disease*, and 136.3 *Pneumocystosis*

A patient with AIDS is admitted to the hospital with severe dehydration and diarrhea. The final diagnosis is Salmonella with dehydration.

Code assignment: 042 *Human immunodeficiency virus (HIV) disease* 003.9 *Salmonella infection, unspecified*, and 276.51 *Dehydration*

A 42-year-old white female who has tested positive for HIV is being seen for a follow-up on the status of her condition. She is presently asymptomatic and has shown no signs or symptoms to date.

Code assignment: V08 *Asymptomatic HIV infection*.

An asymptomatic HIV patient is admitted to undergo Interleukin immunotherapy. The documentation implies that the patient has never had an HIV symptomatic illness.

Code assignment: Code this patient according to the rule for asymptomatic HIV patients - V08. The planned immunotherapy does not interfere with principal/primary diagnosis selection.

045–049 Poliomyelitis and Other Non–arthropod–borne Viral Diseases of Central Nervous System

045 Acute poliomyelitis

Poliomyelitis is an infectious viral disease of the central nervous system that sometimes results in paralysis. The World Health Organization (WHO) declared the Western Hemisphere polio-free in 1994. Today, polio is most prevalent in areas of Africa, the Middle East, and South Asia.

Three types of poliovirus have been identified: the Brunhilde (type I), Lansing (type II), and Leon (type III) strains. Immunity to one strain does not provide protection against the other two. Type I causes 85 percent of paralytic infection, type II causes 5 percent, and type III causes 10 percent.

Polio enters the body through the digestive tract and spreads along nerve cells to affect various parts of the central nervous system. The incubation period ranges from four days to 35 days. Symptoms include fatigue, headache, fever, vomiting, constipation, and stiffness of the neck. Polio infection can cause permanent paralysis. However, nonparalytic cases far outnumber paralytic cases of polio. No drug has proven effective against polio infection, so treatment is symptomatic.

A third of patients who recover from poliomyelitis develop post-polio syndrome (PPS) 30 to 40 years later. PPS causes fatigue, muscle weakness, and muscle and joint pain.

The following fifth-digit subclassification is for use with category 045:

0   poliovirus, unspecified type — unknown
1   poliovirus type I — Brunhilde
2   poliovirus type II — Lansing
3   poliovirus type III — Leon

045.0 ⌐sth   Acute paralytic poliomyelitis specified as bulbar — *infection at site where brain merges with spinal cord*
045.1 ⌐sth   Acute poliomyelitis with other paralysis — *infection of peripheral or spinal nerves*
045.2 ⌐sth   Acute nonparalytic poliomyelitis — *pain, stiffness, or paresthesia without paralysis*
045.9 ⌐sth   Acute unspecified poliomyelitis — *unknown type*

Coding Clarification

Late effects of polio, including PPS, deformities, or paralysis in non-active disease, are reported with 138. Sequence first the manifestation, for example, progressive muscular atrophy (335.21), then report the late effect.

Congenital polio is reported with 771.2.

Do not report personal history of poliomyelitis (V12.02) in patients with active disease.

Exposure to poliovirus is reported with V01.2, and prophylactic vaccination is reported with V04.0. Routine immunization is largely responsible for the eradication of poliomyelitis in the United States.

046 Slow virus infection of central nervous system

Jakob-Creutzfeldt disease is a progressive, fatal disease causing dementia and seizures in adults. Transmission occurs from contaminated humans or human cadavers, although 10 percent of cases are familial in origin. Jakob-Creutzfeldt disease is related to mad cow disease, another form of spongiform encephalopathy with European outbreaks. A type of the disease has emerged called the new variant Creutzfeldt-Jakob disease (nvCJD). This form of Creutzfeldt-Jakob disease is exhibited by people who have eaten meat from infected cows.

Kuru is limited exclusively to New Guinea natives, where the disease has nearly been eradicated. The disease is linked to cannibalism and Fore tribal rituals.

Subacute sclerosing panencephalitis (SSPE) is a rare, progressive, and grave disorder, occurring months or years following measles or measles vaccination, and usually before age 20. Mental faculties are diminished, seizures occur, and the patient deteriorates until death, usually within three years.

The meninges constitute the three layers that cover the brain and spinal cord: the dura mater, pia mater, and arachnoid

046.0	Kuru — *New Guinea-based neural disease*	
046.1	Jakob-Creutzfeldt disease — *spongiform encephalopathy similar to "mad cow" disease*	
046.2	Subacute sclerosing panencephalitis — *Dawson's, Van Bogaert's, Bodechtel-Guttmann disease*	
046.3	Progressive multifocal leukoencephalopathy — *cerebral cortex infection in immunosuppressed*	
046.8	Other specified slow virus infection of central nervous system — *not elsewhere classified*	
046.9	Unspecified slow virus infection of central nervous system — *unknown slow virus infection of CNS*	

Coding Clarification
All slow virus infections in this rubric may present with manifestations that should be reported in addition to the infection source. Dementia should be reported with 294.11, with behavioral disturbance, or 294.10, without behavioral disturbance.

047 Meningitis due to enterovirus
AHA: Jan-Feb, 1987, 6

Meningitis is the inflammation of the membranes surrounding the brain or spinal cord, in this case, due to an aseptic, abacterial, or a viral enterovirus infection not included in other rubrics in this section of ICD-9-CM.

Viral infections must be differentiated from bacterial and other infections. Typically, a viral infection of the central nervous system is suspected by default, when a culture fails to grow bacteria. A virus may be isolated in spinal fluid or other tissues, but viruses causing aseptic meningitis are identified in less than half of all cases.

Coxsackie virus causes symptoms resembling polio, but without paralysis. It is most commonly seen in children during warm months.

ECHO virus is an acronym for enteric cytopathic human orphan virus and is also most prevalent during warm months.

047.0	Meningitis due to coxsackie virus — *coxsackievirus*	
047.1	Meningitis due to ECHO virus — *echovirus*	
047.8	Other specified viral meningitis — *not elsewhere classified*	
047.9	Unspecified viral meningitis — *unknown type*	

048 Other enterovirus diseases of central nervous system ✓

This rubric represents all enterovirus disease of the central nervous system not elsewhere classified. Among these is Boston exanthem, a mild illness with a rash and fever caused by echovirus 16. It is named after an epidemic that occurred in Boston, Mass.

049 Other non-arthropod-borne viral diseases of central nervous system

049.0	Lymphocytic choriomeningitis — *arenavirus*	
049.1	Meningitis due to adenovirus — *adenovirus*	
049.8	Other specified non-arthropod-borne viral diseases of central nervous system — *not elsewhere classified*	
049.9	Unspecified non-arthropod-borne viral disease of central nervous system — *unknown type*	

Coding Clarification
Late effects of viral encephalitis are reported with 139.0. A code for the residual condition or nature of the late effect should be assigned first, followed by 139.0.

050–057 Viral Diseases Accompanied by Exanthem

050 Smallpox
Smallpox is a highly contagious human disease caused by the virus viriolae, of which there are two strains: viriole major, which has severe symptoms and a mortality rate of 20 percent to 40 percent; and

viriole minor, which has less severe symptoms and a 1 percent mortality rate. Smallpox can spread from person to person and through infected blankets, linens, and clothing. An infection is usually through the respiratory tract and local lymph nodes from where the virus enters the blood (primary viremia). Internal organs are infected; the virus reenters the blood (secondary viremia) and spreads to the skin. Symptoms appear about 12 days after exposure and mimic a gastrointestinal illness — nausea, vomiting, headache, and backache. Severe abdominal pain and disorientation follows. About two to three days after the onset of illness, the true smallpox rash appears. It begins as macules, which enlarge and become raised papules. By the third day, the papules progress into blisters, 6.0 mm in diameter and deep in the skin. In two more days, the fluid inside becomes turbid; the papules shrink and dry up in the skin. Toxemia may cause death before the rash is fully developed, but more commonly death, if it occurs, is between the 11th and 15th day of the rash. In severe cases the rash may cover the entire body. Secondary infections can include hemorrhaging and gangrene.

Diagnosis is difficult due to variations from the characteristic pattern.

In people exposed to smallpox, the vaccine can lessen the severity of or even prevent illness if given within four days after exposure. There is no proven treatment for smallpox but research to evaluate new antiviral agents is ongoing. Patients with smallpox can benefit from supportive therapy (intravenous fluids, medicine to control fever or pain, etc.) and antibiotics for any secondary bacterial infections that occur.

The vaccine is 100 percent effective if administered before exposure. Unfortunately, considering recent events, the WHO's vaccination campaign ended in 1980 when the disease was officially declared eradicated. No one in the United States has been inoculated since 1972 and since immunity after vaccination lasts up to 10 years, it is unlikely that anyone in the United States is protected against the disease.

Complications of antibiotics may include nausea, diarrhea, CNS disturbance, local IV site reactions, and abnormalities of hepatic enzymes, eosinophilia, headache, rash, restlessness, vomiting, abdominal pain/discomfort, headache, rash, and restlessness.

050.0	Variola major — *severe form*
050.1	Alastrim — *mild form*
050.2	Modified smallpox — *reinfection form*
050.9	Unspecified smallpox — *unknown type*

Coding Clarification
Rubric 050 is only used for patients with smallpox. If exposure to smallpox has been substantiated, report V01.3 *Contact with or exposure to communicable diseases.* If there is only a suspicion that the patient has been exposed, report V73.1 *Special screening for smallpox.*

Another code that may become appropriate as a result of bioterrorism includes V04.1 *Vaccination against smallpox.*

If smallpox was contracted as a result of terrorist acts, E997.1 *Injury due to biological warfare* may be reported in addition to the appropriate code from rubric 050.

If the patient is isolated for contact with smallpox, report V07.0 *Isolation of individual after contact with infectious diseases.*

Code first the symptoms of the adverse effect and then the E code for Adverse Effects of a Drug in Therapeutic Use. Other coding issues may include reactions to vaccination, such as anaphylactic shock due to serum 999.4, and other serum reaction 999.5. See Complications, vaccination.

051 Cowpox and paravaccinia

Cowpox is also called vaccinia because it is closely related to variola, the causative virus of smallpox, and infection by cowpox renders the patient immune to smallpox. Cowpox infection is due to Poxvirus bovis infection from milking cattle, and is much milder than smallpox, with hard lesions and low fever.

051.0	Cowpox — *vaccinia from cattle*
051.1	Pseudocowpox — *paravaccinia infection*
051.2	Contagious pustular dermatitis — *Poxvirus from sheep or goats*
051.9	Unspecified paravaccinia — *unknown paravaccinia infection*

Coding Clarification
Vaccinia as a result of inoculation is reported with 999.0, not with 051.1.

052 Chickenpox

Varicella zoster virus causes chickenpox and herpes zoster. Chickenpox is the initial, acute phase of the disease, and herpes zoster is a reactivation of the virus in a latent stage.

Chickenpox is highly contagious and usually mild, but it may be severe in infants, adults, or the immunosuppressed. More than 95 percent of Americans have been infected by chickenpox by the

Infectious and Parasitic Diseases

time they reach adulthood. In the United States, four million people are infected with chickenpox each year. Chickenpox has a characteristic itchy rash, which then forms blisters that dry into scabs. An infected person may have anywhere from only a few lesions to more than 500 lesions.

An adult bout of chickenpox is more likely to have complications than a childhood infection. Complications occur when the varicella zoster virus inflames the brain, spinal cord, lung, or other organ, or when infection is accompanied by manifestations of high fever, or when the patient is immunosuppressed. Secondary infections are also considered complications.

052.0	Postvaricella encephalitis	*— with inflammation of brain*
052.1	Varicella (hemorrhagic) pneumonitis	*— with lung infection*
052.2	Postvaricella myelitis	*— with inflammation of spinal cord*
052.7	Chickenpox with other specified complications	*— complications not listed above*
	AHA: Q1, 2002, 3	
052.8	Chickenpox with unspecified complication	*— unknown complication*
052.9	Varicella without mention of complication	*— no complications mentioned*

Coding Clarification
If the complication to chickenpox cannot be described in the codes presented in this rubric, report a code from rubric 052 first, and codes describing the complications or manifestations secondarily, as in the case of myocarditis (422.0) or arthritis (711.50-711.59).

Inoculation against chickenpox is reported with V05.4.

Correct code assignment for myelitis depends upon the underlying disease process contributing to the condition. ICD-9-CM has classified myelitis due to specific viral infections (varicella, herpes, zoster, herpes simplex, tuberculosis, and syphilis) to Chapter 1, Infectious and Parasitic Diseases. Myelitis due to other infectious diseases is classified under inflammatory disorders of the nervous system. The more serious acute transverse myelitis is classified with the demyelinating diseases section of Chapter 6, Nervous System. The numerous new subterms in the index will help direct the coder to the appropriate choice.

053 Herpes zoster
Varicella zoster virus causes chickenpox and herpes zoster. Chickenpox is the initial, acute phase of the disease, and herpes zoster is a reactivation of the virus in a latent stage. Herpes zoster is often referred to as shingles or zona. In herpes zoster, the virus causes unilateral eruptions and painful neuralgia along a nerve path. Herpes zoster myelitis, inflammation of the spinal cord, is a rare complication following an acute attack of chickenpox in which the herpes zoster virus becomes dormant in cranial and spinal ganglia in a noninfectious state. The virus later reactivates in a ganglion and causes a localized, unilateral eruption of shingles, or zona, resulting in the neurologic sequela of myelitis, which typically develops days to weeks after the appearance of the rash. Common symptoms of myelitis include loss of spinal cord function, low back pain, weakness of the muscles, or altered sensations in the feet and toes. These symptoms can progress in severity and may include paralysis, urinary retention, and loss of bowel or bladder control. The disease is classified according to site.

053.0	Herpes zoster with meningitis	*— inflammation of brain and/or spinal cord*
053.10	Herpes zoster with unspecified nervous system complication	*— unknown nervous system complication*
053.11	Geniculate herpes zoster	*— affecting facial nerve*
053.12	Postherpetic trigeminal neuralgia	*— causing oral or nasal pain*
053.13	Postherpetic polyneuropathy	*— multiple nerve involvement*
053.14	Herpes zoster myelitis	*— with inflammation of spinal cord*
053.19	Other herpes zoster with nervous system complications	
053.20	Herpes zoster dermatitis of eyelid	*— unilateral, eyelid*
053.21	Herpes zoster keratoconjunctivitis	*— unilateral in cornea and conjunctiva*
053.22	Herpes zoster iridocyclitis	*— unilateral in iris and ciliary body*
053.29	Other ophthalmic herpes zoster complications	*— other eye complication*
053.71	Otitis externa due to herpes zoster	
053.79	Other specified herpes zoster complications	
053.8	Unspecified herpes zoster complication	
053.9	Herpes zoster without mention of complication	

Coding Clarification
Correct code assignment for myelitis depends upon the underlying disease process contributing to the condition. ICD-9-CM has classified myelitis due to specific viral infections (varicella, herpes, zoster, herpes simplex, tuberculosis, and syphilis) to Chapter 1, Infectious and Parasitic Diseases. Myelitis due to other infectious diseases is classified under inflammatory disorders of the nervous system. The more serious acute transverse myelitis

is classified with the demyelinating diseases section of Chapter 6, Nervous System. The numerous new subterms in the index will help direct the coder to the appropriate choice.

054 Herpes simplex

Herpes simplex is an infection of the herpes simplex virus (HSV), including HSV-1 and HSV-2. The infection causes multiple clusters of fluid-filled, inflamed blisters on the skin or mucous membranes and is usually transmitted by direct contact. HSV-1 is commonly seen about the mouth, lips, and conjunctiva. HSV-2 usually affects genitals and is often transmitted through sexual contact. However, either type of HSV can occur in either site.

The virus can remain dormant and be reactivated by emotional stress, fever, or photosensitivity. Typically, the virus is localized, and code selection is based on the anatomy affected. Herpes simplex infections of the lips or mouth are considered the most benign form of the disease and are reported as "uncomplicated," with 054.9. Systemic manifestations can occur, especially in infants and in the immunosuppressed. Although both strains of HSV may remain dormant in the nervous system and cause neurological sequelae, such as herpes simplex myelitis, or inflammation of the spinal cord with possible permanent damage to the myelin, this is more commonly associated with HSV-2 infection.

054.0	Eczema herpeticum — *invading pre-existing skin inflammation*	
054.10	Unspecified genital herpes — *unknown site* AHA: Jan-Feb, 1987, 15-16	
054.11	Herpetic vulvovaginitis — *vulva and vagina* AHA: Jan-Feb, 1987, 15-16	
054.12	Herpetic ulceration of vulva — *vulva* AHA: Jan-Feb, 1987, 15-16	
054.13	Herpetic infection of penis — *penis* AHA: Jan-Feb, 1987, 15-16	
054.19	Other genital herpes — *other specified site* AHA: Jan-Feb, 1987, 15-16	
054.2	Herpetic gingivostomatitis — *oral mucosa*	
054.3	Herpetic meningoencephalitis — *inflammation of brain and spinal cord*	
054.40	Unspecified ophthalmic complication herpes simplex — *unknown eye complication*	
054.41	Herpes simplex dermatitis of eyelid — *inflammation and lesions on lid*	
054.42	Dendritic keratitis — *inflammation and ulcers of cornea*	
054.43	Herpes simplex disciform keratitis — *inflammation and edema of cornea*	
054.44	Herpes simplex iridocyclitis — *inflammation of iris and ciliary body*	
054.49	Herpes simplex with other ophthalmic complications — *eye complication not elsewhere classified*	
054.5	Herpetic septicemia — *herpes simplex disseminated through bloodstream* AHA: Q2, 2000, 5	
054.6	Herpetic whitlow — *painful herpes lesion on fingertip; "herpetic felon"*	
054.71	Visceral herpes simplex — *infection of thoracic or abdominal organ*	
054.72	Herpes simplex meningitis — *inflammation of lining of brain or spinal cord*	
054.73	Herpes simplex otitis externa — *inflammation and lesions of external ear*	
054.74	Herpes simplex myelitis — *with inflammation of spinal cord*	
054.79	Other specified herpes simplex complications — *complication not elsewhere classified*	
054.8	Unspecified herpes simplex complication — *unknown complications*	
054.9	Herpes simplex without mention of complication — *uncomplicated "fever blister"*	

Coding Clarification

This rubric excludes congenital herpes simplex, which is reported with 771.2.

Correct code assignment for myelitis depends upon the underlying disease process contributing to the condition. ICD-9-CM has classified myelitis due to specific viral infections (varicella, herpes, zoster, herpes simplex, tuberculosis, and syphilis) to Chapter 1, Infectious and Parasitic Diseases. Myelitis due to other infectious diseases is classified under inflammatory disorders of the nervous system. The more serious acute transverse myelitis is classified with the demyelinating diseases section of Chapter 6, Nervous System. The numerous new subterms in the index will help direct the coder to the appropriate choice.

055 Measles

Measles is an acute infection caused by paramyxovirus and presents with a hacking cough, rash, and fevers. German measles (rubella) is a different infection, reported with codes from the 056 rubric.

Measles is usually transmitted from person to person via airborne respiratory droplets. Pharyngitis is common. Koplik's spots are white, grainy spots that can occur in the buccal mucosa and are an early symptom of measles.

In the United States, measles outbreaks have been greatly reduced by government immunization programs. Measles has a low mortality rate in healthy individuals, and the disease generally follows a normal course with high fever, Koplik's spots, generalized rash, and cough.

Patients with measles are susceptible to streptococcal infection, worsening of tuberculosis, or reactivation of an inactive mycobacterial infection. Sequence the measles code first, followed by codes for the secondary infection.

Measles are classified according to complication. In most cases, the complication occurs after the symptoms of the measles have diminished. Pneumonia as a complication is most common in infants.

055.0	Postmeasles encephalitis — *brain infection*
055.1	Postmeasles pneumonia — *lung infection*
055.2	Postmeasles otitis media — *middle ear infection*
055.71	Measles keratoconjunctivitis — *inflammation of cornea and conjunctiva*
055.79	Other specified measles complications — *complication not elsewhere classified*
055.8	Unspecified measles complication — *unknown complication*
055.9	Measles without mention of complication — *typical course of rash, fever, and cough*

Coding Clarification
Prophylactic vaccination against measles is reported with V04.2 as a separate inoculation, or V06.4 for measles-mumps-rubella (MMR) inoculation. Measles that follow a normal course should be reported with code 055.9.

056 Rubella

Rubella is also called German measles or three-day measles. It is a highly contagious virus, but the symptoms are mild and short-lived in most people. Symptoms include malaise, arthralgia, rash, headache, and fever. Rubella during pregnancy, however, can result in abortion, stillbirth, or in congenital defects. Because of its highly contagious nature and effect upon the fetus, rubella is considered a serious health threat.

Rubella codes are selected according to complication. Consult the index to report rubella during pregnancy.

056.00	Unspecified rubella neurological complication — *unknown nervous complication*
056.01	Encephalomyelitis due to rubella — *inflammation of brain and spinal cord*
056.09	Other neurological rubella complications — *nervous complication not elsewhere classified*
056.71	Arthritis due to rubella — *inflammation of joint*
056.79	Rubella with other specified complications — *complication not elsewhere classified, not nervous system*
056.8	Unspecified rubella complications — *unknown complication*
056.9	Rubella without mention of complication — *typical course of rash and fever*

Coding Clarification
If the infection runs its normal course, report rubella without complication with 056.9.

This rubric excludes congenital rubella, which is reported with 771.0.

Exposure to rubella is reported with V01.4.

Prophylactic vaccination against rubella is reported with V04.3 as a separate inoculation or V06.4 for measles-mumps-rubella (MMR) inoculation.

057 Other viral exanthemata

This rubric captures rash-causing viruses that are not specifically outlined in rubrics 050-056.

057.0	Erythema infectiosum (fifth disease) — *contagious rash, livid on cheeks*
057.8	Other specified viral exanthemata — *including fourth disease, sixth disease, roseola infantum, monkeypox*
057.9	Unspecified viral exanthem — *unknown viral exanthemata*

Coding Clarification
Report 057.0 for fifth disease, also called Sticker's disease or erythema infectiosum.

Report 057.8 for any of the following: Dukes (-Filatow) disease, exanthema subitum or sixth disease, fourth disease, parascarlatina, pseudoscarlatina, roseola infantum, and Zahorsky's disease.

060–066 Arthropod–borne Viral Diseases

Insects are the carriers that carry the diseases classified to this section of ICD-9-CM. Early attempts to classify these diseases were made along geographic lines and according to the insect believed to be the carrier. An arbovirus is a common shortened name for arthropod-borne virus.

Mosquitoes are the most common carrier, or transmitting agent, for arboviruses. The bite of a mosquito often transmits the disease from bird to mosquito. The bite of a mosquito to man transmits the disease to man. In equine disease, the mosquitoes transmit disease to horses, or from horses to man. Seldom is the disease carried from man to mosquito to man.

060 Yellow fever

Yellow fever is transmitted from mosquito to man. In cities, the bite of an *Aedes aegypti* mosquito causes the infection; in the jungle (sylvan), *Haemagogus* and other forest canopy mosquitoes acquire the virus from jungle primates and transmit the virus to man. In the United States, cases of yellow fever are usually limited to people who have been abroad. Yellow fever is most commonly seen in Central Africa, South America, and Central America.

Yellow fever causes high fever, headache, jaundice, and hemorrhage. The pulse is slow. Mortality rate can be as high as 10 percent.

060.0	Sylvatic yellow fever — (Use additional code to identify any associated meningitis, 321.2) — *origin in jungle or woods; usually transmitted animal to man, by mosquito*
060.1	Urban yellow fever — (Use additional code to identify any associated meningitis, 321.2) — *origin in city or town; usually transmitted man to man, by mosquito*
060.9	Unspecified yellow fever — (Use additional code to identify any associated meningitis, 321.2) — *unknown*

Coding Clarification

Prophylactic inoculation against yellow fever is reported with V04.4.

061 Dengue ☒

Dengue is transmitted to man by the bite of the Aedes mosquito. The disease is endemic throughout tropical and subtropical regions, and is usually seen in the United States only when people come to this country already infected with the virus.

Dengue causes chills, headache, backache, and prostration. Joint and leg aches and onset of high fever are rapid.

Coding Clarification

This rubric excludes hemorrhagic fever caused by dengue, which is reported with 065.4.

062 Mosquito-borne viral encephalitis

These diseases cause central nervous system symptoms such as tremors, convulsion, coma, confusion, as well as headache, vomiting, and fever. Geographic differences are significant among the varieties. Japanese encephalitis is seen in the Far East. Eastern equine encephalitis (EEE) is most common in the Atlantic and Gulf Coast states, upper New York, and western Michigan. Western equine encephalitis (WEE) is seen in areas west of the Mississippi. St. Louis encephalitis is most common in the United States and Caribbean. Australian encephalitis is usually limited to New Guinea and Australia, and California encephalitis.

062.0	Japanese encephalitis — (Use additional code to identify any associated meningitis, 321.2) — *Flavivirus; Japanese B*
062.1	Western equine encephalitis — (Use additional code to identify any associated meningitis, 321.2) — *Alphavirus; WEE*
062.2	Eastern equine encephalitis — (Use additional code to identify any associated meningitis, 321.2) — *Alphavirus; EEE*
062.3	St. Louis encephalitis — (Use additional code to identify any associated meningitis, 321.2) — *Flavivirus; in United States*
062.4	Australian encephalitis — (Use additional code to identify any associated meningitis, 321.2) — *Flavivirus; in Australia*
062.5	California virus encephalitis — (Use additional code to identify any associated meningitis, 321.2)
062.8	Other specified mosquito-borne viral encephalitis — (Use additional code to identify any associated meningitis, 321.2) — *including Ilheus virus*
062.9	Unspecified mosquito-borne viral encephalitis — (Use additional code to identify any associated meningitis, 321.2) — *unknown*

Coding Clarification

Report Venezuelan equine encephalitis with 066.2.

Report West Nile virus with 066.40-066.49.

063 Tick-borne viral encephalitis

In tick-borne encephalitis, a tick is the carrier instead of a mosquito. Included in this rubric are diseases limited to Russia, Central Europe, and Great Britain. Only Powassan encephalitis is commonly found in North America, both in New York and in Canada. Any other variety is likely to be found among travelers.

063.0	Russian spring-summer (taiga) encephalitis — (Use additional code to identify any associated meningitis, 321.2) — *Russia, central Europe*
063.1	Louping ill — (Use additional code to identify any associated meningitis, 321.2) — *British Isles*

063.2	Central European encephalitis — (Use additional code to identify any associated meningitis, 321.2) — *central Europe*	
063.8	Other specified tick-borne viral encephalitis — (Use additional code to identify any associated meningitis, 321.2) — *including Langat and Powassan (New York)*	
063.9	Unspecified tick-borne viral encephalitis — (Use additional code to identify any associated meningitis, 321.2)	

Coding Clarification
Powassan encephalitis is reported with 063.8

064 Viral encephalitis transmitted by other and unspecified arthropods OK

Report viral encephalitis not otherwise specified, unknown carrier, with 049.9, reserving this code for encephalitis caused by an unidentified arbovirus.

065 Arthropod-borne hemorrhagic fever

This rubric specifies a hemorrhagic fever. If hemorrhage is not a component, seek other codes.

Hemorrhagic fever is not endemic to the United States. Codes in this category may apply to infections obtained while abroad, primarily in Russia and Asia.

065.0	Crimean hemorrhagic fever (CHF Congo virus) — (Use additional code to identify any associated meningitis, 321.2) — *Crimea and Russian Don and Volga river valleys*
065.1	Omsk hemorrhagic fever — (Use additional code to identify any associated meningitis, 321.2) — *Siberia*
065.2	Kyasanur Forest disease — (Use additional code to identify any associated meningitis, 321.2) — *India*
065.3	Other tick-borne hemorrhagic fever — (Use additional code to identify any associated meningitis, 321.2) — *other*
065.4	Mosquito-borne hemorrhagic fever — (Use additional code to identify any associated meningitis, 321.2) — *Dengue hemorrhagic; Chikungunya hemorrhagic*
065.8	Other specified arthropod-borne hemorrhagic fever — (Use additional code to identify any associated meningitis, 321.2) — *including mite-borne hemorrhagic*
065.9	Unspecified arthropod-borne hemorrhagic fever — (Use additional code to identify any associated meningitis, 321.2) — *unknown hemorrhagic arbovirus*

Coding Clarification
Hemorrhagic Dengue fever is reported with 065.4; for dengue fever without mention of hemorrhage, report 061.

Hemorrhagic Chikungunya fever is reported with 065.4; for Chikungunya fever without mention of hemorrhage, report 066.3.

In all cases, with or without hemorrhage, yellow fever is reported with 060.0-060.9.

066 Other arthropod-borne viral diseases

This rubric captures arbovirus infections not classified as hemorrhagic, and not the specific infections of yellow fever or dengue. Colorado tick fever is the arbovirus in this section that would likely be seen in the United States, and causes fever, malaise, headaches, and myalgia. This is a different infection than Rocky Mountain spotted fever, a *Rickettsia* infection that causes a petechial rash in addition to fever, malaise, headache, and myalgia.

West Nile fever is an arbovirus, transmitted to humans by an arthropod; in this case, an infected mosquito. West Nile fever was first isolated 65 years ago in Uganda but was not reported in the continental United States until 1999. It affects humans, birds, and some mammals, including horses, cats, bats, skunks, chipmunks, squirrels, and rabbits. It can cause fatal inflammation of the brain, encephalitis, or of the lining of the brain or spinal cord, meningitis. It can cause other neurological symptoms as well, including tremors, convulsions, coma, and paralysis.

066.0	Phlebotomus fever — (Use additional code to identify any associated meningitis, 321.2) — *sandfly-borne; Asia, Mideast, South America*
066.1	Tick-borne fever — (Use additional code to identify any associated meningitis, 321.2) — *American mountain; Colorado*
066.2	Venezuelan equine fever — (Use additional code to identify any associated meningitis, 321.2)
066.3	Other mosquito-borne fever — (Use additional code to identify any associated meningitis, 321.2) — *Bunyamwera; O'nyong-nyong; Rift valley*
066.40	West Nile fever, unspecified
066.41	West Nile fever with encephalitis
AHA: Q4, 2004, 51
066.42	West Nile fever with other neurologic manifestation — (Use additional code to specify the neurologic condition.)
AHA: Q4, 2004, 51
066.49	West Nile fever with other complications — (Use additional code to specify the neurologic condition.)
066.8	Other specified arthropod-borne viral diseases — (Use additional code to identify any associated meningitis, 321.2) — *including Chandipura and Piry fever*
066.9	Unspecified arthropod-borne viral disease — (Use additional code to identify any associated meningitis, 321.2) — *unknown arbovirus*

Coding Clarification
Colorado tick fever is reported with 066.1.

Rocky Mountain spotted fever is reported with 082.0.

Use an additional code with 066.42 and 066.49 to specify the other conditions.

070–079 Other Diseases Due to Viruses and Chlamydiae

This rubric covers a broad spectrum of infection not elsewhere classified.

070 Viral hepatitis
AHA: Q4, 1991, 26-28

Hepatitis is an inflammation or infection of the liver. Symptoms of hepatitis range from flu-like illness to liver failure and death. Initially, nausea and malaise are common. Later in the course of the disease, jaundice and an enlarged liver are common.

Hepatitis A (HAV) is spread through fecal contamination or by eating contaminated, raw shellfish and is considered to be a milder form of hepatitis. Exposure to hepatitis B (HBV) is limited to direct contact with contaminated blood or blood products, or through sexual congress. HBV is the source of many chronic liver ailments. The hepatitis C virus (HCV) causes 80 percent of hepatitis cases resulting from blood transfusions, and also is associated with more chronic and severe liver ailments. The hepatitis E virus (HEV) is associated with fecal contamination and is a milder form of the disease.

The following fifth-digit subclassification is for use with categories 070.2 and 070.3:

0   acute or unspecified, without mention of hepatitis delta
1   acute or unspecified, with hepatitis delta
2   chronic, without mention of hepatitis delta
3   chronic, with hepatitis delta

Code	Description
070.0	Viral hepatitis A with hepatic coma
070.1	Viral hepatitis A without mention of hepatic coma
070.2 ✓5th	Viral hepatitis B with hepatic coma
070.3 ✓5th	Viral hepatitis B without mention of hepatic coma
	AHA: Q1, 1993, 28
070.41	Acute hepatitis C with hepatic coma
070.42	Hepatitis delta without mention of active hepatitis B disease with hepatic coma
070.43	Hepatitis E with hepatic coma
070.44	Chronic hepatitis C with hepatic coma
070.49	Other specified viral hepatitis with hepatic coma
070.51	Acute hepatitis C without mention of hepatic coma
070.52	Hepatitis delta without mention of active hepatitis B disease or hepatic coma
070.53	Hepatitis E without mention of hepatic coma
070.54	Chronic hepatitis C without mention of hepatic coma
	AHA: Q2, 2006, 13
070.59	Other specified viral hepatitis without mention of hepatic coma
070.6	Unspecified viral hepatitis with hepatic coma
070.70	Unspecified viral hepatitis C without hepatic coma
	AHA: Q4, 2004, 52
070.71	Unspecified viral hepatitis C with hepatic coma
	AHA: Q4, 2004, 52
070.9	Unspecified viral hepatitis without mention of hepatic coma

Documentation Issues

Physician documentation should support answers to the following questions for accurate code selection to be made:

1. Is the hepatitis viral or non-viral?
2. What type of viral hepatitis does the patient have?
3. Is this an acute or chronic phase of the condition?
4. Did the patient experience hepatic coma?
5. Is the patient asymptomatic?

Coding Clarification

Chronic Active Hepatitis: ICD-9-CM classifies hepatitis along two axes, viral and non-viral. Viral forms of the disease are classified to category 070 *Viral hepatitis,* in the Infectious and Parasitic Disease chapter. Non-viral and unspecified hepatitis are classified to category 571 *Chronic liver disease and cirrhosis,* in the Digestive System chapter. Further, hepatitis caused by other specific viruses such as Epstein-Barr or cytomegaloviruses are considered separately, and do not fall into the general accepted usage of the phrase "viral hepatitis." Viral hepatitis is considered to be hepatitis caused by the hepatitis virus and this rubric covers acute and chronic stages of that disease.

If the diagnostic statement is documented as chronic active hepatitis, a code from category 571 should be selected because the type (viral or non-viral) of hepatitis is unspecified. This category specifically excludes viral forms of hepatitis and an excludes note is provided in the tabular section that references codes 070.0-070.9. For example, the diagnostic statement specifically indicates chronic active viral hepatitis B, it should be assigned one code, 070.30 *Viral hepatitis B, without mention of* hepatic coma, acute or unspecified, without mention of hepatitis delta.

General Guidelines: Code selection is based on serotype, acute or chronic phase, and whether it is documented as with or without hepatic coma (code range: 070.0-070.9).

Viral hepatitis is classified into the following major forms:

- Hepatitis A virus or "infectious hepatitis" is caused by the Hepatitis A Virus and is found to be the generally milder disease transmitted by the fecal oral route. This type of viral hepatitis is less likely to progress to chronic forms of hepatitis or cirrhosis.
- Hepatitis B virus or "serum hepatitis" is the more serious virus. This type is transmitted parenterally (through blood products, injections, and sexual contact) and in a high number of cases progresses into chronic liver disease.
- Hepatitis C virus has been identified as the virus responsible for most cases of parenteral non-A, non-B hepatitis. Although typically associated with blood transfusions, it has been proven to result from other types of exposure (e.g., occupational-health care related, sexual contact). It has been noted that up to 40 percent of cases with this form have no recognized cause for the infection. Patients with hepatitis C are more likely to develop chronic liver disease and chronic manifestations such as chronic active hepatitis and/or cirrhosis.
- Hepatitis D, formally known as "Hepatitis Delta virus," is an incomplete virus and requires the presence of hepatitis B surface antigen (HBSAg) to replicate. Spread mainly by needles and blood, hepatitis delta may present itself as a co-infection during acute infection with hepatitis B, and in these cases is more likely to develop into a fulminant hepatitis than hepatitis B infection alone. Delta hepatitis causes acute and/or chronic liver disease in patients with a concurrent hepatitis B infection. A large number of these patients develop fulminant hepatitis and/or chronic active hepatitis and cirrhosis. Chronic delta infection is a frequent event and manifests as severe forms of chronic hepatitis with accelerated progression to cirrhosis and a high mortality rate.
- Hepatitis E virus or enteric "fecal-oral hepatitis" is serologically different from the other known hepatitis viruses. It is clearly produced by a different type of virus than that causing non-A non-B parenteral hepatitis. This type has been identified during investigations of large epidemics in ill-developing countries. The disease is also a clinically distinct entity as one of the foremost causes of acute viral hepatitis in young to middle-aged adults in developing countries and carries a high case-fatality rate among pregnant women. Chronic liver disease has not been reported in these cases.

Acute and Chronic: Both acute and chronic stages of viral hepatitis are classified to category 070 *Viral hepatitis*. When coding viral hepatitis, keep in mind that the fourth-digit subclassification only provides for identifying serotypes with and without mention of coma. Fifth digits are provided in the viral hepatitis categories to differentiate between acute and chronic viral hepatitis. If the diagnostic statement states that the patient has both, then a code for each should be assigned.

Carrier Status: A carrier is defined as a person who has hepatitis B, C, or D in his/her blood even after all of the symptoms (with the exception of fatigue) have disappeared. If the virus is present in the blood it can be transmitted to others. Codes for carrier or suspected carrier of viral hepatitis would be located in the V Codes chapter, category V02.

Pregnancy and Viral Hepatitis: Use code 647.6x *Other viral diseases*, with an additional code to identify the specific form of viral hepatitis. To identify pregnant women who are carriers, use the code that identifies the carrier state as a secondary diagnosis code with OB code 648.9x *Other current conditions classifiable elsewhere*.

Prophylactic Vaccinations: Currently, prophylactic administration of hepatitis vaccines is being provided to newborns upon parental approval. Since hepatitis B vaccination is recommended for all newborns, V05.3 may be used as an additional code on hospital newborn records. Hospitals assign procedure code 99.55 *Prophylactic administration of vaccine against other diseases*.

Coding Scenario

A 49-year-old female is seen in the office for a pre-employment screening and tested positive for hepatitis B. The patient has shown no symptoms for hepatitis. The patients' past medical history shows a long history of IV drug use.

Code assignment: V70.5 *Health examination of defined subpopulations* and V02.61 *Hepatitis B carrier*

A 29-year-old male patient is admitted to the hospital with severe hepatic encephalopathy and jaundice. The patient is diagnosed with viral hepatitis B and hepatic encephalopathy.

Code assignment: 070.20 *Viral hepatitis B with hepatic coma, acute or unspecified, without hepatitis delta*

A patient is seen in the office for treatment of chronic viral hepatitis, type C.

Code assignment: 070.54 *Chronic hepatitis C without mention of hepatic coma*

A patient is admitted to the hospital with acute fulminant hepatitis and liver failure due to chronic viral hepatitis type B.

Code assignment: 070.32 *Viral hepatitis B without mention of hepatic coma, chronic, without mention of hepatitis delta* and 570 *Acute and subacute necrosis of liver*

071 Rabies OK

Rabies, or hydrophobia, is an acute infectious disease caused by a neurotropic virus found in the saliva of rabid mammals. Canine vaccination has nearly eliminated canine rabies in the United States and cases of wild animal bites causing rabies are rare. Rabies causes restlessness, fever, excessive salivation, and painful laryngeal spasms.

Exposure to rabies is usually treated successfully with immediate local wound cleansing and administration of rabies immune globulin.

If the patient develops rabies, the diagnosis is no longer an imminent death sentence. Supportive treatment of respiratory system, circulatory system, and central nervous system complications can result in a positive outcome for the symptomatic rabies patient. Rabies is often described as urban or sylvan, depending on the source of infection.

Coding Clarification
This code is used to report active rabies infection, not simple exposure to rabies.

If a person has been exposed to rabies, but infection status is unknown or an infection has not developed, report V01.5.

To report inoculation against rabies, whether following exposure or as a prophylactic measure for high-risk individuals such as wildlife handlers, report V04.5.

Whether the carrier is from the city or the wilderness, rabies infection is reported with 071.

072 Mumps

Mumps presents as an acute infection of the salivary glands, usually the parotids, caused by paramyxovirus. Inhaling respiratory droplets from an infected person can spread the disease. Most cases occur in children two years of age or older. Mumps causes painful swelling of the salivary glands, pain upon chewing, and high fever. Complications may occur, especially in adults.

072.0	Mumps orchitis — *inflammation of testis*
072.1	Mumps meningitis — *inflammation of lining of brain and/or spinal cord*
072.2	Mumps encephalitis — *inflammation of brain*
072.3	Mumps pancreatitis — *inflammation of pancreas*
072.71	Mumps hepatitis — *inflammation of liver*
072.72	Mumps polyneuropathy — *inflammation of nerves*
072.79	Mumps with other specified complications — *specified inflammation not elsewhere classified*
072.8	Unspecified mumps complication — *complication not elsewhere classified*
072.9	Mumps without mention of complication — *normal course of mumps*

Coding Clarification
Code selection for mumps is determined by complication. In cases that follow the normal uncomplicated course of swollen parotid glands and high fever, report 072.9.

Prophylactic vaccination against mumps is reported with V04.6 as a separate inoculation or V06.4 for measles-mumps-rubella (MMR) inoculation.

073 Ornithosis

Ornithosis is also called psittacosis. The disease is caused by *Chlamydia psittaci* and transmitted most commonly by parrots, parakeets, or lovebirds, but sometimes by domestic birds such as pigeons, turkeys, or canaries, or by some seabirds. Infection usually occurs when dust or droppings are inhaled by man or, rarely, by a bird bite. Ornithosis can also be transmitted from man to man, but this is very rare.

Symptoms include fever, malaise, and cough, in the case of lung infection. Ornithosis has a 30 percent mortality rate without treatment, but responds well to antibiotics.

073.0	Ornithosis with pneumonia — *pulmonary infection*
073.7	Ornithosis with other specified complications — *complication not elsewhere classified*
073.8	Ornithosis with unspecified complication — *complication not specified*
073.9	Unspecified ornithosis — *no complications*

Coding Clarification
Code selection for ornithosis is based on type of complication. Report any significant symptoms, such as cough or shortness of breath, secondarily.

Infectious and Parasitic Diseases

074 Specific diseases due to Coxsackievirus

Coxsackie virus commonly causes infection in summer and fall and is transmitted man-to-man via oral secretions, feces, or blood. Herpangina is an acute infection of Coxsackie virus, causing throat lesions, fever, and vomiting, generally seen in children during the summer months. Epidemic pleurodynia is a Coxsackie infection causing severe paroxysmal pain in the chest and fever, usually limited to young adults and children. It is also called Bornholm disease or devil's grip.

Coxsackie carditis is infection of the heart. Code selection is based on whether the infection occurs in the outer lining of the heart, the heart cavities, or the heart muscle. In infants, a Coxsackie infection of the heart muscle can be life-threatening, but this infection can occur at any age.

Hand, foot, and mouth disease is a Coxsackie infection of the hands, feet, and oral mucosa, most commonly seen in preschool children. It is usually a mild infection.

074.0	Herpangina — *vesicular pharyngitis; typically children in summer*	
074.1	Epidemic pleurodynia — *chest pain with fever; typically children and young adults*	
074.20	Coxsackie carditis, unspecified — *inflammation of heart unspecified*	
074.21	Coxsackie pericarditis — *inflammation of outer lining of heart*	
074.22	Coxsackie endocarditis — *inflammation of within the heart cavities*	
074.23	Coxsackie myocarditis — *inflammation of muscle of heart*	
074.3	Hand, foot, and mouth disease — *lesions on hands, feet, and mouth; typically preschoolers*	
074.8	Other specified diseases due to Coxsackievirus — *including acute lymphonodular pharyngitis*	

Coding Clarification

Report Coxsackie meningitis with 047.0 and Coxsackie enteritis with 008.67.

Coxsackie virus infection of the nervous system, not elsewhere classified, is reported with 048.

075 Infectious mononucleosis

AHA: March-April, 1987, 8; Q3, 2001, 13

Infectious mononucleosis is an active infection by the Epstein-Barr virus, causing fever, sore throat, enlarged lymph glands and spleen, and fatigue. It is most commonly seen in teens and young adults, and runs a mild course in most cases.

Coding Clarification

In mononucleosis with hepatitis, report 075 and 573.1.

076 Trachoma

Trachoma is caused by infection with the organism *Chlamydia trachomatis*. It begins slowly as a mild conjunctivitis that develops into a severe onset infection. The initial stage lasts several weeks and is followed by a chronic stage in which the lids remain swollen, and the cornea becomes eroded, scarred, and vascularized. The lids develop contractures and may turn outward, pulling away from the eye. Eventually, the eyelashes turn in, rubbing on the cornea at the front of the eye. The scarring on the cornea leads to severe vision loss and blindness, usually by age 40 to 50.

076.0	Initial stage trachoma — *mild inflammation of conjunctiva with pain*
076.1	Active stage trachoma — *acute inflammation of conjunctiva with pain*
076.9	Unspecified trachoma — *stage unknown*

Coding Clarification

Report late effects of trachoma with 139.1. Code the sequelae first, as in vision loss (369.00-369.9), followed by 139.1.

077 Other diseases of conjunctiva due to viruses and Chlamydiae

Codes in this rubric are organized by infective agent and symptoms. Inclusion conjunctivitis is caused by Chlamydia trachomatis, and adenovirus type B causes epidemic keratoconjunctivitis and pharyngoconjunctival fever.

077.0	Inclusion conjunctivitis — *due to Chlamydia trachomatis*
077.1	Epidemic keratoconjunctivitis — *shipyard eye; due to adenovirus type B*
077.2	Pharyngoconjunctival fever — *due to adenovirus type B*
077.3	Other adenoviral conjunctivitis — *acute adenoviral follicular conjunctivitis*
077.4	Epidemic hemorrhagic conjunctivitis
077.8	Other viral conjunctivitis — *including Newcastle conjunctivitis*
077.98	Unspecified diseases of conjunctiva due to Chlamydiae
077.99	Unspecified diseases of conjunctiva due to viruses — *unknown virus*

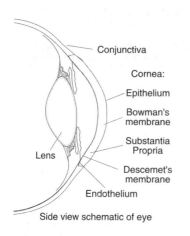

Side view schematic of eye

Coding Clarification

Other diseases and infections of the conjunctiva can be found in the Nervous System chapter under rubrics 372 and 373, as well as under specific infective agents, for example, herpes zoster keratoconjunctivitis (053.21) or trachoma (076.0-076.9).

078 Other diseases due to viruses and Chlamydiae

This rubric addresses specific viral and chlamydial diseases not specified elsewhere.

More than 50 types of human papilloma viruses (HPV) cause plantar and genital warts in humans. These infections may be asymptomatic or produce warts or mucosal lesions.

Commonly, human papilloma virus causes viral warts. They may be documented as condyloma, verruca, or verruca vulgaris. Viral warts caused by condylomata acuminata are sexually transmitted genital warts, distinct from other viral warts in that they are associated with cervical dysplasia and carcinoma of the cervix, penis, and vulva.

Cytomegaloviral disease (CMV) is a human salivary gland virus and member of the herpes group. It affects only humans, and can range in symptoms from being a benign and asymptomatic infection to causing significant impairment or death in infants and the immunosuppressed. In symptomatic cases, fatigue, lymphadenopathy, and low fever may be present.

CMV is a most common and serious organ transplant infection complication.

Code	Description
078.0	Molluscum contagiosum — *poxvirus causing small bumps on skin or conjunctiva*
078.10	Unspecified viral warts — *horny skin wars; human papilloma virus* **AHA:** Q4, 1993, 22; Q2, 1997, 9
078.11	Condyloma acuminatum — *clusters of lesions on genitalia; STD* **AHA:** Q4, 1993, 22; Q2, 1997, 9
078.19	Other specified viral warts — *including Verruca plantaris, Verruca plana; fig wart* **AHA:** Q4, 1993, 22; Q2, 1997, 9
078.2	Sweating fever — *sweating disease; miliary fever*
078.3	Cat-scratch disease — *mild and benign lymphoreticulosis*
078.4	Foot and mouth disease — *aphthous fever; ulcers on mouth, legs and feet*
078.5	Cytomegaloviral disease — (Use additional code to identify manifestation: 484.1, 573.1) — *CMV* **AHA:** Q1, 1989, 9; Q2, 1993, 11; Q3, 1998, 4; Q1, 2003, 10
078.6	Hemorrhagic nephrosonephritis — *Russia and Korea*
078.7	Arenaviral hemorrhagic fever — *Argentina and Bolivia*
078.81	Epidemic vertigo — *dizziness*
078.82	Epidemic vomiting syndrome — *winter vomiting disease*
078.88	Other specified diseases due to Chlamydiae — *not elsewhere classified* **AHA:** Q4, 1996, 22
078.89	Other specified diseases due to viruses — *including Marburg disease, Lassa fever; green monkey disease, pseudorabies, tanapox, and Aujeszky's disease*

Documentation Issues

Condyloma acuminatum are commonly called genital warts on the patient record, but, unless condyloma acuminatum is specifically noted, the patient record does not substantiate use of code 078.11.

Coding Clarification

Viral warts may be documented as condyloma, verruca, or verruca vulgaris and are reported with 078.10.

Viral warts caused by condylomata acuminata are reported with 078.11.

If CMV infection follows transplant, assign a code from category 996.8 to identify the transplanted organ, and 078.5 to report the infection.

When appropriate, an additional code is used to identify the manifestation of CMV infection, as in hepatitis (573.1) or pneumonia (484.1).

For congenital cytomegaloviral infection, report 771.1.

079 Viral and chlamydial infection in conditions classified elsewhere and of unspecified site

HIV-2, generally not seen in the United States, is on the rise elsewhere in the world.

Respiratory syncytial virus (RSV) is a common cause of respiratory disease in winter in the United States. Infants are most vulnerable to the disease. Each year, RSV causes 4,500 U.S. deaths and 90,000 hospitalizations.

Hantavirus is an arbovirus that causes severe respiratory distress in its victims. The mortality rate for *Hantavirus* is about 50 percent, with treatment. Most commonly transmitted to humans when they inhale dust from feces of infected mice, most cases are seen in the Four Corners area of the United States.

SARS (severe acute respiratory syndrome) is a form of respiratory infection that is spreading rapidly through Southeast Asia and other parts of the world. Patients start out with a fever and often have chills, headache, malaise, body aches, and placid respiratory symptoms. In the early stage, patients have decreased white blood cell counts and some also have diarrhea. After three to seven days, the patient usually develops a dry, non-productive cough that increases in severity. As the disease progresses, chest x-rays show significant congestion in the lungs. Eventually, not enough oxygen gets to the blood and, in 10 to 20 percent of cases, patients will require mechanical ventilation. The severity of illness among patients is variable, ranging from mild symptoms to death. Only patients who have traveled within 10 days of the onset of symptoms to an area with suspected SARS cases, or have had contact with a person suspected of having SARS, are considered possible carriers of the disease.

079.0	Adenovirus infection in conditions classified elsewhere and of unspecified site — (Note: This code is to be used as an additional code to identify the viral agent in diseases classifiable elsewhere and viral infection of unspecified nature or site)
079.1	ECHO virus infection in conditions classified elsewhere and of unspecified site — (Note: This code is to be used as an additional code to identify the viral agent in diseases classifiable elsewhere and viral infection of unspecified nature or site)
079.2	Coxsackievirus infection in conditions classified elsewhere and of unspecified site — (Note: This code is to be used as an additional code to identify the viral agent in diseases classifiable elsewhere and viral infection of unspecified nature or site)
079.3	Rhinovirus infection in conditions classified elsewhere and of unspecified site — (Note: This code is to be used as an additional code to identify the viral agent in diseases classifiable elsewhere and viral infection of unspecified nature or site)
079.4	Human papilloma virus in conditions classified elsewhere and of unspecified site — (Note: This code is to be used as an additional code to identify the viral agent in diseases classifiable elsewhere and viral infection of unspecified nature or site) AHA: Q4, 1993, 22; Q2, 1997, 9
079.50	Unspecified retrovirus in conditions classified elsewhere and of unspecified site — (Note: This code is to be used as an additional code to identify the viral agent in diseases classifiable elsewhere and viral infection of unspecified nature or site)
079.52	Human t-cell lymphotrophic virus, type II (HTLV-II), in conditions classified elsewhere and of unspecified site
079.53	Human immunodeficiency virus, type 2 (HIV 2), in conditions classified elsewhere and of unspecified site — (Note: This code is to be used as an additional code to identify the viral agent in diseases classifiable elsewhere and viral infection of unspecified nature or site)
079.59	Other specified retrovirus, in conditions classified elsewhere and of unspecified site — (Note: This code is to be used as an additional code to identify the viral agent in diseases classifiable elsewhere and viral infection of unspecified nature or site)
079.6	Respiratory syncytial virus (RSV) — (Note: This code is to be used as an additional code to identify the viral agent in diseases classifiable elsewhere and viral infection of unspecified nature or site) AHA: Q4, 1996, 27, 28
079.81	Hantavirus infection — (Note: This code is to be used as an additional code to identify the viral agent in diseases classifiable elsewhere and viral infection of unspecified nature or site)
079.82	SARS-associated coronavirus — (Note: This code is to be used as either an additional code to identify the viral agent in diseases classifiable elsewhere or to describe the viral infection of unspecified nature or site) — *severe acute respiratory syndrome* AHA: Q4, 2003, 46
079.88	Other specified chlamydial infection, in conditions classified elsewhere and of unspecified site — (Note: This code is to be used as an additional code to identify the viral agent in diseases classifiable elsewhere and viral infection of unspecified nature or site)
079.89	Other specified viral infection, in conditions classified elsewhere and of unspecified site — (Note: This code is to be used as an additional code to identify the viral agent in diseases

079.98 classifiable elsewhere and viral infection of unspecified nature or site)
Unspecified chlamydial infection, in conditions classifiable elsewhere and of unspecified site — (Note: This code is to be used as an additional code to identify the viral agent in diseases classifiable elsewhere and viral infection of unspecified nature or site)

079.99 Unspecified viral infection, in conditions classifiable elsewhere and of unspecified site — (Note: This code is to be used as an additional code to identify the viral agent in diseases classifiable elsewhere and viral infection of unspecified nature or site)

Coding Clarification
For some respiratory infections, report the infection first and RSV as the infective agent secondarily, as in tracheobronchitis due to RSV, with 466.0 and 079.6. If respiratory syncytial virus is noted with acute bronchitis, two codes are required: 466.0 *Acute bronchitis* and 079.6 *Respiratory syncytial virus (RSV)*.

Some respiratory infection codes identify RSV as the infective agent, so only one code is necessary. Bronchiolitis due to RSV is reported with a single code, 466.11, and pneumonia due to RSV is reported with a single code, 480.1.

Report 079.81 secondarily to pneumonia or other infection code from the Respiratory System chapter of ICD-9-CM.

Report HIV-2 with 079.53 and HIV-1 with 042.

Severe adult respiratory syndrome (SARS) reported without a definitive diagnosis of pneumonia should be reported using code 079.82.

080–088   Rickettsioses and Other Arthropod–borne Diseases

Rickettsial diseases are usually perpetuated by a cycle from animal to insect carrier to man. The illnesses are sudden in onset and include fever, myalgia, malaise, headache, and sometimes rash. In some cases, rickettsioses produce a localized ulcer or lesion at the site of the insect bite.

080   Louse-borne (epidemic) typhus OK
Rickettsia prowazekii is transmitted by feces from the human body louse (*Pediculus humanus*), through a break in the skin, often from scratching, or by entry of the louse droppings into mucus membranes. Epidemic typhus causes headache, rash, and high fever, and is most dangerous to people older than 50.

Coding Clarification
Report 080 for primary typhus infection.

081   Other typhus
Other varieties of typhus are classified by infective agent and by carrier.

081.0	Murine (endemic) typhus	— *Rickettsia typi (mooseri); rat flea*
081.1	Brill's disease	— *R. prowazekii* recurrence
081.2	Scrub typhus	— *R. tsutsugamushi; chigger*
081.9	Unspecified typhus	— unknown

Coding Clarification
Brill's disease is a reoccurrence of epidemic typhus (080) and is reported with 081.1.

082   Tick-borne rickettsioses
These diseases typically begin with a tick bite in which a lesion develops at the site of the bite. This may be called an eschar, or, in boutonneuse fever, a tache noire. Lymphadenopathy, low fever, and a rash usually follow.

Rocky Mountain spotted fever is endemic to the United States. Colorado tick fever is a different infection than Rocky Mountain spotted fever, which causes a petechial rash in addition to fever, malaise, headache, and myalgia.

Boutonneuse fever, caused by *Rickettsia conorii*, occurs in Africa, India, Europe, the Mideast, and near the Caspian, Black, and Mediterranean seas. Normally, boutonneuse fever, Queensland tick typhus, and North Asian tick fever are seen in the United States only among travelers who return with an infection.

Ehrlichiosis is likely caused by various *Ehrlichia* species and code selection is based on the species. Infection resembles Rocky Mountain spotted fever, without a rash, and illness may extend for weeks or months. The infection responds to antibiotics.

082.0	Spotted fevers	— Rocky Mountain spotted fever
082.1	Boutonneuse fever	— *Africa, India, Mediterranean*
082.2	North Asian tick fever	— *Siberia*
082.3	Queensland tick typhus	— *Australia*
082.40	Ehrlichiosis, unspecified	— unknown type
	AHA: Q4, 2000, 38	
082.41	Ehrlichiosis chaffeensis [E. chaffeensis]	
082.49	Other ehrlichiosis	— other than E. chaffeensis
	AHA: Q4, 2000, 38	
082.8	Other specified tick-borne rickettsioses	
082.9	Unspecified tick-borne rickettsiosis	

083   Other rickettsioses
These specific varieties of rickettsioses infection do not fall into the previous rubric classifications.

083.0	Q fever	— *Coxiella burnetii*
083.1	Trench fever	— *Quintan, Wolhynian, Werner-His fever*

Infectious and Parasitic Diseases

083.2	Rickettsialpox — *Rickettsia akari; mite*	
083.8	Other specified rickettsioses — *not elsewhere classified*	
083.9	Unspecified rickettsiosis — *unknown*	

Coding Clarification
Report 083.9 for an infection known to be rickettsioses, but of unknown type and unknown carrier.

084 Malaria
Malaria is a mosquito-borne protozoan infection endemic to the tropics. It is transmitted man to mosquito to man and has largely been eradicated in the United States through insecticide programs and drugs. Most cases of malaria in the United States are seen in people who have traveled abroad. Sometimes, these infected travelers may even spawn a stateside epidemic of malaria. Rarely, malaria may be transmitted through a blood transfusion or shared needle.

Malaria causes malaise and headache with intermittent fever and chill. Jaundice usually develops. Some varieties, most notably Blackwater fever, can cause more serious complications including hemolysis.

084.0	Falciparum malaria (malignant tertian) — *Plasmodium falciparum*
084.1	Vivax malaria (benign tertian) — *P. vivax*
084.2	Quartan malaria — *P. malariae*
084.3	Ovale malaria — *P. ovale*
084.4	Other malaria — *monkey malaria*
084.5	Mixed malaria — *more than one parasite*
084.6	Unspecified malaria — *unknown*
084.7	Induced malaria — *therapeutically induced*
084.8	Blackwater fever — *P. falciparum; with hemoglobinuria*
084.9	Other pernicious complications of malaria — (Use additional code to identify complication: 573.2, 581.81) — *including algid and cerebral malaria*

Coding Clarification
Malaria is coded according to species of *Plasmodium*: *P. falciparum*, *P. malariae*, *P. ovale*, *P. vivax*, or mixed species. A code is also provided in this rubric for therapeutically induced malaria (084.7), regardless of species.

Do not report personal history of malaria (V12.03) in patients with active disease.

085 Leishmaniasis
Leishmaniasis is an infection by *Leishmania*, a genus of parasitic protozoa, usually seen in developing nations and rare in the United States, though seen in parts of South America. The focus of infection and the infective agent are variables that create a broad spectrum of disease associated with leishmaniasis.

085.0	Visceral leishmaniasis (kala-azar) — *L. donovani; systemic; in Far East, USSR, Africa, Mediterranean, South and Central America*
085.1	Cutaneous leishmaniasis, urban — *L. tropica minor; dry/ulcerating lesions; boils*
085.2	Cutaneous leishmaniasis, Asian desert — *L. tropica major; wet/necrotizing skin lesions*
085.3	Cutaneous leishmaniasis, Ethiopian — *L. aethiopica; widespread skin lesions*
085.4	Cutaneous leishmaniasis, American — *L. mexicana; L. tegumentaria diffusa; skin lesions*
085.5	Mucocutaneous leishmaniasis, (American) — *L. braziliensis; called espundia, uta, chiclero ulcer*
085.9	Unspecified leishmaniasis — *unknown Leishmania species*

086 Trypanosomiasis
Trypanosomiasis is caused by protozoa *Trypanosoma* and causes chronic disease with symptoms including fever, lymphadenopathy, headache, and edema. Complications can affect the central nervous system and major organs and can be fatal. International travelers may return to the United States with a trypanosomiasis infection, but the protozoa is endemic only in Africa and South America, so it is seldom seen in North America.

086.0	Chagas' disease with heart involvement — *Trypanosoma cruzi; heart involvement*
086.1	Chagas' disease with other organ involvement — *T. cruzi; other organ involvement*
086.2	Chagas' disease without mention of organ involvement — *T. cruzi; no organ infection*
086.3	Gambian trypanosomiasis — *T. brucei gambiense*
086.4	Rhodesian trypanosomiasis — *T. brucei rhodesiense*
086.5	African trypanosomiasis, unspecified — *sleeping sickness*
086.9	Unspecified trypanosomiasis — *unknown trypanosomiasis*

Coding Clarification
Report the trypanosomiasis code first, followed by any manifestation codes that may apply, for example, encephalitis (323.2), meningitis (321.3). However, cardiomyopathy from Chagas' disease requires only 086.0, and other specific forms of Chagas' disease are reported with 078.88.

087 Relapsing fever
Relapsing fever is an infection caused by *Borrelia* and the symptoms are episodic and may include fever and arthralgia. Code selection is based on the carrier.

087.0	Louse-borne relapsing fever — *lice as carrier*
087.1	Tick-borne relapsing fever — *tick as carrier*
087.9	Unspecified relapsing fever — *unknown carrier*

Coding Clarification
Report 087.9 if the carrier is unknown.

088 Other arthropod-borne diseases
This category identifies arthropod-borne diseases not elsewhere classified.

Bartonellosis is in infection of *Bartonella bacilliformis*, transmitted by sandflies in the Andes mountains of South America. Cases in the United States are rare.

Babesiosis identifies a group of tick-borne diseases infected with the *Babesia* protozoa. Rare in humans, it causes fever, chills, anemia, splenomegaly, and muscle pain. People with a history of splenectomy have a high mortality rate for babesiosis. In others, it resolves within weeks.

Lyme disease is caused by the bite of a tick infected with *Borrelia burgdorferi* and causes joint disorders, skin lesions, and flu-like symptoms. It is endemic to most parts of the United States as well as in Russia, Australia, and the Far East.

088.0	Bartonellosis — *Bartonella bacilliformis*; sandflies; Andes
088.81	Lyme disease — *Borrelia burgdorferi*; ticks, United States AHA: Q2, 1989, 10; Q3, 1990, 14; Q4, 1991, 15
088.82	Babesiosis — *Babesia*; ticks AHA: Q4, 1993, 23
088.89	Other specified arthropod-borne diseases — *not elsewhere classified*
088.9	Unspecified arthropod-borne disease — *unknown*

Coding Scenario
A patient with recently diagnosed Lyme disease is seen in the office for follow-up. She is now complaining of joint pain and swelling in the knees. The physician states that arthritis due to the Lyme disease is now present.

Code assignment: 088.81 *Lyme disease and* 711.86 *Arthropathy associated with other infectious and parasitic diseases, lower leg*

090–099 Syphilis and Other Venereal Diseases
It is estimated that 400,000 people seek treatment for syphilis in the United States each year. Syphilis is caused by the spirochete *Treponema pallidum*. The disease is divided into four categories: congenital syphilis and the three stages of acquired syphilis: early syphilis, a contagious stage with mild symptoms; latent syphilis, asymptomatic and infectious; and the late or tertiary stage, with significant symptoms but not contagious. Infection is transmitted by an infected mother to her fetus or by sexual contact. Rare instances of infection from kissing or close bodily contact have been documented, as the spirochete enters the body through the mucous membranes or skin. Syphilis responds to antibiotic treatment.

The disease can manifest itself in any stage, and may be asymptomatic for years. Usually, the first symptoms are lymphadenopathy and a localized chancre. However, the variety of manifestations can make clinical recognition of syphilis difficult.

Syphilis codes are classified as congenital, early, or latent. The disease is further classified according to its manifestations.

090 Congenital syphilis
Up to 80 percent of syphilitic mothers pass the infection to their fetus. Symptoms do not develop in most neonates, so diagnosis in the hospital nursery is usually the result of tests performed on the infant because of the mother's medical history.

Early congenital syphilis may manifest itself within two years of birth with a rash on the patient's palms and soles, swollen lymph glands, an enlarged spleen, and/or characteristic syphilitic chancres near mucous membranes. Other symptoms may include osteochondritis, epiphysitis, periostitis, chronic coryza, or choroiditis. Syphilis is confirmed with serologic tests. Early symptomatic syphilis is sometimes called Wegner's disease.

Latent early congenital syphilis has no clinical manifestations and is diagnosed through serologic testing within the first two years of life. If a test of spinal fluid is positive for syphilis, the disease is not considered latent, even if the patient does not show symptoms. Instead, the condition is reported as congenital syphilitic meningitis (090.42).

090.0	Early congenital syphilis, symptomatic — *from birth to two years old, symptoms*
090.1	Early congenital syphilis, latent — *from birth to two years old, no symptoms*
090.2	Unspecified early congenital syphilis — *from birth to two years, symptoms unknown*
090.3	Syphilitic interstitial keratitis — *congenital corneal infection*
090.40	Unspecified juvenile neurosyphilis — (Use additional code to identify any associated mental disorder) — *unknown site of infection*
090.41	Congenital syphilitic encephalitis — (Use additional code to identify any associated mental disorder) — *infection of brain*
090.42	Congenital syphilitic meningitis — (Use additional code to identify any associated

Infectious and Parasitic Diseases

	mental disorder) — *infection of the lining of the brain or spinal cord*	091.69	Early syphilis, secondary syphilis of other viscera — *secondary inflammation of other abdominal organs within two years of initial infection*
090.49	Other juvenile neurosyphilis — (Use additional code to identify any associated mental disorder) — *not elsewhere classified*	091.7	Early syphilis, secondary syphilis, relapse — *return of symptoms after asymptomatic period within two years of initial infection*
090.5	Other late congenital syphilis, symptomatic — *older than two years with symptoms*	091.81	Early syphilis, acute syphilitic meningitis (secondary) — *sudden, severe inflammation of lining of the brain or spinal cord within two years of initial infection*
090.6	Late congenital syphilis, latent — *older than two years, no symptoms*		
090.7	Late congenital syphilis, unspecified — *older than two years, symptoms unknown*	091.82	Early syphilis, syphilitic alopecia — *secondary loss of hair within two years of initial infection*
090.9	Congenital syphilis, unspecified — *unknown age in child with unknown symptoms*	091.89	Early syphilis, other forms of secondary syphilis — *other secondary manifestation within two years of initial infection*

Coding Clarification
Report exposure to syphilis with V01.6, and carrier of syphilis with V02.8.

091.9	Early syphilis, unspecified secondary syphilis

If neurological manifestations are present, use codes from the 090.4 series of codes rather than 090.0.

Coding Clarification
Report exposure to syphilis with V01.6, and carrier of syphilis with V02.8.

091 Early syphilis, symptomatic
Generally, early syphilis is the period from initial infection and the first two years of the disease. Early syphilis can be further divided into primary or secondary syphilis. In primary syphilis, a painless chancre appears at the site of infection and regional swelling of lymph nodes occurs as the spirochetes invade the lymphatic system. The lymphadenopathy is sometimes called bubo. In secondary syphilis, the infection spreads to secondary sites. Codes in this section are selected based on whether the infection is primary or secondary and then by anatomic site.

If early syphilis has complications involving the heart or nervous system, report codes in the 093 or 094 rubrics instead.

092 Early syphilis, latent
Latent early syphilis has no clinical manifestations and is diagnosed through serologic testing within the first two years of infection. If a test of spinal fluid is positive for syphilis, the disease is not considered latent, even if the patient does not show symptoms. Instead, the condition is reported with a code from the 094 rubric for neurosyphilis.

091.0	Genital syphilis (primary) — *genital lesion in new case of syphilis*
091.1	Primary anal syphilis — *anal lesion in new case of syphilis*
091.2	Other primary syphilis — *lesion in new case of syphilis, not genital or anal*
091.3	Secondary syphilis of skin or mucous membranes — *secondary lesions within two years of initial infection*
091.4	Adenopathy due to secondary syphilis — *secondary lymph gland inflammation within two years of initial infection*
091.50	Early syphilis, syphilitic uveitis, unspecified — *secondary inflammation of uvea in eye within two years of initial infection*
091.51	Early syphilis, syphilitic chorioretinitis (secondary) — *secondary inflammation of retina and choroid of eye within two years of initial infection*
091.52	Early syphilis, syphilitic iridocyclitis (secondary) — *secondary inflammation of iris and ciliary body of eye within two years of initial infection*
091.61	Early syphilis, secondary syphilitic periostitis — *secondary inflammation of outer layers of bone within two years of initial infection*
091.62	Early syphilis, secondary syphilitic hepatitis — *secondary inflammation of liver within two years of initial infection*

092.0	Early syphilis, latent, serological relapse after treatment — *other than congenital; results positive-negative-positive within first two years*
092.9	Early syphilis, latent, unspecified — *other than congenital; within first two years, no symptoms*

Coding Clarification
Report exposure to syphilis with V01.6, and carrier of syphilis with V02.8.

093 Cardiovascular syphilis
This rubric is reserved for any syphilitic infection of the cardiovascular system, except congenital infection, which is reported with 090.5 instead. Select the code based on anatomic site of infection. Clinical diagnosis is based on echocardiography (ECG) and serologic test for syphilis. Syphilis infection within the heart may lead to congestive heart failure, which is reported in addition to syphilis with 428.0.

093.0	Aneurysm of aorta, specified as syphilitic — *dilation of syphilitic aorta*
093.1	Syphilitic aortitis — *inflammation of main artery leading from heart*
093.20	Unspecified syphilitic endocarditis of valve — *inflammation of unknown heart valve*

Coders' Desk Reference for Diagnoses

093.21	Syphilitic endocarditis, mitral valve — *inflammation of mitral valve*
093.22	Syphilitic endocarditis, aortic valve — *inflammation of aortic valve*
093.23	Syphilitic endocarditis, tricuspid valve — *inflammation of tricuspid valve*
093.24	Syphilitic endocarditis, pulmonary valve — *inflammation of pulmonary value*
093.81	Syphilitic pericarditis — *inflammation of outer lining of heart*
093.82	Syphilitic myocarditis — *inflammation of muscle of heart*
093.89	Other specified cardiovascular syphilis — *other inflammation of heart, including Babinski-Vaquez syndrome*
093.9	Unspecified cardiovascular syphilis

Coding Clarification
Report exposure to syphilis with V01.6, and carrier of syphilis with V02.8.

Cardiovascular complications occur in tandem with neurosyphilis and, in these cases, report codes from both the 093 and 094 rubrics.

094 Neurosyphilis
In neurosyphilis, spirochetes infect the nerves, spinal cord, or brain. Codes in this rubric are organized by anatomy and severity. Tabes dorsalis is a progressive degeneration of nerves and general paresis describes progressive degeneration of brain. Both conditions are considered the most severe and systemic forms of neurosyphilis.

Most symptomatic neurosyphilis is a form of late syphilis, meaning the patient has been infected for more than two years. Any presence of infection in the spinal fluid is considered a form a neurosyphilis, even if the patient is otherwise asymptomatic.

Disorders including dementia and some forms of arthropathy are associated with some forms of neurosyphilis and should be reported in addition to the neurosyphilis code.

094.0	Tabes dorsalis — (Use additional code to identify any associated mental disorder. Use additional code to identify manifestation, 713.5) — *progressive degeneration of nerves in long-term syphilis*
094.1	General paresis — (Use additional code to identify any associated mental disorder) — *degeneration of brain in long-term syphilis*
094.2	Syphilitic meningitis — (Use additional code to identify any associated mental disorder) — *inflammation of lining of the brain and/or spinal cord*
094.3	Asymptomatic neurosyphilis — (Use additional code to identify any associated mental disorder) — *positive spinal fluid, but no symptoms*
094.81	Syphilitic encephalitis — (Use additional code to identify any associated mental disorder) — *inflammation of the brain in neurosyphilis*
094.82	Syphilitic Parkinsonism — (Use additional code to identify any associated mental disorder) — *tremors, decreased motor function, muscular rigidity*
094.83	Syphilitic disseminated retinochoroiditis — (Use additional code to identify any associated mental disorder) — *inflammation of retina and choroid*
094.84	Syphilitic optic atrophy — (Use additional code to identify any associated mental disorder) — *degeneration of the eye and its nerves*
094.85	Syphilitic retrobulbar neuritis — (Use additional code to identify any associated mental disorder) — *inflammation of the posterior optic nerve*
094.86	Syphilitic acoustic neuritis — (Use additional code to identify any associated mental disorder) — *inflammation of acoustic nerve*
094.87	Syphilitic ruptured cerebral aneurysm — (Use additional code to identify any associated mental disorder) — *rupture of blood vessel in brain*
094.89	Other specified neurosyphilis — (Use additional code to identify any associated mental disorder) — *including Argyll Robertson's syndrome, erosion of spine, Heubner's disease*
094.9	Unspecified neurosyphilis — (Use additional code to identify any associated mental disorder)

Coding Clarification
Report exposure to syphilis with V01.6, and carrier of syphilis with V02.8.

Asymptomatic neurosyphilis can be an early or late form of the disease, and is reported with 094.3.

095 Other forms of late syphilis, with symptoms
This rubric covers symptomatic syphilitic infections of more than two years organized by site of secondary infection. Cardiovascular syphilis (093) and neurosyphilis (094) are excluded from this rubric.

095.0	Syphilitic episcleritis — *inflammation of external surface of sclera*
095.1	Syphilis of lung — *pulmonary infection*
095.2	Syphilitic peritonitis — *inflammation of the abdominal membrane lining*
095.3	Syphilis of liver — *hepatic infection*
095.4	Syphilis of kidney — *inflammation of one or both kidneys*
095.5	Syphilis of bone — *infection of bone*
095.6	Syphilis of muscle — *myositis from syphilis*
095.7	Syphilis of synovium, tendon, and bursa
095.8	Other specified forms of late symptomatic syphilis
095.9	Unspecified late symptomatic syphilis

Infectious and Parasitic Diseases

Coding Clarification
Report exposure to syphilis with V01.6, and carrier of syphilis with V02.8.

096 Late syphilis, latent ✓

In latent late syphilis, a positive serologic test has indicated the patient has the disease, but there are no symptoms after an infection of two or more years. The spinal fluid is clear.

Coding Clarification
Report exposure to syphilis with V01.6, and carrier of syphilis with V02.8.

For asymptomatic late syphilis with infected spinal fluid, 094.3 is reported instead.

097 Other and unspecified syphilis

This rubric contains nonspecific codes for use in cases when the timetable of syphilitic infection or the specific site of secondary infection is unknown. These codes are not to be used for patients younger than 2 years of age. See the codes in rubric 090 for congenital and juvenile syphilis.

097.0	Unspecified late syphilis — *after first two years, unknown symptoms*
097.1	Unspecified latent syphilis
097.9	Unspecified syphilis — *unknown acquired syphilis*

Coding Clarification
Report exposure to syphilis with V01.6, and carrier of syphilis with V02.8.

098 Gonococcal infections

Gonorrhea is an acute infection caused by *Neisseria gonorrhoeae*, usually transmitted sexually. Women are often asymptomatic, while men tend to develop urinary symptoms from gonococcus rather quickly. Diagnosis is based on bacteriologic examination of discharge or urine. Gonorrhea responds to antibiotic treatment, though several courses may be required to eradicate the disease.

Gonococcal infection is classified by site. In the most common site of infection, the genitourinary system, a further distinction is made between chronic and acute cases. Report chronic infection codes when the infection has continued for two months or longer.

098.0	Gonococcal infection (acute) of lower genitourinary tract — *sudden onset; bartholinitis, urethritis, vulvovaginitis*
098.10	Gonococcal infection (acute) of upper genitourinary tract, site unspecified — *sudden onset, upper genitourinary tract site unknown*
098.11	Gonococcal cystitis (acute) — *sudden onset; bladder*
098.12	Gonococcal prostatitis (acute) — *sudden onset; prostate*
098.13	Gonococcal epididymo-orchitis (acute) — *sudden onset; epididymis, testis*
098.14	Gonococcal seminal vesiculitis (acute) — *sudden onset; seminal vesicle*
098.15	Gonococcal cervicitis (acute) — *sudden onset; cervix*
098.16	Gonococcal endometritis (acute) — *sudden onset; uterus*
098.17	Gonococcal salpingitis, specified as acute — *sudden onset; fallopian tubes*
098.19	Other gonococcal infections (acute) of upper genitourinary tract — *sudden onset; upper genitourinary tract not elsewhere classified*
098.2	Gonococcal infections, chronic, of lower genitourinary tract — *persistent infection; bartholinitis, urethritis, vulvovaginitis*
098.30	Chronic gonococcal infection of upper genitourinary tract, site unspecified — *persistent infection, upper genitourinary tract site unknown*
098.31	Gonococcal cystitis, chronic — *persistent infection; bladder*
098.32	Gonococcal prostatitis, chronic — *persistent infection; prostate*
098.33	Gonococcal epididymo-orchitis, chronic — *persistent infection; epididymis, testis*
098.34	Gonococcal seminal vesiculitis, chronic — *persistent infection; seminal vesicle*
098.35	Gonococcal cervicitis, chronic — *persistent infection; cervix*
098.36	Gonococcal endometritis, chronic — *persistent infection; uterus*
098.37	Gonococcal salpingitis (chronic) — *persistent infection; fallopian tubes*
098.39	Other chronic gonococcal infections of upper genitourinary tract — *persistent infection; upper genitourinary tract not elsewhere classified*
098.40	Gonococcal conjunctivitis (neonatorum) — *infection of conjunctiva at birth*
098.41	Gonococcal iridocyclitis — *inflammation of iris and ciliary body*
098.42	Gonococcal endophthalmia — *inflammation and infection of the contents of the eyeball*
098.43	Gonococcal keratitis — *inflammation and infection of cornea*
098.49	Other gonococcal infection of eye — *other infection of eye due to gonorrhea*
098.50	Gonococcal arthritis — *inflammation of joint*
098.51	Gonococcal synovitis and tenosynovitis — *inflammation of viscid fluid of joint, causing pain and swelling*
098.52	Gonococcal bursitis — *inflammation of sac-like cavities in joint*
098.53	Gonococcal spondylitis — *inflammation of vertebrae*
098.59	Other gonococcal infection of joint — *gonococcal rheumatism; other joint inflammation not elsewhere classified*
098.6	Gonococcal infection of pharynx — *inflammation of pharynx*
098.7	Gonococcal infection of anus and rectum — *proctitis*
098.81	Gonococcal keratosis (blennorrhagica) — *skin lesions*

Code	Description
098.82	Gonococcal meningitis — *inflammation of the lining of the brain or spinal cord*
098.83	Gonococcal pericarditis — *inflammation of the outer lining of the heart*
098.84	Gonococcal endocarditis — *inflammation of the tissues lining the cavities of the heart*
098.85	Other gonococcal heart disease — *heart inflammation, not elsewhere classified*
098.86	Gonococcal peritonitis
098.89	Gonococcal infection of other specified sites — *other infection, not elsewhere classified*

Coding Clarification
If the patient is infected with a penicillin-resistant form of gonorrhea, report V09.0 *Infection with microorganisms resistant to penicillins,* in addition to the code for chronic gonorrhea.

Chlamydial infections frequently occur with gonorrhea and should be reported in addition to the gonorrhea code, with *Chlamydia* codes from the 099 rubric.

Report exposure to gonorrhea with V01.6, and carrier of gonorrhea with V02.7.

Coding Scenario
A patient is seen for UTI. After examination and testing, a diagnosis of acute gonococcal cystitis is confirmed.

Code assignment: Code 098. 11 *Acute gonococcal cystitis*

099 Other venereal diseases
This category identifies sexually transmitted diseases not elsewhere classified.

Chancroid is a localized infection by *Haemophilus ducreyi,* causing genital ulcers and infecting the inguinal lymph nodes. Care must be taken to distinguish chancroid infection from herpes simplex infection. This diagnosis is made via cultures or microscopic examination.

The most common sexually transmitted disease in the United States is chlamydial infection, and its most common manifestation is urethritis. At least 50 percent of nongonococcal urethritis cases in the United States are due to *Chlamydia.*

Code	Description
099.0	Chancroid — *STD of H. ducreyi; skin lesions*
099.1	Lymphogranuloma venereum — *STD of C. trachomatis; skin lesions*
099.2	Granuloma inguinale — *STD of Calymmatobacterium granulomatis; anogenital skin ulcers*
099.3	Reiter's disease — *(Use additional code for associated condition: 372.33, 711.1) — STD of unknown etiology; urethritis, conjunctivitis*
099.40	Unspecified nongonococcal urethritis (NGU) — *STD, nonspecific NGU*
099.41	Nongonococcal urethritis (NGU) due to Chlamydia trachomatis — *STD, NGU from C. trachomatis*
099.49	Nongonococcal urethritis (NGU) due to other specified organism — *STD, NGU from other specified organism*
099.50	Chlamydia trachomatis infection of unspecified site — *STD, unknown site*
099.51	Chlamydia trachomatis infection of pharynx — *STD, throat*
099.52	Chlamydia trachomatis infection of anus and rectum — *STD, proctitis*
099.53	Chlamydia trachomatis infection of lower genitourinary sites — (Use additional code to specify site of infection: 595.4, 616.0, 616.11) — *STD, excluding urethra*
099.54	Chlamydia trachomatis infection of other genitourinary sites — (Use additional code to specify site of infection: 604.91, 614.9) — *STD, including pelvic inflammatory disease, testis*
099.55	Chlamydia trachomatis infection of unspecified genitourinary site — *STD, unknown site*
099.56	Chlamydia trachomatis infection of peritoneum — *STD, including perihepatitis*
099.59	Chlamydia trachomatis infection of other specified site — *STD, specified site not elsewhere classified*
099.8	Other specified venereal diseases — *STD, other disease, not elsewhere classified*
099.9	Unspecified venereal disease — *STD, unknown*

Coding Clarification
In the past, chlamydial urethritis was reported generically as NGU. As a result, a specific code for NGU due to chlamydial infection falls under rubric 099.4 *Other nongonococcal urethritis,* rather than under 099.5 *Other venereal diseases due to C. trachomatis.* Codes in the 099.5 rubric exclude urethral infection.

In cases of genitourinary infection, other than urethra and due to *C. trachomatis,* an additional code may be required to specify the site of genitourinary infection. For example, sequence 099.54 *Chlamydia trachomatis infection of other genitourinary site* first and 614.9 *Unspecified inflammatory disease of female pelvic organs and tissues* second to report pelvic inflammatory disease due to *Chlamydia.*

Trachoma, a chlamydial infection of the eye, is not venereal and is reported in the rubric 076.

For Reiter's disease (099.3) use a second code to report manifestations of the infection, such as conjunctivitis (372.33).

100–104 Other Spirochetal Diseases
These spirochetal diseases are not classified as sexually transmitted diseases because they are

transmitted from person to person through general body contact.

100 Leptospirosis
Leptospirosis is an infection due to any serotype of *Leptospira*. Dogs and rats are the most common carriers of leptospirosis and, in the United States, the most common source of infection is swimming in contaminated water. The infection usually enters the host through mucous membranes or injured skin. Less than 100 cases are reported in the United States annually.

100.0	Leptospirosis icterohemorrhagica — *Weil's, Mathieu's, Wassilieff's disease*
100.81	Leptospiral meningitis (aseptic) — *inflammation of membranes of brain and spinal cord*
100.89	Other specified leptospiral infections — *including Fort Bragg fever; swamp fever*
100.9	Unspecified leptospirosis — *unknown*

101 Vincent's angina OK
Vincent's angina is an infection of the oral mucosa causing painful bleeding, salivation, edema, and breath odor, caused by fusiform bacillus and a spirochete.

102 Yaws
Yaws is an infection by *Treponema pallidum pertenue* causing lesions of the skin, bone, and soft tissue. Upon infection, a lesion develops at the site and the yaws spirochete enters the body. This lesion is called the "mother yaw." Yaws is endemic to equatorial countries with high humidity, so cases in the United States are limited to travelers.

102.0	Initial lesions of yaws — *initial, mother yaw*
102.1	Multiple papillomata and wet crab yaws due to yaws — *butter, plantar, palmar yaws*
102.2	Other early skin lesions due to yaws — *cutaneous, less than five years since onset*
102.3	Hyperkeratosis due to yaws — *overgrowth of skin on palms and bottoms of feet*
102.4	Gummata and ulcers due to yaws — *rubbery lesions and dead skin*
102.5	Gangosa due to yaws — *massive, mutilating lesions of nose and oral cavity*
102.6	Bone and joint lesions due to yaws — *goundou, bone gumma, osteitis*
102.7	Other manifestations due to yaws — *mucosal, juxta-articular nodules*
102.8	Latent yaws — *asymptomatic with positive test*
102.9	Unspecified yaws — *including parangi*

103 Pinta
Pinta is an infection by *Treponema pallidum carateum* confined to the skin and causing progressive lesions. Pinta is confined to the Indians of Mexico, and Central and South America, so cases in the United States are limited to travelers.

103.0	Primary lesions of pinta — *first stage, early disease*
103.1	Intermediate lesions of pinta — *pigmented lesions, mid-disease*
103.2	Late lesions of pinta — *vitiligo, late in disease*
103.3	Mixed lesions of pinta
103.9	Unspecified pinta

104 Other spirochetal infection
Nonvenereal endemic syphilis is an infection of *Treponema pallidum endemicum* found in the eastern Mediterranean region and Africa. It initially causes skin lesions that may progress to soft tissue and bone lesions.

104.0	Nonvenereal endemic syphilis — *lesions on skin and mucosa, not from STD*
104.8	Other specified spirochetal infections — *including bronchospirochetosis, Castellani's bronchitis*
104.9	Unspecified spirochetal infection — *unknown*

110–118 Mycoses
These diseases are usually considered chronic and may be present for years before a diagnosis is made. Seldom are the symptoms acute, except with immunocompromised hosts. In the immunocompromised host, also report the health problem that causes the immune deficiency. Clinical manifestations of mycoses can be fever, anorexia, malaise, and/or depression. Many of the infections are geographically limited; each has a typical clinical course.

110 Dermatophytosis
Dermatophytoses are superficial fungal infections of the skin. Ringworm, though no worm is present, and athlete's foot are common names for the disease. Dermatophytosis is classified according to the site of the lesion. This rubric includes infections by species of *Epidermophyton*, *Microsporum*, and *Trichophyton tinea*.

110.0	Dermatophytosis of scalp and beard — (Use additional code to identify manifestation: 321.0-321.1, 380.15, 711.6) — *kerion, sycosis, black dot tinea of scalp*
110.1	Dermatophytosis of nail — (Use additional code to identify manifestation: 321.0-321.1, 380.15, 711.6) — *onychomycosis, tinea unguium*
110.2	Dermatophytosis of hand — (Use additional code to identify manifestation: 321.0-321.1, 380.15, 711.6) — *tinea manuum*
110.3	Dermatophytosis of groin and perianal area — (Use additional code to identify manifestation: 321.0-321.1, 380.15, 711.6) — *Dhobie itch, tinea cruris, Baerensprung's disease*
110.4	Dermatophytosis of foot — (Use additional code to identify manifestation: 321.0-321.1, 380.15, 711.6) — *athlete's foot; tinea pedis*

110.5	Dermatophytosis of the body — (Use additional code to identify manifestation: 321.0-321.1, 380.15, 711.6) — *herpes circinatus; tinea imbricata*	112.2	Candidiasis of other urogenital sites — (Use additional code to identify manifestation: 321.0-321.1, 380.15, 711.6) — *other than vulva and vagina*
110.6	Deep seated dermatophytosis — (Use additional code to identify manifestation: 321.0-321.1, 380.15, 711.6) — *Majocchi's granuloma*		**AHA:** Q4, 1996, 33; Q4, 2003, 105
		112.3	Candidiasis of skin and nails — (Use additional code to identify manifestation: 321.0-321.1, 380.15, 711.6) — *intertrigo, onychia, perionyxis*
110.8	Dermatophytosis of other specified sites — (Use additional code to identify manifestation: 321.0-321.1, 380.15, 711.6) — *not elsewhere classified*	112.4	Candidiasis of lung — (Use additional code to identify manifestation: 321.0-321.1, 380.15, 711.6) — *pneumonia*
			AHA: Q2, 1998, 7
110.9	Dermatophytosis of unspecified site — (Use additional code to identify manifestation: 321.0-321.1, 380.15, 711.6) — *unknown site*	112.5	Disseminated candidiasis — (Use additional code to identify manifestation: 321.0-321.1, 380.15, 711.6) — *grave, systemic infection associated with immunosuppression*

111 Dermatomycosis, other and unspecified

These superficial fungal infections of the skin are fungal infections other than ringworm, not elsewhere classified, or have an unknown fungal infectious agent.

AHA: Q2, 1989, 10; Q2, 2000, 5

		112.81	Candidal endocarditis — (Use additional code to identify manifestation: 321.0-321.1, 380.15, 711.6) — *infection of lining of cavities of heart*
111.0	Pityriasis versicolor — (Use additional code to identify manifestation: 321.0-321.1, 380.15, 711.6) — *Malassezia (Pityrosporum) furfur; tinea flava, tinea versicolor*	112.82	Candidal otitis externa — (Use additional code to identify manifestation: 321.0-321.1, 380.15, 711.6) — *infection of outer ear*
111.1	Tinea nigra — (Use additional code to identify manifestation: 321.0-321.1, 380.15, 711.6) — *Cladosporium infection; pityriasis nigra*	112.83	Candidal meningitis — (Use additional code to identify manifestation: 321.0-321.1, 380.15, 711.6) — *infection of lining of brain or spinal cord*
111.2	Tinea blanca — (Use additional code to identify manifestation: 321.0-321.1, 380.15, 711.6) — *Trichosporon (beigelii) (cutaneum); white piedra, Beigel's morbus*	112.84	Candidiasis of the esophagus — (Use additional code to identify manifestation: 321.0-321.1, 380.15, 711.6) — *infection in throat*
			AHA: Q4, 1992, 19
111.3	Black piedra — (Use additional code to identify manifestation: 321.0-321.1, 380.15, 711.6) — *Piedraia hortae infection*	112.85	Candidiasis of the intestine — (Use additional code to identify manifestation: 321.0-321.1, 380.15, 711.6) — *infection in intestines*
			AHA: Q4, 1992, 19
111.8	Other specified dermatomycoses — (Use additional code to identify manifestation: 321.0-321.1, 380.15, 711.6) — *including acladiosis and chromotrichomycosis*	112.89	Other candidiasis of other specified sites — (Use additional code to identify manifestation: 321.0-321.1, 380.15, 711.6) — *including bronchomoniliasis*
			AHA: Q3, 1991, 20; Q1, 1992, 17
111.9	Unspecified dermatomycosis — (Use additional code to identify manifestation: 321.0-321.1, 380.15, 711.6) — *unknown*	112.9	Candidiasis of unspecified site — (Use additional code to identify manifestation: 321.0-321.1, 380.15, 711.6) — *unknown site*

112 Candidiasis

Candidiasis is a yeast infection caused by *Candida* (usually *C. albicans* but also *C. tropicalis, C. parapsilosis*). Topical infections are quite common in the United States and are found in simple cases of diaper rash and vulvovaginal infection. However, *Candida* is an opportunistic illness and significant, systemic infection is seen among the immunosuppressed. Thrush is considered a clinically significant form of *Candida* infection in adults, as it may be an indicator of AIDS. Thrush, an oral infection, is considered benign in children.

Coding Clarification

Only one code is necessary when reporting a candidal urinary tract infection, 112.2 *Candidiasis of other urogenital sites.*

Candidiasis involving the respiratory system may be considered a clinically defining disease of AIDS. The code for HIV (AIDS) infection (042) should be sequenced first, when it is determined that the patient has AIDS, followed by codes for manifestations of HIV infection.

Candidal Pneumonia is reported with code 112.4 *Candidiasis of lung.*

112.0	Candidiasis of mouth — (Use additional code to identify manifestation: 321.0-321.1, 380.15, 711.6) — *thrush*
112.1	Candidiasis of vulva and vagina — (Use additional code to identify manifestation: 321.0-321.1, 380.15, 711.6) — *vaginal yeast infection*

114 Coccidioidomycosis
AHA: Q4, 1993, 23

Coccidioidomycosis is a fungal disease caused by *Coccidioidomycosis immitis* and common to the Southwestern United States. It is acquired by inhaling contaminated dust. The primary infection is an acute respiratory infection. Progressive disease may infect organs, bones, or nervous system.

Coccidioidomycosis infection is classified by site of infection, and by its primary or progressive form.

114.0	Primary coccidioidomycosis (pulmonary) — (Use additional code to identify manifestation: 321.0-321.1, 380.15, 711.6) — *acute, self-limiting lung infection* **AHA:** Q4, 1993, 23
114.1	Primary extrapulmonary coccidioidomycosis — (Use additional code to identify manifestation: 321.0-321.1, 380.15, 711.6) — *other acute, self-limited infection* **AHA:** Q4, 1993, 23
114.2	Coccidioidal meningitis — (Use additional code to identify manifestation: 321.0-321.1, 380.15, 711.6) — *infection of the lining of the brain or spinal cord* **AHA:** Q4, 1993, 23
114.3	Other forms of progressive coccidioidomycosis — (Use additional code to identify manifestation: 321.0-321.1, 380.15, 711.6) — *including disseminated infection* **AHA:** Q4, 1993, 23
114.4	Chronic pulmonary coccidioidomycosis — (Use additional code to identify manifestation: 321.0-321.1, 380.15, 711.6) — *persisting infection of lung* **AHA:** Q4, 1993, 23
114.5	Unspecified pulmonary coccidioidomycosis — (Use additional code to identify manifestation: 321.0-321.1, 380.15, 711.6) — *lung infection, unknown whether chronic or acute* **AHA:** Q4, 1993, 23
114.9	Unspecified coccidioidomycosis — (Use additional code to identify manifestation: 321.0-321.1, 380.15, 711.6) — *unknown infection, or Posada-Wernicke disease* **AHA:** Q4, 1993, 23

115 Histoplasmosis

Histoplasmosis is a fungal disease caused by *Histoplasma capsulatum* in the United States or *H. duboisii* in Africa. Pulmonary infection and lesion characterize the disease.

H. capsulatum is common to the eastern and Midwestern United States. It is also called small form histoplasmosis, while the African variety is called large form.

Histoplasmosis is classified according to American (small) or African (large) and by site of infection.

Histoplasmosis can present with significant symptoms, including cough or shortness of breath. Also report any significant symptoms secondarily.

The following fifth-digit subclassification is for use with category 115:

0 without mention of manifestation
1 meningitis
2 retinitis
3 pericarditis
4 endocarditis
5 pneumonia
9 other

115.0	⌐5th	Histoplasma capsulatum — (Use additional code to identify manifestation: 321.0-321.1, 380.15, 711.6) — *small form seen in United States*
115.1	⌐5th	Histoplasma duboisii — (Use additional code to identify manifestation: 321.0-321.1, 380.15, 711.6) — *large form seen in Africa*
115.9	⌐5th	Unspecified Histoplasmosis — (Use additional code to identify manifestation: 321.0-321.1, 380.15, 711.6) — *unknown form*

116 Blastomycotic infection

Blastomycosis is a fungal infection common to North American and Africa. Paracoccidioidomycosis is confined to South America. Lobomycosis is an infection by *Loboa loboi*, uncultured yeast that causes keloidal blastomycosis.

116.0	Blastomycosis — (Use additional code to identify manifestation: 321.0-321.1, 380.15, 711.6) — *Blastomyces (Ajellomyces) dermatitidis; Chicago disease*
116.1	Paracoccidioidomycosis — (Use additional code to identify manifestation: 321.0-321.1, 380.15, 711.6) — *Paracoccidioides (Blastomyces) brasiliensis; South American form*
116.2	Lobomycosis — (Use additional code to identify manifestation: 321.0-321.1, 380.15, 711.6) — *Loboa (Blastomyces) loboi; keloidal form*

117 Other mycoses

The fungus *Aspergillus* is commonly found in decaying leaves, stored grain, or bird droppings. It can cause three types of lung disease: as a colonization or aspergilloma in a healed site of previous lung disease (as in tuberculosis or lung abscess); as an invasive infection of the lung parenchyma that may spread via the blood stream to other parts of the body; or as an allergic reaction in people with asthma, cystic fibrosis, or who are immunosuppressed.

Mycotic mycetomas are infections by various genera and species of Ascomycetes and Deuteromycetes, such as *Acremonium (Cephalosporium) falciforme*,

Neotestudina rosatii, Madurella grisea, Madurella mycetomi, Pyrenochaeta romeroi, Leptosphaeria senagalensis, and *Kurtha zopfii.*

Cryptococcosis is an infection by *Cryptococcus neoformans.* The primary infection is respiratory and can be followed by infections in organs, bones, or the nervous system. Cryptococcosis is sometimes called European blastomycosis or torulosis, after its former name, Torula histolytica.

117.0	Rhinosporidiosis — (Use additional code to identify manifestation: 321.0-321.1, 380.15, 711.6) — *Rhinosporidium loboi*
117.1	Sporotrichosis — (Use additional code to identify manifestation: 321.0-321.1, 380.15, 711.6) — *Sporothrix (Sporotrichum) schenckii*
117.2	Chromoblastomycosis — (Use additional code to identify manifestation: 321.0-321.1, 380.15, 711.6) — *Cladosporium carrionii, Fonsecaea compactum, F. pedrosoi, Phialophora verrucosa*
117.3	Aspergillosis — (Use additional code to identify manifestation: 321.0-321.1, 380.15, 711.6) — *Aspergillus fumigatus, A. flavus, A. terreus* groups **AHA:** Q4, 1997, 40
117.4	Mycotic mycetomas — (Use additional code to identify manifestation: 321.0-321.1, 380.15, 711.6) — *various Ascomycetes and Deuteromycetes; Madura foot*
117.5	Cryptococcosis — (Use additional code to identify manifestation: 321.0-321.1, 380.15, 711.6) — *Cryptococcus neoformans; Busse-Buschke's disease*
117.6	Allescheriosis (Petriellidosis) — (Use additional code to identify manifestation: 321.0-321.1, 380.15, 711.6) — *Allescheria (Petriellidium) boydii*
117.7	Zygomycosis (Phycomycosis or Mucormycosis) — (Use additional code to identify manifestation: 321.0-321.1, 380.15, 711.6) — *various Absidia, Basidiobolus, Conidiobolus, Cunninghamella, Entomophthora, Mucor, Rhizopus, Saksenaea*
117.8	Infection by dematiacious fungi (Phaehyphomycosis) — (Use additional code to identify manifestation: 321.0-321.1, 380.15, 711.6) — *various fungi including Cladosporium trichoides (bantianum), Dreschlera hawaiiensis, Phialophora gougerotii, Phialophora jeanselmei*
117.9	Other and unspecified mycoses — (Use additional code to identify manifestation: 321.0-321.1, 380.15, 711.6) — *unknown pneumomycosis*

Coding Clarification
In the case of aspergillosis pneumonia, assign codes 117.3 for aspergillosis infection and 484.6 for the pneumonia. For allergic bronchopulmonary aspergillosis (ABA), report 518.6, along with an appropriate asthma code from the 493.9x series.

Report actinomycotic mycetomas with codes from the 039 rubric.

To properly report a urinary tract infection secondary to noncandidal yeast, use two codes: 599.0 *Urinary tract infection, site not specified* and 117.9 *Other and unspecified mycoses.*

118   Opportunistic mycoses
Use this code to report infection of skin, subcutaneous tissues, or organs by a wide variety of fungi generally considered to be pathogenic to compromised hosts only. Among the opportunistic mycoses would be the species of *Alternaria, Dreschlera,* and *Fusarium.* These infections are most likely to occur in patients after radiation therapy or during therapy with corticosteroids or immunosuppressants. People with AIDS, Hodgkin's lymphoma, or diabetes are susceptible to opportunistic mycoses.

120–129   Helminthiases

Helminthiases are diseases caused by worms. Worms are soft-bodied invertebrates and the infections can arise in a variety of ways, from person-to-person contact, contact with infested water, or ingestion of larvae in undercooked meat. Most helminthiasis infections occur in underdeveloped countries.

Infection by intestinal parasites is rarely life threatening, especially when the victim is in good health and proper treatment is instituted. Instead, discomfort and inconvenience are the more likely problems caused by intestinal parasites. However, helminthiasis is a significant problem in underdeveloped countries since these infections rob their hosts of essential nutrients. They often cause local irritation throughout the gastrointestinal tract. Diagnosis of intestinal parasites is usually done by analysis of stool specimens.

Worm infestations in ICD-9-CM are initially classified by type of worms: flukes, tapeworms, nematodes, and hookworms.

120   Schistosomiasis (bilharziasis)
Schistosomiasis, also known as bilharzia or blood fluke, is a water-borne parasitic disease carried by water snails. It is the major health risk in the rural areas of Central China and Egypt and continues to rank high in other developing countries. The main forms of schistosomiasis are caused by five species, and classification of infection is based on the species. The disease is contracted through contact with infested water.

Infectious and Parasitic Diseases

The eggs of the schistosomes in the excreta of an infected host open on contact with water and release a parasite, the miracidium, which seeks a fresh water snail. Once it has found its snail host, the miracidium produces thousands of new parasites (cercariae). The snail excretes the cercariae into the surrounding water. They penetrate the skin, continuing the biological cycle once they have made their way to the victim's blood vessels as worms.

In intestinal schistosomiasis, the worms reside in the blood vessels lining the intestine. In urinary schistosomiasis, they live in the blood vessels of the bladder. Only about a half of the eggs are excreted in the feces (intestinal schistosomiasis) or in the urine (urinary schistosomiasis). The rest remain in the host, damaging other vital organs. It is the eggs and not the worms that cause damage.

120.0	Schistosomiasis due to schistosoma haematobium — *urinary schistosomiasis; Schistosoma haematobium*
120.1	Schistosomiasis due to schistosoma mansoni — *intestinal schistosomiasis; S. mansoni*
120.2	Schistosomiasis due to schistosoma japonicum — *intestinal schistosomiasis; S. japonicum*
120.3	Cutaneous schistosomiasis
120.8	Other specified schistosomiasis
120.9	Unspecified schistosomiasis — *unknown schistosomiasis*

121 Other trematode infections
Trematodes other than bilharziasis are classified in this rubric. Most are very uncommon in the United States.

121.0	Opisthorchiasis — *Opisthorchis; cat liver fluke*
121.1	Clonorchiasis — *Clonorchis sinensis; oriental liver fluke*
121.2	Paragonimiasis — *Paragonimus; oriental lung fluke*
121.3	Fascioliasis — *Fasciola; sheep liver fluke*
121.4	Fasciolopsiasis — *Fasciolopsis (buski); intestinal fluke*
121.5	Metagonimiasis — *Metagonimus yokogawai*
121.6	Heterophyiasis — *Heterophyes*
121.8	Other specified trematode infections — *other trematode including Dicrocoelium dendriticum, Echinostoma ilocanum; Gastrodiscoides hominis*
121.9	Unspecified trematode infection — *unknown fluke disease*

122 Echinococcosis
Echinococcosis is an infection by the tapeworm *Echinococcus*. Diseases are classified according to serotype — *E. granulosus* or *E. multilocularis* — and by site of infection. Other tapeworm infestations are reported with codes from the 123 rubric.

122.0	Echinococcus granulosus infection of liver — *tapeworm*
122.1	Echinococcus granulosus infection of lung
122.2	Echinococcus granulosus infection of thyroid
122.3	Other echinococcus granulosus infection
122.4	Unspecified echinococcus granulosus infection
122.5	Echinococcus multilocularis infection of liver
122.6	Other echinococcus multilocularis infection
122.7	Unspecified echinococcus multilocularis infection
122.8	Unspecified echinococcus of liver — *unknown type, of liver*
122.9	Other and unspecified echinococcosis

123 Other cestode infection
Tapeworms other than *Echinococcus* are reported under this rubric.

123.0	Taenia solium infection, intestinal form — *adult pork tapeworm*
123.1	Cysticercosis — *larval pork tapeworm* AHA: Q2, 1997, 8
123.2	Taenia saginata infection — *Taenia saginata; beef tapeworm*
123.3	Taeniasis, unspecified — *unknown Taenia infection*
123.4	Diphyllobothriasis, intestinal — *adult fish tapeworm*
123.5	Sparganosis (larval diphyllobothriasis) — *larval fish tapeworm*
123.6	Hymenolepiasis — *rat tapeworm*
123.8	Other specified cestode infection — *dog tapeworm*
123.9	Unspecified cestode infection — *unknown*

Coding Clarification
Neurocysticercosis is caused by an infestation of the larval form of the parasite *Taenia solium*. Brain involvement of the parasite can result in epilepsy, increased intracranial pressure, and other neurologic conditions. Two codes should be indicated: 123.1 to identify the parasitic infection and code 780.3x indicating the convulsions.

124 Trichinosis
Trichinosis is an infection by the roundworm, *Trichinella spiralis*, smallest of the parasitic nematodes. *Trichinella* is found in the muscle of bear and pig and, generally, infection occurs when undercooked meat is eaten. Infection is rare but not unknown in the United States. Patients may be asymptomatic or may have gastrointestinal symptoms, muscle pains, fever, and periorbital edema. Trichinosis is also known as trichinellosis and trichiniasis.

125 Filarial infection and dracontiasis
Worms in the Filaria or Dracunculus family cause diseases in this rubric. Most are uncommon in the United States. Many of the filarial infections cause

congestion in the lymphatic system that can lead to other manifestations, including elephantiasis or chyluria.

In dracontiasis, a threadlike worm up to 120 centimeters long inhabits the subcutaneous and muscle tissues of man. Dracontiasis is limited to Africa, India, and Arabia.

125.0	Bancroftian filariasis — *Wuchereria bancrofti*
125.1	Malayan filariasis — *Brugia (Wuchereria) malayi*
125.2	Loiasis — *African eyeworm; Loa loa*
125.3	Onchocerciasis — *Onchocerca volvulus*
125.4	Dipetalonemiasis — *Acanthocheilonema perstans; Caribbean, Central and South America*
125.5	Mansonella ozzardi infection — *Filaria ozzardi*
125.6	Other specified filariasis — *Acanthocheilonema streptocerca, Dipetalonema streptocerca*
125.7	Dracontiasis — *Guinea worm; Africa, India, Asia; subcutaneous worm up to 120 cm*
125.9	Unspecified filariasis — *unknown variety*

126 Ancylostomiasis and necatoriasis

Rubric 126 classifies varieties of hookworm infection. Several infective agents, the most common being *Ancylostoma duodenale* and *Necator americanus*, can cause hookworm. Symptoms include gastrointestinal pain and anemia, though many patients are asymptomatic. *A. duodenale* is common in the Far East and the Mediterranean. *N. americanus* is more common in tropical areas. Currently, incidence of hookworm is very rare in the United States, though the incidence is thought to be as high as one in four people worldwide.

Hookworm is classified according to the infective agent. In symptomatic infection, eggs from the patient's stool can be examined to identify the type of hookworm.

126.0	Ancylostomiasis and necatoriasis due to ancylostoma duodenale — *hookworm*
126.1	Ancylostomiasis and necatoriasis due to Necator americanus — *hookworm*
126.2	Ancylostomiasis and necatoriasis due to ancylostoma braziliense — *hookworm*
126.3	Ancylostomiasis and necatoriasis due to ancylostoma ceylanicum — *hookworm*
126.8	Ancylostomiasis and necatoriasis due to other specified ancylostoma — *hookworm not elsewhere classified*
126.9	Unspecified ancylostomiasis and necatoriasis — *unknown hookworm*

127 Other intestinal helminthiases

Ascariasis is infection by *Ascaris lumbricoides* and may cause gastrointestinal or pulmonary symptoms. It is seen worldwide.

Strongyloidiasis is threadworm infection, endemic to the tropics that may cause gastric pain, vomiting, and diarrhea.

127.0	Ascariasis — *Ascaris lumbricoides; roundworm*
127.1	Anisakiasis — *larval infection*
127.2	Strongyloidiasis — *Strongyloides stercoralis*
127.3	Trichuriasis — *Trichuris trichiura; whipworm*
127.4	Enterobiasis — *Enterobius vermicularis; pinworm or threadworm*
127.5	Capillariasis — *Capillaria philippinensis*
127.6	Trichostrongyliasis — *Trichostrongylus species*
127.7	Other specified intestinal helminthiasis — *Oesophagostomum apiostomum*
127.8	Mixed intestinal helminthiasis — *not elsewhere classified*
127.9	Unspecified intestinal helminthiasis — *unknown*

128 Other and unspecified helminthiases

Toxocariasis is an invasion of the viscera by *Toxocara canis* or *Toxocara cati*, which normally cause diseases confined to dogs and cats. Symptoms are fever, cough, or skin rash and some patients experience recurring pneumonias. Most cases are seen in the very young or very old.

128.0	Toxocariasis — *visceral larva migrans syndrome*
128.1	Gnathostomiasis — *Gnathostoma spinigerum*
128.8	Other specified helminthiasis — *not elsewhere classified*
128.9	Unspecified helminth infection — *unknown*

Coding Clarification
Report any significant symptoms or manifestations in addition to the toxocariasis.

129 Unspecified intestinal parasitism

Use this code only if the disease is known to be parasitic and the parasite is unknown. If the parasite is known, use the appropriate "not elsewhere classified" code from other rubrics in this section.

130–136 Other Infectious and Parasitic Diseases

The diseases in this section of ICD-9-CM are a mixed bag of infections or parasites. Single-cell organisms, amebae, protozoa, mites and lice, fly larvae, or parasites of unknown etiology may cause the infections. As the last subclassification for infectious and parasitic diseases in this chapter, this section provides a hodgepodge of significant diseases.

130 Toxoplasmosis

Toxoplasmosis is caused by a single-celled parasite, *Toxoplasma gondii*. It is found throughout the world. Millions of people in the United States are infected with the *Toxoplasma* parasite, but very few have symptoms because the immune system usually keeps the parasite from causing illness.

Toxoplasmosis is an opportunistic disease and a danger to the unborn and to the immunocompromised patient. Toxoplasmosis is classified according to site or system infected.

130.0	Meningoencephalitis due to toxoplasmosis — inflammation of brain and its lining
130.1	Conjunctivitis due to toxoplasmosis — inflammation of the mucous lining of the eye
130.2	Chorioretinitis due to toxoplasmosis — infection of the posterior lining of the eye
130.3	Myocarditis due to toxoplasmosis — inflammation of the lining of the heart
130.4	Pneumonitis due to toxoplasmosis — inflammation of the lungs
130.5	Hepatitis due to toxoplasmosis — inflammation of the liver
130.7	Toxoplasmosis of other specified sites — not elsewhere classified
130.8	Multisystemic disseminated toxoplasmosis — multiple organ systems; seen in the immunocompromised patient
130.9	Unspecified toxoplasmosis — unknown

Coding Clarification
Congenital toxoplasmosis is classified to the Congenital Anomalies chapter of ICD-9-CM, with 771.2, and toxoplasmosis in pregnancy is classified to the Pregnancy and Childbirth chapter, with a code from the rubric 655.

If multiple sites or systems are infected, report 130.8 *Multisystem disseminated toxoplasmosis.*

In the case of AIDS, the code for HIV infection (042) should be sequenced first, followed by codes for the toxoplasmosis infection. Any functional disturbance (e.g., visual or mental disorder) may be reported secondarily.

131 Trichomoniasis
Trichomonas vaginalis is parasitic flagellated protozoa infestation that is usually sexually transmitted, although transmission by other routes, such as moist, soiled washcloths, has been documented. Most people infected with trichomoniasis are asymptomatic, and most infections are in the genitourinary system. Symptomatic infections are characterized by a white discharge from the genital tract and itching. Complications of infection can be vaginitis, urethritis, enlargement of the prostate, or epididymitis.

131.00	Unspecified urogenital trichomoniasis — STD with infection of urinary or reproductive organs
131.01	Trichomonal vulvovaginitis — STD with infection of vulva or vagina
131.02	Trichomonal urethritis — STD with infection of urethra
131.03	Trichomonal prostatitis — STD with infection of prostate
131.09	Other urogenital trichomoniasis — STD infection at genitourinary site not elsewhere classified
131.8	Trichomoniasis of other specified sites — infection, not genitourinary or intestinal, site not elsewhere classified
131.9	Unspecified trichomoniasis — unknown

Coding Clarification
This rubric classifies only trichomoniasis from *T. vaginalis.* Intestinal trichomoniasis may be caused by any of several other forms of *Trichomonas,* and is reported with 007.3.

132 Pediculosis and Phthirus infestation
This rubric classifies lice infestations. Lice suck the blood of the host and cause severe itching and loss of sleep. Louse saliva or feces irritate some sensitive hosts, increasing the chance of secondary infection from excessive scratching.

Head lice are *Pediculus capitis,* and they live mainly on the scalp and neck hairs of their human host. Head lice are mainly acquired by direct head-to-head contact with an infested person's hair, but may be transferred with shared combs, hats, and other hair accessories. Infestation is seen most often in children and in whites more frequently than other ethnic groups. Most commonly, epidemics are seen among school children. Head lice do not transmit infectious agents from person to person.

Body lice are Pediculus humanus and are closely related to head lice, but are less frequently encountered in the United States. Body lice feed on the body, though they may be discovered on the scalp and facial hair. They usually remain on clothing near the skin and generally deposit their eggs on or near the seams of garments. Body lice are acquired mainly through direct contact with an infested person or clothing and bedding, and are most commonly found on individuals who infrequently change or wash their clothes. Body lice serve as carriers of certain human pathogens including louse-borne typhus, louse-borne relapsing fever, and trench fever.

Pubic or crab lice are *Phthirus pubis* and have a short crab-like body easily distinguished from that of head and body lice. Pubic lice are most frequently found among the pubic hairs of the infested person, but may also be found elsewhere on the body. The infestation by pubic lice is termed phthiriasis. Pubic lice are acquired mainly through sexual contact or by sharing a bed with an infested person. Public lice do not transmit infectious agents from person to person.

132.0	Pediculus capitis (head louse) — *nits, head lice*
132.1	Pediculus corporis (body louse) — *body lice; may be vector to other disease*
132.2	Phthirus pubis (pubic louse) — *crabs; usually sexually transmitted*
132.3	Mixed pediculosis and Phthirus infestation — *infestation of more than one category above*
132.9	Unspecified pediculosis — *unknown infestation by lice*

133 Acariasis

Acariasis is a mite infestation. Acarid infestation is classified according to the type of mite. Scabies causes intense itching and sometimes, secondary infection. Report any significant secondary manifestations.

133.0	Scabies — *Sarcoptes scabiei*
133.8	Other acariasis — *chiggers and other mites, not elsewhere classified*
133.9	Unspecified acariasis — *unknown mite*

Coding Clarification
Scabies (133.0) is caused by *Sarcoptes scabiei*; all other known mites would be classified to 133.8 and unknown infestation would be classified to 133.9.

134 Other infestation

Myiasis is an infestation by fly larvae (maggots), and is most commonly seen in wound or ulcer sites. Myiasis is usually cutaneous, but is also found in nasal mucosa or in the intestines. Hirudiniasis is an infestation of mucous membranes or skin by leeches. While clinical myiasis and hirudiniasis are occasionally pursued as therapeutic interventions, these codes refer to nonclinical infestations.

134.0	Myiasis — *Dermatobia hominis; maggot infestation*
134.1	Other arthropod infestation — *sand fleas or other infestations not elsewhere classified*
134.2	Hirudiniasis — *leech infestation*
134.8	Other specified infestations — *not elsewhere classified*
134.9	Unspecified infestation — *unknown*

135 Sarcoidosis OK

Sarcoidosis is a disease of unknown etiology that has many presentations. It can have an acute onset and rapid resolution, or it can come upon the patient slowly and become an increasingly debilitating chronic condition. Also called sarcoid, the disorder is characterized by epithelioid tubercles in organs and tissues.

Incidence of sarcoid in the United States exceeds that of tuberculosis. Common symptoms include hilar adenopathy, shortness of breath, weight loss, arthralgia, night sweats, and erythema nodosum. The symptoms will vary according to the organs that are affected by sarcoidosis, though nearly all cases show decreased pulmonary function and mediastinal (hilar) adenopathy. Patients with chronic infection frequently have skin lesions. Tissue biopsy is the best method of diagnosing sarcoidosis.

Coding Clarification
Manifestations of sarcoidosis are reported in addition to the infection. These may include cardiac involvement (425.8), pulmonary involvement (517.8), joint involvement (713.7), or erythema nodosum (695.2).

Multiple codes may be required to complete the clinical picture. Report 135 *Sarcoidosis* first, and the manifestations or symptoms of the infection in descending order of severity.

136 Other and unspecified infectious and parasitic diseases

Most of the diseases in this category are "other," not "unspecified." They are listed here by default. There may be no room remaining in the rubric to which they would normally be classified.

Ainhum is an African disease, seen primarily in black males and causing stricture at a distal joint of a digit on the foot or hand. The stricture is progressive, leading to spontaneous amputation. Another name for the disease is dactylolysis spontanea.

Behcet's syndrome is a disease of unknown etiology causing inflammation and lesions of the mucous membrane, joints, and gastrointestinal and nervous systems. It is most common in men in their third decade in Japan and Mediterranean countries.

Free-living amoeba, *Naegleria,* can cause a grave form of meningoencephalitis. The infection is acquired by swimming in infected lakes.

Pneumocystosis is an infection of *Pneumocystis carinii* fungus, causing pneumonia in immunocompromised patients. It is the leading cause of death among AIDS patients. Patients with intact immune systems are not affected by pneumocystosis.

Sarcosporidiosis is an infection by *Sarcocystis* causing muscle cysts and intestinal inflammation.

| 136.0 | Ainhum — *African; stricture causes loss of digit* |
| 136.1 | Behcet's syndrome — *unknown etiology; inflammation and lesions* |

Infectious and Parasitic Diseases

136.2	Specific infections by free-living amebae — ameba causing meningoencephalitis		137.1	Late effects of central nervous system tuberculosis
136.3	Pneumocystosis — *Pneumocystis jiroveci; pneumocystis carinii, a fungus infection seen in the immunocompromised patient*		137.2	Late effects of genitourinary tuberculosis
			137.3	Late effects of tuberculosis of bones and joints
	AHA: Nov-Dec, 1987, 5-6; Q1, 2003, 15; Q1, 2005, 7		137.4	Late effects of tuberculosis of other specified organs
136.4	Psorospermiasis — *Psorospermic infection*			
136.5	Sarcosporidiosis — *Sarcocystis infection; muscle cysts*			
136.8	Other specified infectious and parasitic diseases — *not elsewhere classified, includes candiru infestation, microsporidiosis*			
136.9	Unspecified infectious and parasitic diseases — *unknown*			
	AHA: Q2, 1991, 8			

138 Late effects of acute poliomyelitis OK
This category is used to indicate conditions classifiable to 045 as the cause of the late effects, which are classified elsewhere. The conditions are reported first, with the late effect code being reported secondarily. Late effects include sequelae or complications due to old or inactive polio. When using late effect codes from this category, there should be no evidence of active disease.

Coding Clarification
If the source of infection is found nowhere else in ICD-9-CM and a thorough search of the index does not give better direction, report 136.8 for candiru infestation, microsporidiosis, or an infectious disease not yet classified to ICD-9-CM. If the source of infection remains undiagnosed, report 136.9.

139 Late effects of other infectious and parasitic diseases
This category is to be used to indicate conditions classifiable to 001-009, 020-041, or 046-136 as the cause of the late effects, which are classified elsewhere. The conditions are reported first, with the late effect code being reported secondarily. Late effects include sequelae or complications due to old or inactive infection. When using late effects codes from this category, there should be no evidence of active infection.

137–139 Late Effects of Infectious and Parasitic Diseases
A late effect is a residual effect of a condition that is no longer acute or an illness that has resolved. There is no time frame associated with a late effect; it can be reported at any time after the condition has resolved. Two codes are required to report late effects: one code for residual condition and the second code for the cause of the late effect. Never report the acute condition that caused the late effect with a late effect code.

139.0	Late effects of viral encephalitis
139.1	Late effects of trachoma
139.8	Late effects of other and unspecified infectious and parasitic diseases
	AHA: Q2, 2006, 17

Coding Scenario
A patient who was treated five years ago for Lyme disease is now seen in the office for residual arthritic pain. After examination, the physician's diagnostic statement indicates that the patient has arthritis secondary to Lyme disease. The medical record identifies that the patient is cured of the Lyme disease, but still has the residual arthritis of multiple sites from the disease.

137 Late effects of tuberculosis
This category is used to indicate conditions classifiable to 010-018 as the cause of the late effects, which are classified elsewhere. The conditions are reported first, with the late effect code being reported secondarily. Late effects include sequelae, or complications due to old or inactive TB. When using late effect codes from this category, there should be no evidence of active disease.

> Code assignment: 139.8 *Late effect of other and unspecified infectious and parasitic diseases* and 711.89 *Arthropathy associated with other infectious and parasitic diseases, multiple sites*

137.0	Late effects of respiratory or unspecified tuberculosis — *sequelae*

140–239

Neoplasms

Neoplasms in ICD-9-CM are classified as malignant, carcinoma in situ, uncertain, unknown, or benign. In most cases, anatomic location of the neoplasm is specified in code selection.

In malignancy, the neoplasm invades surrounding tissue or sheds cells that seed malignancies in other body sites. Malignant neoplasms are, therefore, classified as primary, for the original site; or secondary, a seeded site. Classifications within malignant neoplasms also specify certain malignancies as leukemias, Kaposi's sarcoma, melanoma, lymphomas, and carcinoma in situ.

A benign neoplasm may grow, but does not invade, and remains a lesion confined to an area. Uncertain behavior is undetermined and unspecified behavior is unknown.

Because of the nature of malignancy, this chapter classifies anatomy differently than other chapters of ICD-9-CM. In this chapter, malignancies are often classified according to contiguous anatomic site rather than by distinct organ system. Therefore, body parts that in other chapters may be classified separately are grouped together here. For example, soft tissue malignancies, whether blood vessels, tendons, or nerves, are classified under a single rubric for connective and soft tissue.

All neoplasms are classified to this chapter, whether or not they are functionally active. A functionally active neoplasm is a growth that performs functions ascribed to surrounding tissue, as in a thyroid tumor that secretes thyroxine and causes hyperthyroidism in the patient.

The index of ICD-9-CM provides a complex and complete table of neoplasms for easy code lookup. The index is organized alphabetically by anatomy. Find the anatomical site, and the table will identify the codes for primary, secondary, and carcinoma in situ, as well as the codes for benign, uncertain, and unspecified behaviors. After looking up the anatomical site and finding the appropriate code, refer to the tabular section of ICD-9-CM to see appropriate includes and excludes notes and instructions for use of that code. Kaposi's sarcoma is excluded from the index and can be found in the alphabetized index under Kaposi's.

ICD-Oncology Classification

The ICD-Oncology identifies the morphology of neoplasms. These are published by the World Health Organization (WHO) and consist of five digits. The first four identify the histological type of neoplasm, and the fifth digit indicates its behavior as benign (/0); uncertain (/1); carcinoma in situ (/2); malignant, primary (/3); malignant, secondary (/6); or malignant, uncertain (/9). These M codes are used in reporting malignancies to the national cancer registry. In many cases, the index to ICD-9-CM can help in M code selections, which are based on morphology and histology rather than anatomic site.

The ICD-9-CM classification system includes a complete list of the morphology codes, found in Appendix A: Morphology of Neoplasm.

Personal History of Malignant Neoplasm

Codes from the V10 rubric describe personal history of malignant neoplasm, but these codes should never be assigned to patients who have active or recurring disease or are still receiving treatment for their malignancy, except when that disease is secondary. When a previously excised malignant neoplasm recurs at the same site, it is still considered a primary malignancy of that site. If the malignant neoplasm recurs at a different site, it is reported as a secondary malignant neoplasm and an additional code to identify a history of the malignancy of the primary site is reported from the V10 rubric.

Furthermore, when assigning a personal history code, the site should reflect the site of the primary malignant neoplasm, not a metastatic site. Rubric V10 reports only the primary malignancy. There is no method for reporting a history of malignancy in a secondary site.

Sequencing issues

The main rule for sequencing malignancies and their manifestations is to sequence first the reason for the encounter.

In cases of a metastasized malignancy, if a secondary malignancy causes a functional problem, sequence the codes as follows: (1) the functional problem; (2) the secondary malignant neoplasm causing the problem; and (3) the site of the original, metastasized neoplasm (primary site). For example, if a patient with prostate cancer comes to the physician with acute abdominal pain and is found to have a blocked bowel, the result of a secondary malignancy in the ileum, the following codes would be reported in this sequence:

560.89   Other intestinal obstruction without mention of hernia

197.4   Secondary malignant neoplasm of small intestine, including duodenum

185   Malignant neoplasm of the prostate

If the patient is being treated for a condition unrelated to the neoplasm, report the reason for treatment first, followed by the neoplasm only if it could affect the course of care. For example, if a patient with breast cancer fractures her hip, the fracture would be sequenced first, followed by the code for the cancer. However, if the patient's breast neoplasm is known to be benign, only the hip fracture would be reported, since the neoplasm would not affect care, unless the benign neoplasm were discovered in the course of care for the hip fracture. In that case, it would be reported as a secondary diagnosis.

If a patient is seen solely for chemotherapy or radiotherapy, either on an inpatient or outpatient basis, V58.11 *Encounter or admission for antineoplastic chemotherapy*, V58.12 *Encounter for antineoplastic immunotherapy*, or V58.0 *Encounter or admission for radiotherapy* should be sequenced first, and the code for the malignancy reported secondarily. If the patient receives other care related to the malignancy at the time of the therapy, the therapy would not be sequenced first, but secondary to the malignant neoplasm code.

Codes from the signs and symptoms chapter of ICD-9-CM should never be sequenced first when reporting malignancies. If manifestations cannot be specified with other codes, report the malignancy first, followed by any appropriate signs or symptoms.

140–149   Malignant Neoplasm of Lip, Oral Cavity, and Pharynx

This section of ICD-9-CM classifies malignancies of the mouth and throat. The pharynx (throat) is a tube that begins at the internal nares, behind the nasal cavity, and ends at the larynx. While malignant neoplasms of the pharynx are classified in this subsection of ICD-9-CM, malignant neoplasms of the larynx are found in the respiratory section, under rubric 161.

140   Malignant neoplasm of lip
AHA: Q2, 1990, 7

The lips, or labia, contain skeletal muscles. The primary muscle is the orbicularis oris, the sphincter muscle that encircles the mouth and lies between the outer skin (integument) and the mucous membranes of the lips. The labial glands, which are similar to salivary glands, lie between the muscle and mucous membrane tissues. The lips also have many sensory nerves and abundant capillary vessels that produce the normal reddish color. The external margin of the lips, the vermilion border, marks the boundary between the skin of the face and the mucous membrane that lines the alimentary canal of the digestive system.

Anatomically, the lips are divided into two distinct segments. The vermilion border is the pigmented, fleshy, outer lip, and may be described in the medical record as the lipstick area or external lip. The interior aspect is the second segment. Lined in buccal mucosa, the interior aspect may be described as the mucosa, buccal aspect, or frenulum. The commissure of the lip is the juncture of the upper and lower lips, whether at the vermilion border or interior aspect.

140.0	Malignant neoplasm of upper lip, vermilion border — *pigmented, fleshy margin of upper lip* AHA: Q2, 1990, 7
140.1	Malignant neoplasm of lower lip, vermilion border — *pigmented, fleshy margin of lower lip* AHA: Q2, 1990, 7
140.3	Malignant neoplasm of upper lip, inner aspect — *mucous membrane lined, inner margin, upper lip* AHA: Q2, 1990, 7
140.4	Malignant neoplasm of lower lip, inner aspect — *mucous membrane lined, inner margin, lower lip* AHA: Q2, 1990, 7
140.5	Malignant neoplasm of lip, inner aspect, unspecified as to upper or lower — *mucous membrane lined inner margin* AHA: Q2, 1990, 7

140.6	Malignant neoplasm of commissure of lip — *juncture of upper and lower lip* **AHA:** Q2, 1990, 7
140.8	Malignant neoplasm of other sites of lip — *contiguous or overlapping sites* **AHA:** Q2, 1990, 7
140.9	Malignant neoplasm of lip, vermilion border, unspecified as to upper or lower — *pigmented, fleshy margin* **AHA:** Q2, 1990, 7

Coding Clarification
Malignant neoplasms of the lip are classified according to upper, lower, or commissure of lip and whether it is vermilion border or buccal aspect. For overlapping sites, report 140.8 *Other sites of lip*.

141 Malignant neoplasm of tongue
AHA: Q2, 1990, 7

The tongue is a strong muscle that is attached to the floor of the mouth within the curve of the jawbone. It is anchored to muscles at the rear of the mouth, which attach to the base of the skull and to the hyoid bone. The underside of the tongue is attached to the floor of the mouth by membranes. These form a distinct vertical fold in the centerline, called the frenulum linguae. The tongue contains mucous, serous, and lymph glands. The lymph glands at the back of the tongue form the lingual tonsils.

The surface of the tongue is covered with the lingual membrane, a specialized tissue with a variety of papillae protruding from it. These papillae nodules produce the characteristic rough surface of the tongue. Between the papillae are the taste buds, the sensory nerve organs that provide the sensations of flavor. The muscle fibers of the tongue are also heavily supplied with nerves, to provide for manipulation and safe placement of food in the mouth and between the teeth for chewing. The tongue also aids in swallowing and in the formation of sounds of speech.

141.0	Malignant neoplasm of base of tongue — *fixed, dorsal base* **AHA:** Q2, 1990, 7
141.1	Malignant neoplasm of dorsal surface of tongue — *dorsal surface, anterior two-thirds* **AHA:** Q2, 1990, 7
141.2	Malignant neoplasm of tip and lateral border of tongue — *tip and front edge* **AHA:** Q2, 1990, 7
141.3	Malignant neoplasm of ventral surface of tongue — *anterior two-thirds; frenulum linguae* **AHA:** Q2, 1990, 7
141.4	Malignant neoplasm of anterior two-thirds of tongue, part unspecified — *mobile part of tongue NOS* **AHA:** Q2, 1990, 7
141.5	Malignant neoplasm of junctional zone of tongue — *border of tongue at junction* **AHA:** Q2, 1990, 7
141.6	Malignant neoplasm of lingual tonsil — *lymphoid tissue of tongue* **AHA:** Q2, 1990, 7
141.8	Malignant neoplasm of other sites of tongue — *contiguous or overlapping sites* **AHA:** Q2, 1990, 7
141.9	Malignant neoplasm of tongue, unspecified site

Coding Clarification
Malignant neoplasms of the tongue are classified according to site. If multiple or contiguous sites on the tongue are involved, report 141.8 *Other sites of tongue*. For secondary malignant neoplasm of tongue, report 198.89 and for carcinoma in situ, report 239.0.

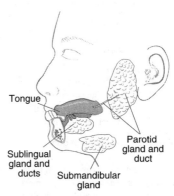

The parotid gland is a common site for malignant lesions. Occurrence is several times the frequency of other major salivary glands

142 Malignant neoplasm of major salivary glands
AHA: Q2, 1990, 7

These codes report malignant neoplasms of major salivary glands, but not of surrounding tissues. Salivary glands secrete saliva to aid in mastication and to keep the mouth moist. The major salivary glands are the parotid, sublingual, and submandibular glands.

The parotid is the most common site of salivary gland tumor, and mucoepidermoid carcinoma is the most common type of parotid cancer.

Symptoms of parotid tumor include pain, enlargement of nodule, and sometimes facial nerve paralysis or lymphadenopathy.

Some types of salivary gland tumors classified as malignant are the following carcinomas: mucoepidermoid, adenoid cystic, epithelial-myoepithelial, primary squamous cell, biphasic malignancy, ex-pleomorphic adenoma, malignant onocytoma, clear cell, or acinic cell.

The minor salivary glands are distributed in the lips, palate, uvula, tongue, peritonsillar area, and cheek.

142.0	Malignant neoplasm of parotid gland — *salivary gland in cheek, in front of ear* AHA: Q2, 1990, 7
142.1	Malignant neoplasm of submandibular gland — *salivary gland at base of mandible* AHA: Q2, 1990, 7
142.2	Malignant neoplasm of sublingual gland — *salivary gland at base of tongue* AHA: Q2, 1990, 7
142.8	Malignant neoplasm of other major salivary glands — *contiguous or overlapping sites* AHA: Q2, 1990, 7
142.9	Malignant neoplasm of salivary gland, unspecified

Coding Clarification
Do not use these codes to report cancers in minor salivary glands. Report malignant neoplasms of minor salivary glands with codes specific to the anatomical site in which they are located.

143 Malignant neoplasm of gum
AHA: Q2, 1990, 7

More than 95 percent of cancers of the oral cavity are squamous cell carcinomas, found most commonly in males, aged 50-70, with a history of tobacco and alcohol use.

143.0	Malignant neoplasm of upper gum — *gingiva, alveolar mucosa, interdental papillae* AHA: Q2, 1990, 7
143.1	Malignant neoplasm of lower gum — *gingiva, alveolar mucosa, interdental papillae* AHA: Q2, 1990, 7
143.8	Malignant neoplasm of other sites of gum — *contiguous or overlapping upper and lower sites* AHA: Q2, 1990, 7
143.9	Malignant neoplasm of gum, unspecified site

Coding Clarification
For malignant neoplasms of contiguous or overlapping sites of the gum, report 143.8 *Other sites of gum.*

144 Malignant neoplasm of floor of mouth
AHA: Q2, 1990, 7

More than 95 percent of cancers of the oral cavity are squamous cell carcinomas, found most commonly in males, aged 50-70, with a history of tobacco and alcohol use. Cancers of the floor of the mouth have a higher incidence of lymph node involvement than do cancers of the lip, palate, or buccal mucosa, which explains their classification separately in ICD-9-CM from other parts of the inside of the mouth.

144.0	Malignant neoplasm of anterior portion of floor of mouth — *anterior to premolar-canine juncture* AHA: Q2, 1990, 7
144.1	Malignant neoplasm of lateral portion of floor of mouth — *on the side* AHA: Q2, 1990, 7
144.8	Malignant neoplasm of other sites of floor of mouth — *overlapping site* AHA: Q2, 1990, 7
144.9	Malignant neoplasm of floor of mouth, part unspecified

Coding Clarification
For malignant neoplasms of contiguous or overlapping sites of the parts of mouth, report 144.8 *Other specified parts of mouth.*

145 Malignant neoplasm of other and unspecified parts of mouth
AHA: Q2, 1990, 7

More than 95 percent of cancers of the oral cavity are squamous cell carcinomas, found most commonly in males, aged 50-70, with a history of tobacco and alcohol use.

The vestibule of the mouth is the part of the oral cavity inside the cheeks and lips and outside the dentoalveolar structures (the teeth and gums). It includes the mucosal and submucosal tissue of the lips and cheeks, and the labial and buccal frenulum, or frenum, the connecting folds of membrane that support and restrain the lips and cheeks. Secretions from the salivary glands lubricate the vestibule.

145.0	Malignant neoplasm of cheek mucosa — *buccal mucosa, inner aspect cheek* AHA: Q2, 1990, 7
145.1	Malignant neoplasm of vestibule of mouth — *buccal sulcus; labial sulcus* AHA: Q2, 1990, 7
145.2	Malignant neoplasm of hard palate — *anterior, rigid* AHA: Q2, 1990, 7
145.3	Malignant neoplasm of soft palate — *posterior, soft* AHA: Q2, 1990, 7

Neoplasms

145.4	Malignant neoplasm of uvula
145.5	Malignant neoplasm of palate, unspecified
145.6	Malignant neoplasm of retromolar area
145.8	Malignant neoplasm of other specified parts of mouth — *overlapping sites* AHA: Q2, 1990, 7
145.9	Malignant neoplasm of mouth, unspecified site

Coding Clarification

Do not use this rubric for reporting neoplasms of the floor of the mouth (144), lips (140), or nasopharyngeal surface of the soft palate (147).

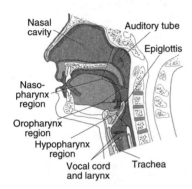

146 Malignant neoplasm of oropharynx
AHA: Q2, 1990, 7

The part of the pharynx that lies posterior to the oral cavity is called the oropharynx. It extends from its upper part at the soft palate down to its lower part that ends at the level of the hyoid bone. The lingual and palatine tonsils are located in the oropharynx. Most oropharyngeal tumors are squamous carcinomas, many with deep infiltrations.

Some tumors of the parapharyngeal space are actually major salivary gland tumors, or carotid body tumors, and should be reported as such. Minor salivary tumors at this site, however, are reported with codes in this rubric.

Oropharyngeal tumors drain bilaterally to lymph nodes, and the incidence of nodal involvement in oropharyngeal malignancy is 70 percent.

146.0	Malignant neoplasm of tonsil — *faucial, palatine* AHA: Sept-Oct, 1987, 8; Q2, 1990, 7
146.1	Malignant neoplasm of tonsillar fossa — *sinus tonsillaris* AHA: Q2, 1990, 7
146.2	Malignant neoplasm of tonsillar pillars (anterior) (posterior) — *faucial pillar, palatoglossal arch* AHA: Q2, 1990, 7
146.3	Malignant neoplasm of vallecula — *Anterior and medial surface of pharyngoepiglottic fold* AHA: Q2, 1990, 7
146.4	Malignant neoplasm of anterior aspect of epiglottis — *glossoepiglottic fold, epiglottis* AHA: Q2, 1990, 7
146.5	Malignant neoplasm of junctional region of oropharynx — *junction of free margin of epiglottis, aryepiglottic fold, and pharyngoepiglottic fold* AHA: Q2, 1990, 7
146.6	Malignant neoplasm of lateral wall of oropharynx — *on the side of the throat* AHA: Q2, 1990, 7
146.7	Malignant neoplasm of posterior wall of oropharynx — *on the back of the throat* AHA: Q2, 1990, 7
146.8	Malignant neoplasm of other specified sites of oropharynx — *contiguous or overlapping sites; brachial cleft* AHA: Q2, 1990, 7
146.9	Malignant neoplasm of oropharynx, unspecified site

147 Malignant neoplasm of nasopharynx
AHA: Q2, 1990, 7

The part of the pharynx that lies behind (posterior) the nasal cavity is called the nasopharynx. The nasopharynx extends from behind the nasal cavity to the soft palate. There are two openings from the nasopharynx to the nose (internal nares) and two openings to the ears (Eustachian tubes). The adenoids (pharyngeal tonsil) are located on the posterior wall of the nasopharynx. The most common tumor of the nasopharynx is squamous cell carcinoma. Lymph node metastases occur in 80 percent of patients with nasopharyngeal cancer.

147.0	Malignant neoplasm of superior wall of nasopharynx — *roof of nasopharynx* AHA: Q2, 1990, 7
147.1	Malignant neoplasm of posterior wall of nasopharynx — *adenoid; pharyngeal tonsil* AHA: Q2, 1990, 7
147.2	Malignant neoplasm of lateral wall of nasopharynx — *pharyngeal recess; fossa of Rosenmüller; opening of auditory tube* AHA: Q2, 1990, 7
147.3	Malignant neoplasm of anterior wall of nasopharynx — *floor of nasopharynx; posterior margin of nasal septum; nasopharyngeal surface of soft palate* AHA: Q2, 1990, 7
147.8	Malignant neoplasm of other specified sites of nasopharynx — *contiguous or overlapping sites* AHA: Q2, 1990, 7

147.9   Malignant neoplasm of nasopharynx, unspecified site

148   Malignant neoplasm of hypopharynx
AHA: Q2, 1990, 7

The lowest part of the pharynx is called the laryngopharynx or hypopharynx. It extends from the hyoid bone and ends at a point where it breaks into two parts, the esophagus and larynx, by blending in with them. More than 95 percent of hypopharyngeal cancers are squamous carcinoma, and the most common site is the periform sinus, which occur on either side of the larynx. These account for 60 percent of hypopharyngeal cancers. Lymphatic involvement is seen in about 70 percent of hypopharyngeal malignancy.

148.0   Malignant neoplasm of postcricoid region of hypopharynx

148.1   Malignant neoplasm of pyriform sinus — *pyriform fossa*
AHA: Q2, 1990, 7

148.2   Malignant neoplasm of aryepiglottic fold, hypopharyngeal aspect — *aryepiglottic fold NOS*
AHA: Q2, 1990, 7

148.3   Malignant neoplasm of posterior hypopharyngeal wall

148.8   Malignant neoplasm of other specified sites of hypopharynx — *overlapping sites*
AHA: Q2, 1990, 7

148.9   Malignant neoplasm of hypopharynx, unspecified site

149   Malignant neoplasm of other and ill-defined sites within the lip, oral cavity, and pharynx
AHA: Q2, 1990, 7

This rubric captures malignant neoplasms in the pharynx and oral cavity that have less specific anatomic boundaries. Waldeyer's ring includes the lymphatic tissues of the lingual, pharyngeal, and palatine tonsils.

149.0   Malignant neoplasm of pharynx, unspecified — *unknown part*
AHA: Q2, 1990, 7

149.1   Malignant neoplasm of Waldeyer's ring — *lymphatic tissues of the lingual, pharyngeal, and palatine tonsils*
AHA: Q2, 1990, 7

149.8   Malignant neoplasm of other sites within the lip and oral cavity — *point of origin cannot be assigned to any one of the categories 140-148*
AHA: Q2, 1990, 7

149.9   Malignant neoplasm of ill-defined sites of lip and oral cavity

Coding Clarification
Report 149.8 if the malignancy is not limited to one of the specific structures, but has invaded contiguous or overlapping structures.

150–159   Malignant Neoplasm of Digestive Organs and Peritoneum

This subsection of ICD-9-CM classifies malignancies of the body parts that carry food through the digestive system where nutrients are absorbed, to the anus where the waste is excreted. These body parts include the esophagus, stomach, intestines, and anus.

Structures that support the digestive process from outside this continuous tube are also included in this system: gallbladder, pancreas, and liver. These organs provide secretions that are critical to food absorption and use by the body.

The digestive system is a group of organs that breaks down and changes food chemically for absorption as simple, soluble substances by blood, lymph systems, and body tissues. The digestive system begins in the mouth, continues in the pharynx and esophagus, the stomach, the small and large intestines, the rectum, and the anus.

Digestion involves mechanical and chemical processes. Mechanical actions include chewing in the mouth, churning action in the stomach, and intestinal peristaltic action. These mechanical forces move the food through the digestive tract and mix it with secretions containing enzymes, which accomplish three chemical reactions: the conversion of carbohydrates to simple sugars, the breakdown of proteins into amino acids, and the conversion of fats into fatty acids and glycerol.

The stomach churns and mixes the food with hydrochloric acid and enzymes and gradually releases materials into the upper small intestine (the duodenum) through the pyloric sphincter.

The majority of the digestive process occurs in the small intestine where most foods are hydrolyzed and absorbed. The products of digestion are actively or passively transported through the wall of the small intestine and assimilated into the body. The stomach and the large intestine (colon) can also absorb water, alcohol, certain salts and crystalloids, and some drugs. Water-soluble digestive products (minerals, amino acids, and carbohydrates) are transferred into the blood system and transported to the liver. Many fats, resynthesized in the intestinal wall, are picked

Neoplasms

up by the lymphatic system and enter the blood stream through the vena caval system, bypassing the liver.

Remaining undigested matter is passed into the large intestine (the colon) where water is extracted. This solid mass (the stool) is propelled into the rectum, where it is held until excreted through the anus.

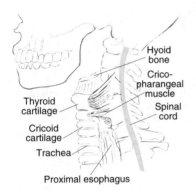

Proximal esophagus

150 Malignant neoplasm of esophagus
AHA: Q2, 1990, 7

The esophagus is the alimentary canal connecting the pharynx to the stomach. Symptoms of carcinoma of the esophagus include difficulty swallowing, weight loss, coughing, and pain. Hoarseness is often seen.

Carcinoma of the esophagus is more common among men and has been linked in the United States to heavy use of alcohol and tobacco. A majority of these cancers are squamous cell or adenocarcinoma. Anatomically, 20 percent occur in the upper third of the esophagus, 30 percent in the mid-esophagus, and 50 percent in the lower esophagus.

Adenocarcinoma is more common in the lower esophagus, while squamous cell carcinoma is common in the mid to the upper esophagus.

150.0	Malignant neoplasm of cervical esophagus — *above the diaphragm* **AHA:** Q2, 1990, 7
150.1	Malignant neoplasm of thoracic esophagus — *within the diaphragm* **AHA:** Q2, 1990, 7
150.2	Malignant neoplasm of abdominal esophagus — *below the diaphragm* **AHA:** Q2, 1990, 7
150.3	Malignant neoplasm of upper third of esophagus — *proximal third* **AHA:** Q2, 1990, 7
150.4	Malignant neoplasm of middle third of esophagus — *middle third* **AHA:** Q2, 1990, 7
150.5	Malignant neoplasm of lower third of esophagus — *distal third* **AHA:** Q2, 1990, 7
150.8	Malignant neoplasm of other specified part of esophagus — *contiguous or overlapping sites of esophagus whose point of origin cannot be determined* **AHA:** Q2, 1990, 7
150.9	Malignant neoplasm of esophagus, unspecified site

Coding Clarification
Cancers in this rubric are classified by site, with one exception. According to ICD-9-CM exclusion notes, if squamous cell carcinoma is present at the distal end of the esophagus (the cardia), report 150.5 *Malignant neoplasm of lower third of esophagus.*

If the malignancy is of contiguous and overlapping sites, report 150.8 *Malignant neoplasm of other specified part of esophagus.*

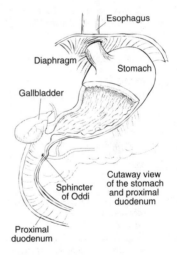

151 Malignant neoplasm of stomach
AHA: Q2, 1990, 7

The stomach has four functions: to act as a reservoir for food, to mix food, to begin the digestive process, and to allow the absorption of some substances.

The stomach begins at the portal between the esophagus and the stomach — the cardia. It ends at the portal to the duodenum — the pylorus. In

Coders' Desk Reference for Diagnoses

between is the corpus, or the body of the stomach. The corpus is divided into the upper portion, the fundus, which is served by the oxyntic gland; the lower portion or the antrum, served by the pyloric gland; and the large midportion, the body. There are no clear demarcations between the segments of the corpus. The lesser and greater curvatures of the stomach refer to the short and long walls of the organ.

Stomach cancer is rarely found before age 40 and is twice as common in men as in women. The most common types of stomach cancers are ulcerating carcinomas, polypoid carcinomas, superficial spreading carcinomas, linitis plastica, and advanced carcinoma.

151.0	Malignant neoplasm of cardia — *cardiac orifice; cardio-esophageal junction* AHA: Q2, 1990, 7
151.1	Malignant neoplasm of pylorus — *pre-pylorus, pyloric canal* AHA: Q2, 1990, 7
151.2	Malignant neoplasm of pyloric antrum — *lower portion of the stomach preceding the pylorus; antrum of stomach* AHA: Q2, 1990, 7
151.3	Malignant neoplasm of fundus of stomach — *upper portion of the stomach proceeding from the cardia* AHA: Q2, 1990, 7
151.4	Malignant neoplasm of body of stomach — *central segment* AHA: Q2, 1990, 7
151.5	Malignant neoplasm of lesser curvature of stomach, unspecified — *not classifiable to 151.1-151.4* AHA: Q2, 1990, 7
151.6	Malignant neoplasm of greater curvature of stomach, unspecified — *not classifiable to 151.0-151.4* AHA: Q2, 1990, 7
151.8	Malignant neoplasm of other specified sites of stomach — *anterior wall, posterior wall, contiguous or overlapping parts* AHA: Q2, 1990, 7
151.9	Malignant neoplasm of stomach, unspecified site — *carcinoma ventriculi, gastric cancer, Brinton's disease* AHA: Q2, 1990, 7; Q2, 2001, 17

Coding Clarification
Cancers in this rubric are classified by site, with the following exceptions: According to ICD-9-CM exclusion notes, if specified as a malignant stromal tumor of the stomach, report with code 171.5 *Malignant neoplasm of connective and other soft tissue of abdomen*. If squamous cell carcinoma is present at the distal end of the esophagus (the cardia), report 150.5 *Malignant neoplasm of lower third of esophagus*.

If the malignancy is of contiguous and overlapping sites, report 151.8 *Malignant neoplasm of other specified sites of stomach.*

152 Malignant neoplasm of small intestine, including duodenum
AHA: Q2, 1990, 7

The small intestine, often called the small bowel, is the portion of the alimentary canal from the pylorus to the cecum and is divided into the upper two-fifths, the jejunum, and the balance (the ileum). There is no demarcation between the two portions of small bowel, but, generally, the jejunum resides to the left side of the peritoneum and the ileum resides to the right and into the pelvis. The duodenum lies between the pylorus valve at the exit of the stomach and the jejunum. The most common form of small intestine malignancy is adenocarcinoma in the proximal jejunum.

152.0	Malignant neoplasm of duodenum — *small intestine immediate to the pylorus* AHA: Q2, 1990, 7
152.1	Malignant neoplasm of jejunum — *middle portion of the small intestine* AHA: Q2, 1990, 7
152.2	Malignant neoplasm of ileum — *distal small intestine that connects to the large intestine* AHA: Q2, 1990, 7
152.3	Malignant neoplasm of Meckel's diverticulum — *abnormal pouch near the terminal part of the ilium near the ileocecal juncture* AHA: Q2, 1990, 7
152.8	Malignant neoplasm of other specified sites of small intestine — *duodenojejunal junction; contiguous or overlapping sites* AHA: Q2, 1990, 7
152.9	Malignant neoplasm of small intestine, unspecified site

Coding Clarification
The small intestine is a common site for melanoma metastases, and these should be classified as secondary cancers rather than with the 152 rubric.

Cancer of the small bowel is classified by site, with one exception: According to ICD-9-CM exclusion notes, if specified as a malignant stromal tumor of the small intestine, report 171.5 *Malignant neoplasm of connective and other soft tissue of abdomen*. If the malignancy is of contiguous or overlapping sites, report 152.8 *Malignant neoplasm of other specified sites of small intestine.* Cancer of the ileocecal valve

Neoplasms

is reported with 153.4 *Malignant neoplasm of the cecum.*

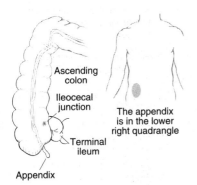

The appendix is in the lower right quadrangle

153 Malignant neoplasm of colon
AHA: Q2, 1990, 7

The large intestine, or colon, extends from the end of the ileum to the rectum. The rectum, however, is excluded from rubric 153 and classified in 154. The right colon consists of the cecum, ascending colon, hepatic flexure, and proximal transverse colon. The left colon consists of the distal transverse colon, the splenic flexure, the descending colon, sigmoid colon, and rectosigmoid colon.

Colon cancer is the third most common form of cancer in the United States. About 150,000 new cases are diagnosed and 60,000 deaths occur each year. Adenocarcinoma is the most common form of colon cancer.

153.0	Malignant neoplasm of hepatic flexure — *juncture of the ascending and transverse colons*	
	AHA: Q2, 1990, 7	
153.1	Malignant neoplasm of transverse colon — *middle portion of the large intestines, between the hepatic and splenic flexures*	
	AHA: Q2, 1990, 7	
153.2	Malignant neoplasm of descending colon — *between the splenic flexure and the sigmoid colon; left colon*	
	AHA: Q2, 1990, 7	
153.3	Malignant neoplasm of sigmoid colon — *S-shaped colon between the descending colon and the rectum*	
	AHA: Q2, 1990, 7	
153.4	Malignant neoplasm of cecum — *pouch at the beginning of the large intestine, including ileocecal valve*	
	AHA: Q2, 1990, 7	
153.5	Malignant neoplasm of appendix — *attached to the cecum*	
	AHA: Q2, 1990, 7	
153.6	Malignant neoplasm of ascending colon — *first portion of the large intestine between the cecum and the hepatic flexure; right colon*	
	AHA: Q2, 1990, 7	
153.7	Malignant neoplasm of splenic flexure — *bend between the transverse and descending colons*	
	AHA: Q2, 1990, 7	
153.8	Malignant neoplasm of other specified sites of large intestine — *not elsewhere classified or contiguous or overlapping sites*	
	AHA: Q2, 1990, 7	
153.9	Malignant neoplasm of colon, unspecified site	

Coding Clarification
If the malignancy is causing obstruction or other manifestation, report the manifestation first, and the neoplasm secondarily.

Coding Scenario
A patient is admitted for blood transfusions for severe anemia. The patient history indicates the patient has colon cancer and chronic obstructive pulmonary disease. The physician documentation specifies the anemia as a chronic simple type.

> Code assignment: 281.9 *Unspecified deficiency anemia,* 153.9 *Malignant neoplasm of colon, unspecified,* and 496 *Chronic airway obstruction, not elsewhere classified*

154 Malignant neoplasm of rectum, rectosigmoid junction, and anus
AHA: Q2, 1990, 7

The rectum begins at the rectosigmoid junction and ends at the anus. The rectum and rectosigmoid junctions are the most common sites for cancer in the colon, accounting for more than 30 percent of cases. In these cancers, the most common symptoms are rectal bleeding with bowel movement and pain upon defecation (tenesmus).

154.0	Malignant neoplasm of rectosigmoid junction — *colon with rectum; rectosigmoid (colon)*
	AHA: Q2, 1990, 7
154.1	Malignant neoplasm of rectum — *rectal ampulla*
	AHA: Q2, 1990, 7
154.2	Malignant neoplasm of anal canal — *including anal sphincter*
	AHA: Q2, 1990, 7; Q1, 2001, 8
154.3	Malignant neoplasm of anus, unspecified site
154.8	Malignant neoplasm of other sites of rectum, rectosigmoid junction, and anus — *anorectum, cloacogenic zone, contiguous or overlapping sites*
	AHA: Q2, 1990, 7

Coding Clarification
Diseases in this rubric are classified according to site. Report 154.8 *Malignant neoplasm of other specified sites* if the malignancy is of contiguous or overlapping sites. If the malignancy is causing bleeding, obstruction, or other manifestation, report the manifestation first, and the malignancy secondarily.

155 Malignant neoplasm of liver and intrahepatic bile ducts
AHA: Q2, 1990, 7

Primary liver cancer is uncommon in the United States; however, the liver is a common site for metastases, and would be reported with 197.7 *Secondary malignant neoplasm of the mediastinum*. About 80 percent of primary liver cancers are hepatomas.

155.0	Malignant neoplasm of liver, primary — including all lobes; hepatoblastoma, liver carcinoma **AHA:** Q2, 1990, 7
155.1	Malignant neoplasm of intrahepatic bile ducts — canaliculi biliferi, interlobular bile ducts; intrahepatic biliary passages, gall duct; intrahepatic bile ducts **AHA:** Q2, 1990, 7
155.2	Malignant neoplasm of liver, not specified as primary or secondary — *unknown whether a metastasis* **AHA:** Q2, 1990, 7

Coding Clarification
For cancers of the hepatic duct, report 156.1 *Malignant neoplasm of extrahepatic bile ducts*.

156 Malignant neoplasm of gallbladder and extrahepatic bile ducts
AHA: Q2, 1990, 7

Gallbladder cancer is uncommon and usually seen only in the elderly. Bile duct tumors are somewhat more common, but still usually limited to older patients. Most of these cancers are adenocarcinomas.

156.0	Malignant neoplasm of gallbladder
156.1	Malignant neoplasm of extrahepatic bile ducts — *biliary, common bile, cystic, hepatic duct; sphincter of Oddi* **AHA:** Q2, 1990, 7
156.2	Malignant neoplasm of ampulla of Vater — *area of dilation at the juncture of common bile and pancreatic ducts near their opening into the lumen of the duodenum* **AHA:** Q2, 1990, 7
156.8	Malignant neoplasm of other specified sites of gallbladder and extrahepatic bile ducts — *not elsewhere classified or of contiguous or overlapping sites* **AHA:** Q2, 1990, 7
156.9	Malignant neoplasm of biliary tract, part unspecified site — *unknown or involving both intrahepatic and extrahepatic bile ducts* **AHA:** Q2, 1990, 7

Coding Clarification
Disease is classified according to site. If the malignancy is of contiguous and overlapping sites, report 156.8 *Other specified sites of gallbladder and extrahepatic bile ducts*.

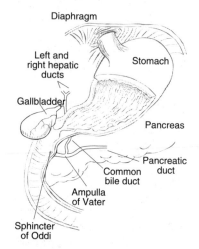

Location of the gallbladder in relation to select surrounding structures

157 Malignant neoplasm of pancreas
AHA: Q2, 1990, 7

The pancreas is a slender organ lying behind the stomach in the abdomen. The head of the pancreas is curved near the duodenum; the body is the main portion, and the tail is the portion that abuts the spleen. There are no clear demarcations between the parts of the pancreas.

The pancreas produces pancreatic juice, enzymes that assist in digestion. It also creates insulin, which regulates blood glucose levels.

Pancreatic cancer is one of the most prevalent cancers in the United States, after lung cancer and colon cancer. It is most common in people aged 50-70. Symptoms include weight loss, jaundice, and abdominal or back pain. Pancreatic cancer is most common in the head of the gland, with 66 percent of malignancies occurring there. Ductal adenocarcinoma is the most common type of malignancy in pancreatic cancer.

If the cancer is in the islets of Langerhans, insulin regulation could be affected.

157.0	Malignant neoplasm of head of pancreas — Bard-Pic's syndrome AHA: Q2, 1990, 7; Q4, 2000, 40; Q2, 2005, 9
157.1	Malignant neoplasm of body of pancreas — main portion AHA: Q2, 1990, 7
157.2	Malignant neoplasm of tail of pancreas
157.3	Malignant neoplasm of pancreatic duct — Santorini, Wirsung ducts AHA: Q2, 1990, 7
157.4	Malignant neoplasm of islets of Langerhans — (Use additional code to identify any functional activity) — *structures in the pancreas that produce insulin, somatostatin, or glucagon* AHA: Q2, 1990, 7
157.8	Malignant neoplasm of other specified sites of pancreas — *ectopic tissue, contiguous or overlapping sites* AHA: Q2, 1990, 7
157.9	Malignant neoplasm of pancreas, part unspecified

Coding Clarification
Any functional activity resulting from the malignancy should be separately reported. If the cancer occurs in overlapping or contiguous portions of the pancreas, report 157.8 *Other specified sites of pancreas.*

158 Malignant neoplasm of retroperitoneum and peritoneum
AHA: Q2, 1990, 7

The retroperitoneum is the space behind the peritoneum and in front of the spine. The peritoneum is the membrane that holds the abdominal organs. A majority of peritoneal malignancies are secondary, with the exception of peritoneal mesothelioma, a rare cancer arising in the mesodermal lining of the peritoneum. Retroperitoneal tumors are usually of mesodermal tissue.

158.0	Malignant neoplasm of retroperitoneum — periadrenal, perirenal, perinephric, retrocecal tissues AHA: Q2, 1990, 7
158.8	Malignant neoplasm of specified parts of peritoneum — *Douglas cul-de-sac, mesentery; mesocolon; omentum; peritoneum; rectouterine pouch; or contiguous or sites* AHA: Q2, 1990, 7
158.9	Malignant neoplasm of peritoneum, unspecified

Coding Clarification
If the malignancy spans both the peritoneum and retroperitoneum, ICD-9-CM instructs to report this condition with 158.8 *Malignant neoplasm of specified parts of peritoneum.*

159 Malignant neoplasm of other and ill-defined sites within the digestive organs and peritoneum
AHA: Q2, 1990, 7

This rubric is reserved for nonspecific malignancies of digestive sites and the peritoneum.

159.0	Malignant neoplasm of intestinal tract, part unspecified
159.1	Malignant neoplasm of spleen, not elsewhere classified — *angiosarcoma, fibrosarcoma of spleen* AHA: Q2, 1990, 7
159.8	Malignant neoplasm of other sites of digestive system and intra-abdominal organs — *point of origin cannot be assigned to any one of the categories 150-158* AHA: Q2, 1990, 7
159.9	Malignant neoplasm of ill-defined sites of digestive organs and peritoneum — *generalized "alimentary canal," "gastrointestinal tract"* AHA: Q2, 1990, 7

Coding Clarification
When a digestive malignancy has progressed so that the point of origin cannot be assigned to a specific code in rubrics 150-158, report 159.8 *Malignant neoplasm of other sites of digestive system and intra-abdominal organs.*

160–165 Malignant Neoplasm of Respiratory and Intrathoracic Organs

The respiratory system can be divided into two main sections: the upper and the lower respiratory tracts. The upper respiratory tract is located outside the thorax (the chest cavity), and is composed of the nose and the pharynx (nasopharynx, oropharynx, and hypopharynx). Malignant neoplasms of this upper portion of respiratory anatomy are classified in 140-149, as part of the oral cavity. This subsection includes the larynx and the lower respiratory tract contained within the thorax, which consists of the trachea, bronchial tree, lungs, and pleura. Also classified to this subsection because of their anatomic locations are malignant neoplasms of the heart, thymus, and mediastinum. However, great vessels are classified to 171.4.

The respiratory system functions as follows: air enters the body through the nose, where it is warmed, filtered, and humidified as it passes through the nasal cavity. The air passes into the pharynx and from the pharynx into the trachea (the "windpipe"). The epiglottis in the pharynx prevents food from entering the trachea. The upper part of the trachea contains the three parts of the larynx and the vocal chords. At its base, the trachea divides into the left and right primary bronchi. Each bronchus divides into smaller branches known as segmental bronchi. These divide into tiny bronchioles that terminate in the microscopic ducts and alveoli sacs of the lungs where gas exchange takes place.

The lungs are large, paired organs in the thorax. The right lung has three lobes. The left lung cavity contains two lobes and encloses the heart. Thin sheets of epithelium (the pleura) separate the inside of the chest cavity from the outer surface of the lungs and the heart.

The respiratory system functions as an air distributor and gas exchanger, to supply oxygen and remove carbon monoxide from the body's cells. All parts of the respiratory system, except the microscopic alveoli of the lungs, function as air distributors. Only the alveoli sacks and ducts serve as gas exchangers. In addition to air distribution and gas exchange, the respiratory system and its structures provide for such functions as yawning, sneezing, coughing, hiccups, sound production (including speech), and the sense of smell (olfaction). The respiratory system also assists in homeostasis (regulation of pH in the body).

Coding Clarification
Malignancies in this section are classified according to anatomic site. If malignancies are found in multiple sites within an anatomic system, a code for "other sites" is in most cases appropriate to report multiple sites. If the malignancy results in functional abnormalities, report the malignancy first, followed by the functional problem. For nonspecific or multiple thoracic or intrathoracic malignancies, report 195.1 *Malignant neoplasm of the thorax*. If the malignancy is carcinoma in situ, report with codes from the 231 rubric instead. If respiratory or thoracic malignancies are secondary, see codes in the 196-199 rubrics.

160 Malignant neoplasm of nasal cavities, middle ear, and accessory sinuses
AHA: Q2, 1990, 7

The nasal cavity opens into the vestibule that is just inside of the nostrils and continues to the respiratory area where bone in three shelves (formed by the nasal cavity) called the superior, middle, and inferior nasal turbinates (nasal conchae) are located. The turbinates come close to the nasal septum and subdivide the nasal cavity into passageways.

160.0   Malignant neoplasm of nasal cavities — *nasal cartilage, septum, conchae, fossa, mucosa, internal nose*
AHA: Q2, 1990, 7

160.1   Malignant neoplasm of auditory tube, middle ear, and mastoid air cells — *eustachian tube, inner ear, middle ear, antrum tympanicum, tympanic cavity*
AHA: Q2, 1990, 7

160.2   Malignant neoplasm of maxillary sinus — *sinus behind cheekbones; maxillary antrum and Highmore antrum*
AHA: Q2, 1990, 7

160.3   Malignant neoplasm of ethmoidal sinus — *sinus between the eyes on either side of the nose*
AHA: Q2, 1990, 7

160.4   Malignant neoplasm of frontal sinus — *sinus above the eyes*
AHA: Q2, 1990, 7

160.5   Malignant neoplasm of sphenoidal sinus — *sinus behind the eyes on either side of the nose*
AHA: Q2, 1990, 7

160.8   Malignant neoplasm of other sites of nasal cavities, middle ear, and accessory sinuses — *contiguous or overlapping sites of nasal cavities, middle ear, and accessory sinuses*
AHA: Q2, 1990, 7

160.9   Malignant neoplasm of site of nasal cavities, middle ear, and accessory sinus, unspecified site

161 Malignant neoplasm of larynx
AHA: Q2, 1990, 7

The larynx has several functions: speech, protection of the airways, respiration, and fixation of the chest. It is commonly called the "voicebox." Most laryngeal malignancies are squamous cell carcinomas and 90 percent of laryngeal cancers occur in males. Hoarseness and throat pain are common symptoms.

161.0   Malignant neoplasm of glottis — *true vocal cord including intrinsic larynx, commissure*
AHA: Q2, 1990, 7

161.1   Malignant neoplasm of supraglottis — *false vocal cord including aryepiglottic fold, epiglottis, extrinsic larynx, ventricular bands*
AHA: Q2, 1990, 7

161.2   Malignant neoplasm of subglottis — *larynx below the vocal cords and above the trachea*
AHA: Q2, 1990, 7

161.3   Malignant neoplasm of laryngeal cartilages — *including arytenoid, cricoid, cuneiform, thyroid cartilage*
AHA: Q2, 1990, 7

161.8   Malignant neoplasm of other specified sites of larynx — *contiguous or overlapping sites of*

Neoplasms

larynx whose point of origin cannot be determined
AHA: Q2, 1990, 7

161.9 Malignant neoplasm of larynx, unspecified site

Coding Clarification
Malignant neoplasms of the larynx are classified according to site. If the malignancy spans two sites of the larynx, ICD-9-CM instructs to report this condition with 161.8 *Malignant neoplasm of other specified sites of larynx*. Do not use codes in this rubric to report malignancies of the epiglottis (146.4) or hypopharynx (rubric 148).

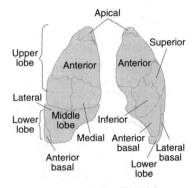

Anterior view of lungs. The left lung is divided into superior and inferior lobes. The right lung has three segments. The subdivisions are defined by the areas served by bronchial divisions

162 Malignant neoplasm of trachea, bronchus, and lung
AHA: Q2, 1990, 7

Lung cancer is the most common cancer in the United States, with more than 150,000 cases diagnosed and more than 100,000 dying from the disease annually. Malignant tumors of the lung may be squamous cell, adenocarcinoma, small cell, large cell, adenosquamous, carcinoma, or bronchial gland carcinoma. Lung cancer is considered one of the most lethal forms of cancer, with only 20 percent of patients surviving one year after diagnosis. Symptoms include wheezing, pneumonia, and pain, as well as symptoms from metastatic sites of disease. The most common site of metastatic lung cancer is the liver; however, brain, kidney, and adrenal gland are also common sites.

162.0 Malignant neoplasm of trachea — *breathing tube anterior to the esophagus and extending from the larynx to the right and left bronchi.*
AHA: Q2, 1990, 7

162.2 Malignant neoplasm of main bronchus — *carina and hilus of lung*
AHA: Q2, 1990, 7

162.3 Malignant neoplasm of upper lobe, bronchus, or lung — *Cuiffini-Pancoase syndrome, Hare's syndrome, Tobias' syndrome*
AHA: Q2, 1990, 7; Q1, 2004, 4

162.4 Malignant neoplasm of middle lobe, bronchus, or lung — *Middle lobe, bronchus or lung*
AHA: Q2, 1990, 7

162.5 Malignant neoplasm of lower lobe, bronchus, or lung — *Lower lobe, bronchus or lung*
AHA: Q2, 1990, 7

162.8 Malignant neoplasm of other parts of bronchus or lung — *contiguous or overlapping sites of bronchus or lung whose point of origin cannot be determined*
AHA: Q2, 1990, 7

162.9 Malignant neoplasm of bronchus and lung, unspecified site

Coding Clarification
Lung cancer is classified according to the lobe of the lung. Report 162.8 if the cancer invades contiguous or overlapping sites in the lung or bronchus if the point of origin cannot be determined.

Coding Scenario
A patient is admitted with an esophageal obstruction due to esophageal metastasis from the lung.

> Code assignment: 530.3 *Stricture and stenosis of esophagus*, 197.8 *Secondary malignant neoplasm of other respiratory and digestive organs*, and 162.9 *Malignant neoplasm of bronchus, and lung, unspecified*

A 49-year-old female is admitted for severe dehydration. The patient is known to have lung cancer with generalized metastases. The patient is treated with IV fluids for the dehydration. The patient's cancer is not treated during this admission.

> Code assignment: 276.5 *Dehydration*, 162.9 *Malignant neoplasm of bronchus and lung, unspecified*, and 199.0 *Malignant neoplasm, disseminated*

A patient is admitted for chemotherapy requiring placement of a Hickman catheter for treatment of lung cancer metastases.

> Code assignment: V58.1 *Encounter for chemotherapy*, 162.9 *Malignant neoplasm of bronchus and lung, unspecified*, and 199.1 *Malignant neoplasm without specification of site, other*

A patient develops agranulocytosis associated with the chemotherapy treatment he has been receiving for lung cancer.

Code assignment: 288.03 *Drug induced neutropenia*, 162.9 *Malignant neoplasm of bronchus and lung, unspecified*, and E933.1 *Adverse effects in therapeutic use, antineoplastic and immunosuppressive drugs*

163 Malignant neoplasm of pleura
AHA: Q2, 1990, 7

The pleura line the lung and localized mesothelioma. Diffuse malignant mesothelioma is the most common form of pleural malignancy. Cancers of the pleura are classified according to site. The parietal pleura are the outer lining of the lung, and the visceral pleura are the inner lining.

163.0	Malignant neoplasm of parietal pleura — *outer lining of the lung* **AHA:** Q2, 1990, 7	
163.1	Malignant neoplasm of visceral pleura — *inner lining of the lung* **AHA:** Q2, 1990, 7	
163.8	Malignant neoplasm of other specified sites of pleura — *contiguous or overlapping sites of pleura whose point of origin cannot be determined* **AHA:** Q2, 1990, 7	
163.9	Malignant neoplasm of pleura, unspecified site	

Coding Clarification
Report 163.8 if the malignancy is overlapping or in contiguous parts of the pleura.

164 Malignant neoplasm of thymus, heart, and mediastinum
AHA: Q2, 1990, 7

The thymus is a bilateral, lymph-rich organ that produces T lymphocytes that circulate throughout the body to provide an immune function. The organ is anterior to the heart, in the upper mediastinum, and is a common site for neoplasms. The most common type of thymoma is epithelial, accounting for 45 percent of cases. Since some lymphomas and Hodgkin's granulomas arise in thymus tissue, check documentation to be sure of appropriate use of codes from this rubric.

The mediastinum is the compartment between the sternum and lungs/heart (anterior), and the spine and lungs/heart (posterior). Because of the general nature of the mediastinum in anatomical descriptions, care should be taken that a more specific site is overlooked when coding malignant neoplasm of the mediastinum. The thymus (164.0) and parathyroid (194.1) reside in the mediastinum, but are reported with more specific codes, as are neurogenic tumors in the mediastinum (classify to nerve).

The heart is the muscle responsible for circulation of blood throughout the body. It is divided into four cavities: the right and left atria and the right and left ventricles. The left atrium receives oxygenated blood from the lung and passes it along to the left ventricle, which pushes the blood through the circulatory system to nourish the body's cells. The right atrium receives the blood that has completed its circuit through the body. From the right atrium, the blood is circulated to the right ventricle, which pumps it back into the lungs for reoxygenation. Four major valves separate the chambers and prevent backflow of blood. The valves consist of flaps called cusps; the ends of the cusps between the atria and ventricles extend into the ventricles where they are connected to the papillary muscles by fibrous cords called the chordae tendineae.

Malignant neoplasms of the heart are rarely seen as primary neoplasms. When primary cancer of the heart occurs, it occurs most commonly in children. The most common cardiac malignancy is cardiac sarcoma, accounting for 30 percent of the cases. Complications from cardiac cancer can be grave and include heart failure, hemorrhagic pericardial effusion with tamponade, and arrhythmia. A primary cancer of the heart is also prone to metastasize to the spine and other major organs.

164.0	Malignant neoplasm of thymus — *lymphoid and endocrine organ behind the sternum* **AHA:** Q2, 1990, 7
164.1	Malignant neoplasm of heart — *endocardium, epicardium, myocardium and pericardium* **AHA:** Q2, 1990, 7
164.2	Malignant neoplasm of anterior mediastinum — *soft and connective tissue between the lungs, in the cavity between the heart and the sternum* **AHA:** Q2, 1990, 7
164.3	Malignant neoplasm of posterior mediastinum — *soft and connective tissue between the lungs, in the cavity between the heart and the spinal column* **AHA:** Q2, 1990, 7
164.8	Malignant neoplasm of other parts of mediastinum — *contiguous or overlapping sites of thymus, heart, and mediastinum* **AHA:** Q2, 1990, 7
164.9	Malignant neoplasm of mediastinum, part unspecified

Coding Clarification
Report malignant neoplasms of the great vessels with 171.4 *Malignant neoplasm of the thorax*. If the malignancy is overlapping or in contiguous parts of the heart and mediastinum, report 164.8 *Malignant neoplasm of other parts of mediastinum*.

Neoplasms

165 Malignant neoplasm of other and ill-defined sites within the respiratory system and intrathoracic organs
AHA: Q2, 1990, 7

This rubric is reserved for nonspecific malignancies of respiratory and intrathoracic organs.

165.0	Malignant neoplasm of upper respiratory tract, part unspecified — *the respiratory organs above the diaphragm* **AHA:** Q2, 1990, 7
165.8	Malignant neoplasm of other sites within the respiratory system and intrathoracic organs — *point of origin cannot be assigned to any one of the categories 160-164* **AHA:** Q2, 1990, 7
165.9	Malignant neoplasm of ill-defined sites within the respiratory system — *respiratory tract not otherwise specified* **AHA:** Q2, 1990, 7

Coding Clarification
When a respiratory malignancy has progressed to a point that it cannot be assigned to a specific code in rubrics 160-164, report 165.8 *Malignant neoplasm of other sites within the respiratory system and intrathoracic organs.*

170–176 Malignant Neoplasm of Bone, Connective Tissue, Skin, and Breast

Codes in this section of ICD-9-CM refer to malignancies in the bone, connective tissue, skin, and breast.

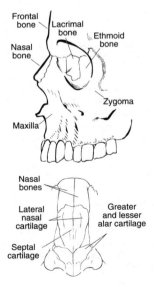

170 Malignant neoplasm of bone and articular cartilage
AHA: Q2, 1990, 7

Primary malignancies of the bone are uncommon compared to the incidence of metastases to the bone.

Multiple myeloma is the most common bone malignancy, occurring usually in older adults. Osteosarcoma is most commonly seen in children and young adults. Pain, swelling, limit to range of motion, or pathological fracture are common symptoms.

170.0	Malignant neoplasm of bones of skull and face, except mandible — *ethmoid, frontal, turbinate, malar, occipital, orbital, zygomatic, sphenoid, temporal* **AHA:** Q2, 1990, 7
170.1	Malignant neoplasm of mandible — *inferior maxilla, lower jaw bone* **AHA:** Q2, 1990, 7
170.2	Malignant neoplasm of vertebral column, excluding sacrum and coccyx — *meaning bony spine, vertebra* **AHA:** Q2, 1990, 7
170.3	Malignant neoplasm of ribs, sternum, and clavicle — *costal cartilage, costovertebral joint, xiphoid process* **AHA:** Q2, 1990, 7
170.4	Malignant neoplasm of scapula and long bones of upper limb — *acromion, radius, ulna, humerus* **AHA:** Q2, 1990, 7; Q2, 1999, 9
170.5	Malignant neoplasm of short bones of upper limb — *bones of hand and wrist; carpal, cuneiform, scaphoid, semilunar of lunate, navicular, phalanges, unciform, trapezoid, pisiform* **AHA:** Q2, 1990, 7
170.6	Malignant neoplasm of pelvic bones, sacrum, and coccyx — *coccygeal vertebra, ilium, ischium, pubic bone, sacral vertebra* **AHA:** Q2, 1990, 7
170.7	Malignant neoplasm of long bones of lower limb — *femur, fibula, tibia* **AHA:** Q2, 1990, 7
170.8	Malignant neoplasm of short bones of lower limb — *bones of knee, foot and ankle; astragalus talus, calcaneus, cuboid, navicular of knee, patella, phalanges, tarsal, metatarsal* **AHA:** Q2, 1990, 7
170.9	Malignant neoplasm of bone and articular cartilage, site unspecified

Coding Clarification
For metastasized cancers, see 198.5 *Secondary malignant neoplasm of the bone and bone marrow.* Malignancies of the bone are classified in ICD-9-CM according to anatomic site and type of bone (long or short). Articular cartilage and periosteum

malignancies are classified to the appropriate bone code. Connective and soft tissue malignancies are classified to the 171 rubric, as connective tissue.

171 Malignant neoplasm of connective and other soft tissue
AHA: Q2, 1990, 7

Malignant neoplasms of the connective tissue and other soft tissue are classified according to site rather than specific type of tissue. These codes can be used to classify malignant neoplasms of blood vessels; bursa; fascia; fat; ligament (except uterine); muscle; peripheral, sympathetic, and parasympathetic nerves; synovia; or tendons. Malignant stromal tumors, connective tissue cell tumors, are also included in this rubric.

Excluded from this rubric are malignant neoplasms of articular cartilage, cartilage of the larynx and nose, and connective tissue of the breast, heart, uterine ligament, and internal organs (except stromal tumors).

Cartilage is a type of dense connective tissue (hyaline, elastic, and fibrocartilage) that is found in joints. Hyaline cartilage is located at joints over the ends of long bones; fibrocartilage is found at other body sites, such as the pubic symphysis, intervertebral discs, menisci of the knee, and the point where the hip bones fuse anteriorly.

Soft tissue generally includes the deep fascia, muscles, tendons, and ligaments. Deep fascia lies beneath the second layer of subcutaneous tissue (hypodermis) of the integumentary system. Deep fascia in the musculoskeletal system lines extremities and holds together groups of muscles. There are three types of muscle tissue: skeletal, cardiac, and visceral. Muscle tissue consists of specialized cells that allow contraction to produce voluntary or involuntary movement of body parts.

Tendons are fibrous cords that vary in length. They are found at the ends of muscles and connecting muscles to bones. Ligaments are bands of fibrous tissue that connect two or more bones or cartilage.

171.0	Malignant neoplasm of connective and other soft tissue of head, face, and neck — *blood vessel, fascia, fat, muscle, cartilage of eye and ear, ligament, and peripheral, sympathetic, and parasympathetic nerve and ganglia* **AHA:** Q2, 1990, 7; Q2, 1999, 6
171.2	Malignant neoplasm of connective and other soft tissue of upper limb, including shoulder — *blood vessel, fascia, fat, muscle, ligament, and peripheral, sympathetic, and parasympathetic nerve and ganglia* **AHA:** Q2, 1990, 7
171.3	Malignant neoplasm of connective and other soft tissue of lower limb, including hip — *blood vessel, fascia, fat, muscle, ligament, and peripheral, sympathetic, and parasympathetic nerve and ganglia* **AHA:** Q2, 1990, 7
171.4	Malignant neoplasm of connective and other soft tissue of thorax — *blood vessel, fascia, fat, muscle, ligament, and peripheral, sympathetic, and parasympathetic nerve and ganglia* **AHA:** Q2, 1990, 7
171.5	Malignant neoplasm of connective and other soft tissue of abdomen — *blood vessel, fascia, fat, muscle, ligament, and peripheral, sympathetic, and parasympathetic nerve and ganglia* **AHA:** Q2, 1990, 7
171.6	Malignant neoplasm of connective and other soft tissue of pelvis — *blood vessel, fascia, fat, muscle, ligament, and peripheral, sympathetic, and parasympathetic nerve and ganglia* **AHA:** Q2, 1990, 7
171.7	Malignant neoplasm of connective and other soft tissue of trunk, unspecified site — *blood vessel, fascia, fat, muscle, ligament, and peripheral, sympathetic, and parasympathetic nerve and ganglia* **AHA:** Q2, 1990, 7
171.8	Malignant neoplasm of other specified sites of connective and other soft tissue — *contiguous or overlapping sites of connective tissue whose point of origin cannot be determined* **AHA:** Q2, 1990, 7
171.9	Malignant neoplasm of connective and other soft tissue, site unspecified

Coding Clarification
If the malignant neoplasm is of contiguous or overlapping soft tissue sites and the point of origin cannot be determined, report 171.8.

172 Malignant melanoma of skin
AHA: Q2, 1990, 7

The integumentary system is a diverse and complex organ forming the boundary and barrier between the internal environment of the body and the outside world. Although quite thin, the skin (or cutaneous membrane) is the largest human organ, usually 12 to 20 square feet in area and composing 12 percent of the total body weight. The depth of the skin varies from 0.5 mm in thin areas such as the eyelids to 5.0 mm or more at its thickest over the back.

There are three integrated layers in the skin: the thinner outer layer (epidermis), the dense connective layer (dermis), and the loose subcutis or subcutaneous layer (also called the hypodermis or superficial fascia), which is composed of fat and areolar tissue.

Neoplasms

The epidermis consists of three distinct cell types: keratinocytes that provide structure, melanocytes that contribute color and filter ultraviolet light, and Langerhans cells that contribute to the immune response. These cells form up to five strata over the dermal epidermal junction or basement membrane. Beneath the epidermal junction lies the dermis, composed of a papillary and a reticular layer. The dermis is rich in skin receptor nerves, blood vessels, and in sweat glands. It provides attachment for smooth and skeletal muscle fibers and the hair follicles. The lipocyte cells of the subcutis, joined to the bottom of the dermis, produce lipids for the subcutaneous tissue to make the fatty, insulating layer that cushions the body against shocks and provides an energy source.

Melanomas are skin cancers that are usually pigmented but otherwise vary in size and presentation. They are among the most invasive of the cancers. Change is the hallmark of melanoma; adjacent tissue is usually transformed. The most common type of melanoma is superficial spreading melanoma, accounting for 65 percent of all melanomas. They are most common on women's legs, or men's trunks. Other types of melanoma include nodular, with dark papules or plaques, and solar lentigo, arising as a flat tan macule on areas of skin that have had long-term sun exposure, especially on the hands and forehead.

172.0	Malignant melanoma of skin of lip — *skin only, outer aspect only* AHA: Q2, 1990, 7
172.1	Malignant melanoma of skin of eyelid, including canthus
172.2	Malignant melanoma of skin of ear and external auditory canal — *auricle, external canal, tragus, helix, pinna, concha, pinna* AHA: Q2, 1990, 7
172.3	Malignant melanoma of skin of other and unspecified parts of face — *external cheek and nose, chin but not neck, forehead, but not scalp* AHA: Q2, 1990, 7
172.4	Malignant melanoma of skin of scalp and neck — *but not chin or forehead* AHA: Q2, 1990, 7
172.5	Malignant melanoma of skin of trunk, except scrotum — *axilla, breast, buttock, groin, perianal skin, perineum, umbilicus* AHA: Q2, 1990, 7
172.6	Malignant melanoma of skin of upper limb, including shoulder — *shoulder, arm, and hand* AHA: Q2, 1990, 7
172.7	Malignant melanoma of skin of lower limb, including hip — *hip, leg, and foot* AHA: Q2, 1990, 7
172.8	Malignant melanoma of other specified sites of skin — *contiguous or overlapping sites of skin* AHA: Q2, 1990, 7
172.9	Melanoma of skin, site unspecified

Coding Clarification

Melanoma begins as a skin cancer, but aggressively metastasizes to other systems or organs. These secondary sites are not classified in ICD-9-CM as melanomas, but as secondary malignant neoplasms, classified by site in rubrics 196-199.

Do not report personal history of malignant melanoma of skin (V10.83) in patients with a recurrence; instead, report the active disease. The personal history code is reserved for patients who have completed treatment and are without recurrence of melanoma.

173   Other malignant neoplasm of skin
AHA: Q2, 1990, 7; Q2, 1996, 12; Q1, 2000, 18

Skin cancers other than melanoma may be basal cell or squamous cell carcinomas. No distinction is made between basal and squamous cells in ICD-9-CM classification. Basal cell carcinoma is usually small, shiny, and firm, but may also be crusty and ulcerous. A squamous cell carcinoma is often more pigmented, but it, too, is highly variable in appearance.

173.0	Other malignant neoplasm of skin of lip — *skin only, outer aspect only* AHA: Q2, 1990, 7; Q2, 1996, 12; Q1, 2000, 18
173.1	Other malignant neoplasm of skin of eyelid, including canthus
173.2	Other malignant neoplasm of skin of ear and external auditory canal — *auricle, external canal, tragus, helix, pinna, concha, pinna* AHA: Q2, 1990, 7; Q2, 1996, 12; Q1, 2000, 18
173.3	Other malignant neoplasm of skin of other and unspecified parts of face — *external cheek and nose, chin but not neck, forehead, but not scalp* AHA: Q2, 1990, 7; Q2, 1996, 12; Q1, 2000, 3; Q1, 2000, 18
173.4	Other malignant neoplasm of scalp and skin of neck — *but not chin or forehead* AHA: Q2, 1990, 7; Q2, 1996, 12; Q1, 2000, 18
173.5	Other malignant neoplasm of skin of trunk, except scrotum — *axilla, breast, buttock, groin, perianal skin, perineum, umbilicus* AHA: Q2, 1990, 7; Q2, 1996, 12; Q1, 2000, 18; Q1, 2001, 8
173.6	Other malignant neoplasm of skin of upper limb, including shoulder — *shoulder, arm and hand* AHA: Q2, 1990, 7; Q2, 1996, 12; Q1, 2000, 18
173.7	Other malignant neoplasm of skin of lower limb, including hip — *hip, leg and foot* AHA: Q2, 1990, 7; Q2, 1996, 12; Q1, 2000, 18

173.8	Other malignant neoplasm of other specified sites of skin — *contiguous or overlapping sites of skin* **AHA:** Q2, 1990, 7; Q2, 1996, 12; Q1, 2000, 18	174.5	Malignant neoplasm of lower-outer quadrant of female breast
		174.6	Malignant neoplasm of axillary tail of female breast
173.9	Other malignant neoplasm of skin, site unspecified	174.8	Malignant neoplasm of other specified sites of female breast — *ectopic sites or overlapping sites* **AHA:** Q4, 1989, 11; Q2, 1990, 7; Q3, 1997, 8

Coding Clarification

Skin cancers in this rubric are classified according to location. For melanoma, see codes in rubric 172; for Kaposi's sarcoma, see rubric 176. Cancers of the skin of the genitalia are reported with genitalia codes, 184.0-184.9 and 187.1-187.9.

174 Malignant neoplasm of female breast
AHA: Q4, 1989, 11; Q2, 1990, 7; Q3, 1997, 8

The mammary glands are accessory organs of the female reproductive system. Each breast contains glandular tissue consisting of secreting cells and ducts. The smaller ducts unite into a single milk-carrying duct for each lobe and these converge toward the nipple. The glandular tissue is contained within dense connective tissue that attaches to the pectoral muscle, and with suspensory ligaments that extend from the skin to the pectoral muscle to provide support. Surrounding the nipple is the circular area of pigmented and irregular surfaced skin called the areola.

The function of the mammary gland is lactation — secretion of colostrum and subsequently milk for the nourishment of newborn infants. Successful lactation relies on pre- and postnatal production of hormones including progesterone, estrogen, prolactin, and oxytocin.

Malignant neoplasms of the female breast are classified according to site. The upper, outer quadrant of the breast is the most likely site for a malignancy; a full 50 percent of breast disease occurs in this quadrant. This is followed by 18 percent in the nipple; 15 percent in the upper, inner quadrant; 6 percent in the lower, inner quadrant; and 1 percent in the lower, outer quadrant. The remaining percentage (10 percent) is distributed in the axillary tail and in multiple sites.

174.0	Malignant neoplasm of nipple and areola of female breast
174.1	Malignant neoplasm of central portion of female breast
174.2	Malignant neoplasm of upper-inner quadrant of female breast
174.3	Malignant neoplasm of lower-inner quadrant of female breast
174.4	Malignant neoplasm of upper-outer quadrant of female breast **AHA:** Q1, 2004, 3

174.9	Malignant neoplasm of breast (female), unspecified site **AHA:** Q3, 2005, 11

Coding Clarification

If a malignancy is found in several sites of the breast, report 174.8 *Malignant neoplasm of other specified sites of female breast,* which includes multiple sites. Do not code each site separately. If the malignancy is in the skin of the breast, report 172.5 (melanoma) or 173.5 (other skin malignancy).

An additional code should be assigned to identify estrogen receptor status (V86.0, V86.1).

Coding Scenario

A 49-year-old female patient is seen in the hospital ambulatory surgery center for a biopsy of a breast lump at the patient's previous mastectomy site. Pathology report confirms a recurrent breast carcinoma.

> Code assignment: 174.9 *Malignant neoplasm of breast (female), unspecified*

A 63-year-old female is diagnosed with an intraductal comedo carcinoma with focal stromal microinvasion, upper inner quadrant right breast.

> Code assignment: 174.2 *Malignant neoplasm of upper-inner quadrant of female breast*

A 49-year-old female with recent radical mastectomy for breast carcinoma is seen for radiation therapy.

> Code assignment: V58.0 *Encounter for radiotherapy* and 174.9 *Malignant neoplasm of breast (female), unspecified*

175 Malignant neoplasm of male breast
AHA: Q2, 1990, 7

Malignant neoplasms of the male breast are classified by site: both nipple and areola or other.

175.0	Malignant neoplasm of nipple and areola of male breast
175.9	Malignant neoplasm of other and unspecified sites of male breast — *ectopic sites* **AHA:** Q2, 1990, 7

Coding Clarification

If the malignancy is in the skin of the breast, report 172.5 (melanoma) or 173.5 (other skin malignancy) instead. Breast cancer in men occurs at only 1 percent of the rate it occurs in women.

An additional code should be assigned to identify estrogen receptor status (V86.0, V86.1).

176 Kaposi's sarcoma
AHA: Q2, 1990, 7; Q4, 1991, 24

Kaposi's sarcoma is a malignancy characterized by numerous vascular skin tumors. Kaposi's sarcoma was once found only rarely, in aging men, usually of Italian or Jewish decent. Today, incidence is common in the United States, as a manifestation of Acquired Immune Deficiency Syndrome (AIDS).

A diagnosis of Kaposi's sarcoma of the skin is significant because it is often the first clinical manifestation of AIDS in a Human Immunodeficiency Virus (HIV) positive patient, though Kaposi's sarcoma itself is rarely a cause of death. Disseminated Kaposi's sarcoma can involve lymph nodes, viscera, and the gastrointestinal tract.

176.0	Kaposi's sarcoma of skin — *any site* AHA: Q2, 1990, 7; Q4, 1991, 24
176.1	Kaposi's sarcoma of soft tissue — *blood vessel, connective tissue, fat, fascia, ligament, muscle and lymphatic tissue NEC* AHA: Q2, 1990, 7; Q4, 1991, 24
176.2	Kaposi's sarcoma of palate — *hard or soft* AHA: Q2, 1990, 7; Q4, 1991, 24
176.3	Kaposi's sarcoma of gastrointestinal sites — *stomach, intestine, anus, liver, spleen, pancreas* AHA: Q2, 1990, 7; Q4, 1991, 24
176.4	Kaposi's sarcoma of lung — *any site* AHA: Q2, 1990, 7; Q4, 1991, 24
176.5	Kaposi's sarcoma of lymph nodes — *any site, but excluding lymphatic channels* AHA: Q2, 1990, 7; Q4, 1991, 24
176.8	Kaposi's sarcoma of other specified sites — *external genitalia, scrotum, vulva, and oral cavity not elsewhere specified* AHA: Q2, 1990, 7; Q4, 1991, 24
176.9	Kaposi's sarcoma of unspecified site — *viscera not otherwise specified* AHA: Q2, 1990, 7; Q4, 1991, 24

Coding Clarification
Kaposi's syndrome is classified according to site of lesion. More than one code may be required to describe disseminated sarcoma, and Kaposi's is never reported with secondary neoplasm codes.

Do not reference the table of neoplasms to assign codes for Kaposi's sarcoma; Kaposi's sarcoma codes are omitted from the table. Instead, refer to Kaposi's sarcoma in the index of ICD-9-CM where a complete indexing is provided.

179–189 Malignant Neoplasm of Genitourinary Organs

Codes in this subsection of ICD-9-CM are classified according to site of malignant neoplasm in the female or male reproductive system or in the urinary system.

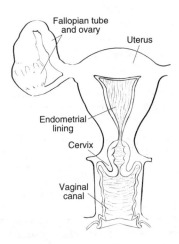

179 Malignant neoplasm of uterus, part unspecified
AHA: Q2, 1990, 7

Use this valid three-digit code to report a malignant neoplasm of the uterus when the specific location is unknown. Use a more specific code whenever possible, as this code is nonspecific and its use may cause reimbursement delays.

Coding Clarification
Use 182.8 *Malignant neoplasm of other specified sites of body of uterus* when the neoplasm is of contiguous or overlapping sites of the uterus.

180 Malignant neoplasm of cervix uteri
AHA: Q2, 1990, 7

Cancer of the cervix uteri may be asymptomatic or may cause vaginal discharge, pain, or postcoital bleeding. Most cervical cancers are squamous cell cancers.

Cervical cancer is classified as either of the endocervix, which opens into the uterus, or the exocervix, the part that protrudes into the vagina.

180.0	Malignant neoplasm of endocervix — *cervical canal opening into uterus* AHA: Q2, 1990, 7		182.0	Malignant neoplasm of corpus uteri, except isthmus — *cornu, endometrium, myometrium, fundus* AHA: Q2, 1990, 7
180.1	Malignant neoplasm of exocervix — *cervical canal opening into vagina* AHA: Q2, 1990, 7		182.1	Malignant neoplasm of isthmus — *narrow portion of the uterus between the cervix and the main body of the uterus.* AHA: Q2, 1990, 7
180.8	Malignant neoplasm of other specified sites of cervix — *cervical stump, squamocolumnar junction of cervix, or contiguous or overlapping sites* AHA: Q2, 1990, 7		182.8	Malignant neoplasm of other specified sites of body of uterus — *contiguous or overlapping sites* AHA: Q2, 1990, 7
180.9	Malignant neoplasm of cervix uteri, unspecified site			

Coding Clarification
Report other specified site, 180.8, if the malignancy is of the cervical stump following hysterectomy, of the squamocolumnar junction of the cervix, or if the malignancy is of contiguous or overlapping sites of the endocervix and exocervix.

181 Malignant neoplasm of placenta
AHA: Q2, 1990, 7

The placenta is an organ of pregnancy, operating as an exchange point for waste from the fetus and nourishment from the mother. In rare cases, an anomalous placenta may develop when no viable fetus exists, as in the case of hydatidiform mole. Use this valid three-digit code to report choriocarcinoma, also called chorioepithelioma. Hydatidiform mole or pregnancy precedes choriocarcinoma. It is an epithelial malignancy that metastasizes rapidly.

Coding Clarification
Do not use this code to report a hydatidiform mole (630), malignant hydatidiform mole (236.1), or chorioadenoma (236.1).

182 Malignant neoplasm of body of uterus
AHA: Q2, 1990, 7

The uterus is the muscular female organ where the fetus develops until delivery. Normally only three inches long and the shape of a pear, the uterus expands greatly during pregnancy.

Malignant neoplasms of the body of the uterus are classified according to site: the body of the uterus, including the fundus and endometrium; and the isthmus of the uterus, the narrow, distal portion of the uterus between the main body and the cervix. Endometrial carcinoma is a common malignancy that affects primarily postmenopausal women. Symptoms include postmenopausal bleeding, though symptoms may not be present until metastases become symptomatic.

Coding Clarification
Endometrial carcinoma is reported with 182.0 *Malignant neoplasm of corpus uteri, except isthmus.*

Report 182.8 *Malignant neoplasm of other specified site of body of uterus* if the malignancy is of contiguous or overlapping sites of the uterus. See codes in the 183 rubric to report cancer of the uterine ligaments.

183 Malignant neoplasm of ovary and other uterine adnexa
AHA: Q2, 1990, 7

The ovary is the female gonad and produces the ova. The organs are situated on either side of the uterus and lie near bilateral fallopian tubes, which carry the ova from the ovary to the uterus. Ligaments secure the female reproductive organs in the abdominal cavity.

Ovarian malignancies often present as an abdominal mass. Common types of ovarian malignancies include mucinous cystadenocarcinoma and endometrioid carcinoma. Other ovarian cancers are hormone producing and include Sertoli-Leydig cell tumors, adrenal cell rest tumors, and granulosa-theca cell tumors. Use an additional code to report any functional activity associated with the ovarian malignancy. If the ovarian malignancy is bilateral, it is usually metastasized disease, rather than a primary malignancy.

183.0	Malignant neoplasm of ovary — (Use additional code to identify any functional activity) — *female gonad* AHA: Q2, 1990, 7
183.2	Malignant neoplasm of fallopian tube — *oviduct, uterine tube* AHA: Q2, 1990, 7
183.3	Malignant neoplasm of broad ligament of uterus — *fold of peritoneum extending from the side of the uterus to the wall of the pelvis; mesovarium, parovarian region* AHA: Q2, 1990, 7

Neoplasms

183.4	Malignant neoplasm of parametrium of uterus — *connective tissue between the uterus and the broad ligament; uterosacral ligament* **AHA:** Q2, 1990, 7
183.5	Malignant neoplasm of round ligament of uterus — *ligament between the uterus and the wall of the pelvis* **AHA:** Q2, 1990, 7; Q3, 1999, 5
183.8	Malignant neoplasm of other specified sites of uterine adnexa — *tubo-ovarian, utero-ovarian, or contiguous or overlapping sites of ovary and other uterine adnexa* **AHA:** Q2, 1990, 7
183.9	Malignant neoplasm of uterine adnexa, unspecified site

Coding Clarification
This rubric excludes Douglas' cul-de-sac, reported with 158.8. If the malignancy is of contiguous or overlapping sites of ovary and uterine adnexa, report 183.8 *Malignant neoplasm of other specified sites of uterine adnexa.*

Coding Scenario
A patient is admitted for treatment of anemia due to malignant neoplasm of the pancreas.

> Code assignment: 285.22 *Anemia in neoplastic disease,* 157.9 *Malignant neoplasm of pancreas, part unspecified*

A patient has a known ovarian cancer currently in the terminal phase. She is admitted at this time to the hospice care facility for palliative care. Treatment is solely for pain management.

> Code assignment: 183.0 *Malignant neoplasm of ovary* and V66.7 *Encounter for palliative care*

184 Malignant neoplasm of other and unspecified female genital organs
AHA: Q2, 1990, 7

Malignancies of external female genitalia and the vagina are classified to this rubric.

184.0	Malignant neoplasm of vagina — *Gartner's duct, vaginal vault* **AHA:** Q2, 1990, 7
184.1	Malignant neoplasm of labia majora — *outer fold of skin and fat on either side of the vagina, including Bartholin's gland* **AHA:** Q2, 1990, 7
184.2	Malignant neoplasm of labia minora — *inner fold of skin between the labia major and the vagina* **AHA:** Q2, 1990, 7
184.3	Malignant neoplasm of clitoris
184.4	Malignant neoplasm of vulva, unspecified site — *specific site in vulva unknown* **AHA:** Q2, 1990, 7
184.8	Malignant neoplasm of other specified sites of female genital organs — *Mullerian duct; contiguous or overlapping sites of female genital organs* **AHA:** Q2, 1990, 7
184.9	Malignant neoplasm of female genital organ, site unspecified

Coding Clarification
If the malignancy affects both labia majora and labia minor, report 184.8 for contiguous or overlapping sites, rather than 184.4 for unspecified vulva.

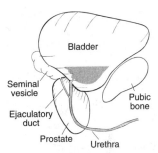

Side view schematic of prostate and related structures

185 Malignant neoplasm of prostate
AHA: Q2, 1990, 7; Q3, 1992, 7; Q3, 1999, 5; Q3, 2003, 13

The prostate is a singular, walnut-sized gland in the male. It surrounds the neck of the bladder and its ducts empty into the prostatic portion of the urethra. The prostate contributes fluid that helps to liquefy semen.

Adenocarcinoma of the prostate is the most common form of cancer in males older than 50 in the United States. Symptoms are uncommon until late in the disease course, when ureteral obstruction and hematuria may occur.

Coding Clarification
For cancer of the seminal vesicles, see 187.8 *Malignant neoplasm of other specified sites of male genital organs.*

Coding Scenario
A 69-year-old male is admitted with urinary retention and undergoes a TURP procedure. The final diagnosis is benign prostatic hypertrophy with urinary obstruction. The pathology report identifies microscopic foci of adenocarcinoma and confirms the benign prostatic hypertrophy.

> Code assignment: 600.01 *Hypertrophy (benign) of prostate with urinary obstruction and other lower urinary tract symptoms (LUTS),* 185

Malignant neoplasm of prostate, and 599.69 Urinary obstruction, not elsewhere classified, and 788.20 Retention of urine, unspecified

186 Malignant neoplasm of testis
AHA: Q2, 1990, 7

The testes are a pair of male gonads found in the scrotum and produce spermatozoa for fertilization. Leydig cells in the testes produce testosterone.

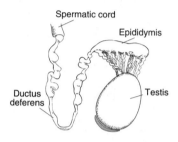

Most testicular masses are malignant and testicular cancer is more common among males with a history of undescended testes, even if the condition has been corrected surgically.

186.0 Malignant neoplasm of undescended testis — (Use additional code to identify any functional activity) — *ectopic, retained*
AHA: Q2, 1990, 7

186.9 Malignant neoplasm of other and unspecified testis — (Use additional code to identify any functional activity) — *descended, scrotal*
AHA: Q2, 1990, 7

Coding Clarification
Testicular tumors rarely cause functional problems. If functional problems occur, however, use an additional code to report it.

187 Malignant neoplasm of penis and other male genital organs
AHA: Q2, 1990, 7

The penis has two functions in males: sexual and excretory. The urethra may convey semen or urine. The tip of the penis is called the glans penis, and is covered in mucous membrane. The prepuce, or foreskin, is a fold of skin at the juncture where the body of the penis meets the glans penis; this extra skin is removed in circumcision. The corpora cavernosa are twin cylinders that extend the length of the organ called the body of the penis. Cancer of the penis usually occurs in uncircumcised males and human papillomavirus infection has been linked to penile cancer rates.

187.1 Malignant neoplasm of prepuce — *foreskin*
AHA: Q2, 1990, 7

187.2 Malignant neoplasm of glans penis — *head, distal end*
AHA: Q2, 1990, 7

187.3 Malignant neoplasm of body of penis — *corpus cavernosum, shaft*
AHA: Q2, 1990, 7

187.4 Malignant neoplasm of penis, part unspecified — *skin of penis not otherwise specified*
AHA: Q2, 1990, 7

187.5 Malignant neoplasm of epididymis — *tube in which sperm is stored*
AHA: Q2, 1990, 7

187.6 Malignant neoplasm of spermatic cord — *tube that carries sperm to the ejaculatory duct; vas deferens*
AHA: Q2, 1990, 7

187.7 Malignant neoplasm of scrotum — *pouch of skin and muscle, but not the contents (testes)*
AHA: Q2, 1990, 7

187.8 Malignant neoplasm of other specified sites of male genital organs — *seminal vesicle, Mullerian duct, tunica vaginalis, and contiguous or overlapping sites of penis and other male genital organs*
AHA: Q2, 1990, 7

187.9 Malignant neoplasm of male genital organ, site unspecified

Coding Clarification
Report 187.8 *Malignant neoplasm of male genital organs* if the malignancy is of contiguous or overlapping sites of the penis or other male reproductive organs.

Neoplasms

188 Malignant neoplasm of bladder
AHA: Q2, 1990, 7

The bladder lies in front (anterior) of the rectum in men and in front (anterior) of the vagina in women. As the bladder fills with urine, impulses from both voluntary and involuntary nerves signal that the bladder is full. When full, the bladder releases the urine it has stored through urination (voiding) via a tube called the urethra that connects the bladder floor to the outside of the body. Internal and external urinary muscle sphincters control the urine flow and stops the urine.

Malignant neoplasms of the bladder are classified by site. The dome of the bladder is the ceiling and the trigone is the triangular lower portion of the bladder bounded by the ureteral and urethral openings. Symptoms of malignant neoplasm of the bladder include hematuria, urinary urgency or frequency, or secondary infection at the tumor site. Pain or urinary retention may be present.

Males are twice as likely to develop bladder cancers as are females, and more than 90 percent of these cancers are transitional cell carcinomas. The most common site for cancer in the bladder is in the trigone.

188.0 Malignant neoplasm of trigone of urinary bladder — *lower portion of the bladder, bounded by a triangle created by the points at which the urethra and two ureters attach to the bladder*
AHA: Q2, 1990, 7

188.1 Malignant neoplasm of dome of urinary bladder — *top wall of the bladder*
AHA: Q2, 1990, 7

188.2 Malignant neoplasm of lateral wall of urinary bladder — *side wall of the bladder*
AHA: Q2, 1990, 7

188.3 Malignant neoplasm of anterior wall of urinary bladder — *front wall of the bladder*
AHA: Q2, 1990, 7

188.4 Malignant neoplasm of posterior wall of urinary bladder — *back wall of the bladder*
AHA: Q2, 1990, 7

188.5 Malignant neoplasm of bladder neck — *internal urethral orifice*
AHA: Q2, 1990, 7

188.6 Malignant neoplasm of ureteric orifice — *bladder surrounding the ureter's opening*
AHA: Q2, 1990, 7

188.7 Malignant neoplasm of urachus — *remnant of the fetal urinary tract*
AHA: Q2, 1990, 7

188.8 Malignant neoplasm of other specified sites of bladder — *contiguous or overlapping sites of bladder*
AHA: Q2, 1990, 7

188.9 Malignant neoplasm of bladder, part unspecified

Coding Clarification
If the malignancy is of contiguous and overlapping sites and the point of origin cannot be determined, report 188.8 *Malignant neoplasm of other specified sites of bladder.*

189 Malignant neoplasm of kidney and other and unspecified urinary organs
AHA: Q2, 1990, 7

The kidneys are paired organs between the parietal peritoneum and the posterior abdominal wall (retroperitoneal). They are located in the area of the last thoracic vertebrae to the third lumbar vertebrae.

Think of the kidneys as the body's blood filter. Items no longer needed are removed from the blood by the filter (kidneys) and eliminated in the form of urine, and elements needed are put back into the blood to be used by the cells and tissues of the body. Some of the blood the heart outputs with each cardiac cycle is sent to the kidneys to be filtered via two renal arteries (one to each kidney). In the kidneys, the renal arteries drain into other small arteries, then into even smaller arterioles and capillary networks called glomeruli where filtration takes place. Once the blood has been filtered and cleaned in the kidneys, it goes through venous capillaries that change into small veins called venules. Venules drain into larger veins that finally drain into the renal veins. The renal veins return the blood that has been filtered to the heart via the inferior vena cava.

Cup-like projections in each of the kidneys, called the renal calyces, drain the urine. Urine that has collected in the renal pelvis is transported via a process called peristalsis to storage in the bladder. The ureters enter the bladder (one at each side) at its base (top) and deposit the urine they carry into the bladder. Each ureter includes a valve that prevents urine that has been placed into the bladder from backing up into the ureters and the renal pelvis.

189.0	Malignant neoplasm of kidney, except pelvis — *parenchyma, Wilms' tumor* AHA: Q2, 1990, 7; Q2, 2004, 4; Q2, 2005, 4
189.1	Malignant neoplasm of renal pelvis — *portal of the kidney from which the ureters collect urine; renal calyces, ureteropelvic junction* AHA: Q2, 1990, 7
189.2	Malignant neoplasm of ureter — *one of a pair of tubes that transport urine from the kidneys to the bladder* AHA: Q2, 1990, 7
189.3	Malignant neoplasm of urethra — *tube that eliminates urine from the bladder, and in males, serves as a genital duct* AHA: Q2, 1990, 7
189.4	Malignant neoplasm of paraurethral glands — *glands and ducts of the urethra* AHA: Q2, 1990, 7
189.8	Malignant neoplasm of other specified sites of urinary organs — *contiguous or overlapping sites of kidney and other urinary organs* AHA: Q2, 1990, 7
189.9	Malignant neoplasm of urinary organ, site unspecified

Coding Clarification
Wilms' tumor is nephroblastoma, a childhood malignancy of the kidney and reported with 189.0. The tumor begins in utero and may be asymptomatic for years, though it is usually diagnosed before age 5.

If a patient is diagnosed with recurrent renal cell cancer of the kidney bed and is status post nephrectomy, query the physician to determine whether the cancer is a local recurrence of the primary cancer or a metastasis to the retroperitoneum. The answer will determine code assignment.

190–195 Malignant Neoplasm of Other and Unspecified Sites

Anatomical sites that don't fall under other rubrics are classified here for malignant neoplasms. Cancers of the eye, the brain, the central nervous system, and glands, as well as undefined locations are reported in this section of ICD-9-CM.

Secondary malignant neoplasms are also reported in this section. Secondary malignancies are sites to which the primary cancer has spread. They are usually classified by anatomical site.

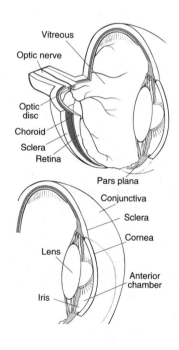

Neoplasms

190 Malignant neoplasm of eye
AHA: Q2, 1990, 7

The eye is the organ of sight and has a complex physiology. The eyeball rests in fatty tissue in the bony orbit of the skull where it is protected from jarring actions. A malignant neoplasm of the orbit lies in these fatty and other tissues between the eyeball and the skull. The eyeball can be divided into several segments: the anterior segment, which includes the lens and all tissue anterior to the lens in the eyeball; and the posterior segment, which includes everything in the eyeball that is situated behind the lens. The eye is basically a fluid-filled ball. Intraocular pressure in the anterior segment of the eye is maintained through the flow of aqueous humor, or tears. The lacrimal system provides these tears and is also an agent in their disposal. Tears are produced in the lacrimal glands, located bilaterally behind the eyebrow, and the lacrimal ducts carry the tears to the eye or away from the eye to the nose. Pressure in the posterior segment of the eye is maintained by gel-like vitreous humor.

A thin, vascular, mucous membrane covers the inner eyelids and the white outer shell of the eye (sclera). This membrane is called the conjunctiva. The cornea is the bulging "window" through which we see, and the retina is the light-sensitive "viewing screen" at the back of the eye. The choroid is a vascular layer of the inside of the eyeball.

190.0	Malignant neoplasm of eyeball, except conjunctiva, cornea, retina, and choroid — *ciliary body, sclera, lens, iris, uveal tract* **AHA:** Q2, 1990, 7
190.1	Malignant neoplasm of orbit — *tissue between the sclera of the eyeball and the orbital bone; retrobulbar tissue, extraocular muscle* **AHA:** Q2, 1990, 7
190.2	Malignant neoplasm of lacrimal gland — *tear-producing gland located behind the eyebrow; excludes lacrimal duct, sac* **AHA:** Q2, 1990, 7
190.3	Malignant neoplasm of conjunctiva — *mucous membrane lining the anterior eyeball and the inner aspect of the eyelid* **AHA:** Q2, 1990, 7
190.4	Malignant neoplasm of cornea — *clear dome that covers the anterior segment of the eye* **AHA:** Q2, 1990, 7
190.5	Malignant neoplasm of retina — *light-sensitive lining of the posterior segment of the eye* **AHA:** Q2, 1990, 7
190.6	Malignant neoplasm of choroid — *vascular layer of the globe of the eye* **AHA:** Q2, 1990, 7
190.7	Malignant neoplasm of lacrimal duct — *passage that carries tears to the eye and nose; lacrimal sac, nasolacrimal duct* **AHA:** Q2, 1990, 7
190.8	Malignant neoplasm of other specified sites of eye — *contiguous or overlapping sites of eye* **AHA:** Q2, 1990, 7
190.9	Malignant neoplasm of eye, part unspecified

Coding Clarification
A congenital cancer that is usually detected before age two, retinoblastoma is reported with 190.5 *Malignant neoplasm of retina*. Retinoblastoma is a malignancy of the retina and occurs bilaterally in 25 percent of patients with the disease.

If the malignant neoplasm is of the skin of the eyelid, it should be reported with codes for malignant neoplasm of the skin (172.1, 173.1). A malignancy of the optic nerve is reported with 192.0 *Malignant neoplasm of cranial nerves*, and of the orbital bone, 170.0 *Malignant neoplasm of skull and face, except mandible*. If the malignant neoplasm is of contiguous or overlapping parts of the eye, report 190.8 *Malignant neoplasm of other specified sites of eye*.

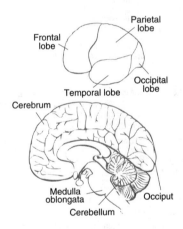

191 Malignant neoplasm of brain
AHA: Q2, 1990, 7

All brain tumors are "malignant" in that they may lead to death as they compromise the circulation of fluids in the brain through compression or obstruction. However, neoplasms classified to this rubric must also be of a metastasizing nature: a true malignancy. The incidences of benign and malignant neoplasms of the brain are about the same at 50 percent.

Symptoms of a neoplasm of the brain include headache, seizures, personality changes, impaired mental or physical functions, or in children, an enlarged head. Use an additional code to report any manifestations associated with the malignancy.

191.0	Malignant neoplasm of cerebrum, except lobes and ventricles — *including basal ganglia, globus pallidus; cerebral cortex; hypothalamus; corpus striatum; thalamus, cerebrum, internal capsule* **AHA:** Q2, 1990, 7
191.1	Malignant neoplasm of frontal lobe of brain — *frontal lobe* **AHA:** Q2, 1990, 7; Q4, 2005, 118
191.2	Malignant neoplasm of temporal lobe of brain — *hippocampus, uncus* **AHA:** Q2, 1990, 7
191.3	Malignant neoplasm of parietal lobe of brain — *parietal lobe* **AHA:** Q2, 1990, 7
191.4	Malignant neoplasm of occipital lobe of brain — *occipital lobe* **AHA:** Q2, 1990, 7
191.5	Malignant neoplasm of ventricles of brain — *choroid plexus, floor of ventricle* **AHA:** Q2, 1990, 7
191.6	Malignant neoplasm of cerebellum NOS — *cerebellopontine angle* **AHA:** Q2, 1990, 7
191.7	Malignant neoplasm of brain stem — *cerebral peduncle, midbrain, medulla oblongata, pons, stem* **AHA:** Q2, 1990, 7
191.8	Malignant neoplasm of other parts of brain — *corpus callosum, tapetum, and contiguous or overlapping sites of brain* **AHA:** Q2, 1990, 7
191.9	Malignant neoplasm of brain, unspecified site

Coding Clarification
Malignant neoplasms of the brain are classified according to location. Symptoms usually correspond to site. Malignant neoplasms of contiguous or overlapping sites in the brain are reported with 191.8. Do not use codes in this rubric to report cancers of the cranial nerves (192.0), of the retrobulbar area (190.1), or of the pituitary gland (194.3).

192 Malignant neoplasm of other and unspecified parts of nervous system
AHA: Q2, 1990, 7

Malignant neoplasms of the spine, meninges, cranial nerves, or sites unknown in the nervous system are classified in this rubric. Primary malignancies arising at these sites are much more rare than malignancies of the brain.

The tentorium is a dural sheath that divides the cranial cavity and supports the occipital lobes

192.0	Malignant neoplasm of cranial nerves — *olfactory bulb* **AHA:** Q2, 1990, 7
192.1	Malignant neoplasm of cerebral meninges — *dura mater, falx, meninges, tentorium* **AHA:** Q2, 1990, 7
192.2	Malignant neoplasm of spinal cord — *cauda equina* **AHA:** Q2, 1990, 7
192.3	Malignant neoplasm of spinal meninges — *lining of the spinal cord* **AHA:** Q2, 1990, 7
192.8	Malignant neoplasm of other specified sites of nervous system — *contiguous or overlapping sites of other parts of nervous system* **AHA:** Q2, 1990, 7
192.9	Malignant neoplasm of nervous system, part unspecified

Coding Clarification
Report 192.8 *Malignant neoplasm of other specified sites of nervous system* if the neoplasm is of overlapping or contiguous sites of the nervous system. Peripheral, sympathetic, or parasympathetic nerve malignancies are classified in rubric 171.

193 Malignant neoplasm of thyroid gland
AHA: Q2, 1990, 7

The thyroid gland is located just below the cricoid cartilage near the larynx and its purpose is to secrete thyroxine and triiodothyronine. Thyroxine and triiodothyronine increase the rate of cell metabolism.

Papillary adenocarcinoma accounts for 85 percent of thyroid cancers and usually appears in young adults. Though the only symptom of thyroid cancer may be a palpable node, some patients with thyroid cancer present with symptoms of hypothyroidism or hyperthyroidism.

Coding Clarification
Use an additional code to report any functional activity associated with the malignancy.

194 Malignant neoplasm of other endocrine glands and related structures
AHA: Q2, 1990, 7

The parathyroid glands come in pairs — the superior and inferior pair — that are embedded in the posterior thyroid. The adrenal glands are situated above each kidney, and the pituitary gland is located in the sella turcica of the sphenoid bone. The pineal gland, located at the base of the corpus callosum, secretes melatonin; the carotid body, located in the fork of the carotid artery, monitors blood oxygen. The aortic body at the aortic arch and right subclavian artery regulates reflex respiration.

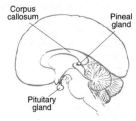

Malignancies of the endocrine glands can create functional activities in those glands. For example, adrenal tumors can cause virilizing or feminizing symptoms. Pituitary cancers can cause gigantism, Cushing's disease, amenorrhea or galactorrhea, or acromegaly. Report these functional activities in addition to the cancer.

Neuroblastoma is a common tumor of childhood that may affect the adrenal gland, retroperitoneum, central nervous system, or thoracic cavity. Usually seen in children younger than age 5, neuroblastomas present with a complex of symptoms according to the site of malignancy. A majority of the neuroblastomas arise in the adrenal gland.

194.0 Malignant neoplasm of adrenal gland — (Use additional code to identify any functional activity) — *cortex, medulla, suprarenal gland*
AHA: Q2, 1990, 7

194.1 Malignant neoplasm of parathyroid gland — (Use additional code to identify any functional activity) — *superior and inferior*
AHA: Q2, 1990, 7

194.3 Malignant neoplasm of pituitary gland and craniopharyngeal duct — (Use additional code to identify any functional activity) — *craniobuccal pouch, Rathke's pouch, hypophysis, sella turcica*
AHA: July-Aug, 1985, 9; Q2, 1990, 7

194.4 Malignant neoplasm of pineal gland — (Use additional code to identify any functional activity) — *located at the base of the corpus callosum*
AHA: Q2, 1990, 7

194.5 Malignant neoplasm of carotid body — (Use additional code to identify any functional activity) — *located at the fork in the carotid artery*
AHA: Q2, 1990, 7

194.6 Malignant neoplasm of aortic body and other paraganglia — (Use additional code to identify any functional activity) — *located at aortic arch and right subclavian artery; coccygeal body, para-aortic body, glomus jugulare*
AHA: Q2, 1990, 7

194.8 Malignant neoplasm of other endocrine glands and related structures — (Use additional code to identify any functional activity. Note: If the sites of multiple involvements are known, they should be coded separately.) — *if the sites of multiple involvements are known, they should be coded separately.*
AHA: Q2, 1990, 7

194.9 Malignant neoplasm of endocrine gland, site unspecified — (Use additional code to identify any functional activity)

Coding Clarification
An additional code from Chapter Three may be reported to identify functional activity associated with any neoplasm, for example, catecholamine-producing malignant pheochromocytoma of adrenal, 194.0 for neoplasm and 255.6 for adrenal hypofunction.

The ICD-9-CM index identifies 194.0 *Malignant neoplasm of adrenal gland* as the code for neuroblastoma for unspecified site. However, if a site other than adrenal gland is specified, consult the Neoplasm Table in ICD-9-CM for the correct code as classified by site.

195 Malignant neoplasm of other and ill-defined sites
AHA: Q2, 1990, 7

Use this rubric only as a last resort when the specific site of primary cancer cannot be identified or when the primary cancer has grown to invade two anatomic areas that would normally be reported with two codes and the point of origin cannot be determined.

195.0	Malignant neoplasm of head, face, and neck — cheek, jaw, nose, supraclavicular region AHA: Q2, 1990, 7; Q4, 2003, 107
195.1	Malignant neoplasm of thorax — axilla, chest wall, or intrathoracic region AHA: Q2, 1990, 7
195.2	Malignant neoplasm of abdomen — intraabdominal AHA: Q2, 1990, 7; Q2, 1997, 3
195.3	Malignant neoplasm of pelvis — groin; sacrococcygeal, inguinal, or presacral regions; rectovaginal or rectovesical septums; or overlapping sites AHA: Q2, 1990, 7
195.4	Malignant neoplasm of upper limb — shoulder, arm, or hand AHA: Q2, 1990, 7
195.5	Malignant neoplasm of lower limb — hip, leg, or foot AHA: Q2, 1990, 7
195.8	Malignant neoplasm of other specified sites — not elsewhere classified, including back, flank, and trunk AHA: Q2, 1990, 7

196–199 Secondary and Unspecified Malignant Neoplasms

All cancers shed cells into the patient's circulation. When these cells adhere to the vascular endothelium and begin to multiply into new tumors, the cancer is said to have metastasized. The new cancers are considered secondary malignancies, the primary malignancy being the "mother" site.

When a cancer recurs at the site of the original malignancy, it is still considered a primary malignancy and should not be reported with secondary malignancy codes. If the cancer recurs at a different site, these codes are appropriate, along with an additional code from the V10 rubric to identify a history of the malignancy of the primary site.

The secondary malignancy is sequenced first in coding if the patient is receiving treatment solely for the secondary malignancy. Otherwise, the code for the secondary site follows the code for the primary malignancy site.

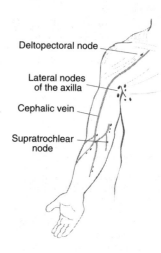

196 Secondary and unspecified malignant neoplasm of lymph nodes
AHA: May-June, 1985, 3; Q2, 1990, 7; Q2, 1992, 3

Secondary malignancies are classified according to site in this rubric. Metastases of cancers to lymphatic sites are fairly common since lymphatic fluid circulates the body and is filtered in the lymph nodes. The primary cancer may be near the affected lymph tissue or distant from it.

196.0	Secondary and unspecified malignant neoplasm of lymph nodes of head, face, and neck — cervicofacial, supraclavicular AHA: May-June, 1985, 3; Q2, 1990, 7; Q2, 1992, 3
196.1	Secondary and unspecified malignant neoplasm of intrathoracic lymph nodes — bronchopulmonary, mediastinal, intercostal, tracheobronchial, intrathoracic, Virchow's AHA: May-June, 1985, 3; Q2, 1990, 7; Q2, 1992, 3
196.2	Secondary and unspecified malignant neoplasm of intra-abdominal lymph nodes — aortic, intestinal, retroperitoneal, mesenteric, AHA: May-June, 1985, 3; Q2, 1990, 7; Q2, 1992, 3; Q4, 2003, 111
196.3	Secondary and unspecified malignant neoplasm of lymph nodes of axilla and upper limb — axillary, brachial, infraclavicular, epitrochlea, pectoral AHA: May-June, 1985, 3; Q2, 1990, 7; Q2, 1992, 3
196.5	Secondary and unspecified malignant neoplasm of lymph nodes of inguinal region and lower limb

Neoplasms

	— *Cloquet, femoral, popliteal, groin, Rosenmueller's, tibial* **AHA:** May-June, 1985, 3; Q2, 1990, 7; Q2, 1992, 3
196.6	Secondary and unspecified malignant neoplasm of intrapelvic lymph nodes — *hypogastric, obturator, iliac, parametrial* **AHA:** May-June, 1985, 3; Q2, 1990, 7; Q2, 1992, 3
196.8	Secondary and unspecified malignant neoplasm of lymph nodes of multiple sites — *lymphatic channel or vessel not elsewhere classified* **AHA:** May-June, 1985, 3; Q2, 1990, 7; Q2, 1992, 3
196.9	Secondary and unspecified malignant neoplasm of lymph nodes, site unspecified

197 Secondary malignant neoplasm of respiratory and digestive systems
AHA: May-June, 1985, 3; Q2, 1990, 7

Secondary malignancies are classified according to site in this rubric.

197.0	Secondary malignant neoplasm of lung — *bronchus* **AHA:** May-June, 1985, 3; Q2, 1990, 7; Q2, 1999, 9; Q1, 2006, 4
197.1	Secondary malignant neoplasm of mediastinum — *soft tissue between sternum and the spinal column, between the lungs* **AHA:** May-June, 1985, 3; Q2, 1990, 7
197.2	Secondary malignant neoplasm of pleura — *lining of the lung* **AHA:** May-June, 1985, 3; Q4, 1989, 11; Q2, 1990, 7; Q4, 2003, 110
197.3	Secondary malignant neoplasm of other respiratory organs — *trachea* **AHA:** May-June, 1985, 3; Q2, 1990, 7
197.4	Secondary malignant neoplasm of small intestine including duodenum — *duodenum, ilium, jejunum* **AHA:** May-June, 1985, 3; Q2, 1990, 7
197.5	Secondary malignant neoplasm of large intestine and rectum — *colon, rectum* **AHA:** May-June, 1985, 3; Q2, 1990, 7
197.6	Secondary malignant neoplasm of retroperitoneum and peritoneum — *mesentery, mesocolon, omentum, retroperitoneal tissue* **AHA:** May-June, 1985, 3; Q4, 1989, 11; Q2, 1990, 7; Q2, 2004, 4
197.7	Secondary malignant neoplasm of liver **AHA:** Q2, 2005, 9; Q1, 2006, 4
197.8	Secondary malignant neoplasm of other digestive organs and spleen — *spleen, pancreas, gall bladder/duct, ampulla of Vater, sphincter of Oddi* **AHA:** May-June, 1985, 3; Q2, 1990, 7; Q2, 1992, 3; Q2, 1997, 3

Coding Clarification
Report metastases to lymph nodes with codes from the rubric 196.

Coding Scenario
A patient is admitted with an esophageal obstruction due to esophageal metastasis from the lung.

> Code assignment: 197.8 *Secondary malignant neoplasm of other respiratory and digestive organs and spleen*, 162.9 *Malignant neoplasm of bronchus and lung, unspecified*, and 530.3 *Stricture and stenosis of esophagus*

198 Secondary malignant neoplasm of other specified sites
AHA: May-June, 1985, 3; Q2, 1990, 7

Secondary malignancies are classified according to site in this rubric.

198.0	Secondary malignant neoplasm of kidney — *parenchyma, calyx, hilus, pelvis* **AHA:** May-June, 1985, 3; Q2, 1990, 7
198.1	Secondary malignant neoplasm of other urinary organs — *bladder, ureter, urethra, prostate utricle* **AHA:** May-June, 1985, 3; Q2, 1990, 7
198.2	Secondary malignant neoplasm of skin — *skin of breast and except genital* **AHA:** May-June, 1985, 3; Q2, 1990, 7
198.3	Secondary malignant neoplasm of brain and spinal cord — *brain and spinal cord nerve root* **AHA:** May-June, 1985, 3; Q2, 1990, 7; Q3, 1999, 7
198.4	Secondary malignant neoplasm of other parts of nervous system — *meninges, parasympathetic, sympathetic, peripheral nerves and ganglia* **AHA:** May-June, 1985, 3; Jan-Feb, 1987, 7; Q2, 1990, 7
198.5	Secondary malignant neoplasm of bone and bone marrow — *bone and associated cartilage or marrow* **AHA:** May-June, 1985, 3; Q4, 1989, 10; Q2, 1990, 7; Q1, 1991, 16; Q2, 1992, 3; Q3, 1999, 5; Q4, 2003, 110
198.6	Secondary malignant neoplasm of ovary — *female gonad* **AHA:** May-June, 1985, 3; Q2, 1990, 7
198.7	Secondary malignant neoplasm of adrenal gland — *suprarenal gland* **AHA:** May-June, 1985, 3; Q2, 1990, 7
198.81	Secondary malignant neoplasm of breast — *male or female* **AHA:** May-June, 1985, 3; Q2, 1990, 7
198.82	Secondary malignant neoplasm of genital organs — *Mullerian duct, oviduct, cervical stump, endometrial stroma* **AHA:** May-June, 1985, 3; Q2, 1990, 7

198.89 Secondary malignant neoplasm of other specified sites — *pharynx, tongue, thyroid, salivary pituitary, connective tissue*
AHA: May-June, 1985, 3; Q2, 1990, 7; Q2, 1997, 4; Q2, 2005, 4

Coding Clarification
Report metastases to lymph nodes with codes from the rubric 196.

199 Malignant neoplasm without specification of site
AHA: Q2, 1990, 7

Secondary malignancies in this rubric are general, though they do have some specific uses. Up to 7 percent of cancer patients are diagnosed with a secondary malignancy for which the primary site cannot be found (e.g., UPO [unknown primary origin]).

199.0 Disseminated malignant neoplasm — *carcinomatosis, multiple in unspecified site*
AHA: Q4, 1989, 10; Q2, 1990, 7

199.1 Other malignant neoplasm of unspecified site — *unspecified primary or secondary site; Eaton-Lambert syndrome*
AHA: Q2, 1990, 7; Q1, 2006, 4

Coding Clarification
In these cases, report the secondary malignancy first, followed by 199.1 *Other malignant neoplasm of unspecified site* to report the unknown primary site. In cases where laboratory results indicate metastases to an unknown site, report the secondary malignancy with the same code, 199.1.

200–208 Malignant Neoplasm of Lymphatic and Hematopoietic Tissue

Malignant neoplasms of the lymphatic and hematopoietic tissues are considered primary neoplasms and do not spread to secondary sites. The malignant cells circulate to other areas through the lymphatic or blood systems.

Cancers of the lymphatic system are called lymphomas and they are more common after age 50. They occur most frequently in the groin (inguinal), neck (cervical), and armpit (axillary) nodes.

Some of the types of neoplasms that are included in this section are lymphosarcomas, Hodgkin's disease, lymphomas, malignant histiocytosis, multiple myeloma, myeloid leukemia, acute leukemia, and chronic leukemia. These diseases are classified by type, by site, and, in some cases, by status of remission or chronic or acute phase.

Do not use codes in this series to report secondary or unspecified lymph node malignancies, secondary bone marrow malignancies, or spleen cancer.

If the encounter is solely for the purpose of chemotherapy, the V code for chemotherapy (V58.1) should be sequenced first and the malignancy sequenced secondarily.

Behavior Classification: Code categories 200-208 identify neoplastic disorders of the blood-forming tissues and neoplasms arising in the reticuloendothelial and lymphatic systems acknowledged or assumed to be primary malignancies. The difference between lymphohematopoietic system malignancies and other malignancies is that the tumor cells typically circulate in large numbers in the bloodstream.

Malignant neoplasms classified by code categories 200-208 that are identified as metastatic or secondary are still classified within the 200-208 categories and would not be classified to category 196. Do not use codes from code range 200-208 to classify secondary sites or metastatic neoplasms when the primary site is not classified within this code range.

Indications for Transplant: The following are clinical indications for the various forms of bone marrow transplants.

- Autologous-Refractory acute leukemia, Burkitt's lymphoma, undifferentiated lymphoma, diffuse histiocytic lymphoma, refractory acute leukemia, melanoma, central nervous system malignancies, soft tissue sarcomas, central axis Ewing's sarcoma, and carcinomas of breast, ovary, lung, and testes.

- Syngeneic-Acute myelogenous leukemia, acute lymphoblastic leukemia, chronic myelogenous leukemia, non-Hodgkin's lymphoma, Ewing's sarcoma, and hairy cell leukemia.

- Allogeneic-Acute myelogenous leukemia, acute lymphoblastic leukemia, chronic myelogenous leukemia, non-Hodgkin's lymphoma, severe combined immunodeficiency disease, Wiskott-Aldrich syndrome, and aplastic anemia.

Bone marrow transplantation is typically performed on patients whose condition is in the state of remission. Patients in remission are better able to tolerate the bone marrow transplant. They are receiving active treatment for the leukemia during the remission phase; therefore codes in the V10 "History of" category are not appropriate. A code from the 204-208 series would be used to designate the type of leukemia.

Neoplasms

200 Lymphosarcoma and reticulosarcoma
AHA: Nov-Dec, 1986, 5; Q2, 1990, 7; Q2, 1992, 3

Lymphosarcoma is a form of non-Hodgkin's lymphoma in which the cells are either a small or large lymphocyte.

Reticulosarcoma (200.1x) along with histiocytic sarcoma is a form of non-Hodgkin's lymphoma derived from the histiocyte, a macrophage present in connective tissue.

Burkitt's tumor or lymphoma is a form of non-Hodgkin's lymphoma characterized by an undifferentiated B-cell tumor. There are two variants: endemic (African) and sporadic. The endemic variant is associated with Epstein-Barr virus infection and has a variable diagnosis. The sporadic variant has a very poor prognosis. Jaw and orbital involvement is typical in endemic Burkitt's lymphoma and abdominal disease predominates in sporadic Burkitt's lymphoma.

> The following fifth-digit subclassification is for use with categories 200-202:
> 0   unspecified site, extranodal and solid organ sites
> 1   lymph nodes of head, face, and neck
> 2   intrathoracic lymph nodes
> 3   intra-abdominal lymph nodes
> 4   lymph nodes of axilla and upper limb
> 5   lymph nodes of inguinal region and lower limb
> 6   intrapelvic lymph nodes
> 7   spleen
> 8   lymph nodes of multiple sites

- **200.0** ✓5th Reticulosarcoma — *reticulum cell sarcoma; pleomorphic cell type*
  AHA: Nov-Dec, 1986, 5; Q2, 1990, 7; Q2, 1992, 3
- **200.1** ✓5th Lymphosarcoma — *lymphoblastoma, prolymphocytic*
  AHA: Nov-Dec, 1986, 5; Q2, 1990, 7; Q2, 1992, 3
- **200.2** ✓5th Burkitt's tumor or lymphoma — *malignant lymphoma*
  AHA: Nov-Dec, 1986, 5; Q2, 1990, 7; Q2, 1992, 3
- **200.8** ✓5th Other named variants of lymphosarcoma and reticulosarcoma — *mixed cell type; reticulolymphosarcoma; lymphoplasmacytoid*
  AHA: Nov-Dec, 1986, 5; Q2, 1990, 7; Q2, 1992, 3

201 Hodgkin's disease
AHA: Nov-Dec, 1986, 5; Q2, 1990, 7; Q2, 1992, 3

Hodgkin's disease is the most common type of lymphoma, and most commonly affects young and middle-aged adults. Hodgkin's disease is a painless, progressive replacement of lymph nodes, spleen, and other lymphatic tissue with tumor tissue consisting of atypical histiocytes together with lymphocytes, eosinophils, plasma cells, and fibrous tissue. In Hodgkin's lymphoma, Reed-Sternberg cells are present.

> The following fifth-digit subclassification is for use with categories 200-202:
> 0   unspecified site, extranodal and solid organ sites
> 1   lymph nodes of head, face, and neck
> 2   intrathoracic lymph nodes
> 3   intra-abdominal lymph nodes
> 4   lymph nodes of axilla and upper limb
> 5   lymph nodes of inguinal region and lower limb
> 6   intrapelvic lymph nodes
> 7   spleen
> 8   lymph nodes of multiple sites

- **201.0** ✓5th Hodgkin's paragranuloma
- **201.1** ✓5th Hodgkin's granuloma
- **201.2** ✓5th Hodgkin's sarcoma
- **201.4** ✓5th Hodgkin's disease, lymphocytic-histiocytic predominance
- **201.5** ✓5th Hodgkin's disease, nodular sclerosis — *cellular phase*
  AHA: Nov-Dec, 1986, 5; Q2, 1990, 7; Q2, 1992, 3
- **201.6** ✓5th Hodgkin's disease, mixed cellularity
- **201.7** ✓5th Hodgkin's disease, lymphocytic depletion — *lymphocytic depletion; diffuse fibrosis; reticular type*
  AHA: Nov-Dec, 1986, 5; Q2, 1990, 7; Q2, 1992, 3
- **201.9** ✓5th Hodgkin's disease, unspecified type — *Paltauf-Sternberg disease*
  AHA: Nov-Dec, 1986, 5; Q2, 1990, 7; Q2, 1992, 3

Coding Scenario
A patient is admitted to the facility with Hodgkin's disease. The final diagnostic statement identifies Hodgkin's disease with lymphocytic depletion (numerous Reed-Sternberg cells) with extensive body involvement.

Code assignment: 201.78 *Hodgkin's disease, lymphocytic depletion, lymph nodes of multiple sites*

202 Other malignant neoplasms of lymphoid and histiocytic tissue
AHA: Nov-Dec, 1986, 5; Q2, 1990, 7; Q2, 1992, 3

Nodular lymphoma is a non-Hodgkin's lymphoma in which lymphoma cells are clustered into identifiable nodules or follicles, and malignant histiocytosis presents with progressive, abnormal histiocytes in the blood. Mycosis fungoides is an uncommon, chronic T-cell lymphoma affecting the skin and sometimes internal organs, usually in patients 50 years or older. T-cell lymphoma often appears as a rash and goes undiagnosed for a period. Sezary disease is an extension of mucosus fungoides that affects the blood. Leukemic reticuloendotheliosis is a chronic leukemia with preponderance of large, mononuclear cells with hairy appearance in the marrow, spleen, liver, and bone. In Letterer-Siwe disease, reticuloendotheliosis occurs in early childhood and presents with skin eruptions, anemia, and enlarged liver, spleen, and lymph nodes.

The following fifth-digit subclassification is for use with categories 200-202:

0   unspecified site, extranodal and solid organ sites
1   lymph nodes of head, face, and neck
2   intrathoracic lymph nodes
3   intra-abdominal lymph nodes
4   lymph nodes of axilla and upper limb
5   lymph nodes of inguinal region and lower limb
6   intrapelvic lymph nodes
7   spleen
8   lymph nodes of multiple sites

202.0 ⌐sth Nodular lymphoma — *Brill-Symmers disease; lymphosarcoma*
AHA: Nov-Dec, 1986, 5; Q2, 1990, 7; Q2, 1992, 3

202.1 ⌐sth Mycosis fungoides — *cutaneous T-cell lymphoma*
AHA: Nov-Dec, 1986, 5; Q2, 1990, 7; Q2, 1992, 3; Q2, 1992, 4

202.2 ⌐sth Sezary's disease — *mycosis fungoides infecting blood*
AHA: Nov-Dec, 1986, 5; Q2, 1990, 7; Q2, 1992, 3; Q2, 1999, 7

202.3 ⌐sth Malignant histiocytosis — *histiocytic medullary reticulosis; malignant reticuloendotheliosis/reticulosis*
AHA: Nov-Dec, 1986, 5; Q2, 1990, 7; Q2, 1992, 3

202.4 ⌐sth Leukemic reticuloendotheliosis — *hairy cell leukemia*
AHA: Nov-Dec, 1986, 5; Q2, 1990, 7; Q2, 1992, 3

202.5 ⌐sth Letterer-Siwe disease — *acute differentiated progressive histiocytosis; histiocytosis X; infantile reticuloendotheliosis*
AHA: Nov-Dec, 1986, 5; Q2, 1990, 7; Q2, 1992, 3

202.6 ⌐sth Malignant mast cell tumors — *mast cell sarcoma; mastocytoma; mastocytosis*
AHA: Nov-Dec, 1986, 5; Q2, 1990, 7; Q2, 1992, 3

202.8 ⌐sth Other malignant lymphomas — *NOS, diffuse*
AHA: Nov-Dec, 1986, 5; Q2, 1990, 7; Q2, 1992, 3; Q2, 1992, 4; For code 202.80: Q2, 2006, 20

202.9 ⌐sth Other and unspecified malignant neoplasms of lymphoid and histiocytic tissue — *Follicular dendritic cell carcinoma, interdigitating dendric cell sarcoma, Langerhans cell sarcoma, malignant neoplasm of bone marrow NOS*
AHA: Nov-Dec, 1986, 5; Q2, 1990, 7; Q2, 1992, 3

Coding Clarification

Cutaneous T-cell Lymphoma with Sezary Syndrome: Cutaneous T-cell lymphoma is synonymous with mycosis fungoides and can be found in the alphabetic index under the main term, Mycosis, fungoides. Use subcategory code 202.1x to report this condition with the appropriate fifth digit. Also code the Sezary disease with 202.2x. When two conditions are present from the same category, as long as the fourth digits are different, it is appropriate to code them both.

Retroperitoneal Follicular Center Cell: Report with code 202.8x *Other malignant lymphomas*, with the fifth digit that identifies the site of the lymphoma.

Coding Scenario

A 59-year-old patient is admitted with intractable bone pain. The patient had been previously diagnosed with malignant lymphoma of the bone. The patient is found to have a lymph node in the chest positive for lymphoma and a biopsy of the bone in the pelvis reveals the same lymphoma cell type.

Code assignment: 202.88 *Other malignant lymphomas, lymph nodes of multiple sites*

A patient is admitted with Sezary syndrome, diagnosed fairly recently, and with cutaneous T-cell lymphoma, diagnosed four years previous.

Code assignment: Code both 202.2x *Sezary disease* and 202.1x *Mycosis fungoides, for cutaneous T-cell lymphoma with Sezary syndrome*. It is permissible to code more than one condition from the same three digit-category, so long as the fourth digits are different.

203 Multiple myeloma and immunoproliferative neoplasms
AHA: Q2, 1990, 7; Q4, 1991, 26

Multiple myeloma is an uncontrolled proliferation of plasma cells and results in a number of organ

Neoplasms

dysfunctions and symptoms of bone pain or fracture, renal failure, infection, anemia, hypercalcemia, as well as clotting and neurologic or vascular abnormalities.

Multiple myeloma is often described as metastatic to the bone, but because this is part of the disease, the bone metastases should not be reported separately as a secondary malignant neoplasm.

> The following fifth-digit subclassification is for use with categories 203, 204, 205, 206, 207, and 208:
>
> 0 without mention of remission
>
> 1 in remission

203.0 ⌐sth Multiple myeloma — *Kahler's disease; myelomatosis*
AHA: Q4, 1989, 10; Q2, 1990, 7; Q4, 1991, 26; Q1, 1996, 16

203.1 ⌐sth Plasma cell leukemia — *plasmacytic leukemia*
AHA: Sept-Oct, 1986, 12; Q2, 1990, 7; Q4, 1990, 26; Q4, 1991, 26

203.8 ⌐sth Other immunoproliferative neoplasms

Coding Clarification
When a patient with multiple myelomas develops a complication from the disease, the complication is generally sequenced first, followed by the myeloma. For example, if a patient with multiple myeloma sustains a stress fracture of the femur, the codes would be sequenced:

733.14 Pathologic fracture of the neck of femur

203.00 Multiple myeloma without mention of remission

204 Lymphoid leukemia
AHA: Q2, 1990, 7; Q3, 1993, 4

Lymphoid leukemia is a malignant proliferation of immature lymphocytes called lymphoblasts. The acute condition is common in children and fatal if untreated. The chronic condition is a generalized, progressive form of lymphocytic leukemia predominantly affecting men older than age 50. It is the least malignant form of leukemia.

> The following fifth-digit subclassification is for use with categories 203, 204, 205, 206, 207, and 208:
>
> 0 without mention of remission
>
> 1 in remission

204.0 ⌐sth Acute lymphoid leukemia — *lymphoblastic, usually in childhood*
AHA: Q2, 1990, 7; Q3, 1993, 4; Q3, 1999, 6

204.1 ⌐sth Chronic lymphoid leukemia — *lymphoblastic, more mature, usually in middle/old age*
AHA: Q2, 1990, 7; Q3, 1993, 4

204.2 ⌐sth Subacute lymphoid leukemia

204.8 ⌐sth Other lymphoid leukemia — *aleukemic leukemia*
AHA: Q2, 1990, 7; Q3, 1993, 4

204.9 ⌐sth Unspecified lymphoid leukemia

Documentation Issues
If the physician documentation specifies that the patient's leukemia has been completely cured, use code V10.6x.

Only when documentation specifically indicates the leukemia is in remission should it be coded as such.

If the physician documentation states the diagnosis of leukemia associated with lymphoma, two codes should be used to identify each as separate entities.

Coding Clarification
Bone Marrow Donor: If the patient has been admitted to donate his/her own marrow for bone marrow transplantation, code V59.3 *Bone marrow donor* would still be appropriate. Use an additional code to identify the specific type of leukemia from code series 204-208. Keep in mind that code V59.3 is only used when the admission is solely for donor purposes.

Coding Scenario
An acute lymphoblastic leukemia patient presents with extreme abdominal pain, having finished his course of chemotherapy the previous week. His laboratory findings are as follows: profound neutropenia — white count of .2, absolute neutrophil count of 20. The hematologist has diagnosed acute neutropenic enterocolitis due to chemotherapy. Abdominal surgery is not required.

> Code assignment: The physician must be queried as to the nature of the enterocolitis — infectious versus noninfectious.

If the enteritis is infectious, the codes are as follows: 288.03 *Drug induced neutropenia;* 009.1 *Colitis, enteritis, and gastroenteritis, of presumed infectious origin;* E933.1 *Adverse effect of antineoplastic drugs;* and 204.00 *Lymphoid leukemia, acute, without mention of remission.*

If the enteritis is non-infectious, the codes are as follows: 288.03 *Drug induced neutropenia,* 558.9 *Other and unspecified noninfectious gastroenteritis and colitis,* E933.1 *Adverse effect of antineoplastic and immunosuppressive drugs,* and 204.00 *Acute lymphoid leukemia, without mention of remission.*

205 Myeloid leukemia
AHA: May-June, 1985, 18; Q2, 1990, 7; Q4, 1990, 3; Q4, 1991, 26; Q3, 1993, 3

Myeloid leukemia is a rapid and malignant proliferation of immature myelocytes called myeloblasts. The acute condition is common in children and fatal if untreated. The chronic condition is a fatal disease characterized by abnormal proliferation of premature granulocytes called myeloblasts, promyelocytes, metamyelocytes, and myelocytes, in bone marrow, peripheral blood, and body tissues.

The following fifth-digit subclassification is for use with categories 203, 204, 205, 206, 207, and 208:
0   without mention of remission
1   in remission

205.0 ⌐sth   Acute myeloid leukemia — *acute promyelocytic; differentiated cell populations*
AHA: May-June, 1985, 18; Q2, 1990, 7; Q4, 1990, 3; Q4, 1991, 26; Q3, 1993, 3; **For code 205.00:** Q2, 2006, 20

205.1 ⌐sth   Chronic myeloid leukemia — *more granulocytic cells; usually in young adults, eosinophilic/neutrophilic*
AHA: July-Aug, 1985, 13; May-June, 1985, 18; Q2, 1990, 7; Q4, 1990, 3; Q4, 1991, 26; Q3, 1993, 3; Q1, 2000, 6

205.2 ⌐sth   Subacute myeloid leukemia

205.3 ⌐sth   Myeloid sarcoma — *chloroma, granulocytic carcoma, green malignancy arising from bone marrow*
AHA: May-June, 1985, 18; Q2, 1990, 7; Q4, 1990, 3; Q4, 1991, 26; Q3, 1993, 3

205.8 ⌐sth   Other myeloid leukemia — *aleukemic*
AHA: May-June, 1985, 18; Q2, 1990, 7; Q4, 1990, 3; Q4, 1991, 26; Q3, 1993, 3

205.9 ⌐sth   Unspecified myeloid leukemia

Documentation Issues
If the physician documentation specifies that the patient's leukemia has been completely cured, use code V10.6x.

Only when documentation specifically indicates the leukemia is in remission should it be coded as such.

If the physician documentation states the diagnosis of leukemia associated with lymphoma, two codes should be used to identify each as separate entities.

Coding Clarification
Blast Crisis: This condition is noted by an abrupt, severe change in the course of chronic myelocytic leukemia that resembles that in acute myelocytic leukemia, with an increase in the proportion of myeloblasts. In some cases, the cells may be lymphoblasts. There is no code to identify the blast crisis as it identifies the progression to chronic myelogenous leukemia. If, for example, the diagnostic statement indicates chronic myelogenous leukemia with blast crisis, it would be coded 205.10 *Chronic myeloid leukemia without mention of remission* and additional codes would be used to identify conditions such as severe anemia due to blood loss (280.0) and thrombocytopenia (287.4). Although a fever may be noted, do not use code 780.6, since it classifies fever of unknown etiology.

Bone Marrow Donor: If the patient has been admitted to donate his/her own marrow for bone marrow transplantation code V59.3 *Bone marrow donor* would still be appropriate. Use an additional code to identify the specific type of leukemia from code series 204-208. Code V59.3 is only used when the admission is solely for donor purposes.

Coding Scenario
A patient is admitted for treatment of chronic myelogenous leukemia with blastic exacerbation.

Code assignment: 205.10 *Chronic myeloid leukemia, without mention of remission*

A patient with myeloblastic leukemia in the remission stage is admitted for bone marrow transplantation.

Code assignment: 205.91 *Unspecified myeloid leukemia, in remission*

206 Monocytic leukemia
AHA: Q2, 1990, 7

The following fifth-digit subclassification is for use with categories 203, 204, 205, 206, 207, and 208:
0   without mention of remission
1   in remission

206.0 ⌐sth   Acute monocytic leukemia — *uncommon; monocytes as predominant cells*
AHA: Q2, 1990, 7

206.1 ⌐sth   Chronic monocytic leukemia

206.2 ⌐sth   Subacute monocytic leukemia

206.8 ⌐sth   Other monocytic leukemia — *aleukemic*
AHA: Q2, 1990, 7

206.9 ⌐sth   Unspecified monocytic leukemia — *Schilling-type*
AHA: Q2, 1990, 7

Documentation Issues
If the physician documentation specifies that the patient's leukemia has been completely cured, use code V10.6x.

Only when documentation specifically indicates the leukemia is in remission should it be coded as such.

If the physician documentation states the diagnosis of leukemia associated with lymphoma, two codes should be used to identify each as separate entities.

Coding Clarification
When a patient has an acute exacerbation of chronic monocytic leukemia, assign 206.10 *Chronic monocytic leukemia, without mention of remission* since the acute exacerbation is included in the code for chronic leukemia. The "acute" designation in this rubric is reserved for an uncommon form of myelogenous leukemia with monocytes as predominant cells.

Bone Marrow Donor: If the patient has been admitted to donate his/her own marrow for bone marrow transplantation, code V59.3 *Bone marrow donor* would still be appropriate. Use an additional code to identify the specific type of leukemia from code series 204-208. Code V59.3 is only used when the admission is solely for donor purposes.

207 Other specified leukemia
AHA: Q2, 1990, 7

This rubric is reserved for several leukemias that do not classify to the other rubrics.

The following fifth-digit subclassification is for use with categories 203, 204, 205, 206, 207, and 208:
0 without mention of remission
1 in remission

- 207.0 ✓5th Acute erythremia and erythroleukemia — *acute erythremic myelosis; Di Guglielmo's disease; erythremic myelosis*
  AHA: Q2, 1990, 7
- 207.1 ✓5th Chronic erythremia — *Heilmeyer-Schöner disease*
  AHA: Q2, 1990, 7
- 207.2 ✓5th Megakaryocytic leukemia — *megakaryocytic myelosis; thrombocytic leukemia*
  AHA: Q2, 1990, 7
- 207.8 ✓5th Other specified leukemia — *lymphosarcoma cell leukemia*
  AHA: Q2, 1990, 7

Documentation Issues
If the physician documentation specifies that the patient's leukemia has been completely cured, use code V10.6x.

Only when documentation specifically indicates the leukemia is in remission should it be coded as such.

If the physician documentation states the diagnosis of leukemia associated with lymphoma, two codes should be used to identify each as separate entities.

Coding Clarification
Leukemias of unspecified cell types are classified to rubric 208.

Bone Marrow Donor: If the patient has been admitted to donate his/her own marrow for bone marrow transplantation, code V59.3 *Bone marrow donor* would still be appropriate. Use an additional code to identify the specific type of leukemia from code series 204-208. Keep in mind that code V59.3 is only used when the admission is solely for donor purposes.

208 Leukemia of unspecified cell type
AHA: Q2, 1990, 7

Use these leukemia codes when documentation does not provide sufficient information or when the patient's specific diagnosis has not yet been established although leukemia is certain.

The following fifth-digit subclassification is for use with categories 203, 204, 205, 206, 207, and 208:
0 without mention of remission
1 in remission

- 208.0 ✓5th Acute leukemia of unspecified cell type — *acute leukemia NOS; stem cell leukemia; blast cell leukemia*
  AHA: Q2, 1990, 7
- 208.1 ✓5th Chronic leukemia of unspecified cell type — *not otherwise specified*
  AHA: Q2, 1990, 7
- 208.2 ✓5th Subacute leukemia of unspecified cell type — *not otherwise specified*
  AHA: Q2, 1990, 7
- 208.8 ✓5th Other leukemia of unspecified cell type
- 208.9 ✓5th Unspecified leukemia — *Bennett's disease*
  AHA: Q2, 1990, 7

Documentation Issues
If the physician documentation specifies that the patient's leukemia has been completely cured, use code V10.6x.

Only when documentation specifically indicates the leukemia is in remission should it be coded as such.

If the physician documentation states the diagnosis of leukemia associated with lymphoma, two codes should be used to identify each as separate entities.

Coding Clarification
Bone Marrow Donor: If the patient has been admitted to donate his/her own marrow for bone marrow transplantation, code V59.3 *Bone marrow donor* would still be appropriate. Use an additional code to identify the specific type of leukemia from

code series 204-208. Code V59.3 is only used when the admission is solely for donor purposes.

210–212 Benign Neoplasms of Digestive and Respiratory System and Intrathoracic Organs

Benign neoplasms are tumors characterized by dividing cells that adhere to each other, so that the mass remains a circumscribed lesion. Benign neoplasms are classified according to site. Many cysts and embryonic cysts are excluded from this classification.

210 Benign neoplasm of lip, oral cavity, and pharynx
AHA: Q2, 1990, 7

Neoplasms are classified by site in this rubric. Excluded from this rubric are cysts, ranulas, and radicular cysts.

210.0	Benign neoplasm of lip — *frenulum labii, inner aspect, mucosa* AHA: Q2, 1990, 7
210.1	Benign neoplasm of tongue — *lingual tonsil* AHA: Q2, 1990, 7
210.2	Benign neoplasm of major salivary glands — *parotid, sublingual, submandibular; Warthin's tumor* AHA: Q2, 1990, 7
210.3	Benign neoplasm of floor of mouth — *floor of mouth* AHA: Q2, 1990, 7
210.4	Benign neoplasm of other and unspecified parts of mouth — *gingiva, oral mucosa, palate, uvula, labial commissure* AHA: Q2, 1990, 7
210.5	Benign neoplasm of tonsil — *faucial, palatine* AHA: Q2, 1990, 7
210.6	Benign neoplasm of other parts of oropharynx — *mesopharynx, tonsillar fossa/pillars, vallecula, brachial cleft, anterior epiglottis* AHA: Q2, 1990, 7
210.7	Benign neoplasm of nasopharynx — *adenoid, pharyngeal tonsil, posterior nasal septum, choana* AHA: Q2, 1990, 7
210.8	Benign neoplasm of hypopharynx — *arytenoid fold, pyriform fossa, postcricoid region, laryngopharynx* AHA: Q2, 1990, 7
210.9	Benign neoplasm of pharynx, unspecified — *site specified only as "throat"* AHA: Q2, 1990, 7

211 Benign neoplasm of other parts of digestive system
AHA: Q2, 1990, 7

Neoplasms are classified by site in this rubric with the exception of benign stromal tumors of the digestive system, which are reported with code 215.5 *Other benign neoplasm of connective and other soft tissue, abdomen.*

211.0	Benign neoplasm of esophagus
211.1	Benign neoplasm of stomach — *cardia, body, fundus, pylorus* AHA: Q2, 1990, 7
211.2	Benign neoplasm of duodenum, jejunum, and ileum — *small intestine* AHA: Q2, 1990, 7
211.3	Benign neoplasm of colon — *large intestine, appendix, cecum, ileocecal valve, Cronkhite-Canada syndrome* AHA: Q2, 1990, 7; Q4, 2001, 56; Q2, 2005, 16; Q3, 2005, 17
211.4	Benign neoplasm of rectum and anal canal — *sphincter, rectosigmoid junction* AHA: Q2, 1990, 7
211.5	Benign neoplasm of liver and biliary passages — *ampulla of Vater, gallbladder, sphincter of Oddi, hepatic or cystic or common bile duct* AHA: Q2, 1990, 7
211.6	Benign neoplasm of pancreas, except islets of Langerhans — *head, tail, or body, except insulin-producing cells* AHA: Q2, 1990, 7
211.7	Benign neoplasm of islets of Langerhans — (Use additional code to identify any functional activity) — *insulin producing cells* AHA: Q2, 1990, 7
211.8	Benign neoplasm of retroperitoneum and peritoneum — *mesentery, mesoappendix, mesocolon, omentum, retroperitoneal tissue* AHA: Q2, 1990, 7
211.9	Benign neoplasm of other and unspecified site of the digestive system — *spleen and generalized sites* AHA: Q2, 1990, 7

Coding Clarification
Benign neoplasms of the digestive system are primarily classified by site in these rubrics. The margin of the anus is excluded from this rubric and would be reported with 216.5 *Benign neoplasm of skin of trunk, except scrotum.* Also excluded are benign stromal tumors of the digestive system, which are reported with code 215.5 *Other benign neoplasm of connective and other soft tissue, abdomen.*

Neoplasms

Coding Scenario
A patient diagnosed with a nonmalignant gastric lymphoma (pseudolymphoma) returns for a follow up visit.

> Code assignment: 211.1 *Benign neoplasm of stomach*

212 Benign neoplasm of respiratory and intrathoracic organs
AHA: Q2, 1990, 7

Neoplasms are classified by site in this rubric.

212.0	Benign neoplasm of nasal cavities, middle ear, and accessory sinuses — *sinus, eustachian tube, septum, nasal cartilage* **AHA:** Q2, 1990, 7
212.1	Benign neoplasm of larynx — *vocal cords including laryngeal cartilage, suprahyoid epiglottis, glottis* **AHA:** Q2, 1990, 7
212.2	Benign neoplasm of trachea
212.3	Benign neoplasm of bronchus and lung — *carina, hilus* **AHA:** Q2, 1990, 7
212.4	Benign neoplasm of pleura — *membrane surrounding lung* **AHA:** Q2, 1990, 7
212.5	Benign neoplasm of mediastinum — *thoracic soft tissue not elsewhere classified* **AHA:** Q2, 1990, 7
212.6	Benign neoplasm of thymus — *lymphoid tissue in upper, anterior mediastinum* **AHA:** Q2, 1990, 7
212.7	Benign neoplasm of heart — *myocardium, pericardium, endocardium* **AHA:** Q2, 1990, 7
212.8	Benign neoplasm of other specified sites of respiratory and intrathoracic organs — *not elsewhere classified* **AHA:** Q2, 1990, 7
212.9	Benign neoplasm of respiratory and intrathoracic organs, site unspecified

Coding Clarification
Classify thoracic or intrathoracic benign neoplasms, not otherwise specified to 229.8.

213-215 Benign Neoplasms of Bone, Connective, and Soft Tissues

Neoplasms in this rubric include lipomas and are classified by site.

213 Benign neoplasm of bone and articular cartilage
AHA: Q2, 1990, 7

Bone and cartilage are not differentiated in this rubric. Code selection is based on anatomic site.

213.0	Benign neoplasm of bones of skull and face — *cranial bone, turbinates, orbit, patella* **AHA:** Q2, 1990, 7
213.1	Benign neoplasm of lower jaw bone — *mandible* **AHA:** Q2, 1990, 7
213.2	Benign neoplasm of vertebral column, excluding sacrum and coccyx — *intervertebral cartilage or disc* **AHA:** Q2, 1990, 7
213.3	Benign neoplasm of ribs, sternum, and clavicle — *xiphoid process, costal cartilage* **AHA:** Q2, 1990, 7
213.4	Benign neoplasm of scapula and long bones of upper limb — *long bones, upper extremity* **AHA:** Q2, 1990, 7
213.5	Benign neoplasm of short bones of upper limb — *short bones, upper extremity* **AHA:** Q2, 1990, 7
213.6	Benign neoplasm of pelvic bones, sacrum, and coccyx — *acetabulum, cuboid* **AHA:** Q2, 1990, 7
213.7	Benign neoplasm of long bones of lower limb — *long bones, lower extremity* **AHA:** Q2, 1990, 7
213.8	Benign neoplasm of short bones of lower limb — *short bones, lower extremity* **AHA:** Q2, 1990, 7
213.9	Benign neoplasm of bone and articular cartilage, site unspecified

Coding Clarification
Benign neoplasms for some cartilage sites are classified elsewhere: ear, eyelid, nose (212.0), larynx (212.1), synovia (215.0-215.9), and exostosis NOS (726.91).

214 Lipoma
AHA: Q2, 1990, 7

A lipoma is a soft nodule of fat that can occur subcutaneously or in any organ system. Treatment is not usually required, unless the lipoma is causing discomfort or compression. Other words used to describe lipomas are angiolipoma, fibrolipoma, hibernoma, myelolipoma, and myxolipoma. Lipomas are classified by site.

214.0	Lipoma of skin and subcutaneous tissue of face — *also called angiolipoma, fibrolipoma, hibernoma, or myelolipoma* **AHA:** Q2, 1990, 7
214.1	Lipoma of other skin and subcutaneous tissue — *excluding face* **AHA:** Q2, 1990, 7

214.2 Lipoma of intrathoracic organs — *intrathoracic, mediastinum, thymus*
AHA: Q2, 1990, 7

214.3 Lipoma of intra-abdominal organs — *peritoneum, retroperitoneum, stomach, kidney*
AHA: Q2, 1990, 7

214.4 Lipoma of spermatic cord — *also called angiolipoma, fibrolipoma, hibernoma, or myelolipoma*
AHA: Q2, 1990, 7

214.8 Lipoma of other specified sites — *not elsewhere classified, including muscle*
AHA: Q2, 1990, 7; Q3, 1994, 7

214.9 Lipoma of unspecified site

215 Other benign neoplasm of connective and other soft tissue
AHA: Q2, 1990, 7

Soft tissue includes blood vessel; bursa; fascia; ligament; muscle; peripheral, sympathetic, or parasympathetic nerve and ganglia; synovia; and tendon.

215.0 Other benign neoplasm of connective and other soft tissue of head, face, and neck — *blood vessel, bursa, fascia, ligament, muscle, or peripheral, sympathetic, and parasympathetic nerve*
AHA: Q2, 1990, 7

215.2 Other benign neoplasm of connective and other soft tissue of upper limb, including shoulder — *blood vessel, bursa, fascia, ligament, muscle, or peripheral, sympathetic, and parasympathetic nerve*
AHA: Q2, 1990, 7

215.3 Other benign neoplasm of connective and other soft tissue of lower limb, including hip — *blood vessel, bursa, fascia, ligament, muscle, or peripheral, sympathetic, and parasympathetic nerve*
AHA: Q2, 1990, 7

215.4 Other benign neoplasm of connective and other soft tissue of thorax — *blood vessel, bursa, fascia, ligament, muscle, or sympathetic and parasympathetic nerve*
AHA: Q2, 1990, 7

215.5 Other benign neoplasm of connective and other soft tissue of abdomen — (Includes benign stromal tumors of abdomen) — *blood vessel, bursa, fascia, ligament, muscle, or sympathetic and parasympathetic nerve*
AHA: Q2, 1990, 7

215.6 Other benign neoplasm of connective and other soft tissue of pelvis — *blood vessel, bursa, fascia, ligament, muscle, or sympathetic and parasympathetic nerve*
AHA: Q2, 1990, 7

215.7 Other benign neoplasm of connective and other soft tissue of trunk, unspecified — *blood vessel, bursa, fascia, ligament, muscle, or sympathetic and parasympathetic nerve*
AHA: Q2, 1990, 7

215.8 Other benign neoplasm of connective and other soft tissue of other specified sites — *not elsewhere classified*
AHA: Q2, 1990, 7

215.9 Other benign neoplasm of connective and other soft tissue of unspecified site

Coding Clarification
Classify benign neoplasm of cartilage to rubric 212 or 213, and of breast to 217. Classify connective tissue of internal organs to the appropriate organ, except for hemangioma or lipoma.

216–217 Benign Neoplasms of Integumentary System

216 Benign neoplasm of skin
AHA: Q2, 1990, 7; Q1, 2000, 21

Codes in this rubric report such benign neoplasms as blue nevus, dermatofibroma, hydrocystoma, pigmented nevus, syringoadenoma, and syringoma.

216.0 Benign neoplasm of skin of lip — *blue nevus, pigmented nevus, dermatofibroma, syringoadenoma, hydrocystoma*
AHA: Q2, 1990, 7; Q1, 2000, 21

216.1 Benign neoplasm of eyelid, including canthus — *blue nevus, pigmented nevus, dermatofibroma, syringoadenoma, hydrocystoma*
AHA: Q2, 1990, 7; Q1, 2000, 21

216.2 Benign neoplasm of ear and external auditory canal — *blue nevus, pigmented nevus, dermatofibroma, syringoadenoma, hydrocystoma*
AHA: Q2, 1990, 7; Q1, 2000, 21

216.3 Benign neoplasm of skin of other and unspecified parts of face — *blue nevus, pigmented nevus, dermatofibroma, syringoadenoma, hydrocystoma*
AHA: Q2, 1990, 7; Q1, 2000, 21

216.4 Benign neoplasm of scalp and skin of neck — *blue nevus, pigmented nevus, dermatofibroma, syringoadenoma, hydrocystoma*
AHA: Q2, 1990, 7; Q3, 1991, 12; Q1, 2000, 21

216.5 Benign neoplasm of skin of trunk, except scrotum — *blue nevus, pigmented nevus, dermatofibroma, syringoadenoma, hydrocystoma*
AHA: Q2, 1990, 7; Q1, 2000, 21

216.6 Benign neoplasm of skin of upper limb, including shoulder — *blue nevus, pigmented nevus, dermatofibroma, syringoadenoma, hydrocystoma*
AHA: Q2, 1990, 7; Q1, 2000, 21

216.7 Benign neoplasm of skin of lower limb, including hip — *blue nevus, pigmented nevus,*

Neoplasms

	dermatofibroma, syringoadenoma, hydrocystoma
	AHA: Q2, 1990, 7; Q1, 2000, 21
216.8	Benign neoplasm of other specified sites of skin — *not elsewhere classified*
	AHA: Q2, 1990, 7; Q1, 2000, 21
216.9	Benign neoplasm of skin, site unspecified

217 Benign neoplasm of breast OK
AHA: Q2, 1990, 7; Q1, 2000, 4

Benign neoplasms of the connective, glandular, or soft parts of the male or female breast are classified to this rubric.

Coding Clarification
Adenofibrosis of the breast is reported with 610.2 *Fibroadenosis of breast.* Benign cyst of the breast is reported with 610.0 *Solitary cyst of breast.* Fibrocystic disease is reported with 610.1 *Diffuse cystic mastopathy* and benign lesion of the skin of the breast with 216.5 *Benign neoplasm of skin of trunk, except scrotum.* Consult the ICD-9-CM index for more information.

218–222 Benign Neoplasms of Genital Organs

218 Uterine leiomyoma
AHA: Q2, 1990, 7

Most leiomyomas are detected during the course of routine pelvic exam; there are often no symptoms. If there are symptoms, they might include abdominal discomfort, urinary frequency, and constipation.

Uterine leiomyomas usually occur in multiples. They are classified according to where they establish within the wall of the uterus. They may be called by alternate names such as uterine fibromyoma or, simply, myoma.

218.0	Submucous leiomyoma of uterus — *Submucous fibroid, fibroma, myoma*
	AHA: Q2, 1990, 7
218.1	Intramural leiomyoma of uterus — *interstitial fibroid, fibroma, myoma*
	AHA: Q2, 1990, 7
218.2	Subserous leiomyoma of uterus — *fibroid, fibroma, myoma on serous membrane*
	AHA: Q2, 1990, 7
218.9	Leiomyoma of uterus, unspecified

219 Other benign neoplasm of uterus
This rubric classifies all benign neoplasms of the uterus, other than leiomyomas, according to site of neoplasm.

219.0	Benign neoplasm of cervix uteri — *cervical stump, internal and external os*
219.1	Benign neoplasm of corpus uteri — *endometrium, fundus, myometrium*
219.8	Benign neoplasm of other specified parts of uterus — *not elsewhere classified*
219.9	Benign neoplasm of uterus, part unspecified

220 Benign neoplasm of ovary OK
AHA: Q2, 1990, 7

The ovary is the female gonad and produces the ova. Some ovarian neoplasms are hormone-producing. Use an additional code to report any functional activity associated with the ovarian neoplasm.

221 Benign neoplasm of other female genital organs
AHA: Q2, 1990, 7

221.0	Benign neoplasm of fallopian tube and uterine ligaments — *oviduct, parametrium, round and broad ligaments*
	AHA: Q2, 1990, 7
221.1	Benign neoplasm of vagina
221.2	Benign neoplasm of vulva — *clitoris, Bartholin's gland, labia (majora) (minora), pudendum*
	AHA: Q2, 1990, 7
221.8	Benign neoplasm of other specified sites of female genital organs — *not elsewhere classified, including Mullerian duct (female)*
	AHA: Q2, 1990, 7
221.9	Benign neoplasm of female genital organ, site unspecified

Coding Clarification
Excluded from this rubric is a cyst of the Bartholin's gland or duct, which is classified to 616.2 *Cyst of Bartholin's gland.*

222 Benign neoplasm of male genital organs
AHA: Q2, 1990, 7

The testes are a pair of male gonads found in the scrotum and produce spermatozoa for fertilization. Leydig cells in the testes produce testosterone. Few testicular masses are malignant. Testicular tumors may cause functional activity problems.

222.0	Benign neoplasm of testis — (Use additional code to identify any functional activity) — *male gonad*
	AHA: Q2, 1990, 7
222.1	Benign neoplasm of penis — *corpus cavernosum, foreskin, prepuce, glans penis*
	AHA: Q2, 1990, 7
222.2	Benign neoplasm of prostate — *median or lateral lobes*
	AHA: Q2, 1990, 7
222.3	Benign neoplasm of epididymis — *parorchis*
	AHA: Q2, 1990, 7
222.4	Benign neoplasm of scrotum — *skin, not contents*
	AHA: Q2, 1990, 7

222.8	Benign neoplasm of other specified sites of male genital organs — *not elsewhere classified, including Mullerian duct (male), seminal vesicle, spermatic cord* AHA: Q2, 1990, 7
222.9	Benign neoplasm of male genital organ, site unspecified

Coding Clarification

If functional activity problems occur, use an additional code to report it.

Benign hyperplasia of the prostate is reported with codes in rubric 600. The codes in rubric 600 describe conditions including adenoma, fibroma, myoma, polyp, cyst, or hyperplasia of prostate.

223 Benign neoplasm of kidney and other urinary organs
AHA: Q2, 1990, 7

223.0	Benign neoplasm of kidney, except pelvis — *parenchyma* AHA: Q2, 1990, 7
223.1	Benign neoplasm of renal pelvis — *calyx, hilus* AHA: Q2, 1990, 7
223.2	Benign neoplasm of ureter — *except orifice of bladder* AHA: Q2, 1990, 7
223.3	Benign neoplasm of bladder — *dome, neck, orifice, sphincter, trigone, urachus, wall* AHA: Q2, 1990, 7
223.81	Benign neoplasm of urethra — *except orifice of bladder* AHA: Q2, 1990, 7
223.89	Benign neoplasm of other specified sites of urinary organs — *paraurethral gland* AHA: Q2, 1990, 7
223.9	Benign neoplasm of urinary organ, site unspecified

Coding Clarification

Excluded from this rubric are congenital cyst of the kidney (753.11), polycystic kidney (753.12-753.14), and multiple cysts of the kidney (753.19).

224–225 Benign Neoplasms of Nervous System

Benign neoplasms of the brain, eye, spine, meninges, cranial nerves, or sites unknown in the nervous system are classified to rubrics 224 and 225. Peripheral, sympathetic, or parasympathetic nerves are classified to codes in rubric 215.

224 Benign neoplasm of eye
AHA: Q2, 1990, 7

The eye is basically a fluid-filled ball and benign neoplasms can pose two major dangers to sight: neoplasms can disrupt the visual field and cause compression that disrupts the flow of blood or aqueous, leading to permanent tissue damage. In addition, a benign neoplasm can result in significant irritation or pain.

Intraocular pressure in the anterior segment of the eye is maintained through the flow of aqueous humor, or tears. The lacrimal system provides these tears and is also an agent in their disposal. Tears are produced in the lacrimal glands, located bilaterally behind the eyebrow, and the lacrimal ducts carry the tears to the eye, or away from the eye to the nose. Pressure in the posterior segment of the eye is maintained by gel-like vitreous humor.

A thin, vascular, mucous membrane covers the inner eyelids and the white outer shell of the eye (sclera). This membrane is called the conjunctiva. The cornea is the bulging "window" through which we see and the retina is the light-sensitive "viewing screen" at the back of the eye. The choroid is a vascular layer of the inside of the eyeball.

224.0	Benign neoplasm of eyeball, except conjunctiva, cornea, retina, and choroid — *ciliary body, iris, sclera, uveal tract* AHA: Q2, 1990, 7
224.1	Benign neoplasm of orbit — *soft tissue between eyeball and bony orbit* AHA: Q2, 1990, 7
224.2	Benign neoplasm of lacrimal gland — *excluding other parts of lacrimal apparatus* AHA: Q2, 1990, 7
224.3	Benign neoplasm of conjunctiva — *of sclera or inner aspect of eyelid* AHA: Q2, 1990, 7
224.4	Benign neoplasm of cornea — *limbus* AHA: Q2, 1990, 7
224.5	Benign neoplasm of retina — *pars optica, pars ciliaris, pars iridica* AHA: Q2, 1990, 7
224.6	Benign neoplasm of choroid — *choroidea, chorioidea* AHA: Q2, 1990, 7
224.7	Benign neoplasm of lacrimal duct — *canaliculi, nasal duct, punctum, sac* AHA: Q2, 1990, 7
224.8	Benign neoplasm of other specified parts of eye
224.9	Benign neoplasm of eye, part unspecified

225 Benign neoplasm of brain and other parts of nervous system
AHA: Q2, 1990, 7

All brain tumors are "malignant" in that they may lead to death as they compromise the circulation of fluids in the brain through compression or obstruction. However, neoplasms classified to this rubric are not of a metastasizing nature; they are circumscribed lesions. The incidence of benign and malignant neoplasms of the brain is about the same at 50 percent.

Symptoms of a neoplasm of the brain include headache, seizures, personality changes, impaired mental or physical functions, or in children, an enlarged head. Use an additional code to report any manifestations associated with the neoplasm.

225.0	Benign neoplasm of brain — *cerebrum, cerebellum, hypothalamus, basal ganglia, stem, medulla oblongata* **AHA:** Q2, 1990, 7
225.1	Benign neoplasm of cranial nerves — *acoustic neuroma; cranial, trigeminal, trochlear, vagus nerve* **AHA:** Q2, 1990, 7; Q4, 2004, 113
225.2	Benign neoplasm of cerebral meninges — *meninges, meningioma* **AHA:** Q2, 1990, 7
225.3	Benign neoplasm of spinal cord — *cauda equina* **AHA:** Q2, 1990, 7
225.4	Benign neoplasm of spinal meninges — *meningioma* **AHA:** Q2, 1990, 7
225.8	Benign neoplasm of other specified sites of nervous system
225.9	Benign neoplasm of nervous system, part unspecified

Coding Clarification
Acoustic neuroma is a common benign tumor of the acoustic nerve, which can cause hearing interruption, dizziness, and tinnitus. It is classified to 225.1 *Benign neoplasm of cranial nerves.*

226–228 Benign Neoplasms of Other and Unspecified Sites

226 Benign neoplasm of thyroid glands
AHA: Q2, 1990, 7

The thyroid gland is located just below the cricoid cartilage near the larynx. Its purpose is to secrete thyroxine and triiodothyronine, which increase the rate of cell metabolism.

Benign thyroid tumors are adenomas, cysts, or involutional nodules. A majority is follicular.

In many cases, the patient with a benign thyroid growth undergoes surgery because of suspicion of cancer, to improve cosmetic appearance, or to correct a functional activity. Use an additional code to report any functional activity associated with the neoplasm.

227 Benign neoplasm of other endocrine glands and related structures
AHA: Q2, 1990, 7

The parathyroid glands come in pairs — the superior and inferior pair — and they are embedded in the posterior thyroid. The adrenal glands are situated above each kidney, and the pituitary gland is located in the sella turcica of the sphenoid bone. The pineal gland, located at the base of the corpus callosum, secretes melatonin; and the carotid body, located in the fork of the carotid artery, monitors blood oxygen. The aortic body at the aortic arch and right subclavian artery regulates reflex respiration.

Benign neoplasms of the endocrine glands can create functional activities in those glands. For example, adrenal tumors can cause virilizing or feminizing symptoms. Pituitary cancers can cause gigantism, Cushing's disease, amenorrhea or galactorrhea, or acromegaly. Report these functional activities in addition to the neoplasm.

227.0	Benign neoplasm of adrenal gland — (Use additional code to identify any functional activity) — *suprarenal gland* **AHA:** Q2, 1990, 7
227.1	Benign neoplasm of parathyroid gland — (Use additional code to identify any functional activity) — *inferior or superior* **AHA:** Q2, 1990, 7
227.3	Benign neoplasm of pituitary gland and craniopharyngeal duct (pouch) — (Use additional code to identify any functional activity) — *craniobuccal pouch, Rathke's pouch, hypophysis, sella turcica* **AHA:** Q2, 1990, 7
227.4	Benign neoplasm of pineal gland — (Use additional code to identify any functional activity) — *pineal body* **AHA:** Q2, 1990, 7
227.5	Benign neoplasm of carotid body — (Use additional code to identify any functional activity) — *glomus caroticum* **AHA:** Q2, 1990, 7
227.6	Benign neoplasm of aortic body and other paraganglia — (Use additional code to identify any functional activity) — *coccygeal body, para-aortic body, glomus jugulare* **AHA:** Nov-Dec, 1984, 17; Q2, 1990, 7
227.8	Benign neoplasm of other endocrine glands and related structures — (Use additional code to identify any functional activity) — *not elsewhere specified* **AHA:** Q2, 1990, 7
227.9	Benign neoplasm of endocrine gland, site unspecified — (Use additional code to identify any functional activity)

Coding Clarification
An additional code from Chapter 3 may be reported to identify functional activity associated with any neoplasm, for example, basophil adenoma of pituitary with Cushing's syndrome, 227.3 for neoplasm and 255.0 for Cushing's syndrome.

228 Hemangioma and lymphangioma, any site
AHA: Q2, 1990, 7; Q1, 2000, 21

Hemangiomas are neoplasms arising from vascular tissue or malformations of vascular structures. Many are congenital. They can occur topically (on the skin) or within any organ system. Common topical hemangiomas include strawberry nevus, nevus vasculosus, capillary hemangioma, port wine stain, and nevus flammeus. Classify hemangiomas according to site.

A lymphangioma is a benign, congenital malformation in the lymphatic system.

228.00		Hemangioma of unspecified site
228.01		Hemangioma of skin and subcutaneous tissue — *any site*
		AHA: Jan-Feb, 1985, 19; Q2, 1990, 7; Q1, 2000, 21
228.02		Hemangioma of intracranial structures — *brain, brain meninges*
		AHA: Jan-Feb, 1985, 19; Q2, 1990, 7; Q1, 2000, 21
228.03		Hemangioma of retina
228.04		Hemangioma of intra-abdominal structures — *peritoneum, retroperitoneum*
		AHA: Jan-Feb, 1985, 19; Q2, 1990, 7; Q1, 2000, 21
228.09		Hemangioma of other sites — *choroid, heart, iris, spinal meninges, spinal cord; systemic angiomatosis*
		AHA: Jan-Feb, 1985, 19; Q2, 1990, 7; Q3, 1991, 20; Q1, 2000, 21
228.1		Lymphangioma, any site — *congenital lymphangioma, lymphatic nevus*
		AHA: Q2, 1990, 7; Q1, 2000, 21

Coding Clarification
Lymphangiomas may be superficial or deep and all lymphangiomas classify to 228.1 *Lymphangioma, any site.*

229 Benign neoplasm of other and unspecified sites
AHA: Q2, 1990, 7

Lymphangiomas are excluded from rubric 229.

229.0	Benign neoplasm of lymph nodes — *any site*
	AHA: Q2, 1990, 7
229.8	Benign neoplasm of other specified sites — *thoracic or intrathoracic, not otherwise specified*
	AHA: Q2, 1990, 7
229.9	Benign neoplasm of unspecified site

Coding Clarification
For intrathoracic or thoracic site not otherwise specified, report 229.8 *Benign neoplasm of other specified sites.*

230–234 Carcinoma In Situ

Carcinoma in situ is defined as a carcinoma that has not invaded neighboring tissue. Once microscopic extension of malignant cells is found in tissue adjacent to carcinoma in situ, it is no longer "in situ," and malignant neoplasm codes should be used.

230 Carcinoma in situ of digestive organs
AHA: Q2, 1990, 7

Carcinoma in situ in this rubric is classified by site within the digestive system.

230.0	Carcinoma in situ of lip, oral cavity, and pharynx — *alveolus, gingiva, palate, pharynx, salivary glands, tongue*
	AHA: Q2, 1990, 7
230.1	Carcinoma in situ of esophagus — *distal, proximal, middle*
	AHA: Q2, 1990, 7
230.2	Carcinoma in situ of stomach — *body, cardia, fundus, pylorus, cardiac orifice*
	AHA: Q2, 1990, 7
230.3	Carcinoma in situ of colon — *appendix, cecum, ileocecal valve, large intestine*
	AHA: Q2, 1990, 7
230.4	Carcinoma in situ of rectum — *rectosigmoid junction*
	AHA: Q2, 1990, 7
230.5	Carcinoma in situ of anal canal — *anal sphincter*
	AHA: Q2, 1990, 7
230.6	Carcinoma in situ of anus, unspecified
230.7	Carcinoma in situ of other and unspecified parts of intestine — *duodenum, jejunum, ileum, small intestine*
	AHA: Q2, 1990, 7
230.8	Carcinoma in situ of liver and biliary system — *ampulla of Vater, gallbladder, common bile duct, hepatic duct, cystic duct, and sphincter of Oddi*
	AHA: Q2, 1990, 7
230.9	Carcinoma in situ of other and unspecified digestive organs — *pancreas, spleen, not elsewhere specified*
	AHA: Q2, 1990, 7

231 Carcinoma in situ of respiratory system
AHA: Q2, 1990, 7

Carcinoma in situ in this rubric is classified by site within the respiratory system.

Neoplasms

231.0	Carcinoma in situ of larynx — *voice box including cartilage, epiglottis* **AHA:** Q2, 1990, 7			
231.1	Carcinoma in situ of trachea — *trachea* **AHA:** Q2, 1990, 7			
231.2	Carcinoma in situ of bronchus and lung — *carina, hilus* **AHA:** Q2, 1990, 7			
231.8	Carcinoma in situ of other specified parts of respiratory system — *accessory sinus, middle ear, nasal cavities, pleura* **AHA:** Q2, 1990, 7			
231.9	Carcinoma in situ of respiratory system, part unspecified			

232 Carcinoma in situ of skin
AHA: Q2, 1990, 7

Carcinoma in situ in this rubric is classified by site within the skin.

232.0	Carcinoma in situ of skin of lip — *excluding vermilion border, mucosal tissue* **AHA:** Q2, 1990, 7
232.1	Carcinoma in situ of eyelid, including canthus
232.2	Carcinoma in situ of skin of ear and external auditory canal — *antitragus, triangular fossa, tragus, lobule, helix, and concha* **AHA:** Q2, 1990, 7
232.3	Carcinoma in situ of skin of other and unspecified parts of face — *chin and forehead, but not neck or scalp* **AHA:** Q2, 1990, 7
232.4	Carcinoma in situ of scalp and skin of neck — *scalp and neck, but not chin and forehead* **AHA:** Q2, 1990, 7
232.5	Carcinoma in situ of skin of trunk, except scrotum — *perianal skin, skin of back, breast, buttock, chest, groin, perineum, umbilicus* **AHA:** Q2, 1990, 7
232.6	Carcinoma in situ of skin of upper limb, including shoulder — *arm, hand, shoulder* **AHA:** Q2, 1990, 7
232.7	Carcinoma in situ of skin of lower limb, including hip — *leg, foot* **AHA:** Q2, 1990, 7
232.8	Carcinoma in situ of other specified sites of skin — *not elsewhere classified* **AHA:** Q2, 1990, 7
232.9	Carcinoma in situ of skin, site unspecified

233 Carcinoma in situ of breast and genitourinary system
AHA: Q2, 1990, 7

Carcinoma in situ in this rubric is classified by site within the genitourinary system.

In situ carcinoma of the vulva and vagina are linked to human papilloma virus and occur frequently in premenopausal women.

Dysplasias of the cervix are cellular deviations from the normal structure and function of the cells of the cervix of the uterus. Dysplasias are considered a precursor to carcinoma. Cervical dysplasia is classified to one of three levels of cervical intraepithelial neoplasm.

233.0	Carcinoma in situ of breast — *male or female* **AHA:** Q2, 1990, 7
233.1	Carcinoma in situ of cervix uteri — *cervical stump, internal and external os, severe dysplasia* **AHA:** Q2, 1990, 7; Q1, 1991, 11; Q3, 1992, 7; Q3, 1992, 8
233.2	Carcinoma in situ of other and unspecified parts of uterus — *endometrium, fundus, and myometrium* **AHA:** Q2, 1990, 7
233.3	Carcinoma in situ of other and unspecified female genital organs — *other and unspecified female genital organs* **AHA:** Q2, 1990, 7
233.4	Carcinoma in situ of prostate — *median or lateral lobes* **AHA:** Q2, 1990, 7
233.5	Carcinoma in situ of penis — *corpus cavernosum, foreskin, prepuce, glans penis* **AHA:** Q2, 1990, 7
233.6	Carcinoma in situ of other and unspecified male genital organs
233.7	Carcinoma in situ of bladder — *trigone, ureteral orifice, urethral orifice, urachus, sphincter* **AHA:** Q2, 1990, 7
233.9	Carcinoma in situ of other and unspecified urinary organs — *not elsewhere classified or unknown* **AHA:** Q2, 1990, 7

Coding Clarification
CIN I is reported with 622.11 *Mild dysplasia of cervix*. CIN II is reported with 622.12 *Moderate dysplasia of cervix*. Report low grade squamous intraepithelial lesion (LGSIL) with 795.03. Report high grade squamous intraepithelial lesion (HGSIL) with 795.04, while CIN III, cervical intraepithelial glandular neoplasia, is reported with 233.1 *Carcinoma in situ of cervix uteri* with the exception of stromal tumors of uncertain behavior of the digestive system, which are reported with code 238.1 *Neoplasm of uncertain behavior of connective and other soft tissue*. Vulvar intraepithelial neoplasm VIN III is classified to 233.3 *Carcinoma in situ of other and unspecified female genital organs*.

Cytologic evidence of malignancy without histologic confirmation is reported with code 795.06 *Papanicolaou smear of cervix with cytologic evidence of malignancy.*

234 Carcinoma in situ of other and unspecified sites
AHA: Q2, 1990, 7

Carcinoma in this rubric is classified by site as the eye, other, or unspecified.

234.0	Carcinoma in situ of eye — *retina, conjunctiva, globe, choroid, iris, ciliary body, cornea* **AHA:** Q2, 1990, 7
234.8	Carcinoma in situ of other specified sites — *endocrine glands* **AHA:** Q2, 1990, 7
234.9	Carcinoma in situ, site unspecified

Coding Clarification

Classify all parts of the eye to 234.0 *Carcinoma in situ of eye,* except eyelid skin (232.1) and eyelid cartilage, optic nerve, or orbital bone (234.8). Carcinomas in situ of the adrenal, parathyroid, pituitary, pineal glands, and the carotid and pineal bodies are classified to 234.8 *Carcinoma in situ of other specified sites.*

235–238 Neoplasms of Uncertain Behavior

Uncertain behavior is a histomorphological determination, as distinguished from unspecified behavior, which indicates a lack of documentation to support a more specific code assignment. Neoplasms of uncertain behavior are classified by site or organ system. Neurofibromatosis, polycythemia vera, and mast cell tumors are classified in this series of rubrics.

235 Neoplasm of uncertain behavior of digestive and respiratory systems
AHA: Q2, 1990, 7

Neoplasms in this rubric are classified by site within the digestive or respiratory systems with the exception of benign stromal tumors of the digestive system, which are reported with code 215.5 *Other benign neoplasm of connective and other soft tissue, abdomen.*

235.0	Neoplasm of uncertain behavior of major salivary glands — *parotid, sublingual, submandibular glands* **AHA:** Q2, 1990, 7
235.1	Neoplasm of uncertain behavior of lip, oral cavity, and pharynx — *gingiva, alveolus, pharynx, tongue, minor salivary glands* **AHA:** Q2, 1990, 7
235.2	Neoplasm of uncertain behavior of stomach, intestines, and rectum — *ilium, jejunum, cardia, colon, sigmoid, duodenum* **AHA:** Q2, 1990, 7
235.3	Neoplasm of uncertain behavior of liver and biliary passages — *ampulla of Vater, gallbladder, bile ducts, liver* **AHA:** Q2, 1990, 7
235.4	Neoplasm of uncertain behavior of retroperitoneum and peritoneum — *abdominal soft tissue other than organs* **AHA:** Q2, 1990, 7
235.5	Neoplasm of uncertain behavior of other and unspecified digestive organs — *esophagus, pancreas, spleen, anus* **AHA:** Q2, 1990, 7
235.6	Neoplasm of uncertain behavior of larynx — *voice box* **AHA:** Q2, 1990, 7
235.7	Neoplasm of uncertain behavior of trachea, bronchus, and lung — *all lobes, trachea, bronchi* **AHA:** Q2, 1990, 7
235.8	Neoplasm of uncertain behavior of pleura, thymus, and mediastinum — *thoracic soft tissue other than heart, lungs* **AHA:** Q2, 1990, 7
235.9	Neoplasm of uncertain behavior of other and unspecified respiratory organs — *accessory sinus, middle ear, nasal cavities* **AHA:** Q2, 1990, 7

236 Neoplasm of uncertain behavior of genitourinary organs
AHA: Q2, 1990, 7

Neoplasms in this rubric are classified by site within the genitourinary system. If a neoplasm of the testis or ovary causes functional changes in hormone levels, report the functional activity in addition to the neoplasm of uncertain behavior.

236.0	Neoplasm of uncertain behavior of uterus — *endometrium, fundus, myometrium* **AHA:** Q2, 1990, 7
236.1	Neoplasm of uncertain behavior of placenta — *chorioadenoma destruens, malignant hydatidiform mole* **AHA:** Q2, 1990, 7
236.2	Neoplasm of uncertain behavior of ovary — (Use additional code to identify any functional activity) — *female gonad* **AHA:** Q2, 1990, 7
236.3	Neoplasm of uncertain behavior of other and unspecified female genital organs — *not elsewhere classified or unknown* **AHA:** Q2, 1990, 7
236.4	Neoplasm of uncertain behavior of testis — (Use additional code to identify any functional activity) — *male gonad* **AHA:** Q2, 1990, 7
236.5	Neoplasm of uncertain behavior of prostate — *median or lateral lobes* **AHA:** Q2, 1990, 7

Neoplasms

236.6	Neoplasm of uncertain behavior of other and unspecified male genital organs — *not elsewhere classified or unknown* **AHA:** Q2, 1990, 7
236.7	Neoplasm of uncertain behavior of bladder — *trigone, ureteral orifice, urethral orifice, urachus, sphincter* **AHA:** Q2, 1990, 7
236.90	Neoplasm of uncertain behavior of urinary organ, unspecified
236.91	Neoplasm of uncertain behavior of kidney and ureter — *calyx, hilus, pelvis of kidney* **AHA:** Q2, 1990, 7
236.99	Neoplasm of uncertain behavior of other and unspecified urinary organs — *urethra* **AHA:** Q2, 1990, 7

237 Neoplasm of uncertain behavior of endocrine glands and nervous system
AHA: Q2, 1990, 7

If a neoplasm causes functional changes in hormone levels or nervous system functions, report the functional activity or manifestation in addition to the neoplasm of uncertain behavior.

237.0	Neoplasm of uncertain behavior of pituitary gland and craniopharyngeal duct — (Use additional code to identify any functional activity) — *pituitary body, fossa, lobe* **AHA:** Q2, 1990, 7
237.1	Neoplasm of uncertain behavior of pineal gland — *pineal body* **AHA:** Q2, 1990, 7
237.2	Neoplasm of uncertain behavior of adrenal gland — (Use additional code to identify any functional activity) — *suprarenal gland* **AHA:** Q2, 1990, 7
237.3	Neoplasm of uncertain behavior of paraganglia — *aortic body, coccygeal body, carotid body, glomus jugulare* **AHA:** Nov-Dec, 1984, 17; Q2, 1990, 7
237.4	Neoplasm of uncertain behavior of other and unspecified endocrine glands — *parathyroid gland, thyroid gland* **AHA:** Q2, 1990, 7
237.5	Neoplasm of uncertain behavior of brain and spinal cord — *frontal lobe, thalamus, cerebrum, cerebellum, temporal lobe and stem* **AHA:** Q2, 1990, 7
237.6	Neoplasm of uncertain behavior of meninges — *cerebral or spinal* **AHA:** Q2, 1990, 7
237.70	Neurofibromatosis, unspecified — *type unknown* **AHA:** Q2, 1990, 7
237.71	Neurofibromatosis, Type 1 (von Recklinghausen's disease) — *"elephant man" syndrome* **AHA:** Q2, 1990, 7
237.72	Neurofibromatosis, Type 2 (acoustic neurofibromatosis) — *bilateral 8th nerve masses* **AHA:** Q2, 1990, 7
237.9	Neoplasm of uncertain behavior of other and unspecified parts of nervous system — *cranial, parasympathetic, sympathetic, peripheral nerves or unknown* **AHA:** Q2, 1990, 7

238 Neoplasm of uncertain behavior of other and unspecified sites and tissues
AHA: Q2, 1990, 7

Although myeloproliferative disorders and myelodysplastic syndrome are now recognized as hematologic malignancies, for data consistency reasons these are maintained with the neoplasms of uncertain behavior of other lymphatic and hematopoietic tissues in ICD-9-CM.

Essential thrombocythemia, also known as essential thrombocytosis, idiopathic thrombocythemia, and primary thrombocytosis is a myeloproliferative disorder causing an abnormal elevation in the number of platelets made in the blood and bone marrow. Symptoms include headaches, altered sensation or appearance (burning, tingling, redness, or warmth) of the hands or feet, and difficulties with vision or hearing. The platelets become sticky and may clump together, resulting in increased risk of stroke, heart attack, or bleeding.

Myelodysplastic syndromes are diseases in which the bone marrow functions abnormally. The immature stem cells formed in the bone marrow do not mature into normal red and white blood cells and platelets. These immature cells, called blasts, die in the bone marrow or shortly after entering the blood stream, leaving less room for the development of healthy cells. This may result in infection, anemia, or bleeding. Symptoms include shortness of breath, weakness, pallor, easy bruising, petechiae, fever, or frequent infections. Diagnosis of the various forms of myelodysplastic syndrome is based on specific changes in the blood cells and bone marrow.

Cutaneous lesions in myelodysplastic syndromes may indicate transition to acute myeloid leukemia and are associated with poorer prognoses. The most common lesions include petechiae and purpura, cutaneous infections, vasculitis, and neutrophilic dermatoses; a dermal infiltrate of malignant hematopoietic cells, which is the specific cutaneous manifestation of myelodysplastic syndromes, is rare.

Myelofibrosis with myeloid metaplasia, also known as chronic idiopathic myelofibrosis, agnogenic myeloid metaplasia, primary myelofibrosis, and myelosclerosis with myeloid metaplasia, is a disorder in which fibrous tissue replaces the bone marrow. This progressive, chronic disease is manifested by splenomegaly and worsening anemia. Since the bone marrow has been replaced by fibrous tissue, blood is made in organs such as the liver and spleen. Symptoms include pain or a full sensation on the left side beneath the ribs, early satiety, fatigue, shortness of breath, easy bruising, petechiae, fever, night sweats, or loss of weight. Tests used to diagnose this condition may include CBC, bone marrow aspiration and biopsy, cytogenetic analysis, and peripheral blood smear.

238.0	Neoplasm of uncertain behavior of bone and articular cartilage — *long and short ones and associated cartilage* AHA: Q2, 1990, 7; Q4, 2004, 128
238.1	Neoplasm of uncertain behavior of connective and other soft tissue — (Includes stromal tumors of the digestive system) — *peripheral, sympathetic, and parasympathetic nerves and ganglia* AHA: Q2, 1990, 7
238.2	Neoplasm of uncertain behavior of skin — *any site* AHA: Q2, 1990, 7
238.3	Neoplasm of uncertain behavior of breast — *male or female* AHA: Q2, 1990, 7
238.4	Neoplasm of uncertain behavior of polycythemia vera — *Vaquez-Osler disease* AHA: Q2, 1990, 7
238.5	Neoplasm of uncertain behavior of histiocytic and mast cells — *mastocytoma NOS* AHA: Q2, 1990, 7
238.6	Neoplasm of uncertain behavior of plasma cells — *plasmacytoma NOS, solitary myeloma* AHA: Q2, 1990, 7
238.71	Essential thrombocythemia — *essential hemorrhagic thrombocythemia; essential thrombocytosis; idiopathic thrombocythemia; idiopathic hemorrhagic thrombocythemia; primary thrombocytosis*
238.72	Low grade myelodysplastic syndrome lesions — *refractory anemia; refractory anemia with ringed sideroblasts; refractory cytopenia with multilineage dysplasia; refractory cytopenia with multilineage dysplasia and ringed sideroblasts*
238.73	High grade myelodysplastic syndrome lesions — *refractory anemia with excess blasts-1; RAEB-1; refractory anemia with excess blasts-2; RAEB-2*
238.74	Myelodysplastic syndrome with 5q deletion — *5 q minus syndrome*
238.75	Myelodysplastic syndrome, unspecified
238.76	Myelofibrosis with myeloid metaplasia — *primary myelofibrosis; agnogenic myeloid metaplasia; idiopathic myelofibrosis; chronic idiopathic myelofibrosis; myelosclerosis with myeloid metaplasia*
238.79	Other lymphatic and hematopoietic tissues — *acute panmyelosis; panmyelosis; myeloproliferative disease; chronic myeloproliferative disease; megakaryocytic myelosclerosis; lymphoproliferative disease; chronic lymphoproliferative disease* AHA: Q2, 1989, 8; Q2, 1990, 7; Q1, 1997, 5; Q3, 2001, 13
238.8	Neoplasm of uncertain behavior of other specified sites — *eye, heart, nasolacrimal duct, lymph gland, Virchow's gland* AHA: Q2, 1990, 7
238.9	Neoplasm of uncertain behavior, site unspecified

Coding Clarification

Report secondary myelofibrosis and myelofibrosis not otherwise specified with code 289.83. Report constitutional 5q deletion with code 758.39. Myelophthisic anemia and myelophthisis are reported with code 284.2.

ICD-9-CM classifies myeloproliferative disorders and myelodysplastic syndromes to "other specified" neoplasms of uncertain behavior of lymphatic and hematopoietic tissues, even though they are recognized as hematological malignancies. Close attention to all instructional notes and index instructions in this section is critical.

Many factors can manifest as bone marrow function abnormalities. Instructional notes are provided as a guide to correct code selection.

239 Neoplasms of Unspecified Nature

This rubric classifies neoplasms for unknown or undocumented morphology. Classify the neoplasm according to site in this rubric.

239	Neoplasms of unspecified nature AHA: Q2, 1990, 7
239.0	Neoplasm of unspecified nature of digestive system — *mouth, esophagus, stomach, intestine, pancreas, gallbladder* AHA: Q2, 1990, 7
239.1	Neoplasm of unspecified nature of respiratory system — *lungs, pleura, bronchi* AHA: Q2, 1990, 7
239.2	Neoplasms of unspecified nature of bone, soft tissue, and skin — *bone, blood vessels, muscles* AHA: Q2, 1990, 7
239.3	Neoplasm of unspecified nature of breast — *male or female* AHA: Q2, 1990, 7

Neoplasms

239.4	Neoplasm of unspecified nature of bladder	**239.8**	Neoplasm of unspecified nature of other specified sites — *mediastinum, lymph glands, eye, heart, thymus*
239.5	Neoplasm of unspecified nature of other genitourinary organs — *male or female*		**AHA:** Q2, 1990, 7
	AHA: Q2, 1990, 7	**239.9**	Neoplasm of unspecified nature, site unspecified
239.6	Neoplasm of unspecified nature of brain — *including cerebellum, cerebrum, stem*		
	AHA: Q2, 1990, 7		
239.7	Neoplasm of unspecified nature of endocrine glands and other parts of nervous system — *thyroid, pituitary, pineal gland*		
	AHA: Q2, 1990, 7		

Coding Clarification

Do not use codes from this rubric to classify a "mass." Instead, consult "mass" in the index. Use of any code in this rubric may cause delays in claims processing due to the nonspecific nature of these codes.

240–279

Endocrine, Nutritional and Metabolic Diseases, and Immunity Disorders

The endocrine system is a group of specialized organs and body tissues that produces, stores, and secretes chemical substances known as hormones. Hormones provide information and instructions to regulate development, control the function of various tissues, support reproduction, and regulate metabolism.

Hormones from the endocrine system are secreted into the blood, where proteins bind to them to keep them intact as the hormones are disbursed through the body. The proteins also regulate the release of hormones.

Usually, the changes a hormone produces also serve to regulate that hormone's secretion. For example, parathyroid hormone causes the body to increase the level of calcium in the blood. As calcium levels rise, the secretion of parathyroid hormone decreases. Other changes in the body also influence hormone secretions. For example, during illness, the adrenal glands increase the secretions of certain hormones to help the body overcome the stress of illness. The normal regulation of hormone secretion is suspended, allowing for a tolerance of higher levels of hormone in the blood until the illness is resolved.

Nutritional deficiencies in this chapter cover deficiencies in vitamins, minerals, and protein-calorie malnutrition. Deficiencies of anemia are classified to Chapter Four Disease of the Blood and Blood-Forming Organs.

Metabolic diseases in this chapter cover a wide range of diseases, including problems with amino-acid transport, carbohydrate transport, lipoid metabolism, plasma protein metabolism, gout, mineral metabolism, and fluid, electrolyte, and acid-base imbalances. Also covered are cystic fibrosis, porphyrin, purine and pyrimidine metabolism, and obesity.

240–246 Disorders of Thyroid Gland

The thyroid gland is attached to the trachea by loose connective tissue and derives its blood supply from the superior and interior thyroid arteries. The function of the thyroid is to create, store, and secrete thyroxine and triiodothyronine. The thyroid gland secretes hormones in response to stimulation by thyroid stimulating hormone (TSH) from the pituitary gland. The thyroid hormones regulate growth and metabolism and play a role in brain development during childhood.

240 Simple and unspecified goiter

In simple goiter, the thyroid gland is enlarged, but the hormone secretions of the thyroid are still within normal limits. Simple goiter can have several causes. Iodine is essential to thyroid hormone secretion. The thyroid of a person whose diet has insufficient iodine will actually become enlarged so that it can produce more thyroid hormone. Iodine deficiency is the most common cause of simple goiter, but as there is no deficiency in the United States, this cause is rarely seen here. Simple goiter can also occur during puberty, pregnancy, or during menses as a result of hormonal imbalances. If a goiter has enough mass, it may cause compression that may lead to airway restriction, swallowing difficulty, or problems with venous flow.

240.0	Goiter, specified as simple — *not affecting hormone production*
240.9	Goiter, unspecified — *extent unknown*

241 Nontoxic nodular goiter

In nontoxic nodular goiter, the thyroid gland exhibits palpable nodules, though the nodules do not affect thyroid hormone secretion. Goiters in this rubric are classified as having a singular nodule or multiple nodules.

241.0	Nontoxic uninodular goiter — *one node, without clinical hypothyroidism*
241.1	Nontoxic multinodular goiter — *multiple nodes, without clinical hypothyroidism*
241.9	Unspecified nontoxic nodular goiter — *struma nodosa (simplex)*

Coding Clarification
Benign neoplasms of the thyroid are reported with codes in the 226 rubric.

242 Thyrotoxicosis with or without goiter

Thyrotoxicosis is an over-secretion of thyroid hormone, and is also called hyperthyroidism. Symptoms include tachycardia, nervousness, tremor, weight loss, heat intolerance, goiter, and fatigue. Thyrotoxicosis is eight to 10 times more common in women than in men.

The causes of thyrotoxicosis are varied. Increased hormone secretion can be related to a thyroid nodule or to ectopic thyroid tissue. Thyrotoxicosis can also be the result of a more systemic problem, as in the case of Grave's disease, an autoimmune disorder.

A thyrotoxic storm is a sudden, life-threatening crisis in which symptoms of hyperthyroidism are exacerbated and new symptoms develop. It is most likely to occur at the time of infection, surgical procedure, or trauma in a patient with undertreated hyperthyroidism. The patient may develop a fever, emotional instability or psychosis, heart complications, and an enlarged liver.

Diseases in this rubric are classified first by the cause of hyperthyroidism, and second, by the status of thyrotoxic storm.

The following fifth-digit subclassification is for use with category 242:
0   without mention of thyrotoxic crisis or storm
1   with mention of thyrotoxic crisis or storm

242.0 ⌐sth	Toxic diffuse goiter — *Grave's disease, Basedow's disease, Marsh's disease, Parry's syndrome, Parson's disease; exophthalmic goiter*
242.1 ⌐sth	Toxic uninodular goiter — *single nodule, toxic, or with hyperthyroidism*
242.2 ⌐sth	Toxic multinodular goiter — *multiple nodules, toxic, or with hyperthyroidism*
242.3 ⌐sth	Toxic nodular goiter, unspecified type — *nodular, unknown type, with hyperthyroidism or toxic; Plummer's disease*
242.4 ⌐sth	Thyrotoxicosis from ectopic thyroid nodule — *aberrant thyroid tissue as cause*
242.8 ⌐sth	Thyrotoxicosis of other specified origin — (Use additional E code to identify cause, if drug-induced) — *overproduction of TSH; thyroid toxicosis factitia*
242.9 ⌐sth	Thyrotoxicosis without mention of goiter or other cause — *not elsewhere specified; Leopold-Levi's syndrome*

Coding Clarification
If a neoplasm is causing the functional activity, report the appropriate neoplasm code in addition to the hyperthyroidism code. Sequencing varies according to the encounter.

Neonatal thyrotoxicosis is reported with 775.3.

243 Congenital hypothyroidism

The most common cause of congenital hypothyroid is absence of a thyroid gland at birth. This requires lifelong hormone therapy since thyroxine regulates metabolism and growth. Untreated, congenital hypothyroidism causes serious problems in the central nervous system, developmental delay, and problems with somatic growth. Screening programs exist in the United States to test newborns for this disorder. By providing replacement thyroid hormones, almost all of the complications of congenital hypothyroidism are avoidable.

Coding Clarification
Congenital goiter with an enzyme defect in synthesis of thyroid hormone is reported with 246.1.

244 Acquired hypothyroidism

Hypothyroidism is a deficiency of thyroid hormone. Primary hypothyroidism usually develops in older adults, usually after age 40, and causes lethargy, fatigue, and mental sluggishness.

244.0	Postsurgical hypothyroidism — *athyroidism or part of thyroid removed*
244.1	Other postablative hypothyroidism — *following irradiation*
244.2	Iodine hypothyroidism — (Use additional E code to identify drug) — *resulting from high iodide intake*
244.3	Other iatrogenic hypothyroidism — (Use additional E code to identify drug) — *resulting from: PAS, phenylbutazone, resorcinol*
244.8	Other specified acquired hypothyroidism — *not elsewhere classified, Gull's disease* AHA: July-Aug, 1985, 9
244.9	Unspecified hypothyroidism — *Brissaud-Meige syndrome; Strumipriva cachexia; Hoffmann's syndrome* AHA: Q4, 1996, 29; Q3, 1999, 19

Coding Clarification
For hypothyroidism complicating pregnancy, see rubric 648.

Coding Scenario
A patient in for laboratory testing was recently diagnosed with iron deficiency anemia due to hypothyroidism.

> Code assignment: 280.9 *Iron deficiency anemia, unspecified* and 244.9 *Unspecified hypothyroidism*

245 Thyroiditis
Diseases in this rubric are classified as acute, subacute, chronic, and iatrogenic. The most common form of thyroiditis in the United States is Hashimoto's thyroiditis (245.2), a chronic condition that usually leads to chronic hypothyroidism and lifetime treatment with synthetic hormone. Hashimoto's thyroiditis is an autoimmune disorder that often presents with other forms of autoimmune disease, including Type 1 diabetes mellitus, hypoparathyroidism, or Addison's disease. Schmidt's syndrome is Addison's disease with hypothyroidism secondary to Hashimoto's thyroiditis, and is reported with 258.1 *Other combinations of endocrine dysfunction*. In diabetes with hypothyroidism, report both conditions rather than this combination code since, as a significant systemic disease, diabetes should always be coded separately.

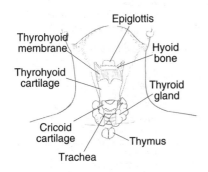

245.0	Acute thyroiditis — (Use additional code to identify organism) — *abscess, pyogenic, suppurative, nonsuppurative*
245.1	Subacute thyroiditis — *de Quervain's, giant cell, granulomatous*
245.2	Chronic lymphocytic thyroiditis — *Hashimoto's disease*
245.3	Chronic fibrous thyroiditis — *Riedel's thyroiditis; struma fibrosa*
245.4	Iatrogenic thyroiditis — (Use additional code to identify cause) — *due to medical treatment other than radiation or excision*
245.8	Other and unspecified chronic thyroiditis — *not elsewhere classified*
245.9	Unspecified thyroiditis

246 Other disorders of thyroid
This rubric captures other disorders of the thyroid, with the exception of neoplasms, which are found in Chapter 2.

246.0	Disorders of thyrocalcitonin secretion — *hypersecretion of calcitonin or thyrocalcitonin*
246.1	Dyshormonogenic goiter — *enzyme defect; congenital dyshormonogenic*
246.2	Cyst of thyroid
246.3	Hemorrhage and infarction of thyroid
246.8	Other specified disorders of thyroid — *atrophy, TBG defect, degeneration* **AHA:** Q2, 2006, 5
246.9	Unspecified disorder of thyroid

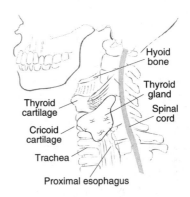

250–259 Diseases of Other Endocrine Glands
Included in this section are diseases associated with insulin-producing cells of the pancreas, the islets of Langerhans, parathyroid, pituitary, hypothalamus, adrenals, ovaries, and testes.

250 Diabetes mellitus
AHA: Nov-Dec, 1985, 11; Q2, 1990, 22; Q3, 1991, 3; Q2, 1992, 5; Q4, 1993, 19; Q3, 1996, 5; Q2, 1997, 14; Q4, 1997, 32; Q2, 1998, 15; Q2, 2001, 16; Q2, 2002, 13; Q2, 2004, 17; Q4, 2004, 56

The pancreas is positioned in the upper abdomen, just under the stomach. The major part of the pancreas, called the exocrine pancreas, secretes digestive enzymes into the gastrointestinal tract.

Distributed through the pancreas are clusters of endocrine cells that secrete insulin, glucagon, and somatostatin. These hormones all participate in regulating energy and metabolism in the body.

Diabetes is a systemic disease and, as such, should be coded even in the absence of documented, active intervention during the patient encounter.

Diabetes mellitus has two forms. Diabetes mellitus Type I is caused by inadequate secretion of insulin by the pancreas. Diabetes mellitus Type II is caused by the body's inability to respond to insulin, called insulin resistance. Both have similar symptoms, including excessive thirst, hunger, and urination as well as weight loss. Laboratory tests that detect glucose in the urine and elevated levels of glucose in the blood usually confirm the diagnosis.

Treatment of diabetes mellitus Type I requires regular injections of insulin. Type II can be treated with diet, exercise, oral medication, or insulin injection.

Only about 10 percent of diabetics are Type I, also known as juvenile-onset. This type is seen at a young age, sometimes in early adulthood, and requires regular insulin due to the autoimmune destruction of pancreatic beta cells, which cease to produce insulin. Type II accounts for 90- to 95 percent of all cases and is usually diagnosed in adulthood as the pancreas gradually loses the ability to produce insulin, or the body becomes more resistant to that which is being produced. An increasing number of children are being diagnosed with Type II diabetes.

The primary factor that distinguishes Type I from Type II is the absence of naturally occurring insulin within the body. Type I diabetics require insulin injections to survive. Type II diabetics may improve their health with insulin injections, and may even come to require insulin, but the administration of insulin has no bearing on code selection for diabetes. nor does the age of onset. A patient with Type II diabetes is always coded as having Type II, even when the medical record states the patient requires insulin.

In this rubric, diabetes is classified according to type of complication, as selected by the fourth digit, and by Type I or Type II status and the presence of diabetic control, selected by the fifth digit.

Diabetes can cause a variety of complications, including kidney problems, pain due to nerve damage, blindness, and coronary heart disease.

Recent studies have shown that controlling blood sugar levels reduces the risk of developing diabetes complications.

The following fifth-digit subclassification is for use with category 250:

0   type II or unspecified type, not stated as uncontrolled
1   type I [juvenile type], not stated as uncontrolled
2   type II or unspecified type, uncontrolled
3   type I [juvenile type], uncontrolled

250.0 ⌐sth   Diabetes mellitus without mention of complication — *no complications arising from disease*
AHA: Nov-Dec, 1985, 11; Q2, 1990, 22; Q3, 1991, 3; Q3, 1991, 3,12; Q2, 1992, 5; Q4, 1993, 19; Q3, 1996, 5; Q2, 1997, 14; Q4, 1997, 32; Q2, 1998, 15; Q2, 2001, 16; Q2, 2002, 13; Q4, 2004, 55; Q1, 2005, 15; Q1, 2006, 14

250.1 ⌐sth   Diabetes with ketoacidosis — *ketosis, acidosis, without coma*
AHA: Nov-Dec, 1985, 11; Q2, 1990, 22; Q3, 1991, 3; Q3, 1991, 6; Q2, 1992, 5; Q4, 1993, 19; Q3, 1996, 5; Q2, 1997, 14; Q4, 1997, 32; Q2, 1998, 15; Q2, 2001, 16; Q2, 2002, 13; Q2, 2006, 19

250.2 ⌐sth   Diabetes with hyperosmolarity — *increased osmolarity of the body fluids as a complication of diabetes*
AHA: Nov-Dec, 1985, 11; Q2, 1990, 22; Q3, 1991, 3; Q3, 1991, 7; Q2, 1992, 5; Q4, 1993, 19; Q3, 1996, 5; Q2, 1997, 14; Q4, 1997, 32; Q2, 1998, 15; Q2, 2001, 16; Q2, 2002, 13

250.3 ⌐sth   Diabetes with other coma — *arising from ketoacidosis or hypoglycemia*
AHA: Nov-Dec, 1985, 11; Q2, 1990, 22; Q3, 1991, 3; Q3, 1991, 7, 12; Q2, 1992, 5; Q4, 1993, 19; Q3, 1996, 5; Q2, 1997, 14; Q4, 1997, 32; Q2, 1998, 15; Q2, 2001, 16; Q2, 2002, 13

250.4 ⌐sth   Diabetes with renal manifestations — (Use additional code to identify manifestation: 585.1-585.9) —*chronic kidney disease*
AHA: Sept-Oct, 1984, 3; Nov-Dec, 1985, 11; Sept-Oct, 1987, 9; Q2, 1990, 22; Q3, 1991, 3; Q3, 1991, 8,12; Q2, 1992, 5; Q4, 1993, 19; Q3, 1996, 5; Q2, 1997, 14; Q4, 1997, 32; Q2, 1998, 15; Q2, 2001, 16; Q2, 2002, 13

250.5 ⌐sth   Diabetes with ophthalmic manifestations — (Use additional code to identify manifestation: 362.01-362.07, 362.83, 365.44, 366.41, 369.0-369.9) — *ocular disease*
AHA: Sept-Oct, 1985, 11; Nov-Dec, 1985, 11; Q2, 1990, 22; Q3, 1991, 3; Q3, 1991, 8; Q2, 1992, 5; Q4, 1993, 19; Q3, 1996, 5; Q2, 1997, 14; Q4, 1997, 32; Q2, 1998, 15; Q2, 2001, 16; Q2, 2002, 13; Q4, 2005, 67

250.6 ⌐sth   Diabetes with neurological manifestations — (Use additional code to identify manifestation:

337.1, 354.0-355.9, 357.2, 358.1, 713.5) — nerve damage or disease
AHA: Nov-Dec, 1984, 9; Nov-Dec, 1985, 11; Q2, 1990, 22; Q3, 1991, 3; Q3, 1991, 9; Q2, 1992, 5; Q2, 1992, 15; Q2, 1993, 6; Q4, 1993, 19; Q3, 1996, 5; Q2, 1997, 14; Q4, 1997, 32; Q2, 1998, 15; Q2, 2001, 16; Q2, 2002, 13; Q2, 2004, 7

250.7 ✓sth Diabetes with peripheral circulatory disorders — (Use additional code to identify manifestation: 443.81, 785.4) — blood vessel damage or disease
AHA: Nov-Dec, 1985, 11; Q2, 1990, 22; Q3, 1990, 15; Q3, 1991, 3; Q3, 1991, 10,12; Q2, 1992, 5; Q4, 1993, 19; Q2, 1994, 17; Q3, 1994, 5; Q1, 1996, 10; Q3, 1996, 5; Q2, 1997, 14; Q4, 1997, 32; Q2, 1998, 15; Q2, 2001, 16; Q2, 2002, 13; Q1, 2004, 14

250.8 ✓sth Diabetes with other specified manifestations — (Use additional code to identify manifestation: 707.10-707.9, 731.8. Use additional E code to identify cause, if drug-induced) — including hypoglycemic shock
AHA: Nov-Dec, 1985, 11; Q2, 1990, 22; Q3, 1991, 3; Q3, 1991, 10; Q2, 1992, 5; Q4, 1993, 19; Q4, 1993, 20; Q3, 1996, 5; Q2, 1997, 14; Q2, 1997, 16; Q4, 1997, 32; Q4, 1997, 43; Q2, 1998, 15; Q4, 2000, 44; Q2, 2001, 16; Q2, 2002, 13; Q1, 2004, 14

250.9 ✓sth Diabetes with unspecified complication

Documentation Issues

If the type of diabetes is not documented in the medical record, the default is to code type II. The documentation may indicate conditions "with" diabetes, but this does not necessarily mean the condition is due to diabetes. Although diabetic patients are vulnerable to chronic conditions affecting other body systems (e.g., renal, ophthalmologic, vascular), this does not indicate a direct correlation. Clarification must be obtained from the physician as to the cause and effect relationship of the condition. Documentation should identify a direct relation by statements such as "due to," "caused by," or "secondary to" before diabetic complication codes are assigned.

For example, the documentation states neurogenic bowel in a diabetic patient. Before a code is assigned, consult with the physician on whether the diabetes is the cause of the neurogenic bowel. If the neurogenic bowel is due to the diabetes, use codes 250.6x, 337.1, and 564.81.

When coding inpatient claims, if the documentation indicates that the patient only has diabetes and does not indicate a complication, the admission would be considered questionable. Clarification should be made with the physician for a more complete diagnosis to substantiate the necessity for the admission.

Documentation must specify that the patient is Type I to allow use of the fifth digit 1 or 3. The patient may be receiving insulin but may not be a true insulin-dependent diabetic. Verify status with the physician if clarification is needed.

Fifth digits specifying uncontrolled diabetes should not be assigned based on blood glucose levels. These codes should only be used if the physician documents uncontrolled diabetes in the medical record.

If the documentation in the record indicates that the patient has metabolic acidosis and diabetes, clarify with the physician if there is a cause and effect relationship. Note that code 276.2 has an exclusion note for diabetic acidosis and references code 250.1x.

When the patient has had a pancreatic transplant, the diabetes code would apply solely if the physician documents diabetes and/or manifestations of the diabetes.

When the physician documents "pseudodiabetes" of newborn, use code 775.1 *Neonatal diabetes mellitus*. This condition is also known as "transient neonatal diabetes," which occurs in the newborn of a diabetic mother.

If the physician documents that the patient has diabetes with a hyperosmolar coma, it does not necessarily mean the patient is in an unconscious state. This condition involves an altered state of consciousness without notable ketosis, with hyperosmolarity and dehydration. Typically this condition occurs in noninsulin dependent diabetics. Use code 250.2x *Diabetes with hyperosmolarity* to identify this condition.

Diabetes mellitus should not be coded as out of control unless the physician specifically indicates it as such in the final diagnostic statement and/or in the body of the medical record. If the record identifies the uncontrolled state and the final diagnostic statement does not, clarification must be obtained from the physician.

Coding Clarification

For diabetic pregnancy, two codes are required: the pregnancy code from the rubric 648 and also a code from the 250 rubric.

Secondary diabetes should not be reported with this rubric. Instead, the condition causing the diabetes should be reported. For example, in post-pancreatectomy diabetes, assign 251.3 *Postsurgical insulinemia.*

Diabetes is one of a number of the ICD-9-CM classification categories that is used as a primary code to classify both the disease and its major manifestations. Additional codes should be used to provide more specificity in defining the manifestations. When a cause and effect relationship between renal failure and diabetes has been established, the diabetes code 250.4x is listed first and the appropriate renal failure code is listed as an additional code. Accordingly, if the diagnosis does not indicate a cause and effect relationship between the diabetes and renal failure, the code for the specified type of renal failure may be listed first.

Atherosclerosis: Diabetic atherosclerosis is coded as 250.7x *Diabetes with peripheral circulatory disorders* and 440.2x *Atherosclerosis of native arteries of extremities.* If the diagnosis is diabetes with ischemic heart disease or cerebrovascular disease, code them as separate entities.

Coexisting or Chronic Conditions: Coexisting or chronic conditions that are treated on an ongoing basis should be coded and reported as many times as the patient receives treatment, management, and additional care for the conditions. Conditions such as diabetes that are considered systemic diseases should be coded, even in the absence of documented active intervention.

End Stage Renal Disease: Diabetes is one of the many diseases that may cause end stage renal disease in chronic kidney disease due to the progressive nature of the disease. Due to the cause and effect relationship between these conditions, always sequence code 250.4x first and the renal manifestation second. If the documentation does not indicate the cause and effect relationship of the chronic kidney disease and the diabetes, the renal condition may be listed as the initial code and the diabetes may be listed as secondary.

Foot Ulcers: Diabetic patients may develop foot ulcers from conditions such as diabetic neuropathy (250.6x), diabetic peripheral vascular disease (250.7x), or superimposed infection. If it is due to the superimposed infection, the foot ulcer would not be coded as a diabetic complication. Use codes 250.0x *Diabetes mellitus* and 707.1x *Ulcer of lower limbs, except decubitus* and an additional code for the causative organism of the infection, if known. If the cause of the diabetic ulcer is not known, use code 250.8x *Diabetes with other specified manifestations* and 707.1x *Ulcer of lower limbs.*

Gangrene: Gangrene noted in the diabetic patient is always coded as a diabetic complication. The exception to this guideline is if there is a history of trauma such as an open wound. If the patient has an open wound that has developed an infection that has progressed to gangrene, use the complicated open wound code with code 785.4 for the gangrene and 250.0x for the diabetes.

Gastroparesis Due to Diabetes: Two codes are required to identify this condition: 250.6x. *Diabetes mellitus with neurological manifestations,* and 536.3 *Gastroparesis.*

Impotence: When coding diabetic impotence, the diabetic condition that caused the impotence would be listed first (e.g., peripheral vascular disease, peripheral neuropathy) followed by the code for the impotence, 607.84. If the cause of the diabetic impotence is not known, use codes 250.8x *Diabetes with other specified manifestations* and 607.84 *Impotence of organic origin.*

Multiple Coding: Multiple coding is required for diabetic complications. Instructions for these conditions appear in the alphabetic index as well as the tabular list of the ICD-9-CM code book. In the alphabetic index, in many cases, both codes are listed with the subentry term. The second code is in brackets. Both codes should be assigned in the same sequence in which they appear in the alphabetic index. In the tabular listing, review instructional terms, such as "Use additional code to identify manifestation" and "Code first the underlying disease." Apply multiple coding instructions throughout the classification where appropriate, whether or not multiple coding directions appear in the alphabetic index. Take steps to avoid indiscriminate multiple coding or irrelevant information, such as symptoms or signs characteristic of the diabetic condition (e.g., acute metabolic complications associated with the diabetes itself).

Ophthalmic Manifestations: Diabetic cataracts, true diabetic cataracts, or those known as "snowflake cataracts" are rare and are found in Type I diabetics. Use codes 250.51 *Diabetes with ophthalmic manifestations* and 366.41 *Diabetic cataract.* Senile cataracts, although commonly seen in diabetics, are not classified as such because they are not caused by the diabetes. Use codes 250.0x

Diabetes mellitus without mention of complication and 366.10 *Senile cataract, unspecified.*

Codes for diabetic retinopathy (250.5x and 362.0x) include:

- Background or simple diabetic retinopathy with microaneurysms, hemorrhages, and/or cotton wool spots (362.01)
- Mild, moderate, severe, and unspecified nonproliferative retinopathy (362.03-362.06)
- Malignant or proliferative diabetic retinopathy (e.g., retinal neovascularization with or without retinal hemorrhages) (362.02)
- Macular edema in branch retinal vein occlusion
- Macular edema resulting in leakage within the retina

Macular edema (362.07) must be reported with a code for diabetic retinopathy (362.01-362.06)

For nondiabetic proliferative retinopathy, assign code 362.29 *Other nondiabetic proliferative retinopathy.*

Osteomyelitis: Diabetic osteomyelitis requires three codes to accurately identify the condition: 250.8x *Diabetes with other specified manifestations,* 731.8 *Other bone involvement in diseases classified elsewhere,* and a code from category 730 *Osteomyelitis, periostitis and other infections involving bone.*

Pregnancy: When coding a condition that is either a complication of pregnancy or that is complicating the pregnancy, always list the code for the obstetric complication first. Additional codes are assigned as needed to provide specificity. Essentially all pregnant diabetics have complications, either with the diabetes or the pregnancy, therefore two codes (648.0x and 250.0x) are always assigned.

Gestational diabetes is not a true diabetes but is often confused as such. Gestational diabetes is a condition that refers to abnormal glucose tolerance during pregnancy. In this condition, the patient may require treatment for control of blood glucose levels, but returns to normal glucose tolerance after childbirth. Use code 648.8x *Abnormal glucose tolerance for gestational diabetes.*

Secondary Diabetes: Secondary diabetes codes should not be selected from category 250. When it has been substantiated that the diabetes is secondary to another condition, code the underlying condition. For example, for postpancreatectomy diabetes, assign code 251.3 *Postsurgical hypoinsulinemia.*

Type I vs. Type II: The primary factor that distinguishes between the Type I and Type II is the absence or presence of insulin that the body can or cannot produce on its own. The Type I diabetic requires insulin to survive; however, there may be short symptom free periods also known as "honeymoon periods" during which insulin is not required. Type II diabetics can produce sufficient amounts but may receive insulin to assist the body in using the insulin that is present in the body. The Type II diabetic is not dependent on insulin to survive. The administration of insulin or age of the patient does not confirm the type of diabetes. Only the type (I or II) of diabetes influences the fifth-digit assignment for diabetic codes.

Use of Insulin: Some patients with type II diabetes mellitus are unable to control their glucose level through diet and oral medication alone and require insulin. For type II patients who routinely use insulin, code V58.67 Long-term (current) use of insulin, should also be assigned to indicate that the patient uses insulin. Code V58.67 should not be assigned if insulin is given temporarily to bring a type II patient's blood glucose level under control during an encounter. If the documentation in a medical record does not indicate the type of diabetes but does indicate that the patient uses insulin, the appropriate fifth digit for type II must be used because the use of insulin does not mean that a patient is a type I diabetic. Assigning V58.67 is unnecessary for type I diabetics because all type I diabetics must use insulin to replace what their bodies do not produce.

Diabetic Complication: Diabetic atherosclerosis of the extremities is coded as 250.7x *Diabetes with peripheral circulatory disorders* and 440.2x *Atherosclerosis of native arteries of extremities.* If the diagnosis is diabetes with ischemic heart disease or cerebrovascular disease, they are coded as separate entities.

When the documentation identifies a diabetic patient with cardiomyopathy, these conditions are coded as separate entities. The diabetic complication code 250.7x does not include cardiomyopathy.

Insulin Pump Malfunction: An underdose of insulin due to mechanical failure of a pump that results in manifestation of symptoms of the disease are considered a manifestation of the diabetes rather than an adverse effect of insulin. An underdose of insulin due to an insulin pump failure should be assigned 996.57 Mechanical complication due to insulin pump, as the principal or first-listed code, followed by the appropriate diabetes mellitus code based on documentation. Overdose of insulin due to insulin pump failure is considered a poisoning. The principal or first-listed code for an encounter due to an insulin pump malfunction resulting in an overdose of insulin should also be 996.57 Mechanical complication due to insulin pump, followed by code 962.3 Poisoning by insulins and antidiabetic agents, and the appropriate diabetes mellitus code based on documentation.

Coding Scenario

A patient is admitted with chronic renal failure for dialysis. The patient history indicates the patient is a Type II diabetic controlled by insulin.

> Code assignment: V56.0 *Encounter for extracorporeal dialysis*, 585 *Chronic kidney disease, unspecified*, and 250.00 *Diabetes mellitus without mention of complication, Type II or unspecified type, not stated as uncontrolled* and V58.67 *Long-term (current) use of insulin*

A 59-year-old male is seen in the physician's office for episodes of dizziness. He is found to have an elevated blood sugar level. Additional testing is done that shows a minimally elevated glucose tolerance test. The physician documentation specifically indicates that diabetes mellitus was ruled out.

> Code assignment: 790.22 *Elevated glucose tolerance test (oral)* and 780.4 *Dizziness and giddiness*

A 48-year-old female is seen in the clinic for her neurogenic bladder disorder secondary to diabetes. Documentation specifically indicates that she is an insulin-requiring Type II diabetic.

> Code assignment: 250.60 *Diabetes with neurological manifestations, Type II or unspecified type, not stated as uncontrolled*, 337.1 *Peripheral autonomic neuropathy in disorders classified elsewhere*, and 596.54 *Syndrome with neurogenic bladder* and V58.67 *Long-term (current) use of insulin*

A 55-year-old male is admitted with hypertension due to hypervolemia as a direct result of his chronic kidney disease. Patient history indicates that the patient is a Type I diabetic with renal failure.

> Code assignment: 250.41 *Diabetes with renal manifestations, Type I, not stated as uncontrolled*, 405.99 *Other secondary hypertension*, 276.6 *Fluid overload*, and 585.9 *Chronic kidney disease, unspecified*

A 28-year-old male is seen at a clinic for his chronic pseudo-obstruction of the intestine, which is related to his Type II diabetes.

> Code assignment: 250.80 *Diabetes with other specified manifestations, Type II or unspecified, not stated as uncontrolled* and 564.89 *Other functional disorders of intestine*

A patient is admitted with diabetic neuropathy with secondary diabetes. Patient history identifies a previous history of a partial pancreatectomy that has caused the diabetic condition.

> Code assignment: 251.3 *Postsurgical hypoinsulinemia* and 357.4 *Polyneuropathy in other diseases classified elsewhere*

A Type I diabetic female is seen in the emergency department and is diagnosed with hypoglycemia. The physician identifies that the patient has been compliant with her prescribed insulin dosage.

> Code assignment: 250.81 *Diabetes with other specified manifestations, Type I, not stated as uncontrolled*, E932.3 *Adverse effect of insulin and antidiabetic agents* and V58.67 *Long-term use of insulin*

A Type II diabetic comes into the emergency department after an accidental overdose of insulin. The patient is admitted with hypoglycemic shock.

> Code assignment: 962.3 *Poisonings by hormones and synthetic substitutes, insulin and antidiabetic agents*, 250.80 *Diabetes with other specified manifestations, Type II or unspecified, not stated as uncontrolled*, and V58.67 *Long-term (current) use of insulin*, and E858.0 *Accidental poisoning by hormones and synthetic substitutes*

A patient is seen in the office for an eye examination that reveals a small snowflake cataract. This patient is a known Type I diabetic since 10 years of age. Verification with the physician confirms this is a diabetic cataract.

> Code assignment: 250.51 *Diabetes with ophthalmic manifestations, Type I, not stated as uncontrolled* and 366.41 *Diabetic cataract*

A Type II diabetic is admitted for a severe chronic left heel ulcer. The patient's history clarifies that the patient's foot ulcer is secondary to diabetic peripheral neuropathy. The final diagnostic statement confirms the diagnosis as diabetic peripheral autonomic neuropathy with chronic left heel ulcer.

> Code assignment: 250.60 *Diabetes with neurological manifestations, Type II or unspecified, not stated as uncontrolled*, 337.1 *Peripheral autonomic neuropathy in disorders classified elsewhere*, and 707.14 *Ulcer of heel and midfoot*

Endocrine, Nutritional and Metabolic Diseases, and Immunity Disorders

A patient is admitted for gangrene of the left leg secondary to diabetic arteriosclerosis. Record documentation identifies that the patient is a Type I diabetic requiring insulin.

Code assignment: 250.71 *Diabetes with peripheral circulatory disorders, Type I, not stated as uncontrolled* and 440.24 *Atherosclerosis of the extremities with gangrene*

The physician's final diagnosis states hypertensive renal disease with chronic renal failure due to diabetes, Type II.

Code assignment: 250.40 *Diabetes with renal manifestations, Type II or unspecified, not stated as uncontrolled* and 403.90 *Hypertensive chronic kidney disease, unspecified, with chronic kidney disease stage I through stage IV or unspecified*, and 585.9 *Chronic kidney disease, unspecified*

A patient is admitted for hemodialysis. The patient is a true insulin-dependent diabetic, Type I, with progressive nephropathy. The physician also documents chronic renal failure in the medical history.

Code assignment: V56.0 *Encounter for extracorporeal dialysis*, 250.41 *Diabetes with renal manifestations, Type I, not stated as uncontrolled*, 583.81 *Nephritis and nephropathy, not specified as acute or chronic, in diseases classified elsewhere*, and 585.9 *Chronic kidney disease, unspecified*.

An elderly patient is transferred from an extended care facility for treatment of a sacral decubitus ulcer. The physician also identifies the patient is a Type II diabetic with related progressive peripheral vascular disease.

Code assignment: 707.03 *Decubitus ulcer, lower back*, 250.70 *Diabetes with peripheral circulatory disorders, Type II or unspecified, not stated as uncontrolled*, and 443.81 *Peripheral angiopathy in diseases classified elsewhere*.

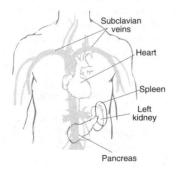

251 Other disorders of pancreatic internal secretion

Diabetes insipidus is caused by a deficiency of vasopressin, one of the antidiuretic hormones (ADH) secreted by the pituitary gland. Symptoms include increased thirst and urination. Treatment is with drugs, such as synthetic vasopressin, that help the body maintain water and electrolyte balance.

251.0 Hypoglycemic coma — (Use additional E code to identify drug, if drug induced) — *Non-diabetic insulin coma*
AHA: March-April, 1985, 8

251.1 Other specified hypoglycemia — (Use additional E code to identify drug, if drug induced) — *including hyperplasia of pancreatic islet beta cells NOS; Harris' syndrome*
AHA: Q1, 2003, 10

251.2 Hypoglycemia, unspecified — *not otherwise specified, including McQuarrie's syndrome*
AHA: March-April, 1985, 8

251.3 Postsurgical hypoinsulinemia — *following complete or partial pancreatectomy*
AHA: Q3, 1991, 6

251.4 Abnormality of secretion of glucagon — *hyperplasia of islet alpha cells with glucagon excess*

251.5 Abnormality of secretion of gastrin — *hyperplasia of alpha cells with gastrin excess; Zollinger-Ellison syndrome*

251.8 Other specified disorders of pancreatic internal secretion — *sclerotic islands of Langerhans*
AHA: Q3, 1991, 6; Q2, 1998, 15

251.9 Unspecified disorder of pancreatic internal secretion — *not elsewhere classified*

252 Disorders of parathyroid gland

The parathyroid glands are four small glands located at the four corners of the thyroid gland. The hormone secreted, parathyroid hormone, regulates the level of calcium in the blood.

Hyperparathyroidism is an excessive secretion of the parathyroid hormone (PTH) from one or more of the parathyroid glands. The parathyroid glands are four pea-sized glands located in the neck on the thyroid. In 85% of cases, a benign tumor, called an adenoma, is found on a gland that causes it be overactive. Most other cases of primary hyperparathyroidism result from enlargement or hyperplasia of two or more glands that also causes overactive hormone production.

Primary hyperparathyroidism is caused by a disorder of the parathyroid glands themselves that results in their secreting too much parathyroid hormone (PTH).

Secondary hyperparathyroidism results from releasing increased levels in response to deconditioning of the body to PTH due to another disease process, such as renal failure. PTH helps regulate the levels of calcium and phosphorus in the body, induces the release of calcium from bone, the amount of calcium taken from food, intestinal absorption of calcium, and the excretion of calcium in the urine. Hypercalcemia, or increased levels of calcium in the blood, is a sign of hyperparathyroidism, when accompanied by a concurrent increase in the level of PTH hormone.

252.00	Hyperparathyroidism, unspecified
252.01	Primary hyperparathyroidism
252.02	Secondary hyperparathyroidism, non-renal **AHA:** Q4, 2004, 57-59
252.08	Other hyperparathyroidism
252.1	Hypoparathyroidism — *low secretion of parathyroid hormones causing a severe convulsive disorder known as tetany; parathyroiditis; parathyroid tetany*
252.8	Other specified disorders of parathyroid gland — *cyst, hemorrhage, or infarct*
252.9	Unspecified disorder of parathyroid gland

Coding Clarification
Code 252.02 reports hyperparathyroidism from non-renal causes. Report 588.81 for secondary hyperparathyroidism of renal origin.

Coding Scenario
A 65-year-old woman has come to her physician with fatigue, constipation and increased urination and thirst. The doctor orders urine and blood tests, which come back high for calcium and orders a blood test to check for PTH levels, which also returns high. Blood sugar levels are normal. Once the diagnosis is established that she has primary hyperparathyroidism, the doctor has her follow up with a bone density exam and an abdominal radiograph to assess for kidney stones. The condition of an overactive, enlarged gland or benign tumor is discussed with surgical option of removal in the future.

Code assignment: 252.01 *Primary hyperparathyroidism*

253 Disorders of the pituitary gland and its hypothalamic control

The hypothalamus controls the pituitary gland from deep within the brain. Acting as liaison between the brain and the pituitary gland, the hypothalamus is the primary link between the endocrine and nervous systems.

The pituitary, located in the base of the brain, secretes several hormones that regulate the function of the other endocrine glands. The pituitary gland is divided into two parts, the anterior and posterior lobes, each having separate functions. The anterior lobe regulates the activity of the thyroid, adrenal, and reproductive glands. It also regulates the body's growth and stimulates milk production in women who are breast-feeding. Hormones secreted by the anterior lobe include adrenocorticotropic hormone (ACTH), thyrotropic hormone (TSH), luteinizing hormone (LH), follicle-stimulating hormone (FSH), growth hormone (GH), and prolactin. The anterior lobe also secretes endorphins, chemicals that act on the nervous system to reduce sensitivity to pain.

The posterior lobe of the pituitary gland contains the nerve endings (axons) from the hypothalamus, which stimulate or suppress hormone production. This lobe secretes antidiuretic hormones (ADH), which control water balance in the body, and oxytocin, which controls muscle contractions in the uterus.

253.0	Acromegaly and gigantism — *acromegaly describes unusual growth beginning in middle age; gigantism usually begins in childhood. Both are caused by overproduction of pituitary growth hormone; Erdheim's, Launois', Marie's, syndromes*
253.1	Other and unspecified anterior pituitary hyperfunction — *Forbes-Albright and Argonz-Del Castillo syndromes* **AHA:** July-Aug, 1985, 9
253.2	Panhypopituitarism — *organic pituitary dysfunction leading to impaired sexual function, fatigue, bradycardia, depression, and impaired growth in children; including cachexia, necrosis, insufficiency; Sheehan's, hypopituitarism, or postpartum-panhypopituitary syndromes*
253.3	Pituitary dwarfism — *with persistence of infantile physical characteristics due to under-secretion of growth hormone and gonadotropin deficiency; HGH deficiency, Lorain-Levi dwarfism, Burnier's syndrome, Nebecourt's syndrome*
253.4	Other anterior pituitary disorders — *isolated or partial deficiency of an anterior pituitary hormone, other than growth hormone; prolactin deficiency; Kallmann's syndrome* **AHA:** July-Aug, 1985, 9
253.5	Diabetes insipidus — *insufficient diuretic hormone release; symptoms include frequent urination, thirst, and weight loss; vasopressin deficiency*
253.6	Other disorders of neurohypophysis — *syndrome of inappropriate secretion of antidiuretic hormone [ADH] and Schwartz-Bartter syndrome*
253.7	Iatrogenic pituitary disorders — *(Use additional E code to identify cause) — drug therapy, radiation therapy, or surgery, causing mild to severe symptoms*

Endocrine, Nutritional and Metabolic Diseases, and Immunity Disorders

253.8	Other disorders of the pituitary and other syndromes of diencephalohypophysial origin — *abscess of pituitary; adiposogenital dystrophy; Rathke's pouch, pituitary or intrasellar cyst, empty sella; or hypophyseal, Launois-Cléret syndrome, Fröhlich's syndrome, Rénon-Delille syndrome*
253.9	Unspecified disorder of the pituitary gland and its hypothalamic control

254 Diseases of thymus gland

The thymus gland is comprised of lymphatic and epithelial tissue (Hassall's corpuscles) and is located in the anterior, superior mediastinum. The thymus processes white blood cells (WBC) known as lymphocytes, which kill foreign cells and stimulate other immune cells to produce antibodies. The role of the thymus is not entirely understood, though it seems to be most important during infancy and until puberty, when the lymphatic tissue is chiefly replaced by fat. In adults, the thymus can be removed without significant impact on health.

Thymic disease in this rubric is classified as abscess, hyperplasia, or other specified disease.

254.0	Persistent hyperplasia of thymus — *continued, abnormal growth of the twin lymphoid lobes that produce T lymphocytes in the anterior superior mediastinum*
254.1	Abscess of thymus — *pocket of liquid puris caused by infection in the thymus*
254.8	Other specified diseases of thymus gland — *atrophy, cyst, hemorrhage, necrotic tissue, inflammation, thymicolymphaticus shunt, Kopp's asthma, hyperthymism*
254.9	Unspecified disease of thymus gland

Coding Clarification

Excluded from this rubric are aplasia, dysplasia, or hypoplasia of the thymus with immunodeficiency (279.2), myasthenia gravis (358.0), thymoma (212.6), and DiGeorge anomaly (279.11). Congenital absence of the thymus is classified to 759.2 Anomalies of other endocrine glands.

255 Disorders of adrenal glands

Located on the kidneys, the adrenal glands have two distinct parts. The outer, called the adrenal cortex, produces a variety of hormones called corticosteroids. Chief among the corticosteroids is cortisol, which regulates salt and water balance in the body, prepares the body for stress, regulates metabolism, interacts with the immune system, and influences sexual function. The inner part, the adrenal medulla, produces catecholamines, such as epinephrine, also called adrenaline, which increases the blood pressure and heart rate during times of stress.

Addison's disease is caused by decreased function of the adrenal cortex. Weakness, fatigue, abdominal pains, nausea, dehydration, fever, and hyperpigmentation (tanning without sun exposure) are among the possible symptoms. Treatment involves providing the body with replacement corticosteroid hormones as well as dietary salt.

Primary Cushing's syndrome is caused by excessive secretion of glucocorticoids, the subgroup of corticosteroid hormones that includes hydrocortisone, by the adrenal glands. Symptoms may develop over many years prior to diagnosis and may include obesity, physical weakness, easily bruised skin, acne, hypertension, and psychological changes. Treatment may include surgery, radiation therapy, chemotherapy, or blockage of hormone production with drugs.

Acromegaly and gigantism both are caused by a pituitary tumor that stimulates production of excessive growth hormone, causing abnormal growth in particular parts of the body. Acromegaly is rare and usually develops over many years in adult subjects. Gigantism occurs when the excess of growth hormone begins in childhood.

255.0	Cushing's syndrome — *(Use additional E code to identify cause, if drug-induced) — oversecretion of adrenal cortisol or use of glucocorticoid medications causing fat deposits in the head and neck and kyphosis; adrenal hyperplasia, ectopic ACTH syndrome*
255.10	Hyperaldosteronism, unspecified — *primary aldosteronism, unspecified*
255.11	Glucocorticoid-remediable aldosteronism — *inherited as an autosomal dominant trait, with moderate to severe hypertension, moderate hypersecretion of aldosterone, suppressed plasma renin activity, with rapid reversal of these abnormalities with glucocorticoids. Familial type.*
255.12	Conn's syndrome — *an aldosteronoma (benign adrenal tumor), usually less than 2 cm in diameter, benign, golden yellow, causing headaches, nocturia, plyuria, fatigue, hypertension, hypokalemic alkalosis, potassium depletion, hypervolemia, decreased renin activity*
255.13	Bartter's syndrome — *found in children, hypokalemia alkalosis, elevated rennin, elevated angiotensin, low or normal blood pressure, no edema, retarded growth. Secondary hyperaldosteronism with juxtaglomerular hyperplasia, hyperaldosteronism with hypokalemic alkalosis*
255.14	Other secondary aldosteronism — *due to extra-adrenal disorders, increased renin, increased aldosterone, sodium retention, hypertensive state, secondary reninism due to decreased renal perfusion*

255.2	Adrenogenital disorders — *congenital or acquired disorders of the genitals due to adrenal dysfunction; Achard-Thiers syndrome, Apert-Gallais syndrome, Cooke-Apert-Gallais syndrome, Corticosexual syndrome, and Hercules syndrome*
255.3	Other corticoadrenal overactivity — *acquired benign adrenal androgenic overactivity; Schroeder's syndrome or Slocum's syndrome*
255.4	Corticoadrenal insufficiency — *underproduction of adrenal hormones causing low blood pressure; Addisonian crisis, Bernard-Sergent syndrome*
255.5	Other adrenal hypofunction — *adrenal medullary insufficiency*
255.6	Medulloadrenal hyperfunction — *catecholamine secretion by pheochromocytoma*
255.8	Other specified disorders of adrenal glands — *abnormality of cortisol-binding globulin, Adrenal collapse; adrenal/suprarenal cyst; adrenal obesity, inflammation, necrosis, sclerosis, swelling*
255.9	Unspecified disorder of adrenal glands

Coding Clarification

A secondary form of the disease can occur as a side effect of drug therapy, and is reported with the same code, 255.0 *Cushing's syndrome.*

Coding Scenario

A 49-year-old patient is seen in the clinic for adrenal-pituitary insufficiency secondary to steroids. The patient is a known steroid-dependent asthmatic.

Code assignment: 255.4 *Corticoadrenal insufficiency*, 493.90 *Asthma, type unspecified*, and E932.0 *Drug causing adverse effects in therapeutic use, adrenal cortical steroids*

256 Ovarian dysfunction
AHA: Q4, 2000, 51

Female gonads secrete sex hormones in response to stimulation from the pituitary gland. Located in the pelvis, the ovaries produce eggs. They also secrete female sex hormones, estrogen and progesterone, which regulate development of the reproductive organs, female secondary sex characteristics, and menstruation and pregnancy.

256.0	Hyperestrogenism — *over-secretion by the ovary of estrogen* **AHA:** Q4, 2000, 51
256.1	Other ovarian hyperfunction — *hypersecretion of ovarian androgens* **AHA:** Q3, 1995, 15; Q4, 2000, 51
256.2	Postablative ovarian failure — (Use additional code for states associated with artificial menopause, 627.4) — *iatrogenic, postsurgical, postirradiation* **AHA:** Q4, 2000, 51; Q2, 2002, 12
256.31	Premature menopause
256.39	Other ovarian failure — *delayed menarche, ovarian hypofunction, and primary ovarian failure NOS* **AHA:** Q4, 2000, 51; Q4, 2001, 41
256.4	Polycystic ovaries — *containing multiple follicular cysts filled with serous fluid; isosexual virilization; Stein-Leventhal syndrome* **AHA:** Q4, 2000, 51
256.8	Other ovarian dysfunction — *hyperthecosis, ovary* **AHA:** Q4, 2000, 51
256.9	Unspecified ovarian dysfunction

Coding Clarification
The rubric excludes the acquired absence of an ovary (V45.77) and artificial menopause NOS (627.4).

257 Testicular dysfunction
Male gonads produce sperm and secrete androgens. The androgens, the most important of which is testosterone, regulate development of the reproductive organs, male secondary sex characteristics, and muscle.

257.0	Testicular hyperfunction — *over-secretion by the testicles of testosterone*
257.1	Postablative testicular hypofunction — *iatrogenic, postsurgical, postirradiation*
257.2	Other testicular hypofunction — *eunuchoidism; defective biosynthesis of testicular androgen; failure of Leydig's cell, adult; fertile eunuch*
257.8	Other testicular dysfunction
257.9	Unspecified testicular dysfunction

258 Polyglandular dysfunction and related disorders

Autoimmune disorders affecting endocrine glands often occur in multiples. Hashimoto's thyroiditis, for example, often presents with Type I diabetes mellitus, hypoparathyroidism, or Addison's disease.

258.0	Polyglandular activity in multiple endocrine adenomatosis — *abnormal production of hormones by two or more endocrine glands due to hyperplasia; caused by genetic defects; Wermer's syndrome*
258.1	Other combinations of endocrine dysfunction — *Lloyd's syndrome, Schmidt's syndrome, Pierre Mauriac's syndrome*
258.8	Other specified polyglandular dysfunction — *atrophy pluriglandular; polyglandular sclerosis*
258.9	Unspecified polyglandular dysfunction

Coding Clarification
Schmidt's syndrome is Addison's disease with hypothyroidism secondary to Hashimoto's thyroiditis, and is reported with 258.1 *Other combinations of endocrine dysfunction*. In diabetes with hypothyroidism, report both conditions rather than this combination code since, as a significant

Endocrine, Nutritional and Metabolic Diseases, and Immunity Disorders

systemic disease, diabetes should always be codified separately.

259 Other endocrine disorders

The parathyroid glands are four small glands located at the four corners of the thyroid gland. The hormone secreted, parathyroid hormone, regulates the level of calcium in the blood.

259.0	Delay in sexual development and puberty, not elsewhere classified — *delayed puberty*
259.1	Precocious sexual development and puberty, not elsewhere classified — *cryptogenic, constitutional, idiopathic*
259.2	Carcinoid syndrome — *Argentaffin syndrome, Björk (-Thorson) syndrome, Cassidy (-Scholte) syndrome, Hedinger's syndrome*
259.3	Ectopic hormone secretion, not elsewhere classified — *arising from an abnormal site or tissue: antidiuretic hormone secretion [ADH], hyperparathyroidism* **AHA:** Nov-Dec, 1985, 4
259.4	Dwarfism, not elsewhere classified — *constitutional*
259.5	Androgen insensitivity syndrome — *partial androgen insensitivity; Reifenstein syndrome* **AHA:** Q4, 2005, 53
259.8	Other specified endocrine disorders — *pineal dysfunction, pineal calcification; Werner's syndrome, Donohue's syndrome, Gilford (-Hutchinson) syndrome, Pellizzi's, Progeria trigeminal plate syndrome; progeria, leprechaunism*
259.9	Unspecified endocrine disorder

Coding Clarification
Obesity due to underlying endocrine disease is reported with 259.9 *Unspecified endocrine disorder*.

260–269 Nutritional Deficiencies

In the United States, nutritional and vitamin deficiencies usually are the result of poverty, prolonged parenteral feeding, chronic substance abuse, food fads, or extreme diets. Malnutrition results from insufficiency in the body's total intake of energizing nutrients and proteins, and vitamin or mineral deficiencies are the result of insufficient intake of very specific nutrients. While patients with malnutrition may also commonly have vitamin or mineral deficiencies, it is also possible to develop a vitamin or mineral deficiency without malnutrition.

Coding Clarification
This group of rubrics excludes deficiency anemias, which are reported with 280.0-281.9.

260 Kwashiorkor

Kwashiorkor is an African word meaning "first-child, second-child." It refers to the protein-deficit illness that affects the first child when it is weaned to make room for the second child. Instead of protein-rich breast milk, the first child is fed a thin gruel made from sweet potato, banana, or cassava. The gruel is starchy, so there is no energy deficit, but the lack of protein causes edema, lethargy, and impaired growth. Kwashiorkor is considered a third-degree malnutrition disorder.

261 Nutritional marasmus
AHA: Q2, 2006, 12

Marasmus results from near starvation with a deficit in protein and nonprotein intake. Typically, marasmus is a childhood disease in underdeveloped countries, and occurs when the mother is unable to breast-feed. The child is very thin, with little muscle or body fat. Marasmus is considered a third-degree malnutrition disorder.

262 Other severe protein-calorie malnutrition
AHA: July-Aug, 1985, 12; Q4, 1992, 24

Classify malnutrition to this rubric if there is nutritional edema without mention of dyspigmentation of skin and hair.

263 Other and unspecified protein-calorie malnutrition
AHA: Q4, 1992, 24

Malnutrition results from inadequate intake or malabsorption of nutrients. Infants and children are at highest risk for malnutrition, since there is a high demand for nutrients during the growth years. Pregnancy and old age also pose other significant risks for malnutrition, as does the presence of chronic disease or adherence to some diets. Substance abuse is also a risk factor for malnutrition.

263.0	Malnutrition of moderate degree — *second degree malnutrition characterized by superimposed biochemical changes in electrolytes, lipids, blood plasma.* **AHA:** July-Aug, 1985, 1; Q4, 1992, 24
263.1	Malnutrition of mild degree — *first degree malnutrition characterized by tissue wasting in an adult or growth failure in a child, but few or no biochemical changes.* **AHA:** July-Aug, 1985, 1; Q4, 1992, 24
263.2	Arrested development following protein-calorie malnutrition — *physical retardation due to malnutrition* **AHA:** Q4, 1992, 24
263.8	Other protein-calorie malnutrition — *not elsewhere specified* **AHA:** Q4, 1992, 24
263.9	Unspecified protein-calorie malnutrition

264 Vitamin A deficiency

Vitamin A is found in green, leafy vegetables, fish, and dairy products, and serious deficiency can cause growth retardation in children, blindness, and increased susceptibility to infection. Vitamin A deficiency is common in kwashiorkor and is endemic in areas in which rice is the staple.

264.0	Vitamin A deficiency with conjunctival xerosis — *conjunctival dryness*
264.1	Vitamin A deficiency with conjunctival xerosis and Bitot's spot — *conjunctival dryness and superficial spots of keratinized epithelium; Bitot's spot in young child*
264.2	Vitamin A deficiency with corneal xerosis — *corneal dryness*
264.3	Vitamin A deficiency with corneal ulceration and xerosis — *corneal dryness and epithelial ulceration*
264.4	Vitamin A deficiency with keratomalacia — *corneal dryness progressing to corneal insensitivity, softness, necrosis; usually bilateral*
264.5	Vitamin A deficiency with night blindness — *failure of vision in dim light*
264.6	Vitamin A deficiency with xerophthalmic scars of cornea — *corneal scars caused by dryness*
264.7	Other ocular manifestations of vitamin A deficiency — *xerophthalmia*
264.8	Other manifestations of vitamin A deficiency — *follicular keratosis, xeroderma, phrynoderma*
264.9	Unspecified vitamin A deficiency

265 Thiamine and niacin deficiency states

Alcoholism is the main cause of thiamine deficiency in the United States. In other countries, it can result from eating a diet of highly polished rice. Infants can develop a thiamine deficiency when breast-fed by thiamine-deficient mothers. Thiamine deficiency causes beriberi, with its manifestations of neuritis, edema, and heart disease.

Niacin deficiency is called pellagra, and is characterized by a light-sensitive rash, diarrhea, glossitis, and psychosis. Pellagra is most common in countries in which corn is the main food source, and is rare in the United States.

265.0	Beriberi — *vitamin B1 deficiency characterized by neuritis, edema, and heart disease*
265.1	Other and unspecified manifestations of thiamine deficiency — *Gayet-Wernicke's syndrome*
265.2	Pellagra — *niacin deficiency causing disturbances in skin, digestion, psyche*

266 Deficiency of B-complex components

Ariboflavinosis is riboflavin, or vitamin B2, deficiency that causes inflammation of the lips, tongue fissures, corneal vascularization, and anemia. Ariboflavinosis is associated with deficiency of milk in the diet, though the disease can also occur secondarily in patients with chronic diseases affecting nutritional absorption.

Vitamin B6 is important in blood, the central nervous system, and skin metabolism. It is uncommon to find a primary deficiency in vitamin B6, but secondary deficiency can result in chronic diseases affecting nutritional absorption, in patients using oral contraceptives, or in alcoholism.

266.0	Ariboflavinosis — *vitamin B2 deficiency causing inflammation of the lips, tongue fissures, corneal vascularization, anemia.* **AHA:** Sept-Oct, 1986, 10
266.1	Vitamin B6 deficiency — *skin, lip, and tongue disturbances, peripheral neuropathy, and in infants, convulsions*
266.2	Other B-complex deficiencies — *B12, burning feet syndrome, Gopalan's syndrome*
266.9	Unspecified vitamin B deficiency

Coding Clarification
Report vitamin B6 responsive sideroblastic anemia with 285.0.

267 Ascorbic acid deficiency

Vitamin C, or ascorbic acid, is essential for wound healing and connective tissue health and it facilitates absorption of iron. A deficiency in this vitamin is commonly called scurvy or Cheadle-Moller-Barlow syndrome. Vitamin C is common to many fruits and vegetables. Symptoms of scurvy include bleeding gums, weight loss, myalgias, and slowing of the healing process. The symptoms are reversed with ascorbic acid therapy.

Coding Clarification
Anemia related to vitamin C deficiency is reported with 281.8 *Anemia associated with other specified nutritional deficiency.*

268 Vitamin D deficiency

Vitamin D is found in yeast, eggs, and dairy products, fish liver oils, and is also created when skin is exposed to sunlight. Deficiency is commonly called "rickets" in children and osteomalacia in adults. The disease is rare in the United States, though seen occasionally in immigrants from India. Demineralization of bone and bone deformity are the most common side effects of vitamin D deficiency.

Diseases in this rubric are classified as active or late effect, and as rickets or adult osteomalacia.

268.0	Rickets, active — *vitamin D deficiency causing metabolic bone disease in children; rosary, rachitic*
268.1	Rickets, late effect — (Use additional code to identify the nature of late effect) — *distorted or demineralized bones as a result of vitamin D*

	deficiency and stated to be a late effect or sequela of rickets
268.2	Osteomalacia, unspecified — *vitamin D deficiency causing metabolic bone disease in adults; Looser-Debray syndrome, Milkman-Looser syndrome, Miller's disease*
268.9	Unspecified vitamin D deficiency — *viosterol deficiency*

Coding Clarification

Renal rickets is reported with 588.0 *Renal osteodystrophy* and celiac rickets is reported with 579.0 *Celiac disease.*

Rickets or osteomalacia can also be caused by a metabolic resistance to absorb vitamin D, rather than a deficiency in intake. If this is the case, report the resistance with 275.3 *Disorders of phosphorus metabolism.*

269 Other nutritional deficiencies

269.0	Deficiency of vitamin K
269.1	Deficiency of other vitamins — *including vitamins E and P*
269.2	Unspecified vitamin deficiency — *multiple vitamin deficiency not specified*
269.3	Mineral deficiency, not elsewhere classified — *dietary calcium, iodine*
269.8	Other nutritional deficiency — *not elsewhere classified*
269.9	Unspecified nutritional deficiency

Coding Clarification

Vitamin K deficiencies associated with hypoprothrombinemia and depression of coagulation are reported with 286.7. Vitamin K deficiency of the newborn is reported with 776.0 *Hemorrhagic disease of newborns.*

Do not use codes from this rubric to report failure to thrive or feeding problems. These conditions are classified to rubric 783. Deficiencies of calcium, potassium, and sodium are classified to rubrics 275 or 276.

270–279 Other Metabolic and Immunity Disorders

Use an additional code to identify any associated mental retardation.

270 Disorders of amino-acid transport and metabolism

270.0	Disturbances of amino-acid transport — (Use additional code to identify any associated mental retardation) — *cystinosis, renal glycinuria, cystinuria, Hartnup disease, Fanconi (-de Toni)*
270.1	Phenylketonuria (PKU) — (Use additional code to identify any associated mental retardation) — *inherited error of metabolism affecting phenylalanine; early diagnosis through screening blood test prevents mental retardation; hyperphenylalaninemia*
270.2	Other disturbances of aromatic amino-acid metabolism — (Use additional code to identify any associated mental retardation) — *albinism, hypertyrosinemia, alkaptonuria, Oasthouse urine disease, Mende's syndrome, Smith-Strang disease, van der Hoeve-Halbertsma-Waardenburg syndrome*

AHA: Q3, 1999, 20

270.3	Disturbances of branched-chain amino-acid metabolism — (Use additional code to identify any associated mental retardation) — *of leucine, isoleucine, and valine; hypervalinemia; intermittent branched-chain ketonuria; leucine-induced hypoglycemia; methylmalonic aciduria*

AHA: Q3, 2000, 8

270.4	Disturbances of sulphur-bearing amino-acid metabolism — (Use additional code to identify any associated mental retardation) — *cystathioninuria, cystathioninuria; disturbances of metabolism of methionine, homocystine, cystathionine, homocystinuria, and hyperhomocyteinemia.*

AHA: Q1, 2004, 6

270.5	Disturbances of histidine metabolism — (Use additional code to identify any associated mental retardation) — *carnosinemia, histidinemia, hyperhistidinemia, imidazole aminoaciduria*
270.6	Disorders of urea cycle metabolism — (Use additional code to identify any associated mental retardation) — *argininosuccinic aciduria; citrullinemia; disorders of metabolism of ornithine, citrulline, argininosuccinic acid, arginine, and ammonia*
270.7	Other disturbances of straight-chain amino-acid metabolism — (Use additional code to identify any associated mental retardation) — *glucoglycinuria; hyperglycinemia and other disturbances of metabolism of glycine, threonine, serine, glutamine, and lysine; pipecolic acidemia, methylmalonic aciduria with glycinemia*

AHA: Q3, 2000, 8

270.8	Other specified disorders of amino-acid metabolism — (Use additional code to identify any associated mental retardation) — *alaninemia, aminoacidopathy, ethanolaminuria, prolinemia, glycoprolinuria, prolinuria, hydroxyprolinemia, sarcosinemia familial iminoglycinuria, and Lowe-Terrey-MacLachlan syndrome*
270.9	Unspecified disorder of amino-acid metabolism — (Use additional code to identify any associated mental retardation)

Coding Clarification

Excluded from this rubric are abnormal findings without manifest disease (790.0 796.9), disorders of purine and pyrimidine metabolism (277.1-277.2), and gout (274.0-274.9).

271 Disorders of carbohydrate transport and metabolism

271.0 Glycogenosis — (Use additional code to identify any associated mental retardation) — *excessive storage of glycogen; amylopectinosis, glucose-6-phosphatase deficiency, McArdle's disease, Pompe's disease, von Gierke's disease*
AHA: Q1, 1998, 5

271.1 Galactosemia — (Use additional code to identify any associated mental retardation) — *galactose-1-phosphate uridyl transferase deficiency, galactosuria*

271.2 Hereditary fructose intolerance — (Use additional code to identify any associated mental retardation) — *essential benign fructosuria, fructosemia*

271.3 Intestinal disaccharidase deficiencies and disaccharide malabsorption — (Use additional code to identify any associated mental retardation) — *intolerance or malabsorption: glucose, lactose, or sucrose*

271.4 Renal glycosuria — (Use additional code to identify any associated mental retardation) — *abnormally large amount of sugar in the urine with normal blood sugar, caused by failure of the renal tubules to reabsorb glucose; renal diabetes*

271.8 Other specified disorders of carbohydrate transport and metabolism — (Use additional code to identify any associated mental retardation) — *essential benign pentosuria, mannosidosis, fucosidosis, oxalosis, xylosuria, Bird's disease, glycolic aciduria*

271.9 Unspecified disorder of carbohydrate transport and metabolism — (Use additional code to identify any associated mental retardation)

Coding Clarification
Excluded from this rubric are abnormality of secretion of glucagon (251.4), diabetes mellitus (rubric 250), hypoglycemia not otherwise specified (251.2), and mucopolysaccharidosis (277.5).

272 Disorders of lipoid metabolism

Cholesterol is a waxy fat that is present in the human body. Two sources contribute to the amount of cholesterol in the human body. First, the liver manufactures about 80 percent of it. Second, people consume it by eating animal products such as meat, eggs, and dairy products. Cholesterol is carried through the bloodstream by certain proteins (apolipoproteins). When these proteins wrap around cholesterol and other types of fats (lipids) to transport them through the bloodstream, they combine and are called lipoproteins.

There are three different types of lipoproteins that carry cholesterol through the bloodstream:

- High-density lipoproteins (HDL), which are associated with "good" cholesterol
- Low-density lipoproteins (LDL), which are associated with "bad" cholesterol
- Very low-density lipoproteins (VLDL), which are associated with "very bad" cholesterol

High levels of LDL cholesterol have been associated with arteriosclerosis (hardening of the arteries) and coronary artery disease. In contrast, high levels of HDL cholesterol have been shown to reduce some of the harmful effects of LDL cholesterol.

The following are cholesterol levels (all measurements are in milligrams per deciliter): Total cholesterol levels less than 200 are desirable; total cholesterol levels between 200 and 239 are borderline-high; total cholesterol levels that are 240 or higher are high and considered to be hypercholesterolemia.

272.0 Pure hypercholesterolemia — (Use additional code to identify any associated mental retardation) — *high cholesterol in the blood; familial, Fredrickson Type II A hyperlipoproteinemia; low-density-lipoid-type [LDL] hyperlipoproteinemia*
AHA: Q4, 2005, 71

272.1 Pure hyperglyceridemia — (Use additional code to identify any associated mental retardation) — *elevated level of glyceride, a natural fatty acid, in the blood; endogenous hyperglyceridemia; Fredrickson Type IV hyperlipoproteinemia; very-low-density-lipoid-type [VLDL] hyperlipoproteinemia*

272.2 Mixed hyperlipidemia — (Use additional code to identify any associated mental retardation) — *elevated level of lipoprotein, a complex of fats and proteins, in the blood due to an inherited lipoprotein metabolism disorder; Fredrickson Type IIb or III hyperlipoproteinemia, hypercholesterolemia with endogenous hyperglyceridemia; tubo-eruptive xanthoma*

272.3 Hyperchylomicronemia — (Use additional code to identify any associated mental retardation) — *Bürger-Grütz syndrome; Fredrickson type I or V hyperlipoproteinemia; Hyperlipidemia, Group D*

272.4 Other and unspecified hyperlipidemia — (Use additional code to identify any associated mental retardation) — *elevated level of chylomicrons in the blood. Chylomicrons are a form of lipoproteins which transport dietary cholesterol and triglycerides from the small intestine to the blood; Seeley-Klionsky disease*
AHA: Q1, 2005, 17

272.5 Lipoprotein deficiencies — (Use additional code to identify any associated mental retardation) — *abnormally low level of lipoprotein, a complex of fats and proteins, in the blood; abetalipoproteinemia, hypoalphalipoproteinemia; Bassen-Kornzweig syndrome; high-density lipoid deficiency*

272.6 Lipodystrophy — (Use additional code to identify any associated mental retardation. Use additional E code to identify cause, if iatrogenic)

Endocrine, Nutritional and Metabolic Diseases, and Immunity Disorders

272.7 Lipidoses — (Use additional code to identify any associated mental retardation) — *chemically-induced; Anderson's disease, Fabry's disease, Gaucher's disease, Niemann-Pick disease, pseudo-Hurler's or mucolipidosis III disease, Wolman's disease; Ruiter-Pompen (-Wyers) syndrome, sea-blue histiocyte syndrome*

— *disturbance in fat metabolism causing abnormal distribution of the body's fatty tissue; Barraquer-Simons disease, Simons' syndrome*

272.8 Other disorders of lipoid metabolism — (Use additional code to identify any associated mental retardation) — *Hoffa's, Launois-Bensaude's, Anders' syndrome, Dercum's syndrome, Farber*

272.9 Unspecified disorder of lipoid metabolism — (Use additional code to identify any associated mental retardation)

Coding Clarification
Excluded from this rubric is localized cerebral lipidoses (330.1).

273 Disorders of plasma protein metabolism

Waldenström's is a rare chronic form of lymphoma that affects plasma cells. Abnormal plasma cells grow out of control and invade bone marrow, lymph nodes and spleen. The cells cause a thickening of the blood by producing an increased amount of an antibody called IgM. This disease affects men more often than women and may cause few symptoms in the early stages.

Alpha-1 is one of the most common and serious hereditary diseases seen in nearly every population. The cases that have been diagnosed are estimated to be less than 10% of those predicted to have Alpha-1. Millions of people are carriers of the deficient gene that causes Alpha-1 and may pass it on to the next generation.

A person with Alpha-1-antitrypsin deficiency carries a gene that produces an abnormal AAT protein that cannot be secreted by the liver. This results in a severe reduction of the circulating levels of the protein as well as damaging accumulation within the liver. The deficiency also results in lung disease, since the protein is designed to protect the lungs from destructive enzymatic activity.

Since Alpha-1 begins in the liver and is a hereditary problem, liver involvement is often seen in children more than in adults, although chronic liver disease can occur at any time in life. Alpha-1 deficiency is the leading genetic cause of liver transplantation in children. This disease is also a major cause of lung transplantation. Lung disease is usually seen in adults, often striking in the prime of life with debilitating lung damage.

273.0 Polyclonal hypergammaglobulinemia — (Use additional code to identify any associated mental retardation) — *elevated level of gamma globulins in the blood, frequently observed in patients with chronic infectious diseases, including Waldenström's*

273.1 Monoclonal paraproteinemia — (Use additional code to identify any associated mental retardation) — *presence of abnormal proteins in the blood plasma; benign monoclonal hypergammaglobulinemia [BMH], monoclonal gammopathy associated with lymphoplasmacytic dyscrasias, paraproteinemia secondary to malignant or inflammatory disease*

273.2 Other paraproteinemias — (Use additional code to identify any associated mental retardation) — *cryoglobulinemic purpura, vasculitis, mixed cryoglobulinemia*

273.3 Macroglobulinemia — (Use additional code to identify any associated mental retardation) — *elevated level of macroglobulins in the blood. Macroglobulins are plasma globulins with an unusually high molecular weight; Waldenström's macroglobulinemia*

273.4 Alpha-1-antitrypsin deficiency

273.8 Other disorders of plasma protein metabolism — (Use additional code to identify any associated mental retardation) — *bisalbuminemia; hyperglobulinemia; hypoalbuminemia; hypoproteinemia; pyroglobulinemia*
AHA: Q2, 1998, 11

273.9 Unspecified disorder of plasma protein metabolism — (Use additional code to identify any associated mental retardation)

Coding Clarification
Excluded from this rubric are agammaglobulinemia and hypogammaglobulinemia (279.0-279.2), coagulation defect (286.0-286.9), and hereditary hemolytic anemias (282.0-282.9).

Coding Scenario
A patient is seen at the clinic for symptoms of peripheral neuropathy. The physician's diagnosis states peripheral neuropathy secondary to POEMS syndrome.

Code assignment: 273.8 *Other disorders of plasma protein metabolism* and 357.4 *Polyneuropathy in other diseases classified elsewhere*

An adult with a history of untreatable asthma and chronic respiratory infections undergoes pulmonary function testing that indicates decreased lung function. X-rays are taken that show a flattened diaphragm, and gas exchange testing shows that pulmonary emphysema is beginning. The physician orders a blood test for Alpha-1 levels, which return at 11 μ M/L. The levels are phenotyped and the patient is diagnosed with Alpha-1-antitrypsin deficiency emphysema (also known as "genetic" or "inherited" emphysema). Weekly replacement intravenous therapy for protein augmentation of Alpha-1 is initiated.

Code assignment: 273.4 *Alpha-1-antitrypsin deficiency*

274 Gout
AHA: Q2, 1995, 4

Deposits of monosodium urate or monohydrate crystals cause gout. The most common site for these deposits is around the joints, especially around the big toe. However, these deposits may be found in organ systems, too. Gout is classified according to site.

274.0	Gouty arthropathy — (Use additional code to identify any associated mental retardation) — *acute inflammatory arthritis caused by deposits of monosodium urate monohydrate crystals in the joints* **AHA:** Q2, 1995, 4
274.10	Gouty nephropathy, unspecified — (Use additional code to identify any associated mental retardation) — *any kidney disease characterized by abnormal production and excretion of uric acid* **AHA:** Nov-Dec, 1985, 15; Q2, 1995, 4
274.11	Uric acid nephrolithiasis — (Use additional code to identify any associated mental retardation) — *with sodium urate stones in the kidney* **AHA:** Q2, 1995, 4
274.19	Other gouty nephropathy — (Use additional code to identify any associated mental retardation) — *not otherwise specified* **AHA:** Q2, 1995, 4
274.81	Gouty tophi of ear — (Use additional code to identify any associated mental retardation) — *deposit of sodium urate inflaming external ear* **AHA:** Q2, 1995, 4
274.82	Gouty tophi of other sites — (Use additional code to identify any associated mental retardation) — *heart* **AHA:** Q2, 1995, 4
274.89	Gout with other specified manifestations — (Use additional code to identify any associated mental retardation. Use additional code to identify manifestations: 357.4, 364.11) — *dermatitis, eczema, episcleritis, iritis, neuritis, phlebitis* **AHA:** Q2, 1995, 4
274.9	Gout, unspecified — (Use additional code to identify any associated mental retardation) — *podagra, thesaurismosis urate, uric acid diathesis* **AHA:** Q2, 1995, 4

Coding Clarification
Pseudogout is classified to rubric 275. Excluded from this rubric is lead gout, which is classified to 984.0-984.9.

Coding Scenario
A 62-year-old male patient is seen by his physician complaining of pain in the left great toe. An x-ray is negative. Uric acid level is elevated. A diagnosis of gout is made and the patient is prescribed allopurinal.

Code assignment: 274.0 *Gouty arthropathy*

275 Disorders of mineral metabolism
Hypercalcemia includes symptoms of nausea, vomiting, anorexia, fever, and constipation. Pseudogout is chondrocalcinosis, a disorder of calcium metabolism. Joint disease is due to deposits of dicalcium phosphate or pyrophosphate crystals.

275.0	Disorders of iron metabolism — (Use additional code to identify any associated mental retardation) — *bronzed diabetes, pigmentary cirrhosis, hemochromatosis, Troisier-Hanot-Chauffard syndrome, von Recklinghausen-Applebaum disease* **AHA:** Q2, 1997, 11
275.1	Disorders of copper metabolism — (Use additional code to identify any associated mental retardation) — *hepatolenticular degeneration; Wilson's disease; amyostatic syndrome, chorea-athetosis-agitans syndrome, Westphal-Strümpel syndrome*
275.2	Disorders of magnesium metabolism — (Use additional code to identify any associated mental retardation) — *hypermagnesemia, hypomagnesemia*
275.3	Disorders of phosphorus metabolism — (Use additional code to identify any associated mental retardation) — *familial hypophosphatemia, vitamin*
275.40	Unspecified disorder of calcium metabolism — (Use additional code to identify any associated mental retardation)
275.41	Hypocalcemia — (Use additional code to identify any associated mental retardation) — *low level of calcium in the blood with possible symptoms including muscle or abdominal cramps, tendon reflex anomalies, or carpopedal spasms* **AHA:** Q4, 1997, 33
275.42	Hypercalcemia — (Use additional code to identify any associated mental retardation) — *elevated level of calcium in the blood with possible symptoms including fatigue, nausea, constipation, depression* **AHA:** Q4, 1997, 33; Q4, 2003, 110
275.49	Other disorders of calcium metabolism — (Use additional code to identify any associated mental retardation) — *nephrocalcinosis; pseudohypoparathyroidism; pseudopseudohypoparathyroidism; and Martin-*

	Albright syndrome, Seabright-Bantam syndromes **AHA:** Q4, 1997, 33
275.8	Other specified disorders of mineral metabolism — (Use additional code to identify any associated mental retardation) — *not elsewhere classified*
275.9	Unspecified disorder of mineral metabolism — (Use additional code to identify any associated mental retardation)

Coding Clarification

Iron Overload due to Transfusions: If a sickle cell patient is admitted with an iron overload (hemochromatosis) due to transfusion, three codes would be required: 275.0 *Disorders of iron metabolism* for the hemochromatosis, 282.60 for the sickle cell, and E934.7 *Drugs, medicinal and biological substances causing adverse effects in therapeutic use, natural blood and blood products*, to identify the adverse reaction of the iron overload from the blood.

Patients being treated with chronic transfusions necessitated by their sickle cell anemia are often treated with prophylactic therapy to prevent iron overload. If the patient is noncompliant with this therapy and is admitted for a high dose infusion to prevent an overload, then two codes would be necessary: 282.60 *Sickle-cell disease, unspecified* and V15.81 *Noncompliance with medical treatment*.

276 Disorders of fluid, electrolyte, and acid-base balance

Dehydration is characterized by excessive free water loss and plasma volume contraction disproportionate to the loss of sodium. Solutes become imbalanced resulting in hypernatremia (increased concentration of serum sodium) as an indicator for true dehydration. Blood volume can be replaced, but the plasma solutes must be correctly balanced as well. Gradual volume restoration is imperative to restore optimal fluid balance slowly.

Dehydration may follow bouts of diarrhea, vomiting, or profuse sweating. It is often a manifestation of the patient's illness (e.g., gastroenteritis), and in such cases, the code for dehydration would not be sequenced first. However, if the patient's dehydration becomes significant enough to warrant separate treatment for rehydration, the dehydration code would be sequenced first.

Volume depletion is the loss of total body water and contraction of the total intravascular plasma while hypovolemia is the depletion of the volume of plasma, or total blood volume.

276.0	Hyperosmolality and/or hypernatremia — (Use additional code to identify any associated mental retardation) — *sodium [Na] excess or overload*
276.1	Hyposmolality and/or hyponatremia — (Use additional code to identify any associated mental retardation) — *sodium [Na] deficiency*
276.2	Acidosis — (Use additional code to identify any associated mental retardation) — *accumulation of acid or depletion of alkali in blood and body tissues; metabolic or respiratory* **AHA:** Jan-Feb, 1987, 15
276.3	Alkalosis — (Use additional code to identify any associated mental retardation) — *accumulation of base or loss of acid without relative loss of base in body fluids, caused by increased arterial plasma bicarbonate concentration or by abnormal loss of carbon dioxide due to hyperventilation; metabolic or respiratory*
276.4	Mixed acid-base balance disorder — (Use additional code to identify any associated mental retardation) — *hypercapnia with mixed acid-base disorder*
276.50	Volume depletion, unspecified — (Use additional code to identify any associated mental retardation) **AHA:** Q2, 1988, 9; Q4, 1997, 30; Q3, 2002, 21; Q2, 2005, 9; Q4, 2005, 54
276.51	Dehydration — (Use additional code to identify any associated mental retardation) — *Luetscher's syndrome* **AHA:** Q4, 2005, 54
276.52	Hypovolemia — (Use additional code to identify any associated mental retardation) — *depletion of volume of plasma* **AHA:** Q2, 1988, 9; Q4, 1997, 30; Q3, 2002, 21; Q4, 2005, 54
276.6	Fluid overload — (Use additional code to identify any associated mental retardation) — *fluid retention*
276.7	Hyperpotassemia — (Use additional code to identify any associated mental retardation) — *elevated level of potassium in the blood with symptoms including abnormal EKG readings and weakness; often associated with defective renal excretion; hyperkalemia, potassium [K] intoxication* **AHA:** Q2, 2001, 12; Q1, 2005, 9
276.8	Hypopotassemia — (Use additional code to identify any associated mental retardation) — *decreased level of potassium in the blood with symptoms including neuromuscular disorders; often associated with potassium loss through vomiting and diarrhea; hypokalemia*
276.9	Electrolyte and fluid disorders not elsewhere classified — (Use additional code to identify any associated mental retardation) — *electrolyte imbalance, hypochloremia, hyperchloremia, disequilibrium syndrome* **AHA:** Jan-Feb, 1987, 15

Documentation Issues

Sequencing: Because dehydration is often the result of another condition as well as a difficult management issue in itself, it causes confusion for coders when sequencing the codes. The decision of when dehydration is listed first is dependent upon the documented reason for the admission/visit as determined by the physician. If, after study, dehydration is determined to be the condition chiefly responsible for occasioning the admission of the patient to the hospital, or the primary reason for the outpatient visit, then the dehydration should be listed first.

If the physician has documented that the patient was being treated for gastroenteritis on an outpatient basis, and the patient's dehydration became so severe he/she was admitted to the hospital for IV rehydration, the dehydration code (276.51) should be listed first followed by the code for the gastroenteritis (558.9) on the hospital claim.

If the physician indicates in the documentation that the patient was admitted for treatment of severe burns and dehydration secondary to the burns, the burn code would be listed first and the dehydration code would be listed second.

If the documentation in the record indicates that the patient has metabolic acidosis and diabetes, clarify with the physician if there is a direct cause and effect relationship. Note that code 276.2 has an exclusion note for diabetic acidosis and references code 250.1x.

If the documentation does not identify the reason chiefly responsible for the admission/encounter, clarification must be obtained from the physician. Be sure the physician clearly documents the reason for the admission/encounter in the medical record.

Coding Clarification

Etiology: Dehydration is the depletion or deprivation of water, disproportionate to sodium loss, causing an imbalance in homeostasis. Symptoms and signs of dehydration may be a direct result of inadequate intake of fluid, diarrhea, vomiting, sweating, or polyuria. In severe cases, patients may be lethargic, weak, and obtunded. Conditions such as shock and coma may also occur. Many conditions are accompanied by dehydration, such as gastroenteritis, intestinal disorders, burns, renal failure, urinary tract infections, cryptosporidiosis, ascites, and diabetic glycosuria.

When reporting any type of volume depletion due to chemotherapy, also report E933.1 *Drugs, medicinal,* and biological substances, causing adverse effects in therapeutic use, antineoplastic and immunosuppresive drugs.

Dialysis Disequilibrium Syndrome: This condition is reported with code 276.9 *Electrolyte and fluid disorder not elsewhere classified.* Code also the underlying disease such as chronic kidney disease (585.1-585.9), and also report the renal dialysis status (V45.1).

Coding Scenario

A 19-year-old patient is admitted to the hospital for IV rehydration. The physician documents that the patient is currently being treated with Kaopectate for his diarrhea but his dehydration became so severe that it was necessary to admit for IV therapy. The final diagnosis is documented as dehydration due to viral gastroenteritis.

> Code assignment: 276.51 *Dehydration* and 008.8 *Intestinal infection due to other organism, not elsewhere classified*

A patient with known HIV is admitted with a diagnosis of diarrhea and dehydration. The physician's final diagnosis was cryptosporidiosis with dehydration secondary to HIV disease.

> Code assignment: 042 *Human immunodeficiency virus [HIV] disease,* 007.4 *Cryptosporidiosis,* and 276.51 *Dehydration*

A 49-year-old female is admitted for severe dehydration. The patient is known to have lung cancer with generalized metastases. The patient is treated with IV fluids for the dehydration. The patient's cancer is not treated during this admission.

> Code assignment: 276.51 *Dehydration,* 162.9 *Malignant neoplasm of bronchus and lung, unspecified,* and 199.0 *Malignant neoplasm, disseminated*

277 Other and unspecified disorders of metabolism

Cystic fibrosis is a hereditary disorder in which the body secretes thick, sticky mucus that clogs organs and leads to problems with breathing and digestion. About 30,000 children and young adults in the United States have cystic fibrosis. The disease affects one in 2,500 Caucasians and one in 17,000 African-Americans.

Cystic fibrosis is caused by a defect in the manufacture of cystic fibrosis transmembrane conductance regulator (CFTR). Normally, CFTR forms a channel through which chloride ions traverse the cells lining the lungs, pancreas, sweat glands, and small intestine. With cystic fibrosis,

Endocrine, Nutritional and Metabolic Diseases, and Immunity Disorders

malfunctioning CFTR precludes chloride from entering or leaving cells, resulting in production of thick, sticky mucus. In the lungs, this mucus blocks airways. In the digestive system, the mucus prevents enzymes produced in the pancreas from reaching the intestines, impairing digestion. In addition, the malfunctioning CFTR causes excessive amounts of salt to escape in the sweat.

Cystic fibrosis is an autosomal recessive genetic disorder. To have cystic fibrosis, both parents must carry the disease. One in 31 people in the United States carries the gene. With two carriers, there is a 25 percent chance of producing a child with cystic fibrosis.

Cystic fibrosis symptoms may be apparent soon after birth, or the symptoms may go undiagnosed for years. In 20 percent of cases, the first symptom is meconium ileus, intestinal blockage in newborns, which may require surgery.

Amyloidosis is a condition in which abnormal proteins, called amyloid, deposit in various tissues such as heart and brain tissue. These proteins, or fibrils, are produced in excess and deposited in different organs and slowly replace normal tissue. The deposits damage the tissues and interfere with the function of the involved organ. Amyloidosis occurs in multiple forms: spontaneous, hereditary, and resulting from a cancer of the blood cells called myeloma. Hereditary amyloidosis is an inherited form that is transmitted as an autosomal dominant trait.

Familial Mediterranean fever (FMF) is characterized by attacks of recurrent high fevers accompanied by pain and inflammation in the lining of the chest and abdominal cavities, skin or joints, and blood vessels (vasculitis). Onset of attacks usually presents in childhood or adolescence. An attack can persist for 12 to 72 hours, and vary in intensity. The intervals between attacks are unpredictable, occurring days, or even months, apart. Although the underlying cause is seemingly genetic, the catalyst for onset of the attacks is unknown. However, stress, physical trauma, and exertion have been reported by patients as possible precipitates or contributive factors. If untreated, kidney damage can result as a complication of amyloidosis, whereby the overproduction of amyloid protein has a destructive effect on renal tissues.

Disorders of fatty acid oxidation are genetic metabolic disorders that render the body incapable of breaking down fatty acids to make that energy available. Different types of specific enzyme deficiencies, in which one may be missing or improperly functioning, may manifest themselves as the cause. If undiagnosed, fatty acid oxidation disorders can result in serious complications of the liver, heart, eyes, and muscle development, and may lead to coma and possibly death, especially if metabolic crisis arises after a fasting period, such as during an infection or flu. Other signs include chronic bouts of low blood sugar, vomiting, diarrhea, lethargy, and even seizures.

Medium-chain acyl-CoA dehydrogenase deficiency (MCAD) is a disorder of the enzyme involved in mitochondrial fatty acid B-oxidation. This is usually diagnosed when a child is between three and 24 months of age, but may present later. Once the diagnosis is made, the child will require increased feedings to prevent long periods of fasting.

Peroxisomal disorders are problems at the subcellular level involving the improper formation or functioning of peroxisomes. These are special compartments within cells, called organelles, that are bound by their own membrane and contain certain enzymes. These peroxisomes help to do a number of jobs that are needed for digestion, producing certain hormones, and making the nervous system work properly. Peroxisomal disorders occur when a defect in the assembly of the peroxisome happens, such as when needed proteins fail to transport inside the peroxisome membrane, or a defect in a specific, single function of the peroxisome arises.

Mitochondria are another of the subcellular compartment organelles separated from the rest of the cell by its own membrane and containing its own DNA. The mitochondrion is responsible for handling the energy considerations of the cell. Many different clinical problems can present with mitochondrial metabolism disorders, especially involving neurological problems, such as mitochondrial encephalopathies and myoclonus with epilepsy.

277.00		Cystic fibrosis without mention of meconium ileus — (Use additional code to identify any associated mental retardation) — *genetic disorder causing pancreatic and respiratory deficiencies.*
		AHA: Q3, 1990, 18; Q4, 1990, 16; Q2, 2003, 12
277.01		Cystic fibrosis with meconium ileus — (Use additional code to identify any associated mental retardation) — *inherited disorder causing pancreatic and respiratory deficiencies; with meconium ileus present at birth*
		AHA: Q3, 1990, 18; Q4, 1990, 16

277.02	Cystic fibrosis with pulmonary manifestations — (Use additional code to identify any associated mental retardation. Use additional code to identify any infectious organism present)
277.03	Cystic fibrosis with gastrointestinal manifestations — (Use additional code to identify any associated mental retardation)
277.09	Cystic fibrosis with other manifestations — (Use additional code to identify any associated mental retardation)
277.1	Disorders of porphyrin metabolism — (Use additional code to identify any associated mental retardation) — *hematoporphyria, hematoporphyrinuria, hereditary coproporphyria, porphyrinuria, protocoproporphyria, Günther's syndrome*
277.2	Other disorders of purine and pyrimidine metabolism — (Use additional code to identify any associated mental retardation) — *hypoxanthine-guanine-phosphoribosyltransferase deficiency [HG-PRT deficiency], Lesch-Nyhan syndrome, xanthinuria*
277.30	Amyloidosis, unspecified — *not otherwise specified*
277.31	Familial Mediterranean fever — *benign paroxysmal peritonitis; hereditary amyloid nephropathy; periodic familial polyserositis; recurrent polyserositis*
277.39	Other amyloidosis — *hereditary cardiac amyloidosis; inherited systemic amyloidosis; neuropathic amyloidosis; Portuguese amyloidosis; Swiss amyloidosis; secondary amyloidosis* **AHA:** Q1, 1996, 16
277.4	Disorders of bilirubin excretion — (Use additional code to identify any associated mental retardation) — *hyperbilirubinemia; Dubin-Johnson syndrome, Gilbert's syndrome, Rotor's syndrome, Crigler-Najjar syndrome*
277.5	Mucopolysaccharidosis — (Use additional code to identify any associated mental retardation) — *gargoylism; osteochondrodystrophy; lipochondrodystrophy; Morquio-Brailsford disease, Hunter's syndrome, Hurler's syndrome, Sanfilippo's syndrome, Scheie's syndrome, Maroteaux-Lamy syndrome*
277.6	Other deficiencies of circulating enzymes — (Use additional code to identify any associated mental retardation) — *hereditary angioedema*
277.7	Dysmetabolic Syndrome X — (Use additional code for associated manifestations: 278.00, 278.01, 414.00-414.07. Use additional code to identify any associated mental retardation.)
277.81	Primary carnitine deficiency — (Use additional code to identify any associated mental retardation) — *decreased carnitine, impairs fatty acid oxidation, not associated with another identifiable systemic illness*
277.82	Carnitine deficiency due to inborn errors of metabolism — (Use additional code to identify any associated mental retardation) — *one or more missing enzyme(s) for metabolic process or partial enzyme processing. Cannot break down fats, sugars, proteins for energy. Malaise, cardiomyopathy, seizures, developmental delay, slow growth, slow weight gain, hypoglycemia*
277.83	Iatrogenic carnitine deficiency — (Use additional code to identify any associated mental retardation) — *may be caused by dialysis, ingestion of valproic acid, pivampicillin, emetine, zidovudine, ketogenic diet*
277.84	Other secondary carnitine deficiency — (Use additional code to identify any associated mental retardation) — *Medical conditions decreasing levels of carnitine in plasma or tissues - cirrhosis, chronic renal failure, diabetes mellitus, heart failure, Alzheimer disease*
277.85	Disorders of fatty acid oxidation—genetic deficiencies that prevent the body from breaking down fatty acids to make energy
277.86	Peroxisomal disorders—rare congenital diseases characterized by the absence of normal metabolic catalytic enzymes in the body; adrenoleukodystrophy, Zellweger syndrome
277.87	Disorders of mitochondrial metabolism (Use additional code for associated conditions) - Defects in mitochondrial or nuclear DNA; Kearns-Sayre, MELAS, MERRF, MNGIE, NARP **AHA:** Q4, 2004, 62
277.89	Other specified disorders of metabolism — (Use additional code to identify any associated mental retardation) — *Chronic histiosytosis, chronic histiosytosis X, acatalasemia, reticulohistiocytoma, craniohypophyseal xanthomatosis, Christian's syndrome, Hand-Schuller-Christian syndrome*
277.9	Unspecified disorder of metabolism — (Use additional code to identify any associated mental retardation)

Coding Scenario

A 5-year-old patient is admitted with acute bronchitis and possible cystic fibrosis. A chest x-ray is performed, confirming the diagnosis of cystic fibrosis. The diagnosis at discharge is acute bronchitis and cystic fibrosis.

Code assignment: 466.0 *Acute bronchitis* and 277.02 *Cystic fibrosis with pulmonary manifestations*

A 1-year-old presents to the emergency room for anorexia with vomiting, lethargy, and fever. Initial blood test shows the child to be very hypoglycemic. A complete metabolic profile, CBC with differential, and carnitine level testing is run. The child is immediately started on a glucose IV to raise and maintain blood sugar levels. The physician diagnoses medium-chain acyl-CoA dehydrogenase deficiency (MCAD). Diet requirements and eating habits are established and discussed with the patient's parents.

Code assignment: 277.85 *Disorders of fatty acid oxidation*

278 Overweight, obesity and other hyperalimentation

A person is generally considered overweight if he or she has a body mass index (BMI) between 25 and 29.9 kg/m2. Obesity is defined as a BMI of 30 or higher. A man is considered obese when he is 20 percent over his maximum optimal weight while a woman is considered obese when she is 25 percent over her maximum optimal weight. Any person greater than 100 lbs overweight is also considered morbidly obese.

Over the past 30 years, the number of overweight children has doubled. In the 6 to 19 age group, more than 30 percent are considered overweight; of these, 15 percent are considered obese. Excess weight and obesity during childhood has been proven to be an indicator of obesity in adulthood. Factors contributing to this increased incidence of pediatric obesity including lack of physical activity, sedentary lifestyle, heredity, social and economic status, eating habits, environmental factors, and underlying genetic, hormonal, or metabolic conditions.

Obesity in children is linked to multiple health issues, including liver disease, heart disease, cancers, vascular disease, orthopaedic problems, specific sleep disorders, and hypercholesterolemia. Obese children are almost 10 times as likely to have hypertension, and 85 percent of children who are diagnosed with Type 2 diabetes are obese.

The terms "overweight" and "obese" are differentiated by the severity of the condition and potential outcomes. Treatment for these conditions and the associated health risks differ in relationship to their progression and severity. To more effectively treat and manage the effect of weight problems in the health care industry, new codes were added in October 2005 to provide a mechanism of severity measurement based on adult body mass indexes (BMI). The American Academy of Pediatrics (AAP) proposed the creation of new codes for pediatric BMI that utilize the value ranges for children (ages 2 to 20 years) as currently represented in the CDC growth charts.

The CDC provides four weight classifications for children:

- "Underweight" refers to a weight that is under the fifth percentile for the child's age.
- "Healthy" refers to a weight between the fifth and 85th percentile.
- "At risk" refers to a weight between the 85th and 95th percentile for the child's age. This corresponds to a BMI of 25, which is considered overweight for an adult.
- "Overweight" refers to a weight ranking above the 95th percentile for the child's age. This is the most severe level of childhood obesity, corresponding to a BMI of at least 30. This is the same indicator used to classify adult obesity.

BMI is a calculation based on height and weight that is found by dividing a persons weight in kilograms by height in meters squared: weight (kg)/height squared (m2). It can also be calculated by multiplying a patient's weight in kilograms by 704.5, and dividing the result by the patient's height in inches twice. BMI measurements are a guideline to categorize weight in a more specific manner than relying solely on outdated "overweight" or "obesity" terminology.

Obesity is epidemic in the United States. It is more common among women than among men and more common among African-Americans than Caucasians. Obesity occurs when caloric intake chronically outpaces the energy required. Obesity puts patients at risk for diabetes, hypertension, and coronary artery disease.

278.00	Obesity, unspecified — (Use additional code to identify Body Mass Index (BMI), if known: V85.0-V85.54) — *not elsewhere classified* AHA: Q1, 1999, 5,6; Q4, 2001, 42; Q4, 2005, 97
278.01	Morbid obesity — (Use additional code to identify Body Mass Index (BMI), if known: V85.0-V85.54) — *100 pounds or more over normal body weight* AHA: Q3, 2003, 6-8; Q2, 2006, 5; Q4, 2005, 97
278.02	Overweight — (Use additional code to identify Body Mass Index (BMI), if known: V85.0-V85.54) AHA: Q4, 2005, 55; Q4, 2005, 97
278.1	Localized adiposity — (Use additional code to identify any associated mental retardation) — *fat pad* AHA: Q2, 2006, 10
278.2	Hypervitaminosis A — (Use additional code to identify any associated mental retardation)
278.3	Hypercarotinemia — (Use additional code to identify any associated mental retardation) — *elevated blood carotene levels due to ingestion of excessive amounts of carotenoids or from an inability to convert carotenoids to vitamin A*
278.4	Hypervitaminosis D — (Use additional code to identify any associated mental retardation) — *ingestion of an excessive amount of vitamin D resulting in weakness, fatigue, loss of weight, and other symptoms.*
278.8	Other hyperalimentation — (Use additional code to identify any associated mental retardation) —

cardiopulmonary obesity syndrome, Pickwickian syndrome

279 Disorders involving the immune mechanism

279.00 Unspecified hypogammaglobulinemia — (Use additional code to identify any associated mental retardation) — *abnormally low levels of immunoglobulins in the blood; agammaglobulinemia or antibody deficiency syndrome*

279.01 Selective IgA immunodeficiency — (Use additional code to identify any associated mental retardation)

279.02 Selective IgM immunodeficiency — (Use additional code to identify any associated mental retardation)

279.03 Other selective immunoglobulin deficiencies — (Use additional code to identify any associated mental retardation) — *selective deficiency of IgG*

279.04 Congenital hypogammaglobulinemia — (Use additional code to identify any associated mental retardation) — *Bruton's type, x-linked agammaglobulinemia, congenital antibody deficiency syndrome*

279.05 Immunodeficiency with increased IgM — (Use additional code to identify any associated mental retardation) — *autosomal recessive and x-linked immunodeficiency with hyper-IgM*

279.06 Common variable immunodeficiency — (Use additional code to identify any associated mental retardation) — *dysgammaglobulinemia and hypogammaglobulinemia*

279.09 Other deficiency of humoral immunity — (Use additional code to identify any associated mental retardation) — *transient hypogammaglobulinemia of infancy*

279.10 Unspecified immunodeficiency with predominant T-cell defect — (Use additional code to identify any associated mental retardation)

279.11 DiGeorge's syndrome — (Use additional code to identify any associated mental retardation) — *pharyngeal pouch syndrome and thymic hypoplasia*

279.12 Wiskott-Aldrich syndrome — (Use additional code to identify any associated mental retardation) — *eczema-thrombocytopenia syndrome*

279.13 Nezelof's syndrome — (Use additional code to identify any associated mental retardation) — *cellular immunodeficiency with abnormal immunoglobulin deficiency*

279.19 Other deficiency of cell-mediated immunity — (Use additional code to identify any associated mental retardation) — *not elsewhere classified*

279.2 Combined immunity deficiency — (Use additional code to identify any associated mental retardation) — *agammaglobulinemia; severe combined immunodeficiency [SCID]; thymic alymphoplasia, aplasia or dysplasia with immunodeficiency*

279.3 Unspecified immunity deficiency — (Use additional code to identify any associated mental retardation)

279.4 Autoimmune disease, not elsewhere classified — (Use additional code to identify any associated mental retardation) — *not elsewhere classified*

279.8 Other specified disorders involving the immune mechanism — (Use additional code to identify any associated mental retardation) — *single complement [C1-C9] deficiency or dysfunction, hypocomplementemia*

279.9 Unspecified disorder of immune mechanism — (Use additional code to identify any associated mental retardation)

Coding Clarification

Transplant failure or rejection is classified to the rubric 996 rather than to this rubric.

280–289

Diseases of the Blood and Blood-Forming Organs

This chapter classifies diseases and disorders of blood and blood-forming (hemopoietic) organs, including anemias, coagulation defects, purpura and other hemorrhagic conditions, diseases of white blood cells, other diseases of blood, and blood-forming organs.

Bone marrow is the principal site for hemopoietic cell proliferation and differentiation. One of the largest organs in the human body, hemopoietic tissue is responsible for producing erythrocytes (red blood cells), neutrophils, eosinophils, basophils, monocytes, platelets, and lymphocytes.

The term "anemia" refers to a lower than normal erythrocyte count or level of hemoglobin in the circulating blood. A clinical sign rather than a diagnostic entity, anemia can be classified by three morphological variations of the erythrocyte: size (volume), hemoglobin content, and shape. These variations give clinicians clues to the specific type of anemia.

In laboratory blood tests, erythrocyte size is gauged by estimating the volume of red cells in the circulating blood. Red cell volume, or mean corpuscular volume, is estimated by dividing the patient's hematocrit (percentage of red blood cells in whole blood) by the red blood cell (count) (RBC). Normal values are normocytic, abnormally low values are microcytic, and abnormally high values are macrocytic.

Hemoglobin content refers to the average amount of hemoglobin in each red blood cell. This value, called the mean cell hemoglobin, is calculated by dividing the patient's hemoglobin by the number of red blood cells. Normal values are normochromic, less than normal values are hypochromic, and greater than normal values are hyperchromic.

Shape is determined by microscopy. Normally, red blood cells have a smooth concave shape.

Erythrocytes with irregular shapes are called poikilocytes, a general term meaning abnormally shaped. Terms referring to specific abnormal cell shapes include acanthocytes, leptocytes, nucleated erythrocytes, macro-ovalocytes, schistocytes, helmet cells, teardrop cells, sickle cells, and target cells.

Once the cell morphology is determined, the anemia can be further classified based on certain physiological and pathological criteria. For example, constitutional aplastic anemia (284.0) is classified physiologically as an anemia of hypoproliferation and pathologically as inborn error of heredity.

The term "coagulation defect" refers to deficiencies or disorders of hemostasis. A complicated process involving substances in the injured tissues, formed elements of blood (platelets, monocytes), and the coagulation proteins, coagulation requires the production of thrombin, a substance that stabilizes the platelet plug and forms the fibrin clot. Together, they mechanically block the extravasation of blood from ruptured vessels.

The coagulation process can be interrupted by a genetic or disease-caused protein deficiency, by an increase in the catabolism of coagulation proteins, or by antibodies directed against the coagulation proteins. There are many proteins involved in coagulation, many of which are identified by the term "factor" followed by a Roman numeral. The appropriate Roman numeral followed by the suffix "a" indicates the activated form of a coagulation factor. For example, when the protein Factor II (prothrombin) is activated by the enzyme thrombin, it is designated Factor IIa.

The term "purpura" refers to a condition characterized by hemorrhage, or extravasation of blood, into the tissues, producing bruises and small red patches on the skin. Purpura may be associated with thrombocytopenia or can occur in a nonthrombocytopenic form. Thrombocytopenia is a decrease of the number of platelets in the circulating blood and may be primary (hereditary or idiopathic) or secondary to a known cause.

Diseases of white blood cells refers to increases, decreases, or genetic or idiopathic anomalies of white blood cells not associated with malignant disease classified to categories 200-208.

Excluded from this rubric is anemia complicating pregnancy and the puerperium, classified to category 648.2x.

280 Iron deficiency anemias

Classified to this rubric are chronic hypochromic and microcytic anemias characterized by small, pale erythrocytes and a depletion of iron stores. In adults, iron deficiency anemia is almost always due to blood loss, with loss of as little as 2-4 ml of blood per day enough to deplete iron stores. This condition also is known as hypoferric anemia, hypochromic or microcytic anemia, and chlorosis.

Signs and symptoms of iron deficiency anemias include pallor, lassitude, somnolence, pica, pagophagia, vertigo, headache, tinnitus, behavioral changes, dyspnea, palpitations, anginal chest pains, and brittle hair and nails. Blood work shows hypochromia, microcytosis, and erythrocyte count less reduced than hemoglobin, serum ferritin below 12 ng/ml, low serum iron, and increased total iron-binding capacity. Bone marrow biopsy shows absence of hemosiderin. Associated conditions include Plummer-Vinson syndrome, glossitis, cheilosis, and koilonychia. Therapies include iron supplementation, either dietary (ferrous sulfate, ferrous gluconate) or parenteral (iron dextran, such as Imferon or similar agent), and blood or blood product transfusion in severe cases.

280.0 Iron deficiency anemia secondary to blood loss (chronic) — *normocytic anemia due to blood loss*
AHA: Q4, 1993, 34

Subcategory 280.0 classifies iron deficiency anemia due to prolonged blood loss, usually from a chronically bleeding lesion in the gastrointestinal tract, such as a gastric ulcer or diverticulitis, or a urologic or gynecologic site.

Signs and symptoms of iron deficiency anemias secondary to blood loss (chronic) include history of a chronically bleeding lesion, pallor, lassitude, somnolence, pica, pagophagia, vertigo, headache, tinnitus, behavioral changes, dyspnea, palpitations, anginal chest pains, and brittle hair and nails. Guaiac test reveals occult bleeding. Blood work shows hypochromia, microcytosis, erythrocyte count less reduced than hemoglobin, serum ferritin below 12 ng/ml, low serum iron, and increased total iron-binding capacity. Bone marrow biopsy shows absence of hemosiderin. Therapies include endoscopy to determine the bleeding site, iron supplementation, either dietary (ferrous sulfate, ferrous gluconate) or parenteral (iron dextran, such as Imferon or similar agent), and blood or blood product transfusion in severe cases.

Coding Clarification
Excluded from this rubric are acute posthemorrhagic anemia (285.1) and familial microcytic anemia (282.4).

280.1 Iron deficiency anemia secondary to inadequate dietary iron intake — *dietary anemia*

Subcategory 280.1 classifies iron deficiency anemia due to excretion of iron that exceeds normal dietary intake. Iron is recycled metabolically so that less than 1 milligram is lost through excretion per day. A normal diet consists of 12-15 mg of iron, of which 0.6-1.5 mg are absorbed. Neonates and young children may develop iron deficiency anemia due to new blood formation and increased iron utilization that exceeds dietary intake.

280.8 Other specified iron deficiency anemias — *Paterson-Kelly syndrome, Plummer-Vinson syndrome, Waldenström-Kjellberg syndrome; sideropenic dysphagia*

Subcategory 280.8 classifies iron deficiency anemias of other specified types and causes, such as gastrectomy, excessive blood donation, and upper small-bowel malabsorption syndromes.

280.9 Unspecified iron deficiency anemia — *achlorhydric, chlorotic, idiopathic hypochromic Witt's anemias; sideropenia, Hayem-Faber syndrome*

Use subcategory 280.9 only when other, more specific codes are not appropriate. Typically classified to 280.9 are microcytic or hypochromic anemias, not otherwise specified and iron deficiency anemia due to impaired iron absorption, not otherwise specified.

281 Other deficiency anemias

281.0 Pernicious anemia — *chronic progressive anemia caused by failure to absorb vitamin B12; Addison's anemia, Biermer's anemia; Dana-Putnam syndrome, Lichtheim's syndrome, Runeberg's disease*
AHA: Nov-Dec, 1984, 1; Sept-Oct, 1984, 16

Use subcategory 281.0 to report chronic, progressive anemia of vitamin B12 deficiency due to an absorption defect. Also known as Addison or Biermer anemia, it rarely occurs before the fourth decade of life. The condition may be due to an inherited genetic defect characterized by a deficiency of intrinsic factor, a substance essential for B12 absorption.

Signs and symptoms of pernicious anemia include anorexia, dyspepsia, pallor with trace of jaundice, weakness, numbness and tingling of extremities, gingival bleeding, and a smooth sore tongue. Blood work reveals oval macrocytes, pancytopenia, hypersegmented neutrophils, elevated serum gastrin, elevated LDH, high serum iron, and absent haptoglobin. Gastric analysis shows no free gastric acid, and reveals a pH above 7. Schilling test measures absorption of vitamin B12. Bone marrow aspiration and analysis shows bone marrow to be megaloblastic. Therapies include parenteral vitamin B12.

281.1 Other vitamin B12 deficiency anemia — *vegan's anemia; selective vitamin B12 malabsorption with proteinuria; Imerslund's syndrome, Imerslund-Gräsbeck syndrome*

Use subcategory 281.1 only when other, more specific codes are not appropriate. Clinical vitamin B12 deficiency may be caused by dietary deficiency, gastrectomy, regional ileitis, diseases of malformation involving the ileum, ileum resection, and fish tapeworm disease.

281.2 Folate-deficiency anemia — (Use additional E code to identify drug) — *congenital, dietary, drug-induced, Zuelzer-Ogden syndrome*

Use subcategory 281.2 to report anemia due to deficient stores of folic acid (pteroylmonoglutamic acid), a water-soluble B complex vitamin essential for cell growth and reproduction. Folate is a salt of folic acid.

Signs and symptoms of folate-deficiency anemia include history of poor nourishment or alcoholism, weight loss, glossitis, and a blunt masklike face. Blood work reveals low serum folate levels, decreased red cell folate levels, and peripheral blood smear shows megaloblastic anemia. Therapies include oral or parenteral folic acid.

Associated conditions include nontropical sprue, malabsorption syndrome, alcoholism, and complicated pregnancy.

Folate deficiency can be the result of drug therapy. If a drug causes the folate deficiency anemia, use an additional E code to identify that drug.

281.3 Other specified megaloblastic anemias not elsewhere classified — *predominance of megaloblasts in bone marrow with few normoblasts; combined B12 and folate-deficiency anemia*

281.4 Protein-deficiency anemia — *amino-acid-deficiency anemia*

281.8 Anemia associated with other specified nutritional deficiency — *scorbutic anemia and achrestic anemia*

281.9 Unspecified deficiency anemia

282 Hereditary hemolytic anemias

282.0 Hereditary spherocytosis — *genetic hemolytic anemia characterized by jaundice, splenomegaly, and abnormally fragile sphere-shaped erythrocytes; acholuric (familial) jaundice; congenital hemolytic anemia (spherocytic); congenital spherocytosis; Minkowski-Chauffard syndrome; spherocytosis (familial)*

282.1 Hereditary elliptocytosis — *genetic hemolytic anemia characterized by an excessive proportion of abnormally fragile rod-shaped erythrocytes; elliptocytosis, ovalocytosis, Dresbach's syndrome*

282.2 Anemias due to disorders of glutathione metabolism — *6-phosphogluconic dehydrogenase deficiency; drug-induced enzyme deficiency; erythrocytic glutathione deficiency; glucose-6-phosphate dehydrogenase [G-6-PD] deficiency; disorder of pentose phosphate pathway; favism*

282.3 Other hemolytic anemias due to enzyme deficiency — *hemolytic nonspherocytic (hereditary), type II; hexokinase deficiency; pyruvate kinase [PK] deficiency; triosephosphate isomerase deficiency*

282.4 ✓5th Thalassemias — *hereditary anemias characterized by impaired or decreased synthesis of the polypeptide chains of hemoglobin, occurring primarily in Mediterranean or Southeast Asian populations*
AHA: Q4, 2003, 51

282.41 Sickle-cell thalassemia without crisis — *inheritance of a sickle gene from one parent and a gene for either hemoglobin C or beta-thalassemia from the other parent*

282.42 Sickle-cell thalassemia with crisis — (Use additional code for type of crisis: 289.52, 517.3) — *inheritance of a sickle gene from one parent and a gene for either hemoglobin C or beta-thalassemia from the other parent*

Coding Clarification
Sickled cells interfere with oxygen transport, obstructing capillary blood flow. Acidosis, dehydration, and/or decreased prevailing oxygen may bring on a crisis. Crises are attacks of pain that affect any part of the body, without warning, lasting hours or days. Carriers may have frequent infections and high fevers.

282.49 Other thalassemia — *thalassemia minor- one inherited gene thalassemia major - two inherited gene trait Cooley's anemia, erythroblastic anemia, Dameshek's syndrome, erythroblastic anemia, high fetal gene thalassemia, hemoglobin thalassemia, Mediterranean* disease, anemia or syndrome, microdrepanocytosis, mixed hemoglobinopathy, hereditary leptocytosis, Lepore hemoglobin syndrome, Rietti-Greppi- Micheli syndrome, Hb-Bart's disease, Hb-S disease, silvestroni-Bianco syndrome

Coding Clarification
The severity, treatment, and prognosis of thalassemia depend on the globin gene arrangement and deletion type. Thalassemia major, the most severe form, is evident soon after birth and requires lifelong blood transfusions. Life expectancy rarely exceeds the second decade.

282.5	Sickle-cell trait — Hb-AS genotype

Coding Clarification
This subcategory reports a heterozygous carrier of both the hemoglobin S and hemoglobin A genes. The condition rarely is associated with a clinical disorder. Couples in which both individuals carry the sickle-cell trait should be counseled about the possibility of having a child with sickle-cell disease.

Excluded from this subcategory is sickle-cell trait with other hemoglobinopathy (282.60-282.69) or that with thalassemia (282.4x).

Sickle-cell anemia is a severe, chronic, and incurable form of anemia occurring in patients who inherit hemoglobin S genes from both their parents. Less severe variations of the disease occur when the patient inherits one hemoglobin S gene from one parent and one hemoglobin C, D, or E gene from the other.

Signs and symptoms of sickle-cell anemia include joint pain, fever, lethargy, weakness, and splenomegaly. Blood work reveals a hematocrit of 20 to 30 percent, a hemoglobin of 6.5-10 g/dl, and a reticulocyte count markedly elevated at 10 to 25 percent. Microscopic exam of erythrocytes reveals characteristic "sickling" deformity. Screening tests, such as sodium metabisulfite test and dithionite solubility test, detect sickle-cell anemia or trait. Hemoglobin electrophoresis or chromatography reveal specific hemoglobin abnormalities such as hemoglobin S. Therapies include IV hydration, analgesics for pain, oxygen for hypoxemia, antibiotics for concomitant infection, blood transfusions, and experimental drugs, such as hydroxyurea, to induce fetal hemoglobin synthesis.

Associated conditions include frequent concomitant infections, dehydration, peripheral vaso-occlusion, and multisystem involvement, e.g., bone (aseptic necrosis), spleen (splenic infarction), pulmonary (pneumonia), neurological (cerebral ischemia), and ophthalmic (retinopathy).

Sickle-cell crisis refers to recurring acute episodes of pain involving any body system, but usually the chest, bones, or abdomen. In children, vaso-occlusive crisis is the most common form, although the term "sickle-cell crisis" may refer to any one of a variety of sudden and potentially serious conditions.

Excluded from this subcategory are sickle-cell thalassemia (282.4x) and sickle-cell trait (282.5).

282.60	Sickle-cell disease, unspecified
282.61	Hb-SS disease without crisis — Herrick's syndrome
282.62	Hb-SS disease with crisis — (Use additional code for type of crisis: 289.52, 517.3) — acute abdominal pain, arthralgia, and leg ulcers in sickle cell anemia; atrophy of the spleen may occur with increased susceptibility to bacterial infection; sickle-cell crisis
	AHA: Q2, 1991, 15; Q2, 1998, 8; Q4, 2003, 56
282.63	Sickle-cell/Hb-C disease without crisis — Hb-S/Hb-C disease without crisis
282.64	Sickle-cell/Hb-C disease with crisis — (Use additional code for type of crisis: 289.52, 517.3) — Sickled cells interfere with oxygen transport, obstructing capillary blood flow, fever, severe pain in joints and abdomen. Acidosis, dehydration and/or decreased prevailing oxygen may bring on a crisis. Hb-S/Hb-C disease with crisis, Sickle-cell/Hb-C disease with vaso-occlusive pain
	AHA: Q4, 2003, 51
282.68	Other sickle-cell disease without crisis — Hb-S/Hb-D disease without crisis, Hb-S/Hb-E disease without crisis, Sickle-cell/Hb-D disease without crisis, Sickle-cell/Hb-E disease without crisis
	AHA: Q4, 2003, 51
282.69	Other sickle-cell disease with crisis — (Use additional code for type of crisis: 289.52, 517.3) — Hb-S/Hb-D with crisis; Hb-S/Hb-E with crisis. Other sickle-cell disease with vaso-occlusive pain, sickle-cell/Hb-D disease with crisis, sickle-cell/Hb-E disease with crisis
282.7	Other hemoglobinopathies — congenital Heinz-body anemia; hemoglobin C [Hb-C], hemoglobin D [Hb-D], hemoglobin E [Hb-E], hemoglobin Zurich [Hb-Zurich]

Coding Clarification
Excluded from this subgroup are familial polycythemia (289.6), hemoglobin M (Hb-M) disease (289.7), and high-oxygen-affinity hemoglobin (289.0).

282.8	Other specified hereditary hemolytic anemias — stomatocytosis
282.9	Unspecified hereditary hemolytic anemia

Diseases of the Blood and Blood-Forming Organs

283 Acquired hemolytic anemias
AHA: Nov-Dec, 1984, 1

This rubric reports anemia characterized by the premature destruction of erythrocytes, exclusive of an inherited erythrocyte disorder. Hemolytic anemias may be acquired through infection, injury, drugs, blood transfusions (autoimmune), or other intrinsic or extrinsic causes. Hemolytic uremic syndrome (hemolytic anemia and thrombocytopenia occurring with acute renal failure) is a common manifestation of nonautoimmune hemolytic anemia.

283.0	Autoimmune hemolytic anemias — (Use additional E code to identify cause, if drug-induced) — *hemolytic anemia: cold, warm, or drug-induced* AHA: Nov-Dec, 1984, 1
283.10	Unspecified non-autoimmune hemolytic anemia — (Use additional E code to identify cause)
283.11	Hemolytic-uremic syndrome — (Use additional E code to identify cause)
283.19	Other non-autoimmune hemolytic anemias — (Use additional E code to identify cause) — *mechanical, microangiopathic, toxic; erythrocyte fragmentation syndrome, Lederer-Brill syndromes* AHA: Nov-Dec, 1984, 1; Q4, 1993, 25
283.2	Hemoglobinuria due to hemolysis from external causes — (Use additional E code to identify cause) — *acute intravascular hemolysis; hemoglobinuria from exertion or due to hemolysis; Marchiafava-Micheli syndrome, Murri's disease* AHA: Nov-Dec, 1984, 1
283.9	Acquired hemolytic anemia, unspecified

Coding Clarification
Use an additional E code to identify the cause, as appropriate. Excluded from this rubric are Evan's syndrome (287.32) and hemolytic disease of newborn (773.0-773.5).

284 Aplastic anemia and other bone marrow failure syndromes
AHA: Nov-Dec, 1984, 1; Sept-Oct, 1984, 16; Q1, 1991, 14

This rubric reports failure of bone marrow to generate blood cells, resulting in a deficiency of all of the formed elements of the blood (erythrocytes, platelets, and leukocytes).

The aplastic anemias include various bone marrow disorders. Constitutional red blood cell aplasia, also known as constitutional pure red cell aplasia or CPRCA, is a syndrome of failed erythropoiesis (formation of red blood cells), and is most often diagnosed within the first year of life. Also known as Blackfan-Diamond syndrome, this is a rare idiopathic blood disorder that is present at birth and distinguished by red blood cell deficiency. Other symptoms and physical findings vary greatly from case to case but may include slow growth, atypical weakness and fatigue, pallor, distinctive facial abnormalities, protruding scapulae, abnormal shortening or webbing of the neck caused by fusion of cervical vertebrae, hand malformations, and congenital heart defects. Blackfan-Diamond syndrome may be inherited as either an autosomal dominant or recessive genetic trait. Diagnosed by blood tests and bone marrow biopsy, treatment includes transfusions and bone marrow transplantation.

Other forms of constitutional aplastic anemia include Fanconi anemia (FA), which is the most frequently reported of the rare inherited bone marrow failure syndromes. Symptoms of bone marrow failure, which is the major cause of death in FA, often present during childhood and include easy bruising, petechiae, thrombocytopenia, fatigue, and paleness caused by anemia, and infections due to neutropenia. Pancytopenia due to aplastic anemia occurs in over 90 percent of patients with Fanconi anemia and is often fatal. Leukemia, myelodysplastic syndrome, and solid tumors are also associated with Fanconi anemia. Age of diagnosis has ranged from birth to 48 years, with a median age of 7 to 8 years. The majority of patients have characteristic birth defects, such as hyper- or hypopigmented skin, short stature, musculoskeletal abnormalities, gonadal anomalies, microencephaly, eye/ear abnormalities, and systemic defects. Diagnostic tools include CBC, flow cytometry, specific imaging studies, molecular diagnostic approaches, and bone marrow biopsy. Treatment options include stem cell transplant, blood transfusions, androgenic agents, granulocyte colony-stimulating factor (G-CSF), and corticosteroids. Surgical treatment is often required for associated musculoskeletal, cardiovascular, or gastrointestinal abnormalities.

Although the majority of aplastic anemias include a component of pancytopenia, which is a reduction in all cell types, pancytopenia can also be caused by other factors, including vitamin B12 or folate deficiency, systemic lupus erythematosus, paroxysmal nocturnal hemoglobinuria, severe infections, brucellosis, sarcoidosis, pregnancy, Fanconi's anemia, primary bone marrow disorders, or splenic disorders. Symptoms may include weakness, fatigue, bleeding or easy bruising, splenomegaly, or lymphadenopathy. Diagnostic tools include CBC, peripheral blood smears, and bone marrow biopsy. Treatment may include transfusions or stem cell transplant.

Myelophthisis is also known as leukoerythroblastic anemia or myelophthisic anemia. The most common underlying causes of myelophthisis include metastatic carcinomas, lymphoma, granulomatous diseases such as miliary tuberculosis, and rare disorders such as Gaucher disease. Fungal infections, sarcoidosis, sickle cell disease, septicemia, and congenital osteopetrosis may also be causative factors. Observed more frequently in countries where access to medical care is not readily available and diseases are more likely to progress to advanced stages, in the United States this disorder occurs most commonly during the advanced stages of cancer. Outcome is highly dependent upon the patient's access to medical care.

Physical findings will usually reflect the underlying disease process. Symptoms may also include pallor, petechiae or ecchymoses, fever, and various infective processes. Diagnostic workup is focused on establishing this underlying condition and may consist of blood tests, imaging studies, and bone marrow aspiration and biopsy. Treatment is diverse and directed toward the underlying disease. Anemia is treated with blood transfusions, and patients with low erythropoietin levels may respond to supplemental erythropoietin therapy.

Associated conditions include concomitant infections.

284.01	Constitutional red blood cell aplasia — Blackfan-Diamond syndrome; familial hypoplastic anemia; congenital red cell aplasia; primary red cell aplasia; red cell aplasia of infants; congenital erythropoiesis
284.09	Other constitutional aplastic anemia — Fanconi's anemia; pancytopenia with malformations; congenital bone marrow absence; hereditary bone marrow absence
	AHA: Nov-Dec, 1984, 1; Sept-Oct, 1984, 16; Q1, 1991, 14

Coding Clarification
Constitutional aplastic anemia is an inherited form of aplastic anemia, both planocellular and unicellular. The etiology is believed to be a fundamental intrinsic abnormality of the stem cells.

284.1	Pancytopenia
284.2	Myelophthisis — (Code first the underlying disorder) — leukoerythroblastic anemia; myelophthisic anemia
284.8	Other specified aplastic anemias — (Use additional E code to identify cause) — aplastic

anemias due to drugs, infection, radiation, toxins, infections, chronic system disease
AHA: Nov-Dec, 1984, 1; Sept-Oct, 1984, 16; March-April, 1985, 14; Q1, 1991, 14; Q1, 1992, 15; Q1, 1997, 5; Q3, 2005, 11

Coding Clarification
When the underlying cause for pancytopenia (284.1) is determined, assign the code for the underlying condition and do not assign 284.1 since the pancytopenia is considered an integral part of the underlying condition. If no underlying condition is identified and the diagnosis is pancytopenia (acquired) and not otherwise specified, assign code 284.1.

Congenital pancytopenia is considered a constitutional aplastic anemia, 284.09.

Code 284.2 *Myelophthisis* is a new code and contains the instruction to code the underlying disease first. The etiology/manifestation mandatory dual coding convention applies. Myelophthisis is bone marrow suppression and is a manifestation of the underlying condition. Code the underlying condition first followed by the code for myelophthisis. Code 284.2 should never be sequenced first or reported alone.

Note that the exclusion terms send coders in the appropriate code assignment of various forms of myelofibrosis.

Subcategory 284.8 reports acquired or secondary forms of aplastic anemia. Etiologies include radiation, chronic systemic disease, infections, drugs, toxic chemicals, and red cell aplasia secondary to thymoma.

284.9	Unspecified aplastic anemia

285 Other and unspecified anemias
AHA: Nov-Dec, 1984, 1; Q1, 1991, 14

285.0	Sideroblastic anemia — (Use additional E code to identify cause, if drug-induced) — *pyridoxine-responsive anemia, sideroblastic anemia, sideroblastic hypochromic with iron loading anemia*
	AHA: Nov-Dec, 1984, 1; Q1, 1991, 14
285.1	Acute posthemorrhagic anemia — *secondary to acute blood loss*
	AHA: Nov-Dec, 1984, 1; Q1, 1991, 14; Q2, 1992, 15

Coding Clarification
Refractory sideroblastic anemia is not reported with code 285.0; rather, it is reported with code 238.72.

Code 285.1 reports anemia due to frank, rapid blood loss. The etiology may be trauma, spontaneous rupture of a blood vessel, surgical procedures involving major blood vessels, pathology such as bleeding peptic ulcers or neoplasms, or extravasation secondary to a bleeding diathesis such as hemophilia. The anemia is usually normochromic and normocytic in an otherwise healthy patient; blood cells can show morphological changes indicative of other concomitant forms of anemia since the condition can occur with any other form of anemia.

Signs and symptoms of acute posthemorrhagic anemia include faintness, dizziness, thirst, weakness, rapid pulse, rapid respirations, orthostatic changes in blood pressure, and hypovolemic shock. Blood work during and immediately after the hemorrhage may reveal high erythrocyte, hemoglobin, and hematocrit levels due to vasoconstriction. Within a few hours, blood work shows evidence of hemodilution with abnormally low blood indices, polymorphonuclear leukocytosis, and increased thrombocyte production.

Therapies include rapid identification of the bleeding site and establishment of hemostasis, blood transfusions and IV hydration to restore blood volume, iron supplementation, and monitoring for hypovolemic shock.

Postoperative blood loss anemia due to an expected blood loss integral to a procedure, does not qualify for coding to 285.1. The physician must document anemia as a complication of the surgery to support coding/reporting.

Associated conditions include angina and hypovolemic shock. Excluded from this rubric is anemia due to chronic blood loss or not specified as acute blood loss (280.0).

Report these codes in conjunction with codes describing the underlying disease as chronic kidney disease, neoplastic disease, or other chronic illness. Sequencing of the codes depends on the presenting patient complaint and clinical circumstances.

Anemia of chronic disease is often the primary reason and focus of a health care encounter. When the anemia is the reason for the encounter and treatment is directed at the anemia rather than the underlying condition, the anemia of chronic disease code (285.22-285.29) is sequenced first, and the code for the underlying condition should also be assigned. This advice supersedes previous advice for coding anemia of chronic disease. Coding anemia due to chemotherapy or antineoplastic treatment follows previous coding guidelines.

285.21	Anemia in chronic kidney disease — *anemia in end stage renal disease [ESRD]* **AHA:** Nov-Dec, 1984, 1; Q1, 1991, 14; Q4, 2000, 39
285.22	Anemia in neoplastic disease — *secondary to neoplastic disease* **AHA:** Nov-Dec, 1984, 1; Q1, 1991, 14; Q4, 2000, 39
285.29	Anemia of other chronic disease — *secondary to other chronic illness* **AHA:** Nov-Dec, 1984, 1; Q1, 1991, 14; Q4, 2000, 39
285.8	Other specified anemias — *not elsewhere classified, von Jaksch's anemia, and Brühl's disease; dyserythropoietic anemia, infantile pseudoleukemia* **AHA:** Nov-Dec, 1984, 1; Q1, 1991, 14; Q1, 1991, 16
285.9	Unspecified anemia

Coding Clarification

Use code 285.9 to report normochromic, normocytic anemia of unspecified type, including anemia of chronic disease characterized by shortened red cell survival, suboptimal marrow compensation (sometimes referred to as "relative marrow failure"), defective reutilization of iron, and, occasionally, reduced production of erythropoietin. Such anemias normally do not require treatment unless other characteristics develop, such as iron deficiency anemia (code 280.9) or folic acid deficiency anemia (code 281.2).

Excluded from this rubric are anemias due to chronic blood loss (280.0) or iron deficiency anemia (280.0-280.9).

286 Coagulation defects

Use an additional E code if the coagulation defect is drug induced.

286.0	Congenital factor VIII disorder — *abnormal coagulation characterized by subcutaneous and intramuscular hemorrhage and caused by a mutant gene on the X chromosome; classical, familial, hereditary hemophilia A*
286.1	Congenital factor IX disorder — *abnormality of coagulation characterized by subcutaneous and intramuscular hemorrhage and caused by a mutant gene on the X chromosome; Christmas disease, hemophilia B*
286.2	Congenital factor XI deficiency — *Rosenthal's disease; hemophilia C*
286.3	Congenital deficiency of other clotting factors — *congenital afibrinogenemia; Owren's disease, Stuart-Prower disease; dysfibrinogenemia, parahemophilia*
286.4	Von Willebrand's disease — *angiohemophilia (A) (B); factor VIII deficiency with vascular defect*

286.5	Hemorrhagic disorder due to intrinsic circulating anticoagulants — (Use additional E code to identify cause, if drug-induced) — *acquired abnormality of coagulation caused by presence of tissue factor activity (TFA) which initiates coagulation. Manifestation may be blood clot formation (subacute) or serious bleeding (acute)* **AHA:** Q3, 1990, 14; Q3, 1992, 15		287.30	Primary thrombocytopenia, unspecified — *reduced number of platelets in the circulating blood as the principle disease or condition; megakaryocytic hypoplasia* **AHA:** Q1, 1991, 14; Q4, 2005, 56
286.6	Defibrination syndrome — *consumption coagulopathy; disseminated intravascular coagulation [DIC syndrome], ICF syndrome, IVC syndrome; pathologic fibrinolysis* **AHA:** Q4, 1993, 29		287.31	Immune thrombocytopenic purpura — idiopathic thrombocytopenic purpura, tidal platelet dysgenesis **AHA:** Q4, 2005, 56, 57
			287.32	Evans' syndrome **AHA:** Q4, 2005, 56
286.7	Acquired coagulation factor deficiency — (Use additional E code to identify cause, if drug-induced) — *deficiency of coagulation factor due to liver disease or vitamin K deficiency* **AHA:** Q4, 1993, 29		287.33	Congenital and hereditary thrombocytopenic purpura — congenital and hereditary thrombocytopenic purpura, thrombocytopenia with absent radii (TAR) syndrome **AHA:** Q4, 2005, 56
286.9	Other and unspecified coagulation defects — *delay in coagulation or hemostasis disorder* **AHA:** Q4, 1993, 29; Q4, 1999, 22		287.39	Other primary thrombocytopenia — Kasabach-Merritt syndrome, thrombopenia-hemangioma syndrome, Werlhof-Wichmann syndrome **AHA:** Q4, 2005, 56

287 Purpura and other hemorrhagic conditions
AHA: Q1, 1991, 14

Excluded from this rubric are hemorrhagic thrombocythemia (238.79) and purpura fulminans (286.6).

287.0	Allergic purpura — *small hemorrhage into the skin, mucous membrane, or serosal surface caused by sensitization to foods, drugs, insect bites; peliosis rheumatica rheumataica; Schönlein-Henoch purpura* **AHA:** Q1, 1991, 14

The definition of allergic purpura is acute and chronic vasculitis. Also known as anaphylactoid purpura and Schönlein-Henoch purpura, allergic purpura affects small vessels of the skin, joints, gastrointestinal tract, and kidneys.

Signs and symptoms of allergic purpura include a rash on the extensor surfaces of the arms, legs, and feet and across the buttocks, fever, polyarthralgia, tenderness and swelling of joints, edema of the hands and feet, colicky abdominal pain, tenderness, melena, hematuria, and proteinuria. Therapies include corticosteroids to control edema and joint and abdominal pain, as well as eliminating the offending drug.

Excluded from this subgroup are hemorrhagic purpura (287.39) and purpura annularis telangiectodes (709.1).

287.1	Qualitative platelet defects — *thrombasthenia; thrombocytasthenia, and Bernard-Soulier thrombopathy* **AHA:** Q1, 1991, 14
287.2	Other nonthrombocytopenic purpuras — *Diamond-Gardener syndrome* **AHA:** Q1, 1991, 14

Megakaryocytic hypoplasia coded to 287.30 is a form of unspecified primary thrombocytopenia in which the megakaryocytes, the cells that mature into platelets, are underdeveloped.

Evan's syndrome is autoimmune hemolytic anemia with immune thrombocytopenia, and sometimes combined with neutropenia, having no known underlying etiology, and varying in their onset, course, and duration. Spontaneous remission and exacerbation occur with autoantibodies acting against specific antigens to different blood components: red blood cells, platelets, and neutrophils. Some research suggests that patients with Evan's syndrome also have autoimmune lymphoproliferative syndrome, and decreased levels of serum immunoglobulins that may be related to T-cell abnormalities.

Thrombocytopenia with absent radius, also known as TAR syndrome, coded to 287.33, is a rare congenital abnormality that affects both blood and bone structure, specifically presenting with low platelet counts through childhood and the absence of the radius in both arms. The thumb is, however, present without the radius.

Tidal platelet dysgenesis, or periodic thrombocytopenia, reported with 287.31, is a rare condition in which platelet counts oscillate from normal to very low values between periods of 20 to 40 days. Many cases of this disorder involve the autoimmune destruction of circulating platelets.

Code 287.31 also reports an abnormally small number of platelets in the circulating blood as a result of increased platelet destruction without an identifiable exogenous cause or underlying disease.

Diseases of the Blood and Blood-Forming Organs

The condition, also known as idiopathic thrombocytopenia purpura (ITP), is characterized by the sudden onset of signs and symptoms.

Signs and symptoms of primary thrombocytopenia include petechiae, epistaxis, hematuria or abnormal bleeding of gums, vagina, gastrointestinal tract, and bruising easily. Blood work shows a decreased platelet count, abnormal bleeding time, normal prothrombin time (PT), and partial thromboplastin time (PTT). Bone marrow biopsy and analysis reveal increased megakaryocytes without surrounding platelets. Therapies include drugs such as corticosteroids, immunosuppressive therapy (e.g., vincristine or vinblastine) or IV immunoglobulin, splenectomy, and avoidance of any activity that would expose the patient to bleeding.

Associated conditions include fatal cerebral hemorrhage, hemorrhage of other sites, acute leukemia, macroglobulinemia, and hematoma formation occasionally causing nerve damage. Excluded from this subgroup are thrombotic thrombocytopenic purpura (446.6) and transient thrombocytopenia of newborn (776.1).

287.4	Secondary thrombocytopenia — (Use additional E code to identify cause) — *reduced number of platelets in the circulating blood as a consequence of an underlying disease or condition; posttransfusion purpura, thrombocytopenia due to drugs, extracorporeal circulation of blood, or platelet alloimmunization* **AHA:** March-April, 1985, 14; Q1, 1991, 14

This subgroup reports thrombocytopenia due to an identifiable exogenous cause or underlying condition, such as congestive splenomegaly, Felty's syndrome, Gaucher's disease, tuberculosis, sarcoidosis, myelofibrosis, lupus erythematosus, Wiskott-Aldrich syndrome, chronic alcoholism, and scurvy. It also may occur as a result of overhydration, blood transfusions, or drug therapy. Use an additional E code to identify the cause.

Coding Clarification
Transient thrombocytopenia of newborn (776.1) is not classified here.

287.5	Unspecified thrombocytopenia
287.8	Other specified hemorrhagic conditions — *capillary fragility (hereditary) and vascular pseudohemophilia* **AHA:** Q1, 1991, 14
287.9	Unspecified hemorrhagic conditions

288 Diseases of white blood cells
AHA: Q1, 1991, 14

Excluded from this rubric is leukemia, reported with codes from the series 204.0-208.9.

Subcategory 288.0 reports neutropenia. Also known as granulocytopenia or agranulocytosis, neutropenia is a condition in which the neutrophil or granulocyte count in the blood is diminished, resulting in an increased susceptibility to bacterial and fungal infections.

Neutropenia may be acute, occurring over a few days, often when the production of neutrophils is impaired, or chronic, most often arising from reduced neutrophil production or in instances in which the spleen sequesters too many neutrophils. Chronic neutropenia may last for months or years. Neutropenia may be caused by an intrinsic defect in the myeloid progenitors or it may be secondary to extrinsic factors.

Intrinsic forms may include cyclic neutropenia, which is an uncommon disorder that is present from birth and manifested by sporadic, intermittent variations in the amount of peripheral neutrophils. Kostmann's syndrome is a severe, rare, congenital disorder in which myeloid maturation is arrested. Chronic idiopathic neutropenia consists of a group of disorders involving stem cells of the myeloid series in which RBCs and platelet precursors are present in normal numbers and splenomegaly is absent.

One of the most common causes of secondary neutropenia is drugs. There are various forms of drug-induced neutropenia, including immune-mediated, toxic, idiosyncratic, or hypersensitivity. Other underlying causes of secondary neutropenia include infections such as sepsis or viral diseases. Radiotherapy, vitamin B12 deficiency, or folate deficiency, malignancy, myelodysplasia, or bone marrow failure can also result in secondary neutropenia.

Signs and symptoms of cyclic neutropenia or severe congenital neutropenia often consist of ulcers of the mouth, stomatitis, or pharyngitis associated with enlargement of the lymph nodes. Pneumonia and chronic periodontitis is often seen. Secondary neutropenia due to malignancy or chemotherapy often manifests with significant bacterial infections resulting from the compromised immune system. Pyogenic infections with fever often include cutaneous cellulitis, liver abscess, pneumonia, septicemia, or furunculosis. Inflammation of the perirectal area, colon, mouth, ears, gums, and sinuses also often occurs.

Methods of diagnosis include WBC and differential counts, bone marrow aspiration and biopsy, cytogenetic analysis, and special stains for detecting leukemia or other malignant disorders. Treatment varies based on the type and underlying cause of the neutropenia and may include antibiotics, administration of G-CSF, corticosteroids, or splenectomy.

288.00		Neutropenia, unspecified AHA: Q3, 2005, 11
288.01		Congenital neutropenia — Kostmann's syndrome; congenital agranulocytosis; infantile genetic agranulocytosis AHA: Q3, 2005, 11
288.02		Cyclic neutropenia — periodic neutropenia; cyclic hematopoiesis AHA: Q3, 2005, 11
288.03		Drug induced neutropenia — (Use additional E code to identify drug) AHA: Q3, 2005, 11
288.04		Neutropenia due to infection AHA: Q3, 2005, 11
288.09		Other neutropenia — immune neutropenia; toxic neutropenia; agranulocytosis AHA: Q1, 1991, 14; Q2, 1996, 6; Q3, 1996, 16; Q2, 1999, 9; Q3, 1999, 6; Q3, 2005, 11

Coding Clarification

Subcategory 288.0 excludes transitory neonatal neutropenia (776.7) and neutropenic splenomegaly (289.53). Any associated fever should be assigned an additional code of 780.6.

Neutropenia (288.0), previously called agranulocytosis, has a "Use additional code" note at the subcategory level as a reminder to code fever associated with the neutropenia. This instruction applies to all the codes within the subcategory. Neutropenia increases the susceptibility of the body to infection, which may cause fever, but the fever is not inherent to the neutropenia. Coding the fever is important as an indicator of the severity of the neutropenia or the compromised state of the individual. If the neutropenia is drug induced, assign the E code to identify the drug causing the condition.

288.1	Functional disorders of polymorphonuclear neutrophils — chronic childhood granulomatous disease, congenital dysphagocytosis, Job's syndrome, lipochrome histiocytosis, and progressive septic granulomatosis AHA: Q1, 1991, 14
288.2	Genetic anomalies of leukocytes — Alder's (-Reilly) syndrome, Chédiak-Steinbrinck (-Higashi) syndrome, Jordan's syndrome, May-Hegglin syndrome, Pelger-Huet syndrome; Döhle body-panmyelopathic syndrome AHA: Q1, 1991, 14

288.3	Eosinophilia — elevated proportion of a type of white blood cell readily stained with eosin; allergic, hereditary, idiopathic, secondary AHA: Q1, 1991, 14; Q3, 2000, 11

Subcategory 288.3 reports an absolute eosinophilcount of more than 500/cu ml. Counts of 500-1,000/cu ml are nonspecific and normally are not viewed as a clinical problem. Associated conditions include allergic disorders, parasitic infestation with tissue invasion, skin diseases, tumors, Hodgkin's disease, granulomatous disease, eosinophilic leukemia, fibroplastic endocarditis, systemic vasculitis, and tropical eosinophilia.

Excluded from this rubric are Loffler's syndrome and pulmonary eosinophilia (518.3).

288.4	Hemophagocytic syndromes — macrophage activation syndrome; familial hemophagocytic lymphohistiocytosis; familial hemophagocytic reticulosis; histiocytic syndrome; infection-associated hemophagocytic syndrome

Hemophagocytic syndrome, also known as infection- or virus-associated hemophagocytic syndrome (VAHS), is a secondary form of hemophagocytic lymphohistiocytosis. It is an aggressive disorder associated with systemic viral infection and is manifested by the infiltration of hemophagocytic histiocytes into the lymphoreticular tissues of multiple organs. Associated viruses include Epstein-Barr, cytomegalovirus, adenovirus, and Herpes simplex virus. Association has also been made to various nonviral infections.

The primary form of hemophagocytic lymphohistiocytosis, familial hemophagocytic lymphohistiocytosis (FHL), is thought to be a genetically transmitted disease. Affecting infants and young children, symptoms include fever, enlargement of the liver and spleen, and pancytopenia. Diagnosis may be made by laboratory analysis or biopsy of skin, lymph nodes, bone marrow, or liver. Treatment options include bone marrow transplant, IVIG, cyclosporine, or corticosteroids.

Macrophage activation syndrome (MAS) is a hemophagocytic syndrome caused by excessive creation and production of T cells and macrophages and is often a life-threatening complication of systemic-onset juvenile rheumatoid arthritis. Symptoms of MAS include prolonged fever, enlarged liver and spleen, bleeding, generalized adenomegaly, rash, and jaundice.

Coding Clarification
Because of the rare nature of hemophagocytic syndromes, all forms are included under a single new code, 288.4 *Hemophagocytic syndromes.*

288.5 ✓5th Decreased white blood cell count

A decrease in the white blood cell count may be manifested as leukocytopenia (reduction in the circulating leukocytes), lymphocytopenia (reduction in the lymphocytes in the blood), or as monocytopenia or plasmacytopenia (reduction in monocytes or plasma cells). The presence of these conditions may indicate an increased risk of infection, malignancy, myelofibrosis, or aplastic anemia, and further workup may need to be undertaken. Decreases in white blood cell counts can be detected by laboratory measurement of WBCs. Treatment is often dependent upon the underlying cause.

288.50	Leukocytopenia, unspecified — *decreased leukocytes; leukopenia; decreased WBC*
288.51	Lymphocytopenia — *decreased lymphocytes*
288.59	Other decreased white blood cell count — *plasmacytopenia; basophilic leukopenia; monocytopenia; eosinophilic leukopenia*

Coding Clarification
Subcategory 288.5 excludes neutropenia, which is reported with a code from range 288.01-288.09.

288.6 ✓5th Elevated white blood cell coun

An increase in white blood cell count may be manifested as elevated leukocytes (leukocytosis), elevated lymphocytes (lymphocytosis) or as elevations in monocytes, plasma cells, or basophils. A leukemoid reaction is a condition in which leukocytosis occurs as a physiologic response to stress or infection. The presence of these conditions may indicate acute infection, inflammation, hemorrhage, or other disease processes. Increases in white blood cell counts can be detected by laboratory measurement of WBCs. Treatment is often dependent upon the underlying cause.

288.60	Leukocytosis, unspecified — *elevated leukocytes; elevated WBC*
288.61	Lymphocytosis (symptomatic) — *elevated lymphocytes*
288.62	Leukemoid reaction — *basophilic; neutrophilic; lymphocytic; myelocytic; monocytic*
288.63	Monocytosis (symptomatic) — *excluded from this code is infectious mononucleosis (075)*
288.64	Plasmacytosis
288.65	Basophilia
288.69	Other elevated white blood cell count

Coding Clarification
Subcategory 288.6 excludes eosinophilia, which is reported with code 288.3.

288.8	Other specified disease of white blood cells **AHA:** March-April, 1987, 12; Q1, 1991, 14
288.9	Unspecified disease of white blood cells

289 Other diseases of blood and blood-forming organs

289.0 Polycythemia, secondary — *elevated number of red blood cells in the circulating blood occurring as a result to reduced oxygen supply to the tissues; Gaisböck's syndrome*

Polycythemia is an increase in the normal number of red blood cells. Secondary polycythemia is also known as secondary erythrocytosis, spurious polycythemia, and reactive polycythemia. Spurious polycythemia, which is characterized by increased hematocrit and normal or increased erythrocyte total mass, results from a decrease in plasma volume and hemoconcentration. Reactive polycythemia is a condition characterized by excessive production of circulating erythrocytes due to an identifiable secondary condition, such as hypoxia, or an underlying disease, such as a neoplasm.

Excluded from this subcategory are neonatal polycythemia (776.4) and primary polycythemia and polycythemia vera (238.4).

289.1 Chronic lymphadenitis — *persistent inflammation of one or more lymph nodes except mesenteric*

Code 289.1 reports inflammation of the lymph nodes. Any pathogen can cause lymphadenitis. Lymphadenitis may be generalized or restricted to regional lymph nodes and may occur with systemic infections. Acute lymphadenitis (683), mesenteric lymphadenitis (289.2), and enlarged glands not otherwise specified (785.6) are excluded.

289.2 Nonspecific mesenteric lymphadenitis — *inflammation of one or more lymph nodes in the peritoneal fold that encases the abdominal organs; Brennemann's syndrome*

Subcategory 289.2 reports lymphadenitis occurring in a double layer of peritoneum attached to the abdominal wall that encloses a portion or all of one of the mesentery (abdominal viscera).

289.3 Lymphadenitis, unspecified, except mesenteric — *unknown and other than mesenteric*
AHA: Q2, 1992, 8

289.4 Hypersplenism — *cellular components of blood or platelets are removed at an accelerated rate causing deficiency of peripheral blood elements; "big spleen" syndrome; hypoleukemia splenica*

This subgroup reports a clinical syndrome characterized by splenic hyperactivity and splenomegaly. The condition results in a peripheral blood cell deficiency because the spleen traps and destroys the circulating peripheral blood cells.

Signs and symptoms of hypersplenism include history of frequent infection and bruising easily, and abnormal bleeding from mucous membranes, genitourinary tract, or gastrointestinal tract. There may be ulcers of the mouth, legs, or feet, fever, weakness, and palpitations. Blood work reveals mild, normochromic, and normocytic anemia with elevated reticulocyte count and markedly decreased platelets and granulocytes. A radionuclide scan of chromium-labeled erythrocytes or platelets demonstrates increased splenic activity, while splenic angiography demonstrates portal obstruction or hypertension. A biopsy of the spleen reveals the pathology such as infiltrative disease (e.g., lymphoma, Gaucher's amyloidosis).

Therapies include medical treatment of the underlying etiology or splenectomy, if medical treatment is ineffective.

Associated conditions include recurrent infections such as persistent leg ulcers, Gaucher disease, Niemann-Pick disease, congestive cirrhosis (portal hypertension) or thrombosis, hemolytic anemia, polycythemia vera, Felty's syndrome, subacute bacterial endocarditis, Letterer-Siwe disease, tuberculosis, and cystic or neoplastic disease, such as leukemia, lymphoma, myelofibrosis, or Boeck's sarcoidosis.

Excluded from this rubric is primary splenic neutropenia (289.53).

289.50	Unspecified disease of spleen
289.51	Chronic congestive splenomegaly — *syndrome consisting of anemia, splenic enlargement, hemorrhages, cirrhosis of the liver. Banti's syndrome.*
289.52	Splenic sequestration — (Code first sickle-cell disease in crisis: 282.42, 282.62, 282.64, 282.69)
289.53	Neutropenic splenomegaly — *primary splenic neutropenia, Doan-Wiseman syndrome, neutropenic splenomegaly, splenic neutropenia syndrome, splenic neutropenia*

Coding Clarification
Neutropenic splenomegaly has been deleted from subcategory 288.0 *Neutropenia* and reclassified to subcategory 289.5 *Other diseases of spleen*. Code 289.53, specifically reports this and related conditions.

Splenomegaly is indicated when the spleen weighs 400-500 grams. A functionally diverse organ, the spleen normally weighs 150 grams, is not easily palpable, and plays an active role in immunosurveillance and hematopoiesis. As it performs its normal functions, the spleen will, in many instances, become enlarged. A wide variety of disease processes are also associated with splenic enlargement.

Neutropenia is defined as an absolute neutrophil count of less than 2,000. A portion of the marginated granulocyte pool is located in the spleen; an increase in this pool results in neutropenia. Splenic sequestration also may play a role in the origin of neutropenia; the degree of neutropenia resulting from splenic sequestration is proportional to the severity of splenomegaly and the ability of the bone marrow to make up for the reduction in circulating bands and neutrophils.

Doan-Wiseman syndrome, or primary splenic neutropenia, is distinguished by an enlarged spleen, hypercellular bone marrow, severe leukopenia and neutropenia, and susceptibility to infection; anemia and thrombocytopenia are sometimes present.

289.59	Other diseases of spleen — *fibrosis, infarct, rupture, infection, abscess, cyst, atrophy, prolapse, ptosis, torsion, splenocele, wandering spleen*
289.6	Familial polycythemia — *elevation of the number of red blood cells in the blood; benign polycythemia; erythrocytosis*
289.7	Methemoglobinemia — (Use additional E code to identify cause)

Hypercoagulable conditions are inherited and acquired disorders that predispose to venous thromboembolism.

289.81	Primary hypercoagulable state — *activated protein C resistance, antithrombin III deficiency, factor V Leiden mutation, lupus anticoagulant, protein C deficiency, protein S deficiency, prothrombin gene mutation, Antithrombin deficiency hyperhomocystinemia, elevated factor VIII levels dysfibrinogenemia, factor XII deficiency, disorders of plasmin generation*
289.82	Secondary hypercoagulable state — *pregnancy, immobility, trauma, postoperative state, use of oral contraceptives, estrogen, tamoxifen, antiphospholipid syndrome, hyperhomocystinemia, malignancy nephrotic syndrome, myeloproliferative disorders, congestive heart failure, heparin-induced thrombocytopenia with thrombosis, paroxysmal nocturnal hemoglobinuria, Beh_et's disease*
289.83	Myelofibrosis — (Code first the underlying disorder) — *not otherwise specified; secondary myelofibrosis*

Myelofibrosis is a rare disorder in which normal bone marrow is replaced by fibrous tissue. Myelofibrosis occurring as a secondary process is coded to 289.83 and may appear in various other disorders such as malignancies, infections, lipid storage disease, sarcoidosis, and osteoporosis or in individuals who have been exposed to certain toxic

Diseases of the Blood and Blood-Forming Organs

substances, such as benzene and radiation. Common symptoms include anemia, splenomegaly, and hepatomegaly. Immature red blood cells are present, and diagnosis is confirmed by bone marrow biopsy. Patients may remain asymptomatic for years, but the anemia gradually worsens until its severity causes weakness, fatigue, weight loss, and general malaise. Treatment may consist of drug therapy with androgen/steroid combinations to temporarily lessen the severity of the anemia, drugs to stimulate the bone marrow to produce more red blood cells, blood transfusions to treat the anemia, and certain chemotherapy drugs may be used to reduce the size of the liver or spleen.

Coding Clarification
This code excludes myelofibrosis that is specified as idiopathic, primary, or that with myeloid metaplasia. These forms of myelofibrosis are reported with code 238.76.

Myelofibrosis, which is the replacement of bone marrow with fibrous tissue, when stated as secondary or without further specificity is considered a manifestation of the underlying condition. Code the underlying condition first followed by the code for myelofibrosis. Code 289.83 should never be sequenced first or reported alone.

When myelofibrosis is associated with myelosclerosis with myeloid metaplasia, the condition is classified as neoplasm of uncertain behavior of lymphatic and hematopoietic tissues (238.76). Other forms of myelofibrosis, such as not otherwise specified and secondary, are assigned code 289.83, *Myelofibrosis.*

289.89	Other specified diseases of blood and blood-forming organs — *hypergammaglobulinemia, pseudocholinesterase defiency, osteosclerosis, myelosclerosis, osteomyelosclerosis, osteomyelofibrosis, osteosclerotic anemia, activated protein C resistance*
289.9	Unspecified diseases of blood and blood-forming organs

290–319
Mental Disorders

The World Health Organization (WHO) offers the following guidelines that apply to this chapter: when classifying behavioral disorders, organically based illnesses should get precedence over functional ones, and within the functional group, the order then may be psychoses, neuroses, personality disorders, and others. When coding mental illnesses associated with physical conditions, assign as many codes as necessary to fully describe the clinical picture.

290–299 Psychoses
The term "psychoses" has been applied to many non-psychotic mental disorders historically. For this classification, the definition of psychoses includes only conditions that interfere with activities of daily living and include a gross impairment of reality. Codes in this section represent disorders that exhibit delusions, hallucinations, markedly incoherent speech, disorganized behaviors, and the inability on the part of the patient to comprehend the inappropriateness of this behavior.

290–294 Organic Psychotic Conditions
Included in this section are senile and presenile dementia, arteriosclerotic dementia, dementia and hallucinosis associated with substance abuse, and organic brain syndromes. Assign a code from these rubrics only when the specific organic clinical feature of a confused state, dementia, or delirium is present. Do not use a code from these categories to report the organic etiology of a psychotic mental state that is coded elsewhere in this chapter.

290 Dementias
AHA: Q1, 1988, 3

Arteriosclerotic dementia is attributable to degenerative arterial disease of the brain. Symptoms suggesting a focal lesion in the brain are common. There may be a fluctuating or patchy intellectual defect with insight, and an intermittent course is common. Clinical differentiation from senile or presenile dementia, which may coexist with it, may be very difficult or impossible. Cerebral atherosclerosis should also be reported in addition to the code for the psychosis.

Senile dementia usually occurs after the age of 65 in which any cerebral pathology other than that of senile atrophic change can be reasonably excluded. Presenile dementia occurs before age 65, and is usually associated with diffuse or lobar cerebral atrophy.

In delirium, a superimposed reversible episode of acute confusional state exists; in the delusional type, delusions vary from simple, poorly formed, paranoid delusions to highly formed paranoid delusional states. Hallucinations are also present in a progressive disease of persons in advanced age. Senile dementia, depressed type, is characterized by development in advanced old age, progressive in nature, in which depressive features, ranging from mild to severe forms of manic-depressive affective psychosis, are also present. Disturbance of the sleep-waking cycle and preoccupation with the deceased are often particularly prominent.

In addition to the appropriate code from this rubric, also code first any associated neurological condition such as Pick's disease, Alzheimer's disease, or Jakob-Creutzfeldt disease. Pick's disease, while present in the senile period, may primarily affect the frontal and temporal lobes. Alzheimer's disease is due to a large loss of cells from brain areas such as the cerebral cortex. Jakob-Creutzfeldt disease is a rare, progressive, fatal virus of the central nervous system.

290.0 Senile dementia, uncomplicated — (Code first the associated neurological condition) — *senile dementia, not otherwise specified*
AHA: Q4, 1999, 4

290.10 Presenile dementia, uncomplicated — (Code first the associated neurological condition) — *simple type*
AHA: Nov-Dec, 1984, 20

Code	Description
290.11	Presenile dementia with delirium — (Code first the associated neurological condition) — *with acute confusional state* **AHA:** Nov-Dec, 1984, 20
290.12	Presenile dementia with delusional features — (Code first the associated neurological condition) — *paranoid type, including Binswanger's dementia* **AHA:** Nov-Dec, 1984, 20
290.13	Presenile dementia with depressive features — (Code first the associated neurological condition) — *depressed type* **AHA:** Nov-Dec, 1984, 20
290.20	Senile dementia with delusional features — (Code first the associated neurological condition) — *paranoid type or senile psychosis not otherwise specified*
290.21	Senile dementia with depressive features — (Code first the associated neurological condition)
290.3	Senile dementia with delirium — (Code first the associated neurological condition) — *with acute confusional state*
290.40	Vascular dementia, uncomplicated — (Code first the associated neurological condition. Use additional code to identify cerebral atherosclerosis, 437.0) — *simple type*
290.41	Vascular dementia, with delirium — (Code first the associated neurological condition. Use additional code to identify cerebral atherosclerosis, 437.0) — *with acute confusional state*
290.42	Vascular dementia, with delusions — (Code first the associated neurological condition. Use additional code to identify cerebral atherosclerosis, 437.0) — *paranoid type*
290.43	Vascular dementia, with depressed mood — (Code first the associated neurological condition. Use additional code to identify cerebral atherosclerosis, 437.0) — *depressed type*
290.8	Other specified senile psychotic conditions — (Code first the associated neurological condition)
290.9	Unspecified senile psychotic condition — (Code first the associated neurological condition)

Documentation Issues
When the physician documents senile dementia with Alzheimer's disease, both conditions should be coded. Report with codes 290.0 *Senile dementia, uncomplicated* and 331.0 *Alzheimer's disease*.

Coding Clarification
Excluded from this rubric are dementias associated with other cerebral conditions (294.10-294.11), psychoses occurring in old age without dementia or delirium (295.0-298.8), senility with mental changes of nonpsychotic severity (310.1), and transient mental disorders due to conditions classified elsewhere (293.0-293.9).

If mental or behavioral problems are unspecified, report V40.9 *Unspecified mental or behavioral problem*. However, this code is not an acceptable principal diagnosis.

291 Alcohol-induced mental disorders
AHA: Sept-Oct, 1986, 3; Q1, 1988, 3

Alcohol induced mental disorders are organic psychotic states due mainly to excessive consumption of alcohol. Defects of nutrition are thought to play an important role in alcoholic mental disorders. Alcoholic mental disorders are classified according to the complex of presenting symptoms.

Alcohol withdrawal delirium is an acute or subacute organic psychotic state in alcoholics characterized by clouded consciousness, disorientation, fear, illusions, delusions, hallucinations of any kind, notably visual and tactile, and restlessness, tremor, and sometimes fever. Alcohol amnestic syndrome is a syndrome of prominent and lasting reduction of memory span, including striking loss of recent memory, disordered time appreciation, and confabulation, occurring in alcoholics as the sequel to an acute alcoholic psychosis (especially delirium tremens) or, more rarely, in the course of chronic alcoholism. It is usually accompanied by peripheral neuritis and may be associated with Wernicke's encephalopathy.

Code	Description
291.0	Alcohol withdrawal delirium — *delirium tremens* **AHA:** Q2, 1991, 11
291.1	Alcohol-induced persisting amnestic disorder — *Korsakoff's psychosis, alcoholic polyneuritic psychosis*
291.2	Alcohol-induced persisting dementia — *chronic alcoholic brain syndrome*
291.3	Alcohol-induced psychotic disorder with hallucinations — *psychosis with hallucinosis* **AHA:** Q2, 1991, 11
291.4	Idiosyncratic alcohol intoxication — *pathologic drunkenness*
291.5	Alcohol-induced psychotic disorder with delusions — *psychosis, paranoid type*
291.81	Alcohol withdrawal — *withdrawal symptoms or syndrome* **AHA:** July-Aug, 1985, 10; Q2, 1991, 11; Q3, 1994, 13; Q4, 1996, 28
291.82	Alcohol induced sleep disorders — *alcohol induced circadian rhythm sleep disorders, alcohol induced hypersomnia, alcohol induced insomnia, alcohol induced parasomnia*
291.89	Other specified alcohol-induced mental disorders — *not elsewhere specified* **AHA:** July-Aug, 1985, 10; Q3, 1994, 13
291.9	Unspecified alcohol-induced mental disorders — *chronic alcoholism with psychosis, not otherwise specified*

Mental Disorders

Documentation Issues

If the documentation references a history of alcohol abuse it should only be reported if it has an impact on the patient treatment or length of stay.

When the medical record indicates that the patient was admitted for a physical complaint related to the alcohol abuse, follow the instructions in the index for the condition described as due to alcohol and sequence the physical condition first, followed by the code for the alcohol abuse.

If the documentation identifies that the patient experienced withdrawal symptoms or syndrome whether prior to, or after admission, report the withdrawal. Use code 291.81 for alcohol withdrawal.

Coding Clarification
Substance Related Mental Conditions:
Psychoactive substance-induced organic mental syndromes are identified by physical or psychotic symptoms related to such use. These conditions are classified by category, such as 291 *Alcohol-induced mental disorders*. The alcohol abuse should also be reported as an additional code.

Alcohol Withdrawal: The phenomenon of alcohol withdrawal begins when an individual either greatly reduces or ceases consumption of alcohol after a period of prolonged and heavy use of the substance. Seizures as a result of alcohol withdrawal are coded to 780.39, together with 291.81.

Symptoms are hand tremor, nausea or vomiting, fleeting hallucinations (auditory, tactile, or visual), illusions, grand mal seizures, anxiety, insomnia, autonomic hyperactivity, and psychomotor agitation. These symptoms may cause very noticeable impairment of the sufferer's ability to function at work or in social settings, peaking on the second day, and improving markedly by the fourth day. The symptoms of anxiety, insomnia, and autonomic dysfunction can linger for as long as six months.

Coding Scenario
A patient is admitted in alcohol withdrawal, suffering from delirium tremens.

> Code assignment: 291.0 *Alcohol withdrawal with delirium tremens.* Code 291.81 specifically excludes the use of the code in conjunction with delirium, including delirium tremens.

292 Drug induced mental disorders
AHA: Sept-Oct, 1986, 3; Q1, 1988, 3; Q2, 1991, 11; Q3, 2004, 8

Drug induced mental disorders are organic mental syndromes that are due to consumption of drugs (notably amphetamines, barbiturates, opiate, and LSD groups) and solvents. Some of the syndromes in this group are not as severe as most conditions labeled "psychotic," but they are included here for practical reasons. Drug psychoses are classified according to the complex of presenting symptoms. In drug withdrawal syndrome, convulsions, tremor, disorientation, and memory disturbances may occur. In hallucinatory/paranoid states, the patient may experience auditory hallucinations and anxiety.

292.0	Drug withdrawal — (Use additional code for any associated drug dependence: 304.00-304.93. Use additional E code to identify drug) — *abstinence syndrome or symptoms*
292.11	Drug-induced psychotic disorder with delusions — (Use additional code for any associated drug dependence: 304.00-304.93. Use additional E code to identify drug) — *paranoid state induced by drugs*
292.12	Drug-induced psychotic disorder with hallucinations — (Use additional code for any associated drug dependence: 304.00-304.93. Use additional E code to identify drug)
292.2	Pathological drug intoxication — (Use additional code for any associated drug dependence: 304.00-304.93. Use additional E code to identify drug) — *reaction resulting in brief psychotic state*
292.81	Drug-induced delirium — (Use additional code for any associated drug dependence: 304.00-304.93. Use additional E code to identify drug)
292.82	Drug-induced persisting dementia — (Use additional code for any associated drug dependence: 304.00-304.93. Use additional E code to identify drug)
292.83	Drug-induced persisting amnestic disorder — (Use additional code for any associated drug dependence: 304.00-304.93. Use additional E code to identify drug) — *memory loss*
292.84	Drug-induced mood disorder — (Use additional code for any associated drug dependence: 304.00-304.93. Use additional E code to identify drug) — *depressive state induced by drugs*
292.85	Drug induced sleep disorders — (Use additional code for any associated drug dependence: 304.00-304.93. Use additional E code to identify drug) — Drug induced circadian rhythm disorders, drug induced hypersomnia, drug induced insomnia, drug induced parasomnia
292.89	Other specified drug-induced mental disorder — (Use additional code for any associated drug dependence: 304.00-304.93. Use additional E code to identify drug) — *drug-induced organic personality syndrome, amotivational syndrome, and drug flashback syndrome*
292.9	Unspecified drug-induced mental disorder — (Use additional code for any associated drug dependence: 304.00-304.93. Use additional E code to identify drug) — *not otherwise specified*

Documentation Issues

If the documentation references a history of drug abuse, it should only be reported if it has an impact on the patient treatment or length of stay.

When the medical record indicates that the patient was admitted for a physical complaint related to the drug abuse, follow the instructions in the index for the condition described as due to drug abuse and sequence the physical condition first, followed by the code for the drug abuse.

If the documentation identifies that the patient experienced withdrawal symptoms or syndrome whether prior to, or after admission, report the withdrawal. Use code 292.0 for drug withdrawal.

Coding Clarification

Use an additional code from rubric 304 to report any associated drug dependence and an E code to identify the drug.

Substance Related Mental Conditions:

Psychoactive substance-induced organic mental syndromes are identified by physical or psychotic symptoms related to such use. These conditions are classified by category, such as 292 *Drug-induced mental disorders*. The drug abuse should also be reported as an additional code.

293 Transient mental disorders due to conditions classified elsewhere
AHA: Q1, 1988, 3

Transient mental disorders due to conditions classified elsewhere are characterized by clouded consciousness, confusion, disorientation, illusions, and frequently vivid hallucinations. Typically, they are due to some intra- or extracerebral toxic, infectious, metabolic, or other systemic disturbance and generally are reversible.

When using a code from this category, assign an additional code to identify the associated physical or neurological condition.

Acute delirium has an acute or rapid onset and is characterized by extreme disturbances of arousal, attention, orientation, perception, intellectual functions, and affect. These conditions are accompanied commonly by fear and agitation.

Organic affective syndrome is similar to depressive or manic-depressive disorder, but occurs in the presence of specific organic factors such as head trauma, endocranial tumors, exocranial tumors (such as pancreatic carcinoma), steroid overuse, Cushing's syndrome, and other endocrine disorders.

293.0	Delirium due to conditions classified elsewhere — (Code first the associated physical or neurological condition)
293.1	Subacute delirium — (Code first the associated physical or neurological condition) — *organic in origin* **AHA:** Q1, 1988, 3
293.81	Psychotic disorder with delusions in conditions classified elsewhere — (Code first the associated physical or neurological condition) — *transient psychotic condition, paranoid type* **AHA:** Q1, 1988, 3
293.82	Psychotic disorder with hallucinations in conditions classified elsewhere — (Code first the associated physical or neurological condition) — *transient psychotic condition, hallucinatory type* **AHA:** Q1, 1988, 3
293.83	Mood disorder in conditions classified elsewhere — (Code first the associated physical or neurological condition) — *transient psychotic condition, depressive type* **AHA:** Q1, 1988, 3
293.84	Anxiety disorder in conditions classified elsewhere — (Code first the associated physical or neurological condition)
293.89	Other specified transient mental disorders due to conditions classified elsewhere, other — (Code first the associated physical or neurological condition) — *Alice in Wonderland syndrome* **AHA:** Q1, 1988, 3
293.9	Unspecified transient mental disorder in conditions classified elsewhere — (Code first the associated physical or neurological condition)

294 Persistent mental disorders due to conditions classified elsewhere
AHA: March-April, 1985, 12; Q1, 1988, 3

Amnestic syndrome presents with a prominent and lasting reduction of memory span, including striking loss of recent memory, disordered time appreciation, and confabulation. The most common causes are chronic alcoholism (alcohol amnestic syndrome, Korsakoff's alcoholic psychosis), chronic barbiturate dependence, and malnutrition. An amnestic syndrome may be the predominating disturbance in the early states of presenile and senile dementia, arteriosclerotic dementia, and in encephalitis and other inflammatory and degenerative diseases in which there is particular bilateral involvement of the temporal lobes, and certain temporal lobe tumors.

294.0	Amnestic disorder in conditions classified elsewhere — *Korsakoff's psychosis or syndrome (nonalcoholic)* **AHA:** March-April, 1985, 12; Q1, 1988, 3
294.10	Dementia in conditions classified elsewhere without behavioral disturbance — (Code first

Mental Disorders

	any underlying physical condition: 046.1, 094.1, 275.1, 330.1, 331.0, 331.11, 331.19, 331.82, 333.4, 340, 345.00-345.91, 446.0)
294.11	Dementia in conditions classified elsewhere with behavioral disturbance — (Code first any underlying physical condition: 046.1, 094.1, 275.1, 330.1, 331.0, 331.11, 331.19, 331.82, 333.4, 340, 345.00-345.91, 446.0)
294.8	Other persistent mental disorders due to conditions classified elsewhere — (Use additional code for associated epilepsy: 345.00-345.91) — *mixed paranoid and affective organic psychotic state* **AHA:** March-April, 1985, 12; Q1, 1988, 3; Q1, 1988, 5; Q3, 2003, 14
294.9	Unspecified persistent mental disorders due to conditions classified elsewhere — *chronic organic psychosis* **AHA:** March-April, 1985, 12; Q1, 1988, 3

Coding Clarification
Other specified chronic organic brain syndromes include conditions that present a clinical picture of organic psychosis but do not take the shape of a confusional state (293), a nonalcoholic Korsakoff's psychosis (294.0), or dementia due to an underlying physical condition (294.1x).

Alzheimer's Dementia: Two codes are required to report this condition. First code the underlying condition 331.0 *Alzheimer's disease*, and then use an additional code to report the dementia, 294.1x *Dementia in conditions classified elsewhere*.

Coding Scenario
A patient is seen for evaluation of Alzheimer's dementia and is referred to a partial hospitalization program for therapy.

Code assignment: 331.0 *Alzheimer's disease* and 294.1x *Dementia in conditions classified elsewhere*

295-299 Other Psychoses
Use an additional code to identify any associated physical disease, injury, or condition affecting the brain with psychoses classifiable to 295-298.

295 Schizophrenic disorders
AHA: Q1, 1988, 3

Schizophrenia is not diagnosed unless there is characteristic disturbance of at least two of these areas: thought, perception, mood, conduct, and personality. Paranoid type schizophrenia includes delusions of persecution or grandeur, thought disorder and hallucinations with less personality disintegration than in other subtypes of schizophrenia. Latent schizophrenia is sometimes called borderline schizophrenia, and is a condition in which there is potential for developing schizophrenia under emotional distress. This term is not recommended for patient diagnosis because a general consensus of its description has not been reached.

Residual schizophrenia presents with symptoms from the acute phase, but the symptoms have lost their prominence or sharpness. Schizoaffective type schizophrenia is a mixture of symptoms from schizophrenia and affective psychoses.

The following fifth-digit subclassification is for use with category 295:
0 unspecified
1 subchronic
2 chronic
3 subchronic with acute exacerbation
4 chronic with acute exacerbation
5 in remission

295.0	Simple type schizophrenia — (Use additional code to identify any associated physical disease, injury, or condition affecting the brain) — *schizophrenia simplex* **AHA:** Q1, 1988, 3
295.1	Disorganized type schizophrenia — (Use additional code to identify any associated physical disease, injury, or condition affecting the brain) — *hebephrenic type schizophrenia* **AHA:** Q1, 1988, 3
295.2	Catatonic type schizophrenia — (Use additional code to identify any associated physical disease, injury, or condition affecting the brain) — *catatonic schizophrenia* **AHA:** Q1, 1988, 3
295.3	Paranoid type schizophrenia — (Use additional code to identify any associated physical disease, injury, or condition affecting the brain) — *paraphrenic schizophrenia* **AHA:** Q1, 1988, 3
295.4	Schizophreniform disorder — (Use additional code to identify any associated physical disease, injury, or condition affecting the brain) — *oneirophrenia, schizophreniform psychosis, confusional* **AHA:** Q1, 1988, 3
295.5	Latent schizophrenia — (Use additional code to identify any associated physical disease, injury, or condition affecting the brain) — *prodromal, pseudoneurotic, borderline, incipient, prepsychotic* **AHA:** Q1, 1988, 3
295.6	Residual schizophrenia — (Use additional code to identify any associated physical disease, injury, or condition affecting the brain) —

chronic un-differentiated, Restzustand schizophrenia
AHA: Q1, 1988, 3

295.7 ⮑sth Schizo-affective type schizophrenia — (Use additional code to identify any associated physical disease, injury, or condition affecting the brain) — *cyclic, mixed*
AHA: Q1, 1988, 3

295.8 ⮑sth Other specified types of schizophrenia — (Use additional code to identify any associated physical disease, injury, or condition affecting the brain) — *acute, atypical, cenesthopathic*
AHA: Q1, 1988, 3

295.9 ⮑sth Unspecified schizophrenia — (Use additional code to identify any associated physical disease, injury, or condition affecting the brain) — *not otherwise specified, including Morel-Kraepelin disease*
AHA: Q1, 1988, 3; Q3, 1995, 6

296 Episodic mood disorders
AHA: March-April, 1985, 14; Q1, 1988, 3

Episodic mood disorders are recurrent, severe disturbances of mood accompanied by one or more of the following: delusions, perplexity, disturbed attitude to self, disorder of perception and behavior. Patients with affective psychoses have a strong characteristic inclination toward suicide. This category includes mild disorders of mood if the symptoms closely match the descriptions.

Manic disorder, as a single episode, is characterized by elation, excitement, rapid thought process, increased psychomotor activity, and emotional instability. Diminished interest in activities, fatigue, insomnia or hypersomnia, and change in weight characterize a major depressive disorder as a single episode. In bipolar disorder, the patient cycles between the two states: manic and depressive.

The following fifth-digit subclassification is for use with categories 296.0-296.6:
0 unspecified
1 mild
2 moderate
3 severe, without mention of psychotic behavior
4 severe, specified as with psychotic behavior
5 in partial or unspecified remission
6 in full remission

296.0 ⮑sth Bipolar I disorder, single, manic episode — (Use additional code to identify any associated physical disease, injury, or condition affecting the brain) — *hypomania, single episode or unspecified*
AHA: March-April, 1985, 14

296.1 ⮑sth Manic disorder, recurrent episode — (Use additional code to identify any associated physical disease, injury, or condition affecting the brain) — *hypomania, recurrent*
AHA: March-April, 1985, 14

296.2 ⮑sth Major depressive disorder, single episode — (Use additional code to identify any associated physical disease, injury, or condition affecting the brain) — *endogenous depression, single episode or unspecified*
AHA: March-April, 1985, 14

296.3 ⮑sth Major depressive disorder, recurrent episode — (Use additional code to identify any associated physical disease, injury, or condition affecting the brain) — *endogenous depression, recurrent*
AHA: March-April, 1985, 14

296.4 ⮑sth Bipolar I disorder, most recent episode(or current) manic — (Use additional code to identify any associated physical disease, injury, or condition affecting the brain) — *circular manic depressive psychosis, in manic state*
AHA: March-April, 1985, 14

296.5 ⮑sth Bipolar I disorder, most recent episode (or current), depressed — (Use additional code to identify any associated physical disease, injury, or condition affecting the brain) — *circular manic depressive psychosis, in depressed state*
AHA: March-April, 1985, 14; Q1, 2006, 10

296.6 ⮑sth Bipolar I disorder, most recent episode (or current), mixed — (Use additional code to identify any associated physical disease, injury, or condition affecting the brain) — *circular manic depressive psychosis, mixed state*
AHA: March-April, 1985, 14

296.7 Bipolar I disorder, most recent episode (or current) unspecified — (Use additional code to identify any associated physical disease, injury, or condition affecting the brain) — *circular manic depressive psychosis, current state unspecified*
AHA: March-April, 1985, 14

296.80 Bipolar disorder, unspecified — (Use additional code to identify any associated physical disease, injury, or condition affecting the brain) — *atypical manic depressive psychosis, current state unspecified*
AHA: March-April, 1985, 14

296.81 Atypical manic disorder — (Use additional code to identify any associated physical disease, injury, or condition affecting the brain) — *atypical manic only*
AHA: March-April, 1985, 14

296.82 Atypical depressive disorder — (Use additional code to identify any associated physical disease, injury, or condition affecting the brain) — *atypical depressive only*
AHA: March-April, 1985, 14

296.89 Other and unspecified bipolar disorders, other — (Use additional code to identify any associated physical disease, injury, or condition affecting the brain) — *atypical manic depressive psychosis, mixed status*
AHA: March-April, 1985, 14

Mental Disorders

296.90 Unspecified episodic mood disorder — (Use additional code to identify any associated physical disease, injury, or condition affecting the brain) — *not otherwise specified*
AHA: March-April, 1985, 14

296.99 Other specified episodic mood disorder — (Use additional code to identify any associated physical disease, injury, or condition affecting the brain) — *mood swings: brief compensatory, rebound*
AHA: March-April, 1985, 14

297 Delusional disorders
AHA: Q1, 1988, 3

Paranoia is a condition in which patients show persistent distrust and suspiciousness of others. They typically present with four or more of the following:

- Suspicion that others are exploiting, harming, or deceiving him or her; preoccupied with unjustified doubts about the loyalty or trustworthiness of friends or associates
- Unwillingness to confide in others because of an unwarranted fear that the information will be used maliciously against him or her; reads hidden unbecoming or threatening meanings into benign remarks or events
- Persistently bears grudges, e.g., is unforgiving of insults, injuries, or slights
- Perceives attacks on character or reputation that are not apparent to others and is quick to react angrily or counterattacks
- Has recurrent suspicions, without justification, regarding fidelity of spouse or sexual partner

The disorder must have been present at least one week for this diagnosis.

The illness is not due to organic disease of the brain. This disorder usually occurs in the middle or late in adult life and may be chronic; it often includes resentment and anger that may lead to violence. These patients rarely seek medical attention but are brought for care by associates or relatives.

297.0 Paranoid state, simple — (Use additional code to identify any associated physical disease, injury, or condition affecting the brain) — *simple*
AHA: Q1, 1988, 3

297.1 Delusional disorder — (Use additional code to identify any associated physical disease, injury, or condition affecting the brain) — *chronic, Sander's disease, Cotard's syndrome, systematized delusions*
AHA: Q1, 1988, 3

297.2 Paraphrenia — (Use additional code to identify any associated physical disease, injury, or condition affecting the brain) — *involutional paranoid state, late paraphrenia, paraphrenia (involutional)*
AHA: Q1, 1988, 3

297.3 Shared psychotic disorder — (Use additional code to identify any associated physical disease, injury, or condition affecting the brain) — *folie à deux, induced psychosis or paranoid disorder*
AHA: Q1, 1988, 3

297.8 Other specified paranoid states — (Use additional code to identify any associated physical disease, injury, or condition affecting the brain) — *paranoia querulans, sensitiver Beziehungswahn, psyche passionelle; tarantism*
AHA: Q1, 1988, 3

297.9 Unspecified paranoid state — (Use additional code to identify any associated physical disease, injury, or condition affecting the brain) — *Lasegue's disease*
AHA: July-Aug, 1985, 9; Q1, 1988, 3

Coding Clarification
Excluded from this rubric are acute paranoid reaction (298.3), alcoholic jealousy or paranoid state (291.5), and paranoid schizophrenia (295.3).

Cotard's syndrome, characterized by suicidal tendencies and sensory disturbances, is classified to 297.1.

298 Other nonorganic psychoses
AHA: Q1, 1988, 3

Classified to this rubric are a small group of psychotic conditions that are attributable largely to a recent life experience. They should not be used for the wider range of psychoses in which environmental factors play some, but not a major, part in the etiology.

298.0 Depressive type psychosis — (Use additional code to identify any associated physical disease, injury, or condition affecting the brain) — *psychogenic depressive psychosis*
AHA: Q1, 1988, 3

298.1 Excitative type psychosis — (Use additional code to identify any associated physical disease, injury, or condition affecting the brain) — *acute hysterical psychosis; reactive excitation*
AHA: Q1, 1988, 3

298.2 Reactive confusion — (Use additional code to identify any associated physical disease, injury, or condition affecting the brain) — *psychogenic confusion/twilight state*
AHA: Q1, 1988, 3

298.3 Acute paranoid reaction — (Use additional code to identify any associated physical disease, injury, or condition affecting the brain) — *acute psychogenic paranoid psychosis; Bouffée délirante*
AHA: Q1, 1988, 3

298.4	Psychogenic paranoid psychosis — (Use additional code to identify any associated physical disease, injury, or condition affecting the brain)
298.8	Other and unspecified reactive psychosis — (Use additional code to identify any associated physical disease, injury, or condition affecting the brain) — *hysterical psychosis, psychogenic stupor* **AHA:** Q1, 1988, 3
298.9	Unspecified psychosis — (Use additional code to identify any associated physical disease, injury, or condition affecting the brain) — *lycanthropy, nosomania, parergasia, vesania* **AHA:** Q1, 1988, 3

Coding Clarification
Lycanthropy, the delusion that the patient believes himself to be a wolf, is classified in the ICD-9-CM index to 298.9, as is nosomania, a delusion of being infected by disease.

299 Pervasive developmental disorders
AHA: Q1, 1988, 3

Infantile autism is a syndrome present from birth or beginning almost invariably in the first 30 months. Responses to auditory and sometimes to visual stimuli are abnormal, and there are usually severe problems in the understanding of spoken language. Speech is delayed and, if it develops, is characterized by echolalia, the reversal of pronouns, immature grammatical structure, and an inability to use abstract terms. There is generally an impaired social use of both verbal and gestural language. Problems in social relationships are most severe before the age of 5 years and include an impaired development of eye-to-eye gaze, social attachments, and cooperative play. Ritualistic behavior is usual and may include abnormal routines, resistance to change, attachment to odd objects, and stereotyped patterns of play. The capacity for abstract or symbolic thought and for imaginative play is diminished. Intelligence ranges from severely subnormal to normal or above. Performance is usually better on tasks involving rote memory or visuospatial skills than on those requiring symbolic or linguistic skills.

The following fifth-digit subclassification is for use with category 299:
0   current or active state
1   residual state

299.0 ✎5th	Autistic disorder — *childhood autism; Kanner's syndrome* **AHA:** Q1, 1988, 3
299.1 ✎5th	Childhood disintegrative disorder — (Use additional code to identify any associated neurological disorder) — *Heller's syndrome* **AHA:** Q1, 1988, 3
299.8 ✎5th	Other specified pervasive developmental disorders — *atypical childhood psychosis; borderline psychosis of childhood* **AHA:** Q1, 1988, 3
299.9 ✎5th	Unspecified pervasive developmental disorder

Coding Clarification
Excluded from this rubric are adult type psychoses occurring in childhood, as in affective disorders (296.0-296.9), manic-depressive disorders (296.0-296.9), and schizophrenia (295.0-295.9).

300–316   Neurotic Disorders, Personality Disorders, and Other Nonpsychotic Mental Disorders

300   Anxiety, dissociative and somatoform disorders
AHA: Q1, 1988, 3

Neurotic disorders have no obvious evidence of an organic etiology, and there is no lost sense of reality or disorganized personality. Symptoms may include anxiety, hysteria, obsession, compulsion, depression, or phobia. Behavior may be greatly affected although usually remaining within socially acceptable limits.

In psychogenic amnesia, there is a temporary disturbance in the ability to recall important personal information that has already been registered and stored in memory. The sudden onset of this disturbance in the absence of an underlying organic mental disorder, and the extent of the disturbance being too great to be explained by ordinary forgetfulness, are the essential features.

In factitious illness, there are physical or psychological symptoms that are not real, genuine, or natural, which are produced by the individual and are under voluntary control. The presentation of physical symptoms may be fabricated, self-inflicted, an exaggeration or exacerbation of a pre-existing physical condition, or any combination or variation of these.

In phobia, the patient experiences abnormal intense dread of certain objects or specific situations. If the anxiety tends to spread from a specified situation or object to a wider range of circumstances, it becomes akin to or identical with an anxiety state, and should be classified as such.

In obsessive-compulsive behavior, the outstanding symptom is a feeling of subjective compulsion, which must be resisted. The obsessional urge or idea is recognized as alien to the personality but as coming from within the self. Obsessional actions may be quasi-ritual performances designed to relieve anxiety. Attempts to dispel the unwelcome thoughts or urges may lead to a severe inner struggle, with intense anxiety.

Code	Description
300.00	Anxiety state, unspecified — *anxiety neurosis; asphyctic syndrome* **AHA:** Q1, 1988, 3; Q1, 2002, 6
300.01	Panic disorder without agoraphobia — *panic attack* **AHA:** Q1, 1988, 3
300.02	Generalized anxiety disorder
300.09	Other anxiety states — *not elsewhere classified* **AHA:** Q1, 1988, 3
300.10	Hysteria, unspecified
300.11	Conversion disorder — *astasia-abasia; hysterical blindness/deafness; Bergeron's disease* **AHA:** Nov-Dec, 1985, 15; Q1, 1988, 3
300.12	Dissociative amnesia — *hysterical amnesia* **AHA:** Q1, 1988, 3
300.13	Dissociative fugue — *hysterical fugue* **AHA:** Q1, 1988, 3
300.14	Dissociative identity disorder — *dissociative identity disorder* **AHA:** Q1, 1988, 3
300.15	Dissociative disorder or reaction, unspecified
300.16	Factitious disorder with predominantly psychological signs and symptoms — *compensation neurosis; Ganser's hysterical syndrome* **AHA:** Q1, 1988, 3
300.19	Other and unspecified factitious illness — *factitious illness with physical symptoms, NOS* **AHA:** Q1, 1988, 3
300.20	Phobia, unspecified
300.21	Agoraphobia with panic disorder — *fear of open spaces, streets, travel; with panic attacks* **AHA:** Q1, 1988, 3
300.22	Agoraphobia without mention of panic attacks — *fear of open spaces, streets, travel; without mention of panic attacks* **AHA:** Q1, 1988, 3
300.23	Social phobia — *fear of eating, washing, speaking in public* **AHA:** Q1, 1988, 3
300.29	Other isolated or specific phobias — *acrophobia, claustrophobia, animal phobias* **AHA:** Q1, 1988, 3
300.3	Obsessive-compulsive disorders — *anancastic neurosis, any obsessional phobia, compulsive neurosis* **AHA:** Q1, 1988, 3
300.4	Dysthymic disorder — *anxiety depression, reactive depression* **AHA:** Q1, 1988, 3
300.5	Neurasthenia — (Use additional code to identify any associated physical disorder) — *fatigue neurosis, general fatigue, psychogenic asthenia* **AHA:** Q1, 1988, 3
300.6	Depersonalization disorder — *neurotic derealization* **AHA:** Q1, 1988, 3
300.7	Hypochondriasis — *body dysmorphic disorder* **AHA:** Q1, 1988, 3
300.81	Somatization disorder — *Briquet's disorder, severe somatoform disorder* **AHA:** Q1, 1988, 3
300.82	Undifferentiated somatoform disorder — *atypical somatoform disorder* **AHA:** Q1, 1988, 3; Q4, 1996, 29
300.89	Other somatoform disorders — *occupational neurosis, including writers' cramp, psychasthenia, Janet's disease* **AHA:** Q1, 1988, 3
300.9	Unspecified nonpsychotic mental disorder — *neurosis NOS, merergasia, self-mutilation, suicide risk* **AHA:** Q1, 1988, 3

Coding Clarification
Excluded from phobic disorders are anxiety states not associated with a specific situation or object (300.00-300.09) and obsessional phobia (300.3).

301 Personality disorders
AHA: Q1, 1988, 3

A dependent personality disorder allows a patient to permit another individual to take control of his/her life. This patient also allows the needs of that person to supersede personal needs. A borderline personality is characterized by instability in interpersonal relationships, behavior, mood, and perception of self-image.

301.0	Paranoid personality disorder — (Use additional code to identify any associated neurosis or psychosis, or physical condition) — *fanatic personality; paranoid traits* **AHA:** July-Aug, 1985, 9; Q1, 1988, 3
301.10	Affective personality disorder, unspecified — (Use additional code to identify any associated neurosis or psychosis, or physical condition)
301.11	Chronic hypomanic personality disorder — (Use additional code to identify any associated neurosis or psychosis, or physical condition)
301.12	Chronic depressive personality disorder — (Use additional code to identify any associated neurosis or psychosis, or physical condition)
301.13	Cyclothymic disorder — (Use additional code to identify any associated neurosis or psychosis,

Coders' Desk Reference for Diagnoses

or physical condition) — *cycloid personality; cyclothymia*
AHA: Q1, 1988, 3

301.20 Schizoid personality disorder, unspecified — (Use additional code to identify any associated neurosis or psychosis, or physical condition)

301.21 Introverted personality — (Use additional code to identify any associated neurosis or psychosis, or physical condition)

301.22 Schizotypal personality disorder — (Use additional code to identify any associated neurosis or psychosis, or physical condition)

301.3 Explosive personality disorder — (Use additional code to identify any associated neurosis or psychosis, or physical condition) — *excessive emotional instability; pathological emotionality*
AHA: Q1, 1988, 3

301.4 Obsessive-compulsive personality disorder — (Use additional code to identify any associated neurosis or psychosis, or physical condition) — *obsessional personality*
AHA: Q1, 1988, 3

301.50 Histrionic personality disorder, unspecified — (Use additional code to identify any associated neurosis or psychosis, or physical condition) — *not elsewhere classified*
AHA: Q1, 1988, 3

301.51 Chronic factitious illness with physical symptoms — (Use additional code to identify any associated neurosis or psychosis, or physical condition) — *hospital addiction syndrome; Munchausen syndrome*
AHA: Q1, 1988, 3

301.59 Other histrionic personality disorder — (Use additional code to identify any associated neurosis or psychosis, or physical condition) — *emotionally unstable; psychoinfantile; labile*
AHA: Q1, 1988, 3

301.6 Dependent personality disorder — (Use additional code to identify any associated neurosis or psychosis, or physical condition) — *asthenic or passive personality*
AHA: Q1, 1988, 3

301.7 Antisocial personality disorder — (Use additional code to identify any associated neurosis or psychosis, or physical condition) — *amoral or sociopathic personality*
AHA: Sept-Oct, 1984, 16; Q1, 1988, 3

301.81 Narcissistic personality disorder — (Use additional code to identify any associated neurosis or psychosis, or physical condition)

301.82 Avoidant personality disorder — (Use additional code to identify any associated neurosis or psychosis, or physical condition)

301.83 Borderline personality disorder — (Use additional code to identify any associated neurosis or psychosis, or physical condition)

301.84 Passive-aggressive personality — (Use additional code to identify any associated neurosis or psychosis, or physical condition)

301.89 Other personality disorder — (Use additional code to identify any associated neurosis or psychosis, or physical condition) — *eccentric, masochistic or psychoneurotic*
AHA: Q1, 1988, 3

301.9 Unspecified personality disorder — (Use additional code to identify any associated neurosis or psychosis, or physical condition) — *Witzelsucht; psychopathic constitutional*
AHA: Q1, 1988, 3

Coding Clarification
Personality disorders include character neuroses, but exclude nonpsychotic personality disorders associated with organic brain syndromes (310.0-310.9). Use an additional code to identify an associated neurosis or psychosis, or physical condition.

302 Sexual and gender identity disorders
AHA: Q1, 1988, 3

The limits and features of normal sexual behavior have not been stated absolutely in different societies and cultures, but applied broadly serve as approved social and biological purposes. The sexual activities of patients with deviant disorders are directed primarily toward sexual acts not associated with coitus normally, or toward coitus performed under abnormal circumstances.

302.0 Ego-dystonic sexual orientation — *ego-dystonic lesbianism; homosexual conflict disorder*
AHA: Q1, 1988, 3

302.1 Zoophilia
302.2 Pedophilia
302.3 Transvestic fetishism
302.4 Exhibitionism
302.50 Trans-sexualism with unspecified sexual history
302.51 Trans-sexualism with asexual history
302.52 Trans-sexualism with homosexual history
302.53 Trans-sexualism with heterosexual history
302.6 Gender identity disorder in children — *feminism in boys; gender identity disorder of childhood*
AHA: Q1, 1988, 3

302.70 Psychosexual dysfunction, unspecified
302.71 Hypoactive sexual desire disorder
302.72 Psychosexual dysfunction with inhibited sexual excitement — *frigidity or impotence*
AHA: Q1, 1988, 3

302.73 Female orgasmic disorder
302.74 Male orgasmic disorder
302.75 Premature ejaculation
302.76 Dyspareunia, psychogenic
302.79 Psychosexual dysfunction with other specified psychosexual dysfunctions — *not elsewhere classified*
AHA: Q1, 1988, 3

302.81 Fetishism
302.82 Voyeurism

302.83	Sexual masochism
302.84	Sexual sadism
302.85	Gender identity disorder in adolescents or adults — *gender identity disorder of adult life* AHA: Q1, 1988, 3
302.89	Other specified psychosexual disorder — *nymphomania, satyriasis, frotteurism, coprophilia and necrophilia* AHA: Q1, 1988, 3
302.9	Unspecified psychosexual disorder

Coding Clarification
If the anomalous behavior becomes manifest only during psychosis or other mental illness, the condition should be classified under the major illness. Excluded from psychosexual dysfunction are organic causes of impotence (607.84), occasional or transient failures of erection or sexual excitement, or other dysfunction with organic cause.

303 Alcohol dependence syndrome
AHA: Sept-Oct, 1986, 3; Q1, 1988, 3; Q4, 1988, 8; Q2, 1991, 9; Q3, 1995, 6

Alcohol dependence syndrome is both a psychic and physical state, resulting from excessive alcohol consumption. The syndrome is characterized by behavioral and other responses that always include a compulsion to take alcohol on a continuous or periodic basis in order to experience its psychic effects, and sometimes to avoid the discomfort of its absence; tolerance may or may not be present.

The following fifth-digit subclassification is for use with categories 303, 304, and 305.0, 305.2-305.9:

 0   unspecified
 1   continuous
 2   episodic
 3   in remission

303.0 ⌐5th Acute alcoholic intoxication — (Use additional code to identify any associated condition: 291.0-291.9, 304.00-304.93, 331.7, 345.00-345.91, 535.3, 571.1, 571.2, 571.3) — *acute drunkenness in alcoholism*
AHA: Sept-Oct, 1986, 3; Q1, 1988, 3; Q4, 1988, 8; Q2, 1991, 9; Q3, 1995, 6

303.9 ⌐5th Other and unspecified alcohol dependence — (Use additional code to identify any associated condition: 291.0-291.9, 304.00-304.93, 331.7, 345.00-345.91, 535.3, 571.1, 571.2, 571.3) — *chronic alcoholism; dipsomania*
AHA: Sept-Oct, 1986, 3; Q1, 1988, 3; Q4, 1988, 8; Q2, 1989, 9; Q2, 1991, 9; Q3, 1995, 6; Q2, 2002, 4

Documentation Issues
If the documentation references a history of alcohol dependence, only report it if it has an impact on the current patient treatment or length of stay.

When the diagnostic statement of acute and chronic alcoholism is noted, further review of the documentation should be performed to determine if the patient was acutely intoxicated at the time of the encounter for appropriate code assignment. Verify with the physician if necessary as only one code should be assigned.

When the patient is admitted for detoxification and is currently pregnant, a diagnosis code from Chapter 11 Complications of Pregnancy, Childbirth and Puerperium (630-677) is required unless the physician documents that this condition is not affecting the pregnancy. A code specifying the type of dependence may also be used as an additional diagnosis. If the physician documents that the pregnancy is incidental, use code V22.2 *Pregnant state, incidental* in addition to the dependency code.

If the documentation identifies that the patient experienced withdrawal symptoms or syndrome whether prior to or after admission, report it. Use code 291.81 for alcohol withdrawal.

Coding Clarification
A person may be dependent on alcohol and other drugs; if so, also record the diagnosis of drug dependence to identify the agent. If alcohol dependence is associated with alcoholic psychosis or with physical complications, both diagnoses should be recorded. Use an additional code to identify any associated conditions, as in alcoholic psychosis (291.0-291.9), drug dependence (304.0-304.9), or physical complications of alcohol, including gastritis (535.3), cirrhosis (571.2), hepatitis (571.1), or cerebral degeneration (331.7).

Axes in this rubric classify the alcohol dependence as acute or chronic, and according to the nature of the dependence during the episode of care. When drunkenness is not otherwise specified, report with 305.0x, which reports nondependent abuse of alcohol.

Alcohol Dependence: This chronic condition is identified by the patient who is unable to cease alcohol use even with detriments to health, social interactions, and job performance. These patients generally experience physical signs of withdrawal with any sudden cessation of drinking. Alcohol dependence is classified to category 303. Subcategory code 303.0x is reported for acute alcohol intoxication in chronic alcoholism. Subcategory code 303.9x is reported when the patient is treated when not acutely intoxicated and is alcohol dependent.

Coding Scenario
A 62-year-old male patient is seen in the office for a physical exam. The patient has been alcohol dependent for 32 years. He has quit drinking for the second time and has been dry for a four-month duration.

> Code assignment: 303.93 *Alcohol dependence syndrome, other and unspecified alcohol dependence, in remission*

304 Drug dependence
AHA: Sept-Oct, 1986, 3; Q1, 1988, 3; Q4, 1988, 8; Q2, 1991, 10

Drug dependence is both a mental and physical state, resulting from taking a drug. It is characterized by behavioral and other responses that always include a compulsion to take a drug on a continuous or periodic basis in order to experience its psychic effects, and sometimes to avoid the discomfort of its absence. Tolerance may be present. A person may be dependent on more than one drug.

> The following fifth-digit subclassification is for use with categories 303, 304, 305.0, and 305.2-305.9:
> 0   unspecified
> 1   continuous
> 2   episodic
> 3   in remission

304.0 [sth] Opioid type dependence — *heroin, opium alkaloids and their derivatives, meperidine, methadone*
AHA: Sept-Oct, 1986, 3; Q1, 1988, 3; Q4, 1988, 8; Q2, 1991, 10; Q2, 2006, 7

304.1 [sth] Sedative, hypnotic or anxiolytic dependence — *nonbarbiturate sedatives and tranquilizers with similar effect: chlordiazepoxide, meprobamate, diazepam, methaqualone, glutethimide*
AHA: Sept-Oct, 1986, 3; Q1, 1988, 3; Q4, 1988, 8; Q2, 1991, 10

304.2 [sth] Cocaine dependence — *coca leaves, crack cocaine, coke*
AHA: Sept-Oct, 1986, 3; Q1, 1988, 3; Q4, 1988, 8; Q2, 1991, 10

304.3 [sth] Cannabis dependence — *hashish, marijuana, pot*
AHA: Sept-Oct, 1986, 3; Q1, 1988, 3; Q4, 1988, 8; Q2, 1991, 10

304.4 [sth] Amphetamine and other psychostimulant dependence — *methylphenidate, phenmetrazine*
AHA: Sept-Oct, 1986, 3; Q1, 1988, 3; Q4, 1988, 8; Q2, 1991, 10

304.5 [sth] Hallucinogen dependence — *dimethyltryptamine [DMT], lysergic acid diethylamide [LSD], mescaline, psilocybin*
AHA: Sept-Oct, 1986, 3; Q1, 1988, 3; Q4, 1988, 8; Q2, 1991, 10

304.6 [sth] Other specified drug dependence — *absinthe; glue sniffing*
AHA: Sept-Oct, 1986, 3; Q1, 1988, 3; Q4, 1988, 8; Q2, 1991, 10

304.7 [sth] Combinations of opioid type drug with any other drug dependence

304.8 [sth] Combinations of drug dependence excluding opioid type drug

304.9 [sth] Unspecified drug dependence — *drug addiction NOS*
AHA: Sept-Oct, 1986, 3; Q1, 1988, 3; Q4, 1988, 8; Q2, 1991, 10

Documentation Issues
If the documentation references a history of drug dependence, only report it if it has an impact on the current patient treatment or length of stay.

When the patient is admitted for detoxification and is currently pregnant, a diagnosis code from chapter 11 Complications of Pregnancy, Childbirth and Puerperium (630-677) is required unless the physician documents this condition as not affecting the pregnancy. A code specifying the type of dependence may also be used as an additional diagnosis. If the physician documents that the pregnancy is incidental, use code V22.2 *Pregnant state, incidental* in addition to the dependency code.

If the documentation identifies that the patient experienced withdrawal symptoms or syndrome whether prior to or after admission, use code 292.0 for drug withdrawal.

Coding Clarification
This rubric excludes nondependent abuse of drugs, which is reported with codes in the 305 rubric.

Drug Dependence: This chronic mental and physical condition is related to the pattern of the patient's drug or drug combination intake and is characterized by behavioral and physiological reactions. These reactions are the obsession to take the drug, the need to have the feeling of its psychic effects, or the attempt to avoid the discomfort of abstinence. Any sudden cessation typically triggers physical signs of withdrawal.

Mental Disorders

Polydrug Addiction: Report code 304.8x *Combinations of drug dependence excluding opioid type drug* if classifying known combinations not of opium derivatives as well as the polydrug addiction, not otherwise specified. Report code 304.7x *Combinations of opioid type drug with any other drug dependence* when an opioid drug is one of the combinations.

Coding Scenario
A patient is seen for neurogenic bowel disorder secondary to ongoing drug dependence of meperidine and opiates. The physician identifies the neurogenic bowel disorder as constipation in the medical record documentation.

> Code assignment: 304.01 *Drug dependence, Opioid type dependence, continuous* and 564.0 *Constipation, unspecified*

305 Nondependent abuse of drugs
AHA: Sept-Oct, 1986, 3; Q1, 1988, 3; Q4, 1988, 8; Q2, 1991, 10

Drug abuse includes cases where the individual, for whom no other diagnosis is possible, has come under medical care because of the maladaptive effect of a drug on which the patient is not dependent. In nondependent abuse of drugs, the individual generally has taken the drug on personal initiative to the detriment of health or social functioning. When drug abuse is secondary to a psychiatric disorder, record the disorder as a primary diagnosis.

Codes in this rubric are classified according to the drug being abused, and whether the abuse is continuous, episodic, or in remission.

The following fifth-digit subclassification is for use with categories 303, 304, 305.0, and 305.2-305.9:

0 unspecified
1 continuous
2 episodic
3 in remission

305.0 ⌫sth Nondependent alcohol abuse — *drunkenness NOS*
AHA: Sept-Oct, 1986, 3; Q1, 1988, 3; Q4, 1988, 8; Q2, 1991, 10; Q3, 1996, 16

305.1 Nondependent tobacco use disorder — *tobacco dependence*
AHA: Nov-Dec, 1984, 12; Sept-Oct, 1986, 3; Q1, 1988, 3; Q4, 1988, 8; Q2, 1991, 10; Q2, 1996, 10

305.2 ⌫sth Nondependent cannabis abuse — *abuse of hashish, marijuana, pot*
AHA: Sept-Oct, 1986, 3; Q1, 1988, 3; Q4, 1988, 8; Q2, 1991, 10

305.3 ⌫sth Nondependent hallucinogen abuse — *abuse of dimethyltryptamine [DMT], lysergic acid diethylamide [LSD], mescaline, psilocybin*
AHA: Sept-Oct, 1986, 3; Q1, 1988, 3; Q4, 1988, 8; Q2, 1991, 10

305.4 ⌫sth Nondependent barbiturate and similarly acting sedative or hypnotic abuse — *abuse of nonbarbiturate sedatives and tranquilizers with similar effect: chlordiazepoxide, meprobamate, diazepam, methaqualone, glutethimide*
AHA: Sept-Oct, 1986, 3; Q1, 1988, 3; Q4, 1988, 8; Q2, 1991, 10

305.5 ⌫sth Nondependent opioid abuse — *abuse of heroin, opium alkaloids, meperidine, methadone*
AHA: Sept-Oct, 1986, 3; Q1, 1988, 3; Q4, 1988, 8; Q2, 1991, 10

305.6 ⌫sth Nondependent cocaine abuse — *abuse of coca leaves, crack cocaine, coke*
AHA: Sept-Oct, 1986, 3; Q1, 1988, 3; Q4, 1988, 8; Q2, 1991, 10; Q1, 1993, 25; Q1, 2005, 6

305.7 ⌫sth Nondependent amphetamine or related acting sympathomimetic abuse — *abuse of methylphenidate, phenmetrazine*
AHA: Sept-Oct, 1986, 3; Q1, 1988, 3; Q4, 1988, 8; Q2, 1991, 10

305.8 ⌫sth Nondependent antidepressant type abuse
305.9 ⌫sth Other, mixed, or unspecified nondependent drug abuse — *laxative habit, nonprescribed drugs or patent medicinals*
AHA: Sept-Oct, 1986, 3; Q1, 1988, 3; Q4, 1988, 8; Q2, 1991, 10; Q3, 1999, 20

Coding Clarification
Cases in which tobacco is used to the detriment of a person's health or social functioning or in which there is tobacco dependence are classified to code 305.1. Dependence is included here rather than under drug dependence because tobacco differs from other drugs of dependence in its psychotoxic effects. Excluded from the code for tobacco dependence is history of tobacco use, V15.82.

Also excluded is smoking or tobacco use disorder complicating pregnancy, reported with a code from subcategory 649.0.

Alcohol Abuse: Patients who have been identified as having alcohol abuse represent those who have developed a problem with drinking, including those that drink alcohol in excess but have not arrived at a stage of physical dependency. Symptoms include slurred speech, blackouts, driving difficulty, social dysfunction, and temporary mental disturbance. To report, use subcategory code 305.0x. Simple drunkenness is included in this code.

Drug Abuse: Patients who have been identified as drug abusers have developed a problem with drugs including those that take an excess of drugs but have not arrived at a stage of physical dependency. Representing a maladaptive pattern due to drugs, including social, mental, and physical dysfunction, this condition also includes blackouts, slurred speech, driving difficulty, and temporary mental disturbance. Use code range 305.1x-305.9x for the diagnosis of drug abuse.

Poisoning with Abuse: When the diagnosis of drug and/or alcohol abuse has been noted with a poisoning or reaction to the improper use of the substance, the poisoning code is sequenced first, then the code for the manifestation. Also use an additional code to report the specific form of abuse.

Pregnancy Complication: Report with subcategory code 648.4 with an appropriate fifth digit to denote the current episode of care. A code specifying the type of abuse may also be reported as an additional diagnosis.

Rehabilitation: Do not report code V57.89 as the principal/primary diagnosis when reporting alcohol/drug rehabilitation services. This code is solely used as an additional code to indicate whether rehabilitation and/or detoxification services were furnished.

Tobacco Abuse: Report with code 305.1 *Tobacco use disorder*. If the documentation indicates a past history of smoking, now in remission, code V15.82 *History of tobacco use*. No fifth digit is required for code 305.1. Tobacco use disorder complicating pregnancy is reported with 649.0x.

Coding Scenario

A patient is seen in the emergency department with acute respiratory failure due to crack overdose. The patient is placed on ventilation and admitted to the intensive care unit for further stabilization.

> Code assignment: 970.8 *Poisoning by other specified central nervous system stimulants*, 305.60 *Non-dependent abuse of drugs, cocaine abuse, unspecified*, and 518.81 *Acute respiratory failure*

A patient is seen in the outpatient clinic in an acute drunken state. The patient is complaining of feeling numb. The physician's diagnostic statement confirms acute alcohol intoxication.

> Code assignment: 305.00 *Nondependent abuse of drugs, alcohol abuse*

A 17-year-old female is seen in the OB clinic for a prenatal visit. The patient admits to occasional use of cocaine.

> Code assignment: 648.43 *Other current conditions in the mother classifiable elsewhere, but complicating pregnancy, childbirth, or the puerperium, mental disorders, antepartum condition or complication* and 305.60 *Nondependent abuse of drugs, cocaine abuse, unspecified*

A 69-year-old male patient is seen in the physician office for COPD. The patient is currently smoking two packs per day and hasn't had much success with smoking cessation programs.

> Code assignment: 496 *Chronic airway obstruction, not elsewhere classified* and 305.1 *Tobacco use disorder*

306 Physiological malfunction arising from mental factors
AHA: Q1, 1988, 3

This rubric includes psychogenic physical and physiological malfunctions that do not include tissue damage.

Code	Description
306.0	Musculoskeletal malfunction arising from mental factors — *psychogenic paralysis or torticollis* AHA: Q1, 1988, 3
306.1	Respiratory malfunction arising from mental factors — *psychogenic hyperventilation; cough, yawn, or hiccough* AHA: Q1, 1988, 3
306.2	Cardiovascular malfunction arising from mental factors — *cardiac neurosis* AHA: July-Aug, 1985, 14; Q1, 1988, 3
306.3	Skin malfunction arising from mental factors — *psychogenic pruritus or hyperhidrosis* AHA: Q1, 1988, 3
306.4	Gastrointestinal malfunction arising from mental factors — *aerophagy, psychogenic vomiting or diarrhea* AHA: Q1, 1988, 3; Q2, 1989, 11
306.50	Psychogenic genitourinary malfunction, unspecified
306.51	Psychogenic vaginismus — *vaginal spasm* AHA: Q1, 1988, 3
306.52	Psychogenic dysmenorrhea — *painful menstruation* AHA: Q1, 1988, 3
306.53	Psychogenic dysuria — *painful urination* AHA: Q1, 1988, 3
306.59	Other genitourinary malfunction arising from mental factors — *specified psychogenic pain* AHA: March-April, 1987, 11; Q1, 1988, 3
306.6	Endocrine malfunction arising from mental factors — *pancreas, thyroid* AHA: Q1, 1988, 3
306.7	Malfunction of organs of special sense arising from mental factors — *eyes, ears* AHA: Q1, 1988, 3

Mental Disorders

306.8	Other specified psychophysiological malfunction — *bruxism, teeth grinding* **AHA:** Q1, 1988, 3
306.9	Unspecified psychophysiological malfunction — *not otherwise specified* **AHA:** Q1, 1988, 3

Coding Clarification

If there is tissue damage, see rubric 316. Also excluded are hysteria (300.11-300.19) and specific nonpsychotic mental disorders following organic brain damage (310.0-310.9).

307 Special symptoms or syndromes, not elsewhere classified
AHA: Q1, 1988, 3

This category is intended for psychopathology manifested by a single specific symptom or group of symptoms not part of an organic illness or other mental disorder classified elsewhere.

In anorexia nervosa, the symptoms include persistent active refusal to eat and marked loss of weight. The level of activity and alertness is characteristically high in relation to the degree of emaciation. Typically the disorder begins in teenage girls but it may begin before puberty. It rarely occurs in males. Amenorrhea is usual and, in advanced cases, slowed pulse and respiration, low body temperature, dependent edema, and heart rhythm abnormalities. Manifestations of anorexia nervosa should be reported additionally.

Code	Description
307.0	Stuttering
307.1	Anorexia nervosa — *fear of obesity, usually in females, resulting in emaciation* **AHA:** Q1, 1988, 3; Q4, 1989, 11; Q2, 2006, 12
307.20	Tic disorder, unspecified
307.21	Transient tic disorder
307.22	Chronic motor or vocal tic disorder — *blink, shrug, grimace, cough, jerk* **AHA:** Q1, 1988, 3
307.23	Tourette's disorder — *motor-verbal tic disorder; Brissaud's motor-verbal tic* **AHA:** Q1, 1988, 3
307.3	Stereotypic movement disorder — *body-rocking; spasmus nutans; head banging* **AHA:** Q1, 1988, 3
307.40	Nonorganic sleep disorder, unspecified
307.41	Transient disorder of initiating or maintaining sleep — *associated with intermittent emotional reactions or conflicts, adjustment insomnia* **AHA:** Q1, 1988, 3
307.42	Persistent disorder of initiating or maintaining sleep — *associated with anxiety, depression, psychosis, idiopathic insomnia, paradoxical insomnia, primary insomnia, psychophysiological insomnia* **AHA:** Q1, 1988, 3
307.43	Transient disorder of initiating or maintaining wakefulness — *associated with acute or intermittent emotional reactions or conflicts* **AHA:** Q1, 1988, 3
307.44	Persistent disorder of initiating or maintaining wakefulness — *associated with depression, insufficient sleep syndrome, primary hypersomnia* **AHA:** Q1, 1988, 3
307.45	Circadian rhythm sleep disorder of non-organic origin — *jet lag syndrome; shifting sleep-work schedule of nonorganic origin* **AHA:** Q1, 1988, 3
307.46	Sleep arousal disorder — *sleepwalking* **AHA:** Q1, 1988, 3
307.47	Other dysfunctions of sleep stages or arousal from sleep — *nightmares* **AHA:** Q1, 1988, 3
307.48	Repetitive intrusions of sleep — *environmental disturbances or repeated REM- interruptions* **AHA:** Q1, 1988, 3
307.49	Other specific disorder of sleep of nonorganic origin — *subjective "short-sleeper;" pseudoinsomnia* **AHA:** Q1, 1988, 3
307.50	Eating disorder, unspecified
307.51	Bulimia nervosa — *binge/purge* **AHA:** Q1, 1988, 3
307.52	Pica — *perverted appetite of nonorganic origin* **AHA:** Q1, 1988, 3
307.53	Rumination disorder — *regurgitation, of nonorganic origin, of food with reswallowing* **AHA:** Q1, 1988, 3
307.54	Psychogenic vomiting — *no physical cause* **AHA:** Q1, 1988, 3
307.59	Other disorder of eating — *no physical cause of nonorganic origin*
307.6	Enuresis — *of nonorganic origin* **AHA:** Q1, 1988, 3
307.7	Encopresis — *of nonorganic origin* **AHA:** Q1, 1988, 3
307.80	Psychogenic pain, site unspecified
307.81	Tension headache — *stress headache* **AHA:** Nov-Dec, 1985, 16; Q1, 1988, 3
307.89	Other pain disorder related to psychological factors — *(Code first to type or site of pain) — not elsewhere classified* **AHA:** Q1, 1988, 3
307.9	Other and unspecified special symptom or syndrome, not elsewhere classified — *hair plucking, masturbation, lalling, nail-biting, lisping, thumb-sucking* **AHA:** Q1, 1988, 3

Coding Clarification

Some sleep disorders are not due to a substance or known physiological or pathological condition. These disorders are classified as having a non-organic origin and are codeable within this section of codes.. Non-organic conditions are of psychophysiological origin, disturbance in sleep environment, paradoxical conditions that exhibit seemingly contradictable aspects, and/or idiopathic conditions that are self-originated or on unknown etiology.

308 Acute reaction to stress
AHA: Q1, 1988, 3

This rubric is reserved for acute reactions as a response to exceptional physical or mental distress, which usually subside within hours or days. Some examples include catastrophic stress, combat fatigue, or gross stress reaction.

308.0	Predominant disturbance of emotions — *anxiety, emotional crisis, panic* **AHA:** Q1, 1988, 3	
308.1	Predominant disturbance of consciousness as reaction to stress — *fugues* **AHA:** Q1, 1988, 3	
308.2	Predominant psychomotor disturbance as reaction to stress — *agitation or stupor* **AHA:** Q1, 1988, 3	
308.3	Other acute reactions to stress — *brief or acute posttraumatic stress disorder* **AHA:** Q1, 1988, 3	
308.4	Mixed disorders as reaction to stress — *combination of reactions classified to 308* **AHA:** Q1, 1988, 3	
308.9	Unspecified acute reaction to stress — *combat fatigue* **AHA:** Q1, 1988, 3	

Coding Clarification
Excluded from this rubric are adjustment reaction disorders (309.0-309.9) and chronic stress reaction (309.1-309.9).

309 Adjustment reaction
AHA: Q1, 1988, 3

An adjustment or adaptation reaction is a mild or transient disorder lasting longer than acute stress reactions and occurring in individuals of any age without any apparent pre-existing mental disorder. Such disorders are often relatively circumscribed or situation-specific, are generally reversible, and usually last only a few months. They are usually closely related in time and content to stresses such as bereavement, migration, or other experiences. Reactions to major stress that last longer than a few days are also included. In children, such disorders are associated with no significant distortion of development.

309.0	Adjustment disorder with depressed mood — *grief reaction* **AHA:** Q1, 1988, 3
309.1	Prolonged depressive reaction as adjustment reaction
309.21	Separation anxiety disorder — *abnormal stress upon leaving another person* **AHA:** Q1, 1988, 3
309.22	Emancipation disorder of adolescence and early adult life
309.23	Specific academic or work inhibition as adjustment reaction
309.24	Adjustment disorder with anxiety
309.28	Adjustment disorder with mixed anxiety and depressed mood — *adjustment reaction with anxiety and depression* **AHA:** Q1, 1988, 3
309.29	Other adjustment reaction with predominant disturbance of other emotions — *culture shock* **AHA:** Q1, 1988, 3
309.3	Adjustment disorder with disturbance of conduct — *conduct disturbance or destructiveness as an adjustment reaction* **AHA:** Q1, 1988, 3
309.4	Adjustment disorder with mixed disturbance of emotions and conduct
309.81	Posttraumatic stress disorder — *chronic posttraumatic stress disorder; concentration camp syndrome; PTSD* **AHA:** Q1, 1988, 3
309.82	Adjustment reaction with physical symptoms
309.83	Adjustment reaction with withdrawal — *elective mutism, hospitalism* **AHA:** Q1, 1988, 3
309.89	Other specified adjustment reaction — *homesickness* **AHA:** Q1, 1988, 3
309.9	Unspecified adjustment reaction — *adaptation reaction NOS* **AHA:** Q1, 1988, 3

Coding Clarification
Excluded from this rubric are acute reactions to major stress (308.0-308.9) and neurotic disorders (300.1-300.9).

310 Specific nonpsychotic mental disorders due to brain damage
AHA: Q1, 1988, 3

Postconcussion syndrome occurs after generalized contusion of the brain, resembling the overall symptoms found in frontal lobe syndrome or any of the neurotic disorders, but in which headache, giddiness, fatigue, insomnia, and a subjective feeling of impaired intellectual ability are also prominent. Mood may fluctuate, and quite ordinary stress may produce exaggerated fear and apprehension. There may be marked intolerance of mental and physical exertion, undue sensitivity to noise, and hypochondriacal preoccupation. The symptoms are more common in persons who have previously suffered from neurotic or personality disorders. This syndrome is particularly associated with the closed type of head injury when signs of localized brain damage are slight or absent, but it may also occur in other conditions.

Frontal lobe syndrome presents with changes in behavior following damage to the frontal areas of the brain or following interference with the connections of those areas. There is a general diminution of self-control, foresight, creativity, and spontaneity, which may be manifest as increased irritability, selfishness, restlessness, and lack of concern for others. Conscientiousness and powers of concentration are often diminished, but measurable deterioration of intellect or memory is not necessarily present. The overall picture is often one of emotional dullness, lack of drive, and slowness; but, particularly in persons previously with energetic, restless, or aggressive characteristics, there may be a change toward impulsiveness, boastfulness, temper outbursts, silly fatuous humor, and the development of unrealistic ambitions. The direction of change usually depends upon the previous personality. A considerable degree of recovery is possible and may continue over the course of several years.

310.0 Frontal lobe syndrome — *postleucotomy syndrome, Klüver-Bucy (-Terzian) syndrome*
AHA: Q1, 1988, 3

310.1 Personality change due to conditions classified elsewhere — *cognitive or personality change of other type, of nonpsychotic severity; mild memory disturbance; presbyophrenia NOS*
AHA: Q1, 1988, 3; Q2, 2005, 6

310.2 Postconcussion syndrome — *postconcussion syndrome or encephalopathy*
AHA: Q1, 1988, 3; Q4, 1990, 24

310.8 Other specified nonpsychotic mental disorder following organic brain damage — *postencephalitic syndrome*
AHA: Q1, 1988, 3

310.9 Unspecified nonpsychotic mental disorder following organic brain damage

311 Depressive disorder, not elsewhere classified
AHA: Q1, 1988, 3; Q4, 2003, 75

This rubric is reserved for depressive disorders not classified in other sections of this chapter, or depressive orders not assigned a more specific diagnosis.

312 Disturbance of conduct, not elsewhere classified
AHA: Q1, 1988, 3

This rubric is reserved for psychosocial and other conduct disorders not classified in other sections of this chapter, or that cannot be assigned a more specific diagnosis. Conduct disorders mainly involve aggressive and destructive behavior and disorders involving delinquency. Codes in this rubric should be used for abnormal behavior, in individuals of any age, which gives rise to social disapproval although not part of any other psychiatric condition. Minor emotional disturbances may also be present. To be included, the behavior, as judged by its frequency, severity, and type of associations with other symptoms, must be abnormal in its context. Disturbances of conduct are distinguished from an adjustment reaction by a longer duration and by a lack of close relationship in time and content to some stress. They differ from a personality disorder by the absence of deeply ingrained maladaptive patterns of behavior present from adolescence or earlier.

The following fifth-digit subclassification is for use with categories 312.0-312.2:
0 unspecified
1 mild
2 moderate
3 severe

312.0 ✓5th Undersocialized conduct disorder, aggressive type — *aggressive outburst, anger reaction; unsocialized, aggressive disorder*
AHA: Q1, 1988, 3

312.1 ✓5th Undersocialized conduct disorder, unaggressive type — *childhood truancy; tantrums, solitary, stealing; unsocialized*
AHA: Q1, 1988, 3

312.2 ✓5th Socialized conduct disorder — *childhood truancy socialized, group delinquency*
AHA: Q1, 1988, 3

312.30 Impulse control disorder, unspecified
312.31 Pathological gambling
312.32 Kleptomania — *compulsive theft*
AHA: Q1, 1988, 3
312.33 Pyromania — *compulsive fire starting*
AHA: Q1, 1988, 3
312.34 Intermittent explosive disorder
312.35 Isolated explosive disorder
312.39 Other disorder of impulse control — *not elsewhere specified, trichotillomania*
AHA: Q1, 1988, 3

312.4 Mixed disturbance of conduct and emotions — *neurotic delinquency*
AHA: Q1, 1988, 3

312.81	Conduct disorder, childhood onset type
312.82	Conduct disorder, adolescent onset type
312.89	Other specified disturbance of conduct, not elsewhere classified
312.9	Unspecified disturbance of conduct

313 Disturbance of emotions specific to childhood and adolescence
AHA: Q1, 1988, 3

Academic underachievement disorder (313.83) presents as a failure to achieve in most school tasks despite adequate intellectual capacity, a supportive and encouraging social environment, and apparent effort. The failure occurs in the absence of a demonstrable specific learning disability and is caused by emotional conflict not clearly associated with any other mental disorder.

313.0	Overanxious disorder specific to childhood and adolescence — *anxiety and fearfulness in childhood* AHA: Q1, 1988, 3
313.1	Misery and unhappiness disorder specific to childhood and adolescence
313.21	Shyness disorder of childhood
313.22	Introverted disorder of childhood
313.23	Selective mutism
313.3	Relationship problems specific to childhood and adolescence
313.81	Oppositional defiant disorder
313.82	Identity disorder of childhood or adolescence
313.83	Academic underachievement disorder of childhood or adolescence
313.89	Other emotional disturbance of childhood or adolescence
313.9	Unspecified emotional disturbance of childhood or adolescence

Coding Clarification
This rubric excludes adjustment reactions (309.0-309.9), neurotic emotional disorders (300.0-300.9), and isolated symptoms including masturbation, nail biting, and thumb-sucking (307.0-307.9).

314 Hyperkinetic syndrome of childhood
AHA: Q1, 1988, 3

Hyperkinetic syndromes of childhood are disorders in which the essential features are short attention span and distractibility. In early childhood, the most striking symptom is disinhibited, poorly organized, and poorly regulated extreme overactivity but in adolescence this may be replaced by underactivity. Impulsiveness, marked fluctuations in mood, and aggression are also common symptoms. Delays in the development of specific skills are often present and disturbed, poor relationships are common.

314.00	Attention deficit disorder of childhood without mention of hyperactivity
314.01	Attention deficit disorder of childhood with hyperactivity
314.1	Hyperkinesis of childhood with developmental delay — (Use additional code to identify any associated neurological disorder)
314.2	Hyperkinetic conduct disorder of childhood — *without developmental delay* AHA: Q1, 1988, 3
314.8	Other specified manifestations of hyperkinetic syndrome of childhood
314.9	Unspecified hyperkinetic syndrome of childhood

Coding Clarification
If the hyperkinesis is symptomatic of an underlying disorder, the diagnosis of the underlying disorder is recorded instead. This rubric excludes hyperkinesis as a symptom of an underlying disorder.

315 Specific delays in development
AHA: Q1, 1988, 3

This rubric classifies a group of disorders in which a specific delay in development is the main feature. For many, the delay is not explicable in terms of general intellectual delay or of inadequate schooling. In each case, development is related to biological maturation, but it is also influenced by nonbiological factors. A diagnosis of a specific developmental delay carries no etiological implications. A diagnosis of specific delay in development should not be made if it is due to a known neurological disorder.

Code	Description
315.00	Developmental reading disorder, unspecified
315.01	Alexia — *inability to comprehend words* AHA: Q1, 1988, 3
315.02	Developmental dyslexia — *impaired reading ability* AHA: Q1, 1988, 3
315.09	Other specific developmental reading disorder
315.1	Mathematics disorder — *dyscalculia* AHA: Q1, 1988, 3
315.2	Other specific developmental learning difficulties — *spelling difficulty* AHA: Q1, 1988, 3
315.31	Expressive language disorder — *expressive language disorder* AHA: Q1, 1988, 3
315.32	Mixed receptive-expressive language disorder — *receptive, expressive language disorder* AHA: Q4, 1996, 30; Q1, 1988, 3; Q2, 2005, 5;
315.39	Other developmental speech or language disorder — *dyslalia* AHA: Q1, 1988, 3
315.4	Developmental coordination disorder — *clumsiness/dyspraxia syndrome* AHA: Q1, 1988, 3
315.5	Mixed development disorder
315.8	Other specified delay in development
315.9	Unspecified delay in development

Mental Disorders

Coding Clarification
Excluded from this rubric are delays in development that are due to neurological disorders (320.0-389.9).

316 Psychic factors associated with diseases classified elsewhere ✓
AHA: Q1, 1988, 3

This rubric is used to report psychological factors in physical conditions classified elsewhere.

Coding Clarification
Use an additional code to report the associated physical condition, as in psychogenic ulcerative colitis (556.x), eczema (691.8, 692.9), paroxysmal tachycardia (427.2), or psychosocial dwarfism (259.4). Do not use this rubric to report physical symptoms and physiological malfunctions not involving tissue damage or mental origin. For those cases, see 306.0-306.9.

317-319 Mental Retardation

Mental retardation is defined as general intellectual functioning at least two standard deviations below the norm as measured in a standardized intelligence test, when it is accompanied by significant limitation in communication, self-care, home living, interpersonal skills, self-direction, work, leisure, health, or safety. The onset must occur before adulthood.

Use additional codes to identify any associated psychiatric or physical conditions.

317 Mild mental retardation ✓
AHA: Q1, 1988, 3

In mild mental retardation, the patient has an IQ of 50-70. Individuals with this level of retardation are usually educable. During the preschool period, they can develop social and communication skills, have minimal delay in sensorimotor areas, and often are not distinguished from normal children until a later age. During the school age period they can learn academic skills up to approximately the sixth-grade level. During the adult years, they can usually achieve social and vocational skills adequate for minimum self-support, but may need guidance and assistance when under social or economic stress.

318 Other specified mental retardation
AHA: Q1, 1988, 3

In moderate mental retardation, the patient has an IQ of 35-49. Individuals with this level of retardation are usually trainable. During the preschool period they can talk or learn to communicate. They have poor social awareness and fair motor development. During the school age period they can profit from training in social and occupational skills, but they are unlikely to progress beyond the second-grade level in academic subjects. During their adult years they may achieve self-maintenance in unskilled or semi-skilled work under sheltered conditions. They need supervision and guidance when under mild social or economic stress.

In severe mental retardation, the patient has an IQ of 20-34. Individuals with this level of retardation evidence poor motor development, minimal speech, and are generally unable to profit from training and self-help during the preschool period. During the school age period they can talk or learn to communicate, can be trained in elementary health habits, and may profit from systematic habit training. During the adult years they may contribute partially to self-maintenance under complete supervision.

In profound mental retardation, the patient has an IQ under 20. Individuals with this level of retardation evidence minimal capacity for sensorimotor functioning and need nursing care during the preschool period. During the school age period some further motor development may occur, and they may respond to minimal or limited training in self-help.

During the adult years some motor and speech development may occur, and they may achieve very limited self-care and need nursing care.

318.0	Moderate mental retardation — (Use additional code(s) to identify any associated psychiatric or physical condition) — IQ 35-49 AHA: Q1, 1988, 3
318.1	Severe mental retardation — (Use additional code(s) to identify any associated psychiatric or physical condition) — IQ 20-34 AHA: Q1, 1988, 3
318.2	Profound mental retardation — (Use additional code(s) to identify any associated psychiatric or physical condition) — IQ under 20 AHA: Q1, 1988, 3

319 Unspecified mental retardation ✓
AHA: Q1, 1988, 3

This rubric is reserved for patients who evidence obvious mental retardation, but the severity of the condition has not been measured with standardized testing.

320–389

Diseases of the Nervous System and Sense Organs

This chapter classifies diseases and disorders of the nervous system including meninges (the covering of the brain and spinal cord), central nervous system, and peripheral nervous system (the nerves that relay signals between the central nervous system and the organs of the body). This chapter also classifies conditions affecting the eye and ear.

320–326 Inflammatory Diseases of the Central Nervous System

The central nervous system (CNS) comprises the brain, the spinal cord, and associated membranes. The brain can be subdivided into several regions:

- The cerebral hemispheres form the largest part of the brain, occupying the anterior and middle cranial fossae in the skull.
- The diencephalon includes the thalamus, hypothalamus, epithalamus and subthalamus, and forms the central core of the brain.
- The midbrain is located at the junction of the middle and posterior cranial fossae.
- The pons is in the anterior part of the posterior cranial fossa; fibers within the pons connect one cerebral hemisphere with its opposite cerebellar hemisphere.
- The medulla oblongata is continuous with the spinal cord and controls the respiratory and cardiovascular systems.
- The cerebellum overlies the pons and medulla and controls motor functions that regulate muscle tone, coordination, and posture.

The spinal column, which encloses the spinal cord, consists of vertebrae linked by intervertebral disks and held together by ligaments. The spinal cord extends from the first lumbar vertebra to the medulla at the base of the brain. The outer layer of the spinal cord consists of myelin-sheathed nerve fibers bundled that conduct impulses triggered by pressure, pain, heat, and other sensory stimuli or conduct motor impulses activating muscles and glands. The inner layer, or gray matter, is primarily composed of nerve cell bodies. The central canal, within the gray matter, circulates the cerebrospinal fluid. The three meninges wrap around the spinal cord and cover the brain; the pia mater is the innermost layer, the arachnoid lies in the middle, and the dura mater is the outside layer, to which the spinal nerves are attached. The 31 pairs of spinal nerves deliver impulses into the spinal cord, which in turn relays them to the brain. Conversely, motor impulses generated in the brain are relayed by the spinal cord to the spinal nerves, which pass the impulses to muscles and glands. Nerve fibers in the spinal cord usually do not regenerate if injured by accident or disease.

Diseases in this rubric are often the result of bacterial invasion spreading from a nearby infection (i.e., a chronic sinus or middle ear infection). The bloodstream may carry bacteria from other sites to the CNS and, in rare cases, head trauma or surgical procedures may introduce bacteria directly into the CNS.

Bacterial infection of the CNS can result in abscesses and empyemas. CNS infections are classified according to the location where they occur. For example, a spinal epidural abscess is located above the dura mater, and a cranial subdural empyema occurs between the dura mater and the arachnoid. As pus and other material from an infection accumulate, pressure is exerted on the brain or spinal cord. This pressure can damage the nervous system tissue and, without treatment, the infection can be fatal. Specific symptoms of CNS infections depend on location, but may include severe headache or back pain, weakness, sensory loss, and a fever. An individual may complain of a stiff neck, nausea or vomiting, and tiredness or disorientation. There is a potential for seizures, paralysis, or coma. The fatality rate associated with CNS infections ranges from 10 to 40 percent, and those surviving an infection may experience permanent damage, resulting in partial paralysis, speech problems, or seizures.

These categories include meningitis, encephalitis, cerebral abscesses, late effects of infections of the central nervous system, and other types of inflammations such as meningitis due to sarcoidosis and lead poisoning (toxic) encephalitis. However, many infections of the central nervous system are excluded.

320 Bacterial meningitis
AHA: Jan-Feb, 1987, 6

Bacterial meningitis is inflammation of the CNS covering of meninges due to a bacterial organism. Bacterial meningitis can be caused by a variety of pyogenic bacterial organisms, most commonly *Haemophilus influenzae (type B)*, *Streptococcus pneumoniae*, Pneumococcus, Neisseria meningitis, *Staphylococcus aureus*, Klebsiella, *Pseudomonas*, and *Escherichia coli*. Code selection is based upon the infective agent.

Anaerobic bacteria are organisms that thrive only in the absence of free oxygen and can be either gram-negative or gram-positive. *Clostridium tetani* is an example of a gram-positive anaerobe, and *Proteus vulgaris* is an example of a gram-negative anaerobe.

The terms "gram-negative" and "gram-positive" refer to a method of differential staining of bacteria for bacterial taxonomy and identification. Gram-positive bacteria retain the basic dye crystal violet, and gram-negative bacteria lose the crystal violet dye to become colorless. Counterstains color gram-negative bacteria pink to red and leave gram-positive bacteria dark purple.

Signs and symptoms of bacterial meningitis include fever and chills, headache, stiff neck, nausea and vomiting, alterations in sensorium, seizure, positive Kernig's and Brudzinski's signs, and rash. These signs and symptoms, in addition to chronically draining ear, are associated with pneumococcal meningitis.

Diagnostic tests include lumbar puncture to obtain cerebrospinal fluid for verifying elevated fluid pressure. Culture of cerebrospinal fluid is performed to identify the organism and a gram stain of cerebrospinal fluid reveals polymorphonuclear leukocytes, elevated white blood cell count, decreased glucose level, and elevated protein content. In addition, a limulus lysate assay test may be performed to detect endotoxins due to gram-negative bacteria and a cranial CT scan may indicate cerebral edema early and subdural effusion or empyema later. Therapies include isolation, avoidance of temperature extremes, antimicrobials administered intravenously in large doses, IV hydration, medication such as Dilantin to control seizures, diuretics or withdrawal of cerebrospinal fluid through an intraventricular catheter to reduce intracranial pressure, oxygen therapy for hypoxia, and intubation and ventilation for hypoventilation with hypercapnia.

Associated conditions include seizures due to increased intracranial pressure, respiratory distress or failure, altered state of consciousness, vasomotor collapse or shock, intravascular coagulation, syndrome of inappropriate antidiuretic hormone secretion (SIADH), dehydration, or various electrolyte imbalances.

320.0	Hemophilus meningitis — *meningitis due to Hemophilus influenzae (H. influenzae)* **AHA:** Jan-Feb, 1987, 6
320.1	Pneumococcal meningitis — *pneumococcal infection causing inflammation of the membranes enveloping the brain and/or spinal cord* **AHA:** Jan-Feb, 1987, 6
320.2	Streptococcal meningitis — *streptococcal infection causing inflammation of the membranes enveloping the brain and/or spinal cord* **AHA:** Jan-Feb, 1987, 6
320.3	Staphylococcal meningitis — *staphylococcal infection causing inflammation of the membranes enveloping the brain and/or spinal cord* **AHA:** Jan-Feb, 1987, 6
320.7	Meningitis in other bacterial diseases classified elsewhere — (Code first underlying disease: 002.0, 027.0, 033.0-033.9, 039.8) — *actinomycosis, listeriosis, typhoid fever, and whooping cough* **AHA:** Jan-Feb, 1987, 6
320.81	Anaerobic meningitis — *bacteroides (fragilis); gram-negative anaerobes* **AHA:** Jan-Feb, 1987, 6
320.82	Meningitis due to gram-negative bacteria, not elsewhere classified — *Aerobacter aerogenes; Klebsiella pneumoniae; Proteus morganii; Pseudomonas* **AHA:** Jan-Feb, 1987, 6
320.89	Meningitis due to other specified bacteria — *Bacillus pyocyaneus* **AHA:** Jan-Feb, 1987, 6
320.9	Meningitis due to unspecified bacterium

Documentation Issues

If the medical documentation indicates aseptic, viral, or nonbacterial meningitis without further specification, see category 047 *Meningitis due to enterovirus.* When meningitis is a manifestation of another disease process (320.7), code the underlying disease first.

321 Meningitis due to other organisms
AHA: Jan-Feb, 1987, 6

Meningitis due to other organisms is inflammation of the CNS covering of meninges due to organisms other than bacteria. These can be fungal organisms, viruses not classified elsewhere, or other nonbacterial organisms.

Signs and symptoms of meningitis due to other organisms vary according to infectious agent. Therapies include specific treatment depending on the infectious agent (e.g., antifungal agents such as amphotericin B for fungal meningitis and corticosteroids for sarcoid meningitis).

321.0	Cryptococcal meningitis — (Code first underlying disease, 117.5) — *cryptococcus infection causing inflammation of the membranes enveloping the brain and/or spinal cord* AHA: Jan-Feb, 1987, 6	
321.1	Meningitis in other fungal diseases — (Code first underlying disease: 110.0-118)	
321.2	Meningitis due to viruses not elsewhere classified — (Code first underlying disease: 060.0-066.9) AHA: Q4, 2004, 51	
321.3	Meningitis due to trypanosomiasis — (Code first underlying disease: 086.0-086.9) — *trypanosomiasis infection causing inflammation of the membranes enveloping the brain and/or spinal cord* AHA: Jan-Feb, 1987, 6	
321.4	Meningitis in sarcoidosis — (Code first underlying disease, 135) — *sarcoidosis causing inflammation of the membranes enveloping the brain and/or spinal cord* AHA: Jan-Feb, 1987, 6	
321.8	Meningitis due to other nonbacterial organisms classified elsewhere — (Code first underlying disease)	

322 Meningitis of unspecified cause
AHA: Jan-Feb, 1987, 6

322.0	Nonpyogenic meningitis — *meningitis with clear cerebrospinal fluid* AHA: Jan-Feb, 1987, 6
322.1	Eosinophilic meningitis — *presence of cells readily stained with eosin causing inflammation of the membranes enveloping the brain and/or spinal cord* AHA: Jan-Feb, 1987, 6
322.2	Chronic meningitis — *persistent inflammation of the membranes enveloping the brain and/or spinal cord* AHA: Jan-Feb, 1987, 6
322.9	Unspecified meningitis — *leptomeningopathy; ventriculitis, cerebral* AHA: Jan-Feb, 1987, 6

323 Encephalitis, myelitis, and encephalomyelitis

Encephalitis, myelitis, and encephalomyelitis are inflammations of the central nervous system that alter the function of various portions of the brain (encephalitis), spinal cord (myelitis), or both (encephalomyelitis). The inflammation usually results from either a direct invasion of the central nervous system by a virus or postinfection involvement of the central nervous system after a viral disease. Bacteria, medications, toxic substances, and parasites also may cause it. Arthropod-borne viruses as seen in mosquitoes most often cause encephalitis. Myelitis infection results from direct invasion or tick bites classified to categories 062 and 063.

Signs and symptoms of encephalitis, myelitis, and encephalomyelitis, with mild benign forms, are malaise, fever, headache, dizziness, apathy, neck stiffness, nausea and vomiting, ataxia, tremors, hyperactivity, and speech difficulties. With severe central nervous system involvement, there is high fever, stupor, seizures, disorientation, ocular palsies, paralysis, spasticity, and coma that may proceed to death.

Diagnostic tests include lumbar puncture with analysis of cerebrospinal fluid to show lymphocytes, moderate rises in protein, and markedly elevated specific viral antibody titers with acute encephalitis. Cultures (i.e., cerebrospinal fluid, blood, and saliva) may identify the specific virus (except arboviruses that rarely are detected in the blood or spinal fluid). A brain biopsy may rule out herpes simplex.

Therapies include IV hydration and control of temperature. Specific treatment depends on the etiology (e.g., chelation therapy for lead poisoning encephalitis and chloroquine for malarial encephalitis).

323.01	Encephalitis and encephalomyelitis in viral diseases classified elsewhere — (Code first underlying disease: 073.7, 075, 078.3) — *cat-scratch disease, infectious mononucleosis, and ornithosis*
323.02	Myelitis in viral diseases classified elsewhere — (Code first underlying disease: 073.7, 075, 078.3) — *cat-scratch disease, infectious mononucleosis, and ornithosis*

323.1	Encephalitis, myelitis, and encephalomyelitis in rickettsial diseases classified elsewhere — (Code first underlying disease: 080-083.9) — *inflammation of the brain caused by rickettsial disease carried by louse, tick or mite*	
323.2	Encephalitis, myelitis, and encephalomyelitis in protozoal diseases classified elsewhere — (Code first underlying disease: 084.0-084.9, 086.0-086.9) — *malaria and trypanosomiasis*	
323.41	Other encephalitis and encephalomyelitis due to infection classified elsewhere — (Code first underlying disease)	
323.42	Other myelitis due to infection classified elsewhere — (Code first underlying disease)	
323.51	Encephalitis and encephalomyelitis following immunization procedures — (Use additional E code to identify vaccine) — *postimmunization encephalitis; postvaccinal encephalitis; postimmunization encephalomyelitis; postvaccinal encephalomyelitis*	
323.52	Myelitis following immunization procedures — (Use additional E code to identify vaccine) — *postimmunization myelitis; postvaccinal myelitis*	
323.61	Infectious acute disseminated encephalomyelitis (ADEM) — (Code first underlying disease) — *acute necrotizing hemorrhagic encephalopathy*	
323.62	Other postinfectious encephalitis and encephalomyelitis — (Code first underlying disease)	
323.63	Postinfectious myelitis — (Code first underlying disease)	
323.71	Toxic encephalitis and encephalomyelitis — (Code first underlying cause: 961.3, 982.1, 984.0-984.9, 985.0, 985.8)	
323.72	Toxic myelitis — (Code first underlying cause: 961.3, 982.1, 984.0-984.9, 985.0, 985.8)	
323.81	Other causes of encephalitis and encephalomyelitis — *noninfectious acute disseminated encephalomyelitis (ADEM)*	
323.82	Other causes of myelitis — *transverse myelitis, NOS*	
323.9	Unspecified cause of encephalitis, myelitis, and encephalomyelitis — *syringomyelitis* AHA: Q1, 2006, 8	

Coding Clarification

Diseases in this rubric are classified according to causative organism. Sequence the underlying disease first. If the organism is unspecified or if there is a noninfectious or toxic etiology, see subcategories 323.5 and 323.8, and code 323.9.

Acute transverse myelitis (341.2x) is classified with demyelinating diseases of the nervous system. Numerous subterms in the Alphabetic Index help direct the coder to the appropriate choice.

324 Intracranial and intraspinal abscess

Intracranial and intraspinal abscess is the localized collection of pus in a cavity involving the brain or spinal column, respectively.

Intracranial abscess is the localized collection of purulent material and liquified brain tissue involving the many layers of the brain, including the epidural or subdural spaces, or within the substance of the brain itself. The etiology is usually bacterial and occurs through direct extension from a contiguous focus, blood-borne metastases, or by penetrating injury. The most common cause of direct extension in a brain abscess is a contiguous infection such as in the middle ear, mastoid, or sinuses. The most common site of origin for blood-borne metastasis is the lung (empyema, bronchiectasis). When the abscess is due to trauma, a skull fracture or penetrating injury is usually involved. The most common organisms are streptococci, pneumococci, and staphylococci.

Signs and symptoms of intracranial abscess, with brain abscess, include headache, altered sensorium (lethargy, irritability, confusion, or coma), nausea and vomiting, fever, seizures, multiple alternation nerve palsies, and other neurologic deficits. Signs and symptoms of intracranial abscess, with subdural abscess, include headache, sinusitis, altered sensorium (lethargy, obtundation, or coma), seizures, fever and chills, hemiparesis, and aphasia. Signs and symptoms of intracranial abscess, with cerebral epidural abscess, involve limited localized symptoms.

Diagnostic tests include MRI and radionuclide or CT scans to identify the location and size of abscess. With subdural abscess, plain skull x-rays reveal underlying sinus or mastoid disease, while cerebral arteriography shows space between cerebral vessels and the inner surface of the cranium. Therapies include antimicrobials for early abscess, incision and drainage, or excision of abscess.

The definition of intraspinal abscess is the localized collection of pus in a cavity involving the layers of the spinal cord, including the epidura, extradura, and subdura. It is usually bacterial, and the most common organisms are streptococci, pneumococci, and staphylococci. The etiology is usually due to blood-borne spread, direct extension from contiguous sites, or as a consequence of an invasive procedure. Most spinal abscesses are epidural.

Signs and symptoms of intraspinal abscess include spinal ache, root pain, weakness, paresthesias, and eventually paralysis. Diagnostic tests include lumbar puncture with analysis of cerebrospinal fluid to show elevated protein, xanthochromia, and normal glucose. Culture identifies the bacterial agent. Myelography, CT scan, and MRI visualize the abscess. Therapies include antimicrobials for early abscess, incision and drainage, or excision for fully established intraspinal abscess.

324.0	Intracranial abscess — *cerebellar (embolic) abscess; abscess (embolic) of brain (any part)*
324.1	Intraspinal abscess — *abscess (embolic) of spinal cord (any part); epidural, extradural or subdural*
324.9	Intracranial and intraspinal abscess of unspecified site — *extradural or subdural abscess NOS*

325 Phlebitis and thrombophlebitis of intracranial venous sinuses OK

This rubric identifies the inflammation and formation of a blood clot in a vein within the brain or its lining. The principal veins in the cranial cavity are incorporated into the dura mater, which is closely bound to the inner bone of the cavity. The venous sinuses (e.g., the sagittal, cavernous, petrosal, sphenoparietal, sigmoid, and transverse sinuses) are held in an open position and generally occur where there is a wide separation between major anatomical entities. The sinuses contain an endothelial lining continuous into the veins connected to them. There are no valves in the sinuses or in the veins and the majority of the venous blood in the sinus drains from the cranium via the internal jugular vein.

Intracranial venous thrombosis occurs as a complication of intracranial infections and can result in symptoms such as headaches, focal seizures, and focal neurologic signs affecting the legs more than the arm. Massive venous infarction, due to thrombosis, may be fatal. The thrombus can be identified by its signal intensity on MRI and the flow void in the affected sinus is clearly documented on MR angiography.

Septic intracranial thrombophlebitis is an extremely serious complication that even with appropriate therapy is fatal in more that one-third of cases. Deep or superficial septic phlebitis can occur by direct invasion from adjacent non-vascular infections associated with a long-term intravenous cannula being used for chronic administration of fluids or medications. The etiologic agent usually can be cultured both from blood and from any metastatic sites of infection and the organism responsible often can be predicted from the site of infection. The worst complications are in patients with phlebitis due to *Staphylococcus aureus*, often the cause of septic intracranial venous sinus thrombophlebitis.

The injection of contrast material into a central catheter often permits visualization of a catheter-associated thrombus or of an extensive fibrin sheath that extends, cloud-like, away from the catheter. Contrast enhanced CT or magnetic resonance imaging (MRI) can identify the extent of the thrombus, the local anatomy of the affected tissues, and any pockets of purulent material that may require drainage.

Extended high-dose anti-microbial therapy is recommended because of the high risk of septic emboli. Heparin halts the progression of septic thrombophlebitis and eliminates an ongoing source of septic emboli. Because septic phlebitis is associated with a high incidence of secondary infection, high-dose antibiotics are continued for at least six weeks after blood cultures become negative.

Coding Clarification
Excluded from this rubric is phlebitis and thrombophlebitis of intracranial venous sinuses associated with pregnancy (671.5) or of nonpyogenic origin (437.6).

326 Late effects of intracranial abscess or pyogenic infection OK

Late effects of intracranial abscess or pyogenic infection are the late effects of meningitis, encephalitis, myelitis, encephalomyelitis, intracranial and intraspinal abscess, and phlebitis or thrombophlebitis of the intracranial sinuses except when these conditions are manifestations of another disease process identified by italics in the ICD-9-CM tabular list.

Coding Clarification
Use an additional code to describe the condition, as in hydrocephalus (331.4) or paralysis (rubrics 342 and 344).

327 Organic Sleep Disorders

327 Organic sleep disorders
AHA: Q4, 2005, 59-64

Organic sleep disorders listed in this section include various types of specified sleep disorders that are, by definition, the result of a demonstrable anatomic or physiologic abnormality or any pathologic (disease) process, as opposed to a psychological, behavioral, or substance-induced disorder.

327.0 ✓5th	Organic disorders of initiating and maintaining sleep [Organic insomnia]

This range of codes addresses specific insomnia conditions in which there is difficulty in initiating or maintaining sleep due to a known physiologic disturbance or pathogenic origin. This subcategory excludes unspecified insomnia (780.52), insomnia not due to a substance or known physiological condition (307.41-307.42), and insomnia with sleep apnea (780.51).

327.00	Organic insomnia, unspecified
327.01	Insomnia due to medical condition classified elsewhere— (Code first underlying condition)
327.02	Insomnia due to mental disorder — (Code first mental disorder)

This code excludes alcohol or drug induced insomnia, coded to 291.82 and 292.85, respectively.

327.09	Other organic insomnia
327.1 ⊷sth	Organic disorder of excessive somnolence [Organic hypersomnia]

This range of codes addresses specific hypersomnia conditions in which there is excessive sleepiness (somnolence), or excessive time spent in a sleep state due to a known physiologic disturbance or pathogenic origin. This subcategory excludes unspecified hypersomnia (780.54), hypersomnia not due to a substance or known physiological condition (307.43-307.44), and hypersomnia with sleep apnea (780.53).

327.10	Organic hypersomnia, unspecified
327.11	Idiopathic hypersomnia with long sleep time
327.12	Idiopathic hypersomnia without long sleep time
327.13	Recurrent hypersomnia — Kleine-Levin syndrome, menstrual related hypersomnia
327.14	Hypersomnia due to medical condition classified elsewhere — (Code first underlying condition)
327.15	Hypersomnia due to mental disorder — (Code first mental disorder)

This code excludes alcohol or drug induced hypersomnia, coded to 291.82 and 292.85, respectively.

327.19	Other organic hypersomnia
327.2 ⊷sth	Organic sleep apnea

This range of codes addresses specific sleep apnea conditions in which there are transient periods when breathing ceases during sleep due to a known physiologic disturbance or pathogenic origin. Sleep apnea may cause hypoxemia, and result in severely fragmented sleep with arousal occurring many times in any given sleep period. This subcategory excludes Cheyne-Stokes breathing (786.04), hypersomnia with sleep apnea (780.53), insomnia with sleep apnea (780.51), sleep apnea in the newborn (770.81-770.82), and unspecified sleep apnea (780.57).

327.20	Organic sleep apnea, unspecified
327.21	Primary central sleep apnea
327.22	High altitude periodic breathing
327.23	Obstructive sleep apnea (adult) (pediatric)
327.24	Idiopathic sleep related nonobstructive alveolar hypoventilation — sleep related hypoxia
327.25	Congenital central alveolar hypoventilation syndrome
327.26	Sleep related hypoventilation/hypoxemia in conditions classifiable elsewhere — (Code first underlying condition)
327.27	Central sleep apnea in conditions classified elsewhere — (Code first underlying condition)
327.29	Other organic sleep apnea
327.3 ⊷sth	Circadian rhythm sleep disorder — organic disorder of sleep wake cycle or schedule

This range of codes addresses disturbances in the normal sleep-wake cycle rhythm or schedule that have a known physiological or pathogenic origin or due to such conditions as jet lag or shift work. This subcategory excludes alcohol induced circadian rhythm sleep disorder (291.82), circadian rhythm sleep disorder of nonorganic origin (307.45), unspecified disruption of 24-hour sleep wake cycle (780.55), and drug induced circadian rhythm sleep disorder (292.85).

327.30	Circadian rhythm sleep disorder, unspecified
327.31	Circadian rhythm sleep disorder, delayed sleep phase type
327.32	Circadian rhythm sleep disorder, advanced sleep phase type
327.33	Circadian rhythm sleep disorder, irregular sleep-wake type
327.34	Circadian rhythm sleep disorder, free-running type
327.35	Circadian rhythm sleep disorder, jet lag type
327.36	Circadian rhythm sleep disorder, shift work type
327.37	Circadian rhythm sleep disorder in conditions classified elsewhere — (Code first underlying condition)
327.39	Other circadian rhythm sleep disorder
327.4 ⊷sth	Organic parasomnia

This range of codes addresses abnormal behavioral and physiological events disrupting sleep caused by falsely timed activation of physiological systems. This subcategory excludes alcohol-induced parasomnia (291.82), drug -induced parasomnia (282.95), and parasomnia not due to a known physiological condition (307.47).

327.40	Organic parasomnia, unspecified
327.41	Confusional arousals
327.42	REM sleep behavior disorder
327.43	Recurrent isolated sleep paralysis
327.44	Parasomnia in conditions classified elsewhere — (Code first underlying condition)
327.49	Other organic parasomnia
327.5 ⊷sth	Organic sleep related movement disorders

This range of codes addresses movement disorders occurring during sleep, such as teeth grinding, muscle cramping, and limb movement. This subcategory excludes restless legs syndrome (333.94) and unspecified sleep related movement disorder (780.58).

Diseases of the Nervous System and Sense Organs

327.51	Periodic limb movement disorder	
327.52	Sleep related leg cramps	
327.53	Sleep related bruxism — *nocturnal teeth grinding*	
327.59	Other organic sleep related movement disorders	
327.8	Other organic sleep disorders	

Coding Clarification
Sleep disorders or conditions that are not due to a substance or to any known physiological condition cannot be classified as organic and are coded elsewhere, either in the Mental Disorders chapter or the Signs and Symptoms chapter.

Coding Scenario
A 17-year-old boy is brought in to see his physician for complaints of excessive bouts of sleeping that seem to come in episodes lasting weeks and are more than normal teenage sleepiness. He also experiences periods of weeklong eating binges and then doesn't seem to recall the excessiveness of these episodes. The physician diagnoses Kleine-Levin syndrome.

Code assignment: 327.13 *Recurrent hypersomnia*

A 7-year-old female presents to the physician's office for sleep walking. Her mother states that she is often awakened by her child wandering the house at night in an apparent sleep state and noted to mumble incoherently. The mother is assured that most children grow out of these abnormal physiological sleep arousals on their own. Diagnosis is consistent with organic childhood parasomnia.

Code assignment: 327.49 *Other organic parasomnia*

A 32-year-old female visits her dentist with a complaint of generalized jaw aching that encompasses all teeth in the lower jaw. She states that there is definite tenderness on biting down. The dentist examines her mouth and discovers tell-tale grinding marks on her teeth, and diagnoses nocturnal tooth grinding. He discusses the options for wearing nighttime mouth pieces to protect her teeth and learning stress management techniques.

Code assignment: 327.53 *Sleep related bruxism*

330–337 Hereditary and Degenerative Diseases of the Central Nervous System

Excluded from this section are hepatolenticular degeneration (275.1), multiple sclerosis (340), and other demyelinating diseases of the central nervous system (rubric 341).

330 Cerebral degenerations usually manifest in childhood

330.0	Leukodystrophy — (Use additional code to identify associated mental retardation) — *Krabbe's disease; globoid cell or metachromatic leukodystrophy; sulfatide lipidosis*
330.1	Cerebral lipidoses — (Use additional code to identify associated mental retardation) — *amaurotic (familial) idiocy; Batten disease; gangliosidosis; Tay-Sachs disease*
330.2	Cerebral degeneration in generalized lipidoses — (Code first underlying disease, 272.7. Use additional code to identify associated mental retardation) — *Fabry's disease, Gaucher's disease, Niemann-Pick disease*
330.3	Cerebral degeneration of childhood in other diseases classified elsewhere — (Code first underlying disease, 272.7. Use additional code to identify associated mental retardation) — *Hunter's disease, mucopolysaccharidosis*
330.8	Other specified cerebral degenerations in childhood — (Use additional code to identify associated mental retardation)
330.9	Unspecified cerebral degeneration in childhood — (Use additional code to identify associated mental retardation) — *childhood cerebral degeneration NOS*

Coding Clarification
Report Rett's syndrome with 330.8. For 330.2 and 330.3, sequence first the underlying disease, as in Fabry's, Gaucher's, Niemann-Pick, or sphingolipidosis (272.7), or Hunter's disease or mucopolysaccharidosis (277.5).

331 Other cerebral degenerations

331.0	Alzheimer's disease — *chronic, progressive form of dementia, characterized by plaque formations in the brain, eventually leading to total dependence on others* **AHA:** Nov-Dec, 1984, 20; Q4, 1999, 7; Q4, 2000, 41

Alzheimer's disease is a form of presenile dementia caused by the destruction of the subcortical white matter of the brain and characterized by increasing loss of intellectual functioning beginning with minor memory loss and eventually resulting in total loss of ability to function.

Signs and symptoms of Alzheimer's disease include loss of interest in usual pursuits and marked changes of habits. CT scan of the brain shows shrinkage of white matter and an increase in the size of the ventricles. A microscopic exam of brain tissue shows neuronal loss with neurofibrillar and granulovacuolar degeneration and may also show amyloid plaques in the cerebral cortex tissue. Neurochemical studies show changes in the cholinergic system (reduced acetylcholine and choline acetyltransferase) and noradrenergic system (decreased norepinephrine) and may reveal low serotonin levels in caudate and hippocampus nuclei.

Therapies include sedatives, such as chloral hydrate or phenhydramine, for sleep disorders; benzodiazepines, such as lorazepam or oxazepam, for aggressive or assaultive behavior or neuroleptics, such as chlorpromazine or haloperidol, for extreme aggressiveness.

331.11	Pick's disease — (Use additional code for associated behavioral disturbance: 294.10-294.11) — *presenile dementia due to atrophy of frontal and temporal lobes of the brain*
331.19	Other frontotemporal dementia — (Use additional code for associated behavioral disturbance: 294.10-294.11) — *frontal dementia*
331.2	Senile degeneration of brain — *decline in intellectual function due to brain deterioration*
331.3	Communicating hydrocephalus
331.4	Obstructive hydrocephalus — *acquired hydrocephalus NOS* AHA: Q1, 1999, 9; Q4, 2003, 106
331.7	Cerebral degeneration in diseases classified elsewhere — (Code first underlying disease: 140.0-239.9, 244.0-244.9, 265.0, 266.2, 303.00-303.93, 430-438, 741.0, 742.3)
331.81	Reye's syndrome — *occurs in children under age 15, and is marked by acute encephalopathy and fatty infiltrates of multiple organs*
331.82	Dementia with Lewy bodies — (Use additional code for associated behavioral disturbance: 294.10-294.11)
331.83	Mild cognitive impairment, so stated

Mild cognitive impairment (MCI), also known as age-associated memory impairment (AAMI), or benign senescent forgetfulness, is considered to be a strong early predictor of Alzheimer's disease and is described as "the transitional stage between normal aging and dementia." This disorder is widespread among the elderly. These patients do not meet established criteria for dementia but demonstrate impairment beyond that which is normal for age in one or more cognitive areas. Patients with MCI may otherwise function normally in society but may exhibit deficiencies in one or more of the following areas:

- Language: Recall of words may be slower than previously; frequent repetition of statements may occur
- Visuospatial ability: Time or space relationships may pose difficulty, such as the ability to draw a box with the correct proportions
- Executive function: Decision-making ability may be challenged
- Memory: Decrease in recent recall may be present; details of conversations, events and appointments may be impaired

There is no single test to diagnose MCI. Rather, diagnosis is made by excluding other conditions and disorders that could be responsible for the signs and symptoms. No cure for MCI currently exists.

331.89	Other cerebral degeneration — *cerebral ataxia*
331.9	Unspecified cerebral degeneration

Documentation Issues
When the physician documents senile dementia with Alzheimer's disease, both conditions should be coded. Report with codes 331.0 *Alzheimer's disease* and 290.0 *Senile dementia, uncomplicated.*

Coding Clarification
Assign an additional code to identify any mental condition, such as presenile dementia in rubric 290, associated with the current condition.

Alzheimer's Dementia: Two codes are required to report this condition. First code the underlying condition 331.0 *Alzheimer's disease,* and then assign an additional code to report the dementia 294.1x *Dementia in conditions classified elsewhere.*

Feeding Difficulty: As this disease progresses many patients require a feeding tube due to feeding difficulties. When the Alzheimer's patient is admitted for a feeding tube because of the feeding difficulty, report code 331.0 for the Alzheimer's disease and an additional code, 783.3, for the feeding difficulty.

Mild Cognitive Impairment: Code 331.83 *Mild cognitive impairment,* uniquely identifies this disorder and serves to avoid classifying these patients to other codes that are neither appropriate nor accurate. Extensive excludes notes identify those conditions that have associated impairment as an integral characteristic of the disease, and cognitive impairment (331.83) should not be coded in addition. Altered mental status and change in mental status are considered symptoms and not definitive diagnoses.

Coding Scenario
A patient is seen in the clinic with progressive memory loss and disorientation. The physician's diagnostic statement indicates progressive Alzheimer's disease.

Code assignment: 331.0 *Alzheimer's disease*

An elderly patient is seen for evaluation of violent behavior and episodes of wandering off. The physician documents Alzheimer's disease with dementia.

Code assignment: 331.0 *Alzheimer's disease* and 294.11 *Dementia in conditions classified elsewhere with behavioral disturbance*

332 Parkinson's disease

Paralysis agitans is an idiopathic neurological disease causing degeneration and dysfunction of the basal ganglia. This disease, also known as Parkinsonism or Parkinson's disease, is due to a toxic degeneration of the nigral neurons, a group of specialized cells in the midbrain that contain neuromelanin and manufacture the neurotransmitter substance dopamine. When 75 to 80 percent of the dopamine innervation is destroyed, signs and symptoms of Parkinsonism appear.

Signs and symptoms of paralysis agitans include tremor, rigidity, difficulty starting movement or slowness in movement, "pill-rolling" movement of fingers, shuffling gait with short steps and dragging feet, drooling, and problems of articulation.

Therapies include Levodopa or anticholinergic agents, transplantation of catecholamine tissue (autologous adrenal medulla) into brain adjacent to striatum, and surgery to destroy areas controlling specific functions to control severe tremor.

This disease is associated with mental disorders such as dementia, depression, and delirium. True dementia affects 20 to 30 percent of patients.

Secondary Parkinsonism is a neurologic disease similar to paralysis agitans that affects the central nervous system. It is caused by a number of other diseases or by the adverse affect of certain drugs and chemicals.

Associated conditions include Wilson's disease, postencephalic Parkinsonism, midbrain injury or trauma (dementia pugalistica), neoplasms, vascular malformations, Binswanger's disease, etat lacunaire, and hypertensive cerebrovascular disease with normal pressure hydrocephalus. Use the appropriate E code to identify the causative drug or chemical such as carbon monoxide, manganese, methylphenyltetrahydropyridine (MPTP), or reserpine.

332.0	Paralysis agitans — *Parkinson's disease; NOS, idiopathic, primary* **AHA:** March-April, 1987, 7
332.1	Secondary Parkinsonism — (Use additional E code to identify drug, if drug-induced) — *Parkinsonism due to drugs, neuroleptic-induced Parkinsonism*

Coding Clarification

If the medical record documentation indicates Huntington's disease, see 333.4. For progressive supranuclear palsy, striatonigral degeneration, corticodentationigral degeneration with neuronal achromasia, olivopontocerebellar atrophy, Shy-Drager syndrome, or multiple system atrophy, see 333.0. If the Parkinsonism is secondary to syphilis, see 094.82.

333 Other extrapyramidal disease and abnormal movement disorders

333.0	Other degenerative diseases of the basal ganglia — *progressive supranuclear ophthalmoplegia; Parkinsonian syndrome associated with idiopathic orthostatic hypotension or symptomatic orthostatic hypotension* **AHA:** Q3, 1996, 8
333.1	Essential and other specified forms of tremor — (Use additional E code to identify drug, if drug-induced) — *benign essential tremor; familial tremor, medication-induced postural tremor*
333.2	Myoclonus — (Use additional E code to identify drug, if drug-induced) — *familial essential myoclonus; progressive myoclonic epilepsy* **AHA:** March-April, 1987, 12; Q3, 1997, 4
333.3	Tics of organic origin — (Use additional E code to identify drug, if drug-induced)
333.4	Huntington's chorea — *inherited, progressive disease involving CNS, leading to involuntary movements and deterioration of mental faculties ending in dementia*

Coding Clarification

Huntington's chorea is a fatal hereditary disease affecting the basal ganglia and cerebral cortex. The onset varies but usually begins in the fourth decade of life. Death usually follows within 15 years. Signs and symptoms of Huntington's chorea include family history of Huntington's chorea; weight loss; facial grimacing; ceaseless rapid, complex, jerky movements; personality changes, including irritability and indifference; mental deterioration until dementia is reached; and, in children, rigid rather than choreic movements and seizures.

Diagnostic tests include MRI or CT scan of the head to reveal gross atrophy and caudate neuronal loss in with lesser changes elsewhere in the brain. Microscopic exam of tissue identifies gliosis and loss of intrinsic neurons. Neurochemical studies reveal loss of gamma-aminobutyric acid (GABA), acetylcholine, substance P (a tachykinin of 11 amino acids), and enkephalin.

333.5	Other choreas — (Use additional E code to identify drug, if drug-induced) — *hemiballism; paroxysmal choreo-athetosis*

333.6 Genetic torsion dystonia — *deformans progressiva or musculorum deformans dystonia*

Subcategory 333.7 reports acquired torsion dystonia. Dystonia is a condition of abnormal muscle tone, either excessive or inadequate. Involuntary movements and prolonged muscle contractions occur, with resultant tremors, abnormality in posture, and twisting body motions that affect an isolated area or the whole body. Multiple forms of dystonia exist and may be genetic or acquired.

Athetoid, or dyskinetic, cerebral palsy is a form of acquired torsion dystonia manifested by abnormal, uncontrolled, slow and writhing movements, usually affecting the extremities. The muscles of the tongue and face may also be affected, resulting in drooling or grimacing. Symptoms may be exacerbated during times of stress and often disappear during sleep. Acute dystonic reaction due to drugs is another form of acquired torsion dystonia, which is most often a transient occurrence following a one-time exposure.

333.71 Athetoid cerebral palsy — *double athetosis syndrome; Vogt's disease*

333.72 Acute dystonia due to drugs — (Use additional E code to identify drug) — *neuroleptic-induced acute dystonia; acute dystonic reaction due to drugs*

333.79 Other acquired torsion dystonia

333.81 Blepharospasm — *spasmodic contraction of orbicularis oculi muscle caused by a number of conditions*

333.82 Orofacial dyskinesia — *defect in voluntary movement of orofacial muscles*

333.83 Spasmodic torticollis — (Use additional E code to identify drug, if drug-induced) — *impermanent condition in which head tilts to one side*

333.84 Organic writers' cramp — (Use additional E code to identify drug, if drug-induced) — *cramp affecting thumb, index finger and third finger due to prolonged writing*

333.85 Subacute dyskinesia due to drugs — (Use additional E code to identify drug) — *tardive dyskinesia; blepharospasm due to drugs; orofacial dyskinesia due to drugs*

333.89 Other fragments of torsion dystonia — (Use additional E code to identify drug, if drug-induced)

Coding Clarification

Subacute dyskinesia due to drugs is often characterized by rapid, jerking motions such as tongue protrusion, facial grimacing, lip smacking or puckering, and eye blinking. The extremities and trunk may also be involved, as well as the fingers. Other manifestations of drug-induced subacute dyskinesia include blepharospasm (a focal dystonia characterized by increased blinking and involuntary eye closure) or orofacial dyskinesia (involuntary, repetitive movements of the mouth and face). Symptoms may develop after weeks or years of drug exposure.

Orofacial dyskinesia and blepharospasm due to drugs are classified to 333.85 *Subacute dyskinesia due to drugs*.

Infantile cerebral palsy is classified to a separate category 343, Infantile cerebral palsy.

333.90 Unspecified extrapyramidal disease and abnormal movement disorder — (Use additional E code to identify drug, if drug-induced) — *extrapyramidal disorder NOS, medication-induced movement disorder NOS*

333.91 Stiff-man syndrome — *disease of the CNS marked by progressive muscle rigidity and spasms*

333.92 Neuroleptic malignant syndrome — (Use additional E code to identify drug)

333.93 Benign shuddering attacks — *protracted period of convulsive tremors*
AHA: Q4, 1994, 37

333.94 Restless legs syndrome [RLS]

Restless legs syndrome (RLS) is a common but often misdiagnosed neurologic movement disorder whose characteristics include unpleasant sensations deep within the legs that take place at rest and worsen at bedtime or during sleep. An irresistible urge to move the legs, which may temporarily relieve the symptoms, is accompanied by motor restlessness and sensations of pain, burning, prickling, or tingling. Dopaminergic dysfunction is thought to be a factor since RLS has a favorable response to antiparkinsonian medications such as levodopa and dopamine agonists. Symptoms may occur as a result of other underlying conditions, such as pregnancy, end-stage renal disease, various polyneuropathies, or deficiencies in iron, vitamin B12, folate, or magnesium.

Restless legs syndrome can occur at any age but is more prevalent in woman than men and those who are middle aged and older. Patients report an inability to sit still, relax, or get comfortable with an urge to move the legs, accompanied by uncomfortable leg sensations; temporary partial or total relief upon movement, such as walking or stretching; onset or exacerbation of symptoms when inactive or at rest or in the evening and nighttime hours; and sleep disturbances.

333.99 Other extrapyramidal disease and abnormal movement disorder — (Use additional E code to identify drug, if drug-induced) — *neuroleptic-induced acute akathisia*
AHA: Q4, 1994, 37; Q2, 2004, 12; Q4, 2004, 95

Coding Clarification
Benign Shuddering Attacks: This movement disorder is not coded as an epileptic condition; it is a nonepileptic disorder. Use code 333.93 to classify this condition.

Restless Legs Syndrome: The symptoms of restless legs syndrome may worsen at bedtime or during sleep. This syndrome should not be confused with organic sleep disorders that manifest as abnormal movements during sleep, such as periodic limb movement disorder (327.51) or sleep related leg cramps (327.52). RLS is a syndrome and definitive diagnosis, not a symptom.

334 Spinocerebellar disease
334.0	Friedreich's ataxia — *inherited disease marked by dorsal and lateral columnar sclerosis of the spinal cord*
334.1	Hereditary spastic paraplegia — *paralysis of lower half of body marked by increased muscle tone and heightened tendon reflexes*
334.2	Primary cerebellar degeneration — *Sanger-Brown cerebellar ataxia; dyssynergia cerebellaris myoclonica; primary cerebellar degeneration NOS* **AHA:** March-April, 1987, 9
334.3	Other cerebellar ataxia — (Use additional E code to identify drug, if drug-induced) — *cerebellar ataxia NOS*
334.4	Cerebellar ataxia in diseases classified elsewhere — (Code first underlying disease: 140.0-239.9, 244.0-244.9, 303.00-303.93)
334.8	Other spinocerebellar diseases — *ataxia-telangiectasis (Louis-Bar syndrome); corticostriatal-spinal degeneration*
334.9	Unspecified spinocerebellar disease

335 Anterior horn cell disease
335.0	Werdnig-Hoffmann disease — *infantile spinal muscular atrophy; progressive muscular atrophy of infancy*
335.10	Unspecified spinal muscular atrophy — *muscular atrophy of the spine NOS*
335.11	Kugelberg-Welander disease — *familial spinal muscular atrophy*
335.19	Other spinal muscular atrophy — *adult spinal muscular atrophy*
335.20	Amyotrophic lateral sclerosis — *motor neuron disease (bulbar) (mixed type); Lou Gehrig's disease* **AHA:** Q4, 1995, 81
335.21	Progressive muscular atrophy — *Duchenne-Aran muscular atrophy; progressive muscular atrophy (pure)*
335.22	Progressive bulbar palsy — *degeneration of the nuclear cells of lower cranial nerves leading to paralysis*
335.23	Pseudobulbar palsy — *condition in which balance and walking are affected by arteriosclerosis-mediated mini-strokes that damage the pertinent areas of the brain*
335.24	Primary lateral sclerosis — *sclerosis of lateral column of spinal cord*
335.29	Other motor neuron diseases
335.8	Other anterior horn cell diseases
335.9	Unspecified anterior horn cell disease

Coding Scenario
A patient is admitted for chemotherapy treatment for amyotrophic lateral sclerosis.

Code assignment: 335.20 *Amyotrophic lateral sclerosis*

336 Other diseases of spinal cord
336.0	Syringomyelia and syringobulbia — *progressive spinal cord disease marked by cavitation and gliosis of surrounding tissues* **AHA:** Q1, 1989, 10
336.1	Vascular myelopathies — *acute infarction of spinal cord (embolic) (nonembolic); arterial thrombosis of spinal cord; hematomyelia*
336.2	Subacute combined degeneration of spinal cord in diseases classified elsewhere — (Code first underlying disease: 266.2, 281.0, 281.1)
336.3	Myelopathy in other diseases classified elsewhere — (Code first underlying disease: 140.0-239.9)
336.8	Other myelopathy — (Use additional E code to identify cause) — *drug-induced myelopathy; radiation-induced myelopathy*
336.9	Unspecified disease of spinal cord — *cord compression NOS; myelopathy NOS*

337 Disorders of the autonomic nervous system

The nervous system consists of the central nervous system (the brain and the spinal cord) and the peripheral nervous system (the sense organs and the nerves linking the sense organs, muscles, and glands to the central nervous system). The structures of the peripheral nervous system are subdivided into the autonomic nervous system (automatic bodily processes — parasympathetic and sympathetic) and the somatic nervous system. The autonomic nervous system conveys sensory impulses from the blood vessels, the heart, and all of the organs in the chest, abdomen, and pelvis through nerves to other parts of the brain (mainly the medulla, pons, and hypothalamus). These impulses are largely automatic or reflex responses through the efferent autonomic nerves, and cause reactions of the heart, the vascular system, and all the organs of the body to variations in environmental temperature, posture, food intake, stressful experiences, and other changes to which all individuals are exposed.

There are two major components of the autonomic nervous system, the sympathetic and the parasympathetic systems. The parasympathetic division of the autonomic nervous system controls anabolism (energy storage); an anabolic activity occurs in normal, nonstressful situations, such as initiating digestion after eating. In general, sympathetic processes reverse parasympathetic responses. The sympathetic division operates for defense or in response to stress. In defensive situations, catabolism (energy use) produces an increased heart rate, an expansion of the lungs to hold more energy, dilated pupils, and blood flow to the muscles.

Abnormalities of the autonomic nervous system include anxiety disorders, such as muscular tension, hyperventilation, increased heart rate, and high blood pressure that can lead to physiological illnesses such as headaches and digestive problems. At times, parasympathetic responses occur simultaneously, such as involuntary discharge of the bladder and bowels in extremely stressful situations.

Damage to the sympathetic nerve to the eye may result in Horner's syndrome (337.9), which causes a small, regular pupil, ptosis (drooping) of the eyelid on the same side, and occasionally loss of sweat formation on the forehead of the affected eye. The pupil will still react to light stimulus and accommodate to distant vision, but will not enlarge in the dark. The diagnosis of Horner's syndrome is by topical application of liquid cocaine. In many cases there is no treatment that improves or reverses the condition. Treatment in acquired cases is directed toward eradicating the disease that is producing the syndrome.

337.0	Idiopathic peripheral autonomic neuropathy — carotid sinus syncope or syndrome; cervical sympathetic dystrophy or paralysis
337.1	Peripheral autonomic neuropathy in disorders classified elsewhere — (Code first underlying disease: 250.6, 277.30-277.39)

Coding Clarification
Peripheral autonomic neuropathy in disorders classified elsewhere are the chronic and progressive disorders of the peripheral autonomic nerves most often associated with diabetes mellitus, usually insulin dependent or of long-standing duration. Other common etiologies include amyloidosis, botulism, porphyria, and multiple endocrine adenomas.

Signs and symptoms of peripheral autonomic neuropathy in disorders classified elsewhere include impotence, bladder atony, nocturnal diarrhea, orthostatic hypotension, hypersensitivity to cold, and gustatory sweating.

Diagnostic tests include voiding cystometrogram to study urinary neuropathy and motility studies for the esophagus, stomach, and duodenum. Therapies include rigorous control of blood glucose for diabetic autonomic polyneuropathy and symptomatic therapies such as stool bulking agents for diabetic diarrhea, bladder neck resection for urinary bladder dysfunction, and penile implants for impotence.

Associated conditions include foot ulcers, gangrene, other diabetic complications such as diabetic nephropathy, Charcot's joint, or diabetic gastroparesis.

Use codes 250.6x and 337.1 to report diabetic peripheral/cranial neuropathy. For more specific diagnosis identification, more specific codes should be used. For example, orthostatic hypotension secondary to diabetes should be reported with codes 250.6x *Diabetes with neurological manifestations,* 337.1 *Peripheral autonomic neuropathy in disorders classified elsewhere,* and 458.0 *Orthostatic hypotension.*

Gastroparesis, also known as gastroparalysis, requires two codes for accurate reporting: 250.6x *Diabetes mellitus with neurological manifestations,* and 536.3 *Gastroparesis.*

Assign as many codes from category 250 as needed to identify all of the associated conditions that the patient has. The corresponding secondary codes are listed under each of the diabetes codes. Coding guidelines for diabetes instructs coders to assign multiple codes to fully describe the manifestations of diabetes unless specifically directed otherwise by the Index to Disease. For example, in the disease index under the main term "Diabetes, diabetic" is the subterm "gastroparesis" with the coding instruction 250.6 [536.3].

337.20	Unspecified reflex sympathetic dystrophy
337.21	Reflex sympathetic dystrophy of the upper limb
337.22	Reflex sympathetic dystrophy of the lower limb
337.29	Reflex sympathetic dystrophy of other specified site
337.3	Autonomic dysreflexia — (Use additional code to identify the underlying cause: 560.39, 599.0, 707.0)
337.9	Unspecified disorder of autonomic nervous system

338 Pain

338 Pain
This rubric excludes generalized pain (780.96), pain disorder exclusively attributed to psychological

factors (307.80), and localized pain of an unspecified type, which should be coded to pain by site.

Use an additional code (307.89) to identify pain associated with psychological factors. Central pain syndrome is a neurological condition caused by injury to or dysfunction of the central nervous system and has multiple etiologies, including stroke, tumors, epilepsy, brain or spinal cord trauma, multiple sclerosis, or Parkinson's disease. Central pain syndrome may affect a smaller area, such as the hands or feet, or a large portion of the body. Pain is characteristically constant, moderate to severe in intensity, and is frequently made worse by touch, movement, strong emotions, and changes in temperature. Pain sensations vary from "pins and needles" type sensations, to a pressing, lacerating, or aching type of pain, or brief, excruciating bursts of sharp pain. Central pain syndrome often starts soon after the causative injury or damage, but may also be delayed by months or years, particularly if it is related to a previous stroke.

Acute pain is a sensation generated in the nervous system that may be an alert to possible injury, as a response to trauma, or postoperative sequelae. Analgesics are often prescribed to treat acute pain. Other treatment options include heat and cold applications, massage, therapeutic touch, transcutaneous electrical nerve stimulation (TENS), relaxation techniques, guided imagery, hypnosis, music distraction, or cognitive therapies such as art and activity therapy.

Chronic pain is a persistent condition in which the nervous system generates pain signals that may be ongoing for weeks to years. Often occurring as a result of past injuries, infections, or surgical interventions, chronic pain may also be due to ongoing disease processes, such as arthritis, cancer, or recurrent infections. Some patients suffer chronic pain in the absence of past injury or physical damage. A variety of chronic pain conditions affect older adults. Complaints include headache, low back pain, pain related to cancerous neoplasms or arthritis, and neurogenic or psychogenic pain. Treatment options for chronic pain include medications, acupuncture, local electrical stimulation, surgery, psychotherapy, relaxation, and medication therapies, biofeedback, and behavior modification.

338.0	Central pain syndrome — *Dejerine-Roussy syndrome; myelopathic pain syndrome; thalamic pain syndrome*
338.11	Acute pain due to trauma
338.12	Acute post-thoracotomy pain — *post-thoracotomy pain not otherwise specified*
338.18	Other acute postoperative pain — *postoperative pain not otherwise specified*
338.19	Other acute pain — Excludes neoplasm-related acute pain (338.3)
338.21	Chronic pain due to trauma
338.22	Chronic post-thoracotomy pain
338.28	Other chronic postoperative pain
338.29	Other chronic pain
338.3	Neoplasm related pain (acute) (chronic) — *pain due to malignancy; cancer-associated pain; tumor-associated pain*
338.4	Chronic pain syndrome — *chronic pain associated with significant psychological dysfunction*

Coding Clarification
Category 338 contains an instructional note to coders to use an additional code (307.80) to identify pain related to psychological factors. Psychogenic pain, or pain that is exclusively attributed to psychological factors, is to be assigned code 307.80, or to 307.89, sequenced secondary to the site of pain, if known. This type of pain is not to be coded in addition to the 338 category codes.

Generalized pain (780.96) is a symptom and not a definitive diagnosis. Pain specified by site should be coded to the site. Follow the index instruction to code pain to a specific site.

340–349 Other Disorders of the Central Nervous System

340 Multiple sclerosis
Multiple sclerosis is chronic demyelinating disease affecting the white matter of the spinal cord and brain. Multiple sclerosis is characterized by the breaking down of the myelin fibers of the nervous system; patches of scarred nervous fibers develop at these sites. The etiology is unknown, but recent studies suggest the condition may be a cell-mediated autoimmune disease due to an inherited disorder of immune regulation. The disease affects adults between ages 20 and 40 and occurs more often in women.

Signs and symptoms of multiple sclerosis include acute optic neuritis, diplopia, internuclear ophthalmoplegia, frequent dropping of articles, stumbling or falling for no reason, Lhermitte's phenomenon (flexion of the neck producing tingling and paresthesias of legs), and mental changes.

Lab work shows cerebrospinal fluid with five to 100 lymphocytes per cubic millimeter, elevated gamma globulin level (IgG), and abnormal gold curve.

Evoked-potential testing of the visual evoked response, brainstem auditory evoked response, and somatosensory evoked response is abnormally delayed. Therapies include corticosteroids to lessen the intensity and duration of acute exacerbations, physical and occupational therapy to preserve muscle strength and maintain motor function, and muscle relaxant and transcutaneous electrical nerve stimulation (TENS) units to treat spasm and pain. Immunosuppressive therapy with agents such as oral azathioprine and high dose IV cyclophosphamide is in the experimental phase.

Associated conditions include poor bladder tone (atonic and neurogenic) and urinary incontinence.

341 Other demyelinating diseases of central nervous system

341.0 Neuromyelitis optica — *syndrome involving demyelination of spinal cord, optic nerves and optic chiasma*

341.1 Schilder's disease — *Balo's concentric sclerosis; encephalitis periaxialis diffusa*

Subcategory 341.2 reports acute (transverse) myelitis, a focal inflammatory condition of the spinal cord resulting in motor, sensory, and autonomic dysfunction. "Transverse" indicates dysfunction at a specific level across the spinal cord, with altered function below it and normal function above it. Sixty percent of TM cases are idiopathic. Other cases can be linked to known, underlying diseases. The most optimal treatment of ATM is dependent upon a timely and accurate diagnosis. Rapid symptom progression, back pain, and spinal shock predict a poor recovery. ATM tends to peak between the ages of 10 and 19, and 30 and 39 years. In younger patients, transverse myelitis may be a first sign of multiple sclerosis, while in older adults, it may be caused by a spinal cord stroke.

The classic symptoms of transverse myelitis are weakness of the extremities causing stumbling, dragging of one foot, or legs feeling heavier than normal; altered sensation manifesting as numbness, tingling, coldness or burning, and a heightened, painful sensitivity to touch; pain in the back or intense, shooting sensations that radiate down the legs, arms, or around the torso; loss of the ability to feel pain or temperature sensitivity; and bowel or bladder dysfunction.

MRI or myelography may be performed to rule out mass-occupying lesions of the spinal cord. Lumbar puncture is often performed to assess the degree of inflammation. Blood tests, immunoglobulin levels, and protein electrophoresis may also be used to diagnose myelitis. Treatment often consists of intravenous corticosteroids, plasma exchange, and intravenous cyclophosphamide or chemical agents that modify the immune response.

341.20 Acute (transverse) myelitis NOS

341.21 Acute (transverse) myelitis in conditions classified elsewhere — (Code first the underlying condition)

341.22 Idiopathic transverse myelitis

341.8 Other demyelinating diseases of central nervous system — *central demyelination of corpus callosum; central pontine myelinosis*
AHA: Nov-Dec, 1987, 6

341.9 Unspecified demyelinating disease of central nervous system

Coding Clarification

Acute (transverse) myelitis is classified with demyelinating diseases of the nervous system. Numerous subterms in the Alphabetic Index help direct the coder to the appropriate choice. If the condition occurs in conditions classified elsewhere, report with code 341.21, which contains an instructional note to code first the underlying condition. The etiology/manifestation mandatory dual coding convention applies. Code the underlying cause first followed by the code for acute transverse myelitis. Code 341.21 should never be sequenced first or reported alone.

Acute transverse myelitis, NOS is assigned code 341.20. This should not be confused with transverse myelitis NOS (323.82). Idiopathic transverse myelitis is uniquely identified by code 341.22.

342 Hemiplegia and hemiparesis
AHA: Q4, 1994, 38

Flaccid hemiplegia is the loss of muscle tone in paralyzed body parts with absence of tendon reflex. It may be caused by disease or trauma affecting the nerves associated with the involved muscles.

Spastic hemiplegia is muscle spasm within paralyzed parts of the body with increased tendon reflexes. It may be caused by disease or trauma affecting the nerves associated with the involved muscles.

The following fifth-digit subclassification is for use with codes 342.0-342.9:

0   affecting unspecified side
1   affecting dominant side
2   affecting nondominant side

342.0 Flaccid hemiplegia — *hemiplegia (paralysis of half the body) with absent or defective muscle tone*
AHA: Q4, 1994, 38

Diseases of the Nervous System and Sense Organs

342.1 ⌐sth	Spastic hemiplegia — *hemiplegia (paralysis of half the body) with increased muscular tone* **AHA:** Q4, 1994, 38	344.01	Quadriplegia and quadriparesis, C1-C4, complete — *paralysis at least below the level of C4 and lesion transects cord*
342.8 ⌐sth	Other specified hemiplegia — *hemiplegia (paralysis of half the body) NEC* **AHA:** Q4, 1994, 38	344.02	Quadriplegia and quadriparesis, C1-C4, incomplete — *paralysis at least below the level of C4 and does not completely transect the cord*
342.9 ⌐sth	Unspecified hemiplegia — *hemiplegia (paralysis of half the body NOS* **AHA:** Q4, 1994, 38; Q4, 1998, 87	344.03	Quadriplegia and quadriparesis, C5-C7, complete — *paralysis at least below the level of C7 and lesion transects cord*

343 Infantile cerebral palsy

Infantile cerebral palsy is chronic nonprogressive disorders, present from birth, due to damage to the motor function of the brain. The functional impairment may range from disorders of movement or coordination to paresis.

The term "congenital diplegia" is used to include a group of cases characterized by bilateral and symmetrical disturbances of motility present from birth and that remain stationary or tend to improve. Traditionally, the term "diplegia" is used when all four limbs are affected, but weakness and spasticity are more severe in the lower limbs. Quadriplegia or tetraplegia is the term used when all four limbs are affected to an equal extent.

Congenital hemiplegia refers to conditions demonstrated at birth while infantile hemiplegia is the term applied to hemiplegia that develops during the first few years of life. Clinically, the distinction between congenital and infantile hemiplegia is academic.

343.0	Diplegic infantile cerebral palsy — *congenital paraplegia; stiffness is greater in legs than in arms*
343.1	Hemiplegic infantile cerebral palsy — *congenital hemiplegia*
343.2	Quadriplegic infantile cerebral palsy
343.3	Monoplegic infantile cerebral palsy — *infantile cerebral palsy which affects a single limb or a single group of muscles*
343.4	Infantile hemiplegia — *infantile hemiplegia (postnatal) NOS*
343.8	Other specified infantile cerebral palsy — *congenital or infantile triplegia*
343.9	Unspecified infantile cerebral palsy — *cerebral palsy NOS* **AHA:** Q4, 2005, 89

Coding Clarification

Category 343 excludes athetoid cerebral palsy (333.71) and hereditary cerebral paralysis such as Vogt's disease (333.71).

344 Other paralytic syndromes

344.00	Unspecified quadriplegia — *quadriplegia NOS* **AHA:** Q4, 1998, 38; Q4, 2003, 103
344.01	Quadriplegia and quadriparesis, C1-C4, complete — *paralysis at least below the level of C4 and lesion transects cord*
344.02	Quadriplegia and quadriparesis, C1-C4, incomplete — *paralysis at least below the level of C4 and does not completely transect the cord*
344.03	Quadriplegia and quadriparesis, C5-C7, complete — *paralysis at least below the level of C7 and lesion transects cord*
344.04	C5-C7, incomplete — *incomplete; paralysis at least below the level of C7 and does not completely transect the cord*
344.09	Other quadriplegia and quadriparesis
344.1	Paraplegia — *paralysis of both lower limbs; paraplegia (lower)* **AHA:** March-April, 1987, 10; Q4, 2003, 110
344.2	Diplegia of upper limbs — *diplegia (upper); paralysis of both upper limbs*
344.30	Monoplegia of lower limb affecting unspecified side — *paralysis of lower limb NOS*
344.31	Monoplegia of lower limb affecting dominant side
344.32	Monoplegia of lower limb affecting nondominant side
344.40	Monoplegia of upper limb affecting unspecified side — *monoplegia of upper limb NOS*
344.41	Monoplegia of upper limb affecting dominant side
344.42	Monoplegia of upper limb affecting nondominant side
344.5	Unspecified monoplegia
344.60	Cauda equina syndrome without mention of neurogenic bladder
344.61	Cauda equina syndrome with neurogenic bladder — *acontractile bladder; autonomic hyperreflexia of bladder; cord bladder* **AHA:** March-April, 1987, 10; May-June, 1987, 12
344.81	Locked-in state — *victim cannot communicate except sometimes through eye-blinking, that he is fully conscious* **AHA:** Q4, 1993, 24
344.89	Other specified paralytic syndrome — *alternating oculomotor paralysis, Avellis' syndrome, Babinski-Nageotte syndrome, Benedikt's paralysis, Brown-Sequard syndrome, Cestan-Chenais syndrome, tegmental syndrome, triplegia, Weber-Leyden syndrome* **AHA:** Q2, 1999, 4
344.9	Unspecified paralysis

Coding Clarification

Neurogenic Bladder: Many conditions may result in neurogenic bladder including cauda equina syndrome, injury to the spine and spinal cord, spondylitis, neoplasms, fractures, and congenital defects. When the neurogenic bladder is not due to a spinal condition, it is classified to one of the bladder dysfunction categories.

Cauda Equina Syndrome: This condition is due to a compression of the lumbosacral nerve roots. Symptoms include a dull aching pain in the sacral region and/or pain in the legs. There is weakness or paralysis of the muscles. These symptoms slowly progress and a loss of bladder control may eventually occur. When a neurogenic bladder is caused by cauda equina syndrome, code 344.61 is assigned.

Posterior Midline Disk Prolapse: A compression of the nerve roots at the level of L2-3 may result in acute cauda equina syndrome. In these instances, code 722.73 should be reported as well as code 344.61 to indicate both the prolapsed disc and the cauda equina syndrome with neurogenic bladder.

Spondylosis is a compression of any or all of the nerve roots of the cauda equina and causes a variety of sensory and motor deficits. Spondylosis with myelopathy indicates deficits due to nerve compression and would include neurogenic bladder. However, it is appropriate to code lumbar or sacral spondylosis with neurogenic bladder by reporting both codes 721.42 and 344.61.

345 Epilepsy and recurrent seizures
AHA: Q2, 1992, 8; Q4, 1992, 23; Q1, 1993, 24

Epilepsy is a disorder characterized by recurrent transient disturbances of the cerebral function. An abnormal paroxysmal neuronal discharge in the brain usually results in convulsive seizures, but may result in loss of consciousness, abnormal behavior, and sensory disturbances in any combination. Epilepsy may be secondary to prior trauma, hemorrhage, intoxication (toxins), chemical imbalances, anoxia, infections, neoplasms, or congenital defects.

Signs and symptoms of epilepsy include momentary interruption of activity, staring, and mental blankness. More severe symptoms include complete loss of consciousness, sudden momentary loss or contracture of muscle tone, rolling of the eyes, stiffness, violent jerking movements, and incontinence of urine and feces.

Diagnostic tests include lab work such as CBC for signs of infection and serum lead levels for signs of lead poisoning. Lumbar puncture may rule out suspected cerebrospinal infection or trauma, while a CT scan of the brain may rule out intracranial lesions, and an EEG may detect abnormal electrical activity in the brain.

Therapies include anticonvulsives such as phenobarbital, Tegretol, phenytoin (Dilantin), and surgery (temporal lobectomy, extratemporal cortical resections, hemispherectomy, and CT- or MRI-based stereotactic resections of epileptogenic lesions) for severe, intractable, or life-threatening disease.

The following fifth-digit subclassification is for use with categories 345.0, 345.1, and 345.4-345.9:

0   without mention of intractable epilepsy
1   with intractable epilepsy

345.0 ⌐5th   Generalized nonconvulsive epilepsy — *atonic absences; minor epilepsy; petit mal; atonic seizures, Lennox-Gastaut Syndrome*
AHA: Q2, 1992, 8; Q4, 1992, 23; Q1, 1993, 24; Q1, 2004, 18

345.1 ⌐5th   Generalized convulsive epilepsy — *clonic, tonic, myoclonic epileptic seizures; grand mal; major epilepsy*
AHA: Q2, 1992, 8; Q4, 1992, 23; Q1, 1993, 24; Q3, 1997, 4

345.2   Epileptic petit mal status — *epileptic absence status*
AHA: Q2, 1992, 8; Q4, 1992, 23; Q1, 1993, 24

345.3   Epileptic grand mal status — *status epilepticus NOS*
AHA: Q2, 1992, 8; Q4, 1992, 23; Q1, 1993, 24; Q3, 2005, 12

345.4 ⌐5th   Localization-related (focal) (partial) epilepsy and epileptic syndromes with complex partial seizures — *partial epilepsy with impairment of consciousness; — limbic system epilepsy; partial secondarily graded epilepsy; psychomotor epilepsy; epileptic automatism*
AHA: Q2, 1992, 8; Q4, 1992, 23; Q1, 1993, 24

345.5 ⌐5th   Localization-related (focal) (partial) epilepsy and epileptic syndromes with simple partial seizures — *partial epilepsy without impairment of consciousness; — Bravais-Jacksonian epilepsy NOS; motor partial epilepsy; sensory-induced epilepsy; visceral epilepsy; temporal lobe epilepsy*
AHA: Q2, 1992, 8; Q4, 1992, 23; Q1, 1993, 24

345.6 ⌐5th   Infantile spasms — *hypsarrhythmia; lightning spasms*
AHA: Nov-Dec, 1984, 12; Q2, 1992, 8; Q4, 1992, 23; Q1, 1993, 24

345.7 ⌐5th   Epilepsia partialis continua — *Kojevnikov's epilepsy*
AHA: Q2, 1992, 8; Q4, 1992, 23; Q1, 1993, 24

345.8 ⌐5th   Other forms of epilepsy and recurrent seizures — *cursive or gelastic epilepsy*
AHA: Q2, 1992, 8; Q4, 1992, 23; Q1, 1993, 24

345.9 ⌐5th   Unspecified epilepsy — *epileptic convulsions, fits or seizures NOS; recurrent seizures NOS; seizure disorder, NOS*
AHA: Nov-Dec, 1987, 12; Q2, 1992, 8; Q4, 1992, 23; Q1, 1993, 24

Documentation Issues

Diagnoses stated as convulsive disorder, convulsive seizure or fit, or recurrent convulsions should be reported with code 780.39.

The terms grand mal and tonic-clonic seizures in the documentation do not establish the diagnosis of epilepsy.

In cases where repeated admissions for seizures have occurred during the first three years after birth, verify with the physician if the patient's diagnosis of "convulsions" or "seizures" should be classified as infantile spasms, code 345.6x. If the physician does not verify that the condition is infantile spasms and no underlying pathology is found, use code 780.39 for convulsions of unknown etiology.

When the documentation only indicates the diagnosis of posttraumatic seizure disorder, clarify with the physician if the seizure disorder is to be coded seizure (780.39) or epilepsy (345.9x).

Only if the documentation specifically indicates intractable epilepsy should it be coded as such. Documentation of recurrence does not substantiate an intractable epilepsy because all seizures in an epileptic patient are recurrent.

Coding Clarification

Assign a fourth digit to indicate the type of epilepsy. If the physician does not indicate the type of epilepsy in the medical record, report 345.9x with the appropriate fifth digit.

A series of seizures at intervals too brief to allow consciousness between attacks is known as status epilepticus and can result in death. Status epilepticus not otherwise specified is classified to code 345.3x, grand mal status, but status epilepticus can occur in other specified forms of epilepsy.

Benign Shuddering Attacks: This movement disorder is not coded as an epileptic condition; it is a nonepileptic disorder. Use code 333.93 to classify this condition.

Posttraumatic Epilepsy: Posttraumatic epilepsy is classified with a late effect code, 907.0 *Late effect intracranial injury without mention of skull fracture*. When using a code from the late effect categories (905-909), code first the residual condition, then list the late effect code. The late effects include those specified as such, or as sequelae, which may occur at any time after the acute injury.

Recurrent Seizures: Recurrent seizures, not otherwise specified, are now reported with code 345.9 *Epilepsy, unspecified*, as is seizure disorder, not otherwise specified. Diagnoses specified as infantile convulsions, convulsive disorder, recurrent convulsions, convulsive seizures or fit, not otherwise specified are reported with code 780.39 *Other convulsions*.

346 Migraine

The most common type of vascular headache is migraine. The precise cause of a migraine is unclear; however, people who get migraine headaches appear to have blood vessels that overreact to various triggers. According to current thinking, blood flow changes in the vessels may be a nervous system response to a trigger such as stress or an allergic reaction to food in susceptible people by creating a spasm in the arteries at the base of the brain. The spasm constricts several arteries supplying blood to the brain, which reduces blood flow to the brain. Reduced blood flow decreases the brain's supply of oxygen. The arteries within the brain dilate in response to the reduced oxygen supply that, in turn, triggers the release of pain-producing substances called prostaglandins. The result is a throbbing pain in the head.

No medical test exists for migraine, so the diagnosis is based on having some or all of the following symptoms:

- Moderate to severe throbbing pain for up to 72 hours that is frequently on one side of the head (the word migraine comes from the Greek hemicranios, meaning half a head)
- Nausea, with or without vomiting
- Sensitivity to light and sound

About 20 percent of migraine sufferers experience visual and other disturbances about 15 minutes before the head pain. These symptoms, collectively known as "aura," may include flashing lights, bright spots, loss of part of one's field of vision, or numbness or tingling in the hand, tongue, or side of the face. Migraines preceded by an aura are called classic migraines; others are referred to as common migraines of which symptoms beforehand include mental fuzziness, mood changes, fatigue, and unusual retention of fluids. Common migraine pain can last three to four days. In addition to classic and common, migraine headache can take several other forms:

- Patients with hemiplegic migraine have temporary paralysis on one side of the body.
- In ophthalmoplegic migraine, the pain is around the eye and is associated with a droopy eyelid, double vision, and other sight problems.

- Basilar artery migraine involves a disturbance of a major brain artery and occurs primarily in adolescent and young adult women and is often associated with the menstrual cycle.
- Status migrainosus is a rare and severe type of migraine that can last 72 hours or longer, with pain and nausea so intense that people must be hospitalized.

Migraines affect both males and females, and most often the disorder begins between the ages of 5 and 35. The condition is more common in adult women.

Drug therapy, biofeedback training, stress reduction, and cutting certain foods from the diet are the most common methods of preventing and controlling migraine headaches. For infrequent migraines, drugs can be taken at the first sign of a headache, but for most migraine sufferers who get moderate to severe headaches, and for all cluster patients, stronger drugs may be necessary to control the pain.

The following fifth-digit subclassification is for use with category 346:

0 without mention of intractable migraine

1 with intractable migraine, so stated

346.0 ⌐sth Classical migraine — *migraine preceded or accompanied by transient focal neurological symptoms; migraine with aura*
346.1 ⌐sth Common migraine — *atypical migraine; sick headache*
346.2 ⌐sth Variants of migraine — *cluster headache; histamine cephalgia; abdominal migraine; migrainous or ciliary neuralgia*
346.8 ⌐sth Other forms of migraine — *hemiplegic or ophthalmoplegic migraine*
346.9 ⌐sth Unspecified migraine

347 Cataplexy and narcolepsy

Cataplexy is a neurologic condition, often confused with epilepsy. Patients with cataplexy experience sudden loss of muscle tone and fall to the floor because of laughter, stress, or frightening experiences. The cataplectic patient does not lose consciousness but lies without moving for a few minutes until normal body tone returns. Cataplexy can exist by itself, or more commonly, as a feature of narcolepsy. Narcolepsy is a disorder characterized by sudden attacks of irrepressible REM sleep. It is sometimes associated with the following:

- Cataplexy
- Frightening and recurring visual hallucinations when falling to or arousing from sleep
- Paralysis of voluntary musculature while falling asleep

Narcolepsy rarely begins before adolescence. Patients with narcolepsy are easily aroused and become spontaneously alert and are often treated by stimulants such as caffeine, amphetamines, and methylphenidate. These same stimulants are not useful in treating cataplexy, which can be controlled with imipramine or desipramine, given in gradually increasing doses.

347.00 Narcolepsy, without cataplexy
347.01 Narcolepsy, with cataplexy
347.10 Narcolepsy in conditions classified elsewhere, without cataplexy
347.11 Narcolepsy in conditions classified elsewhere, with cataplexy

348 Other conditions of brain

348.0 Cerebral cysts — *arachnoid cyst; pseudoporencephaly*
348.1 Anoxic brain damage — (Use additional E code to identify cause)
348.2 Benign intracranial hypertension — *pseudotumor cerebri*
348.30 Encephalopathy, unspecified — *cerebral or cortical dysrhythmia*
348.31 Metabolic encephalopathy — *organic brain dysfunction from metabolic causes; septic encephalopathy, HIV-1-associated dementia (HAD)*
348.39 Other encephalopathy
348.4 Compression of brain — *brain (stem) compression or herniation*
  AHA: Q4, 1994, 37
348.5 Cerebral edema — *swelling of the brain*
348.8 Other conditions of brain — *cerebral fungus or calcification*
  AHA: Sept-Oct, 1997, 9
348.9 Unspecified condition of brain

349 Other and unspecified disorders of the nervous system

349.0 Reaction to spinal or lumbar puncture — *headache following lumbar puncture*
  AHA: Q3, 1990, 18; Q2, 1999, 9
349.1 Nervous system complications from surgically implanted device
349.2 Disorders of meninges, not elsewhere classified — *meningeal adhesions, (cerebral), (spinal); acquired meningocele; acquired pseudomeningocele*
  AHA: Q3, 1994, 4; Q2, 1998, 18; Q1, 2006, 15
349.81 Cerebrospinal fluid rhinorrhea — *escape of CSF through nose*
349.82 Toxic encephalopathy — (Use additional E code to identify cause) — *toxic metabolic encephalopathy*
349.89 Other specified disorder of nervous system — *nervous system disorders NEC*
349.9 Unspecified disorders of nervous system — *disorder of nervous system (central) NOS*

350–359 Disorders of the Peripheral Nervous System

The Cranial Nerves
Ten of the 12 pairs of cranial nerves originate from the brain stem, but all leave the skull through the foramina of the skull. The nerves are designated by Roman numerals that indicate the order in which the nerves arise from the brain (anterior to posterior), while the name of each pair indicates the function —sensory, motor, or mixed motor/sensory. The name and order of each cranial nerve are as follows: olfactory (I) nerve, optic (II) nerve, oculomotor (III) nerve, trochlear (IV) nerve, trigeminal (V) nerve, abducens (VI) nerve, facial (VII) nerve, vestibulocochlear (VIII) nerve, glossopharyngeal (IX) nerve, vagus (X) nerve, accessory (XI) nerve, and hypoglossal (XII) nerve.

350 Trigeminal nerve disorders
This rubric identifies disorders of the trigeminal (V) nerve, which is a mixed (motor/sensory) cranial nerve and the largest of the cranial nerves. The trigeminal nerve has three branches: ophthalmic, maxillary, and mandibular. Trigeminal neuralgia (350.1) is characterized by intermittent, shooting pain in the gums, teeth, and lower face initiated by shaving, chewing, or a particular jaw motion. The pain may present for weeks or months and then cease spontaneously for a variable period of time. Diagnosis is based on medical history and an exam that rules out other conditions. An enlarged looping artery or vein pressing the trigeminal nerve is the most common cause. A brain tumor identified by magnetic resonance imaging (MRI) may also cause the disorder. Trigeminal neuralgia can occur at any age, though onset is generally 50 years of age or older. Treatment includes medication and surgery (i.e., microvascular decompression, glycerol injections, gamma knife radiation, electrocoagulation, and balloon compression).

350.1	Trigeminal neuralgia — *tic douloureux; trifacial neuralgia*
350.2	Atypical face pain
350.8	Other specified trigeminal nerve disorders — *auriculotemporal syndrome; compression fifth cranial nerve; Frey's syndrome; gustatory sweating syndrome; lesion of gasserian ganglion*
350.9	Unspecified trigeminal nerve disorder

Coding Clarification
A disorder of any of the cranial nerves can produce severe loss of function of which the most common are trigeminal neuralgia (350.1) and Bell's palsy (351.0).

351 Facial nerve disorders
This rubric identifies disorders of the facial (VII) nerve, which is a mixed (motor/sensory) cranial nerve. Its motor fibers originate from the pons and are distributed to facial, scalp, and neck muscles. The sensory fibers convey sensations from the face and scalp and taste buds of the tongue. Bell's palsy (351.0) describes paralysis of muscles on one side of the face that results from temporary damage to the facial nerve. Abnormal tearing from the eye may result when the weakened eyelid can no longer funnel tears into the lacrimal ducts. Severity depends on the extent of nerve damage and although the cause is unknown, a viral infection is suspected. The disorder occurs at all ages, but is most frequent between ages 30 and 60. Ninety percent of patients with Bell's palsy recover without treatment. A cortisone substance may be prescribed to reduce inflammation if the diagnosis is made within the first 48 hours. If eyelid function is compromised, the eye must be covered to prevent drying or injury. Electrophysiologic testing of facial nerve function, though not diagnostic of Bell's palsy, may locate a lesion.

351.0	Bell's palsy — *facial palsy*
351.1	Geniculate ganglionitis — *geniculate ganglionitis NOS*
351.8	Other facial nerve disorders — *facial myokymia; Melkersson's syndrome* AHA: Q3, 2002, 13
351.9	Unspecified facial nerve disorder — *facial nerve disorder NOS*

352 Disorders of other cranial nerves

352.0	Disorders of olfactory (1st) nerve — *disorders of olfactory (1st) nerve*
352.1	Glossopharyngeal neuralgia — *pain between the throat and the ear along the petrosal and jugular ganglia* AHA: Q2, 2002, 8
352.2	Other disorders of glossopharyngeal (9th) nerve
352.3	Disorders of pneumogastric (10th) nerve — *disorders of vagal nerve*
352.4	Disorders of accessory (11th) nerve — *disorder in the nerves affecting the palate, pharynx, larynx, thoracic viscera, and sternocleidomastoid and trapezius muscles*
352.5	Disorders of hypoglossal (12th) nerve — *disorder in the nerves affecting the muscles of the tongue*
352.6	Multiple cranial nerve palsies — *Collet-Sicard syndrome; polyneuritis cranialis*
352.9	Unspecified disorder of cranial nerves

353 Nerve root and plexus disorders

This rubric identifies disorders arising from the nerve networks of the peripheral nervous system. Thoracic outlet syndrome (353.0) is a group of symptoms arising from the upper extremity, the chest, neck, shoulders, and head. The Selmonosky Triad test (e.g., tenderness in the supra clavicular area, tingling and burning sensations in the hand on elevation, and adduction and abduction weakness of fingers) during physical examination may be used for diagnosis. The brachial plexus is a network of nerves formed by fibers located between the shoulder and the neck. Severe shoulder and upper arm pain followed by marked upper arm weakness characterizes Parsonage-Turner Syndrome, also known as brachial plexus neuritis or neuralgic amyotrophy (353.5). Magnetic resonance imaging (MRI) of the shoulder and upper arm musculature may reveal denervation, allowing prompt diagnosis. Electromyography three to four weeks after the onset of symptoms can localize the lesion and confirm the diagnosis. Treatment includes analgesics and physical therapy. Phantom limb syndrome (353.6) is a side effect of the brain's attempt to reorganize following a serious disruption in the sensory information processed in the cerebral cortex, thalamus, and brainstem. Those who have lost limbs through amputation are not the only people who have phantom sensations; those with spinal cord injuries, peripheral nerve injury, diabetic neuropathy, and stroke survivors all report similar feelings.

353.0	Brachial plexus lesions — *cervical rib syndrome; thoracic outlet syndrome; scalenus anticus syndrome*
353.1	Lumbosacral plexus lesions — *acquired defect in tissue along the network of nerves in the lower back, causing corresponding motor and sensory dysfunction*
353.2	Cervical root lesions, not elsewhere classified — *cervicodorsal outlet syndrome*
353.3	Thoracic root lesions, not elsewhere classified
353.4	Lumbosacral root lesions, not elsewhere classified
353.5	Neuralgic amyotrophy — *Parsonage-Aldren-Turner syndrome*
353.6	Phantom limb (syndrome) — *postamputation neural disorder causing itch, ache, or pain as if in the nerves of the amputated limb*
353.8	Other nerve root and plexus disorders
353.9	Unspecified nerve root and plexus disorder

354 Mononeuritis of upper limb and mononeuritis multiplex

Carpal tunnel syndrome is a common disorder that is inflammation of the tendons in the carpal tunnel, which can normally be attributed to repetitive use of the hand and/or wrist.

At the base of the palm is a tight canal or "tunnel" (carpal tunnel) through which tendons and nerves must pass on their way from the forearm to the hand and fingers. The median nerve passes through this narrow tunnel to reach the hand. If anything takes extra room in the canal, things become too tight and the nerve in the canal becomes constricted or "pinched." This pinching of the nerve causes numbness and tingling in the area of the hand that the nerve travels to.

The most common cause of carpal tunnel syndrome is repetitive strain injuries (RSIs). This is caused by long periods of steady hand movement. RSIs tend to come with work that demands repeated grasping, turning, and twisting; they are especially likely to get carpal tunnel syndrome if the work requires repeated twisting or involves repetitive vibration, as in hammering nails or operating a power tool.

A number of sports can bring on repetitive stress injuries: rowing, golf, tennis, downhill skiing, archery, competitive shooting, and rock climbing are examples of activities that stress the hand and wrist joints. Injuries and ailments that cause swelling or compression of soft tissue on nerves, such as sprains, leukemia, and rheumatoid arthritis, can lead to stress injuries. Diabetes, thyroid problems, and other systemic disorders are also associated with discomfort from stressed nerves, as is the fluid accumulation that sometimes accompanies pregnancy. Some clinicians believe that a pyridoxine (vitamin B6) deficiency can also induce the symptoms.

354.0	Carpal tunnel syndrome — *median nerve entrapment; partial thenar atrophy*
354.1	Other lesion of median nerve — *acquired defect in tissue in the ulnar nerve, causing corresponding motor and sensory dysfunction in the forearm and hand; cubital tunnel syndrome; tardy ulnar nerve palsy*
354.2	Lesion of ulnar nerve
354.3	Lesion of radial nerve — *acquired defect in tissue in the radial nerve, causing corresponding motor and sensory dysfunction in the forearm and hand; acute radial nerve palsy* **AHA:** Nov-Dec, 1987, 6
354.4	Causalgia of upper limb — *dysfunction of peripheral nerve of upper limb, usually due to injury, causing burning pain and trophic skin changes*
354.5	Mononeuritis multiplex — *combinations of single conditions classifiable to 354 or 355*
354.8	Other mononeuritis of upper limb — *paralysis nerve phrenic (acquired); paralysis*

	subscapularis; subcostal nerve compression syndrome
354.9	Unspecified mononeuritis of upper limb

355 Mononeuritis of lower limb and unspecified site

355.0	Lesion of sciatic nerve — *acquired defect in tissue in the sciatic nerve, causing corresponding motor and sensory dysfunction in the back, buttock, and leg; pyriformis syndrome* AHA: Q2, 1989, 12
355.1	Meralgia paresthetica — *lateral cutaneous femoral nerve of thigh compression or syndrome*
355.2	Other lesion of femoral nerve
355.3	Lesion of lateral popliteal nerve — *lesion of common peroneal nerve*
355.4	Lesion of medial popliteal nerve
355.5	Tarsal tunnel syndrome — *neuropathy of distal tibial nerve*
355.6	Lesion of plantar nerve — *Morton's metatarsalgia, neuralgia or neuroma*
355.71	Causalgia of lower limb
355.79	Other mononeuritis of lower limb
355.8	Unspecified mononeuritis of lower limb
355.9	Mononeuritis of unspecified site — *causalgia NOS*

356 Hereditary and idiopathic peripheral neuropathy

356.0	Hereditary peripheral neuropathy — *Dejerine-Sottas disease*
356.1	Peroneal muscular atrophy — *Charcot-Marie-Tooth disease; neuropathic muscular atrophy*
356.2	Hereditary sensory neuropathy — *inherited defect in dorsal root ganglia, optic nerve, and cerebellum causing sensory losses, shooting pains, foot ulcers*
356.3	Refsum's disease — *heredopathia atactica polyneuritiformis*
356.4	Idiopathic progressive polyneuropathy — *advancing disease or dysfunction of multiple nerves; cause unknown*
356.8	Other specified idiopathic peripheral neuropathy — *supranuclear paralysis*
356.9	Unspecified hereditary and idiopathic peripheral neuropathy

357 Inflammatory and toxic neuropathy

Inflammatory and toxic neuropathy is pain, swelling, and loss of function of the peripheral nerves in response to another disease process, injury, or unknown etiology (inflammatory neuropathy), or in response to a toxic substance (toxic neuropathy).

357.0	Acute infective polyneuritis — *Guillain-Barré syndrome; postinfectious polyneuritis* AHA: Q2, 1998, 12

Acute infective polyneuritis is polyneuropathy due to an infective organism, usually viral or bacterial. The most common infective organism causing polyneuritis is herpes zoster, which is classified to code 053.13. Guillain-Barré syndrome, the most common diagnosis classified here, is characterized by rapid development of symmetrical weakness or flaccid paralysis affecting the lower extremities. The upper extremities and face are less often affected.

Signs and symptoms of acute infective polyneuritis include history of recent herpesvirus (cytomegalovirus, Epstein-Barr virus) infection or immunization, paresthesia and tingling, depressed respirations in severe disease, weakness of hands and feet, and inability to perform fine movements.

Diagnostic tests include lumbar puncture with analysis of cerebrospinal fluid to show elevated protein level, often in normal cell counts. Therapies include plasmapheresis (plasma exchange), immunoglobulins in high doses, IV corticosteroids, and respiratory assistance.

Use an additional code to identify the organism causing the infection. Human immunodeficiency virus (HIV) is becoming a common cause of acute or infective polyneuropathy and is coded 042, along with code 357.0 or 079.53.

357.1	Polyneuropathy in collagen vascular disease — (Code first underlying disease: 446.0, 710.0, 714.0)
357.2	Polyneuropathy in diabetes — (Code first underlying disease: 250.6)

Polyneuropathy in diabetes is neuropathy involving the long sensory nerves supplying the hands and feet. The axons of the sensory nerves degenerate from the most distal sites and gradually spread more proximally.

Signs and symptoms of polyneuropathy in diabetes include loss of sensation to body part involved, thin and shiny skin, hair loss, "stocking and glove" effect, decreased sensation, and paresthesias.

Therapies include strict control of blood glucose levels, vitamin B and thiamine, drugs such as phenytoin, carbamazepine, amitriptyline, and fluphenazine.

Associated conditions include complications of diabetes mellitus such as diabetic nephropathy, ulcers, gangrene, and frequent infections of hands and feet.

Use codes 250.6x and 357.2 to report diabetic polyneuropathy.

357.3	Polyneuropathy in malignant disease — (Code first underlying disease: 140.0-208.9)
357.4	Polyneuropathy in other diseases classified elsewhere — (Code first underlying disease: 032.0-032.9, 135, 251.2, 265.0, 265.2, 266.0-266.9, 277.1, 277.3x, 585.9, 586)

357.5 Alcoholic polyneuropathy

Alcoholic polyneuropathy, also called polyneuritis potatorum, is due to thiamine and other vitamin deficiency caused by chronic alcohol abuse. In addition, alcohol is believed to be neurotoxic.

Signs and symptoms of alcoholic polyneuropathy are pain, particularly in the midcalf and soles of the feet, tingling, loss of sensation, weakness of hands and feet, inability to perform fine movements, diminished tendon reflexes, excessive perspiration, and atrophy of lower limbs.

Diagnostic tests include EMG to show axonal sensorimotor neuropathy. Lab work reveals low vitamin B levels, anemia (chronic alcoholism interferes with eating balanced meals), and elevated liver enzymes (SGOT, SGPT, and bilirubin). Therapies include control of alcohol intake, correction of nutritional deficiencies, and physiotherapy in severe cases.

Associated conditions include cirrhosis of the liver, foot drop and wrist drop, and Korsakoff's psychosis.

357.6	Polyneuropathy due to drugs — (Use additional E code to identify drug)
357.7	Polyneuropathy due to other toxic agents — (Use additional E code to identify toxic agent)
357.81	Chronic inflammatory demyelinating polyneuritis
357.82	Critical illness polyneuropathy — *acute motor neuropathy*
	AHA: Q4, 203, 111; Q2, 1998, 12; Q4, 2002, 47
357.89	Other inflammatory and toxic neuropathy
357.9	Unspecified inflammatory and toxic neuropathy

Coding Clarification
Toxic Neuropathy: A common toxic effect of anticancer drugs is peripheral neuropathy. To accurately report this condition, use codes 357.6 *Polyneuropathy due to drugs* and E933.1 *Drugs, medicinal and biological substances causing adverse effects in therapeutic use, antineoplastic and immunosuppressive drugs.*

Coding Scenario
A patient is admitted with diabetic neuropathy with secondary diabetes. Patient history identifies the patient has a previous history of a partial pancreatectomy that has caused the diabetic condition.

Code assignment: 251.3 *Postsurgical hypoinsulinemia* and 357.4 *Polyneuropathy in other diseases classified elsewhere*

358 Myoneural disorders

Myasthenia gravis is a disorder of neuromuscular transmission due to the presence of autoimmune antibodies at the neuromuscular junction.

Signs and symptoms of myasthenia gravis include skeletal muscle weakness and fatigability, dysarthria, chewing fatigue, dysphagia, fever, respiratory distress, ptosis, and ocular muscle weakness.

Diagnostic tests include blood serum with AChR-ab (gamma globulin antibody found in 90 percent of patients). CT scan of mediastinum or chest x-ray may show thymoma or prominent thymus gland, while an EMG shows abnormalities in muscle fiber performance. Therapies include drugs such as anticholinesterase, adrenal corticosteroids, and immunosuppressants such as azathioprine, thymectomy, plasmapheresis, and leukoplasmapheresis.

Associated conditions include thymus gland abnormalities, osteoporosis, cataracts, frequent infections, and cholinergic crisis (primarily respiratory depression and paroxysmal atrial tachycardia) due to anticholinesterase medications.

Code	Description
358.00	Myasthenia gravis without (acute) exacerbation — *Goldflam-Erb disease or syndrome, Hoppe-Goldflam disease or syndrome, pseudoparalytica, asthenic bulbar, bulbospinal paralysis*
358.01	Myasthenia gravis with (acute) exacerbation — *crisis includes life-threatening inability to use respiratory muscles*
	AHA: Q4, 2004, 139; Q1, 2005, 4
358.1	Myasthenic syndromes in diseases classified elsewhere — (Code first underlying disease: 005.1, 140.0-208.9, 242.00-242.91, 244.0-244.9, 250.6, 281.0) — *amyotrophy or Eaton-Lambert syndrome from stated cause classified elsewhere*
358.2	Toxic myoneural disorders — (Use additional E code to identify toxic agent)
358.8	Other specified myoneural disorders — *amyotonia congenita; Oppenheim's disease*
358.9	Unspecified myoneural disorders

Coding Clarification
If the documentation states that the patient's myasthenic symptoms are due to another underlying condition, see subcategory 358.1.

359 Muscular dystrophies and other myopathies

Muscular dystrophies and other myopathies are disease processes that are genetic in origin and cause the degeneration of muscle and nerve fibers.

359.0	Congenital hereditary muscular dystrophy — *benign congenital myopathy; central core disease; centronuclear myopathy*
359.1	Hereditary progressive muscular dystrophy — *Gower's or Duchenne's muscular dystrophy*

Hereditary progressive muscular dystrophy is a disease process that is genetic in origin and causes the degeneration of muscle and nerve fibers. This condition usually has an early onset, primarily affects males, and has a relentless progression until death. In the final stages, wasting of the muscles of the diaphragm and respiratory system causes respiratory failure. Classified here are any of the X-linked recessive types of dystrophy such as Duchenne's, Erb's dystrophy, Landouzy-Dejerine disease, or Gower's dystrophy.

Signs and symptoms of hereditary progressive muscular dystrophy include wasting of muscles and deformities of small and large joints.

Diagnostic tests include serum enzyme measurements that may reveal extremely high levels of serum creatine phosphokinase, aldolase, and glutamic-oxaloacetic transaminase in the first two years, diminishing (but not returning to normal) as the disease progresses. A muscle biopsy shows degeneration of muscle fibers, and an EMG reveals a decrease in amplitude and duration of motor unit potentials. Therapies include physical and occupational therapy to maintain muscle function and treatment of complications such as heart failure or concomitant infection.

Associated conditions include atrophy of the liver, frequent infections, contracture deformities, heart failure, and respiratory failure.

359.2	Myotonic disorders — *dystrophia myotonica; Thomsen's disease*
359.3	Familial periodic paralysis — *hypokalemic familial periodic paralysis*
359.4	Toxic myopathy — (Use additional E code to identify toxic agent) — *muscle disorder caused by toxic agent* **AHA:** Q1, 1988, 5
359.5	Myopathy in endocrine diseases classified elsewhere — (Code first underlying disease: 242.00-242.91, 244.0-244.9, 253.2, 255.0, 255.4)
359.6	Symptomatic inflammatory myopathy in diseases classified elsewhere — (Code first underlying disease: 135, 140.0-208.9, 277.3x, 446.0, 710.0, 710.1, 710.2, 714.0)
359.81	Critical illness myopathy
359.89	Other myopathies
359.9	Unspecified myopathy

360–379   Disorders of the Eye and Adnexa

Endophthalmitis is inflammation of the eye that may affect either the anterior or posterior chamber or both, caused by an infection. Noninfectious or sterile endophthalmitis may be a result or retained lens material and/or toxic agents. There are two types of endophthalmitis: endogenous, with results from the hematogenous spread of organisms from a distant source of infection (e.g., endocarditis); and exogenous, which is the result from a direct inoculation, such as a complication of ocular surgery, foreign bodies, or blunt or penetrating ocular trauma. These may also be fungal or candidal in nature.

Endophthalmitis may include white nodules on the lens capsule, iris, retina, or choroid, or inflammation of all of the ocular tissues, which leads to a globe of full, purulent exudates. Inflammation may spread to the orbital soft tissue. Symptoms usually present as acute pain, redness, lid swelling, decreased visual acuity, headache, photophobia, and ocular discharge.

360   Disorders of the globe

360.00	Unspecified purulent endophthalmitis
360.01	Acute endophthalmitis — *sudden, severe infection of the eyeball, with pus*
360.02	Panophthalmitis — *sudden, severe infection throughout the eyeball*
360.03	Chronic endophthalmitis — *persistent infection and inflammation of the eyeball*
360.04	Vitreous abscess — *a pocket of pus in the gel-like fluid that fills the eyeball*
360.11	Sympathetic uveitis — *inflammation of the vascular layer of the uninjured eye following an injury to the patient's other eye*
360.12	Panuveitis — *inflammation of the entire vascular layer of the eye, including the choroid, iris and ciliary body*
360.13	Parasitic endophthalmitis NOS — *inflammation of the entire eye in a parasitic infection*
360.14	Ophthalmia nodosa — *inflammation of the conjunctiva of the eye caused by embedded caterpillar hairs*
360.19	Other endophthalmitis — *not elsewhere classified*

Coding Clarification

Subcategories 360.0 and 360.1 exclude bleb-associated endophthalmitis, which is reported with code 379.63.

360.20	Unspecified degenerative disorder of globe
360.21	Progressive high (degenerative) myopia — *malignant myopia* **AHA:** Q3, 1991, 3
360.23	Siderosis of globe — *deposits of iron pigment within the tissues of the eyeball, caused by high iron content of blood* **AHA:** Q3, 1991, 3
360.24	Other metallosis of globe — *chalcosis* **AHA:** Q3, 1991, 3

360.29	Other degenerative disorders of globe — *not elsewhere classified* **AHA:** Q3, 1991, 3
360.30	Unspecified hypotony of eye
360.31	Primary hypotony of eye — *low intraocular pressure without apparent cause*
360.32	Ocular fistula causing hypotony — *low intraocular pressure due to leak through abnormal passage*
360.33	Hypotony associated with other ocular disorders — *associated with other ocular disorders*
360.34	Flat anterior chamber of eye — *obliteration of the eye, anterior chamber*
360.40	Unspecified degenerated globe or eye
360.41	Blind hypotensive eye — *atrophy of globe; phthisis bulbi*
360.42	Blind hypertensive eye — *absolute glaucoma*
360.43	Hemophthalmos, except current injury — *pool of blood within the eyeball, not from current injury*
360.44	Leucocoria — *reflection from mass behind lens, so that the pupil may look white, often indicative of retinoblastoma*
360.50	Foreign body, magnetic, intraocular, unspecified
360.51	Foreign body, magnetic, in anterior chamber of eye
360.52	Foreign body, magnetic, in iris or ciliary body
360.53	Foreign body, magnetic, in lens
360.54	Foreign body, magnetic, in vitreous
360.55	Foreign body, magnetic, in posterior wall
360.59	Intraocular foreign body, magnetic, in other or multiple sites
360.60	Foreign body, intraocular, unspecified
360.61	Foreign body in anterior chamber
360.62	Foreign body in iris or ciliary body
360.63	Foreign body in lens
360.64	Foreign body in vitreous
360.65	Foreign body in posterior wall of eye
360.69	Foreign body in other or multiple sites of eye
360.81	Luxation of globe — *double whammy syndrome*
360.89	Other disorders of globe — *acquired deformity of globe; adhesion of globe*
360.9	Unspecified disorder of globe

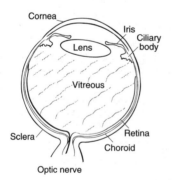

361 Retinal detachments and defects

The retina is sensitive nervous tissue that sends messages via the optic nerve to the brain and one of three layers of the eyeball. The outer, white layer is the sclera, which is the true wall of the eyeball. Lining the sclera is the choroid, a thin membrane that supplies nutrients to part of the retina. The retina, the innermost layer, begins just posterior to the iris, just behind the area called the pars plana, and lines the inner wall of the eye. The central portion of the retina is the macula, which is roughly the area inside of the arcade vessels that extend from the optic nerve and around the macula. The macula is the area of the retina where central vision is the clearest for color and reading vision. The true focal point of the eye is the foveal avascular zone (FAZ), which is only 400 microns wide (0.4mm). The single-layer retinal pigment epithelium (RPE) outside the retina provides nutrients to the photoreceptors; it is also dark with melanin, which decreases light scatter within the eye. The rod and cone are photoreceptors; the cone system dominates vision in daytime, whereas the rod system dominates night vision. Below the RPE is a multi-layered membrane called Bruch's membrane, which separates the RPE and retina from the choroid. The choroid is a vascular layer that provides most of the oxygen to the photoreceptors and RPE. The vitreous is a clear gel-like substance that fills up most of the inner space of the eyeball. It lies behind the lens and is in contact with the retina.

361.00	Retinal detachment with retinal defect, unspecified
361.01	Recent retinal detachment, partial, with single defect
361.02	Recent retinal detachment, partial, with multiple defects
361.03	Recent retinal detachment, partial, with giant tear
361.04	Recent retinal detachment, partial, with retinal dialysis — *dialysis (juvenile) of retina (with detachment)*
361.05	Recent retinal detachment, total or subtotal
361.06	Old retinal detachment, partial — *delimited old retinal detachment*
361.07	Old retinal detachment, total or subtotal

Retinoschisis and retinal cysts involve the splitting of the retina due to microcystoid degeneration (retinoschisis) and development of fluid-filled sacs on the retina (retinal cysts). Retinoschisis often is bilateral and is seen in older persons. Retinal detachment is an occasional complication.

This subcategory excludes juvenile retinoschisis (362.73) and cystic or cytoid degeneration of the retina (362.62).

Diseases of the Nervous System and Sense Organs

361.10	Unspecified retinoschisis		362.01	Background diabetic retinopathy — (Code first diabetes, 250.5) — *diabetic retina microaneurysm*
361.11	Flat retinoschisis — *slowly progressive split of retinal sensory layers*			
361.12	Bullous retinoschisis — *fluid retention between split retinal sensory layers*			**AHA:** Q3, 1991, 8
			362.02	Proliferative diabetic retinopathy — (Code first diabetes, 250.5) — *neovascularization, vitreous hemorrhage and detachment in a diabetic retina*
361.13	Primary retinal cysts — *abnormal fluid-filled cavities or sacs within the retina*			
361.14	Secondary retinal cysts — *abnormal fluid-filled cavities or sacs within the retina, caused by another condition or disease*			**AHA:** Q3, 1991, 8; Q3, 1996, 5
			362.03	Nonproliferative diabetic retinopathy NOS — (Code first diabetes, 250.5)
361.19	Other retinoschisis and retinal cysts — *cyst of ora serrata*		362.04	Mild nonproliferative diabetic retinopathy — (Code first diabetes, 250.5)
361.2	Serous retinal detachment		362.05	Moderate nonproliferative diabetic retinopathy — (Code first diabetes, 250.5)
			362.06	Severe nonproliferative diabetic retinopathy — (Code first diabetes, 250.5)
				AHA: Q4, 2005, 67

Coding Clarification
Serous retinal detachment is separation of the retina from the choroid. Usually spontaneous, although it may be due to a trauma, this condition usually occurs in patients 50 years of age or older. Aging may cause the vitreous to shrink, which causes the retina to tear.

Signs and symptoms of serous retinal detachment include reduced vision, flashing lights (photopsia), vitreous floaters, with total detachment, and no light perception.

Diagnostic tests include exam with an ophthalmoscope and a scleral depressor, which allows visualization of the tear. Therapies include scleral buckling.

Retinal defects that predispose a patient to retinal detachment classified elsewhere include peripheral cystoid degeneration, senile retinoschisis, peripheral chorioretinal degeneration, lattice degeneration, and dialysis of retina.

361.30	Unspecified retinal defect
361.31	Round hole of retina without detachment — *hole of retina*
361.32	Horseshoe tear of retina without detachment — *operculum of retina*
361.33	Multiple defects of retina without detachment
361.81	Traction detachment of retina — *traction detachment with vitreoretinal organization*
361.89	Other forms of retinal detachment — *not elsewhere classified*
	AHA: Q3, 1999, 12
361.9	Unspecified retinal detachment

362 Other retinal disorders

362.0 ⌐5th   Diabetic retinopathy
AHA: Q4, 2005, 65

Diabetic retinopathy is a common complication of diabetes affecting the vasculature of the retina. Leakage and scar tissue from damaged retinal blood vessels distort and blur vision. Diabetic retinopathy is the third most common cause of legal blindness in adults in the United States.

Coding Clarification
Nonproliferative diabetic retinopathy describes the early stage of the disease. In the nonproliferative stage, microaneurysm formation, hemorrhages, and blind spots are characteristic. As the disease progresses, more vessel leakage occurs. The disease progresses from mild to moderate to severe nonproliferative retinopathy and becomes proliferative in its more advanced stage, characterized by new blood vessel formation in the retina due to significant ischemia from the damaged vessels.

According to the American Academy of Ophthalmology's scale, the severity of disease progression is as follows: mild nonproliferative diabetic retinopathy is characterized by microaneurysm formation with small, balloon-like swelling of retinal vessels; moderate nonproliferative diabetic retinopathy is characterized by microaneurysms becoming more pronounced with some vessel blockage occurring; severe nonproliferative diabetic retinopathy is characterized by vascular breakdown within the retina resulting in multiple blockages, and numerous intraretinal hemorrhages in different quadrants.

Proliferative diabetic retinopathy is characterized by ischemic effects of vessel blockages causing new blood vessel formation as compensation. Leakage from the fragile new blood vessels causes loss of vision.

362.07	Diabetic macular edema — (Code first diabetes, 250.5; Code 362.07 must be used with a code for diabetic retinopathy, 362.01-362.06) — *diabetic retinal edema*

Coding Clarification
Leakage from retinal blood vessels can cause the retina to swell, resulting in diabetic macular edema.

When the edematous process occurs, the macula, the central portion of the retina, swells and impairs vision. Exudate or plaques may form in the posterior pole of the retina due to the breakdown of the vasculature and presents a risk for vision loss. Diabetic macular, or retinal, edema is a complication of diabetic retinopathy and can occur at any stage of the disease process; therefore, macular edema must be accompanied by a code specifying the diabetic retinopathy.

Code	Description
362.10	Unspecified background retinopathy **AHA:** Q1, 2006, 12
362.11	Hypertensive retinopathy — *retinal irregularities caused by systemic hypertension* **AHA:** Q3, 1990, 3
362.12	Exudative retinopathy — *Coat's syndrome* **AHA:** Q3, 1999, 12
362.13	Changes in vascular appearance of retina — (Use additional code for any associated atherosclerosis, 440.8) — *vascular sheathing of retina*
362.14	Retinal microaneurysms NOS — *microscopic dilation of retinal vessels in nondiabetic*
362.15	Retinal telangiectasia — *permanent dilation of blood vessels of the retina*
362.16	Retinal neovascularization NOS — *choroidal or subretinal revascularization*
362.17	Other intraretinal microvascular abnormalities — *retinal varices*
362.18	Retinal vasculitis — *Eales' disease; retinal arteritis or endarteritis*
362.21	Retrolental fibroplasia — *Terry's syndrome*
362.29	Other nondiabetic proliferative retinopathy
362.30	Unspecified retinal vascular occlusion
362.31	Central artery occlusion of retina
362.32	Arterial branch occlusion of retina
362.33	Partial arterial occlusion of retina — *Hollenhorst plaque; retinal microembolism*
362.34	Transient arterial occlusion of retina — *amaurosis fugax* **AHA:** Q1, 2000, 16
362.35	Central vein occlusion of retina
362.36	Venous tributary (branch) occlusion of retina
362.37	Venous engorgement of retina — *incipient or partial occlusion of retinal vein*
362.40	Unspecified retinal layer separation
362.41	Central serous retinopathy — *serous-filled blister causing localized detachment of retina from pigment epithelium*
362.42	Serous detachment of retinal pigment epithelium — *exudative detachment of retinal pigment epithelium*
362.43	Hemorrhagic detachment of retinal pigment epithelium — *blood-filled blister causing localized detachment of retina from pigment epithelium*
362.50	Macular degeneration (senile) of retina, unspecified — *Behr's disease*
362.51	Nonexudative senile macular degeneration of retina — *atrophic or dry senile macular degeneration*
362.52	Exudative senile macular degeneration of retina — *Kuhnt-Junius degeneration; disciform or wet senile macular degeneration*
362.53	Cystoid macular degeneration of retina — *cystoid macular edema*
362.54	Macular cyst, hole, or pseudohole of retina — *break or tear in macula*
362.55	Toxic maculopathy of retina — (Use additional E code to identify drug, if drug-induced) — *macular disease caused by toxic substance*
362.56	Macular puckering of retina — *preretinal fibrosis*
362.57	Drusen (degenerative) of retina — *white hyaline deposits on the retinal pigment epithelium*
362.60	Unspecified peripheral retinal degeneration
362.61	Paving stone degeneration of peripheral retina — *spots of retinal thinning through which the choroid can be seen*
362.62	Microcystoid degeneration of peripheral retina — *Blessig's or Iwanoff's cysts*
362.63	Lattice degeneration of peripheral retina — *palisade degeneration of retina*
362.64	Senile reticular degeneration of peripheral retina — *net-like appearance of retina; a sign of degeneration*
362.65	Secondary pigmentary degeneration of peripheral retina — *pseudoretinitis pigmentosa*
362.66	Secondary vitreoretinal degenerations peripheral retina — *non-ocular disease causing vitreoretinal change*
362.70	Unspecified hereditary retinal dystrophy
362.71	Retinal dystrophy in systemic or cerebroretinal lipidoses — (Code first underlying disease: 272.7, 330.1) — *cerebroretinal lipidoses, systemic lipidoses*
362.72	Retinal dystrophy in other systemic disorders and syndromes — (Code first underlying disease: 272.5, 356.3) — *Bassen-Kornzweig syndrome, Refsum's disease*
362.73	Vitreoretinal dystrophies — *juvenile retinoschisis*
362.74	Pigmentary retinal dystrophy — *retinal dystrophy, albipunctate; retinitis pigmentosa*
362.75	Other dystrophies primarily involving the sensory retina — *progressive cone (-rod) dystrophy; Stargardt's disease*
362.76	Dystrophies primarily involving the retinal pigment epithelium — *fundus flavimaculatus; vitelliform dystrophy*
362.77	Retinal dystrophies primarily involving Bruch's membrane — *hyaline or pseudoinflammatory foveal dystrophy; hereditary drusen*
362.81	Retinal hemorrhage — *preretinal, retinal (deep) (superficial) or subretinal hemorrhage* **AHA:** Q4, 1996, 43
362.82	Retinal exudates and deposits — *fatty fluids or denser deposits leaking into the retina*
362.83	Retinal edema — *cotton wool retinal spots; retinal edema (localized) (macular) (peripheral)*
362.84	Retinal ischemia — *abnormal reduction of retinal blood supply*

362.85	Retinal nerve fiber bundle defects — *anomalies within the retinal nerves*		363.15	Disseminated retinitis and retinochoroiditis, pigment epitheliopathy — *acute posterior multifocal placoid pigment epitheliopathy*
362.89	Other retinal disorders — *hyperemia of retina; phakoma; tessellated fundus, retina (tigroid)*		363.20	Unspecified chorioretinitis
362.9	Unspecified retinal disorder		363.21	Pars planitis — *posterior cyclitis*
			363.22	Harada's disease — *uveomeningeal syndrome*

Coding Clarification

Hypertensive Retinopathy: To report this condition accurately, two codes are required, code 362.11 *Hypertensive retinopathy;* and an appropriate code from categories 401-405 to identify the specific type of hypertension.

363 Chorioretinal inflammations, scars, and other disorders of choroid

The choroid is the layer of blood vessels and connective tissue between the sclera and the retina. Blood vessels first appear in the choroid during the 15th week of development, and arteries and veins can be recognized by the 22nd week. Part of the choroid develops into the cores of the ciliary processes. At the posterior end of the optic cup, the choroid forms a sheath around the optic nerve. The choroid, iris, and ciliary body are also referred to as the uvea. The choroid is heavily pigmented, which prevents stray light from reaching the retina. It supplies nutrients to the inner parts of the eye and acts to exchange heat generated by retinal metabolism. The outer layer, which surrounds the choroid, is the sclera. Diseases of the choroid include choroidal melanoma, which is a common form of cancer that primarily affects the adult's eye, and choroiditis, which is the inflammation of the choroid. Melanoma of the uveal tract is the most common primary ocular cancer in adults.

363.00	Unspecified focal chorioretinitis
363.01	Focal choroiditis and chorioretinitis, juxtapapillary
363.03	Focal choroiditis and chorioretinitis of other posterior pole
363.04	Focal choroiditis and chorioretinitis, peripheral
363.05	Focal retinitis and retinochoroiditis, juxtapapillary — *neuroretinitis*
363.06	Focal retinitis and retinochoroiditis, macular or paramacular
363.07	Focal retinitis and retinochoroiditis of other posterior pole
363.08	Focal retinitis and retinochoroiditis, peripheral
363.10	Unspecified disseminated chorioretinitis
363.11	Disseminated choroiditis and chorioretinitis, posterior pole
363.12	Disseminated choroiditis and chorioretinitis, peripheral
363.13	Disseminated choroiditis and chorioretinitis, generalized — (Code first any underlying disease, 017.3)
363.14	Disseminated retinitis and retinochoroiditis, metastatic — *metastatic*

363.30	Unspecified chorioretinal scar
363.31	Solar retinopathy — *macular damage from staring at the sun*
363.32	Other macular scars of chorioretina — *not elsewhere classified*
363.33	Other scars of posterior pole of chorioretina
363.34	Peripheral scars of the chorioretina
363.35	Disseminated scars of the chorioretina
363.40	Unspecified choroidal degeneration
363.41	Senile atrophy of choroid — *wasting away of choroid due to advanced age*
363.42	Diffuse secondary atrophy of choroid — *wasting away of choroid in systemic disease*
363.43	Angioid streaks of choroid — *cracks radiating from the optic disk in the layer separating the choriocapillaris from retinal epithelium*
363.50	Unspecified hereditary choroidal dystrophy or atrophy
363.51	Circumpapillary dystrophy of choroid, partial
363.52	Circumpapillary dystrophy of choroid, total — *helicoid dystrophy of choroid*
363.53	Central dystrophy of choroid, partial — *central areolar choroidal dystrophy; circinate choroidal dystrophy*
363.54	Central choroidal atrophy, total — *central gyrate choroidal dystrophy; serpiginous choroidal dystrophy*
363.55	Choroideremia — *degeneration of choroid, affecting both sexes, leading to blindness in males*
363.56	Other diffuse or generalized dystrophy of choroid, partial — *diffuse choroidal sclerosis*
363.57	Other diffuse or generalized dystrophy of choroid, total — *generalized gyrate atrophy, choroid*
363.61	Unspecified choroidal hemorrhage
363.62	Expulsive choroidal hemorrhage
363.63	Choroidal rupture
363.70	Unspecified choroidal detachment
363.71	Serous choroidal detachment — *blister of serous fluid causing localized detachment of choroid from the sclera*
363.72	Hemorrhagic choroidal detachment — *blood-filled blister causing localized detachment of choroid from the sclera*
363.8	Other disorders of choroid — *not elsewhere classified*
	AHA: Q1, 2006, 12
363.9	Unspecified disorder of choroid

364 Disorders of iris and ciliary body

The ciliary body is formed from the two layers composing the rim of the optic cup, which undergo folding to form the ciliary processes. The ciliary body produces the clear fluid into the eye that goes through the pupil and drains back into the blood stream through a tissue in front of the periphery of the iris. The ciliary body also contains the muscle that attaches to the outside of the lens of the eye and alters the focus of the eye. In turn, the ciliary body is continuous with a pigmented layer, the choroid, which lines the back of the eye outside the light sensitive retina. The iris, which extends partly over the lens, is composed of the two layers forming the edge of the optic cup and a layer of vascularized connective tissue containing the pupillary muscle. The iris muscles can make the pupil larger or smaller and the pigmented layer is responsible for eye color. The iris is continuous with the ring shaped ciliary body behind it. The iris, ciliary body, and choroid ensure that light only enters the eye through the pupil, and blood vessels in the choroid help to nourish the retina.

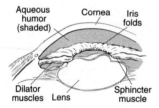

Sideview of iris and lens

Iridocyclitis is a combination of inflammation of the iris and inflammation of the ciliary body. When the iris is inflamed, its blood vessels dilate and the blood vessels of the white of the eye make it reddened. The dilated vessels leak proteins and blood cells into the clear eye fluid, which tends to prevent fluid from going through the pupil. The iris tissue and the ciliary body are richly supplied with sensory nerves so that the inflamed tissue causes pain especially when it moves in bright light or when focusing for near objects.

364.00	Unspecified acute and subacute iridocyclitis
364.01	Primary iridocyclitis — *inflammation of the iris and ciliary body*
364.02	Recurrent iridocyclitis — *repeated bouts of inflammation of the iris and ciliary body*
364.03	Secondary iridocyclitis, infectious — *inflammation of the iris and ciliary body as a result of a primary infection elsewhere*
364.04	Secondary iridocyclitis, noninfectious — *inflammation of the iris and ciliary body as a result of a other systemic disease or disorder; aqueous fibrin or flare*
364.05	Hypopyon — *accumulation of pus between the cornea and the lens*
364.10	Unspecified chronic iridocyclitis — *persistent inflammation of the iris and ciliary body as a result of an underlying disease or condition*
364.11	Chronic iridocyclitis in diseases classified elsewhere — *(Code first underlying disease: 017.3, 135)*
364.21	Fuchs' heterochromic cyclitis — *unilateral inflammation of the ciliary body and iris, making the eyes appear to be different colors*
364.22	Glaucomatocyclitic crises — *uveal inflammation causing acute rise in intraocular pressure*
364.23	Lens-induced iridocyclitis — *immune reaction to proteins in the lens; follows lens trauma or extraction and causes inflammation of the iris*
364.24	Vogt-Koyanagi syndrome — *oculocutaneous syndrome; uveocutaneous syndrome*
364.3	Unspecified iridocyclitis
364.41	Hyphema — *hemorrhage of iris or ciliary body*
364.42	Rubeosis iridis — *neovascularization of iris or ciliary body*
364.51	Essential or progressive iris atrophy — *weakened and defective iris of unknown cause*
364.52	Iridoschisis — *splitting of the iris into two layers*
364.53	Pigmentary iris degeneration — *acquired heterochromia of iris; translucency of iris*
364.54	Degeneration of pupillary margin — *atrophy of sphincter of iris; ectropion of pigment epithelium of iris*
364.55	Miotic cysts of pupillary margin
364.56	Degenerative changes of chamber angle
364.57	Degenerative changes of ciliary body
364.59	Other iris atrophy — *iris atrophy (generalized) (sector shaped)*
364.60	Idiopathic cysts of iris, ciliary body, and anterior chamber — *fluid-filled sacs of the iris or ciliary body of unknown etiology*
364.61	Implantation cysts of iris, ciliary body, and anterior chamber — *epithelial down-growth, anterior chamber; implantation cysts (surgical) (traumatic)*
364.62	Exudative cysts of iris or anterior chamber — *protein or fatty fluid-filled sacs of the iris or ciliary body caused by leak of fluid from blood vessels*
364.63	Primary cyst of pars plana — *fluid-filled sacs of the outermost ciliary ring*
364.64	Exudative cyst of pars plana — *protein or fatty fluid-filled sacs of the outermost ciliary ring, caused by leak of fluid from blood vessels*
364.70	Unspecified adhesions of iris
364.71	Posterior synechiae — *adhesions binding iris to the lens*
364.72	Anterior synechiae — *adhesions binding iris to cornea*

364.73	Goniosynechiae — *peripheral anterior synechiae*	
364.74	Adhesions and disruptions of pupillary membranes — *iris bombe; pupillary occlusion or seclusion*	
364.75	Pupillary abnormalities — *deformed pupil; rupture of pupillary sphincter; ectopic pupil*	
364.76	Iridodialysis — *tear at the base of the iris, separating it from the ciliary body*	
364.77	Recession of chamber angle of eye	
364.8	Other disorders of iris and ciliary body — *hernia of ciliary body; hernia of iris; iridodonesis*	
364.9	Unspecified disorder of iris and ciliary body	

365 Glaucoma

Glaucoma is an increase in intraocular pressure due to an abnormal aqueous humor outflow from the anterior chamber or, rarely, from an above normal rate of aqueous humor production by the ciliary body. If untreated, glaucoma ultimately leads to optic nerve damage and loss of vision.

365.00	Unspecified preglaucoma	
365.01	Borderline glaucoma, open angle with borderline findings — *open angle with cupping of optic discs*	
	AHA: Q1, 1990, 8	
365.02	Borderline glaucoma with anatomical narrow angle — *defect restricting aqueous flow in the anterior segment, possibly resulting in high intraocular pressure*	
	AHA: Q1, 1990, 8	
365.03	Borderline glaucoma with steroid responders	
365.04	Borderline glaucoma with ocular hypertension — *high fluid pressure within the eye due to no apparent cause*	
	AHA: Q1, 1990, 8	

Open-angle glaucoma is an increase in intraocular pressure due to the free access of aqueous humor to the trabecular network in the angle of the anterior chamber. Heredity may play a factor in patients developing primary open-angle glaucoma as well as trauma.

Signs and symptoms of open-angle glaucoma include progressive loss of peripheral vision over a span of years, blurred or foggy vision, seeing halos around lights, reduced night vision, and aching in the eyes.

Diagnostic tests include tonometry using an applanation such as a Schiotz or pneumatic tonometer to measure intraocular pressure. An exam (ophthalmoscope, slit lamp) shows the fundus, optic disk, and anterior structure of the eyes, while a gonioscopy differentiates between chronic open-angle glaucoma and acute closed-angle glaucoma. Perimetry and visual field tests determine the extent of peripheral vision loss and fundus photography records and monitors changes in the optic disk.

Therapies include topical miotic drugs (Pilocarpine, Carcholin), carbonic anhydrase inhibitors (acetazolamide), surgery (iridectomy, trephine procedures, trabeculectomy, posterior lip sclerectomy, thermal sclerotomy) to reduce intraocular pressure, Argon laser trabeculoplasty or iridectomy, and cyclodialysis or cyclocryotherapy.

365.10	Unspecified open-angle glaucoma	
365.11	Primary open-angle glaucoma — *chronic simple glaucoma*	
365.12	Low tension open-angle glaucoma — *comparatively low rise in intraocular pressure*	
365.13	Pigmentary open-angle glaucoma — *high intraocular pressure due to iris pigment granules breaking free and blocking aqueous flow*	
365.14	Open-angle glaucoma of childhood — *infantile or juvenile glaucoma*	
365.15	Residual stage of open angle glaucoma	

Primary angle-closure glaucoma is an increase in intraocular pressure due to the iris occluding the anterior chamber structures and preventing the aqueous humor from reaching its usual outflow channel. Acute angle-closure glaucoma is a medical emergency and requires immediate, definitive treatment.

Signs and symptoms of primary angle-closure glaucoma include progressive loss of peripheral vision over a span of years, blurred or foggy vision, seeing colored halos around lights, severe eye pain and headache, corneal epithelial edema, and nausea and vomiting.

Diagnostic tests include exam (flashlight, slit lamp, or ophthalmoscope) to reveal corneal epithelial edema as a fine rough haziness in light and to allow visualization of the fundus and optic disk. Gonioscopy confirms angle closure and tonometry, using an applanation such as a Schiotz or pneumatic tonometer, measures intraocular pressure. Perimetry and visual field tests determine the extent of peripheral vision loss, and fundus photography records and monitors changes in the optic disk.

Therapies include systemic osmotics (glycerol, mannitol, and acetazolamide) to lower intraocular pressure, topical miotic drugs (Pilocarpine, Carcholin), carbonic anhydrase inhibitors (acetazolamide), argon laser iridotomy, and surgical peripheral iridectomy.

365.20	Unspecified primary angle-closure glaucoma — *interval or subacute angle-closure glaucoma*	

Code	Description
365.21	Intermittent angle-closure glaucoma
365.22	Acute angle-closure glaucoma — *sudden, severe rise in intraocular pressure due to blockage in aqueous drainage*
365.23	Chronic angle-closure glaucoma — *persistent elevation of intraocular pressure due to continued blockage in aqueous drainage* **AHA:** Q2, 1998, 16
365.24	Residual stage of angle-closure glaucoma
365.31	Corticosteroid-induced glaucoma, glaucomatous stage
365.32	Corticosteroid-induced glaucoma, residual stage
365.41	Glaucoma associated with chamber angle anomalies — (Code first associated disorder, 743.44)
365.42	Glaucoma associated with anomalies of iris — (Code first associated disorder: 364.51, 743.45)
365.43	Glaucoma associated with other anterior segment anomalies — (Code first associated disorder, 743.41)
365.44	Glaucoma associated with systemic syndromes — (Code first associated disease: 237.7, 759.6)
365.51	Phacolytic glaucoma — (Use additional code for associated hypermature cataract, 366.18)
365.52	Pseudoexfoliation glaucoma — (Use additional code for associated pseudoexfoliation of capsule, 366.11)
365.59	Glaucoma associated with other lens disorders — (Use additional code for associated disorder: 379.33, 379.34, 743.36)
365.60	Glaucoma associated with unspecified ocular disorder
365.61	Glaucoma associated with pupillary block — (Use additional code for associated disorder, 364.74)
365.62	Glaucoma associated with ocular inflammations — (Use additional code for associated disorder: 364.00-364.3, 364.22)
365.63	Glaucoma associated with vascular disorders of eye — (Use additional code for associated disorder: 362.35, 364.41)
365.64	Glaucoma associated with tumors or cysts — (Use additional code for associated disorder: 190.0-190.9, 224.0-224.9, 364.61)
365.65	Glaucoma associated with ocular trauma — (Use additional code for associated condition: 364.77, 921.3)
365.81	Hypersecretion glaucoma
365.82	Glaucoma with increased episcleral venous pressure
365.83	Aqueous misdirection — *malignant glaucoma* **AHA:** Q4, 2002, 48
365.89	Other specified glaucoma
365.9	Unspecified glaucoma

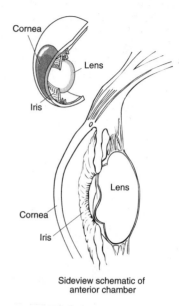

Sideview schematic of anterior chamber

366 Cataract

Cataract is the partial or total opacity of the crystalline lens or lens capsule. Cataracts form gradually and occur bilaterally usually in patients older than 70 years of age, with the exception of traumatic and congenital cataracts. Cataracts are classified by the zones of the lens involved in the opacity: anterior and posterior cortical, equatorial cortical, and supranuclear and nuclear. They are further subdivided into congenital, degenerative, traumatic, secondary, or complicated (due to ocular or systemic disease, radiation, or other external influences), toxic, and after-cataracts (meaning one remaining in the lens or capsule following cataract extraction).

The definition of infantile, juvenile, and presenile cataract is the partial or total opacity of the lens occurring in an infant, a young child, or a young adult. This type of cataract usually is the result of an injury or associated with conditions such as nutritional deficiencies (e.g., galactosemia), previous inflammation, or convulsions.

Signs and symptoms of infantile, juvenile, and presenile cataract include slowly progressing and painless loss of vision, leukocoria, behavioral problems indicative of vision problems, and strabismus.

Senile cataract is partial or total opacity of the lens due to degenerative changes in the lens in patients older than 55 years of age.

Signs and symptoms of senile cataract include slowly progressing and painless loss of vision, leukocoria, difficulty in night driving, altered color perception, and strabismus.

Diagnostic tests include tests of visual acuity to detect any loss of vision sharpness or clarity. An exam (flashlight, slit lamp, or ophthalmoscope) reveals opacity of the lens and pupil, shows the anterior portion of the eye, and detects nuclear cataracts. Refraction and retinoscopy detect nuclear myopia and lenticonus. A-scan and B-scan ultrasound measure thickness and location of the cataract.

Therapies include cataract extraction, intra- or extracapsular, phacoemulsification and aspiration, lensectomy and phacofragmentation, intraocular lens implantation, and cataract glasses postoperatively.

Associated conditions include galactosemia and galactokinase deficiency, hypoglycemia (neonatal), Lowe's syndrome (oculocerebrorenal syndrome), myotonic dystrophy, congenital ichthyosis, Rothmund-Thomson syndrome, rubella, Werner's syndrome, and Hallermann-Streiff-Francois syndrome.

Code	Description
366.00	Unspecified nonsenile cataract
366.01	Anterior subcapsular polar cataract, nonsenile
366.02	Posterior subcapsular polar cataract, nonsenile
366.03	Cortical, lamellar, or zonular cataract, nonsenile
366.04	Nuclear cataract, nonsenile
366.09	Other and combined forms of nonsenile cataract
366.10	Unspecified senile cataract
366.11	Pseudoexfoliation of lens capsule
366.12	Incipient cataract
366.13	Anterior subcapsular polar senile cataract
366.14	Posterior subcapsular polar senile cataract
366.15	Cortical senile cataract
366.16	Nuclear sclerosis
366.17	Total or mature senile cataract
366.18	Hypermature senile cataract
366.19	Other and combined forms of senile cataract
366.20	Unspecified traumatic cataract
366.21	Localized traumatic opacities of cataract
366.22	Total traumatic cataract
366.23	Partially resolved traumatic cataract
366.30	Unspecified cataracta complicata
366.31	Cataract secondary to glaucomatous flecks (subcapsular) — (Code first underlying glaucoma: 365.00-365.9)
366.32	Cataract in inflammatory ocular disorders — (Code first underlying condition: 363.00-363.22)
366.33	Cataract with ocular neovascularization — (Code first underlying condition, 364.10)
366.34	Cataract in degenerative ocular disorders — (Code first underlying condition: 360.21, 360.24, 362.74)
366.41	Diabetic cataract — (Code first diabetes, 250.5)
366.42	Tetanic cataract — (Code first underlying disease: 252.1, 275.4)
366.43	Myotonic cataract — (Code first underlying disorder, 359.2)
366.44	Cataract associated with other syndromes — (Code first underlying condition: 271.1, 756.0)
366.45	Toxic cataract — (Use additional E code to identify drug or other toxic substance)
366.46	Cataract associated with radiation and other physical influences — (Use additional E code to identify cause)
366.50	Unspecified after-cataract
366.51	Soemmering's ring
366.52	Other after-cataract, not obscuring vision
366.53	After-cataract, obscuring vision
366.8	Other cataract
366.9	Unspecified cataract

Documentation Issues
When the documentation states the patient is being seen for an eye examination for cataracts based on long-term use of a high risk medication, and the exam is normal, use codes V58.69 *Long-term (current) use of other medications* and the code for the condition for which the prescribed medication was being taken (e.g., rheumatoid arthritis).

When the documentation identifies a cataract in a diabetic patient, then clarification should be obtained from the physician as to the cause and effect relationship of the cataract and the diabetes. Senile cataracts are commonly seen in diabetics but are not always associated with the diabetes.

Coding Clarification
Diabetic Complication: True diabetic cataracts, or those known as "snowflake cataracts," are rare and are found in Type I diabetics. Use codes 250.51 *Diabetes with ophthalmic manifestations* and 366.41 *Diabetic cataract*. Senile cataracts, although commonly seen in diabetics, are not classified as such because they are not caused by the diabetes. Use codes 250.0x *Diabetes mellitus, without mention of complication* and 366.10 *Senile cataract, unspecified*.

Drug-Induced: Also known as "toxic" cataracts, drug-induced cataracts are noted in patients who have been taking prescribed medications (e.g., steroids) for conditions such as asthma and rheumatoid arthritis. Use code 366.45 *Toxic cataract*, along with a code to identify the condition for which the prescribed medication was being taken (e.g., asthma). In addition, code V58.6x *Long term (current) use of drugs*, should be used. An E-code may also be used to identify the specific drug or other toxic substance that caused the cataract.

Coding Scenario
A patient is seen for steroid-induced cataracts. The patient has a long-standing history of chronic obstructive asthma.

> Code assignment: 366.45 *Toxic cataract*, 493.20 *Chronic obstructive asthma*, and E932.0 *Adverse effect, therapeutic use, adrenal cortical steroids*, V58.65 *Long term (current) use of steroids*

A patient who has completed a high-risk medication regimen for rheumatoid arthritis is given an eye exam. A cataract is noted on the eye exam.

> Code assignment: V67.51 *Follow-up examination following completed treatment with high-risk medications, not elsewhere classified*, 366.45 *Toxic cataract*, 714.0 *Rheumatoid arthritis*

A patient is seen in the office for an eye examination that reveals a small snowflake cataract. This patient is a known insulin-dependent Type I diabetic. Verification with the physician confirms that this is a diabetic cataract.

> Code assignment: 250.51 *Diabetes with ophthalmic manifestations, Type I* and 366.41 *Diabetic cataract*

367 Disorders of refraction and accommodation

A refractive error occurs due to a disorder among the optical components of the eye (i.e., the curvatures, refractive indices, and distances between the cornea, aqueous, crystalline lens, and vitreous) and the overall axial length of the eye. There are four kinds of refractive types: normal eyesight, myopia (nearsightedness), hyperopia (farsightedness), and astigmatism.

In myopia, parallel light rays from an object are focused in front of the retina, with accommodation relaxed. The term nearsightedness comes from the manifestation, which is blurred distance vision. Correction includes concave spectacle or contact lenses or corneal modification to decrease refractive power. In some cases of pseudomyopia, unaided distance vision can be improved with vision therapy.

Myopia can increase the risk for more severe conditions such as retinal breaks or detachment and glaucoma.

In hyperopia, parallel rays of light entering the eye reach a focal point behind the plane of the retina, while accommodation is maintained in a state of relaxation. The additional dioptic power of the converging lenses required to advance the focusing of light rays onto the retina determines the degree of impairment. Corrective lenses may be spherical or spherocylindrical, depending on the nature of the hyperopia and the amount of astigmatic refractive error present.

Astigmatism is due to an elliptically shaped cornea, rather than the normal spherical shape. A point of light, going through an astigmatic cornea, has two points of focus, instead of one sharp image on the retina, resulting in blurred vision. The degree of impairment depends upon the amount and the direction of the astigmatism. A person with myopia or hyperopia may see a dot as a blurred circle, while a person with astigmatism may see the same dot as a blurred oval-shape.

Accommodation is the ability of both eyes to adjust to change in the printed word at various distances and to different print sizes. Tests to check accommodation include negative relative accommodation (NRA) and positive relative accommodation (PRA). In NRA, the patient looks through a phoropter and plus lenses are added binocularly as the patient fixates at 40 centimeters. The PRA is performed immediately after the NRA. In this test, minus lenses are added in front of the eyes until the patient reports a blurred image. The endpoint of both tests is reached when the lenses in front of the eyes provide the first sustained blur.

367.0	Hypermetropia	— *far-sightedness; hyperopia*
367.1	Myopia	— *near-sightedness*
367.20	Unspecified astigmatism	— *light rays are refracted over a diffuse area, rather than over a focus on the retina*
367.21	Regular astigmatism	— *refers to a state of mutual perpendicularity of the sharp (maximum curvatures) and flat (minimum curvatures) of the meridians of the lens and cornea*
367.22	Irregular astigmatism	— *axes are irregular, not usually correctable with spherocylinder lens*
367.31	Anisometropia	— *refractive errors differing by at least one diopter when eyes are compared*
367.32	Aniseikonia	— *unequal retinal image sizes in eyes, usually caused by differing refractive errors*
367.4	Presbyopia	— *loss of elasticity of the elderly lens causing errors of accommodation*
367.51	Paresis of accommodation	— *cycloplegia*
367.52	Total or complete internal ophthalmoplegia	— *large pupil incapable of focus due to total paralysis of ciliary muscle*

Diseases of the Nervous System and Sense Organs

367.53	Spasm of accommodation — *focus dysfunction due to abnormal contraction of ciliary muscle*	368.11	Sudden visual loss
367.81	Transient refractive change — *temporary change in refractive error*	368.12	Transient visual loss — *concentric fading; scintillating scotoma*
367.89	Other disorders of refraction and accommodation — *drug-induced disorders of refraction and accommodation*	368.13	Visual discomfort — *asthenopia; eye strain*
		368.14	Visual distortions of shape and size — *distortions of shape and size, including macropsia; micropsia*
367.9	Unspecified disorder of refraction and accommodation	368.15	Other visual distortions and entoptic phenomena — *photopsia; refractive diplopia; visual halos*

368 Visual disturbances

Amblyopia (368.0), also referred to by the public as "lazy eye," is a unilateral, rarely a bilateral, condition in which the best corrected visual acuity is less than normal (20/20) in the absence of any obvious structural anomalies or ocular disease. Functional amblyopia develops in children up to the age of 6 to 8 years, although it may persist for life once established.

Diplopia (368.2) may be the result of a refractive error, light splitting objects into two images by a defect in the eye's optical system, or it may result from failure of both eyes to point at the object being viewed, a condition referred to as ocular misalignment. If the eyes do not point at the same object, the image seen by each eye is different and cannot be fused. This results in double vision.

Color blindness (368.5) is a lack of perceptual sensitivity to certain colors. There are three types of color receptors in our eyes — red, green, and blue — in addition to black and white receptors. Color blindness is due to a lack of one or more color receptors. Red-green color blindness (368.51) is due to a lack of red receptors. Yellow-blue (368.53) is the second most common form. Lack of all three receptors results in black and white only vision (368.54).

Night blindness (368.6) is an eye disorder in which vision is abnormally impaired in dim light or at night due to a deficiency in rhodopsin (visual purple) in the rods, which is responsible for light sensitivity and the degree of dark adaptation. Night blindness most commonly occurs as a result of retinitis pigmentosa, a degenerative condition of the retina. Visual purple may also decrease if there is a dietary deficiency of its principal component vitamin A.

368.00	Unspecified amblyopia
368.01	Strabismic amblyopia — *suppression amblyopia*
368.02	Deprivation amblyopia — *decreased vision associated with suppression of retinal image of one eye*
368.03	Refractive amblyopia — *decreased vision in one eye associated with uncorrected refractive error*
368.10	Unspecified subjective visual disturbance

368.16	Psychophysical visual disturbances — *visual agnosia; visual hallucinations; disorientation syndrome; Riddoch's syndrome*
368.2	Diplopia — *double vision*
368.30	Unspecified binocular vision disorder
368.31	Suppression of binocular vision
368.32	Simultaneous visual perception without fusion
368.33	Fusion with defective stereopsis
368.34	Abnormal retinal correspondence
368.40	Unspecified visual field defect
368.41	Scotoma involving central area in visual field — *centrocecal scotoma; chiasmatic syndrome*
368.42	Scotoma of blind spot area in visual field — *enlarged angioscotoma; paracecal scotoma*
368.43	Sector or arcuate defects in visual field — *Bjerrum scotoma*
368.44	Other localized visual field defect — *scotoma NOS; nasal step visual field defect*
368.45	Generalized contraction or constriction in visual field
368.46	Homonymous bilateral field defects in visual field — *hemianopsia (altitudinal) (homonymous); quadrant anopia*
368.47	Heteronymous bilateral field defects in visual field — *binasal hemianopsia; bitemporal hemianopsia*
368.51	Protan defect in color vision — *protanomaly; protanopia*
368.52	Deutan defect in color vision — *deuteranomaly; deuteranopia*
368.53	Tritan defect in color vision — *tritanomaly; tritanopia*
368.54	Achromatopsia — *monochromatism (cone) (rod)*
368.55	Acquired color vision deficiencies
368.59	Other color vision deficiencies — *anomalous trichromatopsia (congenital)*
368.60	Unspecified night blindness
368.61	Congenital night blindness — *hereditary night blindness; Oguchi's disease*
368.62	Acquired night blindness
368.63	Abnormal dark adaptation curve — *abnormal threshold of cones or rods; delayed adaptation of cones or rods*
368.69	Other night blindness
368.8	Other specified visual disturbances
368.9	Unspecified visual disturbance **AHA:** Q1, 2004, 15

369 Blindness and low vision

Blindness typically refers to vision loss that is not correctable with eyeglasses or contact lenses, and some people who are considered blind may perceive slowly moving lights or colors. Low vision refers to moderately impaired vision. People with low vision may have a visual impairment that affects only central vision or peripheral vision. Visual acuity and visual field are the two measurements used to assess vision. Visual acuity is the ability to see details (normal vision is 20/20) and visual field refers to peripheral vision (normal visual field is 180 degrees in diameter). Cataract, trachoma, macular degeneration, and glaucoma account for more than 70 percent of all blindness and low vision. Cataracts are not a disease, but a condition affecting the eye. Cataracts usually start as a slight cloudiness that grows more opaque. Light that does reach the retina becomes increasingly blurred and distorted. If left untreated, cataracts can cause blindness. Trachoma is caused by the bacterium Chlamydia trachomatis. It begins in childhood and repeated infections into adulthood irritate and scar the inside of the eyelid and, eventually, the cornea. Scarring on the cornea leads to vision loss. Macular degeneration is a disturbance of the retina and the leading cause of legal blindness in people older than 55 years of age. Glaucoma is a group of conditions related by optic nerve damage, predominantly as a result of elevated intraocular pressure (IOP). The pressure on the optic nerve affects peripheral vision and with glaucoma, central vision is affected as the disease progresses.

Classification		Levels of Visual Impairment				Additional descriptors which may be encountered
"Legal"	WHO	Visual acuity and/or visual field limitation (whichever is worse)				
	(Near-) Normal Vision	Range of Normal Vision 20/10 20/13 20/16 20/20 20/25 2.0 1.6 1.25 1.0 0.8				
		Near-Normal Vision 20/30 20/40 20/50 20/60 0.7 0.6 0.5 0.4 0.3				
	Low Vision	Moderate Visual Impairment 20/70 20/80 20/100 20/125 20/160 0.25 0.20 0.16 0.12				Moderate low vision
Legal Blindness (U.S.A.) Both Eyes	Blindness (WHO) One or Both Eyes	Severe Visual Impairment 20/200 20/250 20/320 20/400 0.10 0.08 0.06 0.05 Visual field: 20 degrees or less				Severe low vision, "Legal" blindness
		Profound Visual Impairment 20/500 20/630 20/800 20/1000 0.04 0.03 0.025 0.02 Count fingers at: less than 3m (10 ft.) Visual field: 10 degrees or less				Profound low vision, Moderate blindness
		Near-Total Visual Impairment Visual acuity: less than 0.02 (20/1000) Count fingers at: 1m (3 ft.) or less Hand movements: 5m (15 ft.) or less Light projection, light perception Visual field: 5 degrees or less				Severe blindness, Near-total blindness
		Total Visual Impairment No light perception (NLP)				Total blindness

Visual acuity refers to best achievable acuity with correction.
Non-listed Snellen fractions may be classified by converting to the nearest decimal equivalent, e.g., 10/200 = 0.05, 6/30 = 0.20.
CF (count fingers) without designation of distance, may be classified to profound impairment.
HM (hand motion) without designation of distance, may be classified to near-total impairment.
Visual field measurements refer to the largest field diameter for a 1/100 white test object.

369.00	Blindness of both eyes, impairment level not further specified — blindness, both eyes		369.08	Better eye: profound vision impairment; lesser eye: profound vision impairment
369.01	Better eye: total vision impairment; lesser eye: total vision impairment		369.10	Profound, moderate or severe vision impairment, not further specified — blindness, one eye, low vision other eye
369.02	Better eye: near-total vision impairment; lesser eye: not further specified		369.11	Better eye: severe vision impairment; lesser eye: blind, not further specified
369.03	Better eye: near-total vision impairment; lesser eye: total vision impairment		369.12	Better eye: severe vision impairment; lesser eye: total vision impairment
369.04	Better eye: near-total vision impairment; lesser eye: near-total vision impairment		369.13	Better eye: severe vision impairment; lesser eye: near-total vision impairment
369.05	Better eye: profound vision impairment; lesser eye: not further specified		369.14	Better eye: severe vision impairment; lesser eye: profound vision impairment
369.06	Better eye: profound vision impairment; lesser eye: total vision impairment		369.15	Better eye: moderate vision impairment; lesser eye: blind, not further specified
369.07	Better eye: profound vision impairment; lesser eye: near-total vision impairment		369.16	Better eye: moderate vision impairment; lesser eye: total vision impairment

Code	Description
369.17	Better eye: moderate vision impairment; lesser eye: near-total vision impairment
369.18	Better eye: moderate vision impairment; lesser eye: profound vision impairment
369.20	Vision impairment, both eyes, impairment level not further specified
369.21	Better eye: severe vision impairment; lesser eye; impairment not further specified
369.22	Better eye: severe vision impairment; lesser eye: severe vision impairment
369.23	Better eye: moderate vision impairment; lesser eye: impairment not further specified
369.24	Better eye: moderate vision impairment; lesser eye: severe vision impairment
369.25	Better eye: moderate vision impairment; lesser eye: moderate vision impairment
369.3	Unqualified visual loss, both eyes
369.4	Legal blindness, as defined in USA — blindness according to U.S.A. definition
369.60	Impairment level not further specified — including blindness one eye
369.61	One eye: total vision impairment; other eye: not specified
369.62	One eye: total vision impairment; other eye: near-normal vision
369.63	One eye: total vision impairment; other eye: normal vision
369.64	One eye: near-total vision impairment; other eye: vision not specified
369.65	One eye: near-total vision impairment; other eye: near-normal vision
369.66	One eye: near-total vision impairment; other eye: normal vision
369.67	One eye: profound vision impairment; other eye: vision not specified
369.69	One eye: profound vision impairment; other eye: normal vision
369.70	Low vision, one eye, not otherwise specified
369.71	One eye: severe vision impairment; other eye: vision not specified
369.72	One eye: severe vision impairment; other eye: near-normal vision
369.73	One eye: severe vision impairment; other eye: normal vision
369.74	One eye: moderate vision impairment; other eye: vision not specified
369.75	One eye: moderate vision impairment; other eye: near-normal vision
369.76	One eye: moderate vision impairment; other eye: normal vision
369.8	Unqualified visual loss, one eye
369.9	Unspecified visual loss

370 Keratitis

Keratitis is inflammation of the cornea, the transparent membrane at the front of the eye, with or without associated conjunctivitis (keratoconjunctivitis). Keratitis usually is due to Type 1 herpes simplex virus (dendritic keratitis, code 054.42), but may be due to bacteria, fungus, amoeba, radiation, trauma, or another source of inflammatory reaction.

Signs and symptoms of keratitis include impaired vision (early) or blindness (late), opacity of the cornea, irritation and tearing, and photophobia.

Diagnostic tests include exam (flashlight, slit lamp) to reveal exudate and hypopyon, which are typical of corneal ulcer, and to confirm keratitis. Instillation of fluorescein dye outlines corneal ulcers. Culture and sensitivity of corneal exudate or hypopyon identify the causative organism. For corneal ulcer, superficial keratectomy may provide culture material.

Therapies include antimicrobials for infection, eye lubricants, plastic bubble eye shield or eye patch, and replacement of cornea from a cadaver (keratoplasty) for corneal scarring.

370.00	Unspecified corneal ulcer
370.01	Marginal corneal ulcer — tissue loss and inflammation in the margins of the cornea
370.02	Ring corneal ulcer — continuous, peripheral tissue loss ringing the cornea
370.03	Central corneal ulcer — corneal tissue loss in the center of the cornea
370.04	Hypopyon ulcer — serpiginous ulcer
370.05	Mycotic corneal ulcer — fungal infection causing corneal tissue loss
370.06	Perforated corneal ulcer — tissue loss through all layers of the cornea
370.07	Mooren's ulcer — painful chronic inflammation and tissue loss at the junction of the cornea and sclera; seen in elderly
370.20	Unspecified superficial keratitis
370.21	Punctate keratitis — Thygeson's superficial punctate keratitis
370.22	Macular keratitis — nummular or areolar keratitis
370.23	Filamentary keratitis — painful and inflamed cornea due to flaking of corneal cells
370.24	Photokeratitis — snow blindness; welders' keratitis **AHA:** Q3, 1996, 6
370.31	Phlyctenular keratoconjunctivitis — (Use additional code for any associated tuberculosis, 017.3)
370.32	Limbar and corneal involvement in vernal conjunctivitis — (Use additional code for vernal conjunctivitis, 372.13)
370.33	Keratoconjunctivitis sicca, not specified as Sjögren's — inadequate tear production causing dry, burning eye
370.34	Exposure keratoconjunctivitis — incomplete closure of eyelid causing dry, inflamed eye **AHA:** Q3, 1996, 6
370.35	Neurotrophic keratoconjunctivitis — corneal and conjunctival inflammation, insensitivity, and nerve damage following injury
370.40	Unspecified keratoconjunctivitis — superficial keratitis with conjunctivitis

Code	Description
370.44	Keratitis or keratoconjunctivitis in exanthema — (Code first underlying condition: 050.0-052.9) — corneal inflammation accompanying infection and rash
370.49	Other unspecified keratoconjunctivitis
370.50	Unspecified interstitial keratitis
370.52	Diffuse interstitial keratitis — *Cogan's syndrome*
370.54	Sclerosing keratitis — *chronic corneal inflammation leading to opaque scarring*
370.55	Corneal abscess — *pocket of pus and inflammation on the cornea*
370.59	Other interstitial and deep keratitis — *other interstitial and deep keratitis*
370.60	Unspecified corneal neovascularization
370.61	Localized vascularization of cornea — *limited infiltration of the cornea by new blood vessels*
370.62	Pannus (corneal) — *shallow infiltration of the cornea by new blood vessels* AHA: Q3, 2002, 20
370.63	Deep vascularization of cornea — *deep infiltration of the cornea by new blood vessels*
370.64	Ghost vessels (corneal) in corneal neovascularization — *transparent, empty blood vessels remaining in cornea after the inflammation that created them has resolved*
370.8	Other forms of keratitis
370.9	Unspecified keratitis

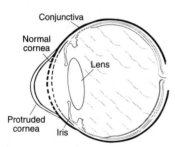

Depiction of keratoconus, a noninflammatory protruding deformity of the cornea

371 Corneal opacity and other disorders of cornea

The cornea is the transparent tissue that covers the front of the eye. It has three layers:

1. The epithelium blocks the passage of foreign material and provides a smooth surface that absorbs oxygen and other needed cell nutrients that are contained in tears.
2. The stroma gives the cornea its strength and elasticity, and the protein fibers of the stroma produce the cornea's light-conducting transparency.
3. The endothelium pumps excess water out of the stroma.

Unlike most tissues in the body, the cornea contains no blood vessels to protect it against infection. The cornea serves as a physical barrier that shields the inside of the eye from germs, dust, and other foreign objects. It also acts as the eye's outermost lens. When light strikes the cornea, it refracts the incoming light onto the crystalline lens. The lens focuses the light onto the retina. Although much thinner than the lens, the cornea provides about 65 percent of the eye's power to bend light. Most of this power resides in the center of the cornea, which is rounder and thinner than the outer part of the tissue and is better suited to bend light waves.

371.00	Unspecified corneal opacity — *corneal sear*
371.01	Minor opacity of cornea — *corneal nebula*
371.02	Peripheral opacity of cornea — *corneal macula not interfering with central vision*
371.03	Central opacity of cornea — *corneal leucoma or macula interfering with central vision*
371.04	Adherent leucoma — *dense, opaque corneal growth adhering to the iris*
371.05	Phthisical cornea — (Code first underlying tuberculosis, 017.3)
371.10	Unspecified corneal deposit
371.11	Anterior pigmentations of cornea — *Stähli's lines*
371.12	Stromal pigmentations of cornea — *hematocornea*
371.13	Posterior pigmentations of cornea — *Krukenberg spindle*
371.14	Kayser-Fleischer ring — *copper deposits forming ring at outer edge of cornea*
371.15	Other deposits of cornea associated with metabolic disorders
371.16	Argentous deposits of cornea — *silver deposits in cornea*
371.20	Unspecified corneal edema
371.21	Idiopathic corneal edema — *corneal swelling and fluid retention of unknown cause*
371.22	Secondary corneal edema — *corneal swelling and fluid retention caused by underlying disease, injury or condition*
371.23	Bullous keratopathy — *small blisters formed on swollen corneal epithelium*
371.24	Corneal edema due to wearing of contact lenses
371.30	Unspecified corneal membrane change
371.31	Folds and rupture of Bowman's membrane — *folds and rupture in the second outermost layer of the cornea*
371.32	Folds in Descemet's membrane — *folds in the second innermost layer of the cornea*
371.33	Rupture in Descemet's membrane — *rupture in the second innermost layer of the cornea*
371.40	Unspecified corneal degeneration
371.41	Senile corneal changes — *arcus senilis; Hassall-Henle bodies*
371.42	Recurrent erosion of cornea
371.43	Band-shaped keratopathy — *horizontal bands of superficial corneal calcium deposits*

371.44	Other calcerous degenerations of cornea
371.45	Keratomalacia NOS — *corneal softening with the development of opacities*
371.46	Nodular degeneration of cornea — *Salzmann's nodular dystrophy*
371.48	Peripheral degenerations of cornea — *marginal degeneration of cornea (Terrien's)*
371.49	Other corneal degenerations — *discrete colliquative keratopathy*
371.50	Unspecified hereditary corneal dystrophy — *unspecified corneal dystrophy*
371.51	Juvenile epithelial corneal dystrophy
371.52	Other anterior corneal dystrophies — *microscopic, cystic corneal dystrophy*
371.53	Granular corneal dystrophy
371.54	Lattice corneal dystrophy
371.55	Macular corneal dystrophy
371.56	Other stromal corneal dystrophies — *crystalline corneal dystrophy*
371.57	Endothelial corneal dystrophy — *combined corneal dystrophy; cornea guttata; Fuchs' endothelial dystrophy*
371.58	Other posterior corneal dystrophies — *polymorphous corneal dystrophy*
371.60	Unspecified keratoconus
371.61	Keratoconus, stable condition
371.62	Keratoconus, acute hydrops
371.70	Unspecified corneal deformity
371.71	Corneal ectasia — *bulging protrusion of a thinned, scarred cornea*
371.72	Descemetocele — *protrusion of Descemet's membrane into the cornea*
371.73	Corneal staphyloma — *protrusion of the cornea into surrounding tissue*
371.81	Corneal anesthesia and hypoesthesia — *decreased or absent sensitivity of the cornea*
371.82	Corneal disorder due to contact lens

Coding Clarification

Corneal disorders can arise due to contact lens use. Complications associated with contact lens use include, but are not limited to, foreign body sensation and irritation, infectious and noninfectious infiltrates, anterior chamber reaction, peripheral vascularization, corneal distortion, corneal perforations, and giant papillary conjunctivitis.

371.89	Other corneal disorder — *hypertrophic cornea* **AHA:** Q3, 1999, 12
371.9	Unspecified corneal disorder

372 Disorders of conjunctiva

Acute conjunctivitis is an inflammation of the mucous membrane covering the anterior surface of the eyeball and the lining of the eyelids. Acute conjunctivitis usually is due to bacteria such as *Staphylococcus aureus*, *Staphylococcus epidermidis*, *Streptococcus pneumoniae*, *Streptococcus pyogenes*, *Moraxella lacunata*, and *Neisseria gonorrhoeae* (098.40). Acute conjunctivitis also may be due to viruses and chlamydiae (rubric 077), and to allergies (atopic).

Signs and symptoms of acute conjunctivitis include hyperemia of conjunctiva, pain and itching, tearing, sticky mucopurulent discharge, injection of bulbar conjunctival vessels, and history of contact lens wear.

Diagnostic tests include culture and sensitivity of discharge to identify the infective organism. Stain may show predominant eosinophils if allergy related, neutrophils if bacterial, and monocytes if caused by a virus (category 077).

Therapies include topical antibiotics for bacterial conjunctivitis, corticosteroid drops, antihistamines and cold compresses for allergic conjunctivitis, and eye lubricants.

372.00	Unspecified acute conjunctivitis — *unspecified acute conjunctivitis*
372.01	Serous conjunctivitis, except viral — *severe conjunctival inflammation with watery discharge*
372.02	Acute follicular conjunctivitis — *conjunctival folliculitis NOS; Parinaud's oculoglandular syndrome*
372.03	Other mucopurulent conjunctivitis — *catarrhal conjunctivitis*
372.04	Pseudomembranous conjunctivitis — *membranous conjunctivitis*
372.05	Acute atopic conjunctivitis — *sudden severe conjunctivitis due to allergies*

Chronic conjunctivitis is chronic inflammation of the conjunctiva characterized by acute exacerbations and remissions occurring over months or years. Degenerative changes or damage may occur from repeated acute attacks. The clinical presentation is similar in most respects to acute conjunctivitis except that it is more innocuous at the onset and runs a more protracted course.

372.10	Unspecified chronic conjunctivitis
372.11	Simple chronic conjunctivitis — *persistent conjunctival inflammation*
372.12	Chronic follicular conjunctivitis — *persistent conjunctival inflammation with dense, localized infiltrations of lymphoid tissues of inner eyelids*
372.13	Vernal conjunctivitis — *persistent seasonal conjunctival inflammation in childhood* **AHA:** Q3, 1996, 8
372.14	Other chronic allergic conjunctivitis
372.15	Parasitic conjunctivitis — (Code first underlying disease: 085.5, 125.0-125.9)
372.20	Unspecified blepharoconjunctivitis
372.21	Angular blepharoconjunctivitis — *inflammation at the junction where the upper and lower eyelids meet; usually blocks lacrimal secretions*

372.22	Contact blepharoconjunctivitis — *inflammation of the eyelid margin and conjunctiva due to an allergic reaction*		373.11	Hordeolum externum — *hordeolum NOS; stye*
			373.12	Hordeolum internum — *infection of meibomian gland; stye*
372.30	Unspecified conjunctivitis		373.13	Abscess of eyelid — *furuncle of eyelid*
372.31	Rosacea conjunctivitis — (Code first underlying rosacea dermatitis, 695.3)		373.2	Chalazion — *meibomian (gland) cyst*
			373.31	Eczematous dermatitis of eyelid — *itchy inflammation of eyelid*
372.33	Conjunctivitis in mucocutaneous disease — (Code first underlying disease: 099.3, 695.1)		373.32	Contact and allergic dermatitis of eyelid — *inflammation of the eyelid due to allergic reaction*
372.39	Other and unspecified conjunctivitis			
372.40	Unspecified pterygium			
372.41	Peripheral pterygium, stationary		373.33	Xeroderma of eyelid — *rough, dry, and scaly skin of the eyelid*
372.42	Peripheral pterygium, progressive			
372.43	Central pterygium		373.34	Discoid lupus erythematosus of eyelid — *swollen eyelids from discoid lupus erythematosus*
372.44	Double pterygium			
372.45	Recurrent pterygium			
372.50	Unspecified conjunctival degeneration		373.4	Infective dermatitis of eyelid of types resulting in deformity — (Code first underlying disease: 017.0, 030.0-030.9, 102.0-102.9)
372.51	Pinguecula — *benign subconjunctival elevation on either side of the cornea*			
372.52	Pseudopterygium		373.5	Other infective dermatitis of eyelid — (Code first underlying disease: 039.3, 051.0, 110.0-111.9, 684, 999.0)
372.53	Conjunctival xerosis — *conjunctival dryness due to insufficient secretions*			
372.54	Conjunctival concretions — *hard masses in the conjunctiva*		373.6	Parasitic infestation of eyelid — (Code first underlying disease: 085.0-085.9, 125.2, 125.3, 132.0)
372.55	Conjunctival pigmentations — *conjunctival argyrosis*		373.8	Other inflammations of eyelids — *inflammations of eyelids NEC*
372.56	Conjunctival deposits		373.9	Unspecified inflammation of eyelid
372.61	Granuloma of conjunctiva — *abnormal dense collection of cells in the conjunctiva*		**374**	**Other disorders of eyelids**
			374.00	Unspecified entropion — *entropion NOS*
372.62	Localized adhesions and strands of conjunctiva — *abnormal fibrous connections in conjunctiva*		374.01	Senile entropion — *eyelid margin curves inward in an elderly eye*
372.63	Symblepharon — *extensive adhesions of conjunctiva*		374.02	Mechanical entropion — *eyelid margin curves inward due to external forces*
372.64	Scarring of conjunctiva — *contraction of eye socket (after enucleation)*		374.03	Spastic entropion — *eyelid margin curves inward intermittently and involuntarily*
372.71	Hyperemia of conjunctiva — *conjunctival blood vessel congestion causing eye redness*		374.04	Cicatricial entropion — *eyelid margin curves inward due to scarring*
372.72	Conjunctival hemorrhage — *hyposphagma; subconjunctival hemorrhage*		374.05	Trichiasis of eyelid without entropion — *eyelashes curve inward, without eyelid margin defect*
372.73	Conjunctival edema — *subconjunctival edema*			
372.74	Vascular abnormalities of conjunctiva — *aneurysm (ata) of conjunctiva*		374.10	Unspecified ectropion — *ectropion NOS*
			374.11	Senile ectropion — *lower eyelid droops away from the elderly eye*
372.75	Conjunctival cysts — *abnormal thin-walled sacs of fluid in the conjunctiva*		374.12	Mechanical ectropion — *lower eyelid droops away from eye due to external forces*
372.81	Conjunctivochalasis			
372.89	Other disorders of conjunctiva		374.13	Spastic ectropion — *lower eyelid droops away from eye intermittently and involuntarily*
372.9	Unspecified disorder of conjunctiva			
			374.14	Cicatricial ectropion — *cicatricial*

373 Inflammation of eyelids

The patient presenting with a chalazion differs from the patient presenting with a hordeolum (stye) in that the chalazion is usually painless after a few days, while discomfort from a hordeolum usually escalates. A chalazion will usually resolve within a few months and can be treated with hot compresses to hasten resolution. Intrachalazion administration of corticosteroid is another method of treatment.

			374.20	Unspecified lagophthalmos — *lagophthalmos NOS*
			374.21	Paralytic lagophthalmos — *full closure of eyelid prevented by nerve defect*
			374.22	Mechanical lagophthalmos — *outside force prevents full closure of eyelids*
			374.23	Cicatricial lagophthalmos — *scar tissue prevents full closure of eyelids*
			374.30	Unspecified ptosis of eyelid
373.00	Blepharitis, unspecified		374.31	Paralytic ptosis — *drooping of upper eyelid due to nerve defect*
373.01	Ulcerative blepharitis — *inflammation of the eyelid with erosion of tissue*		374.32	Myogenic ptosis — *drooping of upper eyelid due to muscular defect*
373.02	Squamous blepharitis — *inflammation of eyelid margin with scaling of tissue*			

Diseases of the Nervous System and Sense Organs

Code	Description
374.33	Mechanical ptosis — *outside force causes drooping of upper eyelid*
374.34	Blepharochalasis — *drooping or relaxation of upper eyelid due to atrophy of intercellular tissue*
374.41	Eyelid retraction or lag
374.43	Abnormal innervation syndrome of eyelid — *jaw-blinking; paradoxical facial movements*
374.44	Sensory disorders of eyelid
374.45	Other sensorimotor disorders of eyelid — *deficient blink reflex*
374.46	Blepharophimosis — *ankyloblepharon*
374.50	Unspecified degenerative disorder of eyelid
374.51	Xanthelasma of eyelid — (Code first underlying condition: 272.0-272.9)
374.52	Hyperpigmentation of eyelid — *chloasma; dyspigmentation*
374.53	Hypopigmentation of eyelid — *vitiligo of eyelid*
374.54	Hypertrichosis of eyelid — *excessive eyelash growth*
374.55	Hypotrichosis of eyelid — *less than normal amount, or absence of, eyelashes; madarosis of eyelid*
374.56	Other degenerative disorders of skin affecting eyelid — *other degenerative skin disorders affecting eyelid NEC*
374.81	Hemorrhage of eyelid — *bleeding eyelid*
374.82	Edema of eyelid — *hyperemia of eyelid*
374.83	Elephantiasis of eyelid — *filarial disease causing dermatitis and enlargement of eyelid*
374.84	Cysts of eyelids — *sebaceous cyst of eyelid*
374.85	Vascular anomalies of eyelid
374.86	Retained foreign body of eyelid
374.87	Dermatochalasis — *loss of elasticity causing skin under eye to sag*
374.89	Other disorders of eyelid — *blepharoplegia; granuloma of eyelid*
374.9	Unspecified disorder of eyelid

375 Disorders of lacrimal system

The lacrimal system produces and distributes the tears that lubricate and clean the eye and keep nasal tissues moist. Excluded from this rubric are congenital disorders of the lacrimal system.

Code	Description
375.00	Unspecified dacryoadenitis
375.01	Acute dacryoadenitis — *severe, sudden inflammation of the lacrimal gland*
375.02	Chronic dacryoadenitis — *persistent inflammation of the lacrimal gland*
375.03	Chronic enlargement of lacrimal gland
375.11	Dacryops — *overproduction and constant flow of tears*
375.12	Other lacrimal cysts and cystic degeneration
375.13	Primary lacrimal atrophy — *wasting away of the lacrimal gland*
375.14	Secondary lacrimal atrophy — *wasting away of the lacrimal gland due to other disease process*
375.15	Unspecified tear film insufficiency — *dry eye syndrome* AHA: Q3, 1996, 6
375.16	Dislocation of lacrimal gland
375.20	Epiphora, unspecified as to cause
375.21	Epiphora due to excess lacrimation — *overflow of tears due to overproduction*
375.22	Epiphora due to insufficient drainage — *overflow of tears due to blocked drainage*
375.30	Unspecified dacryocystitis
375.31	Acute canaliculitis, lacrimal — *sudden, severe inflammation of the tear drainage system*
375.32	Acute dacryocystitis — *acute peridacryocystitis*
375.33	Phlegmonous dacryocystitis — *infection of the tear sac with pockets of pus*
375.41	Chronic canaliculitis — *persistent inflammation of the tear drainage system*
375.42	Chronic dacryocystitis — *persistent inflammation of the tear sac*
375.43	Lacrimal mucocele — *enlarged pocket of mucus in lacrimal system*
375.51	Eversion of lacrimal punctum — *abnormal turning outward of the tear duct*
375.52	Stenosis of lacrimal punctum — *abnormal narrowing of tear duct*
375.53	Stenosis of lacrimal canaliculi — *abnormal narrowing of the tear drainage system*
375.54	Stenosis of lacrimal sac — *abnormal narrowing of tear sac*
375.55	Obstruction of nasolacrimal duct, neonatal — *acquired narrowing of the tear drainage system from the eye to the nose*
375.56	Stenosis of nasolacrimal duct, acquired
375.57	Dacryolith — *concretion of stone anywhere in lacrimal system*
375.61	Lacrimal fistula — *abnormal communication from the lacrimal system*
375.69	Other change of lacrimal passages — *changes of lacrimal passage NOS*
375.81	Granuloma of lacrimal passages — *abnormal nodules within the tear drainage system*
375.89	Other disorder of lacrimal system — *disorders of lacrimal system NOS*
375.9	Unspecified disorder of lacrimal system

376 Disorders of the orbit

This rubric identifies disorders of the orbit, which is the bony housing for the eyeball that expands for the first two years of life as the eye grows. Between the bony housing and the eyeball are other structures such as fat, muscle, blood vessels, and glands. The orbital fat cushioning each globe is divided into central and peripheral compartments. The central space contains the optic, oculomotor, abducent, and nasociliary nerves. The peripheral space contains the trochlear, lacrimal, frontal, and infraorbital nerves.

Codes in subclassification 376.0 are selected by site. In orbital cellulitis, the infection is between the orbital bone and the eyeball. In orbital periostitis, the infection is in the connective tissue covering the orbital bone. In orbital osteomyelitis, the bone is infected; and in tenonitis, the infection is in the

Tenon's capsule, the thin membrane that envelops the eyeball.

376.00	Unspecified acute inflammation of orbit — *acute orbital inflammation NOS*
376.01	Orbital cellulitis — *abscess of orbit*
376.02	Orbital periostitis — *inflammation of connective tissue covering the orbital bone*
376.03	Orbital osteomyelitis — *inflammation of the orbital bone*
376.04	Orbital tenonitis — *inflammation of Tenon's capsule, the thin membrane that envelops the eyeball*
376.10	Unspecified chronic inflammation of orbit — *chronic orbital inflammation NOS*
376.11	Orbital granuloma — *pseudotumor (inflammatory) of orbit*
376.12	Orbital myositis — *painful inflammation of the muscles of the eye*
376.13	Parasitic infestation of orbit — (Code first underlying disease: 122.3, 122.6, 122.9, 134.0)
376.21	Thyrotoxic exophthalmos — *bulging eyes as a result of hyperthyroidism*
376.22	Exophthalmic ophthalmoplegia — *inability to rotate eyes as a result of bulging eyes*
376.30	Unspecified exophthalmos
376.31	Constant exophthalmos — *continuous, abnormal protrusion or bulging of eyeball*
376.32	Orbital hemorrhage — *bleeding behind the eyeball, causing it to bulge forward*
376.33	Orbital edema or congestion — *fluid retention behind eyeball, causing it to bulge forward*
376.34	Intermittent exophthalmos — *separate incidences of abnormal bulging of the eyeball*
376.35	Pulsating exophthalmos — *throbbing bulge or protrusion of the eyeball, usually associated with a carotid-cavernous fistula*
376.36	Lateral displacement of globe of eye — *abnormal displacement of the eyeball away from the nose, toward the temple*
376.40	Unspecified deformity of orbit
376.41	Hypertelorism of orbit — *congenital anomaly in which the eyes are widely placed*
376.42	Exostosis of orbit — *abnormal bony growth of orbit*
376.43	Local deformities of orbit due to bone disease — *acquired abnormalities of the orbit due to bone disease*
376.44	Orbital deformities associated with craniofacial deformities — *congenital malformation of the orbital bone*
376.45	Atrophy of orbit — *wasting away of bone tissue of orbit*
376.46	Enlargement of orbit
376.47	Deformity of orbit due to trauma or surgery
376.50	Enophthalmos, unspecified as to cause — *recession of eyeball deep into eye socket*
376.51	Enophthalmos due to atrophy of orbital tissue — *recession of eyeball deep into eye socket due to atrophy of orbital tissue*
376.52	Enophthalmos due to trauma or surgery
376.6	Retained (old) foreign body following penetrating wound of orbit — *retrobulbar foreign body*
376.81	Orbital cysts — *encephalocele of orbit; mucocele of orbit* **AHA:** Q3, 1999, 13
376.82	Myopathy of extraocular muscles — *disease in one or more of the six muscles that control eyeball movement*
376.89	Other orbital disorder — *emphysema of eye; retrobulbar hemorrhage*
376.9	Unspecified disorder of orbit

Coding Clarification
A second code from Infectious and Parasitic Diseases (001-139) can be reported to identify the infective agent.

Orbital cellulitis (376.01) is the inflammation of the orbital tissues caused by infection that extends from the nasal sinuses or teeth, by metastatic spread from infections elsewhere, or by bacteria introduced via orbital trauma. Exophthalmos (376.30, 376.31) describes the protrusion of one eyeball or both that results from orbital inflammation, edema, tumors, injuries, cavernous sinus thrombosis, or enlargement of the eyeball (as in congenital glaucoma and unilateral high myopia). When an infection or tumor develops, the tissues swell, causing the eye to protrude. Aggressive therapy, including surgical intervention, may be necessary to save the eye and retain functional sight. Hypertelorism (376.41) describes increased space between the eyes and is often associated with other skeletal abnormalities such as an encephalocele or syndromes such as Apert syndrome. Craniofacial surgery is often required for orbital deformities associated with craniofacial deformity (376.44). In congenital or trauma-induced enophthalmos (376.50, 376.51, 376.52), the eyeballs are displaced far back into the orbit.

When an underlying disease causes the orbital disorder, sequence the underlying disease code first and a code from this rubric secondarily.

377 Disorders of optic nerve and visual pathways
The optic nerve is the extent of the visual system pathway from the back of the eyeball up to the optic chiasm. It contains axons of ganglion cells in the retina of the ipsilateral (i.e., same side) eye. Each optic nerve splits and half of its fibers cross over to the other side at the optic chiasm. If the optic nerve is damaged between an eyeball and the optic chiasm, the person may become blind in that eye. If the problem lies farther back in the optic nerve pathway,

both eyes may lose half of the visual fields, a condition called hemianopia. If both eyes lose peripheral vision, the cause may be damage at the optic chiasm. If both eyes lose half of the visual field on the same side, the cause is usually damage to the optic nerve pathway on the opposite side of the brain caused by a stroke, hemorrhage, or tumor. Dysfunction of the optic nerve may be congenital or acquired. If congenital, it is usually hereditary. The acquired type may be due to vascular disturbances, secondary to degenerative retinal disease (e.g., papilledema or optic neuritis), a result of pressure against the optic nerve, or related to metabolic diseases (e.g., diabetes), trauma, glaucoma, or toxicity (to alcohol, tobacco, or other poisons).

Code	Description
377.00	Unspecified papilledema
377.01	Papilledema associated with increased intracranial pressure — *pressure within the brain causes swelling and engorgement of the optic disc and its blood vessels*
377.02	Papilledema associated with decreased ocular pressure — *reduced pressure within the eyeball causes swelling and engorgement of the optic disc and its blood vessels*
377.03	Papilledema associated with retinal disorder — *retinal disease or dysfunction causes swelling and engorgement of optic disc and its blood vessels*
377.04	Foster-Kennedy syndrome — *basofrontal syndrome*
377.10	Unspecified optic atrophy
377.11	Primary optic atrophy — *disc is grayish white with sharp edges*
377.12	Postinflammatory optic atrophy — *eye wastes away due to inflammation*
377.13	Optic atrophy associated with retinal dystrophies — *wasting away of eye due to progressive changes in retinal tissue due to metabolic defects*
377.14	Glaucomatous atrophy (cupping) of optic disc — *wasting away of eye as a result of high intraocular pressure*
377.15	Partial optic atrophy — *temporal pallor of optical disc*
377.16	Hereditary optic atrophy — *Leber's optic atrophy*
377.21	Drusen of optic disc — *glistening white nodules within optic nerve head*
377.22	Crater-like holes of optic disc — *crater-like holes*
377.23	Coloboma of optic disc — *congenital cleft, or defect in continuity of the optic disc*
377.24	Pseudopapilledema — *optic nerve head deformity resembling a choked optic disc*
377.30	Unspecified optic neuritis
377.31	Optic papillitis — *swelling and inflammation of the optic disc*
377.32	Retrobulbar neuritis (acute) — *inflammation of optic nerve in the orbit behind the eye*
377.33	Nutritional optic neuropathy — *optic nerve disorder caused by malnutrition*
377.34	Toxic optic neuropathy — *toxic amblyopia*
377.39	Other optic neuritis — *optic neuritis NEC*
377.41	Ischemic optic neuropathy — *optic nerve disorder due to decreased blood flow*
377.42	Hemorrhage in optic nerve sheaths — *bleeding in optic nerve sheaths*
377.43	Optic nerve hypoplasia

Optic nerve hypoplasia (ONH) is a condition present at birth in which the optic nerve is not fully developed. Bilateral occurrence is more common than unilateral and is one of the three most common causes of impaired vision in children. ONH is not progressive nor is it inherited, and it cannot be cured. In the majority of cases, there is no known cause, although studies have indicated that maternal factors such as diabetes, alcohol abuse, use of antiseizure drugs, and young maternal age (20 years of age or less) may be associated with the condition. Characteristics include photophobia, depressed visual fields, impaired depth perception, and nystagmus. Visual function may range from normal visual acuity to the absence of light perception. There may be generalized loss of detailed vision in both central and peripheral visual fields, or there may be only subtle peripheral field loss. Visual function may improve minimally as the brain undergoes the maturation process.

Diagnosis is made by examination of the optic nerve and observation of its size together with that of the nerve head. Neuroimaging techniques are helpful in diagnosing ONH. There is currently no cure, and treatment is generally directed toward the visual difficulties associated with this disorder.

Code	Description
377.49	Other disorder of optic nerve — *compression of optic nerve*
377.51	Disorders of optic chiasm associated with pituitary neoplasms and disorders — *disruption in nerve chain from retina to brain, caused by abnormal pituitary growth*
377.52	Disorders of optic chiasm associated with other neoplasms — *disruption in nerve chain from retina to brain, caused by abnormal growth, other than pituitary*
377.53	Disorders of optic chiasm associated with vascular disorders — *disruption in nerve chain from retina to brain, caused by a vascular disorder*
377.54	Disorders of optic chiasm associated with inflammatory disorders — *disruption in nerve chain from retina to brain, caused by inflammatory disease*
377.61	Disorders of other visual pathways associated with neoplasms
377.62	Disorders of other visual pathways associated with vascular disorders

377.63	Disorders of other visual pathways associated with inflammatory disorders
377.71	Disorders of visual cortex associated with neoplasms
377.72	Disorders of visual cortex associated with vascular disorders
377.73	Disorders of visual cortex associated with inflammatory disorders
377.75	Disorders of visual cortex associated with cortical blindness — *blindness due to brain disorder, not eye disorder*
377.9	Unspecified disorder of optic nerve and visual pathways

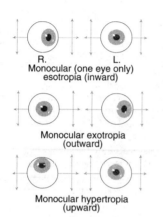

R.   L.
Monocular (one eye only) esotropia (inward)

Monocular exotropia (outward)

Monocular hypertropia (upward)

The various heterophorias present when the visual axis fails upon removal of the fusioning stimuli. The eye then wanders in the indicated direction

378 Strabismus and other disorders of binocular eye movements

Binocular fixation is necessary to see three-dimensionally and to aid in depth perception. A visual defect in which the two eyes fail to work together results in a partial or total loss of binocular depth perception and stereoscopic vision. At least 12 percent of the population has some type of binocular vision disability, of which amblyopia and strabismus are the most common types.

Strabismus is a condition in which the eyes do not point in the same direction. It can also be referred to as a tropia or squint. The disorder occurs in 2 to 5 percent of all children. About half are born with the condition, which causes one or both eyes to turn:

- Esotropia — inward turning of the eye
- Exotropia — outward turning of the eye
- Hypertropia — upward turning of the eye
- Hypotropia — downward turning of the eye

A baby's eyes should be straight and parallel by three or four months of age. A child who develops strabismus after the age of 8 or 9 years is said to have adult-onset strabismus. Most children with strabismus have comitant strabismus, in which the degree of deviation does not change. In incomitant strabismus, the amount of misalignment depends upon which direction the eyes are pointed.

To determine misalignment, the ophthalmologist looks at a flashlight reflection on the cornea when the patient looks in all directions. The light should be reflected on the same portion of the cornea bilaterally or the diagnosis may be made with the cover test, in which each eye is covered in turn as the child looks at an object about 20 feet away. When the eye is covered, the uncovered eye should not move in a normal individual. In those with strabismus, the uncovered eye will move to focus properly on the object. Treatment may be surgical for muscle imbalance, use of refractive lenses, or patching the normal eye to allow the affected eye to regain strength and vision.

There is a genetic basis for several types of inherited strabismus, including those associated with genetic multisystem disorders such as Moebius syndrome, Prader-Willi syndrome, craniofacial dysostoses, and mitochondrial myopathies. It is especially common in children who have brain tumors, hydrocephalus, or genetic disorders (i.e., Down syndrome). In adults, diabetes, head trauma, stroke, or brain tumor may cause strabismus. Untreated strabismus can damage vision in the unused eye and possibly result in amblyopia (lazy eye). Amblyopia involves lowered visual acuity and poor muscle control in one eye. The result is often a loss of stereoscopic vision and binocular depth perception. Other binocular disorders include visual fine motor difficulties, eye movement inefficiencies, and visual perceptual lags that can result in eye strain, headache, double vision, blurred vision, learning related vision problems, and poor eye-hand coordination.

378.00	Unspecified esotropia
378.01	Monocular esotropia — *one eye turns inward*
378.02	Monocular esotropia with A pattern — *one eye turns inward with A pattern*
378.03	Monocular esotropia with V pattern — *one eye turns inward with V pattern*
378.04	Monocular esotropia with other noncomitancies — *monocular esotropia with X or Y pattern*
378.05	Alternating esotropia — *each eye takes turns deviating toward inner eye*
378.06	Alternating esotropia with A pattern — *each eye takes turns deviating toward inner eye with A pattern*

Diseases of the Nervous System and Sense Organs

378.07	Alternating esotropia with V pattern — *each eye takes turns deviating toward inner eye with V pattern*	378.62	Mechanical strabismus from other musculofascial disorders
378.08	Alternating esotropia with other noncomitancies — *each eye takes turns deviating toward inner eye with X or Y pattern*	378.63	Mechanical strabismus from limited duction associated with other conditions
378.10	Unspecified exotropia	378.71	Duane's syndrome — *eye retraction syndrome*
378.11	Monocular exotropia — *one eye turns outward*	378.72	Progressive external ophthalmoplegia — *von Graefe's syndrome*
378.12	Monocular exotropia with A pattern — *one eye turns outward with A pattern*	378.73	Strabismus in other neuromuscular disorders
378.13	Monocular exotropia with V pattern — *one eye turns outward with V pattern*	378.81	Palsy of conjugate gaze — *oculomotor syndrome' Parinaud's syndrome*
378.14	Monocular exotropia with other noncomitancies — *monocular exotropia with X or Y pattern*	378.82	Spasm of conjugate gaze — *muscle contractions impairing parallel movement of eyes*
378.15	Alternating exotropia — *each eye takes turns deviating outward*	378.83	Convergence insufficiency or palsy in binocular eye movement
378.16	Alternating exotropia with A pattern — *each eye takes turns deviating outward with A pattern*	378.84	Convergence excess or spasm in binocular eye movement — *overcompensation in parallel movement of eye*
378.17	Alternating exotropia with V pattern — *each eye takes turns deviating outward with V pattern*	378.85	Anomalies of divergence in binocular eye movement
378.18	Alternating exotropia with other noncomitancies — *each eye takes turns deviating outward with X or Y pattern*	378.86	Internuclear ophthalmoplegia — *eye movement anomaly attributed to brainstem lesion*
378.20	Unspecified intermittent heterotropia — *intermittent esotropia NOS or intermittent exotropia NOS*	378.87	Other dissociated deviation of eye movements — *skew deviation*
378.21	Intermittent esotropia, monocular — *monocular*	378.9	Unspecified disorder of eye movements
378.22	Intermittent esotropia, alternating — *alternating*		
378.23	Intermittent exotropia, monocular — *monocular*		
378.24	Intermittent exotropia, alternating — *alternating*		
378.30	Unspecified heterotropia		
378.31	Hypertropia — *vertical heterotropia (constant) (intermittent)*		
378.32	Hypotropia		
378.33	Cyclotropia		
378.34	Monofixation syndrome — *microtropia*		
378.35	Accommodative component in esotropia		
378.40	Unspecified heterophoria		
378.41	Esophoria		
378.42	Exophoria		
378.43	Vertical heterophoria		
378.44	Cyclophoria		
378.45	Alternating hyperphoria		
378.50	Unspecified paralytic strabismus		
378.51	Paralytic strabismus, third or oculomotor nerve palsy, partial		
378.52	Paralytic strabismus, third or oculomotor nerve palsy, total — *Nothnagel's syndrome; ophthalmoplegia-cerebellar ataxia syndrome* **AHA:** Q2, 1989, 12		
378.53	Paralytic strabismus, fourth or trochlear nerve palsy		
378.54	Paralytic strabismus, sixth or abducens nerve palsy		
378.55	Paralytic strabismus, external ophthalmoplegia — *Tolosa-Hunt syndrome*		
378.56	Paralytic strabismus, total ophthalmoplegia		
378.60	Unspecified mechanical strabismus		
378.61	Mechanical strabismus from Brown's (tendon) sheath syndrome — *unilateral defect in sheath of superior oblique muscle, mimicking palsy*		

379 Other disorders of eye

Aphakia is classified to this rubric.

Scleritis is the inflammation of the sclera (the white, outer wall of the eye) that can be superficial or deep. It is usually associated with autoimmune diseases such as rheumatoid arthritis, lupus erythematosus, infections, or chemical injuries, but sometimes the cause is unknown. It occurs most often in people between the ages of 30 and 60 and is rare in children. Symptoms include severe eye pain, blurred vision, sensitivity to light, and tearing of the eyes.

Staphyloma is a protrusion of the cornea or sclera, consisting of uveal tissue, caused by thinning of the sclera. No treatment has shown its effectiveness and evisceration is usually indicated.

Inflammation of postprocedural blebs is a complication of certain ophthalmologic procedures now occurring on a more frequent basis due to the increased use of antimetabolites in these procedures over the past decade. During certain procedures, an auxiliary drain on the outside of the eyeball, known as a filtering bleb, is created. Most often associated with trabeculectomy for the treatment of glaucoma, filtering blebs may also be created with other procedures, such as full-thickness filtration surgery. Antimetabolites are applied locally to retard healing so that scar formation will be decreased. In addition to producing extensive thin-walled filtration blebs that may be easily invaded by bacteria, antimetabolites such as mitomycin-C and 5-

fluorouracil may also create low pressure or ocular hypotony, and inflammation or infection can occur.

Postprocedural bleb inflammation has three stages of severity. In stage 1, bleb purulence is present with or without mild inflammation of the anterior segment. Treatment usually consists of topical antibiotics. In stage 2, moderate inflammation of the anterior segment is present in addition to bleb purulence. Treatment consists of topical drugs and oral antibiotics; however, subconjunctival antibiotic injection may be required if improvement is not noted within 24 to 48 hours. Stage 3 is characterized by severe pain, vitritis, and obvious anterior chamber reaction. Bleb-related endophthalmitis and acute visual loss may occur. Repeat subconjunctival antibiotic injections may be required, and surgical revision of the bleb may be needed following resolution of the infection.

Code	Description
379.00	Unspecified scleritis — *episcleritis NOS*
379.01	Episcleritis periodica fugax — *inflammation of outermost layer of the sclera, with blood engorgement*
379.02	Nodular episcleritis — *inflammation of outermost layer of the sclera, with nodular formations*
379.03	Anterior scleritis — *scleritis adjacent to corneal limbus*
379.04	Scleromalacia perforans — *softening and thinning of sclera*
379.05	Scleritis with corneal involvement — *scleroperikeratitis*
379.06	Brawny scleritis — *severe scleral inflammation with thickening corneal margins*
379.07	Posterior scleritis — *sclerotenonitis*
379.09	Other scleritis and episcleritis — *scleral abscess; scleral ulcer*
379.11	Scleral ectasia — *scleral staphyloma NOS*
379.12	Staphyloma posticum — *stretched, bulging sclera and uveal tissue at the posterior pole of eye*
379.13	Equatorial staphyloma — *stretched, bulging sclera and uveal tissue midway between anterior and posterior portions of eye*
379.14	Anterior staphyloma, localized — *stretched, bulging sclera and uveal tissue at the anterior pole of eye*
379.15	Ring staphyloma — *stretched, bulging sclera and uveal tissue in ring shape*
379.16	Other degenerative disorders of sclera
379.19	Other scleral disorder
379.21	Vitreous degeneration — *vitreous cavitation, detachment or liquefaction*
379.22	Crystalline deposits in vitreous — *asteroid hyalitis; synchysis scintillans*
379.23	Vitreous hemorrhage — *bleeding into the vitreous* AHA: Q3, 1991, 15
379.24	Other vitreous opacities — *vitreous floaters*
379.25	Vitreous membranes and strands — *membranes and strands*
379.26	Vitreous prolapse — *vitreous slippage from normal position*
379.29	Other disorders of vitreous
379.31	Aphakia — *condition of being without natural optical lens*
379.32	Subluxation of lens — *partial dislocation of natural lens*
379.33	Anterior dislocation of lens — *anterior displacement of natural lens toward iris*
379.34	Posterior dislocation of lens — *backward displacement of natural lens toward vitreous*
379.39	Other disorders of lens
379.40	Unspecified abnormal pupillary function
379.41	Anisocoria — *unequal pupils, differing by 1mm or more*
379.42	Miosis (persistent), not due to miotics — *sustained, abnormal contraction of pupil*
379.43	Mydriasis (persistent), not due to mydriatics — *sustained, abnormal dilation of pupil*
379.45	Argyll Robertson pupil, atypical — *Argyll Robertson phenomenon or pupil, nonsyphilitic*
379.46	Tonic pupillary reaction — *Adie's pupil or syndrome; Saenger's syndrome*
379.49	Other anomaly of pupillary function — *pupillary paralysis*
379.50	Unspecified nystagmus
379.51	Congenital nystagmus — *oscillating eye movements, congenital*
379.52	Latent nystagmus
379.53	Visual deprivation nystagmus — *oscillating eye movements caused by darkness*
379.54	Nystagmus associated with disorders of the vestibular system — *oscillating eye movements due to inner ear disease*
379.55	Dissociated nystagmus — *oscillating eye movements independent of each other*
379.56	Other forms of nystagmus
379.57	Nystagmus with deficiencies of saccadic eye movements — *abnormal optokinetic response*
379.58	Nystagmus with deficiencies of smooth pursuit movements — *dysfunction in normal tracking focus and movement of eyes*
379.59	Other irregularities of eye movements — *opsoclonus*
379.60	Inflammation (infection) of postprocedural bleb, unspecified
379.61	Inflammation (infection) of postprocedural bleb, stage 1
379.62	Inflammation (infection) of postprocedural bleb, stage 2
379.63	Inflammation (infection) of postprocedural bleb, stage 3 — *bleb-associated endophthalmitis*
379.8	Other specified disorders of eye and adnexa
379.90	Unspecified disorder of eye
379.91	Pain in or around eye
379.92	Swelling or mass of eye
379.93	Redness or discharge of eye
379.99	Other ill-defined disorder of eye

Documentation Issues
Assigning the stage of post-procedural bleb inflammation is the responsibility of the physician and should be documented in the medical record. Otherwise, assign code 379.60 *Inflammation (infection) of postprocedural bleb, unspecified.*

Coding Clarification
Report aphakia as a condition warranting treatment with 379.31, while aphakia (pseudophakia) as a post-cataract extraction status is reported with V45.61. Congenital aphakia is reported with 743.35.

Exclusion notes at purulent endophthalmitis (360.0), other endophthalmitis (360.1), and postoperative infection (998.5) help the coder correctly report inflammation and infection of postprocedural bleb to subcategory 379.6X codes, by applicable stage.

380–389   Diseases of the Ear and Mastoid Process

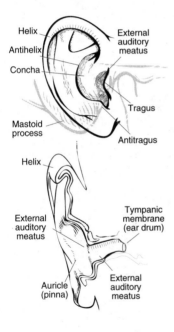

380   Disorders of external ear
Disorders of the external ear include those of the auricle (pinna) and external auditory meatus. The auricle consists of the helix, anthelix, scapha, concha, tragus, antitragus, intertragic notch, and lobule. The auricle is a single, elastic cartilage covered in skin and normal adnexal features (hair follicles, sweat glands, and sebaceous glands). The ridged nature of the auricle is to channel sounds into the acoustic meatus. The semicircular depression leading to the ear is named the concha, Latin for shell. The external auditory meatus consists of cartilaginous and osseous portions with the canal lined with epidermis, hair, and ceruminous glands that extend to the tympanic membrane.

Perichondritis is infection of the skin and tissue layer surrounding the cartilage of the ear and often happens after trauma or another infection has occurred. Chondritis is infection that has progressed into the cartilage itself. Though not a common infection, the recent increase in ear piercing through the cartilage around the outside of the ear has increased this risk. It is also a serious complication following surgery or injury as the damage can be severe, progressing to necrosis, requiring removal and reconstruction of the pinna.

Infective otitis externa is inflammation and infection of the auricle and external meatus. Bacteria, such as Pseudomonas, *Proteus vulgaris, Streptococci,* and *Staphylococcus aureus,* or fungal infections such as Candida albicans can cause this condition.

Signs and symptoms of infective otitis externa include redness and swelling that can obstruct the meatus, serous or purulent drainage, external ear tenderness, and enlarged regional lymph nodes.

Diagnostic tests include culture and sensitivity to identify the infective organism. An otoscopy reveals inflammation and ceruminous impaction.

Therapies include antimicrobials (topically, systemically, or both), heat therapy to relieve pain, and gentle ear cleansing.

380.00	Unspecified perichondritis of pinna
380.01	Acute perichondritis of pinna — *sudden, severe inflammation of the connective tissue of the cartilage of the outer ear*
380.02	Chronic perichondritis of pinna — *persistent inflammation of the connective tissue of outer ear*
380.03	Chondritis of pinna AHA: Q4, 2004, 76
380.10	Unspecified infective otitis externa — *otitis externa (acute), circumscribed; otitis externa (acute), hemorrhagica*
380.11	Acute infection of pinna — *sudden, severe infection of outer ear canal*
380.12	Acute swimmers' ear — *beach ear; tank ear*

380.13	Other acute infections of external ear — (Code first underlying disease: 035, 684, 690.10-690.18)
380.14	Malignant otitis externa — *severe infection of outer ear canal with some tissue destruction*
380.15	Chronic mycotic otitis externa — (Code first underlying disease: 111.9, 117.3)
380.16	Other chronic infective otitis externa — *chronic infective otitis externa NOS*
380.21	Cholesteatoma of external ear — *keratosis obturans of external ear (canal)*
380.22	Other acute otitis externa — *actinic, chemical, contact, eczematoid, reactive*
380.23	Other chronic otitis externa — *chronic otitis externa NOS*
380.30	Unspecified disorder of pinna
380.31	Hematoma of auricle or pinna — *collection of blood in the tissue of the fleshy external ear*
380.32	Acquired deformities of auricle or pinna
380.39	Other noninfectious disorder of pinna — *ossification ear*
380.4	Impacted cerumen — *wax in ear*
380.50	Acquired stenosis of external ear canal unspecified as to cause
380.51	Acquired stenosis of external ear canal secondary to trauma — *narrowing of the external ear canal due to trauma*
380.52	Acquired stenosis of external ear canal secondary to surgery — *postsurgical narrowing of external ear canal*
380.53	Acquired stenosis of external ear canal secondary to inflammation — *narrowing of the external ear canal due to inflammation*
380.81	Exostosis of external ear canal
380.89	Other disorder of external ear — *auricular calcification; cicatrix of auricle; fistula of ear canal*
380.9	Unspecified disorder of external ear

Coding Clarification
Assign a fifth digit to indicate the exact nature and/or location of the inflammation.

When chondritis occurs as a result of a postoperative infection, assign 380.03 and 998.59. When chondritis occurs as sequelae following a burn, assign 906.5 as an additional diagnosis to 380.03.

Coding Scenario
A 16-year-old girl presented to her physician's office with her outer ear severely abscessed and the surrounding tissue beginning to show signs of vascular compromise, following multiple ear piercings. When the physician asked her why she waited so long to come in, she told him her mother had forbidden her to get multiple ear piercings around her ear and she had hoped it would heal with topical antiseptic. A culture was taken which revealed a *Pseudomonas aeruginosa* infection. The physician had her hospitalized where drains were inserted, some wound debridement was done, and she was placed on intravenous antibiotic therapy to stop the approach of gangrene.

Code assignment: 380.03 *Chondritis of pinna* 041.7 *Pseudomonas infection*

381 Nonsuppurative otitis media and Eustachian tube disorders

Suppurative and unspecified otitis media are infections of the middle ear due to pyogenic organisms such as *staphylococci, pneumococci, Haemophilus influenzae, beta-hemolytic streptococci,* and gram-negative bacteria.

Signs and symptoms of suppurative and unspecified otitis media include chills and fever, malaise, deep throbbing ear pain, nausea and vomiting, dulled or impaired hearing, ear drainage, bulging of tympanic membrane, signs of upper respiratory infection, and a tender and swollen mastoid process.

Diagnostic tests include otoscopy to reveal obscured or distorted bony landmarks of the tympanic membrane, with scarring and thickening in chronic otitis media. A pneumatoscope shows decreased tympanic membrane motility. Culture and sensitivity of purulent material identify the infective organism.

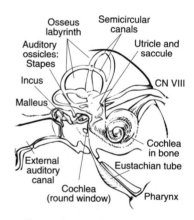

Exposed view of middle and inner ear

Therapies include systemic antibiotics, nasal decongestants, and analgesics such as aspirin to control pain and fever, and myringotomy with aspiration of the middle ear fluid if the tympanic membrane is in danger of rupture. Surgery may be performed (tympanoplasty, myringoplasty, mastoidectomy, excision of cholesteatomas) for chronic otitis media.

Associated conditions include adenoiditis or tonsillitis, colds or sinusitis, cholesteatoma, adhesions or scarring of middle ear structures, conductive hearing loss, abscesses, meningitis, mastoiditis, suppurative labyrinthitis, facial paralysis, otitis externa, sigmoid sinus, and jugular vein thrombosis.

381.00	Unspecified acute nonsuppurative otitis media	
381.01	Acute serous otitis media — *acute or subacute secretory otitis media*	
381.02	Acute mucoid otitis media — *acute or subacute seromucinous otitis media; blue drum syndrome*	
381.03	Acute sanguinous otitis media — *sudden, severe infection of the middle ear, with blood*	
381.04	Acute allergic serous otitis media — *allergic serous*	
381.05	Acute allergic mucoid otitis media — *allergic mucoid*	
381.06	Acute allergic sanguinous otitis media — *allergic sanguinous*	
381.10	Simple or unspecified chronic serous otitis media — *persistent infection of the middle ear, without pus*	
381.19	Other chronic serous otitis media — *serosanguinous chronic otitis media*	
381.20	Simple or unspecified chronic mucoid otitis media	
381.29	Other chronic mucoid otitis media — *mucosanguineous chronic otitis media*	
381.3	Other and unspecified chronic nonsuppurative otitis media — *otitis media, chronic - allergic, exudative, secretory, transudative, with effusion*	
381.4	Nonsuppurative otitis media, not specified as acute or chronic — *allergic, catarrhal, exudative, secretory, serous, transudative, with effusion, otitis media*	
381.50	Unspecified Eustachian salpingitis	
381.51	Acute Eustachian salpingitis — *sudden, severe inflammation of the Eustachian tube*	
381.52	Chronic Eustachian salpingitis — *persistent inflammation of the Eustachian tube*	
381.60	Unspecified obstruction of Eustachian tube — *obstruction of Eustachian tube NOS*	
381.61	Osseous obstruction of Eustachian tube — *obstruction of Eustachian tube from cholesteatoma, polyp, or other osseous lesion*	
381.62	Intrinsic cartilagenous obstruction of Eustachian tube — *Eustachian tube blockage caused by Eustachian cartilage overgrowth*	
381.63	Extrinsic cartilagenous obstruction of Eustachian tube — *compression of Eustachian tube; Eustachian tube blockage caused by other cartilage overgrowth*	
381.7	Patulous Eustachian tube — *distended, oversized*	
381.81	Dysfunction of Eustachian tube	
381.89	Other disorders of Eustachian tube — *adhesion of Eustachian tube; diverticula of Eustachian tube*	
381.9	Unspecified Eustachian tube disorder	

Coding Scenario
A 5-year-old male is seen in the emergency department. His mother states that he suffered a seizure. Upon examination the child is found to have otitis media and a temperature of 104.2. The physician documents the diagnosis as febrile convulsions and acute nonsuppurative otitis media.

Code assignment: 780.31 *Febrile convulsions (simple), unspecified* and 381.00 *Acute nonsuppurative otitis media, unspecified*

382 Suppurative and unspecified otitis media
The middle ear cleft extends from the nasopharyngeal orifice of the eustachian tube to the mastoid air cells. The three main segments are the eustachian tube, middle ear (tympanum), and the air cells of the mastoid, petrosa, and related areas. Suppurative otitis media is a serious bacterial infection of the middle ear that can follow untreated acute otitis media. Infections with *Streptococcus pneumoniae, Haemophilus influenza,* and *Moraxella catarrhalis* are the most common causes of acute suppurative otitis media (382.0). Most complications of otitis media are associated with chronic or subacute disease. Acute and chronic otitis media infection may spread beyond the temporal bone and cause intratemporal (i.e., mastoiditis, petrositis, labyrinthitis, and facial nerve paralysis) and intracranial (i.e., extradural abscess, brain abscess, subdural abscess, sigmoid sinus thrombophlebitis, otic hydrocephalus, and meningitis) complications. The classic signs of acute otitis media are redness and bulging of the tympanic membrane. If the process continues to worsen, necrosis of the tympanic membrane occurs and the effusion passes into the ear canal through a perforation (suppurative otitis media). Diagnosis includes use of a pneumotoscopy when the presence of fluid behind the eardrum is not clear or an otomicroscopy using the operating microscope to visualize depth and three-dimensional structure. Antibiotics are usually prescribed for infection. Once osteitis is diagnosed, mastoidectomy is generally warranted to remove the infected, often necrotic bone. If an abscess is present, surgery is performed for drainage of pus and removal of the infected bone.

382.00	Acute suppurative otitis media without spontaneous rupture of eardrum — *severe inflammation of middle ear, with pus*	
382.01	Acute suppurative otitis media with spontaneous rupture of eardrum — *sudden, severe inflammation of middle ear, with pressure tearing ear drum tissue, with pus*	

Code	Description
382.02	Acute suppurative otitis media in diseases classified elsewhere — (Code first underlying disease: 034.1, 487.8)
382.1	Chronic tubotympanic suppurative otitis media — *benign chronic suppurative otitis media or chronic tubotympanic disease with anterior perforation of ear drum*
382.2	Chronic atticoantral suppurative otitis media — *chronic atticoantral disease or persistent mucosal disease with posterior or superior marginal perforation of ear drum*
382.3	Unspecified chronic suppurative otitis media — *chronic purulent otitis media*
382.4	Unspecified suppurative otitis media — *purulent otitis media NOS*
382.9	Unspecified otitis media — *otitis media NOS, acute otitis media NOS; chronic otitis media NOS*
	AHA: Nov-Dec, 1984, 16

383 Mastoiditis and related conditions

Mastoiditis and related conditions describe inflammation and/or infection of the mastoid bone or an abscess in the mastoid antrum. The infections usually are due to Pneumococcus, *Haemophilus influenzae*, beta-hemolytic *Streptococci*, and gram-negative organisms.

Signs and symptoms of mastoiditis and related conditions include dull ache and tenderness over the mastoid process, low-grade fever, thick and purulent discharge, postauricular edema, erythema, and conductive hearing loss.

Diagnostic tests include x-rays of the mastoid area to reveal hazy signs of infection and an otoscopy to reveal dull and thick edematous tympanic membrane.

Therapies include antibiotics, myringotomy and drainage of purulent fluid, mastoidectomy (simple or radical), sequestrectomy, or debridement of necrotic bone.

Associated conditions include meningitis, facial paralysis, brain abscess, suppurative labyrinthitis, chronic otitis media, and conductive hearing loss.

Code	Description
383.00	Acute mastoiditis without complications — *sudden, severe inflammation of the mastoid air cells*
383.01	Subperiosteal abscess of mastoid — *von Bezold's abscess*
383.02	Acute mastoiditis with other complications — *Gradenigo's syndrome*
383.1	Chronic mastoiditis — *caries of mastoid; fistula of mastoid*
383.20	Unspecified petrositis
383.21	Acute petrositis — *sudden, severe inflammation of the dense bone behind the ear*
383.22	Chronic petrositis — *persistent inflammation of the dense bone behind the ear*
383.30	Unspecified postmastoidectomy complication — *postmastoidectomy complication NOS*
383.31	Mucosal cyst of postmastoidectomy cavity — *mucous-lined cyst cavity following removal of mastoid bone*
383.32	Recurrent cholesteatoma of postmastoidectomy cavity — *cyst-like mass of cell debris in cavity following removal of mastoid bone*
383.33	Granulations of postmastoidectomy cavity — *chronic inflammation of postmastoidectomy cavity*
383.81	Postauricular fistula — *abnormal passage behind mastoid cavity*
383.89	Other disorder of mastoid — *perforation of mastoid (antrum) (cell)*
383.9	Unspecified mastoiditis

384 Other disorders of tympanic membrane

The tympanic membrane (eardrum), which separates the outer ear from the middle ear, is a three-layer structure. The outer layer and inner layer are squamous and respiratory epithelia, which attempt to bridge defects in the middle ear. If there is a poor blood supply, or if there is an infection during the healing process, the squamous and respiratory epithelial layers may interfere with the process of spontaneous repair. A perforated eardrum (384.2x) is a hole or rupture in the eardrum, of which there are several causes, such as a skull fracture, infection, or from pushing a foreign object too far into the ear. Middle ear infections may cause pain, hearing loss, and spontaneous rupture of the eardrum resulting in a perforation. Most eardrum perforations heal spontaneously within weeks after rupture, during which time the ear must be protected from water and trauma. The location of the perforation affects the degree of hearing loss. If severe trauma (e.g., skull fracture) disrupts the bones in the middle ear or causes injury to the inner ear structures, the loss of hearing may be quite severe. Permanent hearing loss occurs in 3 percent of patients operated on for chronic otitis media and is associated with excessive ossicular mobilization, fracture of stapedial foot plate, direct trauma, or introduction of toxic materials.

Code	Description
384.00	Unspecified acute myringitis
384.01	Bullous myringitis — *myringitis bullosa hemorrhagica*
384.09	Other acute myringitis without mention of otitis media
384.1	Chronic myringitis without mention of otitis media — *chronic tympanitis*
384.20	Unspecified perforation of tympanic membrane
384.21	Central perforation of tympanic membrane
384.22	Attic perforation of tympanic membrane — *attic perforation including pars flaccida*
384.23	Other marginal perforation of tympanic membrane

384.24	Multiple perforations of tympanic membrane		385.01	Tympanosclerosis involving tympanic membrane only — *tough fibrous tissue impeding functions of the ear drum*
384.25	Total perforation of tympanic membrane			
384.81	Atrophic flaccid tympanic membrane — *healed perforation of ear drum*		385.02	Tympanosclerosis involving tympanic membrane and ear ossicles — *tough fibrous tissue impeding functions of the eardrum and middle ear bones (stapes, malleus, and incus)*
384.82	Atrophic nonflaccid tympanic membrane			
384.9	Unspecified disorder of tympanic membrane			
			385.03	Tympanosclerosis involving tympanic membrane, ear ossicles, and middle ear — *tough fibrous tissue impeding functions of the ear drum, middle ear bones, and middle ear canal*

Coding Clarification
Myringitis (384.0x) is always associated with otitis media. Bullous myringitis (384.01) is an inflammatory and contagious disorder of the eardrum or tympanum (caused by infection) resulting in painful blisters on the eardrum.

385.09	Tympanosclerosis involving other combination of structures
385.10	Adhesive middle ear disease, unspecified as to involvement

385 Other disorders of middle ear and mastoid

The mastoid is a part of the temporal bone of the skull (e.g., bony bump just behind and slightly above the level of the external ear) that is connected with the middle ear. In the adult, the mastoid portion of the temporal bone contains mastoid air cells that are separated from the brain by thin bony partitions. When there is a collection of fluid in the middle ear, there is usually also a slight collection of fluid within the airspaces of the mastoid. Attached to the eardrum (tympanic membrane) are three ear bones known as the malleus, incus, and stapes. The malleus pushes the incus; the incus pushes the stapes. When sound waves strike the eardrum, it vibrates and sets the bones into a motion that is transmitted to the inner ear, which generates nerve impulses that are sent to the brain. The muscles of the middle ear modify the performance of the middle ear bones and act as safety devices to protect the ear against excessively large vibrations from loud noises. As the noise level rises, one set of muscles tightens to restrict the movement of the malleus thus weakening the vibrations transmitted within the middle ear. At the same time, the stapes muscle contracts to pull the stapes away from the oval window so that less vibration is passed along to the very sensitive inner ear. The middle ear is connected to the nose by the Eustachian tube, which equalizes pressure in the middle ear. A healthy middle ear must contain air at the same atmospheric pressure as outside of the ear, so all these structures can vibrate freely. Tympanosclerosis is a common sequela after acute and chronic otitis media; the pathological calcified plaques are found in the tympanic membrane and the middle ear ossicles, leading to hearing impairment. Treatment is surgery but recurrences are common and there is also a risk for iatrogenic sensorineural hearing loss.

385.11	Adhesions of drum head to incus
385.12	Adhesions of drum head to stapes
385.13	Adhesions of drum head to promontorium
385.19	Other middle ear adhesions and combinations
385.21	Impaired mobility of malleus — *ankylosis of malleus*
385.22	Impaired mobility of other ear ossicles — *ankylosis of ear ossicles, except malleus*
385.23	Discontinuity or dislocation of ear ossicles — *disruption in the auditory chain created by the malleus, incus, and stapes*
385.24	Partial loss or necrosis of ear ossicles — *loss of tissue in the malleus, incus, or stapes*

Coding Clarification
Cholesteatoma of the middle ear and mastoid is an abnormal growth of squamous epithelial cells within the middle ear extending from the external meatus. The dead epithelial tissue, which usually is forced to the exterior of the ear with the movement of the earwax, forms a sac, and produces keratin.

Signs and symptoms of cholesteatoma of the middle ear and mastoid include hearing loss and history of acute or chronic otitis media.

Otoscopy reveals white debris in the middle ear and destruction of the external auditory canal bone; x-rays of the middle ear and mastoid show tumor formation.

Therapies include control of concomitant infection, excision of cholesteatoma in extreme cases, tympanoplasty (reconstruction of ossicles), and myringoplasty.

Associated conditions include acute or chronic otitis media, hearing loss due to bony destruction of the ossicles, middle ear hemorrhage, attic and marginal perforations of the tympanic membrane, aural polyps, purulent labyrinthitis, facial paralysis, and intracranial abscess.

385.00	Tympanosclerosis, unspecified as to involvement		385.30	Unspecified cholesteatoma
			385.32	Cholesteatoma of middle ear — *cystlike mass of cell debris in middle ear*

385.33	Cholesteatoma of middle ear and mastoid — *cyst-like mass of cell debris in middle ear and mastoid air cells behind ear*	
	AHA: Q3, 2000, 10	
385.35	Diffuse cholesteatosis of middle ear and mastoid — *cyst-like masses of cell debris throughout middle ear*	
385.82	Cholesterin granuloma of middle ear — *fatty granulations in the middle ear*	
385.83	Retained foreign body of middle ear	
385.89	Other disorders of middle ear and mastoid — *caries of middle ear; cicatrix of middle ear; hemotympanum; neuralgic mastoid; fistula of middle ear*	
385.9	Unspecified disorder of middle ear and mastoid — *disorder of middle ear or mastoid NOS*	

Schematic of labyrinth and semicircular ducts

386 Vertiginous syndromes and other disorders of vestibular system
AHA: March-April, 1985, 12

The inner ear consists of a system of fluid-filled tubes and sacs called the labyrinth, as well as the nerves that connect the labyrinth to the brain. The labyrinth, which rests inside the bone of the skull, contains the cochlea, and other organs, called the vestibular system, which control balance and eye movements. The first part of the vestibular system is made up of three semicircular canals that respond to angular acceleration of the head. The second part consists of the utricle and the saccule, which contain otoliths, or macular organs that respond to linear acceleration of the head as well as gravity.

Labyrinthitis and neuronitis are bacterial or viral inflammations of the inner ear or the nerves connecting the inner ear to the brain. Inflammation of the cochlea can cause disturbances in hearing, such as tinnitus. Dizziness, unsteadiness or imbalance when walking, and nausea are the most common symptoms of vestibular disorders. Because the vestibular system interacts with other parts of the nervous system, there may be problems with vision, muscles, thinking, and memory. Patients with vestibular disorders often report fatigue and loss of stamina and an inability to concentrate. Diagnosis depends on a variety of tests, including a physical exam to rule out other causes (i.e., cardiovascular disorders), vestibular testing, electronystagmography to record eye movements, and balance testing. Treatment consists of drug therapy, physical therapy, or, in severe cases, surgery.

In many cases, the underlying cause cannot be determined, though head trauma is a frequent cause in individuals younger than age 50. Ear infections such as otitis media and labyrinthitis and conditions that reduce blood flow to the inner ear (i.e., stroke) may damage the vestibular and hearing structures of the inner ear. High doses or long-term use of certain antibiotics can also cause permanent damage to the inner ear. Other drugs, such as aspirin, caffeine, alcohol, nicotine, sedatives, and tranquilizers can cause temporary dizziness but do not result in permanent damage to the vestibular system.

Menier_'s disease is a disorder of the inner ear that causes episodes of vertigo, tinnitus, a feeling of fullness or pressure in the ear, and fluctuating hearing loss, and which can last two to four hours. Menier_'s episodes may occur in clusters, or weeks, months, or years may pass between episodes. Between the acute attacks, most people are free of symptoms or note only mild imbalance and tinnitus. Between attacks, medication may be prescribed to help regulate the fluid pressure in the inner ear, reducing the severity and frequency of episodes. A hydrops diet regimen results in significant improvement in most patients. Surgery (possibly including instillation of gentamicin or other substances) may be performed to relieve the pressure on the inner ear or to block the transmission of information from the affected ear to the brain.

Benign paroxysmal positional vertigo (386.11) is a type of vertigo often induced when a patient turns over in bed, or gets in and out of bed. It is a benign disorder due to calcium impacted inner ear canals and treated with removal of the impaction. Diagnosis is through the Dix Halpike maneuver, which involves moving the patient rapidly from a sitting position, to the head hanging position, below horizontal, such as with a head hanging off the end of an examining table.

Diseases of the Nervous System and Sense Organs

Vestibular neuronitis (386.12) is characterized by a sudden loss of balance that can be so severe that the patient may not be able to walk for several days or weeks. Viral neuronitis or a blood clot in the arterial system may precipitate the disorder. Diagnosis is based on symptoms, a physical exam, and tests, including audiometry, electronystagmography, and magnetic resonance imaging of the head. Treatment depends on the extent of balance loss (e.g., partial or total) and the onset of the disease in relation to treatment. Anticoagulants may be prescribed in conjunction with vasodilators to expand the blood vessels and allow the clot to pass. Corticosteroids may be used to treat a viral infection.

Labyrinthitis is a bacterial or viral infection secondary to acute otitis media or to purulent meningitis. When bacterial, there is a total loss of hearing on the affected side; if tuberculosis or syphilis is the cause, the hearing loss may be only partial. Diagnosis is by clinical exam of the ear and the patient's description of symptoms. Treatment of bacteria-caused labyrinthitis consists of heavy doses of antibiotics. The viral form is usually self-limiting, and the only treatment is bed rest, tranquilizers, and a medication to combat the dizziness.

386.00	Unspecified Meniere's disease — *Menier_'s disease (active); Lermoyez' syndrome* **AHA:** March-April, 1985, 12
386.01	Active Meniere's disease, cochleovestibular
386.02	Active Meniere's disease, cochlear
386.03	Active Meniere's disease, vestibular
386.04	Inactive Meniere's disease — *Menier_'s disease in remission* **AHA:** March-April, 1985, 12
386.10	Unspecified peripheral vertigo
386.11	Benign paroxysmal positional vertigo
386.12	Vestibular neuronitis — *Pedersen's (epidemic) vertigo* **AHA:** March-April, 1985, 12
386.19	Other and unspecified peripheral vertigo — *aural vertigo; otogenic vertigo; otolith syndrome* **AHA:** March-April, 1985, 12
386.2	Vertigo of central origin — *central positional nystagmus; malignant positional vertigo* **AHA:** March-April, 1985, 12
386.30	Unspecified labyrinthitis
386.31	Serous labyrinthitis — *Serous labyrinthitis; diffuse labyrinthitis; inflammation with fluid buildup* **AHA:** March-April, 1985, 12
386.32	Circumscribed labyrinthitis — *focal labyrinthitis; localized inflammation* **AHA:** March-April, 1985, 12
386.33	Suppurative labyrinthitis — *purulent labyrinthitis; inflammation with pus* **AHA:** March-April, 1985, 12
386.34	Toxic labyrinthitis — *inflammation caused by toxic reaction* **AHA:** March-April, 1985, 12
386.35	Viral labyrinthitis — *inflammation caused by virus* **AHA:** March-April, 1985, 12
386.40	Unspecified labyrinthine fistula
386.41	Round window fistula
386.42	Oval window fistula
386.43	Semicircular canal fistula
386.48	Labyrinthine fistula of combined sites
386.50	Unspecified labyrinthine dysfunction
386.51	Hyperactive labyrinth, unilateral — *oversensitivity of labyrinth, one ear* **AHA:** March-April, 1985, 12
386.52	Hyperactive labyrinth, bilateral — *bilateral; oversensitivity of labyrinth, both ears* **AHA:** March-April, 1985, 12
386.53	Hypoactive labyrinth, unilateral — *reduced sensitivity of labyrinth, one ear* **AHA:** March-April, 1985, 12
386.54	Hypoactive labyrinth, bilateral — *reduced sensitivity of labyrinth, both ears* **AHA:** March-April, 1985, 12
386.55	Loss of labyrinthine reactivity, unilateral — *reduced reaction of labyrinth, one ear* **AHA:** March-April, 1985, 12
386.56	Loss of labyrinthine reactivity, bilateral — *bilateral; reduced reaction of labyrinth, both ears* **AHA:** March-April, 1985, 12
386.58	Other forms and combinations of labyrinthine dysfunction
386.8	Other disorders of labyrinth — *caries of labyrinth; hemorrhage of cochlea; otoconia* **AHA:** March-April, 1985, 12
386.9	Unspecified vertiginous syndromes and labyrinthine disorders — *vertiginous syndrome or labyrinthine disorder NOS* **AHA:** March-April, 1985, 12

387 Otosclerosis

Otosclerosis is an inherited disorder involving the growth of abnormal spongy bone in the middle ear, which prevents the stapes from vibrating in response to sound waves. The condition leads to progressive hearing loss and is the most frequent cause of middle ear hearing loss in young adults, most commonly in women, 15 to 30 years old. Risks include a family history of hearing loss in pregnancy, which may trigger the onset. Diagnosis depends on a physical exam to rule out other causes of hearing loss and an audiometry exam to determine the extent of hearing loss. A computed tomography scan or x-ray of the head may be used to distinguish otosclerosis from other causes of hearing loss. Treatment includes medications such as oral fluoride, calcium, or vitamin D to stabilize the hearing loss. Surgery involves removal of the stapes and replacement with a prosthesis; this may be a total replacement (stapedectomy) or a laser may be used to make a hole in the stapes to allow placement of the prosthesis.

387.0	Otosclerosis involving oval window, nonobliterative — *tough, fibrous tissue impeding functions of the oval window*
387.1	Otosclerosis involving oval window, obliterative — *tough, fibrous tissue blocking the oval window*
387.2	Cochlear otosclerosis — *otosclerosis involving otic capsule or round window*
387.8	Other otosclerosis
387.9	Unspecified otosclerosis — *ossification of middle ear; otoporosis; otospongiosis*

388 Other disorders of ear

388.00	Unspecified degenerative and vascular disorders — *degenerative and vascular disorders NOS*
388.01	Presbyacusis — *loss of hearing associated with aging process*
388.02	Transient ischemic deafness — *temporary loss of hearing due to restricted blood flow to auditory organs*
388.10	Unspecified noise effects on inner ear — *effects on inner ear NOS*
388.11	Acoustic trauma (explosive) to ear — *otitic blast injury*
388.12	Noise-induced hearing loss — *noise-induced loss*
388.2	Unspecified sudden hearing loss — *sudden hearing loss NOS*
388.30	Unspecified tinnitus
388.31	Subjective tinnitus — *noises heard only by patient; usually biochemical in nature*
388.32	Objective tinnitus — *noises originating within patient and audible to others*
388.40	Unspecified abnormal auditory perception — *abnormal auditory perception NOS*
388.41	Diplacusis — *cochlear dysfunction causing patient to hear a single auditory stimulus as two sounds*
388.42	Hyperacusis — *acute hearing sensitivity; not necessarily painful*
388.43	Impairment of auditory discrimination — *impairment in ability to distinguish sound*
388.44	Other abnormal auditory perception, recruitment — *impairment in ability to distinguish volume of sound*
388.5	Disorders of acoustic nerve — *acoustic neuritis; degeneration or disorder of acoustic or eighth nerve*
	AHA: March-April, 1987, 8
388.60	Unspecified otorrhea — *discharging ear NOS*
388.61	Cerebrospinal fluid otorrhea — *spinal fluid leakage from ear*
388.69	Other otorrhea — *otorrhagia*
388.70	Unspecified otalgia — *earache NOS*
388.71	Otogenic pain — *ear pain caused by a condition within the ear*
388.72	Referred otogenic pain — *ear pain caused by a condition outside the ear*
388.8	Other disorders of ear — *swelling ear*
388.9	Unspecified disorder of ear — *atrophic ear*

389 Hearing loss

The ear consists of three parts: the outer ear, middle ear, and inner ear. The outer ear is the visible part plus the canals. The canals lead to the eardrum (middle ear), which is attached to the ossicles that amplify and conduct sound to the inner ear. The inner ear consists of the cochlea, which contains hair cells that vibrate when a sound is conducted to them by the eardrum and ossicles. The movement of the hair cells transmits electrical impulses down the auditory nerve to the brain, which is the sound heard.

Conductive hearing loss results from external or middle ear problems, which are often mechanical in nature. There are various causes for conductive hearing loss, including otitis media and otosclerosis. The most common cause of conductive hearing loss in children is otitis media infection in the middle ear cavity. The most common cause of conductive hearing loss in adults is otosclerosis. The loss results from fixation of the stapes (the third bone in the middle ear) so that sounds cannot be transported to the inner ear. Conductive hearing loss can be either temporary or permanent, and is treatable with medication and/or surgery.

Sensory hearing losses are due to disorders in the inner ear, specifically, the cochlea. This type of loss may be congenital, resulting from abnormal cochlea development or inherited conditions, or the loss may be the result of an acquired condition, such as meningitis, an infection of the fluid around the brain often extending into the inner ear.

Neural hearing loss results from a problem with the auditory nerve, often caused by an acoustic neuroma, which is a benign tumor that grows on the vestibular nerve and presses upon the auditory nerve. Early detection and prompt removal of the tumor is curative and may prevent future hearing loss. The acoustic reflex is a way of testing for neural hearing loss. The stapedius is a small muscle attached to the stapes that contracts in response to any loud sound, thus protecting the ear. The level of sound required to elicit this acoustic reflex can be used as a rough measure of hearing sensitivity. If the middle ear is normal, absence of the acoustic reflex may indicate a neural type of hearing loss. Neural hearing loss is also characterized by a greater loss of speech discrimination than experienced with sensory loss.

Sensorineural hearing loss is usually permanent loss of hearing sensitivity, often occuring more in the high frequencies than in the lower frequencies. Involving not only a reduction in sound level, sensorineural hearing loss also affects speech, cognition, and the ability to hear clearly and understand conversations. Damage to the cochlea (inner ear) or to the nerve pathways from the inner ear to the brain cause this type of hearing loss. Underlying causes include birth injury, diseases, toxic drugs, and genetic syndromes. Other causes are head trauma, exposure to noise, viruses, tumors such as acoustic neuroma or meningioma, and aging. Asymmetrical hearing loss is that which is bilateral but more pronounced in one ear, while unilateral hearing loss affects only one side. If a sensorineural cause is suspected, an electrocochleography and auditory brainstem response tests are performed to measure the activity of the cochlea, auditory nerve, and brain.

Central auditory dysfunction refers to auditory impairment resulting from problems in the brain. Fortunately, central problems are uncommon. While they cause communication difficulties, they do not cause deafness because they usually affect only one side of the brain: both sides of the brain are involved in hearing. Central auditory dysfunction can result from aging, from Alzheimer's disease, and from other uncommon problems.

389.00	Unspecified conductive hearing loss
389.01	Conductive hearing loss, external ear
389.02	Conductive hearing loss, tympanic membrane
389.03	Conductive hearing loss, middle ear
389.04	Conductive hearing loss, inner ear
389.08	Conductive hearing loss of combined types
389.10	Unspecified sensorineural hearing loss
389.11	Sensory hearing loss, bilateral
389.12	Neural hearing loss, bilateral
389.14	Central hearing loss, bilateral
389.15	Sensorineural hearing loss, unilateral
389.16	Sensorineural hearing loss, asymmetrical
389.18	Sensorineural hearing loss of combined types, bilateral
389.2	Mixed conductive and sensorineural hearing loss — *deafness or hearing loss of type classifiable to 389.0 with 389.1*
389.7	Deaf mutism, not elsewhere classifiable — *deaf, nonspeaking*
389.8	Other specified forms of hearing loss
389.9	Unspecified hearing loss — *deafness NOS*

AHA: Q1, 2004, 15

390-459

Diseases of the Circulatory System

Coding diseases of the circulatory system can be complex for several reasons, some of which are among the following:

- Interrelationship of conditions
- Specificity of coding guidelines
- Varied medical lexicon used to describe circulatory conditions

390-392 Acute Rheumatic Fever

Acute rheumatic fever is defined as a systemic disease/nonsuppurative acute complication, generally affecting joints (arthritis), subcutaneous tissue (nodules), skin (erythema marginatum), heart (carditis), and brain (chorea). The fever usually follows a throat infection by Group A Streptococci. Therapies include medications such as antibiotics (including subsequent antistreptococcal prophylaxis), analgesics, and anti-inflammatory agents.

Rheumatic fever is classified according to the site of inflammation. In acute rheumatic fever, the infection is active. Excluded from these rubrics are chronic heart conditions caused by rheumatic fever (393.0-398.9).

390 Rheumatic fever without mention of heart involvement OK

This rubric is limited to rheumatic fever that may have acute or subacute arthritis, but no heart involvement.

391 Rheumatic fever with heart involvement

Acute rheumatic pericarditis is an acute rheumatic fever with fibrinous involvement of the pericardium without mention of other cardiac involvement. It is uncommon in adults.

Acute rheumatic endocarditis is an acute rheumatic fever with involvement of the endocardium. This form of acute rheumatic fever principally involves one or more of the heart valves. Echocardiography of a patient with acute rheumatic endocarditis reveals large, friable "vegetations" on the heart valves or chordae tendineae.

Acute rheumatic myocarditis is an acute rheumatic fever with involvement of the heart muscle. Signs and symptoms may include tachycardia out of proportion to fever, cardiac manifestations such as heart blocks and arrhythmias, or a history of recent upper respiratory infection, pharyngitis, or tonsillitis. Diagnostic tests, such as stool and throat cultures, may identify the bacteria present, while endomyocardial biopsy provides a definite diagnosis. Disorders associated with acute rheumatic myocarditis may include cardiac arrhythmias, congestive heart failure, thromboembolism, or pericarditis. Therapies include antibiotics for bacterial infection, anti-arrhythmics for cardiac arrhythmias, and/or anticoagulants for possible thromboembolism.

391.0	Acute rheumatic pericarditis — *sudden, severe inflammation of the lining of the heart*
391.1	Acute rheumatic endocarditis — *sudden, severe inflammation of the heart cavities*
391.2	Acute rheumatic myocarditis — *sudden, severe inflammation of the heart muscle*
391.8	Other acute rheumatic heart disease — *sudden, severe inflammation of multiple sites in heart*
391.9	Unspecified acute rheumatic heart disease — *sudden, severe inflammation of unknown site of heart*

392 Rheumatic chorea

Rheumatic chorea is an inflammatory complication of Group A streptococcal infection involving the central nervous system. It is also known as chorea minor, chorea dance, Sydenham's chorea, and Saint Vitus dance. It generally affects children and young adults. Signs and symptoms may include involuntary, irregular, jerky movements of the face (excluding eyes), neck, or limbs.

| 392.0 | Rheumatic chorea with heart involvement — *involuntary muscle movement and weakness* |
| 392.9 | Rheumatic chorea without mention of heart involvement — *involuntary muscle movement and weakness* |

393–398 Chronic Rheumatic Heart Disease

Chronic rheumatic heart disease is a chronic disease resulting from single or repeated attacks of acute rheumatic fever that produce late effects in the structure of the heart, usually the endocardium. Sequelae include rigidity and deformity of the valvular cusps, fusion of the commissures, or shortening and fusion of the chordae tendinea. Damage also may occur in the myocardium following severe bouts of acute rheumatic myocarditis affecting cardiac performance. Associated conditions may include valvular stenosis and/or insufficiency and, usually, mitral and myocardial damage.

393 Chronic rheumatic pericarditis

Chronic rheumatic pericarditis is a set of conditions such as adhesive pericarditis and constrictive pericarditis when specified as a manifestation following an acute rheumatic infection. Adhesive pericarditis (chronic) occurs when adhesions develop between the two-pericardial layers, or between the pericardium and the heart or other neighboring structures. Constrictive pericarditis (chronic) is a thickening of the pericardial membrane with constriction of the cardiac chambers.

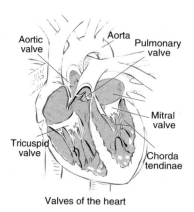

Valves of the heart

394 Diseases of mitral valve

Mitral stenosis, mitral valve disease (unspecified), and mitral valve failure are presumed to be rheumatic in origin for classification purposes and need not be stated as rheumatic. Other manifestations, such as insufficiency, incompetence, or regurgitation (without stenosis) must be specified as due to rheumatic heart disease for classification under rubric 394.

Mitral stenosis is a narrowing of the orifice of the mitral valve due to (presumed) rheumatic heart disease that impedes left ventricular filling. Signs and symptoms include left or combined left and right heart failure, hemoptysis, systematic embolism, hoarseness, atrial fibrillation, or pulmonary rales and increased S1/S2 heart sounds.

Rheumatic mitral insufficiency is a reflux of a portion of blood back into the left atrium instead of forward into the aorta, resulting in increased atrial pressure and decreased forward cardiac output. Signs and symptoms may include dyspnea due to left ventricular failure (which may be combined with right heart failure in severe cases), pulmonary hypertension, holosystolic apical murmur, S3 heart sound, or brisk carotid upstroke. An EKG may show left ventricular hypertrophy and left atrial enlargement in cases of rheumatic mitral insufficiency, and a chest x-ray usually shows heart enlargement and vascular congestion when the insufficiency has resulted in heart failure. Echocardiography may visualize scarring and retraction of the mitral leaflets. Cardiac catheterization with a pulmonary capillary wedge monitor (Swan-Ganz) may reveal systolic volume overload, which is characterized by a large V wave on right heart catheterization, and left ventriculography demonstrates systolic regurgitation of contrast material into the left atrium. Therapies for rheumatic mitral insufficiency may include medications (digitalis, diuretics, or vasodilators) to increase forward cardiac output and reduce pulmonary venous hypertension. Anticoagulants may be prescribed for patients with atrial fibrillation or surgery, such as annuloplasty or replacement of the mitral valve, for chronic mitral valve insufficiency and sometimes in cases demonstrating relatively mild symptoms to forestall significant ventricular muscle dysfunction. Conditions associated with rheumatic mitral insufficiency include atrial fibrillation, pulmonary hypertension, left or congestive heart failure, and systemic embolism.

394.0	Mitral stenosis — *obstruction*
394.1	Rheumatic mitral insufficiency — *incompetence, regurgitation*
	AHA: Q2, 2005, 14

394.2	Mitral stenosis with insufficiency — *obstruction with incompetence or regurgitation*
394.9	Other and unspecified mitral valve diseases — *unknown or not otherwise specified*

395 Diseases of aortic valve

Rheumatic aortic stenosis is a pathological narrowing of the aortic valve orifice due to fibrosis of the commissures and/or degenerative distortion of the aortic valve cusps. Commissural fusion and scarring may be present early in the progression of the disease, and calcification of the valve is often a late complication. The resulting stenosis produces a pressure overload on the left ventricle due to the increased pressure needed to force the blood through the narrowed aortic valve orifice. Signs and symptoms of rheumatic aortic stenosis include angina, syncope, heart failure, delayed carotid upstroke, and/or a sustained forceful apex beat, systolic ejection murmur, or softened singular S2 heart sound with S4 heart sound. An EKG normally shows left ventricular hypertrophy in cases of rheumatic aortic stenosis, and cardiac catheterization provides definitive diagnosis and evaluation of the condition. Echocardiography and fluoroscopy may be of limited value in assessing the severity of the stenosis. Therapies include medications (digitalis, diuretics, and antiarrhythmics) as temporary symptomatic measures, or aortic valve replacement. Associated conditions include left heart failure, mitral valve disease, angina (exertional), heart blocks due to calcification of the conduction system, and atrial and ventricular arrhythmias.

Rheumatic aortic insufficiency is the reflux of blood into the left ventricle during diastole due to an incompetent aortic valve. Chronic aortic insufficiency eventually leads to left ventricular dysfunction and failure. The condition is also known as rheumatic aortic regurgitation and rheumatic aortic incompetence. Signs and symptoms include left ventricular failure, syncope, angina, diastolic murmur along the left sternal border or an Austin Fling murmur, and/or stroke volume increase. An EKG normally shows left ventricular hypertrophy in cases of rheumatic aortic insufficiency. Chest x-rays show cardiac enlargement in severe chronic cases. Echocardiography demonstrates an enlarged left ventricular cavity and frequently reveals diastolic vibration of the mitral valve. Cardiac catheterization and arteriography demonstrate regurgitation of contrast material back into the left ventricle. Therapies include medications (digitalis, diuretics, and vasodilators) for symptomatic relief, and aortic valve replacement in severe cases. Associated conditions include angina and left heart failure, and congestive heart failure.

395.0	Rheumatic aortic stenosis — *obstruction* AHA: Q4, 1988, 8
395.1	Rheumatic aortic insufficiency — *incompetence or regurgitation*
395.2	Rheumatic aortic stenosis with insufficiency — *obstruction with incompetence or regurgitation*
395.9	Other and unspecified rheumatic aortic diseases — *unknown or not otherwise specified*

396 Diseases of mitral and aortic valves
AHA: Nov-Dec, 1987, 8

For more information about the subcategories of this rubric, refer to the detailed descriptions of the individual components of combined aortic and mitral valve disease.

396.0	Mitral valve stenosis and aortic valve stenosis — *narrowing of both valves* AHA: Nov-Dec, 1987, 8
396.1	Mitral valve stenosis and aortic valve insufficiency — *narrowing of mitral valve with incompetence or regurgitation of aortic valve* AHA: Nov-Dec, 1987, 8
396.2	Mitral valve insufficiency and aortic valve stenosis — *incompetence or regurgitation of mitral valve with narrowing of aortic valve* AHA: Nov-Dec, 1987, 8; Q2, 2000, 16
396.3	Mitral valve insufficiency and aortic valve insufficiency — *incompetence or regurgitation of both valves* AHA: Nov-Dec, 1987, 8
396.8	Multiple involvement of mitral and aortic valves — *stenosis and insufficiency of mitral or aortic valve with stenosis or insufficiency, or both, of the other valve* AHA: Nov-Dec, 1987, 8
396.9	Unspecified mitral and aortic valve diseases

Coding Clarification
When both the mitral and aortic valves are involved, ICD-9-CM presumes an etiology of rheumatic heart disease for classification purposes. In all cases, when both the aortic and mitral valves are diseased, the ICD-9-CM index will lead to rubric 396.

397 Diseases of other endocardial structures
This rubric includes chronic rheumatic heart diseases of the tricuspid, pulmonary, and unspecified heart valves. Note that diseases of the tricuspid valve are presumed to be of rheumatic etiology, but diseases of the pulmonary or unspecified heart valves must be stated as due to a late effect of rheumatic heart disease.

Diseases of the tricuspid valve are classified to codes in the 397.0 subclassification and report insufficiency, obstruction, regurgitation, and stenosis of the tricuspid valve. Tricuspid regurgitation may occur secondary to right ventricular pressure overload from left-sided lesions. It also may occur as a result of primary rheumatic heart disease of the tricuspid valve itself. Tricuspid stenosis serves as a mechanical obstruction blocking the return of blood to the right ventricle of the heart.

Rheumatic diseases of pulmonary valves (397.1) include valve insufficiency and stenosis. Pulmonary valve insufficiency is a reflux of blood back into the right ventricle through an incompetent pulmonary valve and may be associated with pulmonary hypertension. Pulmonary valve stenosis is an obstruction of the blood through the pulmonary valve.

397.0	Diseases of tricuspid valve — *insufficiency, obstruction, regurgitation, stenosis* AHA: Q2, 2000, 16
397.1	Rheumatic diseases of pulmonary valve — *insufficiency, obstruction, regurgitation, stenosis*
397.9	Rheumatic diseases of endocardium, valve unspecified — *unknown valve*

Coding Clarification
All diseases of the tricuspid valve not specifically directed to other code categories in the ICD-9-CM index are included in 397.0.

Code 397.1 includes all diseases of the pulmonary valve specified as due to a late effect of rheumatic heart disease not directed to other code categories in the ICD-9-CM index.

398 Other rheumatic heart disease
This rubric includes rare occurrences of chronic rheumatic heart disease not involving the heart valves.

398.0	Rheumatic myocarditis — *myocardium*
398.90	Unspecified rheumatic heart disease
398.91	Rheumatic heart failure (congestive) — *left ventricular failure* AHA: Q3, 1988, 3; Q1, 1995, 6; Q2, 2005, 14
398.99	Other and unspecified rheumatic heart diseases — *not otherwise specified, inactive pancarditis with rheumatic fever*

Coding Clarification
Chronic inflammation of the muscular walls of the heart (myocarditis) specified as due to or a late effect of rheumatic heart disease is reported with 398.0. Code this condition in addition to rheumatic valve disease when indicated. Congestive rheumatic heart failure is reported with 398.91 and includes left heart failure and congestive heart failure due to rheumatic heart disease. Left and congestive heart failure, common in the rheumatic valvular diseases described in rubrics 394-396, may be coded in addition to rheumatic valvular disease when indicated.

401–405 Hypertensive Disease
Hypertensive disease is a condition in which the diastolic pressure exceeds 100 mm Hg in persons 60 years of age or older or 90 mm Hg in persons younger than 60 years of age. The World Health Organization (WHO) defines hypertension as pressures exceeding 160/90 mm Hg, but studies have shown that increased morbidity and mortality are associated with diastolic pressures of just 85 mm Hg. It is generally asymptomatic until complications develop. Complications may include retinal changes, loud aortic sounds and early systolic ejection click heard on auscultation, headache, tinnitus, and palpitations.

Rubrics 401-404 include primary (essential) hypertension of no known cause and account for approximately 90 percent of the population. The remaining 10 percent of the population have secondary hypertension classifiable to 405, due to definitive and diagnosable disease such as Cushing's syndrome. Use the hypertension table in the ICD-9-CM index to distinguish between primary and secondary hypertension and assign the correct code.

Use the fourth digits in categories 401-405 to specify the course of hypertensive disease as malignant, benign, or unspecified. Do not try to make the distinction between benign and malignant without first obtaining physician verification for coding and classification purposes.

401 Essential hypertension
AHA: July-Aug, 1984, 11; Sept-Oct, 1987, 9; Q2, 1989, 12; Q3, 1990, 3; Q2, 1992, 5

High blood pressure, also called hypertension, occurs when the arterioles narrow, causing the blood to exert excessive pressure against the vessel wall and the heart must work harder to maintain the higher pressure. Over time, damage to the brain, eye, and kidney can result ("target organ damage"). Essential or primary hypertension means that there is no underlying condition that is causing the blood pressure to increase. Up to 95 percent of hypertension is the essential type and, unless blood pressure readings are very high, efforts to control blood pressure are usually based on changes in lifestyle (weight loss, exercise, dietary changes, and reducing stress). Use rubric 401 to report all primary

Diseases of the Circulatory System

forms of hypertension without mention of heart or renal disease, including arterial, idiopathic, systemic, and vascular hypertension.

401.0	Essential hypertension, malignant — *severe high arterial blood pressure without apparent organic cause* AHA: July-Aug, 1984, 11; May-June, 1985, 19; Sept-Oct, 1987, 9; Q2, 1989, 12; Q3, 1990, 3; Q2, 1992, 5
401.1	Essential hypertension, benign — *mild elevation in arterial blood pressure without apparent organic cause* AHA: July-Aug, 1984, 11; Sept-Oct, 1987, 9; Q2, 1989, 12; Q3, 1990, 3; Q2, 1992, 5
401.9	Unspecified essential hypertension AHA: Q4, 2004, 78; Q3, 2005, 8; Q4, 2005, 71

Documentation Issues

Unless documentation identifies a cause and effect relationship between hypertension and congestive heart failure they should be coded as separate entities, 428.0 and 401.x. However, if the documentation indicates the congestive heart failure is due to the hypertension, only one code is necessary, 402.91.

The physician must document the type and nature (e.g., malignant, benign) of the hypertension for accurate classification of the condition.

When the documentation identifies a postoperative hypertension, the physician needs to document whether it was caus4ed by inadequate control of pain or patient agitation, and if the hypertension was merely an elevation in blood pressure without mention of hypertension (796.2), or a benign hypertension (401.1).

Documentation indicates the patient has congestive heart failure and hypertension. If the documentation does not identify a cause and effect relationship, verify with the physician. Ask the physician if this was hypertensive heart disease with congestive heart failure (402.91). If no clarification as to the cause and effect relationship is obtained, use codes 428.0 and 401.9.

If the patient is diagnosed as having hypertension and renal failure, request that documentation clarify if the hypertension is malignant or accelerated for accurate code selection.

When documentation identifies hypertension in a patient who is status post-renal transplant for chronic renal failure, more information is required for accurate code selection. Review the medical record or obtain the information necessary from the physician, such as:

- If the hypertension is caused by a complication of the transplant, use codes 996.81 and 405.99.
- If the hypertension is a side effect of the postoperative immunotherapy given after the transplantation, use codes 405.99, E933.1, and V42.0.
- If the hypertension existed prior to the transplant and is still present, use a code from the hypertension code series 401-404.

If the physician documents the diagnosis of hypertensive cardiovascular disease, review the medical record for any reference to coronary arteriosclerosis, angina, or chronic myocardial ischemia. If these conditions are noted, code them in addition to the hypertensive heart disease. If the documentation also notes any myocardial ischemic conditions, they need to be coded separately.

Coding Clarification

Coexisting or Chronic Conditions: Coexisting or chronic conditions that are treated on an ongoing basis should be coded and reported as many times as the patient receives treatment, management, and additional care for the conditions. Conditions such as hypertension that are considered systemic diseases should be coded even in the absence of documented active intervention.

Elevated Blood Pressure: Also known as transient hypertension, this is an elevated blood pressure reading without a diagnosis of hypertension and may be characteristic of older age groups or due to emotional stress. For these cases, report code 796.2 *Elevated blood pressure reading without diagnosis of hypertension.*

Hypertensive Cerebrovascular Disease: Cerebral symptoms resulting in an abrupt elevation in blood pressure, such as confusion, agitation, headaches, obtundation, stupor, and convulsions, are known as cerebral encephalopathy (437.2 and an additional code from categories 401-405). An extended exposure to arterial benign hypertension may cause intracerebral hemorrhage, which may result from a rupture of an arteriosclerotic vessel (431 and an additional code from categories 401-405). Malignant hypertension could result in a cerebral infarction; use codes 434.0 and 401.0.

Malignant Hypertension: Interchangeable terms also identifying malignant hypertension are necrotizing or accelerating hypertension. This condition is distinguished by symptoms of progressive heart failure, impairment of vision, ocular hemorrhage, exudates, and papilledema. By definition, papilledema is always associated with malignant hypertension. More serious outcomes are uremia, cerebral hemorrhage, or heart failure. To report, use code 401.0 *Essential hypertension, malignant.*

Postoperative Hypertension: It is appropriate to use complication code 997.91 *Complications affecting specified body systems, NEC, hypertension* and an additional code to identify the specific type of hypertension. Sequence the complication code first and the hypertension code second. If the physician documents hypertension sometime after the operative episode, but does not indicate it as postoperative or as a complication of surgery, use a code from categories 401-405 only.

Pregnancy Complication: If the hypertension is noted as a mild pre-eclampsia, hypertension in pregnancy with mild proteinuria and edema, use code 642.4x. If the diagnosis states pregnancy with severe proteinuria or severe pre-eclampsia (HELLP syndrome), use code 642.5x. Hypertension that develops in the second half of pregnancy through the last trimester should be reported with code 642.4x and, if stated as severe, code 642.5x. For pregnancy with hypertension secondary to renal disease, use code 642.1x and, if pre-eclampsia or eclampsia is also present, use code 642.7x. If the diagnosis is stated as transient hypertension of pregnancy, use code 642.3x.

Questionable Admission Diagnosis: CMS issued a list of codes to the medical review entities that usually do not warrant inpatient admissions. When these diagnoses appear as the principal diagnoses, the justification for admission is considered questionable. Benign essential hypertension code 401.1 is on this questionable diagnosis list.

Retinopathy: To accurately report this condition, two codes are required: code 362.11 *Hypertensive retinopathy* and an appropriate code from categories 401-405 to identify the specific type of hypertension.

Secondary Hypertension: This condition may be due to a number of underlying causes. Always code the underlying cause first, if indicated as a current condition, and then the secondary hypertension.

Systolic Hypertension: This is typically defined as a systolic pressure higher that 160 mm Hg and a diastolic pressure of less than 95 mm Hg. It is also known as arteriosclerotic hypertension because patients have a tendency to develop arteriosclerosis of the central aorta and its branches. Code 401.1

Benign hypertension should be used to identify this condition as there appears to be no reference to it as a malignant hypertension.

Uncontrolled Hypertension: This does not indicate the hypertension is malignant, only that the condition is in an uncontrolled state. It typically indicates the need for diuretics or other antihypertensive drugs, such as beta-blockers. There is no code to identify this condition so classification would be to its type and nature.

Coding Scenario

A patient previously diagnosed with atherosclerotic hypertension is now seen in the clinic for follow up. Medical record indicates coronary atherosclerosis and benign hypertension. Past medical history is pertinent for CABG five years ago.

> Code assignment: 414.00 *Coronary atherosclerosis of unspecified type of vessel, native or graft*, 401.1 *Essential hypertension, benign*, V45.81 *Aortocoronary bypass status*

A patient is admitted with a diagnosis of hypertension. The physician's final diagnosis at discharge is atherosclerosis of the aorta and generalized arteriosclerosis.

> Code assignment: 440.0 *Atherosclerosis of aorta*, and 440.9 *Generalized and unspecified atherosclerosis*

A patient is seen in the emergency department with uncontrolled hypertension. The patient was previously treated with diuretics. The physician's documentation identifies the hypertension as benign. The patient is discharged to follow up with attending the next day.

> Code assignment: 401.1 *Essential hypertension, benign*

A patient is seen in the outpatient clinic for a follow-up visit for hypertension and angina. The physician prescribes nitroglycerin for the angina and a diuretic for the hypertension. The patient history also identifies the patient had pneumonia six months ago.

> Code assignment: 401.9 *Essential hypertension, unspecified* and 413.9 *Angina pectoris, unspecified*

A patient is admitted and treated for acute renal failure and essential hypertension.

> Code assignment: 584.9 *Acute renal failure, unspecified* and 401.9 *Essential hypertension, unspecified*

402 Hypertensive heart disease
AHA: July-Aug, 1984, 11; Nov-Dec, 1984, 18; Sept-Oct, 1987, 9; Q2, 1989, 12; Q3, 1990, 3; Q2, 1993, 9; Q4, 2002, 49

Use rubric 402 to report heart disease due to the effects of systemic hypertension. It is characterized by concentric hypertrophy of the left ventricle that in time can lead to left ventricular failure.

402.00 Malignant hypertensive heart disease without heart failure — *(Use additional code to specify type of heart failure, 428.0-428.43, if known)* — *severe high blood pressure causing heart complications*
AHA: July-Aug, 1984, 11; Nov-Dec, 1984, 18; Sept-Oct, 1987, 9; Q2, 1989, 12; Q3, 1990, 3; Q2, 1993, 9; Q4, 2002, 49

402.01 Malignant hypertensive heart disease with heart failure — *(Use additional code to specify type of heart failure, 428.0-428.43, if known)* — *severe high blood pressure causing heart complications*
AHA: July-Aug, 1984, 11; Nov-Dec, 1984, 18; Sept-Oct, 1987, 9; Q2, 1989, 12; Q3, 1990, 3; Q2, 1993, 9; Q4, 2002, 49

402.10 Benign hypertensive heart disease without heart failure — *(Use additional code to specify type of heart failure, 428.0-428.43, if known)* — *mild elevation in blood pressure causing heart complications*
AHA: July-Aug, 1984, 11; Nov-Dec, 1984, 18; Sept-Oct, 1987, 9; Q2, 1989, 12; Q3, 1990, 3; Q2, 1993, 9; Q4, 2002, 49

402.11 Benign hypertensive heart disease with heart failure — *(Use additional code to specify type of heart failure, 428.0-428.43, if known)* — *mild elevation in blood pressure causing heart complications*
AHA: July-Aug, 1984, 11; Nov-Dec, 1984, 18; Sept-Oct, 1987, 9; Q2, 1989, 12; Q3, 1990, 3; Q2, 1993, 9; Q4, 2002, 49

402.90 Unspecified hypertensive heart disease without heart failure — *(Use additional code to specify type of heart failure, 428.0-428.43, if known)* — *high blood pressure of unknown degree causing heart complications*
AHA: July-Aug, 1984, 11; Nov-Dec, 1984, 18; Sept-Oct, 1987, 9; Q2, 1989, 12; Q3, 1990, 3; Q2, 1993, 9; Q4, 2002, 49

402.91 Unspecified hypertensive heart disease with heart failure — *(Use additional code to specify type of heart failure, 428.0-428.43, if known)* — *high blood pressure of unknown degree causing heart complications*
AHA: July-Aug, 1984, 11; Nov-Dec, 1984, 18; Sept-Oct, 1987, 9; Q2, 1989, 12; Q3, 1990, 3; Q1, 1993, 19; Q2, 1993, 9; Q4, 2002, 49; Q4, 2002, 52

Documentation Issues
If the documentation indicates that the patient has heart failure, review the record for any hypertensive heart or hypertensive heart and renal disease. If documentation identifies these conditions, a combination code may be used from categories 402 and 404.

Even if the patient is being seen for another condition, if the heart failure is noted in the record and the patient is still under treatment, the heart failure should be coded as a secondary condition.

Note that there must be a stated or implied cause and effect relationship between the heart disease and the hypertension. For example, the statement "benign hypertension with congestive heart failure" is coded to 401.1 and 428.0; but the statement "benign hypertensive heart disease with heart failure" is reported with 402.11.

Coding Clarification
Hypertension and Atherosclerosis: Hypertension frequently accelerates atherosclerosis and if both are documented, code both conditions. Systolic hypertension may be referenced as "arteriosclerotic hypertension" of the elderly. In younger patients, systolic hypertension may be associated with an arteriovenous fistula or thyrotoxicosis, and would be classified as a secondary hypertension.

Hypertensive cardiovascular arteriosclerotic disease with heart failure is coded 402.91. Use an additional code of 414.0x to identify the coronary arteriosclerosis.

Coding Scenario
A patient is admitted with hypertensive cardiovascular disease. Documentation identifies that the patient was having chest pain due to angina. The physician's final diagnosis is hypertensive cardiovascular disease, benign, with angina pectoris.

> Code assignment: 402.10 *Benign hypertensive heart disease, without heart failure* and 413.9 *Other and unspecified angina pectoris*

A patient is seen in the clinic for evaluation of treatment for hypertensive cardiomyopathy. Record documentation identifies that the cardiomyopathy was secondary to hypertensive heart disease.

> Code assignment: 402.90 *Unspecified hypertensive heart disease, without heart failure* and 425.8 *Cardiomyopathy in other diseases classified elsewhere*

Cardiology consultation identifies a benign hypertensive heart disease with left ventricular failure.

Code assignment: 402.11 *Benign hypertensive heart disease, with heart failure* and 428.1 *Left heart failure*

A patient is admitted with fluid overload. Final diagnosis indicates that the patient has heart failure due to hypertensive cardiovascular disease. Documentation also reveals the patient has arteriosclerotic heart disease without previous surgical intervention.

Code assignment: 402.91 *Unspecified hypertensive heart disease, with heart failure*, 428.9 *Heart failure, unspecified*, and 414.01 *Coronary atherosclerosis of native coronary artery*

A 57-year-old male is admitted to the facility with left ventricular failure and benign hypertensive heart disease.

Code assignment: 402.11 *Benign hypertensive heart disease, with heart failure* and 428.1 *Left heart failure*

403 Hypertensive chronic kidney disease
AHA: July-Aug, 1984, 11; Sept-Oct, 1987, 9; Q2, 1989, 12; Q3, 1990, 3; Q2, 1992, 5; Q4, 1992, 22; Q4, 2005, 68

Hypertensive kidney disease is a condition also known as arteriolar nephrosclerosis, and is reported with codes from rubric 403. It is characterized by intimal thickening of the afferent arteriole of the glomerulus and due to long-standing or poorly controlled hypertension. In severe nephrosclerosis, the nephron is deprived of its blood supply, and areas of infarction occur with subsequent scar formation. Renal insufficiency occurs when the kidney is scarred and contracted. In most cases, the patient will eventually develop kidney failure.

This rubric reports chronic kidney disease associated with hypertensive renal disease due to progressive and irreversible destruction of the nephrons and should not be confused with acute renal failure. Acute renal failure is classified to rubric 584 and describes failure of the kidneys to perform their essential function due to trauma, impaired blood flow, toxic substances, bacterial infection, or obstruction of the urinary tract.

Both diabetes mellitus and hypertension have associated kidney manifestations such as chronic kidney disease.

The following fifth-digit subclassification is for use with category 403:

0 with chronic kidney disease stage I through stage IV, or unspecified — (Use additional code to identify the stage of chronic kidney disease: 585.1-585.4, 585.9)

1 with chronic kidney disease stage V or end stage renal disease — (Use additional code to identify the stage of chronic kidney disease: 585.5, 585.6)

403.0 ✓5th Hypertensive chronic kidney disease, malignant — *severe high blood pressure causing kidney malfunctions*
AHA: July-Aug, 1984, 11; Sept-Oct, 1987, 9; Q2, 1989, 12; Q3, 1990, 3; Q2, 1992, 5; Q4, 1992, 22

403.1 ✓5th Hypertensive chronic kidney disease, benign — *mild high blood pressure causing kidney malfunctions*
AHA: July-Aug, 1984, 11; Sept-Oct, 1987, 9; Q2, 1989, 12; Q3, 1990, 3; Q2, 1992, 5; Q4, 1992, 22

403.9 ✓5th Hypertensive chronic kidney disease, unspecified — *high blood pressure of unknown degree causing kidney malfunctions*
AHA: July-Aug, 1984, 11; Sept-Oct, 1987, 9; Q2, 1989, 12; Q3, 1990, 3; Q2, 1992, 5; Q4, 1992, 22; Q1, 2003, 20; Q1, 2004, 14; Q4, 2004, 78; Q4, 2005, 69

Documentation Issues
In cases where the diagnostic statement indicates hypertensive renal failure due to diabetes mellitus, report the diabetes with renal manifestations from the series 250.4x and 403.9x to indicate the hypertensive renal failure, although the code description terminology has been changed to hypertensive chronic kidney disease. Report a code from category 585 to specify the stage of chronic kidney disease. For example, if the chronic hypertensive kidney disease is noted to be in end stage renal disease, report 585.6 in addition to the chronic hypertensive kidney disease (403.91).

For coding and classification purposes, any condition classifiable to categories 585-587 with hypertension is presumed due to hypertension, so no cause and effect relationship need be stated or implied in the diagnostic statement.

Coding Clarification
Hypertensive Chronic Kidney Disease: Category 403 identifies hypertensive chronic kidney disease. The stage of chronic kidney disease is identified with a fifth digit of 0 (stage I through stage IV, or unspecified), or 1 (stage V or end stage renal disease). An additional code should be assigned from category 585 to further denote the stage of chronic kidney disease. In many cases, renal failure is seen in hypertensive kidney disease only when the hypertension becomes malignant or accelerated. In

these cases, code 403.00 *Hypertensive chronic kidney disease, malignant, with chronic kidney disease stage I through stage IV or unspecified* would be assigned together with 585.9 identifying the chronic renal failure as unspecified. Keep in mind that the code for malignant or accelerated hypertension can be assigned only if the physician documents it as such.

Category 403 excludes acute renal failure, which is coded to category 584 *Acute renal failure.*

Nephrosclerosis: This condition is presumed to be a secondary process of hypertensive renal disease and does not require another code in addition.

Coding Scenario
The physician's final diagnosis states hypertensive renal disease with chronic renal failure in end stage due to diabetes, Type II.

> Code assignment: 250.40 *Diabetes with renal manifestations, Type II or unspecified type, not stated as uncontrolled,* 403.91 *Hypertensive chronic kidney disease, unspecified, with chronic kidney disease stage V or end stage renal disease* and 585.6 *End stage renal disease*

A patient is seen for acute renal failure that has an established hypertensive renal nephrosclerosis.

> Code assignment: 584.9 *Acute renal failure, unspecified,* 403.90 *Hypertensive chronic kidney disease, unspecified, with chronic kidney disease stage I through stage IV, or unspecified,* and 585.9 *Chronic kidney disease, unspecified*

404 Hypertensive heart and chronic kidney disease
AHA: July-Aug, 1984, 11; July-Aug, 1984, 14; Sept-Oct, 1987, 9; Q2, 1989, 12; Q3, 1990, 3; Q4, 2002, 49; Q4, 2005, 68

This category is used for combined forms of heart and renal disease as classified in categories 402 and 403.

The following fifth-digit subclassification is for use with category 404:

0   without heart failure and with chronic kidney disease stage I through stage IV, or unspecified — (Use additional code to identify the stage of chronic kidney disease: 585.1)

1   with heart failure and with chronic kidney disease stage I through stage IV, or unspecified — (Use additional code to identify the stage of chronic kidney disease: 585.1-585.4, 585.9)

2   without heart failure and with chronic kidney disease stage V or end stage renal disease — (Use additional code to identify the stage of chronic kidney disease: 585.5, 585.6)

3   with heart failure and with chronic kidney disease stage V or end stage renal disease — (Use additional code to identify the stage of chronic kidney disease: 585.5, 585.6)

404.0   Hypertensive heart and chronic kidney disease, malignant — (Use additional code to specify type of heart failure, 428.0-428.43, if known)

404.1   Hypertensive heart and chronic kidney disease, benign — (Use additional code to specify type of heart failure, 428.0-428.43, if known)

404.9   Hypertensive heart and chronic kidney disease, unspecified — (Use additional code to specify type of heart failure, 428.0-428.43, if known)

Documentation Issues
For coding and classification purposes, the heart disease must be stated or implied as due to hypertension, but the renal disease may be presumed. For example, the statement "hypertensive heart failure and chronic renal failure" would be coded 404.91 and 585.9 even though hypertension is not the stated cause of the chronic renal failure.

Coding Clarification
Hypertensive Heart and Chronic Kidney Disease: Category 404 identifies hypertensive heart and chronic kidney disease. The fifth digit subclassification denotes the presence or absence of heart failure and the stage of chronic kidney disease. An additional code from category 585 should be assigned to further identify the stage of chronic kidney disease. An additional code should also be assigned from range 428.0-428.43 to identify the type of heart failure, if known.

In many cases, renal failure is only seen in hypertensive heart and chronic kidney disease when the hypertension becomes malignant or accelerated. In these cases, 404.00 *Hypertensive heart and chronic kidney disease, malignant, without heart failure and with chronic kidney disease stage I through stage IV or unspecified* would be assigned together with 585.9 identifying the chronic renal failure as unspecified. Keep in mind that the code for malignant or accelerated hypertension can be assigned only if the physician documents it as such.

Category 404 excludes acute renal failure, which is coded to category 584 *Acute renal failure.*

Coding Scenario
A patient is admitted with a diagnosis of congestive failure. Record documentation identifies that the patient has benign hypertensive heart and kidney

disease with chronic renal failure in addition to the heart failure.

Code assignment: 404.11 *Hypertensive heart and chronic kidney disease, benign, with heart failure and chronic kidney disease stage I through stage IV or unspecified*, 585.9 *Chronic kidney disease, unspecified*, and 428.0 *Congestive heart failure, unspecified*

405 Secondary hypertension
AHA: July-Aug, 1984, 11; July-Aug, 1984, 14; Sept-Oct, 1987, 9,11; Q2, 1989, 12; Q3, 1990, 3

Secondary hypertension is a condition caused by renovascular or other diseases. Renovascular hypertension is the obstruction of renal blood flow at the level of the renal artery. The obstruction stimulates the renin-angiotensin system causing an increase in systemic angiotensin, which in turn causes the retention of sodium and water resulting in hypertension. Surgical reconstruction of the renal artery or percutaneous transluminal angioplasty may be performed to relieve the obstruction. Other causes of secondary hypertension include renal parenchymal diseases, oral contraceptives, primary aldosteronism, Cushing's syndrome, pheochromocytoma, hyperparathyroidism, hyperthyroidism, and acromegaly.

405.01	Secondary renovascular hypertension, malignant — *severe high blood pressure as a result of an underlying disease or condition* **AHA:** July-Aug, 1984, 11; July-Aug, 1984, 14; Sept-Oct, 1987, 9,11; Q2, 1989, 12; Q3, 1990, 3
405.09	Other secondary hypertension, malignant — *severe high blood pressure as a result of an underlying disease or condition* **AHA:** July-Aug, 1984, 11; July-Aug, 1984, 14; Sept-Oct, 1987, 9,11; Q2, 1989, 12; Q3, 1990, 3
405.11	Secondary renovascular hypertension, benign — *mild high blood pressure as a result of an underlying disease or condition* **AHA:** July-Aug, 1984, 11; July-Aug, 1984, 14; Sept-Oct, 1987, 9,11; Q2, 1989, 12; Q3, 1990, 3
405.19	Other secondary hypertension, benign — *mild high blood pressure as a result of an underlying disease or condition* **AHA:** July-Aug, 1984, 11; July-Aug, 1984, 14; Sept-Oct, 1987, 9,11; Q2, 1989, 12; Q3, 1990, 3
405.91	Secondary renovascular hypertension, unspecified — *high blood pressure of unknown degree as a result of an underlying disease or condition* **AHA:** July-Aug, 1984, 11; July-Aug, 1984, 14; Sept-Oct, 1987, 9,11; Q2, 1989, 12; Q3, 1990, 3; Q3, 2000, 4
405.99	Other secondary hypertension, unspecified — *high blood pressure of unknown degree as a result of an underlying disease or condition* **AHA:** July-Aug, 1984, 11; July-Aug, 1984, 14; Sept-Oct, 1987, 9,11; Q2, 1989, 12; Q3, 1990, 3; Q3, 2000, 4

Coding Clarification
ICD-9-CM separates only renovascular hypertension from all other etiologies at the fifth-digit level. Renal parenchymal diseases are conditions that reduce kidney function by affecting the kidney's ability to excrete water and sodium and are not the same as renovascular hypertension. Do not code renal parenchymal disease to the neovascular fifth-digit "1."

Secondary Hypertension: Category 405 *Secondary hypertension* does not include renal failure, so two codes are necessary to identify cases of renal failure with secondary hypertension.

Coding Scenario
A 55-year-old male is admitted with hypertension due to hypervolemia as a direct result of his chronic renal failure. Patient history indicates that the patient is an adult onset insulin-dependent diabetic with renal failure.

Code assignment: 250.40 *Diabetes with renal manifestations, Type II, or unspecified type, not stated as uncontrolled*, 405.99 *Other secondary hypertension, unspecified*, 276.6 *Fluid overload*, and 585.9 *Chronic kidney disease, unspecified*, and V58.67 *Long-term (current) use of insulin*

410–414 Ischemic Heart Disease
Ischemic heart disease is an inadequate flow of blood through the coronary arteries to the tissue of the heart. The predominant etiology of the ischemia is arteriosclerosis. Partially obstructed coronary artery blood flow can manifest in angina pectoris; complete

obstruction results in an infarction of the myocardium.

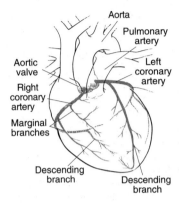

410 Acute myocardial infarction
AHA: July-Aug, 1984, 5; Q3, 1989, 3; Q1, 1991, 14; Q3, 1991, 10,18; Q1, 1992, 10; Q4, 1992, 24; Q3, 1995, 9; Q4, 1997, 37; Q3, 1998, 15; Q3, 2001, 21; Q4, 2005, 69; Q2, 2006, 9

Rubric 410 reports sudden partial or total reduction in the supply of blood to the heart, which results in necrosis of the myocardium. Occlusion of one of the coronary arteries due to thrombosis is believed to be the most common etiology. Other possible precipitating conditions include prolonged coronary artery spasm, subintimal hemorrhage at the site of atheromatous narrowing, and nonocclusive etiologies such as postoperative or traumatic shock, gastrointestinal bleeding with acute blood loss anemia, hypotension, and dehydration.

The inclusion terms of ST elevation (STEMI) and non-ST elevation (NSTEMI) myocardial infarction were added to mirror the national standard guidelines of The American College of Cardiology and the American Heart Association for classifying patients with acute coronary syndrome. The intention is that the expanded classification terminology will help in optimizing clinical care, refining new therapies, and reporting data more congruently with that collected through clinical trial and registries.

Most patients who have ST-segment elevation will ultimately develop a Q-wave acute myocardial infarction. Patients with ST segment elevation may benefit from thrombolytic therapy and may require more aggressive intervention measures than those patients with unstable angina or NSTEMI. STEMI tends to occur in a wide range of anatomical sites.

Myocardial ischemia in a patient without ST elevation on ECG is usually indicative of unstable angina or a non-ST segment myocardial infarction that can develop into a non-Q-wave MI. The non-Q wave infarction tends to occur in mainly a subendocardial or mid-myocardial site, and does not display the usual Q-wave patters seen in STEMIs. NSTEMI, however, can still produce minor, less-dramatic degrees of some ST or T wave abnormalities, but can be termed as "NSTEMI." Totally occlusive thrombus is not usually associated with NSTEMI, and so thrombolytic therapy is not indicated.

The following fifth-digit subclassification is for use with category 410:

0 episode of care unspecified

Use when the source document does not contain sufficient information for the assignment of fifth digit 1 or 2.

1 initial episode of care

Use fifth digit 1 to designate the first episode of care (regardless of facility site) for a newly diagnosed myocardial infarction. The fifth digit 1 is assigned regardless of the number of times a patient may be transferred during the initial episode of care.

2 subsequent episode of care

Use fifth-digit 2 to designate an episode of care following the initial episode when the patient is admitted for further observation, evaluation, or treatment for a myocardial infarction that has received initial treatment, but is still less than eight weeks old.

410.0 Acute myocardial infarction of anterolateral wall
— (Use additional code to identify presence of hypertension: 401.0-405.9) — *coronary artery embolism, occlusion, rupture, thrombosis, ST elevation myocardial infarction (STEMI) of anterolateral wall*
AHA: July-Aug, 1984, 5; Q3, 1989, 3; Q1, 1991, 14; Q3, 1991, 10,18; Q1, 1992, 10; Q4, 1992, 24; Q3, 1995, 9; Q4, 1997, 37; Q3, 1998, 15; Q3, 2001, 21

410.1 Acute myocardial infarction of other anterior wall
— (Use additional code to identify presence of hypertension: 401.0-405.9) — *ST elevation myocardial infarction (STEMI) of other anterior wall*

410.2 Acute myocardial infarction of inferolateral wall
— (Use additional code to identify presence of hypertension: 401.0-405.9) — *coronary artery embolism, occlusion, rupture, thrombosis, ST elevation myocardial infarction (STEMI) of inferolateral*
AHA: July-Aug, 1984, 5; Q3, 1989, 3; Q1, 1991, 14; Q3, 1991, 10,18; Q1, 1992, 10; Q4, 1992, 24; Q3, 1995, 9; Q4, 1997, 37; Q3, 1998, 15; Q3, 2001, 21

410.3 ⌐sth Acute myocardial infarction of inferoposterior wall — (Use additional code to identify presence of hypertension: 401.0-405.9) — *coronary artery embolism, occlusion, rupture, thrombosis, ST elevation myocardial infarction (STEMI) of Inferoposterior wall*
AHA: July-Aug, 1984, 5; Q3, 1989, 3; Q1, 1991, 14; Q3, 1991, 10,18; Q1, 1992, 10; Q4, 1992, 24; Q3, 1995, 9; Q3, 1997, 37; Q3, 1998, 15; Q3, 2001, 21

410.4 ⌐sth Acute myocardial infarction of other inferior wall — (Use additional code to identify presence of hypertension: 401.0-405.9) — *diaphragmatic wall or inferior wall, not otherwise specified; coronary artery embolism, occlusion, rupture, thrombosis, ST elevation myocardial infarction (STEMI) of other inferior wall*
AHA: July-Aug, 1984, 5; Q3, 1989, 3; Q1, 1991, 14; Q3, 1991, 10,18; Q1, 1992, 10; Q4, 1992, 24; Q3, 1995, 9; Q3, 1997, 10; Q4, 1997, 37; Q3, 1998, 15; Q4, 1999, 9; Q1, 2000, 7,26; Q3, 2001, 21

410.5 ⌐sth Acute myocardial infarction of other lateral wall — (Use additional code to identify presence of hypertension: 401.0-405.9) — *apical-lateral, basal-lateral, high lateral, posterolateral; including coronary artery embolism, occlusion, rupture, thrombosis, ST elevation myocardial infarction (STEMI) of other lateral wall*
AHA: July-Aug, 1984, 5; Q3, 1989, 3; Q1, 1991, 14; Q3, 1991, 10,18; Q1, 1992, 10; Q4, 1992, 24; Q3, 1995, 9; Q4, 1997, 37; Q3, 1998, 15; Q3, 2001, 21

410.6 ⌐sth Acute myocardial infarction, true posterior wall infarction — (Use additional code to identify presence of hypertension: 401.0-405.9) — *posterobasal, strictly posterior; including coronary artery embolism, occlusion, rupture, thrombosis, ST elevation myocardial infarction (STEMI) of true posterior wall*
AHA: July-Aug, 1984, 5; Q3, 1989, 3; Q1, 1991, 14; Q3, 1991, 10,18; Q1, 1992, 10; Q4, 1992, 24; Q3, 1995, 9; Q4, 1997, 37; Q3, 1998, 15; Q3, 2001, 21

410.7 ⌐sth Acute myocardial infarction, subendocardial infarction — (Use additional code to identify presence of hypertension: 401.0-405.9) — *nontransmural; including coronary artery embolism, occlusion, rupture, thrombosis, non-ST elevation myocardial infarction (NSTEMI)*
AHA: Q2, 2005, 18; July-Aug, 1984, 5; Q3, 1989, 3; Q1, 1991, 14; Q3, 1991, 10,18; Q1, 1992, 10; Q4, 1992, 24; Q3, 1995, 9; Q4, 1997, 37; Q3, 1998, 15; Q1, 2000, 7; Q3, 2001, 21; Q2, 2005, 19; Q4, 2005, 71

410.8 ⌐sth Acute myocardial infarction of other specified sites — (Use additional code to identify presence of hypertension: 401.0-405.9) — *not otherwise specified, including atrium, papillary muscle, septum alone; including coronary artery embolism, occlusion, rupture, thrombosis, ST elevation myocardial infarction (STEMI) of other specified sites*
AHA: July-Aug, 1984, 5; Q3, 1989, 3; Q1, 1991, 14; Q3, 1991, 10,18; Q1, 1992, 10; Q4, 1992, 24; Q3, 1995, 9; Q4, 1997, 37; Q3, 1998, 15; Q3, 2001, 21

410.9 ⌐sth Acute myocardial infarction, unspecified site — (Use additional code to identify presence of hypertension: 401.0-405.9) — *unknown site; including coronary artery embolism, occlusion, rupture, thrombosis*
AHA: July-Aug, 1984, 5; Q3, 1989, 3; Q1, 1991, 14; Q3, 1991, 10,18; Q1, 1992, 9; Q1, 1992, 10; Q4, 1992, 24; Q3, 1995, 9; Q1, 1996, 17; Q4, 1997, 37; Q3, 1998, 15; Q3, 2001, 21; Q2, 2005, 18

Documentation Issues
A common documentation problem for myocardial infarctions is that the physician does not identify the site of the infarction. The site of the infarction must be documented in the medical record for accurate code selection. Contact the physician for identification and be sure the documentation is updated to identify the site.

Coding Clarification
Use an additional code to identify presence of hypertension (401.0-405.9) with ischemic heart disease.

The fourth digits for rubric 410 identify the site of the acute myocardial infarction as identified on an EKG. One exception to this is the fourth digit 7, which is for subendocardial and nontransmural infarctions regardless of site. A subendocardial infarction is one that involves the pericardium and not the endocardium; a nontransmural infarction is one that fails to extend from the endocardium to the epicardium. "Non-Q-wave" infarctions also are classified here. In some instances, the diagnostic statement will include the term "subendocardial" or "nontransmural" along with a specific site for the infarction.

Acute myocardial infarction is classified as an initial episode of care when the history does not mention a previous infarction. A myocardial infarction of greater than eight weeks duration with persistent symptoms is classified to 414.8.

Duration: When a myocardial infarction is identified as occurring within an eight-week time frame, a code may be selected from category 410 and the appropriate fifth digit would identify the episode of care (e.g., initial, subsequent). If a myocardial infarction is noted of greater than eight weeks duration with persistent symptoms, use code 414.8.

Impending Myocardial Infarction: If the final diagnostic statement indicates an impending myocardial infarction, documentation should be reviewed to ensure that the myocardial infarction did not occur. If not, use code 411.1 *Intermediate coronary syndrome* to identify the condition.

Infarction of the Inferior Wall-Acute, Subsequent Episode: This is coded as 410.42. This is a correction for advice given in *Coding Clinic for ICD-9-CM* Fourth Quarter, 1999, page 9.

Multiple Myocardial Infarctions: The key to correct coding of multiple myocardial infarctions is to code all of the events as long as they occurred at different sites. Do not use two codes in an attempt to describe various sites if the patient had only one infarction. A reinfarction in the same episode occurring at the same site is considered an extension of the original MI and is not coded.

Reinfarction: If a reinfarction occurs at the same site of the myocardial infarction (an extension), it is only coded once. If the reinfarction or extension occurs at a different site of the heart, assign two codes from category 410.

Coding Scenario

A patient is admitted with congestive heart failure directly from the physician's office. Final diagnosis states acute anterior myocardial infarction with benign hypertensive cardiovascular disease and coronary atherosclerosis of native artery.

> Code assignment: 410.11 *Acute myocardial infarction of other anterior wall, initial episode of care*, 402.11 *Benign hypertensive heart disease, with heart failure*, 428.0 *Congestive heart failure, unspecified*, and 414.01 *Coronary atherosclerosis of native coronary artery*

A patient is admitted for cardiac catheterization. History identifies an acute inferior wall infarction three weeks prior. The cardiac catheterization is performed, followed by a percutaneous transluminal coronary angioplasty.

> Code assignment: 410.42 *Acute myocardial infarction of other inferior wall, subsequent episode of care*

A 59-year-old male patient presents to the hospital as an emergency admission. The admitting diagnosis is severe crescendo angina. In an effort to avert an impending myocardial infarction, single vessel PTCA with thrombolic agent administration is performed. Despite these measures, the patient's condition evolves to an inferolateral wall myocardial infarction.

> Code assignment: 410.21 *Acute myocardial infarction of inferolateral wall, initial episode of care*

A 72-year-old female is admitted for observation with chest pain. Later in the day, she is admitted to the coronary care unit with a diagnosis of impending myocardial infarction. Discharge diagnosis states acute diaphragmatic wall myocardial infarction.

> Code assignment: 410.41 *Acute myocardial infarction of other inferior wall, initial episode of care*

A 65-year old male is admitted through the emergency department with an acute MI, initial episode beginning one hour prior to arrival. At discharge, the diagnosis listing is as follows: Subendocardial myocardial infarction, inferior wall 10/1/03, and infarction, inferolateral wall, 10/1/03.

> Code assignment: The patient has suffered two infarctions, so both are coded: 410.71 *Acute myocardial infarction, subendocardial infarction, initial episode of care* and 410.21 *Acute myocardial infarction of inferolateral wall, initial episode of care*

A patient is admitted to the facility via the emergency department with severe chest pain and shortness of breath. The final diagnosis is an acute nontransmural infarction complicated by acute respiratory failure.

> Code assignment: 410.71 *Acute myocardial infarction, subendocardial infarction, initial episode of care* and 518.81 *Acute respiratory failure*

411 Other acute and subacute forms of ischemic heart disease

AHA: July-Aug, 1984, 5; Q3, 1991, 10, 24; Q4, 1994, 55

This rubric includes all acute and subacute forms of ischemic heart disease excluding acute myocardial infarction. Acute forms of ischemia include conditions with a relatively short and severe course, and subacute forms of ischemia denote a course of ischemic disease that falls in between acute and chronic disease.

411.0	Postmyocardial infarction syndrome — (Use additional code to identify presence of hypertension: 401.0-405.9) — *fever, pain, and inflammation within six weeks of MI; Dressler's syndrome* AHA: July-Aug, 1984, 5; Q3, 1991, 10, 24; Q4, 1994, 55
411.1	Intermediate coronary syndrome — (Use additional code to identify presence of

hypertension: 401.0-405.9) — *impending infarction, preinfarction angina, unstable angina*
AHA: July-Aug, 1984, 5; Q4, 1989, 10; Q3, 1990, 6; Q1, 1991, 14; Q3, 1991, 24; Q3, 1991, 10, 24; Q4, 1994, 55; Q2, 1996, 10; Q4, 1998, 86; Q2, 2001, 7, 9; Q3, 2001, 15; Q1, 2003, 12; Q2, 2004, 3; Q4, 2005, 105

411.81 Acute coronary occlusion without myocardial infarction — (Use additional code to identify presence of hypertension: 401.0-405.9) — *interruption of blood flow without death of heart tissue*
AHA: July-Aug, 1984, 5; Q3, 1989, 4; Q1, 1991, 14; Q3, 1991, 18; Q3, 1991, 24; Q3, 1991, 10, 24; Q4, 1994, 55

411.89 Other acute and subacute form of ischemic heart disease — (Use additional code to identify presence of hypertension: 401.0-405.9) — *coronary insufficiency, subendocardial ischemia*
AHA: July-Aug, 1984, 5; Q3, 1989, 4; Q3, 1991, 18; Q3, 1991, 10, 24; Q1, 1992, 9; Q4, 1994, 55; Q3, 2001, 14

Documentation Issues

Often, the diagnosis of "angina" is documented without further details. Clarification should be obtained from the physician as to the specific type of angina, because a patient who is admitted to the hospital would usually be treated for preinfarctional or unstable angina (411.1). If further specification cannot be obtained, the diagnosis of "angina" would be assigned code 413.9 *Other and unspecified angina pectoris*.

Angina identified in the documentation by terms such as preinfarction, crescendo, initial onset, or unstable should be reported with code 411.1 *Intermediate coronary syndrome*.

When documentation indicates "acute ischemic (coronary) heart disease" or "acute myocardial ischemia" and the diagnostic tests reveal no evidence of myocardial infarction and this is verified with the physician, it may be appropriate to use a code from category 411 *Other acute and subacute forms of ischemic heart disease*. Clarification must be obtained from the physician as to whether code 411.1 or 411.8x should be used or if it should be classified to ischemic anginal pain from the 413 category.

Coding Clarification

Postmyocardial infarction syndrome is reported with 411.0 and is a complication occurring several days to several weeks following an acute myocardial infarction. Also known as Dressler's syndrome, this condition is believed to be due to an antibody antigen reaction that takes place in the myocardial tissue during the healing phase of an infarction. Some patients will continue to experience unstable angina pectoris after their recent myocardial infarction because of persistent coronary artery disease. Do not confuse angina due to ischemic heart disease (coronary artery disease) following a myocardial infarction with postmyocardial infarction syndrome. Code postmyocardial angina due to myocardial ischemia to 413.9 or 411.1. Code Dressler's syndrome and postmyocardial angina due to postmyocardial infarction syndrome to 411.0.

Intermediate coronary syndrome is reported with 411.1 and is an intermediate state between angina pectoris of effort and acute myocardial infarction. Since the mortality rate for myocardial infarction is greatest within the first few hours, unstable angina, with its increased likelihood of impeding myocardial infarction, is a medical emergency and requires acute care hospitalization. The term "class III" and "class IV" describing the functional classification of patients with heart disease may be used in conjunction with unstable angina. However, do not assume every patient with class III or class IV angina or heart disease has unstable angina. Code 411.1 cannot be assigned when the condition evolves into a myocardial infarction for which a code from rubric 410 will be assigned.

Acute coronary syndrome (ACS) is a serious condition that requires immediate treatment. If the ACS has not developed into an acute myocardial infarction, code the condition to unstable angina, 411.1. If the underlying cause of ACS is due to CAD, code 414.0x followed by 411.1.

Coronary occlusion without myocardial infarction is reported with 411.81. This code classifies patients with an acute or subacute, complete or incomplete, occlusion of the coronary artery, not associated with acute myocardial infarction. The occlusion may be embolic, thrombotic, other, or unspecified and will usually be associated with some form of angina. This code may be used in conjunction with a diagnosis of stable or unstable angina.

Coding Scenario

A patient is admitted with a severe anginal episode. A cardiac catheterization is performed and a diagnosis of an incomplete coronary artery occlusion is established. Documentation in the record indicates that an infarction did not occur. Final diagnosis is an incomplete coronary artery occlusion with severe angina.

Code assignment: 411.81 *Acute coronary occlusion without myocardial infarction* and 413.9 *Other and unspecified angina pectoris*

A 63-year-old female is admitted with unstable angina. After successful treatment with IV thrombolytic agents, the patient is discharged.

Code assignment: 411.1 *Intermediate coronary syndrome*

A patient is admitted with severe chest pain resembling an acute myocardial infarction and TPA is administered. After the TPA administration, the physician documents aborted myocardial infarction and subsequently transfers the patient to another facility for further diagnostic testing.

Code assignment: 411.1 *Intermediate coronary syndrome*

412 Old myocardial infarction OK
AHA: July-Aug, 1984, 5; Q3, 1990, 7; Q2, 1991, 22; Q3, 1991, 10; Q3, 1998, 15; Q2, 2001, 9; Q2, 2003, 10

This rubric includes diagnoses with a history of myocardial infarction. These patients usually demonstrate EKG changes but currently present no symptoms and warrant no clinical intervention.

Coding Clarification
Patients can have both an acute myocardial infarction and an old myocardial infarction in different sites during the same episode of care. Code both conditions. Also, it is possible that an old myocardial infarction may "reinfarct," extending the degree of necrosis at the site of the old myocardial infarction. In this case, code only the acute myocardial infarction.

Coding Scenario
A patient is admitted for treatment of impending myocardial infarction and CABG with a known history of coronary atherosclerosis, status post myocardial infarction several years ago. After the patient is treated with intravenous thrombolytic agents, the acute myocardial infarction is averted.

Code assignment: 411.1 *Intermediate coronary syndrome*, 414.00 *Coronary atherosclerosis of unspecified type of vessel, native or graft,* and 412 *Old myocardial infarction*

413 Angina pectoris
AHA: July-Aug, 1984, 5; Q3, 1991, 10

Angina pectoris is a clinical syndrome due to myocardial ischemia caused by atherosclerotic heart disease, but may be due to coronary artery spasm, severe aortic stenosis or insufficiency, syphilitic aortitis, vasculitis, marked anemia, paroxysmal tachycardia with rapid ventricular rates, or any disease or disorder that markedly increases metabolic demands. Angina decubitus is a form of angina occurring at night or when the patient is resting quietly. Prinzmetal angina is a variant characterized by chest pain at rest and by sinus tachycardia (ST) segment elevation, rather than depression, during the attack.

413.0	Angina decubitus — (Use additional code to identify presence of hypertension: 401.0-405.9) — *nocturnal angina; occurs only when lying down* AHA: July-Aug, 1984, 5; Q3, 1991, 10
413.1	Prinzmetal angina — (Use additional code to identify presence of hypertension: 401.0-405.9) — *occurs when lying down; associated with ST-segment elevations; variant angina pectoris* AHA: July-Aug, 1984, 5; Q3, 1991, 10
413.9	Other and unspecified angina pectoris — (Use additional code to identify presence of hypertension: 401.0-405.9) — *Heberden's, Likoff's, X syndromes; syncope anginosa, stenocardia* AHA: July-Aug, 1984, 5; Q3, 1990, 6; Q3, 1991, 10; Q3, 1991, 16; Q3, 2002, 4

Documentation Issues
Often, the diagnosis of "angina" is documented without further details. Clarification should be obtained from the physician as to the specific type of angina, because a patient who is admitted to the hospital would usually be treated for preinfarctional or unstable angina (411.1). If further specification cannot be obtained, the diagnosis of "angina" would be assigned code 413.9 *Other and unspecified angina pectoris.*

Angina identified in the documentation by terms such as preinfarction, crescendo, initial onset, or unstable, should be reported with code 411.1 *Intermediate coronary syndrome.*

When documentation indicates "acute ischemic (coronary) heart disease" or "acute myocardial ischemia" and the diagnostic tests reveal no evidence of myocardial infarction and this is verified with the physician, it may be appropriate to use a code from category 411 *Other acute and subacute forms of ischemic heart disease.* Clarification must be obtained from the physician as to whether code 411.1 or 411.8x should be used or if it should be classified to ischemic anginal pain from the 413 category.

If the physician documents a diagnosis of hypertensive cardiovascular disease, review the documentation in the record for any mention of angina pectoris, arteriosclerosis, or chronic myocardial ischemia. If any of these are present, code them in addition.

Only if documentation identifies that angina was a complication of a procedure should it be coded as such.

If the patient is admitted with unstable angina but the documentation states that the condition progressed to a myocardial infarction, only code the infarction.

Angina due to coronary atherosclerosis or coronary artery disease must be documented as such. If the etiology of the angina is not documented, the code for the angina is listed first. When the etiology (e.g., atherosclerosis) is documented, the code for that condition should be listed first.

When a patient is admitted with unstable angina and then has a cardiac catheterization that identifies coronary atherosclerosis as the cause of the angina, the atherosclerosis would be listed as the principal/primary diagnosis and the unstable angina as secondary.

If the diagnosis is documented as atherosclerosis, verify the site of the disease with the physician.

Coding Clarification
Report 413.9 for angina not specified or classified elsewhere, including stable angina pectoris. Angina described with class I or class II heart disease is often classified to 413.9; do not equate these functional classifications of heart disease as synonymous for stable angina.

Assignment of a code from rubric 413 cannot be made in addition to a code from rubric 410 for the same episode of care.

Coexisting Conditions: These conditions should not be coded unless they require or affect patient care treatment or management. In many cases angina may be asymptomatic, but if still being treated it would qualify as a reportable condition and should be coded. Do not code conditions that were previously treated and no longer exist.

Intermediate Coronary Syndrome: This condition is also known as unstable angina, preinfarction angina, or crescendo angina. This condition represents an intermediate stage between angina of effort and acute myocardial infarction. The patient's pain is more acute, longer lasting and more frequent then angina, and more resistant to anti-anginal treatment. This type of angina often results in an acute myocardial infarction. Initial onset of angina is also classified to code 411.1. Code 413.9 excludes preinfarctional angina.

Myocardial Infarction with Angina: Angina is a symptom of the myocardial infarction and should not be coded in addition.

Other and Unspecified: Code 413.9 encompasses the commonly and uncommonly used descriptors that are not specific to codes 413.0 and 413.1 (e.g., anginal syndrome, status anginosus, stenocardia), typically stable forms of angina. Make sure you use the following guidelines:

- Code the significant sign or symptom that prompted the admission if no actual clinical diagnosis is documented
- Code the condition that was concluded after study
- Use a code from category V71 if no other diagnosis was made

Postinfarctional Angina: Code selection is based on the type of angina indicated. If unstable, assign code 411.1 *Intermediate coronary syndrome.* If stable, use code 413.9 *Other and unspecified angina pectoris.*

Coding Scenario
A patient is admitted with hypertensive cardiovascular disease. Documentation identifies that the patient was having chest pain due to angina. The physician's final diagnosis is hypertensive cardiovascular disease, benign, with angina pectoris.

> Code assignment: 402.10 *Benign hypertensive heart disease, without heart failure* and 413.9 *Other and unspecified angina pectoris*

A 59-year-old male is admitted to the facility with chest pain and possible myocardial infarction. After study the patient is diagnosed with an acute anginal attack. The physician indicates in his final diagnosis that the myocardial infarction was ruled out.

> Code assignment: 413.9 *Other and unspecified angina pectoris*

A patient is admitted with a severe anginal episode. A cardiac catheterization is performed and a diagnosis of an incomplete coronary artery occlusion is established. Documentation in the record indicates that an infarction did not occur. Final diagnosis is an incomplete coronary artery occlusion with severe angina.

> Code assignment: 411.81 *Acute coronary occlusion without myocardial infarction* and 413.9 *Other and unspecified angina pectoris*

A patient is admitted via the emergency department with chest pain. The physician's final diagnosis is chest pain, due to either angina or esophageal spasm.

> Code assignment: 786.50 *Chest pain, unspecified,* 413.9 *Other and unspecified angina pectoris,* and 530.5 *Dyskinesia of esophagus*

A 67-year-old male is admitted to the facility with stable angina. After performing a combined left and right cardiac catheterization, the physician determines that the patient has severe atherosclerotic heart disease. The patient has no previous history of bypass grafting.

> Code assignment: 414.01 *Coronary atherosclerosis of native coronary artery* and 413.9 *Other and unspecified angina pectoris*

A patient is seen in the outpatient clinic for a follow-up visit for hypertension and angina. The physician prescribes nitroglycerin for the angina and a diuretic for the hypertension. The patient history also identifies the patient had pneumonia six months ago.

> Code assignment: 401.9 *Essential hypertension, unspecified* and 413.9 *Other and unspecified angina pectoris*

414 Other forms of chronic ischemic heart disease
AHA: July-Aug, 1984, 5; Q3, 1991, 10

This rubric classifies obstruction of blood flow to the heart, usually due to a mechanical obstruction of one or more of the coronary arteries. Obliterative atherosclerosis of the coronary arteries is by far the most common form of ischemic heart disease. In time, the accumulations may calcify throughout the cardiovascular system, leading to the condition known as "hardening of the arteries."

Coronary atherosclerosis is localized, subintimal accumulations of fatty and fibrous tissue caused by proliferation of smooth muscle cells in combination with a disorder of lipid metabolism. Atherosclerotic heart disease eventually leads to acute and subacute forms of ischemic heart disease such as unstable angina and myocardial infarction.

Aneurysm of the heart is a dilatation, stretching, weakening, or bulging of the tissue of the heart or of the coronary arteries. An aneurysm of the heart wall is an aneurysm of heart muscle, known as a cardiac, mural, or ventricular wall aneurysm, which is usually a consequence of myocardial infarction.

Aneurysm of the coronary vessels is a circumscribed dilation of a coronary artery or a blood-containing tumor connecting directly with the lumen of a coronary artery.

414.00 Coronary atherosclerosis of unspecified type of vessel, native or graft — (Use additional code to identify presence of hypertension: 401.0-405.9)
AHA: Q1,2004, 24

414.01 Coronary atherosclerosis of native coronary artery — (Use additional code to identify presence of hypertension: 401.0-405.9) — *ASHD, arteriosclerosis, arteritis, atheroma, sclerosis, stricture in natural heart vessels*
AHA: July-Aug, 1984, 5; Q3, 1990, 7; Q3, 1991, 10; Q1, 1994, 6; Q2, 1994, 13; Q4, 1994, 49; Q2, 1995, 17; Q2, 1996, 10; Q4, 1996, 31; Q2, 1997, 13; Q3, 1997, 15; Q2, 2001, 8,9; Q3, 2001, 15; Q3, 2002, 4-9; Q3, 2003, 9, 14; Q4, 2003, 105, 108; Q2, 2004, 3; Q4, 2005, 71

414.02 Coronary atherosclerosis of autologous vein bypass graft — (Use additional code to identify presence of hypertension: 401.0-405.9) — *plaque deposit in grafted vein originating within patient*
AHA: July-Aug, 1984, 5; Q3, 1990, 7; Q3, 1991, 10; Q1, 1994, 6; Q2, 1994, 13; Q4, 1994, 49; Q2, 1995, 17; Q2, 1997, 13

414.03 Coronary atherosclerosis of nonautologous biological bypass graft — (Use additional code to identify presence of hypertension: 401.0-405.9) — *plaque deposit in grafted vessel originating outside patient*
AHA: July-Aug, 1984, 5; Q3, 1990, 7; Q3, 1991, 10; Q1, 1994, 6; Q2, 1994, 13; Q4, 1994, 49; Q2, 1995, 17; Q2, 1997, 13

414.04 Coronary atherosclerosis of artery bypass graft — (Use additional code to identify presence of hypertension: 401.0-405.9) — *plaque deposit in grafted artery originating within patient*
AHA: July-Aug, 1984, 5; Q3, 1990, 7; Q3, 1991, 10; Q1, 1994, 6; Q2, 1994, 13; Q4, 1994, 49; Q2, 1995, 17; Q4, 1996, 31; Q2, 1997, 13

414.05 Coronary atherosclerosis of unspecified type of bypass graft — (Use additional code to identify presence of hypertension: 401.0-405.9) — *plaque deposit in grafted vessel of unknown origin*
AHA: July-Aug, 1984, 5; Q3, 1990, 7; Q3, 1991, 10; Q1, 1994, 6; Q2, 1994, 13; Q4, 1994, 49; Q2, 1995, 17; Q4, 1996, 31; Q2, 1997, 13; Q3, 1997, 15

414.06 Coronary atherosclerosis, of native coronary artery of transplanted heart — (Use additional code to identify presence of hypertension: 401.0-405.9)

414.07 Coronary atherosclerosis, Of bypass graft (artery) (vein) of transplanted heart — (Use additional code to identify presence of hypertension: 401.0-405.9)

414.10	Aneurysm of heart — (Use additional code to identify presence of hypertension: 401.0-405.9) — *dilation of a wall in the heart* AHA: July-Aug, 1984, 5; Q3, 1991, 10; Q4, 2002, 54	
414.11	Aneurysm of coronary vessels — (Use additional code to identify presence of hypertension: 401.0-405.9) — *dilation of a wall of a coronary vessel* AHA: July-Aug, 1984, 5; Q3, 1991, 10; Q1, 1999, 17; Q4, 2002, 54; Q3, 2003, 10	
414.12	Dissection of coronary artery — (Use additional code to identify presence of hypertension: 401.0-405.9)	
414.19	Other aneurysm of heart — (Use additional code to identify presence of hypertension: 401.0-405.9) — *acquired arteriovenous fistula* AHA: July-Aug, 1984, 5; Q3, 1991, 10; Q4, 2002, 54	
	4AHA: July-Aug, 1984, 5; Q3, 1991, 10; Q4, 2002, 54	
414.8	Other specified forms of chronic ischemic heart disease — (Use additional code to identify presence of hypertension: 401.0-405.9) — *chronic coronary insufficiency, chronic myocardial ischemia* AHA: July-Aug, 1984, 5; Q2, 1990, 19; Q3, 1990, 7,15; Q3, 1991, 10; Q1, 1992, 10; Q3, 2001, 15	
414.9	Unspecified chronic ischemic heart disease — (Use additional code to identify presence of hypertension: 401.0-405.9) — *unknown or not otherwise specified* AHA: July-Aug, 1984, 5; Q3, 1991, 10	

Documentation Issues
If the physician documents both ischemic congestive cardiomyopathy and idiopathic ischemic cardiomyopathy, only one code is necessary as all ischemic cardiomyopathies are classified with code 414.8 *Other specified forms of chronic ischemic heart disease*.

When the documentation identifies a diabetic patient with cardiomyopathy, these conditions are coded as separate entities. The diabetic complication code 250.7x does not include cardiomyopathy.

Coding Clarification
Report 414.11 for abnormal communication between a coronary artery and vein resulting in the formation of an arteriovenous aneurysm, usually resulting from myocardial infarction. Report 414.19 for an arteriovenous fistula of the coronary vessels.

Myocardial Bridge: This condition has been identified as a congenital disorder that develops when the heart muscle wraps around the coronary artery causing constriction. This bridge typically builds over the middle component of the left anterior descending artery. There is increasing evidence that this condition causes conditions such as myocardial infarction, ischemia, ventricular fibrillation, conduction disturbances, and even sudden death. For reporting, use code 746.85 *Myocardial bridge, congenital* and a code that identifies chronic ischemic disease, 414.8.

Hypertension and Atherosclerosis: Hypertension frequently accelerates atherosclerosis and if both are documented, code both conditions. Systolic hypertension may be referenced as "arteriosclerotic hypertension" of the elderly. In younger patients, systolic hypertension may be associated with an arteriovenous fistula or thyrotoxicosis, and would be classified as a secondary hypertension.

Hypertensive cardiovascular arteriosclerotic disease with heart failure is coded 402.91. Use an additional code of 414.0x to identify the coronary arteriosclerosis.

Occlusion of Bypass Grafts: Coronary artery bypass graft occlusions are reported with codes 414.02 (autologous), 414.03 (nonautologous), 414.04 (of artery), 414.05 (unspecified type), and 414.07 (of transplanted heart). If the graft type is unknown, use code 414.05 *Coronary atherosclerosis of unspecified type of bypass graft*.

Post-Coronary Artery Bypass Graft: Although a coronary artery bypass was done, coronary artery disease (CAD) is still present. When a patient is admitted with unstable angina post coronary artery bypass graft, assign code 414.00 *Coronary atherosclerosis of unspecified type of vessel, native or graft* as the principal diagnosis and code 411.1 *Intermediate coronary syndrome*. Use code V45.81 as an additional code to identify the aortocoronary bypass status.

Re-occlusion Post PTCA: A PTCA leaves the coronary artery intact and no grafting is performed. When a PTCA is performed, a balloon device is used to apply pressure inside the vessel, which compresses the arteriosclerotic plaque against the wall of the artery. Re-occlusion is typically caused by progression of the disease or re-expansion of the plaque within the vessel. Assign code 414.0x *Coronary atherosclerosis*, unless the physician specifically indicates that re-occlusion was due to a complication of the procedure. Use code V45.82 as an additional code to identify the angioplasty status.

Peripheral: Arteriosclerosis (occlusive) of the extremities is reported with code 440.2x.

If the documentation indicates the patient has coronary artery disease with diastolic dysfunction, use code 414.9 *Chronic ischemic heart disease, unspecified.*

Ischemic Cardiomyopathy: The term "ischemic" cardiomyopathy is used to specify the condition in which ischemic heart disease causes diffuse fibrosis or multiple infarctions, resulting in heart failure with left ventricular dilation. All ischemic heart diseases are classified to the code series 410-414. Unless more specific documentation is obtained from the physician, ischemic cardiomyopathy is reported with code 414.8 *Other specified forms of chronic ischemic heart disease.*

Coding Scenario

A 56-year-old male is admitted for stent placement and vein allograft of a left anterior descending (LAD) aneurysm. Final diagnostic statement verifies the LAD aneurysm.

> Code assignment: 414.11 *Aneurysm of coronary vessels*

A patient previously diagnosed with atherosclerotic hypertension is now seen in the clinic for follow up. Medical record indicates coronary atherosclerosis and benign hypertension.

> Code assignment: 414.00 *Coronary atherosclerosis of unspecified type of vessel, native or graft* and 401.1 *Benign essential hypertension*

A 67-year-old male is admitted to the facility with stable angina. After performing a combined left and right cardiac catheterization, the physician determines that the patient has severe atherosclerotic heart disease. The patient has no previous history of bypass grafting.

> Code assignment: 414.01 *Coronary atherosclerosis of native coronary artery* and 413.9 *Other and unspecified angina pectoris*

A 63-year-old patient is seen in the office for progression of his coronary atherosclerosis. The patient has a history of a heart transplant five years ago.

> Code assignment: 414.06 *Coronary atherosclerosis of coronary artery of transplanted heart* and V42.1 *Organ or tissue replaced by transplant, heart*

A patient is admitted for treatment of impending myocardial infarction with a known history of coronary atherosclerosis, status post myocardial infarction several years ago and no history of CABG. After the patient is treated with intravenous thrombolytic agents, the acute myocardial infarction is averted.

> Code assignment: 411.1 *Intermediate coronary syndrome,* 414.01 *Coronary atherosclerosis of native coronary artery,* and 412 *Old myocardial infarction*

415–417 Diseases of Pulmonary Circulation

Diseases of the pulmonary circulation include acute pulmonary heart disease (415), chronic pulmonary heart disease (416), and other diseases of the pulmonary circulation (417).

415 Acute pulmonary heart disease

Acute cor pulmonale is a dilation and failure of the right side of the heart due to pulmonary embolism. The condition is usually reversible. Pulmonary embolism and infarction is a condition that occurs when a thrombus, usually forming in the veins of the lower extremities or pelvis but may be secondary to atrial fibrillation or flutter, travels through the right-sided circulation, and becomes lodged in the pulmonary artery. Pulmonary infarction is the consequential hemorrhagic consolidation and necrosis of the lung parenchyma.

415.0	Acute cor pulmonale
415.11	Iatrogenic pulmonary embolism and infarction — *death of lung tissue due to blocked vessels from medical treatment*
	AHA: Q4, 1990, 25; Q4, 1995, 58
415.19	Other pulmonary embolism and infarction — *not otherwise specified*
	AHA: Q4, 1990, 25

416 Chronic pulmonary heart disease

Chronic pulmonary heart disease is a rare increase in pulmonary circulation, often resulting in right ventricular failure or fatal syncope.

Primary pulmonary hypertension is a condition characterized by pulmonary hypertension and raised pulmonary vascular resistance in the lungs in the absence of any other disease of the lungs or heart. It is marked by diffuse narrowing of the pulmonary arterioles and, in moderate to severe cases, formation of pulmonary thrombi and emboli. The clinical picture is similar to pulmonary hypertension from any other cause, and has a poor prognosis with patients developing severe right heart failure within two to three years.

Kyphoscoliotic heart disease arises from a forward and lateral deformity of the spine. It is characterized by difficult breathing, respiratory alkalosis, pulmonary hypertension, and, in severe cases, congestive heart failure. It is a form of chronic secondary pulmonary hypertension.

416.0	Primary pulmonary hypertension — *idiopathic pulmonary arteriosclerosis, pulmonary hypertension, Arrillaga-Ayerza and Cardiacos negros syndromes*
416.1	Kyphoscoliotic heart disease — *high blood pressure within the lungs as a result of curvature of the spine*
416.8	Other chronic pulmonary heart diseases — *pulmonary hypertension, secondary to disease*
416.9	Unspecified chronic pulmonary heart disease

Coding Clarification
Report 416.8 in cases of pulmonary hypertension secondary to a known etiology (excluding kyphoscoliosis), such as chronic bronchitis, chronic obstructive pulmonary disease, obesity-hypoventilation syndrome, chronic mountain sickness, obstructive sleep apnea, and neuromuscular disease.

417 Other diseases of pulmonary circulation
Arteriovenous fistula of the pulmonary vessels is an abnormal communication between a pulmonary artery and vein that may result in embolization or ischemia. It may occur as a result of previous pulmonary infarction. An aneurysm of the pulmonary artery is a dilation of the pulmonary artery or a blood-containing tumor within the lumen of the pulmonary artery.

417.0	Arteriovenous fistula of pulmonary vessels — *abnormal communication between blood vessels within the lung*
417.1	Aneurysm of pulmonary artery — *dilation of the wall of the main artery in the lung*
417.8	Other specified disease of pulmonary circulation — *arteritis; rupture or stricture of pulmonary vessel, endarteritis*
417.9	Unspecified disease of pulmonary circulation

Coding Clarification
Both true and false (pseudo-) aneurysms are reported with 417.1

420–429 Other Forms of Heart Disease
This section covers inflammatory conditions of the pericardium, endocardium, and myocardium, as well as heart valve disorders, cardiomyopathies, and nerve conduction disorders of the heart.

420 Acute pericarditis
Acute pericarditis is inflammation of the fibroserous membrane that surrounds the heart. The inflammation may be described as fibrinous, serous, sanguineous, hemorrhagic, or purulent. Etiologies for acute pericarditis include myocardial infarction, Dressler's syndrome, viral and bacterial infections, collagen vascular disease, adverse reaction to drugs (such as procainamide, hydralazine, and isoniazid), metastatic disease, and uremia.

420.0	Acute pericarditis in diseases classified elsewhere — (Code first underlying disease: 017.9, 039.8, 066.8, 585.9, 586) — *secondary to disease*
420.90	Unspecified acute pericarditis
420.91	Acute idiopathic pericarditis — *inflammation of heart lining, cause unknown*
420.99	Other acute pericarditis — *pneumococcal, purulent, staphylococcal, streptococcal, pneumopyopericardium, pyopericardium*

Coding Clarification
Subclassification 420.0 reports acute pericarditis in diseases classified elsewhere. Report the etiology first, then the manifestation.

Unspecified acute pericarditis, including cases in which the specific infective organism is unknown, or in which the etiology is unknown, is reported with 420.90. This code may also be used to report acute pericarditis due to a malignant neoplasm. Acute idiopathic pericarditis, a benign, nonspecific, or viral pericarditis that often follows upper respiratory infections, is reported with 420.91. Use this code only when other etiologies have been ruled out.

Report 420.99 for acute pericarditis caused by bacterial infection or when the acute pericarditis has no known etiology.

421 Acute and subacute endocarditis
Use this rubric for diseases in which the endocardium is inflamed, usually due to bacterial infection. A variety of organisms may cause endocarditis, but *Staphylococcus aureus* is the most common pathogen. Infection of previously damaged valves is due to *Viridans streptococci* or other organisms comprising normal oral flora and may be secondary to a dental procedure. Infection of a prosthetic valve usually is due to Staphylococci within the first two months of surgery, and Streptococci more than two months after surgery. Infection of normal valves is rare and usually associated with intravenous drug abuse.

421.0	Acute and subacute bacterial endocarditis — (Use additional code to identify infectious organism) — *bacterial, infective, lenta, malignant, purulent, septic, ulcerative, vegetative, SBE* **AHA:** Q1, 1991, 15; Q1, 1999, 12

Diseases of the Circulatory System

421.1 Acute and subacute infective endocarditis in diseases classified elsewhere — (Code first underlying disease: 002.0, 083.0, 116.0) — *sudden, severe inflammation of lining of the heart secondary to other disease*

421.9 Unspecified acute endocarditis

Coding Clarification
Acute endocarditis due to fungal infection is excluded from this rubric, and classified to rubrics 112 and 115.

422 Acute myocarditis
This rubric reports focal or diffuse inflammation of the myocardium that may be due to toxins, adverse reactions to drugs, or viral, bacterial, rickettsial, fungal, or parasitic disease.

In myocarditis in disease classified elsewhere, code first the underlying disease, as in influenza (487.8) or tuberculosis (017.9).

For acute myocarditis secondary to metastatic disease, report 422.99.

422.0 Acute myocarditis in diseases classified elsewhere — (Code first underlying disease: 017.9, 487.8) — *sudden severe inflammation of muscle of the heart secondary to other disease*

422.90 Unspecified acute myocarditis

422.91 Idiopathic myocarditis — *giant cell, isolated, nonspecific, Fiedler's myocarditis*

422.92 Septic myocarditis — (Use additional code to identify infectious organism) — *caused by bacteria, including pneumococcal and staphylococcal*

422.93 Toxic myocarditis — *as a reaction to a toxic substance*

422.99 Other acute myocarditis — *not otherwise specified*

Coding Clarification
Excluded from this rubric are myocarditis due rheumatic fever (391.2), to Coxsackie virus (074.23), diphtheritic infection (032.82), meningococcal infection (036.43), syphilis (093.82), and toxoplasmosis (130.3).

423 Other diseases of pericardium
Hemopericardium is the presence of blood in the pericardial sac. It includes cardiac tamponade due to hemoperitoneum. Emergency pericardiocentesis is usually performed.

Report adhesive pericarditis for adhesions between the two pericardial layers, between the heart and the pericardium, or between the pericardium and other contiguous structures in the chest.

Constrictive pericarditis is a diffuse thickening of the pericardium as a late effect of inflammation. Cardiac output is limited due to the reduced distensibility of the cardiac chambers, and filling pressures are increased in response to the external constrictive force placed on the heart by the pericardium. This condition may be associated with congestive heart failure.

423.0 Hemopericardium — *escape of blood into the lining of the heart*

423.1 Adhesive pericarditis — *adherent, fibrosis, milk spots, obliterative*

423.2 Constrictive pericarditis — *loss of elasticity; Concato's or Pick's disease, Gouley's syndrome*

423.8 Other specified diseases of pericardium — *not elsewhere specified; calcification, fistula, acquired diverticula, cholesterol pericarditis, cyst*
  AHA: Q2, 1989, 12

423.9 Unspecified disease of pericardium

Coding Clarification
Excluded from this rubric is hemopericardium due to trauma, classified as an internal injury of the chest in rubric 860.

Report 423.8 for diseases of the pericardium not reported elsewhere in this rubric, including calcified pericardium, diverticula of pericardium, cyst of pericardium, and fistula of pericardium. Code 423.9 is usually reserved for cardiac tamponade due to nontraumatic pericardial effusion, not specified as hemorrhagic or due to hemopericardium, pericardial compression scarring, and pneumohemopericardium.

424 Other diseases of endocardium
This rubric includes diseases of the heart valves that are specified or presumed to be non-rheumatic in origin, classified to categories 394-397.

424.0 Mitral valve disorders — *incompetence, insufficiency, regurgitation, prolapse; ballooning posterior leaflet syndrome, Barlow's syndrome*
  AHA: Nov-Dec, 1984, 8; Nov-Dec, 1987, 8; Q3, 1998, 11; Q2, 2000, 16

424.1 Aortic valve disorders — *incompetence, insufficiency, regurgitation, stenosis, nonrheumatic*
  AHA: Nov-Dec, 1987, 8; Q4, 1988, 8

424.2 Tricuspid valve disorders, specified as nonrheumatic — *incompetence, insufficiency, regurgitation, stenosis, nonrheumatic*

424.3 Pulmonary valve disorders — *incompetence, insufficiency, regurgitation, stenosis, nonrheumatic*

424.90 Endocarditis, valve unspecified, unspecified cause — *incompetence, insufficiency, regurgitation, stenosis, endocardial tag, nonrheumatic, unknown cause*

424.91 Endocarditis in diseases classified elsewhere — (Code first underlying disease: 017.9, 710.0) — *secondary to underlying disease*

424.99 Other endocarditis, valve unspecified — incompetence, insufficiency, regurgitation, stenosis, nonrheumatic, with specified cause

Coding Clarification
Syphilitic endocarditis is excluded from 424.91 *Endocarditis in diseases classified elsewhere.* For this code, sequence first the underlying disease, for example, tuberculosis (017.9) or disseminated lupus erythematosus (710.0).

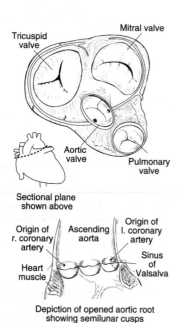

Depiction of opened aortic root showing semilunar cusps

425 Cardiomyopathy
AHA: July-Aug, 1985, 15

Cardiomyopathy is a complex and heterogenous group of diseases of the heart muscle. Rubric 425 includes diseases of the heart muscle itself that are classified to specific etiologies.

Endomyocardial fibrosis is a thickening of the ventricular endocardium due to fibrosis. Occasionally, the tricuspid and mitral valves may be involved and there is thrombus formation.

Hypertrophic obstructive cardiomyopathy, idiopathic hypertrophic subaortic stenosis, and asymmetrical septal hypertrophy are reported with 425.1. The etiology is believed to be an autosomal dominant genetic disorder and is characterized by an excessively hypertrophied interventricular septum. Left ventricular outflow obstruction results when the septum mechanically obstructs the anterior leaflet of the mitral valve.

425.0 Endomyocardial fibrosis — *fibrous tissue invading the muscle of the heart*
AHA: July-Aug, 1985, 15

425.1 Hypertrophic obstructive cardiomyopathy — *abnormal growth of the left ventricle wall causing obstructed blood flow; idiopathic hypertrophic subaortic stenosis*
AHA: July-Aug, 1985, 15

425.2 Obscure cardiomyopathy of Africa — *Becker's disease, South African cardiomyopathy syndrome, idiopathic mural endomyocardial disease*
AHA: July-Aug, 1985, 15

425.3 Endocardial fibroelastosis — *increased elastic tissue production with enlarged left ventricle wall; elastomyofibrosis*
AHA: July-Aug, 1985, 15

425.4 Other primary cardiomyopathies — *congestive, restrictive, familial, hypertrophic, idiopathic, nonobstructive, obstructive, restrictive, cardiovascular collagenosis*
AHA: July-Aug, 1985, 15; Q2, 1990, 19; Q4, 1997, 55; Q1, 2000, 22; Q2, 2005, 14; Q2, 2005, 14

425.5 Alcoholic cardiomyopathy — *heart disease resulting from excessive alcohol consumption*
AHA: Sept-Oct, 1985, 15; July-Aug, 1985, 15

425.7 Nutritional and metabolic cardiomyopathy — (Code first underlying disease: 242.00-242.91, 265.0, 271.0, 277.3x, 277.5) — *secondary to specific underlying disease*
AHA: July-Aug, 1985, 15

425.8 Cardiomyopathy in other diseases classified elsewhere — (Code first underlying disease: 135, 334.0, 359.1, 359.2) — *secondary to specific underlying disease*
AHA: July-Aug, 1985, 15; Q2, 1993, 9

425.9 Unspecified secondary cardiomyopathy

Coding Clarification
Note that the term "cardiomyopathy" often is used for a disease or disorder that should be classified elsewhere. For example, the term, "ischemic cardiomyopathy" should be interpreted as ischemic heart disease and classified to the series 414.8.

Endomyocardial fibrosis is reported with 425.0.

Idiopathic cardiomegaly, idiopathic mural endomyocardial disease, Becker's disease, and South African cardiomyopathy are all types of obscure cardiomyopathy of Africa, reported with 425.2. These conditions are thought to be late effects of an infectious myocarditis, and are rarely encountered in the United States.

Endocardial fibroelastosis (425.3) is a congenital condition characterized by thickening of the endocardium and subendocardium, with malformation of the cardiac valves, hypertrophy of the heart, and proliferation of elastic tissue in the myocardium. It is also called elastomyofibrosis. Many patients with this condition do not survive infancy.

Report 425.4 for unspecified cardiomyopathy and cardiomyopathy of unknown or obscure etiology. Both obstructive cardiomyopathy and hypertrophic cardiomyopathy may be classified to 425.4, but the combined form of hypertrophic obstructive cardiomyopathy is reported with 425.1.

For cardiomyopathy due to underlying disease, code first the underlying disease, then the myopathy with 435.7 or 435.8. Some examples of underlying disease include amyloidosis (277.3), beriberi (265.0), cardiac glycogenesis (271.0), mucopolysaccharidosis (277.5), thyrotoxicosis (242.0-242.9), Friedreich's ataxia (334.0), myotonia atrophica (359.1), and sarcoidosis (135). Subclassification 435.7 excludes gouty tophi of the heart, reported with 274.82, and subclassification 437.8 excludes cardiomyopathy in Chagas' disease (086.0).

Holiday Heart Syndrome: This condition is noted in patients with no known heart disease who develop cardiac arrhythmias due to acute alcohol consumption. The condition may appear in patients who are alcohol dependent (303.00) or nondependent (305.00). Two codes are necessary to identify this condition — one for the specific type of arrhythmia (e.g., atrial fibrillation, atrial flutter) and the other for the acute ingestion of alcohol. If the specific arrhythmia is not known, use code 427.9 *Cardiac dysrhythmia, unspecified.*

This syndrome may also be noted in patients with a diagnosis of chronic alcohol consumption with associated congestive cardiomyopathy. In this situation, three codes are required to accurately report the patient's diagnoses. Code the type of arrhythmia from category 427, the alcoholic cardiomyopathy with code 425.5, and the acute alcoholic intoxication in alcoholism, dependent with 303.00.

Congestive Cardiomyopathy: This condition, also known as congestive dilated cardiomyopathy (425.4), is a heart muscle disease of unknown etiology or a heart muscle disorder secondary to a disease elsewhere in the body. The symptoms are basically the same as those noted in congestive heart failure (CHF). It is possible to have a diagnosis of both congestive cardiomyopathy and congestive heart failure, and both conditions would be reported. In the majority of cases of CHF and cardiomyopathy, patient care revolves around the treatment of the CHF, and in those instances the CHF is listed first.

Diastolic Dysfunction: Cardiomyopathy can result in diastolic dysfunction. If documentation identifies that the diastolic dysfunction is due to cardiomyopathy, use code 425.4 *Other primary cardiomyopathies.*

Hypertensive Cardiomyopathy: If the physician documentation identifies that the hypertensive heart disease is the cause of the cardiomyopathy, use codes 402.9x *Unspecified hypertensive heart disease* and 425.8 *Cardiomyopathy in other diseases classified elsewhere.*

Coding Scenario

A patient is admitted with congestive heart failure and congestive cardiomyopathy.

> Code assignment: 428.0 *Congestive heart failure* and 425.4 *Other primary cardiomyopathies*

A patient is seen in the clinic for evaluation of treatment for hypertensive cardiomyopathy. Record documentation identifies that the cardiomyopathy was secondary to hypertensive heart disease.

> Code assignment: 402.90 *Unspecified hypertensive heart disease without mention of congestive heart failure* and 425.8 *Cardiomyopathy in other diseases classified elsewhere*

A patient's diagnostic condition is documented as idiopathic dilated cardiomyopathy.

> Code assignment: 425.4 *Other primary cardiomyopathies*

A patient is admitted in decompensated congestive failure resulting from end-stage cardiomyopathy. Laboratory findings are metabolic acidosis, elevated BUN/creatine, and elevated liver enzymes. The physician diagnoses both renal and heart failure and liver shock.

> Code assignment: 428.0 *Congestive heart failure, unspecified,* is the principal diagnosis. Assign 570 Subacute necrosis of the liver for the liver shock. Assign code 584.9 *Acute renal failure, unspecified* and 425.4 *Other primary cardiomyopathies*

426 Conduction disorders

Nerve conduction disorders include a group of conditions in which the transmission of cardiac electrical impulses controlling heart rhythm is abnormal, slowed, or interrupted.

Complete atrioventricular block is the most advanced form of heart block. Usually, there is a lesion distal to the bundle of His and is associated with bilateral bundle branch block. Some patients may go through periods of transition between partial and complete heart block.

426.0	Atrioventricular block, complete — third degree atrioventricular block, Lev's and Rytand-Lipsitch syndrome **AHA:** Q2, 2006, 14
426.10	Unspecified atrioventricular block — AV block, incomplete or partial
426.11	First degree atrioventricular block — first degree incomplete AV block; prolonged P-R interval not specified elsewhere **AHA:** Q2, 2006, 14
426.12	Mobitz (type) II atrioventricular block — incomplete AV block, Mobitz Type II, second degree **AHA:** Q2, 2006, 14
426.13	Other second degree atrioventricular block — incomplete AV block, Mobitz, Type I, second degree; Wenckebach's phenomenon
426.2	Left bundle branch hemiblock — left anterior or posterior fascicular block
426.3	Other left bundle branch block — complete, main stem, anterior fascicular with posterior fascicular, not otherwise specified
426.4	Right bundle branch block
426.50	Unspecified bundle branch block
426.51	Right bundle branch block and left posterior fascicular block
426.52	Right bundle branch block and left anterior fascicular block
426.53	Other bilateral bundle branch block — bifascicular block not otherwise specified; right bundle ranch with left bundle brand block
426.54	Trifascicular block
426.6	Other heart block — intraventricular, diffuse, myofibrillar, sinoatrial, sinoauricular block
426.7	Anomalous atrioventricular excitation — accelerated, accessory, pre-excitation; including bundle of Kent syndrome, Wolff-Parkinson-White syndrome
426.81	Lown-Ganong-Levine syndrome — short P-R interval, normal QRS complexes, and supraventricular tachycardias
426.82	Long QT syndrome **AHA:** Q4, 2005, 72
426.89	Other specified conduction disorder — AV, interference, isorhythmic dissociation, nonparoxysmal AV nodal tachycardia
426.9	Unspecified conduction disorder

Coding Clarification

Long QT syndrome: A serious and potentially fatal condition that can be precipitated by vigorous exertion, emotional upset, or startling moments. The Q-T interval is the time it takes for the duration of electrical activity that controls the pumping action of the heart's ventricles, measured in fractions of a second. When the interval is longer than normal, it is identified as long QT syndrome. This imbalance in electrical timing makes the patient susceptible to recurrent episodes of syncope and rapid arrhythmias that can become malignant, leading to sudden death.

427 Cardiac dysrhythmias
AHA: July-Aug, 1985, 15

Cardiac dysrhythmias are disturbances in cardiac rate and rhythm, including abnormalities in the rate, regularity, and sequence of atrial and/or ventricular contractions. Cardiac dysrhythmias can take many forms; the clinical significance of each depends on the extent to which they lower blood pressure and reduce cardiac output with resulting hypoperfusion of vital organs such as the brain, kidneys, and the heart. Cardiac dysrhythmias may be benign or malignant, depending on the severity of the dysrhythmia and the patient's ability to tolerate it.

The etiology of cardiac dysrhythmia may be idiopathic, due to heart disease such as arteriosclerosis and rheumatic heart disease or due to other noncardiac etiologies such as thyrotoxicosis, alcoholism, trauma, and intravenous drug abuse. Many cardiac dysrhythmias are chronic, but acute dysrhythmias also can occur in cases of acute infection or digitalis toxicity. Symptoms may include fatigue, light-headedness, decreased exercise tolerance, or syncope, but often, there are no symptoms.

427.0	Paroxysmal supraventricular tachycardia — very rapid atrial rhythm; including PAT, AV, junctional, nodal **AHA:** July-Aug, 1985, 15
427.1	Paroxysmal ventricular tachycardia — very rapid ventricular rhythm **AHA:** July-Aug, 1985, 15; March-April, 1986, 11; Q3, 1995, 9; Q2, 2006, 15
427.2	Unspecified paroxysmal tachycardia — Bouveret-Hoffmann syndrome, essential paroxysmal tachycardia **AHA:** July-Aug, 1985, 15
427.31	Atrial fibrillation — irregular, rapid atrial contractions **AHA:** July-Aug, 1985, 15; Q3, 1995, 9; Q2, 1999, 17; Q1, 2003, 8; Q4, 2003, 95, 105; Q3, 2004, 7; Q4, 2004, 78, 121; Q3, 2005, 8
427.32	Atrial flutter — regular, rapid atrial contractions **AHA:** July-Aug, 1985, 15; Q4, 2003, 94

Diseases of the Circulatory System

427.41	Ventricular fibrillation — *irregular, rapid ventricular contractions*	
	AHA: July-Aug, 1985, 15; Q3, 2002, 5	
427.42	Ventricular flutter — *regular, rapid ventricular contractions*	
	AHA: July-Aug, 1985, 15	
427.5	Cardiac arrest — *heart stops and atrial blood pressure flattens*	
	AHA: July-Aug, 1985, 15; Q2, 1988, 8; Q3, 1995, 8; Q2, 2000, 12; Q3, 2002, 5	
427.60	Unspecified premature beats — *ectopic beats, extrasystolic arrhythmia, premature contractions; unknown site*	
	AHA: July-Aug, 1985, 15	
427.61	Supraventricular premature beats — *ectopic beats, extrasystolic arrhythmia, premature contractions; atrial*	
	AHA: July-Aug, 1985, 15	
427.69	Other premature beats — *ectopic beats, extrasystolic arrhythmia, premature contractions, site not otherwise specified*	
	AHA: July-Aug, 1985, 15; Q4, 1993, 42	
427.81	Sinoatrial node dysfunction — *persistent or severe sinus bradycardia; including sick sinus syndrome*	
	AHA: July-Aug, 1985, 15; Q3, 2000, 8	
427.89	Other specified cardiac dysrhythmias — *not otherwise specified, including bigeminy, trigeminy, split heart sounds, wandering pacemaker, gallop rhythm*	
	AHA: July-Aug, 1985, 15	
427.9	Unspecified cardiac dysrhythmia	

Coding Clarification

Holiday Heart Syndrome: This condition is noted in patients with no known heart disease who develop cardiac arrhythmias due to acute alcohol consumption. The condition may appear in patients who are alcohol dependent (303.00) or nondependent (305.00). Two codes are necessary to identify this condition — one for the specific type of arrhythmia (e.g., atrial fibrillation, atrial flutter) and the other for the acute ingestion of alcohol. If the specific arrhythmia is not known use code 427.9 *Cardiac dysrhythmia, unspecified*.

This syndrome may also be noted in patients with a diagnosis of chronic alcohol consumption with associated congestive cardiomyopathy. In this situation, three codes are required to accurately report the patient's diagnoses. Code the type of arrhythmia from category 427, the alcoholic cardiomyopathy with code 425.5, and the acute alcoholic intoxication in alcoholism, dependent with 303.00.

Postural Orthostatic Tachycardia Syndrome (POTS): This condition is classified as a specified cardiac dysrhythmia, other, code 427.89. If orthostatic hypotension is noted, assign code 458.0. If the documentation identifies that any neurological factors are present, they should be coded also.

Ventricular Dysfunction: This condition is not a cardiac arrhythmia. The alphabetic index entry, Dysfunction, heart, 427.9, refers to dysrhythmia. The appropriate code for ventricular dysfunction, if a more definitive diagnosis cannot be established, is 428.9 *Unspecified heart failure.*

Coding Scenario

A patient receives ambulatory cardiac monitoring. The patient is being treated with antiarrhythmic drug therapy for paroxysmal tachycardia. Monitoring is being performed for effectiveness of drug therapy.

Code assignment: 427.2 *Unspecified paroxysmal tachycardia*

A 59-year-old male is seen in the emergency department after passing out at an office party. The patient is extremely intoxicated but states that his heart is racing. The patient has a known alcohol dependency. EKG findings indicate atrial fibrillation. The physician's diagnosis states holiday heart syndrome with atrial fibrillation and acute alcoholic42 intoxication in alcoholism.

Code assignment: 427.31 *Atrial fibrillation* and 303.00 *Acute alcoholic intoxication in alcoholism, unspecified use*

The diagnosis is documented as ventricular tachycardia secondary to holiday heart syndrome secondary to acute alcohol intoxication. The final diagnosis also indicates chronic alcoholism with alcoholic cardiomyopathy.

Code assignment: 427.0 *Paroxysmal supraventricular tachycardia,* 425.5 *Alcoholic cardiomyopathy,* and 303.00 *Acute alcoholic intoxication in alcoholism, unspecified use*

428 Heart failure

AHA: Q3, 1988, 3; Q2, 1989, 10; Q2, 1990, 16, 19; Q3, 1998, 5; Q4, 2002, 49

Congestive heart failure is a mechanical inability of the heart to pump blood efficiently, thus compromising circulation and causing systemic complications due to congestion and edema of fluids in the tissues. Etiologies fall into three groups: disorders that decrease contractile function, disorders than increase myocardial overload, and abnormalities in myocardial preload.

Contractile function of the heart decreases when the myocardium has been damaged as in myocardial infarction, thus reducing the ventricles' ability to contract forcefully.

Increased myocardial afterload refers to the increased force that the myocardium must generate to contract the ventricles. For example, in acute and severe systemic hypertension, the force exerted upon the ventricle by increased blood pressure exceeds the force the ventricle must generate to contract, leading to pulmonary congestion.

Myocardial preload refers to the stretching of the myocardial fibers prior to myocardial contraction. Although this stretching increases the force-generating capabilities of the ventricles, eventually pulmonary congestion occurs when the ventricular filling pressure concomitantly increases.

In ICD-9-CM, congestive heart failure also is defined as right ventricular failure or right ventricular failure due to left ventricular failure. Right ventricular failure is most frequently due to failure of the left ventricle, but may occur independently of left ventricular failure. Chronic obstructive pulmonary disease can produce a pressure overload in the right ventricle independent of any failure on the left side.

428.0	Congestive heart failure, unspecified — *right heart failure; decreased efficiency of heart output causing fluid collection in lungs, hypertension, and congestion of the vessels* **AHA:** Q3, 1988, 3; Q2, 1989, 10; Q2, 1989, 12; Q2, 1990, 16, 19; Q3, 1991, 18, 19; Q3, 1996, 9; Q3, 1997, 10; Q4, 1997, 55; Q3, 1998, 5; Q1, 1999, 11; Q4, 1999, 4; Q1, 2000, 22; Q2, 2000, 16; Q4, 2000, 48; Q2, 2001, 13; Q4, 2002, 49; Q4, 2002, 52; Q1, 2003, 9; Q4, 2003, 109; Q3, 2004, 7; Q4, 2004, 140; Q1, 2005, 5, 9; Q4, 2005, 120
428.1	Left heart failure — *decreased efficiency of the left ventricle of the heart causing fluid in lungs* **AHA:** Q3, 1988, 3; Q2, 1989, 10; Q2, 1990, 16, 19; Q3, 1998, 5; Q4, 2002, 49
428.20	Unspecified systolic heart failure
428.21	Acute systolic heart failure
428.22	Chronic systolic heart failure **AHA:** Q4, 2005, 120
428.23	Acute on chronic systolic heart failure
428.30	Unspecified diastolic heart failure
428.31	Acute diastolic heart failure
428.32	Chronic diastolic heart failure
428.33	Acute on chronic diastolic heart failure
428.40	Unspecified combined systolic and diastolic heart failure
428.41	Acute combined systolic and diastolic heart failure **AHA:** Q4, 2004, 140
428.42	Chronic combined systolic and diastolic heart failure
428.43	Acute on chronic combined systolic and diastolic heart failure
428.9	Unspecified heart failure — *unknown whether right or left* **AHA:** Nov-Dec, 1985, 14; Q3, 1988, 3; Q2, 1989, 10; Q2, 1990, 16, 19; Q3, 1998, 5; Q4, 2002, 49

Documentation Issues

If the documentation indicates that the patient has congestive heart failure, review the record for any hypertensive heart or hypertensive heart and renal disease. If documentation identifies these conditions, a combination code may be used from categories 402 and 404.

Even if the patient is being seen for another condition, if the heart failure is noted in the record and the patient is still under treatment, the heart failure should be coded as a secondary condition.

Unless documentation identifies a cause and effect relationship between hypertension and congestive heart failure, they should be coded as separate entities, 428.0 and 401.x. However, if the documentation indicates the heart failure is due to the hypertension, only one code is necessary, 402.91.

If fluid overload is identified in conjunction with congestive heart failure, it is not coded separately because it is a component of the congestive heart failure.

When the documentation states an acute and chronic heart failure, check with the physician to see if the diagnosis refers to congestive heart failure, such as a congestive heart failure that has become decompensated. If so, use code 428.0. If no clarification can be obtained, use code 428.9 *Unspecified heart failure.*

Coding Clarification

Documentation of an impaired heart muscle or left ventricular dysfunction does not indicate heart failure unless symptoms of fatigue, shortness of breath, and fluid retention are documented. Documentation indicating impaired heart muscle implies definitive causes, such as virus or drug abuse. Documentation of idiopathic or dilated congested cardiomyopathy indicates only that there is four-chamber enlargement of the heart, which may occur without heart failure. Classify compensated and decompensated heart failure to 428.0.

Ventricular Dysfunction: This condition is not a cardiac arrhythmia. The alphabetic index entry, Dysfunction, heart 427.9, refers to dysrhythmia. The appropriate code for ventricular dysfunction, if a more definitive diagnosis cannot be established, is 428.9 *Unspecified heart failure*.

If the congestive heart failure occurs as a result of the patient noncompliance to diet, medication, or dialysis treatment, code the congestive heart failure (428.0) and use an additional code to identify the noncompliance (V15.81).

Etiology: In general, heart failure is defined as an abnormality of heart function and is accountable for the inability of the heart to pump blood at a rate adequate for tissue metabolism or can do so only from an abnormal filling pressure.

Congestive heart failure (CHF) is a typical manifestation of an underlying organic heart condition (e.g., arteriosclerotic, rheumatic, congenital) defined as the inability of the heart to supply adequate output relative to the body's requirement. Uncompensated congestive heart failure results in pulmonary edema.

Heart Transplant Complications: If the patient develops an illness that affects the transplanted organ it is coded as a complication of the transplanted organ (e.g., 996.83 *Complications of transplanted organ, heart*), and an additional diagnosis code is used to identify the illness that affected the organ (e.g., 428.0 *Congestive heart failure, unspecified*).

Myocardial Infarction with CHF: Congestive heart failure is a typical manifestation of a myocardial infarction and would be sequenced as a secondary diagnosis if an infarction is detected.

Pleural Effusion: Pleural effusion is typically noted in cases of heart failure because there is usually some collection of fluid in the pleural space. If pleural effusion is identified with heart failure, it should only be coded if it is specifically evaluated and treated.

Rheumatic: When heart failure is present with rheumatic aortic and mitral valve insufficiency, the heart failure is always classified as rheumatic.

Two codes are required to report congestive heart failure with systolic or diastolic heart failure, since congestive heart failure is not an inherent part of either condition.

Types of Heart Failure

Right vs. Left-sided Heart Failure

- Right-sided heart failure is caused by liver hypertrophy, systemic venous congestion, pitting edema, or ascites due to congestion of fluid behind the left ventricle.
- Left-sided heart failure is demonstrated by paroxysmal nocturnal dyspnea, cardiac asthma, dyspnea, orthopnea, and/or acute pulmonary edema caused by the collection of excess fluid behind the left ventricle.

Low Output vs. High Output Heart Failure

- Low output can be defined as either left or right-sided heart failure. It may be due to ischemic heart disease, cardiomyopathy, hypertension, or valvular or pericardial disease.
- High output can develop with anemia, hyperthyroidism, arteriovenous fistulas, or beriberi and Paget's disease.

Compensated vs. Decompensated Heart Failure

- Compensated heart failure describes the state achieved when the heart develops compensatory mechanisms on a chronic basis such as increased force of contraction, elevated atrial pressures, hypertrophy, and ventricular dilation.
- Decompensated heart failure occurs when these measures are unable to handle the additional workload.

Coding Scenario

A patient is admitted with congestive heart failure and congestive cardiomyopathy.

> Code assignment: 428.0 *Congestive heart failure, unspecified* and 425.4 *Other primary cardiomyopathies*

A patient is admitted in decompensated congestive failure resulting from end-stage cardiomyopathy. Laboratory findings are: metabolic acidosis, elevated BUN/creatine, and elevated liver enzymes. The physician diagnosis both renal and heart failure and liver shock.

> Code assignment: 428.0 *Congestive heart failure, unspecified,* is the principal diagnosis. Assign 570 *Subacute necrosis of the liver* for the liver shock. Assign code 584.9 *Acute renal failure, unspecified* and 425.4 *Other primary cardiomyopathies*

A patient arrives in the emergency department with acute respiratory failure. The patient is found to have cardiogenic pulmonary edema and respiratory failure. Subsequently the patient is intubated in the emergency department and then admitted for treatment.

> Code assignment: 518.81 *Acute respiratory failure* and 428.0 *Congestive heart failure, unspecified*

429 Ill-defined descriptions and complications of heart disease

429.0	Unspecified myocarditis — (Use additional code to identify presence of arteriosclerosis) — *inflammation, cause unknown, but not rheumatic*
429.1	Myocardial degeneration — (Use additional code to identify presence of arteriosclerosis) — *Beau's syndrome, softening, fatty, mural, muscular disease*
429.2	Unspecified cardiovascular disease — (Use additional code to identify presence of arteriosclerosis) — *ASCVD, specifics unknown*
429.3	Cardiomegaly — *enlargement of the heart; dilation, hypertrophy, dilatation*
429.4	Functional disturbances following cardiac surgery — *or due to prosthesis* **AHA:** Nov-Dec, 1985, 6; Q2, 2002, 12
429.5	Rupture of chordae tendineae — *torn tissue between heart valves and papillary muscles*
429.6	Rupture of papillary muscle — *torn muscle between chordae tendineae and heart wall*
429.71	Acquired cardiac septal defect — (Use additional code to identify the associated myocardial infarction: with onset of 8 weeks of less, 410.00-410.92; with onset of more than 8 weeks, 414.8)
429.79	Other certain sequelae of myocardial infarction, not elsewhere classified — (Use additional code to identify the associated myocardial infarction: with onset of less, 410.00-410.92; with onset of more than 8 weeks, 414.8) — *mural thrombus following MI, not otherwise specified* **AHA:** Q3, 1989, 5; Q1, 1992, 10
429.81	Other disorders of papillary muscle — *atrophy, degeneration, dysfunction, incompetence, incoordination, scarring*
429.82	Hyperkinetic heart disease — *abnormally increased motor function of the heart*
429.83	Takotsubo syndrome — *broken heart syndrome; reversible left ventricular dysfunction following sudden emotional stress; stress-induced cardiomyopathy; transient left ventricular apical ballooning syndrome*

Takotsubo syndrome is a form of stress cardiomyopathy, also known as broken heart syndrome and left ventricular apical balloon syndrome. The majority of cases are diagnosed in women. Heart muscles are temporarily weakened in patients without a known history of coronary artery disease, and the symptoms can easily be confused with a heart attack. A sudden, massive surge of adrenalin stuns the heart, greatly reducing the ability to pump blood. The common treatment of administering adrenalin to support blood pressure during a heart attack is therefore not appropriate for this condition.

Takotsubo syndrome is a reversible left ventricular dysfunction in patients without coronary disease, precipitated by emotional or physiological stress. The word "tako-tsubo" refers to a Japanese fishing pot used for trapping octopus. The shape of this pot mimics that of the heart abnormalities characteristic in the syndrome. Clinical signs and symptoms include chest pain that mimics acute myocardial infarction, ST-segment elevation in the precordial leads similar to AMI, slight elevation of cardiac enzyme and biomarker levels, and transient apical systolic left ventricular dysfunction or failure. An intense tako-tsubo episode is usually transient though severe, but it can become lethal if not properly treated and allowed to progress to cardiogenic shock.

429.89	Other ill-defined heart disease — *not specified elsewhere, including carditis, hemorrhage of heart, ventricular asynergy, ventricular dyssynergia* **AHA:** Q1, 1992, 10; Q3, 2005, 14; Q2, 2006, 18
429.9	Unspecified heart disease — *unknown type or site* **AHA:** Q1, 1993, 19

Coding Clarification
The inclusion terms listed with code 429.83 indicate the reversible nature of this stress-induced syndrome, as opposed to the non-stress-induced, more permanent ventricular dysfunctions associated with cardiomyopathy (category 425), heart failure (category 428), or hypertensive heart disease (categories 402 and 404).

430–438 Cerebrovascular Disease

This section of ICD-9-CM classifies the acute, organic conditions of the cerebrovascular system. Conditions coded to this section are nontraumatic in origin and include hemorrhages, thromboses, embolisms, transient cerebral ischemia, other ill-defined cerebrovascular diseases, and the late effects of cerebrovascular disease.

430 Subarachnoid hemorrhage
AHA: March-April, 1985, 6; Q2, 1989, 8; Q3, 1990, 3; Q3, 1991, 10; Q1, 1993, 27; Q4, 2004, 77

A subarachnoid hemorrhage is an extravasation of blood into the subarachnoid space. The episodes usually are sudden in nature and account for 5 to 10 percent of all cerebrovascular accidents. The etiology may be secondary to head trauma and classified to

Diseases of the Circulatory System

the injury chapter, or due to primary disease such as arteriosclerotic aneurysm, arteriovenous malformation, or hemorrhagic diathesis.

Coding Clarification
This rubric excludes syphilitic ruptured cerebral aneurysm (094.87).

431 Intracerebral hemorrhage OK
AHA: March-April, 1985, 6; Q2, 1989, 8; Q3, 1990, 3; Q3, 1991, 10; Q1, 1993, 27; Q4, 2004, 77

An intracerebral hemorrhage is a spontaneous extravasation of blood within the brain. Etiologies include hypertension with microaneurysmal formation, bleeding diathesis (leukemia, thrombocytopenia, hemophilia), disseminated intravascular coagulation, anticoagulant therapy, liver disease, cerebral amyloid angiopathy, AV malformation, and brain neoplasms.

432 Other and unspecified intracranial hemorrhage
AHA: March-April, 1985, 6; Q2, 1989, 8; Q3, 1990, 3; Q3, 1991, 10; Q1, 1993, 27; Q4, 2004, 77

This rubric classifies nontraumatic extradural (epidural) and subdural hemorrhage of the cerebrovascular system.

432.0	Nontraumatic extradural hemorrhage — (Use additional code to identify presence of hypertension) — *bleeding between the skull and the lining of the brain* AHA: March-April, 1985, 6; Q2, 1989, 8; Q3, 1990, 3; Q3, 1991, 10; Q1, 1993, 27
432.1	Subdural hemorrhage — (Use additional code to identify presence of hypertension) — *bleeding between the outermost and other layers of the lining of the brain* AHA: March-April, 1985, 6; Q2, 1989, 8; Q3, 1990, 3; Q3, 1991, 10; Q1, 1993, 27
432.9	Unspecified intracranial hemorrhage — (Use additional code to identify presence of hypertension) — *unknown site* AHA: March-April, 1985, 6; Q2, 1989, 8; Q3, 1990, 3; Q3, 1991, 10; Q1, 1993, 27

Coding Clarification
Excluded from this rubric is extradural and subdural hemorrhage as a spinal cord vascular disease.

433 Occlusion and stenosis of precerebral arteries
AHA: March-April, 1985, 6; Q2, 1989, 8; Q3, 1990, 3,16; Q3, 1991, 10; Q1, 1993, 27; Q2, 1995, 14

The precerebral arteries — basilar, carotid, and vertebral — extend from the aortic arch. Blood is supplied to the brain by the internal carotid arteries and vertebral arteries. The right and left vertebral arteries come together at the base of the brain to form the basilar artery. The right common carotid originates in the innominate artery and the left common carotid is normally the second branch from the aortic arch. The common carotids have no branches until their terminal bifurcation. The internal carotid artery ascends through the base of the skull to give rise to the anterior and middle cerebral arteries. The external carotid artery supplies blood to the face and scalp. The vertebral arteries arise from the subclavian arteries and emerge from the posterior base of the skull to form the basilar artery. Occasionally, the basilar splits into two vessels that reunite. The vertebral artery takes blood to the basilar artery, and from there the blood goes to the circle of Willis, which controls blood pressure in the brain and allows a continued supply of oxygenated blood to the brain in the event that a vessel becomes occluded.

Syndromes of the aortic arch, also referred to as vertebral-basilar artery disease, carotid artery occlusive syndrome, and subclavian steal syndrome, are associated with structural defects resulting from atherosclerosis, trauma, blood clots, or congenital abnormalities of vessel structure. Atherosclerotic occlusive disease of the external portion of the carotid artery is the most common cause of a stroke. Strokes can result from a blocked blood vessel due to an embolism or a constriction or narrowing of an artery in the head or neck (stenosis). Bleeding of a blood vessel is called hemorrhagic stroke. Symptoms include neurologic changes (i.e., dizziness, blurred vision, or weakness), blood pressure changes, and reduced pulse. An embolism can obstruct the vessels causing damage from the lack of blood supply reaching the brain and can occur as a result of surgery if multiple punctures are required or if an atherosclerotic plaque becomes dislodged by the catheter or guidewire. Occlusion of the posterior cerebral arteries can result in loss of pain information from the face and vertigo. Occlusion of the superior cerebellar arteries interferes with the major output of the cerebellum.

The following fifth-digit subclassification is for use with categories 433 and 434:

0   without mention of cerebral infarction

1   with cerebral infarction

433.0 ✓5th Occlusion and stenosis of basilar artery — (Use additional code to identify presence of hypertension) — *embolism, narrowing, obstruction, thrombosis*
AHA: Q4, 2004, 77; March-April, 1985, 6; Q2, 1989, 8; Q3, 1990, 3,16; Q3, 1991, 10; Q1, 1993, 27; Q2, 1995, 14

433.1 ✓5th Occlusion and stenosis of carotid artery — (Use additional code to identify presence of hypertension) — *embolism, narrowing, obstruction, thrombosis*
AHA: Q4, 2004, 77; March-April, 1985, 6; Q2, 1989, 8; Q3, 1990, 3,16; Q3, 1991, 10; Q1, 1993, 27; Q2, 1995, 14; Q1, 2000, 16; Q1, 2006, 17

433.2 ✓5th Occlusion and stenosis of vertebral artery — (Use additional code to identify presence of hypertension) — *embolism, narrowing, obstruction, thrombosis*
AHA: March-April, 1985, 6; Q2, 1989, 8; Q3, 1990, 3,16; Q3, 1991, 10; Q1, 1993, 27; Q2, 1995, 144

433.3 ✓5th Occlusion and stenosis of multiple and bilateral precerebral arteries — (Use additional code to identify presence of hypertension) — *embolism, narrowing, obstruction, thrombosis*
AHA: March-April, 1985, 6; Q2, 1989, 8; Q3, 1990, 3,16; Q3, 1991, 10; Q1, 1993, 27; Q2, 1995, 14; Q2, 2002, 19; Q1, 2006, 17

433.8 ✓5th Occlusion and stenosis of other specified precerebral artery — (Use additional code to identify presence of hypertension) — *pontine, meningeal, hypophyseal, communicating posterior, choroidal, cerebellar, internal auditory, anterior spinal artery; embolism, narrowing, obstruction, thrombosis*
AHA: March-April, 1985, 6; Q2, 1989, 8; Q3, 1990, 3,16; Q3, 1991, 10; Q1, 1993, 27; Q2, 1995, 14

433.9 ✓5th Occlusion and stenosis of unspecified precerebral artery — (Use additional code to identify presence of hypertension) — *embolism, narrowing, obstruction, thrombosis; unknown site*
AHA: Q4, 2004, 77-78; March-April, 1985, 6; Q2, 1989, 8; Q3, 1990, 3,16; Q3, 1991, 10; Q1, 1993, 27; Q2, 1995, 14

Coding Scenario
A patient is admitted via the emergency department with episodes of syncope, possible CVA. A bilateral cerebral arteriogram identifies bilateral carotid occlusions. The left carotid artery identifies a 75 percent occlusion and the right carotid at 95 percent occlusion. The patient undergoes a bilateral endarterectomy and is discharged in good condition. The final diagnosis is bilateral carotid occlusion.

Code assignment: 433.30 *Occlusion and stenosis of multiple and bilateral precerebral arteries, without mention of cerebral infarction*

434 Occlusion of cerebral arteries
AHA: March-April, 1985, 6; Q2, 1989, 8; Q3, 1990, 3; Q3, 1991, 10; Q1, 1993, 27; Q2, 1995, 14

Cerebrovascular accident (CVA) is a vague term often used to describe a condition best classified to this category.

The following fifth-digit subclassification is for use with categories 433 and 434:
0   without mention of cerebral infarction
1   with cerebral infarction

434.0 ✓5th Cerebral thrombosis — (Use additional code to identify presence of hypertension) — *blood clot*
AHA: March-April, 1985, 6; Q2, 1989, 8; Q3, 1990, 3; Q3, 1991, 10; Q1, 1993, 27; Q2, 1995, 14; Q4, 2004, 77

434.1 ✓5th Cerebral embolism — (Use additional code to identify presence of hypertension) — *complete blockage*
AHA: March-April, 1985, 6; Q2, 1989, 8; Q3, 1990, 3; Q3, 1991, 10; Q1, 1993, 27; Q2, 1995, 14; Q3, 1997, 11; Q4, 2004, 77

434.9 ✓5th Unspecified cerebral artery occlusion — (Use additional code to identify presence of hypertension) — *extent unknown*
AHA: March-April, 1985, 6; Q2, 1989, 8; Q3, 1990, 3; Q3, 1991, 10; Q1, 1993, 27; Q2, 1995, 14; Q4, 1998, 87; Q4, 2004, 77-78

Documentation Issues
Unspecified CVA and stroke have been re-indexed to default to 434.91 instead of 436. For strokes and CVAs that are specified as hemorrhagic, embolic, or thrombotic, the specific codes should be assigned.

When the physician documentation states that the patient had a lacunar infarction, use code 434.91 *Cerebral artery occlusion, unspecified, with cerebral infarction*. Lacunar infarctions occur in small vessels that are due to occlusion of branches of the middle cerebral, posterior cerebral, and basilar arteries.

Coding Clarification
Cerebral Artery: Occlusion of cerebral arteries is classified with a code from category 434 *Occlusion of cerebral arteries*. Review the medical record for information identifying if the occlusion is due to thrombosis (434.0x) or embolism (434.1x). If unspecified, use code 434.9x. Fifth digits are required with category 434 to identify if the event occurred with or without a cerebral infarction during the current admission.

Diseases of the Circulatory System

435 Transient cerebral ischemia
AHA: March-April, 1985, 6; Q2, 1989, 8; Q3, 1990, 3; Q3, 1991, 10; Q1, 1993, 27

Transient cerebral ischemia describes episodes of focal neurological symptoms. Its most common form is known as a transient ischemic attack (TIA). A typical TIA lasts between two and 15 minutes and always resolves within 24 hours. Commonly, the etiology of the TIA is embolization due to cardiac causes such as rheumatic heart disease, cardiac dysrhythmias, mitral valve disease, infective endocarditis, mural thrombi complicating myocardial infarction, and myxoma.

This rubric includes reversible ischemic neurological deficits (RIND), if the patient's neurological deficits are associated with TIA and abate within 24 hours.

435.0	Basilar artery syndrome — (Use additional code to identify presence of hypertension)
435.1	Vertebral artery syndrome — (Use additional code to identify presence of hypertension) — *Verbiest's syndrome* **AHA:** March-April, 1985, 6; Q2, 1989, 8; Q3, 1990, 3; Q3, 1991, 10; Q1, 1993, 27
435.2	Subclavian steal syndrome — (Use additional code to identify presence of hypertension)
435.3	Vertebrobasilar artery syndrome — (Use additional code to identify presence of hypertension)
435.8	Other specified transient cerebral ischemias — (Use additional code to identify presence of hypertension) — *carotid artery insufficiency* **AHA:** March-April, 1985, 6; Q2, 1989, 8; Q3, 1990, 3; Q3, 1991, 10; Q1, 1993, 27
435.9	Unspecified transient cerebral ischemia — (Use additional code to identify presence of hypertension) — *TIA, Alvarez syndrome, impending cerebrovascular accident* **AHA:** March-April, 1985, 6; Nov-Dec, 1985, 12; Q2, 1989, 8; Q3, 1990, 3; Q3, 1991, 10; Q1, 1993, 27

Coding Clarification

RIND also may be associated with other conditions in rubrics 430-437 and should be coded to the underlying condition causing the deficits. RIND may require a second code to classify the specific neurological deficit and the appropriate code from categories 430-437.

Coding Scenario

A patient is admitted with left leg weakness and facial numbness. The physician's final diagnosis indicates transient ischemic attack with RIND. The discharge summary identifies that the neurological deficits have subsided with the exception of minimal weakness.

Code assignment: 435.9 *Unspecified transient cerebral ischemia*

436 Acute, but ill-defined, cerebrovascular disease
AHA: March-April, 1985, 6; Q2, 1989, 8; Q3, 1990, 3; Q3, 1991, 10; Q1, 1993, 27; Q4, 1999, 3; Q4, 2004, 77

Wallenberg syndrome is characterized by difficulty in swallowing and hoarseness due to paralysis of the ipsilateral vocal cord and, in some cases, partial loss of the sense of taste due to associated affects on the tongue. The glossopharyngeal (IX) & vagus (X) are the primary cranial nerves involved in this syndrome. Occlusion of the posterior inferior cerebellar artery (PICA) leads to damage to the posterior region of the medulla, which explains the name "lateral medullary plate syndrome" often used to refer to this disorder.

Documentation Issues

Code 436 should never be used with a code from category 430-435.

Unspecified CVA and stroke have been re-indexed to default to 434.91 instead of 436. For strokes and CVAs that are specified as hemorrhagic, embolic, or thrombotic, the specific codes should be assigned.

437 Other and ill-defined cerebrovascular disease
AHA: March-April, 1985, 6; Q2, 1989, 8; Q3, 1990, 3; Q3, 1991, 10; Q1, 1993, 27

437.0	Cerebral atherosclerosis — (Use additional code to identify presence of hypertension) — *deposits narrowing arteries that branch into the brain* **AHA:** March-April, 1985, 6; Q2, 1989, 8; Q3, 1990, 3; Q3, 1991, 10; Q1, 1993, 27
437.1	Other generalized ischemic cerebrovascular disease — (Use additional code to identify presence of hypertension) — *chronic cerebral ischemia, acute cerebrovascular insufficiency not otherwise specified* **AHA:** March-April, 1985, 6; Q2, 1989, 8; Q3, 1990, 3; Q3, 1991, 10; Q1, 1993, 27
437.2	Hypertensive encephalopathy — (Use additional code to identify presence of hypertension) — *brain disease caused by high blood pressure* **AHA:** July-Aug, 1984, 14; March-April, 1985, 6; Q2, 1989, 8; Q3, 1990, 3; Q3, 1991, 10; Q1, 1993, 27
437.3	Cerebral aneurysm, nonruptured — (Use additional code to identify presence of hypertension) — *dilation of artery in the brain* **AHA:** March-April, 1985, 6; Q2, 1989, 8; Q3, 1990, 3; Q3, 1991, 10; Q1, 1993, 27

Coders' Desk Reference for Diagnoses

437.4 Cerebral arteritis — (Use additional code to identify presence of hypertension) — *inflammation of artery within the brain*
AHA: March-April, 1985, 6; Q2, 1989, 8; Q3, 1990, 3; Q3, 1991, 10; Q1, 1993, 27; Q4, 1999, 21

437.5 Moyamoya disease — (Use additional code to identify presence of hypertension) — *tiny neovacularizations in patients with ischemia*
AHA: March-April, 1985, 6; Q2, 1989, 8; Q3, 1990, 3; Q3, 1991, 10; Q1, 1993, 27

437.6 Nonpyogenic thrombosis of intracranial venous sinus — (Use additional code to identify presence of hypertension)

437.7 Transient global amnesia — (Use additional code to identify presence of hypertension) — *temporary memory loss not due to psychological factors*
AHA: March-April, 1985, 6; Q2, 1989, 8; Q3, 1990, 3; Q3, 1991, 10; Q4, 1992, 20; Q1, 1993, 27

437.8 Other ill-defined cerebrovascular disease — (Use additional code to identify presence of hypertension) — *cerebral hyperemia, hypertensive paralysis, necrotic brain, mollities, cortical or cerebral quadriplegia*
AHA: March-April, 1985, 6; Q2, 1989, 8; Q3, 1990, 3; Q3, 1991, 10; Q1, 1993, 27

437.9 Unspecified cerebrovascular disease — (Use additional code to identify presence of hypertension)

438 Late effects of cerebrovascular disease
AHA: March-April, 1985, 6; March-April, 1986, 7; Nov-Dec, 1986, 12; Q2, 1989, 8; Q3, 1990, 3; Q3, 1991, 10; Q4, 1992, 21; Q1, 1993, 27; Q4, 1997, 35,37; Q4, 1998, 39,88; Q4, 1999, 4,6,7

This rubric classifies conditions in categories 430-437 as the cause of a late effect. ICD-9-CM classifies late effects of cerebrovascular disease according to the neurological deficit.

438.0 Cognitive deficits due to cerebrovascular disease — (Use additional code to identify presence of hypertension) — *thought, memory, perception*
AHA: March-April, 1985, 6; March-April, 1986, 7; Nov-Dec, 1986, 12; Q2, 1989, 8; Q3, 1990, 3; Q3, 1991, 10; Q4, 1992, 21; Q1, 1993, 27; Q4, 1997, 35,37; Q4, 1998, 39,88; Q4, 1999, 4,6,7

438.10 Unspecified speech and language deficit due to cerebrovascular disease — (Use additional code to identify presence of hypertension)

438.11 Aphasia due to cerebrovascular disease — (Use additional code to identify presence of hypertension) — *speech loss or deficit*
AHA: March-April, 1985, 6; March-April, 1986, 7; Nov-Dec, 1986, 12; Q2, 1989, 8; Q3, 1990, 3; Q3, 1991, 10; Q4, 1992, 21; Q1, 1993, 27; Q4, 1997, 36; Q4, 1997, 35,37; Q4, 1998, 39,88; Q4, 1999, 4,6,7; Q4, 2003, 105

438.12 Dysphasia due to cerebrovascular disease — (Use additional code to identify presence of hypertension) — *inability to organize words in their appropriate order*
AHA: March-April, 1985, 6; March-April, 1986, 7; Nov-Dec, 1986, 12; Q2, 1989, 8; Q3, 1990, 3; Q3, 1991, 10; Q4, 1992, 21; Q1, 1993, 27; Q4, 1997, 35,37; Q4, 1998, 39,88; Q4, 1999, 3,9; Q4, 1999, 4,6,7

438.19 Other speech and language deficits due to cerebrovascular disease — (Use additional code to identify presence of hypertension) — *not otherwise specified*
AHA: March-April, 1985, 6; March-April, 1986, 7; Nov-Dec, 1986, 12; Q2, 1989, 8; Q3, 1990, 3; Q3, 1991, 10; Q4, 1992, 21; Q1, 1993, 27; Q4, 1997, 35,37; Q4, 1998, 39,88; Q4, 1999, 4,6,7

438.20 Hemiplegia affecting unspecified side due to cerebrovascular disease — (Use additional code to identify presence of hypertension)

438.21 Hemiplegia affecting dominant side due to cerebrovascular disease — (Use additional code to identify presence of hypertension)

438.22 Hemiplegia affecting nondominant side due to cerebrovascular disease — (Use additional code to identify presence of hypertension)

438.30 Monoplegia of upper limb affecting unspecified side due to cerebrovascular disease — (Use additional code to identify presence of hypertension)

438.31 Monoplegia of upper limb affecting dominant side due to cerebrovascular disease — (Use additional code to identify presence of hypertension)

438.32 Monoplegia of upper limb affecting nondominant side due to cerebrovascular disease — (Use additional code to identify presence of hypertension)

438.40 Monoplegia of lower limb affecting unspecified side due to cerebrovascular disease — (Use additional code to identify presence of hypertension)

438.41 Monoplegia of lower limb affecting dominant side due to cerebrovascular disease — (Use additional code to identify presence of hypertension)

438.42 Monoplegia of lower limb affecting nondominant side due to cerebrovascular disease — (Use additional code to identify presence of hypertension)

438.50 Other paralytic syndrome affecting unspecified side due to cerebrovascular disease — (Use additional code to identify type of paralytic syndrome: 344.81, 344.00-344.09. Use additional code to identify presence of hypertension)

438.51 Other paralytic syndrome affecting dominant side due to cerebrovascular disease — (Use additional code to identify type of paralytic syndrome: 344.81, 344.00-344.09. Use additional code to identify presence of hypertension)

Diseases of the Circulatory System

438.52	Other paralytic syndrome affecting nondominant side due to cerebrovascular disease — (Use additional code to identify type of paralytic syndrome: 344.81, 344.00-344.09. Use additional code to identify presence of hypertension)
438.53	Other paralytic syndrome, bilateral — (Use additional code to identify type of paralytic syndrome: 344.81, 344.00-344.09. Use additional code to identify presence of hypertension)
438.6	Alteration of sensations as late effect of cerebrovascular disease — (Use additional code to identify the altered sensation. Use additional code to identify presence of hypertension)
438.7	Disturbance of vision as late effect of cerebrovascular disease — (Use additional code to identify the visual disturbance. Use additional code to identify presence of hypertension)
438.81	Apraxia due to cerebrovascular disease — (Use additional code to identify presence of hypertension) — *inability to properly use an object or carry out normal tasks* AHA: March-April, 1985, 6; March-April, 1986, 7; Nov-Dec, 1986, 12; Q2, 1989, 8; Q3, 1990, 3; Q3, 1991, 10; Q4, 1992, 21; Q1, 1993, 27; Q4, 1997, 35,37; Q4, 1998, 39,88; Q4, 1999, 4,6,7
438.82	Dysphagia due to cerebrovascular disease — (Use additional code to identify presence of hypertension) — *difficulty in swallowing* AHA: March-April, 1985, 6; March-April, 1986, 7; Nov-Dec, 1986, 12; Q2, 1989, 8; Q3, 1990, 3; Q3, 1991, 10; Q4, 1992, 21; Q1, 1993, 27; Q4, 1997, 35,37; Q4, 1998, 39,88; Q4, 1999, 4,6,7
438.83	Facial weakness as late effect of cerebrovascular disease — (Use additional code to identify presence of hypertension) — *facial droop* AHA: March-April, 1985, 6; March-April, 1986, 7; Nov-Dec, 1986, 12; Q2, 1989, 8; Q3, 1990, 3; Q3, 1991, 10; Q4, 1992, 21; Q1, 1993, 27; Q4, 1997, 35,37; Q4, 1998, 39,88; Q4, 1999, 4,6,7
438.84	Ataxia as late effect of cerebrovascular disease — (Use additional code to identify presence of hypertension)
438.85	Vertigo as late effect of cerebrovascular disease — (Use additional code to identify presence of hypertension)
438.89	Other late effects of cerebrovascular disease — (Use additional code to identify the late effect. Use additional code to identify presence of hypertension) — *not specified elsewhere* AHA: March-April, 1985, 6; March-April, 1986, 7; Nov-Dec, 1986, 12; Q2, 1989, 8; Q3, 1990, 3; Q3, 1991, 10; Q4, 1992, 21; Q1, 1993, 27; Q4, 1997, 35,37; Q4, 1998, 39; Q4, 1998, 39,88; Q4, 1999, 4,6,7; Q1, 2005, 13
438.9	Unspecified late effects of cerebrovascular disease due to cerebrovascular disease — (Use additional code to identify presence of hypertension)

Documentation Issues

If documentation only identifies a previous cerebrovascular accident but no residual neurological deficits are noted, use code V12.59 *Personal history of other diseases of the circulatory system*. Codes from category 438 are not appropriate if no residual neurologic deficit remains.

Coding Clarification

Excluded from this rubric is history of cerebrovascular disease when no neurological deficit is present as a late effect. The appropriate code in that case would be V12.59 *Personal history of other disease of the circulatory system*.

Assign a code from rubric 438 in addition to a code from 430-437 if the patient has a current CVA in addition to deficits from an old CVA.

Neurogenic Bladder: When neurogenic bladder occurs as a result of a cerebrovascular hemorrhage, thrombosis, infarction, or obstruction, it is reported with codes 438.89 *Other late effects of cerebrovascular disease* and 596.54 *Neurogenic bladder NOS*. Two codes are necessary since there is no specific combination code for this condition.

Official Inpatient Coding Guidelines: The residual condition or nature of the late effect is sequenced first, followed by the cause of the late effect, except in those few instances where the code for the late effect is followed by a manifestation code identified in the tabular list and the title of the late effect code has been expanded (at the fourth- and fifth-digit levels) to include the manifestation. Unlike other late effect codes, codes from category 438 should be assigned as principal/primary diagnosis when there is a late effect of CVA:

- Late Effect of Cerebrovascular Disease — Category 438 is used to indicate conditions classifiable to categories 430-437. The neurologic deficits caused by cerebrovascular disease may be present from the onset or may arise at any time after the onset of the condition classifiable to 430-437.

- Codes from category 438 may be assigned along with codes from 430-437, if the patient has a recurrent CVA and deficits from an old CVA. Assign code V12.59 (not a code from category 438) as an additional code for history of cerebrovascular disease when no neurologic deficits are present.

Do not assign a code from category 438 when a current diagnosis classifiable to the 430-437 series is present.

Coding Scenario
A 62-year-old male is seen for speech therapy of his aphasia. This patient has a history of a CVA five months ago.

> Code assignment: V57.3 *Care involving use of rehabilitation procedures, speech therapy* and 438.11 *Late effect of cerebrovascular disease, speech and language deficits, aphasia*

440-448 Diseases of Arteries, Arterioles, and Capillaries

This section includes conditions affecting the arteries, arterioles, and capillaries, including atherosclerosis, aneurysm, peripheral vascular disease, embolism and thrombosis, arteritis, and stricture.

440 Atherosclerosis

Atherosclerosis is a form of arteriosclerosis characterized by irregularly distributed atheromas accumulating within the tunica intima of arteries. The deposits are associated with calcification and fibrosis, reducing the size of the arterial lumen and resulting in obstructive ischemia.

440.0	Atherosclerosis of aorta — *atheroma, degeneration, endarteritis* **AHA:** Q4, 1988, 8; Q2, 1993, 7; Q2, 1993, 8
440.1	Atherosclerosis of renal artery — *atheroma, degeneration, endarteritis*
440.20	Atherosclerosis of native arteries of the extremities, unspecified — *unknown manifestations* **AHA:** March-April, 1987, 6; Q3, 1990, 15; Q4, 1992, 25; Q4, 1993, 27; Q4, 1994, 49
440.21	Atherosclerosis of native arteries of the extremities with intermittent claudication — *Charcot's due to atherosclerosis* **AHA:** March-April, 1987, 6; Q3, 1990, 15; Q4, 1992, 25; Q4, 1993, 27; Q4, 1994, 49
440.22	Atherosclerosis of native arteries of the extremities with rest pain
440.23	Atherosclerosis of native arteries of the extremities with ulceration — (Use additional code for any associated ulceration: 707.10-707.9)
440.24	Atherosclerosis of native arteries of the extremities with gangrene — (Use additional code for any associated ulceration: 707.10-707.9)
440.29	Other atherosclerosis of native arteries of the extremities — *not otherwise specified* **AHA:** March-April, 1987, 6; Q3, 1990, 15; Q4, 1992, 25; Q4, 1993, 27; Q4, 1994, 49
440.30	Atherosclerosis of unspecified bypass graft of extremities — *graft origin unknown* **AHA:** Q4, 1994, 49
440.31	Atherosclerosis of autologous vein bypass graft of extremities — *graft from patient* **AHA:** Q4, 1994, 49
440.32	Atherosclerosis of nonautologous biological bypass graft of extremities — *graft other than from patient* **AHA:** Q4, 1994, 49
440.8	Atherosclerosis of other specified arteries — *not otherwise specified; arteriosclerotic retinitis*
440.9	Generalized and unspecified atherosclerosis — *unknown or disseminated*

Documentation Issues
When documentation identifies that a patient with aortic atherosclerosis has an occlusion of the aortoiliac artery due to an embolus, two codes should be used: 444.0 *Arterial embolism and thrombosis of abdominal aorta* and 440.0 *Atherosclerosis of aorta*. Even though the index assumes aortic occlusions are thromboembolic, if the etiology is specified (e.g., atherosclerosis), then that condition should be coded.

If the documentation states that the patient has an aortoiliac artery occlusion due to a stricture in conjunction with aortic arteriosclerosis, two codes are required: 447.1 *Other disorders of arteries and arterioles, stricture of artery* and 440.0 *Atherosclerosis of aorta*.

When the documentation states gangrene of amputation stump and the patient has diabetic arteriosclerosis, obtain clarification from the physician as to the cause of the gangrene. If it is an actual complication of the amputation, use codes 997.62 *Amputation stump infection* and 785.4 *Gangrene*. If it is due to a natural progression of the diabetic arteriosclerotic disease, use codes 250.7x *Diabetes with peripheral circulatory diseases* and 440.24 *Atherosclerosis of native arteries of the extremities with gangrene*.

Coding Clarification
Peripheral: Arteriosclerosis (occlusive) of the extremities is reported with code 440.2x.

Combination Code Hierarchy: Fifth digits used with subcategory code 440.2 identify additional manifestations of the atherosclerotic peripheral vascular disease. These codes are listed by order of increasing priority. All patients classified to this subcategory who have gangrene (regardless whether they have rest pain, ulceration, and/or intermittent claudication) are coded to 440.24. Patients without gangrene but with ulceration (regardless of whether

Diseases of the Circulatory System

they have rest pain and/or intermittent claudication) are coded to 440.23. Patients without gangrene or ulceration, with rest pain (with or without intermittent claudication) are assigned code 440.22, and those with only intermittent claudication use code 440.21.

Diabetic Complication: Diabetic atherosclerosis of extremities is coded as 250.7x *Diabetes with peripheral circulatory disorders* and 440.2x *Atherosclerosis of native arteries of extremities.* If the diagnosis is diabetes with ischemic heart disease or cerebrovascular disease, they are coded as separate entities.

Gas Gangrene: Arteriosclerosis with gas gangrene is reported with two codes: 440.29 *Other atherosclerosis of native arteries of extremities* and 040.0 *Gas gangrene.* It is inappropriate to use code 440.24; this code only includes ischemic gangrene.

Coding Scenario

A patient is admitted for gangrene of the left leg secondary to diabetic arteriosclerosis. Record documentation identifies that the patient is Type I insulin dependent.

> Code assignment: 250.71 *Diabetes with peripheral circulatory disorders, Type I, not stated as uncontrolled* and 440.24 *Atherosclerosis of native arteries of the extremities with gangrene*

A patient is admitted to the hospital with leg pain and weakness. The final diagnosis indicates peripheral arteriosclerosis with rest pain and intermittent claudication.

> Code assignment: 440.22 *Atherosclerosis of native arteries of the extremities with rest pain*

A 49-year-old female is admitted for occlusion of peripheral artery bypass graft. Her history and physical report indicates that a nonautologous biological bypass graft was performed one year ago. The physician's documentation identifies the occlusion as a progression of the artherosclerotic disease.

> Code assignment: 440.32 *Atherosclerosis of nonautologous biological bypass graft of extremities*

A patient is admitted with a diagnosis of hypertension. The physician's final diagnosis at discharge is atherosclerosis of the aorta and generalized arteriosclerosis.

> Code assignment: 440.0 *Atherosclerosis of aorta,* and 440.9 *Generalized and unspecified atherosclerosis*

Inpatient consultation is provided for a 69-year-old female with pain and weakness in both legs. The patient undergoes a peripheral vascular plethysmography for confirmation of arterial occlusion. The physician's diagnosis states atherosclerosis of bilateral extremities with intermittent claudication.

> Code assignment: 440.21 *Atherosclerosis of native arteries of the extremities with intermittent claudication*

A 53-year-old male is admitted for atherosclerosis. The discharge summary states the final diagnosis as aortoiliac artery occlusion secondary to stricture and aortic atherosclerosis.

> Code assignment: 447.1 *Other disorders of arteries and arterioles, stricture of artery* and 440.0 *Atherosclerosis of aorta*

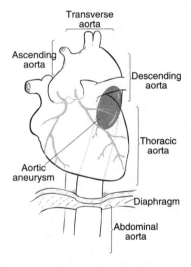

441 Aortic aneurysm and dissection

Aortic aneurysms are circumscribed dilations of the aorta or a blood-containing tumor connecting directly within the lumen of the aorta. Generally, an aneurysm is considered clinically significant if its diameter is twice that of the normal artery. A dissecting aneurysm is characterized by blood entering through a split or tear in the intima of the artery wall or by interstitial hemorrhage. Dissecting aortic aneurysms may rupture, constituting a medical emergency. This condition is most frequently seen in men between 40 and 60 years of age.

Coders' Desk Reference for Diagnoses

Code	Description
441.00	Dissecting aortic aneurysm (any part), unspecified site — *dilation and split of aorta lining, site unknown* **AHA:** Q4, 1989, 10
441.01	Dissecting aortic aneurysm (any part), thoracic — *dilation and split of aorta lining in the chest cavity* **AHA:** Q4, 1989, 10
441.02	Dissecting aortic aneurysm (any part), abdominal — *dilation and split of aorta lining in the abdomen* **AHA:** Q4, 1989, 10
441.03	Dissecting aortic aneurysm (any part), thoracoabdominal — *dilation and split of aorta lining in chest and abdomen* **AHA:** Q4, 1989, 10
441.1	Thoracic aneurysm, ruptured — *dilation and tear in aorta in chest*
441.2	Thoracic aneurysm without mention of rupture — *dilation in aorta in chest* **AHA:** Q3, 1992, 10
441.3	Abdominal aneurysm, ruptured — *dilation and tear of aorta in abdomen*
441.4	Abdominal aneurysm without mention of rupture — *dilation of aorta in abdomen* **AHA:** Q3, 1992, 10; Q1, 1999, 15,16,17; Q4, 2000, 64
441.5	Aortic aneurysm of unspecified site, ruptured — *dilation and tear of aorta in unknown site*
441.6	Thoracoabdominal aneurysm, ruptured — *dilation and tear of aorta in abdomen and chest*
441.7	Thoracoabdominal aneurysm without mention of rupture — *dilation of aorta in abdomen and chest* **AHA:** Q2, 2006, 16
441.9	Aortic aneurysm of unspecified site without mention of rupture — *dilation of aorta, site and rupture status unknown*

Documentation Issues
If the documentation states Type I, Type II, Type III abdominal aortic aneurysm, the condition is still classified to 441.0x *Dissection of aorta*. The fifth-digit for this category identifies the site of the aneurysm (e.g., abdominal, thoracic, thoracoabdominal).

Coding Clarification
Aneurysms of Adjoining Sites: When an aneurysm develops at an adjoining site, code each site separately unless a code is 44provided that identifies the adjoining site. For example, aortoiliac aneurysm requires two codes: 441.4 and 442.2; for a dissecting thoracoabdominal aneurysm one code is required: 441.03.

Coding Scenario
A 68-year-old female patient was admitted with a possible myocardial infarction. After study, the patient was diagnosed with a dissecting thoracoabdominal aortic aneurysm.

Code assignment: 441.03 *Dissection of aorta, thoracoabdominal*

A 43-year-old patient is admitted with thoracic aneurysm and hypertension. The physician documents the final diagnosis as a dissecting aneurysm of the thoracic aorta with nonmalignant systemic hypertension.

Code assignment: 441.01 *Dissection of aorta, thoracic* and 401.1 *Essential hypertension, benign*

442 Other aneurysm

Code	Description
442.0	Aneurysm of artery of upper extremity — *dilation; brachial, radial, interosseous, ulnar, superficial palmar arch*
442.1	Aneurysm of renal artery — *dilation*
442.2	Aneurysm of iliac artery — *dilation* **AHA:** Q1, 1999, 16,17
442.3	Aneurysm of artery of lower extremity — *dilation; femoral, popliteal artery, medial plantar, posterior tibial, anterior tibial* **AHA:** Q1, 1999, 16; Q3, 2002, 24-26
442.81	Aneurysm of artery of neck — *dilation; internal, external, common carotid*
442.82	Aneurysm of subclavian artery — *dilation*
442.83	Aneurysm of splenic artery — *dilation*
442.84	Aneurysm of other visceral artery — *dilation; celiac, gastroduodenal, hepatic, pancreaticoduodenal, superior mesenteric, gastroepiploic*
442.89	Aneurysm of other specified artery — *dilation; mediastinal, spinal artery*
442.9	Other aneurysm of unspecified site

443 Other peripheral vascular disease

Code	Description
443.0	Raynaud's syndrome — (Use additional code to identify gangrene, 785.4) — *construction of arteries of the digits caused by cold or stress*
443.1	Thromboangiitis obliterans (Buerger's disease) — *inflammation and swelling in distal arteries, causing occlusions*
443.21	Dissection of carotid artery
443.22	Dissection of iliac artery
443.23	Dissection of renal artery
443.24	Dissection of vertebral artery
443.29	Dissection of other artery
443.81	Peripheral angiopathy in diseases classified elsewhere — (Code first underlying disease, 250.7) — *secondary to underlying disease* **AHA:** Q3, 1991, 10; Q1, 2004, 14
443.82	Erythromelalgia **AHA:** Q4, 2005, 73
443.89	Other peripheral vascular disease — *not otherwise specified, Crocq's, Gerhardt's, Weir Mitchell's disease, acrocyanosis, erythrocyanosis, Schultz's acroparesthesia, Nothnagel's vasomotor acroparesthesia*

Diseases of the Circulatory System

443.9 Unspecified peripheral vascular disease

Coding Clarification
Erythromelalgia: A rare condition in which maldistribution of blood flow causes redness, pain, increased skin temperature, and burning sensations in various parts of the body, most frequently occurring in the extremities but also the torso, ears, and face. The condition may manifest itself on one or both sides of the body, externally as well as affecting internal organs. Heat exposure may trigger a flare. Patients generally have heat intolerance, sensitivity to alcohol, and spicy foods. Body positioning may also contribute to experiencing symptoms. Onset and progression vary from gradual to rapid and severity may be mild to debilitating episodes. The cause of primary erythromelalgia is unknown.

Coding Scenario
An elderly patient is transferred from an extended care facility for treatment of a decubitus ulcer of the buttock. The physician also identifies the patient as a Type I insulin dependent diabetic with related progressive peripheral vascular disease.

Code assignment: 707.05 *Decubitus ulcer, buttock*, 250.71 *Diabetes with peripheral circulatory disorders, Type I, not stated as uncontrolled*, and 443.81 *Peripheral angiopathy in diseases classified elsewhere*

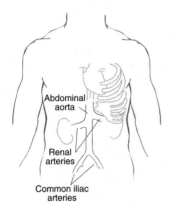

444 Arterial embolism and thrombosis
AHA: Q4, 1990, 27; Q2, 1992, 11

An arterial embolism is a partial or complete obstruction of an artery due to the migration of a blood clot or other foreign material. An arterial thrombosis is the formation of a blood clot within the lumen of an artery. In each case, infarction of the tissues perfused by the artery is a potential complication.

444.0 Embolism and thrombosis of abdominal aorta — *aortic bifurcation and Leriche's syndromes, saddle embolus, aortoiliac obstruction*
AHA: Q4, 1990, 27; Q2, 1992, 11; Q2, 1993, 7

444.1 Embolism and thrombosis of thoracic aorta — *embolism of thrombosis of thoracic aorta*
AHA: Q4, 1990, 27; Q2, 1992, 11

444.21 Embolism and thrombosis of arteries of upper extremity — *brachial, radial, interosseous, ulnar, superficial palmar arch*
AHA: March-April, 1987, 6; Q4, 1990, 27; Q2, 1992, 11

444.22 Embolism and thrombosis of arteries of lower extremity — *femoral, popliteal artery, medial plantar, posterior tibial, anterior tibial*
AHA: March-April, 1987, 6; Q3, 1990, 16; Q4, 1990, 27; Q2, 1992, 11; Q1, 2003, 17; Q3, 2003, 10

444.81 Embolism and thrombosis of iliac artery

444.89 Embolism and thrombosis of other specified artery — *hepatic and splenic arteries*
AHA: Q4, 1990, 27; Q2, 1992, 11

444.9 Embolism and thrombosis of unspecified artery

Documentation Issues
When documentation identifies that a patient with aortic atherosclerosis has an occlusion of the aortoiliac artery due to an embolus, two codes should be used: 444.0 *Arterial embolism and thrombosis of abdominal aorta* and 440.0 *Atherosclerosis of aorta*. Even though the index assumes aortic occlusions are thromboembolic, if the etiology is specified (e.g., atherosclerosis), then that condition should be coded.

445 Atheroembolism
AHA: Q4, 2002, 57

Atheroembolism occurs when fragments of atherosclerotic plaques break off from their location in an artery and travel to another site, such as the kidney, where the embolus then gets lodged. This may occur spontaneously but often happens as a result of manipulation in the aorta, such as during cardiac catheterization.

445.01 Atheroembolism of upper extremity
445.02 Atheroembolism of lower extremity
445.81 Atheroembolism of kidney — (Use additional code for any associated acute renal failure or chronic kidney disease: 584, 585)
445.89 Atheroembolism of other site

446 Polyarteritis nodosa and allied conditions
446.0 Polyarteritis nodosa — *inflammation of small and medium size arteries causing tissue death; disseminated necrotizing periarteritis, necrotizing angiitis, Harkavy's syndrome*

446.1	Acute febrile mucocutaneous lymph node syndrome (MCLS) — *inflammatory disease causing fever, skin eruptions, and edema; including Kawasaki disease*		447.3	Hyperplasia of renal artery — *overgrowth of cells in the muscular lining of the renal artery*
			447.4	Celiac artery compression syndrome — *compression of the celiac artery by the median arcuate ligament; celiac axis, Marable's, medial arcuate ligament syndromes*
446.20	Unspecified hypersensitivity angiitis — *unknown inflammatory disease of vessels caused by antigen sensitivity*			
			447.5	Necrosis of artery — *death of arterial tissue*
446.21	Goodpasture's syndrome — (Use additional code to identify renal disease, 583.81) — *antiglomerular basement membrane antibody-mediated nephritis with pulmonary hemorrhage*		447.6	Unspecified arteritis
			447.8	Other specified disorders of arteries and arterioles — *not otherwise specified; fibromuscular hyperplasia of nonrenal artery; Dego's, Wright's, or popliteal artery entrapment syndromes; dilation, hyperabduction, hypertrophy, papulosis*
446.29	Other specified hypersensitivity angiitis — *not otherwise specified* **AHA:** Q1, 1995, 3			
446.3	Lethal midline granuloma — *tumor that begins midface and leads to death; malignant granuloma of face*		447.9	Unspecified disorders of arteries and arterioles

Documentation Issues
If the documentation states that the patient has an aortoiliac artery occlusion due to a stricture in conjunction with aortic arteriosclerosis, two codes are required: 447.1 *Stricture of artery* and 440.0 *Atherosclerosis of aorta.*

446.4	Wegener's granulomatosis — *necrotizing granulomatous inflammation of vessels of respiratory tract; Churg-Strauss syndrome* **AHA:** Q3, 2000, 11
446.5	Giant cell arteritis — *giant cells and inflammation in large artery, leading to occlusion; including cranial arteritis, Horton's disease, Bagratuni's syndrome*
446.6	Thrombotic microangiopathy — *blockages in the smallest arteries and arterioles; including Moschcowitz's syndrome, Baehr-Schiffrin disease*
446.7	Takayasu's disease — *progressive inflammation of brachiocephalic truck and left common carotid arteries above source in aortic arch; including Martorell-Fabre, Raeder-Harbitz, young female syndromes, pulseless disease*

Coding Scenario
A 53-year-old male is admitted for atherosclerosis. The discharge summary states the final diagnosis as aortoiliac artery occlusion secondary to stricture and aortic atherosclerosis.

Code assignment: 447.1 *Stricture of artery* and 440.0 *Atherosclerosis of aorta*

448 Disease of capillaries
Arterioles entering tissue that branch into vessels are called capillaries. Nutrients and wastes are exchanged between the blood and body through the walls of the capillaries, which, before leaving the tissues, reunite to form the venules. Although found near almost every cell in the body, their distribution is regulated by the activity of the tissue (i.e., capillary supplies are dense in the liver, kidneys, lungs, muscles, and nervous system and less extensive in tendons and ligaments). Telangiectasia is the permanent dilatation of groups of superficial capillaries and venules that can be caused by dermatoses, rosacea, and collagen vascular diseases. A nevus flammeus is a flat capillary hemangioma that is present at birth and varies from pale red to deep reddish purple. It rarely causes any problems.

Coding Clarification
Polyarteritis nodosa is a systemic disease characterized by segmental inflammation with infiltration and necrosis of medium-sized or small arteries. It is most common in males and produces symptoms related to involvement of arteries in the kidneys, muscles, gastrointestinal tract, and heart, and is reported with 446.0.

Septic Leukocytoclastic Vasculitis: Two codes are required to report this condition: 446.29 *Other specified hypersensitivity angiitis* and a code from category 682 *Other cellulitis and abscess.*

447 Other disorders of arteries and arterioles

447.0	Arteriovenous fistula, acquired — *communication between an artery and vein caused by error in healing*
447.1	Stricture of artery — *structurally narrow section of an artery* **AHA:** March-April, 1987, 6; Q2, 1993, 8
447.2	Rupture of artery — *tearing of artery with bleeding, not associated with aneurysm, but caused by erosion, (not arteriovenous) fistula or ulcer*
448.0	Hereditary hemorrhagic telangiectasia
448.1	Nevus, non-neoplastic — *araneus, senile, spider, stellar*
448.9	Other and unspecified capillary diseases — *not otherwise specified, or unknown; thrombosis, rupture, hemorrhage, hyperpermeability, telangiectasia*

451–459 Diseases of Veins and Lymphatics, and Other Diseases of Circulatory System

451 Phlebitis and thrombophlebitis
AHA: Q1, 1992, 16

Phlebitis is inflammation of a vein. Thrombophlebitis is a partial or complete obstruction of a vein with secondary inflammatory reaction in the wall of the vein.

451.0	Phlebitis and thrombophlebitis of superficial vessels of lower extremities — (Use additional code to identify drug, if drug-induced) — *inflammation and formation of a blood clot in the superficial veins of the legs and feet; including greater and lesser saphenous veins* **AHA:** Q3, 1991, 16; Q1, 1992, 16
451.11	Phlebitis and thrombophlebitis of femoral vein (deep) (superficial) — (Use additional E code to identify drug, if drug-induced) — *inflammation and formation of a femoral blood clot* **AHA:** Q3, 1991, 16; Q1, 1992, 16
451.19	Phlebitis and thrombophlebitis of other deep vessels of lower extremities — (Use additional E code to identify drug, if drug-induced) — *inflammation and formation of a blood clot in the femoropopliteal, tibia, popliteal veins; blue phlebitis* **AHA:** Q3, 1991, 16; Q1, 1992, 16
451.2	Phlebitis and thrombophlebitis of lower extremities, unspecified — (Use additional E code to identify drug, if drug-induced) **AHA:** Q4, 2004, 80
451.81	Phlebitis and thrombophlebitis of iliac vein — (Use additional E code to identify drug, if drug-induced) — *inflammation and formation of a blood clot* **AHA:** Q1, 1992, 16
451.82	Phlebitis and thrombophlebitis of superficial veins of upper extremities — (Use additional E code to identify drug, if drug-induced) — *inflammation and formation of a blood clot in the antecubital, basilic, cephalic veins* **AHA:** Q1, 1992, 16
451.83	Phlebitis and thrombophlebitis of deep veins of upper extremities — (Use additional E code to identify drug, if drug-induced) — *inflammation and formation of a blood clot in the brachial, radial, ulnar veins* **AHA:** Q1, 1992, 16
451.84	Phlebitis and thrombophlebitis of upper extremities, unspecified — (Use additional E code to identify drug, if drug-induced)
451.89	Phlebitis and thrombophlebitis of other site — (Use additional E code to identify drug, if drug-induced) — *not otherwise specified, axillary, jugular, subclavian, hepatic, umbilical veins* **AHA:** Q1, 1992, 16
451.9	Phlebitis and thrombophlebitis of unspecified site — (Use additional E code to identify drug, if drug-induced)

Coding Clarification
This rubric excludes thrombophlebitis that is due to or following an implant or a catheter device (996.61-996.62) or infusion, perfusion, or transfusion (999.2).

Classify phlebitis and thrombophlebitis according to the vessel. Use an additional E code to identify the drug, if the condition is drug induced.

Deep Venous Thrombosis and Thrombophlebitis:
The correct way to code a diagnosis of thrombosis and thrombophlebitis is to report only the thrombophlebitis. Thrombosis is the formation of a clot within a blood vessel. Thrombophlebitis is inflammation of a vein associated with thrombus formation. Thrombophlebitis has the characteristic signs of swelling, pain, induration, and redness.

Often the term "DVT," or deep venous thrombosis, is used as a synonym for thrombophlebitis. If the signs and symptoms described above are seen in the documentation, query the physician and obtain an addendum to the record if the physician states that the patient has thrombophlebitis. It will then be appropriate to code the thrombophlebitis as the only code. An excludes note gives direction to assign only a code from category 451 if both conditions are present.

Deep Vein Category: The femoropopliteal vein, the tibial vein, and the popliteal vein belong to the "deep" category.

Codes in category 451 distinguish between the superficial, deep, and unspecified veins of the upper and lower extremities. The need for this specificity arose with the increasing use of catheters and cannulas, which are often placed in the arm. Included in the deep vessels of the upper extremities are the following veins: branchial vein, radial vein, and ulner vein.

Coding Scenario
The patient is diagnosed with DVT and thrombophlebitis of the superficial femoral vein.

> Code assignment: 451.11 *Phlebitis and thrombophlebitis of femoral vein (deep) (superficial)*

A 24-year-old female is discharged with a diagnostic statement of "DVT of the basilic vein." The nursing notes state that the arm is reddened, indurated, painful, and swollen.

> Code assignment: Code the case as 453.8 *Embolism and thrombosis of other specified veins*. Documentation from the physician must determine thrombophlebitis in order to assign a code from 451

452   Portal vein thrombosis ✓

This type of thrombosis describes inflammation and blood clot in the main vein of the liver.

Coding Clarification

The classification excludes hepatic vein thrombosis (453.0) and phlebitis of portal vein (572.1).

453   Other venous embolism and thrombosis
AHA: Q1, 1992, 16

Budd-Chiari syndrome is a thrombus in the main vein that leaves the liver. Symptoms of this syndrome include ascites, jaundice and abnormal liver function tests.

The formation of a blood clot, or thrombus, in the deep veins of the leg not only impedes blood circulation, but also may become life-threatening if the clot or pieces of the blood clot break loose and travel to the lungs where they lodge in an artery, causing pulmonary embolism. The American Heart Association estimates that up to 2 million people a year are affected by DVT, and up to 200,000 die from developing pulmonary embolism—that is more than breast cancer and AIDS combined, and accounts for one of the nation's leading, but preventable causes of death.

People develop deep vein thrombosis from prolonged sitting, immobility, or bed rest that may be occasioned by long distance traveling, major injuries, paralysis, surgery, or pregnancy. Surgery that involves the legs or pelvis, existing heart or circulation problems, hormone replacement therapy, obesity, age, and certain genetic conditions that make blood clotting more likely than usual increase the risk. When a thrombus forms, blood flow back to the heart is impeded, causing redness, swelling, and pain in the leg below the clot that may be perceived as aching or tightness.

Deep vein thrombosis may be associated with inflammation, phlebitis, and thrombophlebitis.

453.0	Budd-Chiari syndrome — *hepatic vein thrombosis with liver enlargement and severe hypertension* AHA: Q1, 1992, 16
453.1	Thrombophlebitis migrans — *spontaneous, recurring inflammation of veins with blood clots; including Trousseau's and carcinogenic thrombophlebitis syndromes* AHA: Q1, 1992, 16
453.2	Embolism and thrombosis of vena cava — *blockage and clotting of vena cava* AHA: Q1, 1992, 16
453.3	Embolism and thrombosis of renal vein — *blockage and clotting of major kidney vein* AHA: Q1, 1992, 16
453.40	Venous embolism and thrombosis of unspecified deep vessels of lower extremity
453.41	Venous embolism and thrombosis of deep vessels of proximal lower extremity AHA: Q4, 2004, 79
453.42	Venous embolism and thrombosis of deep vessels of distal lower extremity
453.8	Embolism and thrombosis of other specified veins — *not otherwise specified; iliac, femoral axillary veins; Paget-Schroetter syndrome* AHA: March-April, 1987, 6; Q3, 1991, 16; Q1, 1992, 16
453.9	Embolism and thrombosis of unspecified site

Documentation Issues

If the documentation states that the thrombus is not associated with inflammation, assign the appropriate code from rubric 453. If the signs and symptoms associated with inflammation (swelling, erythema, pain, induration) are documented, query the physician as to whether the condition is thrombophlebitis and, if it is, assign a code from rubric 451 instead.

Coding Clarification

Report code from rubric 451 for thrombosis with thrombophlebitis.

Coding Scenario

A 56-year-old female, who has recently undergone back surgery, presents to her physician's office complaining of pain and tenderness in her right leg. The physician notes swelling and redness developing in the lower half of her upper leg. As a deep vein thrombosis is suspected, with a greater risk of developing pulmonary embolism from its location, she is taken to the hospital where doppler ultrasound and venography are done that confirm a thrombus in the femoral vein. She is admitted, the leg is held in elevated position, and she is monitored closely as intravenous heparin is administered.

> Code assignment: 453.41 *Venous embolism and thrombosis of deep vessels of proximal lower extremity*

454 Varicose veins of lower extremities
AHA: Q2, 1991, 20

Varicose veins are dilated, elongated, and tortuous networks in the subcutaneous venous system resulting from valvular incompetence. Other etiologies include congenital or acquired arteriovenous fistulas and valve damage following deep venous thrombophlebitis. The condition develops predominantly in the lower extremities. Most commonly, the long saphenous vein and its tributaries are involved, but the short saphenous vein also may be affected. Symptoms include night cramps, localized pain, edema, inflammation, or hemorrhage and a dull aching or fatigue exacerbated by standing in place.

454.0	Varicose veins of lower extremities with ulcer — *incompetent vein valves allow reversed blood flow and erosion of tissue* **AHA:** Q2, 1991, 20; Q4, 1999, 18
454.1	Varicose veins of lower extremities with inflammation — *incompetent vein valves allow reversed blood flow and inflammation* **AHA:** Q2, 1991, 20
454.2	Varicose veins of lower extremities with ulcer and inflammation — *incompetent vein valves allow reversed blood flow, erosion of tissue, and inflammation* **AHA:** Q2, 1991, 20
454.8	Varicose veins of the lower extremities with other complications — *Edema, pain, swelling* **AHA:** Q2, 1991, 20; Q4, 2002, 58
454.9	Asymptomatic varicose veins

Coding Clarification
Stasis Dermatitis: Determine which of the following diagnoses is appropriate: stasis dermatitis with varicosity, with or without ulceration; stasis dermatitis with venous peripheral insufficiency, and previous deep venous thrombosis. While stasis dermatitis often occurs with varicosity, it also appears after a deep venous thrombosis and may appear as a singular entity (venous peripheral insufficiency).

When consulting the index, a basic coding rule is the requirement for further research if the code title suggested by the index is in contradiction to the condition. In the example for chronic venous insufficiency and previous deep vein thrombosis, the user must reject the suggestion of the index (varicose veins) because they are not the clinical entity at issue.

The codes that may be used to describe stasis dermatitis are: 454.1 *Varicose veins of lower extremity with inflammation,* 454.2 *Varicose veins of lower extremity with ulcer and inflammation,* 459.1x *Post phlebitic syndrome,* and 459.81 *Venous insufficiency, unspecified.*

Varicose vein with ulceration and hemorrhage:
When coding ulcerated varicose veins that have ruptured and are hemorrhaging, the coder does not need to code the hemorrhage as a separate clinical entity. Also, the term "ruptured" is a non-essential modifier. Typically after rupture of a varicose vein, bleeding will occur.

Coding Scenario
An 80-year-old presents to the emergency department with stasis dermatitis on the right lower extremity. The physical examination reveals varicosities on the same extremity that have ulcerated.

> Code assignment: 454.2 *Varicose veins of lower extremities with ulcer and inflammation*

A patients presents to the emergency department for control of bleeding from an ulcerated varicose vein of the right lower extremity. The diagnostic statement reads "Varicose veins with ulceration and hemorrhage."

> Code assignment: 454.0 *Varicose veins of lower extremities with ulcer.* Do not assign a separate code for the hemorrhage.

455 Hemorrhoids
Hemorrhoids are dilated veins of the hemorrhoidal plexus in the lower rectum. External hemorrhoids are on the outer side of the external sphincter, covered by skin of the anal canal. Internal hemorrhoids are within the external sphincter, covered with rectal mucosa.

Internal hemorrhoids may be classified as first, second, third, or fourth degree. Fourth-degree hemorrhoids are the most severe and are characterized as both incarcerated and prolapsed; third-degree hemorrhoids are prolapsed. Both third- and fourth-degree hemorrhoids should be classified as complicated.

455.0	Internal hemorrhoids without mention of complication — *reversed blow flow and dilation of vein; contained within rectum* **AHA:** Q3, 2005, 17
455.1	Internal thrombosed hemorrhoids — *reversed blow flow and clotted blood in vein; contained within rectum*
455.2	Internal hemorrhoids with other complication — *reversed blow flow with strangulation, ulcer, prolapse, or bleeding; contained within rectum* **AHA:** Q1, 2003, 8; Q3, 2005, 17

455.3	External hemorrhoids without mention of complication — *reversed blow flow and dilation of vein; extending beyond anus*	
	AHA: Q3, 2005, 17	
455.4	External thrombosed hemorrhoids — *reversed blow flow and clotted blood in vein; extending beyond anus*	
455.5	External hemorrhoids with other complication — *reversed blow flow with strangulation, ulcer, prolapse, or bleeding; extending beyond anus*	
	AHA: Q1, 2003, 8; Q3, 2005, 17	
455.6	Unspecified hemorrhoids without mention of complication — *reversed blow flow and dilation of vein; unknown site*	
455.7	Unspecified thrombosed hemorrhoids — *reversed blow flow and clotted blood in vein; unknown site*	
455.8	Unspecified hemorrhoids with other complication — *reversed blow flow with strangulation, ulcer, prolapse, or bleeding; unknown site*	
455.9	Residual hemorrhoidal skin tags — *redundant tissue remains in anus or rectum following treatment of hemorrhoids*	

456 Varicose veins of other sites

Varicose veins may occur at sites other than the lower extremities. Esophageal varices are the most clinically significant and comprise longitudinal venous varices located in the distal end of the esophagus.

456.0	Esophageal varices with bleeding — *distended, tortuous veins of the esophagus, with leaking of blood*	
456.1	Esophageal varices without mention of bleeding — *distended, tortuous veins of the esophagus, without bleeding*	
456.20	Esophageal varices with bleeding in diseases classified elsewhere — (Code first underlying disease: 571.0-571.9, 572.3) — *secondary to underlying disease*	
	AHA: Nov-Dec, 1985, 14	
456.21	Esophageal varices without mention of bleeding in diseases classified elsewhere — (Code first underlying disease: 571.0-571.9, 572.3) — *secondary to underlying disease*	
	AHA: Q2, 2002, 4; Q3, 2005, 15	
456.3	Sublingual varices — *distended, tortuous veins beneath the tongue*	
456.4	Scrotal varices — *distended, tortuous veins of the scrotum*	
456.5	Pelvic varices — *distended, tortuous veins within the pelvic region*	
456.6	Vulval varices — *distended, tortuous veins of the external female genitalia*	
456.8	Varices of other sites — *distended, tortuous veins of sites not otherwise specified, including orbit, pharynx, renal papilla, spine, spleen, urethra, vocal cord, nasal septum*	
	AHA: Q2, 2002, 4	

Coding Clarification
Varicose veins are almost always due to portal hypertension (456.2). Code the portal hypertension first, followed by 456.20, if bleeding is present, or 456.21, without bleeding.

457 Noninfectious disorders of lymphatic channels

Lymphatic vessels originate in spaces between cells called lymph capillaries, which originate throughout the body (excluding avascular tissue, the central nervous system, splenic pulp, and bone marrow). The vessels contain lymph nodes at various intervals. The lymphatics of the skin converge with the lymphatics of the viscera to form the lymphatic channels (the thoracic duct and the right lymphatic duct). The thoracic duct receives lymph from the left side of the head, neck, and chest, the left upper extremity, and the entire body below the ribs. The right lymphatic duct collects lymph from the right jugular trunk, which drains the right side of the head and neck; from the right subclavian trunk, which drains the right upper extremity; and from the right bronchomediastinal trunk, which drains the right side of the thorax, right lung, right side of the heart, and part of the convex surface of the liver. Skeletal muscle contractions and respiratory movements are factors maintaining lymph flow.

Postmastectomy syndrome is a form of lymphedema due to excision of the axillary lymphatic structures during mastectomy.

457.0	Postmastectomy lymphedema syndrome — *edema in arms and hands caused by pooling in interstitial fluids, due to reduced lymphatic circulation*	
	AHA: Q2, 2002, 12	
457.1	Other noninfectious lymphedema — *other retention of fluids due to reduced lymphatic circulation; including elephantiasis, lymphedema*	
	AHA: Q3, 2004, 5	
457.2	Lymphangitis — *subacute or chronic inflammation of the lymph glands*	
457.8	Other noninfectious disorders of lymphatic channels — *not otherwise specified, including sclerotic lymph gland, chylocele, or lymph node fistula, cyst infarction, or rupture*	
	AHA: Q3, 2003, 17; Q1, 2004, 5	
457.9	Unspecified noninfectious disorder of lymphatic channels	

458 Hypotension

458.0	Orthostatic hypotension — *abnormally low blood pressure worsened when the seated patient stands*	
	AHA: Q3, 1991, 9; Q3, 2000, 8	

Diseases of the Circulatory System

458.1	Chronic hypotension — *persistent abnormally low blood pressure*		459.10	Postphlebitic syndrome without complications
458.2 ⟋sth	Iatrogenic hypotension — *abnormally low blood pressure as a result of medical treatment* AHA: Q4, 1995, 57; Q3, 2002, 12; Q4, 2003, 60		459.11	Postphlebitic syndrome with ulcer
			459.12	Postphlebitic syndrome with inflammation
			459.13	Postphlebitic syndrome with ulcer and inflammation
458.21	Hypotension of hemodialysis — *intra-dialytic hypotension* AHA: Q4, 2003, 61		459.19	Postphlebitic syndrome with other complication
			459.2	Compression of vein — *stricture of vein; vena cava syndrome*
458.29	Other iatrogenic hypotension — *postoperative hypotension*		459.3 ⟋sth	Chronic venous hypertension — *stasis edema* AHA: Q4, 2002, 59
458.8	Other specified hypotension — *not otherwise specified* AHA: Q4, 1997, 37		459.30	Chronic venous hypertension without complications
			459.31	Chronic venous hypertension with ulcer
458.9	Unspecified hypotension		459.32	Chronic venous hypertension with inflammation
			459.33	Chronic venous hypertension with ulcer and inflammation

Coding Clarification
Orthostatic hypotension is an excessive fall in blood pressure when assuming an erect position. Severe orthostatic hypotension can be associated with a neuropathic disorder known as Shy-Drager syndrome or idiopathic orthostatic hypotension, classified to 333.0. It may also be due to volume depletion.

Iatrogenic hypotension or postoperative hypotension is classified to 458.29. This code fully describes postoperative hypotension and does not require an additional code to indicate complication of surgical or medical care.

Use code 458.8 to code postmyocardial infarction hypotension. Sequence the myocardial infarction code first.

459 Other disorders of circulatory system
Postphlebitic syndrome is a complex of symptoms due to venous hypertension as a consequence of postphlebitic incompetence of communicating veins.

459.0	Unspecified hemorrhage — *spontaneous rupture of blood vessel, not otherwise specified* AHA: Q4, 1990, 26
459.39	Chronic venous hypertension with other complication
459.81	Unspecified venous (peripheral) insufficiency — (Use additional code for any associated ulceration: 707.10-707.9) AHA: Q3, 2004, 5
459.89	Other specified circulatory system disorders — *not otherwise specified*
459.9	Unspecified circulatory system disorder — *unknown site and unknown disorder*

Coding Clarification
Excluded from this rubric are cases of hemorrhage due to trauma.

Coding Scenario
A 45-year-old female, a data entry clerk by occupation, presents with a stasis dermatitis of the left lower extremity. The history reveals that three weeks previously, she suffered a deep venous thrombosis of the same leg. The physician has not documented any varicosity of the extremity.

Code assignment: 459.1x *Postphlebitic syndrome*

460–519

Diseases of the Respiratory System

This chapter classifies diseases and disorders of the nose (external, nasal cavity), sinuses (frontal, ethmoid, sphenoid, maxillary), pharynx (nasopharynx, oropharynx), larynx (true and false vocal cords, glottis), trachea, bronchi (left, right, main, carina), and lungs (intrapulmonary bronchi, bronchioli, lobes, alveoli, pleura).

This complex of organs is responsible for pulmonary ventilation and the exchange of oxygen and carbon dioxide between the lungs and ambient air. The organs of the respiratory system also perform nonrespiratory functions such as warming and moisturizing the air passing into the lungs, providing airflow for the larynx and vocal cords for speech, and releasing excess body heat in the process of thermoregulation for homeostasis. The lungs also perform important metabolic and embolic filtering functions.

460–466 Acute Respiratory Infections

Pneumonia and influenza are excluded from this section and can be found in rubrics 480-487.8.

460 Acute nasopharyngitis (common cold)
AHA: Q1, 1988, 12

This rubric classifies nasopharyngitis, rhinitis, coryza, or nasal catarrh of an acute nature. Acute nasopharyngitis is the most common of the upper respiratory infections, and is characterized by edema of the nasal mucous membrane, discharge, and obstruction.

Coding Clarification
Chronic nasopharyngitis is reported with 472.2.

461 Acute sinusitis

This rubric classifies sinusitis that is sudden and severe, according to the site of infection: frontal, maxillary, ethmoidal, sphenoidal, or multiple sites. Included in the definition of acute sinusitis are abscess, empyema, and suppuration. Acute sinusitis is usually preceded by an acute respiratory infection. A second code from Chapter 1 Infectious and Parasitic Diseases can be reported to identify the infectious agent, which most commonly is streptococci, pneumococci, *H. influenzae*, or staphylococci. In the case of immuno-compromised patients, the infectious agents are more likely to be aspergillosis, candidiasis, or fungal infections of the order Mucorales.

461.0	Acute maxillary sinusitis — *behind cheekbones*
461.1	Acute frontal sinusitis — *above the eyes*
461.2	Acute ethmoidal sinusitis — *between the eyes on either side of the nose*
461.3	Acute sphenoidal sinusitis — *behind the eyes on either side of the nose*
461.8	Other acute sinusitis — *pansinusitis*
461.9	Acute sinusitis, unspecified

Coding Clarification
Chronic sinusitis is excluded from this rubric and is reported with 473.0-473.9.

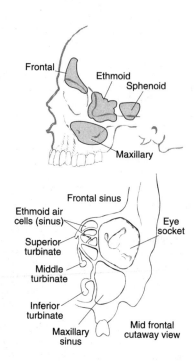

462 Acute pharyngitis OK
AHA: Sept-Oct, 1985, 8; Q4, 1999, 26

Acute pharyngitis is an acute inflammatory disorder of the throat, which may be caused by a virus or bacteria. Frequently, coryza or other communicable disease precedes acute pharyngitis.

Signs and symptoms of acute pharyngitis include history of tobacco or alcohol abuse, sore throat, dysphagia, fever, headache, and muscle and joint pain.

Therapies include warm saline gargles and analgesics such as aspirin to relieve throat discomfort, bed rest, IV hydration in severe cases, and antibiotics for suspected bacterial acute pharyngitis. Associated conditions include dehydration, sinusitis, and allergies.

Coding Clarification
A code from Chapter 1 Infectious and Parasitic Diseases can be reported secondarily to identify the infective agent in pharyngitis. The most common causes are the infectious agents streptococci, *Mycoplasma pneumoniae, Chlamydia pneumoniae,* or a virus.

Do not use this code to report chronic pharyngitis (472.1) or an abscess of the peritonsillar region (475), pharynx (478.29), or retropharynx (478.24). Also excluded is acute pharyngitis due to Coxsackie virus (074.0), gonococcus (098.6), herpes simplex (054.79), flu (487.1), or streptococcus (034.0). Septic pharyngitis is reported with 034.0.

463 Acute tonsillitis OK
AHA: Nov-Dec, 1984, 16

A sudden severe inflammation of the palatine tonsil is classified to this rubric. The infective agent is most commonly streptococcal or viral. Tonsillitis may be accompanied by throat pain, high fever, and, in some cases, vomiting.

Coding Clarification
Excluded from this rubric are chronic tonsillitis (474.0), hypertrophy of tonsil (474.1), streptococcal tonsillitis (034.0), and sore throat, not otherwise specified (462).

464 Acute laryngitis and tracheitis
Sudden and severe inflammation of the larynx, trachea, and epiglottis associated with infection are classified to this rubric, with obstruction of the airway being an axis for code choice. Laryngitis and tracheitis usually follow an upper respiratory infection, but may occur during the course of pneumonia, bronchitis, flu, or measles.

Acute epiglottitis usually is due to an infection by *Haemophilus influenzae,* pneumococci, or group A streptococci and can develop into a laryngeal airway obstruction. Signs and symptoms of acute epiglottitis include history of upper respiratory infection or chronic lung disease, high fever, sore throat, dysphagia, stridor, and respiratory distress.

Diagnostic tests/reports/findings include a throat exam to reveal an enlarged, edematous epiglottis. Laryngoscopy or lateral neck x-rays reveal inflammatory changes and signs of obstruction. Therapies include endotracheal intubation for obstruction, IV hydration to prevent dehydration, antibiotics (parenteral), oxygen therapy, and blood gas monitoring for hypoxia and hypercapnia.

Croup is an acute laryngotracheobronchitis usually seen in early childhood and characterized by stridor, respiratory distress, and swelling. Parainfluenza virus is usually the infective agent, although respiratory syncytial virus can also cause croup.

Diseases of the Respiratory System

464.00	Acute laryngitis, without mention of obstruction
464.01	Acute laryngitis, with obstruction
464.10	Acute tracheitis without mention of obstruction — *sudden, severe inflammation of vocal cords*
464.11	Acute tracheitis with obstruction — *sudden, severe inflammation of vocal cords w/ obstruction*
464.20	Acute laryngotracheitis without mention of obstruction — *sudden, severe inflammation of trachea and vocal cords*
464.21	Acute laryngotracheitis with obstruction — *sudden, severe inflammation of trachea and vocal cords w/ obstruction*
464.30	Acute epiglottitis without mention of obstruction — *sudden, severe inflammation of epiglottis*
464.31	Acute epiglottitis with obstruction — *sudden, severe inflammation of epiglottis w/ obstruction*
464.4	Croup — *barking cough with inflammation of larynx*
464.50	Unspecified supraglottis, without mention of obstruction
464.51	Unspecified supraglottis, with obstruction

Coding Clarification
Excluded from this rubric are cases associated with the flu (487.1) or strep infection (034.0). For chronic laryngitis, see rubric 476; for chronic tracheitis, report 491.8.

If inflammation of the larynx is combined with inflammation of the trachea, report codes from subclassification 464.2 *Acute laryngotracheitis*.

465 Acute upper respiratory infections of multiple or unspecified sites
This rubric is reserved for acute infections of multiple sites or when the site is not otherwise specified.

465.0	Acute laryngopharyngitis — *sudden, severe inflammation of vocal cords and pharynx*
465.8	Acute upper respiratory infections of other multiple sites — *multiple URI*
465.9	Acute upper respiratory infections of unspecified site — *unknown site, URI*

Coding Clarification
Excluded from this rubric are upper respiratory infections due to flu (487.1) or strep (034.0).

466 Acute bronchitis and bronchiolitis
Acute bronchitis is sudden and severe inflammation of the tracheobronchial tree. Acute bronchitis may have an infectious or irritative etiology.

Signs and symptoms of acute bronchitis include a history of upper respiratory infection or exposure to irritants such as dust or fumes, cough, malaise, fever, and pain in the back and chest. Therapies include bed rest and antibiotics such as oral tetracycline when purulent sputum is present. For patients with chronic respiratory disease, therapy includes antipyretics for fever, bronchodilators for bronchial asthma, and monitoring of arterial blood gases (ABGs) in cases of significant underlying chronic respiratory disease.

466.0	Acute bronchitis — *sudden, severe inflammation of bronchial tree main branches* AHA: Q1, 1988, 12; Q4, 1991, 24; Q4, 1996, 28; Q4, 2002, 46; Q1, 2004, 3; Q4, 2004, 137
466.11	Acute bronchiolitis due to respiratory syncytial virus (RSV) — *bronchiolitis, capillary pneumonia due to RSV* AHA: Q4, 1996, 27; Q1, 2005, 10
466.19	Acute bronchiolitis due to other infectious organisms — (Use additional code to identify infectious organism) — *bronchiolitis, capillary pneumonia, other infectious agent*

Documentation Issues
When the documentation identifies acute and chronic bronchitis, report 491.22. If the documentation states chronic bronchitis, with or without mention of centrilobular emphysema (blue bloater), use code 491.2x.

If the physician documentation indicates COPD with asthmatic bronchitis, assign code 493.2x.

If the diagnostic statement specifies only "acute bronchospasm," report with code 519.11.

Coding Clarification
Acute and Chronic Bronchitis: Use two codes (466.0 and 491.9) when reporting acute and chronic bronchitis. This will correspond with the following coding guideline: If the same condition is described as both acute (subacute) and chronic and separate subentries exist in the Alphabetic Index at the same

level, code both and list the acute (subacute) code first.

Acute Bronchitis and Emphysema: Two codes are required (466.0 *Acute bronchitis* and 492.8 *Other emphysema*) to accurately report this condition as per the National Center for Health Statistics.

Respiratory Syncytial Virus (RSV): If respiratory syncytial virus is noted with acute bronchitis, two codes are required: 466.0 *Acute bronchitis* and 079.6 *Respiratory syncytial virus (RSV)*. If the RSV is noted with acute bronchiolitis, use only code 466.11 *Acute bronchiolitis due to respiratory syncytial virus (RSV)*.

Associated conditions include underlying chronic lung disease such as chronic obstructive bronchitis or COPD, pneumonia or bronchopneumonia, or allergies. Excluded from this rubric are acute bronchitis with asthma (493), bronchiectasis (494.1), and COPD (491.21).

If the physician documents acute bronchitis and exacerbation of COPD, assign only the combination code of COPD with acute bronchitis (491.22).

Acute bronchitis represents an infection or inflammation that can occur whether a patient has chronic lung disease or not. An acute exacerbation of COPD is a flare or worsening of a chronic condition and does not imply the presence of acute bronchitis.

Coding Scenario

A 5-year-old patient is admitted with acute bronchitis and possible cystic fibrosis. A chest x-ray is performed, confirming the diagnosis of cystic fibrosis. The diagnosis at discharge is acute bronchitis and cystic fibrosis.

> Code assignment: 466.0 *Acute bronchitis* and 277.02 *Cystic fibrosis with pulmonary manifestations*

470–478 Other Diseases of the Upper Respiratory Tract

Included in this rubric are many chronic inflammatory diseases of the upper respiratory tract.

The upper respiratory tract includes the nasal cavity and the pharynx and any structure connecting to or associated with them (the paranasal sinus cavities, lacrimal apparatus and conjunctival sac, auditory tube, and middle ear). Though these accessory structures are associated with functions other than breathing or gas exchange, they are all lined with mucous membrane that is continuous with the nasal cavity and pharynx, and infections beginning anywhere in that mucous membrane can readily spread to adjacent structures. The larynx, which can be considered with either upper or lower respiratory structures, is the voice box and connects the pharynx with the tracheo-bronchial tree. It is lined with mucous membrane.

The nasal cavity has a mucociliary lining similar to that of the lower respiratory tract. The inside of the nose is lined with hair that filters inhaled particles. Mucous covering the turbinate bones, or baffle plates, captures particles not filtered by nasal hairs. The change in direction of the airway from the sinuses to the pharynx causes a large number of larger particles to impinge on the back of the throat. The adenoids and tonsils are lymphoid organs in the upper respiratory tract that are vital to an immune response to pathogens. A layer of mucous and ciliated cells covers the lower portion of the lower respiratory tract. Single and subepithelial cells secrete mucous. Particles or respiratory pathogens that reach the lower respiratory tract are first trapped in the mucous layer and are driven upwards by ciliary action to the back of the throat. There are two main obstacles a bacterium or virus must overcome in order to initiate an infection in the respiratory tract: the microorganism must avoid the mucous layers of the upper respiratory tract; however, if the microorganism gets past the mucous layers, it can travel to the lower respiratory tract or lung, where it either is destroyed by phagocytosis or multiplies in the phagocytic cell.

Most of the surfaces of the upper respiratory tract (including nasal and oral passages, nasopharynx, oropharynx, and trachea) are colonized by normal flora. These organisms rarely cause disease, but compete with pathogenic organisms for attachment sites.

Normal flora found in the nose, nasopharynx, and sinuses is as follows:

- Staphylococcus epidermidis
- Staph. aureus (especially in hospital staff)
- Streptococci (including *S. pyogenes* and *S. pneumoniae*)
- Haemophilus sp.
- Neisseria sp.

Normal flora found in the mouth and throat is as follows:

- Streptococci (mainly *S. mitis* and *S. salivarius*)
- Diphtheroids

- Anaerobes (e.g., Fusobacterium sp.)
- Staph. epidermidis

470 Deviated nasal septum ✓

Deviated nasal septum is a common disorder that often requires no treatment. However, in some cases, the deviation in the septum, the result of past trauma, causes obstructions in the nasal passages that lead to chronic conditions like sinusitis or epistaxis. If the deviation predisposes the patient to chronic problems, the condition may be treated surgically. When coding, sequence the code for sinusitis or epistaxis first and the deviation secondarily.

Coding Clarification

Excluded from this rubric is congenital deviated septum, which is reported with 754.0.

471 Nasal polyps

Nasal polyps are a natural reaction to chronic sinusitis due to infection or allergy. Polyps most commonly form around the ostia of the maxillary sinus, and are classified according to site. Polyps may be asymptomatic or they may block the nasal airways or promote chronic sinus infection.

471.0	Polyp of nasal cavity — *choanal, nasopharyngeal*	
471.1	Polypoid sinus degeneration — *Woakes' syndrome or ethmoiditis*	
471.8	Other polyp of sinus — *accessory, ethmoidal, maxillary, sphenoidal, frontal, turbinate, mucous membrane*	
471.9	Unspecified nasal polyp	

Coding Clarification

Excluded from this rubric is adenomatous polyps (212.0).

472 Chronic pharyngitis and nasopharyngitis

Persistent inflammation of the pharynx and nasopharynx can be the result of an infective agent or due to an allergy or exposure to an irritant.

472.0	Chronic rhinitis — *persistent ozena, atrophic, granulomatous, purulent, ulcerative*
472.1	Chronic pharyngitis — *persistent sore throat, atrophic, hypertrophic*
472.2	Chronic nasopharyngitis — *persistent inflammation from the nares to the pharynx*

Coding Clarification

Allergic rhinitis (477) is excluded from this rubric, as are all acute forms of pharyngitis or nasopharyngitis.q

473 Chronic sinusitis

Chronic sinusitis includes any persistent abscess, empyema, or infection of the nasal sinuses. It can be caused by an infective agent or by exposure to an allergic agent or irritant. Code selection is based on site: maxillary, frontal, ethmoidal, sphenoidal, or multiple sites.

473.0	Chronic maxillary sinusitis — *persistent inflammation of the sinus cavities behind the cheekbone; cloudy antrum*
473.1	Chronic frontal sinusitis — *persistent inflammation of the sinus cavities above the eyes*
473.2	Chronic ethmoidal sinusitis — *persistent inflammation of the sinus cavities between the eyes on either side of the nose*
473.3	Chronic sphenoidal sinusitis — *persistent inflammation of the sinus cavities behind the eyes on either side of the nose*
473.8	Other chronic sinusitis — *persistent pansinusitis*
473.9	Unspecified sinusitis (chronic) — *persistent sinusitis, unknown site*

Coding Clarification

Excluded from this rubric is acute sinusitis, which is classified to rubric 461.

474 Chronic disease of tonsils and adenoids

474.00	Chronic tonsillitis — *persistent inflammation, tonsil*
	AHA: Q4, 1997, 38
474.01	Chronic adenoiditis — *persistent inflammation, adenoid*
	AHA: Q4, 1997, 38
474.02	Chronic tonsillitis and adenoiditis — *persistent inflammation tonsil and adenoid*
	AHA: Q4, 1997, 38
474.10	Hypertrophy of tonsil with adenoids — *enlargement, tonsil and adenoid*
	AHA: Q2, 2005, 16
474.11	Hypertrophy of tonsils alone — *enlargement, tonsil*
474.12	Hypertrophy of adenoids alone — *enlargement, adenoid*
474.2	Adenoid vegetations — *fungus-like growth*
474.8	Other chronic disease of tonsils and adenoids — *amygdalolith, calculus, cicatrix, tag, ulcer, cyst, plica, necrosis*
474.9	Unspecified chronic disease of tonsils and adenoids

475 Peritonsillar abscess ✓

Use this code to report an abscess of the tonsil, peritonsillar cellulitis, or Quinsy. In peritonsillar abscess, tonsillitis extends beyond tonsillar tissue to include the soft palate or the space between the tonsillar pillars.

Coding Clarification
Excluded from this rubric are chronic tonsillitis (474.0) and acute tonsillitis (463).

476 Chronic laryngitis and laryngotracheitis
Chronic laryngitis and laryngotracheitis are related to allergic reactions, inhalation of irritants, gastroesophageal reflux, or voice overuse. The voice is compromised, hoarse, or absent.

476.0	Chronic laryngitis — *persistent inflammation, vocal cords*	
476.1	Chronic laryngotracheitis — *persistent inflammation, vocal cords and trachea*	

Coding Clarification
Excluded from this rubric are chronic inflammations of the trachea (491.8) and acute laryngitis or tracheitis, classified to 464.00-464.51.

477 Allergic rhinitis
Allergic rhinitis, more commonly referred to as hay fever, is an inflammation of the nasal passages caused by allergic reaction to airborne substances. There are two types of allergic rhinitis: seasonal and perennial. The seasonal type occurs when airborne plant pollens are at highest levels. Home or workplace airborne pollutants are usually the cause of the perennial type. Both types of allergies can develop at any age, although childhood through early adulthood onset is most common. Common allergens include pollen, mold, fungi, animal dander, and dust mites. Oftentimes, the animal need not be present to cause the reaction to animal dander; it can occur upon exposure to the allergens left in a room where the animal has previously been. Common symptoms include inflammation of the nose, or rhinitis, accompanied by sneezing, runny nose, redness, and tenderness. Sinus swelling can constrict the eustachian tube, causing a congested feeling. Allergy tests, including skin testing and provocation testing, can help identify the allergen. When it is not possible to avoid one or more allergens, there are two major forms of medical treatment; drugs and immunotherapy.

477.0	Allergic rhinitis due to pollen — *pollinosis*
477.1	Allergic rhinitis, due to food
477.2	Allergic rhinitis, due to animal (cat) (dog) hair and dander
477.8	Allergic rhinitis due to other allergen
477.9	Allergic rhinitis, cause unspecified — *unknown cause*

AHA: Q2, 1997, 9

Coding Scenario
A 9-year-old girl is brought to see her pediatrician because she has been suffering nasal congestion, runny nose, and itchy eyes that have not subsided and now she appears to be having breathing trouble. The family just adopted a new pet, a cat, and that seems to be when the sneezing started. The doctor recommends finding the cat a new home and doing a thorough cleaning to remove the allergens left behind and diagnoses her with acute allergic rhinitis from cat hair.

Code assignment: 477.2 *Allergic rhinitis due to animal (cat) (dog) dander*

478 Other diseases of upper respiratory tract

478.0	Hypertrophy of nasal turbinates — *overgrowth of nasal cavity bones*
478.11	Nasal mucositis (ulcerative) — (Use additional E code to identify adverse effects of therapy, such as radiation therapy [E879.2] or antineoplastic and immunosuppressive drugs [E930.7, E933.1])

Mucosal tissues are especially vulnerable to damage by chemotherapy, radiation therapy, and immune system diseases. Nasal mucositis is coded in the respiratory chapter, but mucositis can also occur throughout the body at any site where there are mucous membranes, through the entire digestive tract — anywhere from the mouth and esophagus to the rectum, and also in genital areas.

Nasal mucositis causes signs and symptoms such as pain, inflammation, irritation, and decreased sense of smell. Treatment of mucositis involves nasal irrigation, treatment of secondary infections with anti-infective medications (antibiotics, antifungals, etc.) and pain management, either oral or topical, as indicated.

478.19	Other disease of nasal cavity and sinuses — *abscess of nose; abscess of nasal septum; rhinolith; nasal cyst; nasal mucocele; cyst of sinus; mucocele of sinus; ulcer of nose; ulcer of nasal septum; necrosis of nose; necrosis of nasal septum*
478.20	Unspecified disease of pharynx
478.21	Cellulitis of pharynx or nasopharynx — *inflammation of deep, soft tissues*
478.22	Parapharyngeal abscess — *pocket of pus*
478.24	Retropharyngeal abscess — *pocket of pus*
478.25	Edema of pharynx or nasopharynx — *fluid retention*
478.26	Cyst of pharynx or nasopharynx — *fluid-filled sac*

Diseases of the Respiratory System

Tornwaldt's cyst is a superficial nasopharyngeal cyst that causes purulent exudate and drainage, sore throat, and eustachian tube complications. It is reported with 478.26.

478.29	Other disease of pharynx or nasopharynx — *including abscess, hyperactive gag reflex, polyp, Tornwaldt's bursitis, ulcer, perforation, spontaneous rupture*
478.30	Unspecified paralysis of vocal cords or larynx — *unknown side*
478.31	Unilateral partial paralysis of vocal cords or larynx — *one side*
478.32	Unilateral complete paralysis of vocal cords or larynx — *one side*
478.33	Bilateral partial paralysis of vocal cords or larynx — *both sides*
478.34	Bilateral complete paralysis of vocal cords or larynx — *both sides*
478.4	Polyp of vocal cord or larynx — *growth of benign tissue*
478.5	Other diseases of vocal cords — *abscess, cellulitis, granuloma, leukoplakia, chorditis, singer's nodes*
478.6	Edema of larynx — *fluid retention*
478.70	Unspecified disease of larynx
478.71	Cellulitis and perichondritis of larynx — *inflammation of deep soft tissue*
478.74	Stenosis of larynx — *narrowing of the diameter of larynx*
478.75	Laryngeal spasm — *involuntary muscle contraction; laryngismus, Millar's asthma*
478.79	Other diseases of larynx — *abscess, necrosis, obstruction, pachyderma, ulcer, nodule, ossification, sclerosis* **AHA:** Q3, 1991, 20
478.8	Upper respiratory tract hypersensitivity reaction, site unspecified — *site unknown*
478.9	Other and unspecified diseases of upper respiratory tract — *abscess and cicatrix of trachea, not otherwise specified*

Coding Clarification

Excluded from this rubric is ulcerative laryngitis, classified to 464.00-464.01.

Use an additional E code to identify adverse effects of therapy. If applicable, mucositis due to antineoplastic and immunosuppressive drugs or radiation therapies will be identified first, followed by the appropriate causative external causes (E code) sequenced second. Assign the appropriate additional code — E930.7 *Antineoplastic antibiotics,* E933.1 *Antineoplastic and immunosuppressive drugs,* or E879.2 for radiation therapy — as the causative agent.

480–487 Pneumonia and Influenza

Pneumonia and influenza are inflammations in the alveolar parenchyma of the lung caused by microbial infection, irradiation, or physicochemical agents. Microbial agents include viral, bacterial, fungal, protozoal, mycobacterial, mycoplasmal, or rickettsial pathogens. Physicochemical agents may be inhaled or reach the lung via the bloodstream. Inhaled agents include toxic gases, irritant particles, or irritant fluids such as gastric juice. Bleomycin is an example of a blood-borne anticancer agent that can cause pneumonia.

The terms "pneumonia" and "pneumonitis" describe two clinical patterns of inflammatory reaction in the lung. The unqualified term "pneumonia" generally refers to pneumonia with exudation in the air spaces. Inflammatory exudate fills the lung alveoli, which are then rendered airless and solid, in a process called consolidation. The terms "pneumonitis" and "interstitial pneumonia" commonly refer to pneumonia with interstitial exudate.

Signs and symptoms of pneumonia vary according to etiology (e.g., with bacterial pneumonia: coughing, sputum production, pleuritic chest pain, shaking chills, fever; with aspiration pneumonia: chest rales, dyspnea, cyanosis, hypotension, and tachycardia).

In pneumonia, chest x-ray shows infiltration or consolidation. Blood work may show normal, slightly elevated or markedly elevated white blood cell count (WBC), depending on etiology. Smears, cultures, and gram stains of sputum and/or pleural fluid isolate and identify bacteria. Percutaneous aspiration of lung tissue, endoscopic or open lung biopsy identifies difficult nonbacterial agents such as cytomegalovirus.

Therapies include antibiotics for confirmed and suspected bacterial pneumonia, oxygen therapy, complete bed rest, and intubation and ventilatory support for critically ill patients developing respiratory failure. In addition, there is respiratory therapy, which involves suctioning, coughing, and deep breathing exercises.

Associated conditions include pleural effusion, respiratory failure, empyema, atelectasis, and underlying chronic lung disease such as COPD.

To ensure proper code assignment, first refer to the ICD-9-CM index under the main terms "Pneumonia" and "Pneumonitis." Many forms of pneumonia are classified to other chapters of ICD-9-CM because of etiology. For example, candidal pneumonia is classified to code 112.4 and congenital toxoplasmosis pneumonitis is classified to codes 771.2 and 484.8. The pneumonia and influenza subchapter, codes 480-487, excludes aspiration pneumonia of the newborn, which is coded to 770.18

480 Viral pneumonia

480.0	Pneumonia due to adenovirus — *viral infection of lung*
480.1	Pneumonia due to respiratory syncytial virus — *viral infection of lung* AHA: Q1, 1988, 12; Q4, 1996, 28
480.2	Pneumonia due to parainfluenza virus — *viral infection of lung*
480.3	Pneumonia due to SARS-associated coronavirus — *due to severe acute respiratory syndrome; symptoms include fever, dry cough, dyspnea, headache, hypoxemia (low blood oxygen concentration); usual laboratory findings include lymphopenia (reduced lymphocyte numbers), mildly elevated aminotransferase levels, possible respiratory failure and death due to alveolar damage* AHA: Q4, 2003, 46-47
480.8	Pneumonia due to other virus not elsewhere classified — *viral infection*
480.9	Unspecified viral pneumonia — *viral infection of lung, unknown virus* AHA: Q3, 1998, 5

481 Pneumococcal pneumonia (streptococcus pneumoniae pneumonia) OK
AHA: March-April, 1985, 6; Q1, 1988, 13; Q1, 1991, 13; Q1, 1992, 18; Q4, 1992, 19; Q2, 1998, 7

482 Other bacterial pneumonia
AHA: Q4, 1993, 39

482.0	Pneumonia due to Klebsiella pneumoniae — *bacterial infection* AHA: Q4, 1993, 39
482.1	Pneumonia due to Pseudomonas — *bacterial infection of lung* AHA: Q4, 1993, 39
482.2	Pneumonia due to Hemophilus influenzae (H. influenzae) — *bacterial infection of lung* AHA: Q4, 1993, 39; Q2, 2005, 19

This rubric excludes pneumonia due to *Streptococcus pneumoniae* (481).

482.30	Pneumonia due to unspecified Streptococcus — *strep infection of lung, unknown variety* AHA: Q1, 1988, 13; Q4, 1993, 39
482.31	Pneumonia due to Streptococcus, group A — *strep infection of lung* AHA: Q1, 1988, 13; Q4, 1993, 39
482.32	Pneumonia due to Streptococcus, group B — *strep infection of lung* AHA: Q1, 1988, 13; Q4, 1993, 39
482.39	Pneumonia due to other Streptococcus — *strep infection of lung, not otherwise specified* AHA: Q1, 1988, 13; Q4, 1993, 39
482.40	Pneumonia due to Staphylococcus, unspecified — *staph infection of lung, unknown variety* AHA: Q3, 1991, 16; Q4, 1993, 39
482.41	Pneumonia due to Staphylococcus aureus — *staph infection of lung* AHA: Q3, 1991, 16; Q4, 1993, 39
482.49	Other Staphylococcus pneumonia — *staph infection of lung, unknown variety* AHA: Q3, 1991, 16; Q4, 1993, 39
482.81	Pneumonia due to anaerobes — *bacteroides, gram-negative anaerobes* AHA: Q3, 1988, 11; Q4, 1993, 39
482.82	Pneumonia due to Escherichia coli (E. coli)
482.83	Pneumonia due to other gram-negative bacteria — *proteus, Serratia marcescens, gram-negative not otherwise specified* AHA: Q3, 1988, 11; Q4, 1993, 39; Q3, 1994, 9; Q2, 1998, 5
482.84	Legionnaires' disease
482.89	Pneumonia due to other specified bacteria — *not elsewhere classified* AHA: Q3, 1988, 11; Q4, 1993, 39; Q2, 1997, 6
482.9	Unspecified bacterial pneumonia — *bacterial pneumonia, unknown* AHA: Q4, 1993, 39; Q1, 1994, 17; Q2, 1997, 6; Q2, 1998, 6

483 Pneumonia due to other specified organism
AHA: Nov-Dec, 1987, 5

Mycoplasma pneumoniae is also known as Eaton agent pneumonia.

Signs and symptoms of pneumonia due to *Mycoplasma pneumoniae* include history of recent upper respiratory infection or bronchitis, headache, fever, severe and minimally productive cough, harsh or diminished breath sounds, earache, and cervical lymphadenopathy.

Diagnostic tests include gram stain and culture of sputum or throat washing to reveal polymorphonuclear leukocytes with no dominant organism. Other lab work demonstrates fourfold or greater rise in complement-fixing antibodies and elevated cold agglutinins (IgM antibodies binding to the erythrocyte I antigen). Chest x-ray shows pulmonary infiltrates resembling bacterial or viral pneumonia.

Therapies include antibiotics such as erythromycin or tetracycline, bed rest, and high protein diet.

Associated conditions include cold agglutinin induced hemolytic anemia, arthralgia and polyarthritis, skin rashes, Stevens-Johnson syndrome, transverse myelitis, meningoencephalitis, and myocarditis.

483.0	Pneumonia due to Mycoplasma pneumoniae — Eaton's agent, pleuropneumonia-like organism [PPLO]	
	AHA: Nov-Dec, 1987, 5	
483.1	Pneumonia due to Chlamydia	
483.8	Pneumonia due to other specified organism — not elsewhere classified	
	AHA: Nov-Dec, 1987, 5	

484 Pneumonia in infectious diseases classified elsewhere

484.1	Pneumonia in cytomegalic inclusion disease — (Code first underlying disease, 078.5) — infection of lung
484.3	Pneumonia in whooping cough — (Code first underlying disease: 033.0-033.9) — infection of lung
484.5	Pneumonia in anthrax — (Code first underlying disease, 022.1) — infection of lung
484.6	Pneumonia in aspergillosis — (Code first underlying disease, 117.3) — infection of lung
	AHA: Q4, 1997, 40
484.7	Pneumonia in other systemic mycoses — (Code first underlying disease) — infection of lung
484.8	Pneumonia in other infectious diseases classified elsewhere — (Code first underlying disease: 002.0, 083.0) — infection of lung

485 Bronchopneumonia, organism unspecified ☒

486 Pneumonia, organism unspecified ☒
AHA: Q3, 1988, 11; Q3, 1994, 10; Q3, 1997, 9; Q1, 1998, 8; Q2, 1998, 4,5; Q3, 1998, 7; Q3, 1999, 9; Q4, 1999, 6

487 Influenza

Influenza is an acute respiratory infection due to orthomyxoviruses characterized by the abrupt onset of acute tracheobronchitis. The severity of the disease varies from a mild upper respiratory infection to an extensive pneumonia that can be fatal.

Influenza virus type A is the most common and causes epidemics of varying severity. Influenza virus type B is associated with more limited epidemics and has been linked to Reye's syndrome. Influenza virus type C is an uncommon strain that causes very mild upper respiratory symptoms.

Signs and symptoms of influenza include fever, chills, malaise, cough, muscle aches, and excessive catarrh.

Diagnostic tests/reports/findings include blood work that may show leukopenia and proteinuria. Inoculation of embryonated eggs or cell cultures of throat washing isolate the virus. Chest x-ray may show pneumonia, commonly due to secondary pneumococcal or staphylococcal pneumonia.

Therapies include bed rest, antibiotics for secondary bacterial pneumonia, antipyretics for fever, and aerosol ribavirin for influenza type A or B.

Associated conditions include Reye's syndrome, secondary pneumococcal or staphylococcal pneumonia, acute sinusitis, otitis media, and, rarely, circulatory system complications such as pericarditis, myocarditis, and thrombophlebitis.

487.0	Influenza with pneumonia — (Use additional code to identify the type of pneumonia, 480.0-480.9, 481, 482.0-482.9, 483.0-483.8, 485) — flu with any form of pneumonia or bronchopneumonia
487.1	Influenza with other respiratory manifestations — flu with upper respiratory infection [URI], except pneumonia or bronchopneumonia
	AHA: Q4, 1999, 26; Q2, 2005, 18; Q1, 2006, 18
487.8	Influenza with other manifestations — encephalopathy

490–496 Chronic Obstructive Pulmonary Disease and Allied Conditions

490 Bronchitis, not specified as acute or chronic ☒
AHA: Q3, 1988, 5

Coding Clarification
Excluded from this rubric is bronchitis due to allergy (493.9), fumes and vapors (506.0), or with asthma (493.9).

491 Chronic bronchitis
AHA: Q3, 1988, 5

Obstructive chronic bronchitis is chronic bronchitis combined with obstructive lung disease. Chronic bronchitis is defined as a persistent cough with sputum production occurring on most days for at least three months of the year for at least two years. Obstructive lung disease is defined as a chronic or recurrent reduction in expiratory airflow within the lungs. Obstructive chronic bronchitis is characterized by an increased mass of mucous glands in the lungs, resulting in an increase in the thickness of the bronchial mucosa. Its most common etiology is cigarette smoking, but it also may be caused by environmental pollution or inhalation of irritant chemicals.

Signs and symptoms of obstructive chronic bronchitis include history of cigarette smoking or other respiratory irritants, sputum productive cough, exertional dyspnea, weight gain due to edema, cyanosis, tachypnea, rhonchi, wheezing with prolonged expiratory time, use of accessory muscles for respiration, jugular or neck vein distention, and pedal edema.

Diagnostic tests include chest x-ray that may show hyperinflation with increased bronchovascular markings. Pulmonary function tests show increased residual volume, decreased vital capacity, and forced expiratory volumes, normal static compliance, and diffusing capacity; ABGs reveal decreased pO2 and normal or increased pCO2. Culture of sputum reveals many neutrophils and varied organisms.

Therapies include oxygen therapy for hypoxia, antibiotics for concomitant respiratory infections, bronchodilators such as aminophylline to control bronchospasm and promote mucociliary expectoration, diuretics for edema, and ultrasonic or mechanical nebulizer treatments to loosen and help mobilize secretions.

Associated conditions include respiratory failure, atrial arrhythmias, and acute respiratory infections.

Acute bronchitis is sudden and severe inflammation of the tracheobronchial tree. Acute bronchitis may have an infectious or irritative etiology.

Signs and symptoms of acute bronchitis include a history of upper respiratory infection or exposure to irritants such as dust or fumes, cough, malaise, fever, and pain in the back and chest. Therapies include bed rest and antibiotics such as oral tetracycline when purulent sputum is present.

491.0	Simple chronic bronchitis — *persistent, catarrhal, smoker's cough*	
	AHA: Q3, 1988, 5	
491.1	Mucopurulent chronic bronchitis — *persistent, purulent, recurrent*	
	AHA: Q3, 1988, 5; Q3, 1988, 12	
491.20	Obstructive chronic bronchitis, without exacerbation	
491.21	Obstructive chronic bronchitis, with (acute) exacerbation	
	AHA: Q1, 2004, 3	
491.22	Obstructive chronic bronchitis with acute bronchitis	
	AHA: Q4, 2004, 82	
491.8	Other chronic bronchitis — *tracheitis or tracheobronchitis*	
	AHA: Q3, 1988, 5	
491.9	Unspecified chronic bronchitis — *unknown type*	
	AHA: Q3, 1988, 5	

Documentation Issues

If the documentation states chronic bronchitis, with or without mention of centrilobular emphysema (blue bloater), use code 491.2x.

If the physician documentation indicates COPD with asthmatic bronchitis, assign 493.2x.

Assign a fifth digit 0 to indicate obstructive chronic bronchitis without mention of acute exacerbation and fifth digit 1 for obstructive chronic bronchitis with acute exacerbation. Acute exacerbation of chronic obstructive bronchitis is not the same as acute bronchitis.

If the physician documents acute bronchitis and exacerbation of COPD, assign only the combination code of COPD with acute bronchitis (491.22).

Coding Clarification

Excluded from this rubric is chronic obstructive asthma with acute exacerbation, classified to 493.22.

492 Emphysema

AHA: Q3, 1988, 5; Q2, 1991, 21

Emphysema refers to any condition in which air is present in a small area of an organ or tissue, for example, in the interstices of the conjunctival tissue. Emphysema classified to category 492 refers to pulmonary emphysema only.

The definition of emphysematous bleb is a disease characterized by the formation of subpleural, air-filled cyst-like structures that are greater than 1.0 centimeter in diameter. Also known as emphysematous bullae, they can be found in association with other forms of pulmonary emphysema or can occur alone, especially in younger patients. Apical bullae are the most common cause of spontaneous pneumothorax in young patients.

492.0	Emphysematous bleb — *tension pneumatocele, vanishing lung, giant bullous emphysema*
	AHA: Q3, 1988, 5; Q2, 1991, 21; Q2, 1993, 3
492.8	Other emphysema — *pink puffer, MacLeod's syndrome, Swyer-James syndrome*
	AHA: July-Aug, 1984, 17; Q3, 1988, 5; Q2, 1991, 21; Q4, 1993, 41; Q1, 2005, 4

Coding Clarification

Other emphysema is abnormal irreversible enlargement of the air spaces distal to the terminal bronchioli accompanied by destruction of alveolar walls. The condition results in a reduction of the alveolar surface necessary for gas exchange. There are two major types of pulmonary emphysema: centroacinar and panacinar.

Centroacinar or centrilobar, emphysema affects the central parts of the lung acini and destroys the respiratory bronchioli. It often is associated with chronic bronchitis and smoking.

Panacinar, or pan lobar, emphysema destroys the alveolar walls and is distributed uniformly among the lung acini. The disease is more diffuse than centroacinar emphysema. Like centroacinar emphysema, panacinar emphysema occurs in cigarette smokers, but is also found in young adults with a familial history of emphysema.

Signs and symptoms of other emphysema include history of cigarette smoking, barrel-chested appearance, shortness of breath, anorexia, weight loss, breathing abnormalities such as the use of accessory muscles, prolonged expiration, grunting, pursed lip breathing, tachypnea, peripheral cyanosis, and digital clubbing.

Associated conditions include recurrent respiratory infections, cor pulmonale, and respiratory failure.

Other forms of pulmonary emphysema classified to this subcategory are distal acinar or paraseptal emphysema, irregular or paracicatricial emphysema, mixed emphysema, and unclassified forms of emphysema.

Emphysema stated as "with chronic bronchitis" or "chronic obstructive pulmonary disease" is assigned the appropriate code from the 491.20-491.21 range.

493 Asthma

AHA: Nov-Dec, 1984, 17; July-Aug, 1985, 8; Q3, 1988, 5,9; Q1, 1991, 13; Q4, 2000, 42; Q4, 2001, 43; Q4, 2003, 62; Q4, 2004, 137

Asthma is the narrowing of the airways due to increased responsiveness of the trachea and bronchi to various stimuli. Asthma is reversible, changing in severity either spontaneously or as a result of treatment. Asthma is associated with bronchospasm and pathologic features such as increased mucous secretion, mucosal edema and hyperemia, hypertrophy of bronchial smooth muscle, and acute inflammation.

Signs and symptoms of asthma include recurrent or chronic episodes of wheezing, dyspnea, cough, chest tightness, chest pain, tachycardia, tachypnea, increased accessory muscle respiration, and history of familial allergy.

Diagnostic tests include blood work that may show increased WBC during acute attack and eosinophilia. ABGs may show hypoxemia and respiratory alkalosis. Gross exam of sputum demonstrates viscidity, while microscopic exam of sputum reveals mucous casts, eosinophils, and elongated rhomboid crystals. Pulmonary function tests show typical abnormalities of obstructive dysfunction. Chest x-ray may show hyperinflated lungs and skin tests and inhalation bronchial challenge tests identify and evaluate the clinical significance of allergens.

Therapies include bronchodilators such as epinephrine, aminophylline, albuterol; other medications such as cromolyn sodium, anticholinergics, corticosteroids, hyposensitization or "allergy" shots; oxygen therapy; and intubation and ventilation therapy for severe attacks of asthma.

Associated conditions include respiratory failure, eosinophilia, pneumothorax, acute cor pulmonale, and atelectasis.

Triad asthma is a syndrome that occurs in patients with three conditions that can be coded: intrinsic asthma (subclassification 493.0), aspirin sensitivity (apply codes according to ICD-9-CM coding rules regarding adverse reaction), and nasal polyposis (rubric 471).

In ICD-9-CM, asthma is classified as extrinsic, intrinsic, chronic obstructive, or unspecified. Extrinsic asthma is asthma due to allergenic exposure to substances such as pollen, house dust, animal dander, molds, food or beverages, vapors, or drugs. Most prevalent in children, this condition is associated with abnormally high levels of IgE immunoglobulins, indicating an allergic reaction.

Intrinsic asthma is asthma due to nonallergenic factors such as emotional stresses, fatigue, endocrine changes, irritants (nonallergenic) such as dust and chemicals, and acute respiratory infection. More prevalent in adults, intrinsic asthma is associated with normal IgE immunoglobulin levels, indicating a nonallergic reaction.

This differentiation between extrinsic or intrinsic is considered archaic by many clinicians because manifestations of both extrinsic and intrinsic diseases commonly occur in the same patient. It is recommended that hospitals and physician offices develop coding policies for patients diagnosed with both intrinsic and extrinsic asthmatic conditions.

Chronic obstructive asthma is used to identify obstructive forms of asthma (in obstructive lung disease). Patients with chronic obstructive pulmonary disease with asthma have a continuous obstruction to airflow on expiration, which is different than patients with nonobstructive asthma, who wheeze during an asthma attack, but return to normal breathing once the attack subsides. Respiratory insufficiency is included in subcategory 493.2x because it is integral to COPD; do not code separately.

Status asthmaticus refers to a prolonged, severe asthmatic attack or airway obstruction (mucous plug) not relieved by bronchodilators. Symptoms of status asthmaticus are prolonged, severe, intractable wheezing, severe respiratory distress, asthma with respiratory failure, asthma attack with absence of breath sounds, lethargy, confusion, and failure to respond to the usual therapies.

Steroid Dependent Asthma: If there is no mention of side effects due to the steroid therapy, use a code from category 493. If, however, side effects are mentioned, both the asthma and the side effects of the steroid are coded. When the patient is being examined for adverse effects based on the long-term use of steroids, use code V58.65 *Long term (current) use of steroids* and a code from category 493 to identify the asthma.

The following fifth-digit subclassification is for use with category codes 493.0x-493.2x, 493.9x:
0 unspecified
1 with status asthmaticus
2 with acute exacerbation

493.0 ✓sth	Extrinsic asthma — *caused by environmental factor (allergy)*	
	AHA: Nov-Dec, 1984, 17; July-Aug, 1985, 8; Q3, 1988, 5,9; Q1, 1991, 13; Q4, 2000, 42; Q4, 2001, 43	
493.1 ✓sth	Intrinsic asthma — *caused by body's response to infection or other factor*	
	AHA: Nov-Dec, 1984, 17; March-April, 1985, 7; July-Aug, 1985, 8; Q3, 1988, 9; Q3, 1988, 5,9; Q1, 1991, 13; Q4, 2000, 42; Q4, 2001, 43	
493.2 ✓sth	Chronic obstructive asthma — *persistent restriction of airflow and labored breathing*	
	AHA: Nov-Dec, 1984, 17; July-Aug, 1985, 8; Q3, 1988, 5,9; Q2, 1990, 20; Q1, 1991, 13; Q2, 1991, 21; Q4, 2000, 42; Q4, 2001, 43	
493.81	Exercise induced bronchospasm — *physical activity causing spasms of the smooth muscle of the bronchi*	
493.82	Cough variant asthma — *chronic cough (more than three weeks) is the only symptom; nonproductive, nocturnal only cough is common; diagnosis only confirmed when cough resolves with asthma medication*	
493.9 ✓sth	Unspecified asthma — *unknown type*	
	AHA: Nov-Dec, 1984, 17; July-Aug, 1985, 8; Q3, 1988, 5,9; Q1, 1991, 13; Q4, 1997, 40; Q4, 2000, 42; Q4, 2001, 43; Q4, 2004, 137; Q1, 2005, 5	

Documentation Issues
Documentation must always be clear and concise when identifying asthma with other conditions.

The physician must document the presence of "status asthmaticus" to promote coding accuracy. The admission of an asthma patient to the hospital is typically due to the patient's failure to respond to therapy, requiring more intensive therapy. Do not assume that since the patient was admitted, the diagnosis is status asthmaticus. Confirm the patient status with the physician before assigning the fifth digit 1.

Coding Clarification
Asthma with Associated Conditions: The following are common diagnostic statements and their associated code assignments:

- Asthma with COPD (493.2x)
- Asthma (493.0x-493.9x) and acute bronchitis (466.0)
- Chronic obstructive emphysema (492.8) associated with asthma (493.0x-493.9x)
- Either chronic obstructive bronchitis or asthma as comorbidity, such as chronic obstructive bronchitis (491.2x) superimposed on intrinsic asthma (493.10)
- Chronic pneumothorax (512.8) with intrinsic (493.10) or extrinsic (493.00) asthma
- Atelectasis (518.0) associated with asthma (493.0x-493.9x)
- Bronchiectasis (494) associated with asthma (493.0x-493.9x)
- Mediastinal or subcutaneous nontraumatic emphysema (518.1) with asthma (493.00 or 493.10)
- Wheezing (786.07) (commonly noted symptom of COPD with asthma)
- Pneumonia (486) with asthma (493.0x-493.9x)
- Reactive airway disease (493.90 *Asthma, type unspecified, status unspecified*)

Two codes are required when a patient is admitted with acute bronchitis and acute exacerbation of asthma, since both conditions are acute. Sequencing depends on the focus of care.

Coding Scenario
A 49-year-old patient is seen in the clinic for adrenal-pituitary insufficiency secondary to steroids. The patient is a known steroid-dependent asthmatic.

Code assignment: 255.4 *Corticoadrenal insufficiency*, 493.90 *Asthma, type unspecified, status unspecified*, and E932.0 *Drug causing adverse effects in therapeutic use, adrenal cortical steroids*

A 14-year-old male patient is seen in the emergency department with acute shortness of breath. The

Diseases of the Respiratory System

patient is a known asthmatic. The physician's diagnosis is asthma.

Code assignment: 493.90 *Asthma, type unspecified*

A patient is admitted with acute respiratory insufficiency and asthma. The patient's history identifies that the patient has chronic obstructive asthma. The physician's final diagnosis on the discharge summary indicates chronic obstructive asthma with status asthmaticus and acute respiratory failure.

Code assignment: 518.81 *Acute respiratory failure* and 493.21 *Chronic obstructive asthma with status asthmaticus*

Note: Acute respiratory failure may be assigned as the principal diagnosis when the condition is established as chiefly responsible for the admission. While the documentation indicated that the patient was admitted with acute respiratory failure and chronic obstructive asthma with status asthmaticus, both are life-threatening conditions and meet the definition of principal diagnosis. Either may be sequenced first. Coding guidelines give preference to assigning the acute respiratory failure as principal when associated with another respiratory condition.

A 20-year-old female patient, a collegiate track athlete, is admitted after collapsing during a track event with acute exacerbation of asthma. The patient's condition is brought under control with Albuterol and oxygen.

Code assignment: 493.92 *Asthma, unspecified, with acute exacerbation*

494 Bronchiectasis
AHA: Q3, 1988, 5; Q4, 2000, 42

Bronchiectasis is the dilation of bronchi with mucous production and persistent cough. Mounier-Kuhn syndrome is a form of bronchiectasis. Code choice is determined by whether the patient also presents with acute bronchitis (acute exacerbation).

494.0	Bronchiectasis without acute exacerbation — *dilation of bronchi, mucous production, cough* **AHA:** Q3, 1988, 5; Q4, 2000, 42
494.1	Bronchiectasis with acute exacerbation — *dilation of bronchi, mucous production, cough, with sudden worsening of condition* **AHA:** Q3, 1988, 5; Q4, 2000, 42

Coding Clarification
Excluded from this rubric is bronchiectasis as a congenital disorder (748.61) and bronchiectasis in active tuberculosis (011.5).

495 Extrinsic allergic alveolitis
AHA: Q3, 1988, 5

Codes in this rubric report inflammation of the alveoli of the lung due to allergic reaction to the environment, including inhaled organic dust particles of fungal, thermophilic actinomycete, or other origin.

495.0	Farmers' lung — *antigen: Micropolyspora faeni or Thermoactinomyces vulgaris in moldy hay* **AHA:** Q3, 1988, 5
495.1	Bagassosis — *antigen: Micropolyspora faeni or Thermoactinomyces vulgaris in sugarcane waste* **AHA:** Q3, 1988, 5
495.2	Bird-fanciers' lung — *antigen: bird droppings from parakeets, pigeons and chickens* **AHA:** Q3, 1988, 5
495.3	Suberosis — *antigen: moldy cork dust; "cork-handler's lung"* **AHA:** Q3, 1988, 5
495.4	Malt workers' lung — *antigen: Aspergillus clavatus or Aspergillus fumigatus in moldy barley or malt* **AHA:** Q3, 1988, 5
495.5	Mushroom workers' lung — *antigen: Micropolyspora faeni or Thermoactinomyces vulgaris in mushroom compost* **AHA:** Q3, 1988, 5
495.6	Maple bark-strippers' lung — *antigen: Cryptostroma corticale in infected maple bark* **AHA:** Q3, 1988, 5
495.7	"Ventilation" pneumonitis — *antigen: any of numerous organisms growing in ventilation systems* **AHA:** Q3, 1988, 5
495.8	Other specified allergic alveolitis and pneumonitis — *wood asthma, coffee workers' lung, fish meal workers' lung, furrier's lung* **AHA:** Q3, 1988, 5
495.9	Unspecified allergic alveolitis and pneumonitis — *unknown extrinsic alveolitis* **AHA:** Q3, 1988, 5

496 Chronic airway obstruction, not elsewhere classified
AHA: Q3, 1988, 5,56; Q2, 1991, 21; Q2, 1992, 16; Q2, 2000, 15; Q4, 2003, 109

Chronic airway obstruction is a nonspecific condition characterized by a chronic or recurrent reduction in expiratory airflow within the lung. Chronic obstructive pulmonary disease (COPD) and chronic obstructive lung disease (COLD) are the two most common descriptive diagnostic terms assigned to this code category.

Signs and symptoms of chronic airway obstruction, not elsewhere classified, include history of cigarette smoking and frequent respiratory infections, dyspnea on exertion with reduced exercise tolerance, sputum-productive cough, bronchi, decreased intensity of breath sounds, and prolonged expiration. Therapies include bronchodilators such as theophylline, corticosteroids such as prednisone, oxygen therapy and chest physiotherapy, and antibiotics for superimposed acute respiratory infections. Associated conditions include cor pulmonale (chronic pulmonary hypertension), sinus tachycardia, supraventricular arrhythmias, secondary polycythemia, acute bronchitis, pneumonia, left ventricular failure, pulmonary embolism, and acute respiratory insufficiency or failure.

Coding Clarification
Do not assign code 496 with any code from categories 491 through 493.

500–508 Pneumoconioses and Other Lung Diseases Due to External Agents

500 Coal workers' pneumoconiosis OK
Inhaling coal dust for prolonged periods can cause the disabling coal workers' pneumoconiosis, also known as black lung disease, which may produce: 1) asymptomatic anthracosis; 2) simple coal-workers pneumoconiosis (characterized by coal macules and nodules containing carbon-laden macrophages), with little or no pulmonary dysfunction; or 3) complicated coal-workers pneumoconiosis or progressive massive fibrosis (e.g., black scars in the lungs compromising pulmonary function).
Symptoms include shortness of breath and a chronic cough. The diagnosis can be made with chest x-ray or a pulmonary function test. Most affected workers are older than age 50. Although some miners never develop the disease, others may develop the early signs after less than 10 years of mining experience. According to recent studies by the National Institute for Occupational Safety and Health (NIOSH), about one of every 20 miners studied has X-ray evidence of some pneumoconiosis. Pneumoconiosis is not reversible and federal laws require that mine dust levels be controlled to help prevent pneumoconiosis.

501 Asbestosis OK
Asbestosis is a serious lung inflammation caused by asbestos exposure (i.e., installed or removed insulation before 1975) that makes the lungs more susceptible to lung infections, such as the flu or pneumococcus. In addition, asbestosis can lead to mesothelioma, a rare form of cancer in which malignant cells are found in the sac lining of the chest or abdomen. There is no cure for asbestosis, although symptoms can be treated. For example, the coughing can be treated with supplemental oxygen and treatments to remove secretions from the lung. According to the Occupational Safety and Health Administration: "OSHA is aware of no instance in which exposure to a toxic substance has more clearly demonstrated detrimental health effects on humans than has asbestos exposure. The diseases caused by asbestos exposure are life-threatening or disabling. Among these diseases are lung cancer, cancer of the mesothelial lining of the pleura and peritoneum, asbestosis, and gastrointestinal cancer."

502 Pneumoconiosis due to other silica or silicates OK
Silicosis is a pneumoconiosis that usually follows long-term inhalation of small particles of crystalline free silica in such industries as metal mining (lead, hard coal, copper, silver, gold), metal casting, pottery making, and sandstone and granite cutting. The etiology involves alveolar macrophages that engulf particles of free silica and enter the lymphatics and interstitial tissue. The macrophages cause the release of toxic enzymes, and fibrosis of the lung parenchyma occurs. When a macrophage dies, the silica particles are released and engulfed by other macrophages, and the process is repeated. Patients with simple nodular silicosis have no respiratory symptoms and usually no respiratory impairment. They may cough and raise sputum, but these symptoms are due to industrial bronchitis and occur as often in persons with normal x-rays.
Conglomerate silicosis may lead to severe shortness of breath, cough, and sputum, with severity related to the size of the conglomerate in the lungs. Extensive masses can cause severe disability. Exposure of 20 to 30 years is necessary before the disease becomes apparent, although it can develop in less than 10 years when the exposure to dust is extremely high (i.e., in industries such as tunneling, abrasive soap making, and sandblasting). No effective treatment is known other than lung transplantation.

503 Pneumoconiosis due to other inorganic dust OK
Parenchymal lung diseases due to chronic inhalation of inorganic (mineral) dusts are called pneumoconioses. Several inert dusts, including iron oxide, barium, and tin, can produce conditions known as siderosis, baritosis, and stannosis,

respectively. Berylliosis, also called beryllium disease, beryllium poisoning, or beryllium granulomatosis, is generalized granulomatous disease caused by inhalation of dust or fumes containing beryllium compounds and products. Acute berylliosis is a chemical pneumonitis, but other tissues (i.e., skin and conjunctivae) may be affected. Symptoms of chronic berylliosis include cough, chest pain, weight loss, and fatigue, although the patient may not develop any of these until 20 years after exposure has ceased. Diagnosis depends on a history of exposure and clinical manifestations. However, unless special immunologic techniques are used, distinguishing berylliosis from sarcoidosis (reported with ICD-9-CM code 135) is often impossible.

504　Pneumonopathy due to inhalation of other dust OK

505　Unspecified pneumoconiosis OK

506　Respiratory conditions due to chemical fumes and vapors

506.0	Bronchitis and pneumonitis due to fumes and vapors — (Use additional E code to identify cause) — *sudden, severe chemical bronchitis*
506.1	Acute pulmonary edema due to fumes and vapors — (Use additional E code to identify cause) — *sudden, severe edema* AHA: Q3, 1988, 4
506.2	Upper respiratory inflammation due to fumes and vapors — (Use additional E code to identify cause) — *upper respiratory infection [URI] other than what is specified* AHA: Q3, 2005, 10
506.3	Other acute and subacute respiratory conditions due to fumes and vapors — (Use additional E code to identify cause) — *not specified elsewhere*
506.4	Chronic respiratory conditions due to fumes and vapors — (Use additional E code to identify cause) — *emphysema, obliterative bronchiolitis, pulmonary fibrosis*
506.9	Unspecified respiratory conditions due to fumes and vapors — (Use additional E code to identify cause)

507　Pneumonitis due to solids and liquids
AHA: Q3, 1991, 16

Pneumonitis due to solids and liquids is pneumonitis and pneumonia due to aspiration of foreign material into the tracheobronchial tree. Aspiration of inert material such as drinking water may cause asphyxia (category 934), but rarely results in pneumonia or pneumonitis. Aspiration of gastric contents or toxic materials such as petroleum distillates often causes pneumonia or pneumonitis due to an inflammatory response in the lungs and lung parenchyma.

"Cafe coronary syndrome" is an acute condition characterized by obstruction of the trachea or bronchi due to large particulate material such as meat and often results in a necrotizing pneumonitis. Signs and symptoms of pneumonitis due to inhalation of food or vomitus include a history of feeding disorder, convulsive disorder, marked debility or disturbance of consciousness, drug or alcohol intoxication, rales, dyspnea, cyanosis, hypotension, and tachycardia.

Diagnostic tests include chest x-ray to locate areas of multilobar infiltrates. ABGs suggest hypoxemia and gross exam may show blood-tinged sputum. Culture of sputum may reveal gram-positive and gram-negative organisms if infective nasopharyngeal organisms have been aspirated. Associated conditions include dehydration, concomitant bacterial pneumonia, bronchiectasis, pulmonary fibrosis, and acute respiratory failure.

Aspiration of gastric acid with a pH of less than 2.5, which can result in a life-threatening pneumonitis, may be referred to as "chemical pneumonitis." Fetal aspiration pneumonitis is not coded to this category and should be assigned 770.18.

507.0	Pneumonitis due to inhalation of food or vomitus — *aspiration pneumonia from food, saliva, vomit, not otherwise specified* AHA: Q1, 1989, 10; Q3, 1991, 16
507.1	Pneumonitis due to inhalation of oils and essences — *exogenous lipoid pneumonia* AHA: Q3, 1991, 16
507.8	Pneumonitis due to other solids and liquids — *detergent asthma* AHA: Q3, 1991, 16

Coding Clarification

Although chemical pneumonitis usually is classified to rubric 506, when chemical pneumonitis is due to aspiration, assign 507.0.

Aspiration pneumonia or pneumonitis due to — or resulting from the presence of — a nasogastric tube, endotracheal tube, or tracheostomy is classified as a postoperative complication (997.3). The code for aspiration pneumonia may be used as a secondary code to further explain the nature of the respiratory complication. Note that in the case of aspiration pneumonia or pneumonitis following anesthesia, the proper cause and effect relationship needs to be determined. For example, if the aspiration pneumonia or pneumonitis is due to the induction of anesthesia (endotracheal intubation and aspiration, including Mendelson's syndrome), assign 997.3. If the aspiration pneumonia or pneumonitis is due to the anesthetic agent, follow ICD-9-CM coding rules regarding adverse reactions to drugs and chemicals.

Subcategory 507.1 includes lipid (or "lipoid") pneumonia when due to an exogenous source. Lipid pneumonia is a chronic syndrome due to the repeated aspiration of oil-containing substances such as mineral oil, cod liver oil, and oily nose drops. This code excludes endogenous lipid pneumonia, which is caused by retention of lipids in the lung parenchyma released during the breakdown of tissue. Endogenous lipid pneumonia is reported with 516.8.

Subcategory 507.8 includes hydrocarbon pneumonitis and pneumonia due to inhalation or aspiration of solids and liquids. It excludes hydrocarbon pneumonitis and pneumonia due to fumes and vapors, which are classified in rubric 506.

508 Respiratory conditions due to other and unspecified external agents

508.0	Acute pulmonary manifestations due to radiation — (Use additional E code to identify cause) — *radiation pneumonitis* AHA: Q2, 1988, 4
508.1	Chronic and other pulmonary manifestations due to radiation — (Use additional E code to identify cause) — *fibrosis of lung following radiation*
508.8	Respiratory conditions due to other specified external agents — (Use additional E code to identify cause) — *not elsewhere specified*
508.9	Respiratory conditions due to unspecified external agent — (Use additional E code to identify cause)

510–519 Other Diseases of Respiratory System

510 Empyema

Empyema is an infection in the pleural space. It is frequently accompanied by chest pain, shortness of breath, weakness, fever, and hemoptysis.

510.0	Empyema with fistula — (Use additional code to identify infectious organism: 041.00-041.9) — *including thoracic, pleural, mediastinal, hepatopleural, bronchopleural, bronchocutaneous*
510.9	Empyema without mention of fistula — (Use additional code to identify infectious organism: 041.00-041.9) — *with abscess, pyothorax, pyopneumothorax, empyema, fibrinopurulent pleurisy* AHA: Q3, 1994, 6

Coding Clarification
A code for the infective agent in empyema can be found in Chapter 1 Infectious and Parasitic Diseases and should be reported secondarily. Empyema is classified according to whether a fistula is present.

511 Pleurisy

Pleurisy, also called pleuritic chest pain, is the inflammation of the pleura membrane that lines the chest cavity and contains the lung. Most cases are caused by infection, and many are associated with pneumonia in the underlying lung. Some cases are caused by viral infections or it may occur in other diseases such as tuberculosis, systemic lupus erythematosus, rheumatic fever, and kidney failure. Pleurisy may develop in conjunction with a blood clot on the lung; it may also be associated with the development of fluid in the pleural space between the chest wall and the lung. Sharp pain brought on by breathing and coughing is the most common symptom. If considerable fluid accumulates, the pain may subside, but the fluid may compress the lung and the patient may feel short of breath. In acute pleurisy, the pleura become reddened and covered by an exudate of lymph, fibrin, and cellular elements. The disease may advance to the second stage, in which adhesions, usually permanent, unite the inflamed surfaces. Diagnosis includes patient history about symptoms and previous illness and listening to the chest for sounds of irritated pleurae and pleural effusion. A chest x-ray may be required. A sample of fluid may be taken from the pleural space with a needle and syringe for microscopic examination in cases of suspected pleural effusion (fluid accumulation and bacterial infection). Since pleurisy and pleural effusion are symptoms of basic disorders, the treatment requires identifying and treating the underlying disease. The pain is controlled with analgesic drugs. For acute pleurisy accompanied by effusion, treatment includes drugs, including streptokinase and urokinase, cortisone and cefotetan, and fibrinolytic agents, and non-drug therapies such as shunts and chest drainage catheters, mini-invasive surgery, open thoracotomy, and decortication.

The definition of unspecified pleural effusion is abnormal accumulation of fluid in the pleural space, unspecified as to etiology. Included are transudative and exudative pleurisy and pleural effusions without further specification. Pleural effusion is a common manifestation of both systemic and intrathoracic diseases.

Signs and symptoms of unspecified pleural effusion include pleuritic chest pain, dyspnea, decreased tactile fremitus, pleural friction rub, dullness to percussion, egophony, and distant breath sounds. Therapies include thoracentesis (percutaneous) to remove excess fluid and relieve pain, tube thoracostomy for continuous drainage, and pleurodesis or pleurectomy for malignant pleural effusion.

511.0	Pleurisy without mention of effusion or current tuberculosis — *with adhesion, calcification, thickening of pleura* **AHA:** Q3, 1994, 5
511.1	Pleurisy with effusion, with mention of bacterial cause other than tuberculosis — *pneumococcal, staphylococcal, streptococcal*
511.8	Pleurisy with other specified forms of effusion, except tuberculous — *encysted pleurisy, hemopneumothorax, hemothorax, hydropneumothorax, pleurorrhea, hydrothorax* **AHA:** Q1, 1997, 10
511.9	Unspecified pleural effusion

Coding Clarification
Malignant pleural effusion (197.2) and pleurisy with tuberculosis (012.0) are excluded from this rubric.

512 Pneumothorax
Pneumothorax is air or other gas in the pleural space. This gas displaces lung capacity, and is commonly referred to as a "collapsed lung" because of the reduction in lung volume.

An iatrogenic pneumothorax occurs as the result of air introduced into the pleural space or lung puncture during a medical procedure. Most commonly, iatrogenic pneumothorax will occur during thoracentesis, catheter placement, arteriography, or intercostal nerve block.

Pneumothorax is a common risk associated with most thoracic surgery. It is inappropriate to assign the code for iatrogenic pneumothorax, unless it is specified as such by the physician.

Spontaneous pneumothorax is most common in adult males and has a high incidence of occurrence among patients with Marfan's syndrome. Nearly a third of patients with spontaneous pneumothorax have underlying chronic pulmonary disease.

Tension pneumothorax occurs when pressure in the pleural space is not sufficient to displace the mediastinum to the opposite side. Because this compromises venous return, tension pneumothorax is considered a medical emergency.

512.0	Spontaneous tension pneumothorax — *air leaking from the lung, and trapped in the lung lining* **AHA:** Q3, 1994, 5
512.1	Iatrogenic pneumothorax — *air leaking from the lung, following surgery* **AHA:** Q4, 1994, 40
512.8	Other spontaneous pneumothorax — *spontaneous or sucking pneumothorax, or pneumothorax not otherwise specified* **AHA:** Q2, 1993, 3

513 Abscess of lung and mediastinum

513.0	Abscess of lung — *abscess, necrosis, or gangrene* **AHA:** Q2, 1998, 7
513.1	Abscess of mediastinum — *pocket of pus in the tissue between the organs behind the sternum*

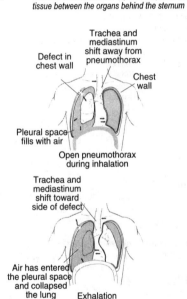

514 Pulmonary congestion and hypostasis
AHA: Q3, 1988, 5; Q2, 1998, 6

Coding Clarification
Hypostatic pneumonia due to or specified as a specific type of pneumonia would not be reported with this code; rather, a code should be assigned based on the type of pneumonia (480.0-480.9, 481, 482.0-482.49, 483.0-483.8, 485, 486, 487.0).

Coders' Desk Reference for Diagnoses

515 Postinflammatory pulmonary fibrosis ✓3

516 Other alveolar and parietoalveolar pneumonopathy

516.0   Pulmonary alveolar proteinosis — *chronic proteinaceous deposits in alveoli; Rosen-Castleman-Liebow syndrome*

516.1   Idiopathic pulmonary hemosiderosis — (Code first underlying disease, 275.0) — *essential brown induration of lung*

516.2   Pulmonary alveolar microlithiasis — *minute concretions in alveoli*

516.3   Idiopathic fibrosing alveolitis — *alveolar capillary block, diffuse pulmonary, Hamman-Rich syndrome*

516.8   Other specified alveolar and parietoalveolar pneumonopathies — *not otherwise classified, including endogenous lipoid pneumonia*
AHA: Q1, 1992, 12; Q2, 2006, 20

516.9   Unspecified alveolar and parietoalveolar pneumonopathy

517 Lung involvement in conditions classified elsewhere

517.1   Rheumatic pneumonia — (Code first underlying disease, 390)

517.2   Lung involvement in systemic sclerosis — (Code first underlying disease, 710.1)

517.3   Acute chest syndrome — (Code first sickle-cell disease in crisis: 282.42, 282.62, 282.64, 282.69)

517.8   Lung involvement in other diseases classified elsewhere — (Code first underlying disease: 135, 277.3, 710.0, 710.2, 710.4) — *not otherwise specified*
AHA: Q2, 2003, 7

Coding Clarification
Codes in this rubric should not be used as the principal or primary diagnosis. Code first the underlying disease.

518 Other diseases of lung

518.0   Pulmonary collapse — *no air in a part of the lung; atelectasis, Brock's syndrome, middle lobe syndrome*
AHA: Q4, 1990, 25

Pulmonary collapse is incomplete expansion of lobules (clusters of alveoli) or lung segments. Also called atelectasis, this condition may result in partial or complete lung collapse, which impairs gas exchange, resulting in hypoxia. Pulmonary collapse may be due to obstructions, such as mucous plugs, neoplasms and foreign bodies, or to external compression of the lungs from conditions such as pleural effusion, enlarged thoracic lymph nodes, and pneumothorax.

Signs and symptoms of pulmonary collapse include asymptomatic with slowly developing or minor atelectasis, decreased breath sounds, dull chest percussions with rapidly developing or massive atelectasis, sudden dyspnea, cyanosis, hypotension, tachycardia, elevated temperature, peripheral circulatory collapse or shock, diaphoresis, and substernal or intercostal retraction. Associated conditions include bronchiectasis, pulmonary fibrosis, infective pneumonitis, pleural effusion, enlarged thoracic lymph nodes, and pneumothorax.

518.1   Interstitial emphysema — *air trapped inappropriately in tissue outside bronchi, alveoli, or bronchioli; mediastinal emphysema or Hamman's syndrome*

518.2   Compensatory emphysema — *overdistension of lung tissue into a void created when adjacent tissue was excised or damaged*

518.3   Pulmonary eosinophilia — *transient infiltrations of lungs by eosinophilia; Löffler's syndrome, PIE syndrome, Weingarten's syndrome*

518.4   Unspecified acute edema of lung — *severe, sudden fluid retention within the lung, including postoperative*

518.5   Pulmonary insufficiency following trauma and surgery — *adult respiratory distress syndrome [ARDS], Woillez's disease*
AHA: Sept-Oct, 1987, 1; Q3, 1988, 3; Q3, 1988, 7; Q4, 2004, 139

518.6   Allergic bronchopulmonary aspergillosis

518.7   Transfusion related acute lung injury (TRALI)

Transfusion related acute lung injury (TRALI) is a relatively rare, but serious, pulmonary complication of blood transfusion. The signs and symptoms that occur post-transfusion include acute respiratory distress, noncardiogenic pulmonary edema, cyanosis, hypoxemia, hypotension, fever, and chills. Onset usually occurs within one to two hours of transfusion, with rapid progression during four to six hours post-transfusion. White blood cell response to antigens leads to increased vascular permeability of the pulmonary microvasculature. This capillary injury results in pulmonary edema.

Treatment of TRALI is the same as for ARDS. Of primary importance is stopping the offending transfusion. Most often, face-mask continuous positive airway pressure and added oxygen or ventilation with hemodynamic support are required. The vast majority of cases resolve within 96 hours if properly treated and often with complete resolution and little sequelae. Renal failure or other antibody-related organ damage has occurred in some cases.

TRALI can be prevented by avoiding unnecessary transfusion, carefully screening donors for leukocyte antibodies, and using commercially available pooled plasma preparations instead of single-donor fresh-frozen plasma.

518.8 ⌐sth   Other diseases of lung

Coding Clarification

Respiratory failure is failure of oxygenation and/or ventilation that is severe enough to impair or threaten the functioning of vital organs. With failure of oxygenation, the tissues of the lung are not functioning properly. An example of failure of oxygenation would be an acute exacerbation of bronchial asthma in a patient with emphysema. With failure of ventilation, airflow in and out of the lungs is impaired, for example, by compression of the trachea caused by metastatic carcinoma of the thoracic lymph nodes.

Signs and symptoms of respiratory failure include headache, cyanosis, dyspnea, impaired motor function, restlessness, confusion, anxiety, delirium, and occasionally symptoms of depressed consciousness, tachypnea, tachycardia, and tremor. Associated conditions include chronic obstructive lung disease such as chronic obstructive bronchitis, emphysema, cystic fibrosis, acute obstructive lung disease such as asthma, pneumonia, and acute bronchitis.

Diagnosis of respiratory failure based on ABG values is not absolute and may be adjusted according to the patient's baseline blood gas levels. Since some COPD patients have chronically abnormal values, the diagnosis of respiratory failure is made based on further decompensation from the patient's baseline.

518.81	Acute respiratory failure — *not otherwise specified* **AHA:** Sept-Oct, 1987, 1; Q3, 1988, 7; Q3, 1988, 10; Q2, 1990, 20; Q4, 1990, 25; Q2, 1991, 3; Q3, 1991, 14; Q4, 1998, 41; Q1, 2003, 15; Q4, 2004, 139; Q1, 2005, 3-8; Q2, 2005, 19; Q4, 2005, 96
518.82	Other pulmonary insufficiency, not elsewhere classified — *acute respiratory distress not elsewhere classified* **AHA:** Q3, 1988, 7; Q2, 1991, 21; Q4, 2003, 105
518.83	Chronic respiratory failure — *persistent* **AHA:** Q4, 2003, 103, 111; Q4, 2005, 96
518.84	Acute and chronic respiratory failure — *sudden, severe*
518.89	Other diseases of lung, not elsewhere classified — *cyst, degeneration, scarring, pulmolithiasis, calcification, broncholithiasis, or occlusion* **AHA:** Q4, 1988, 6; Q3, 1990, 18

Documentation Issues

When reviewing the documenta5tion for supporting evidence of respiratory failure, the arterial blood gas pH is a helpful tool in making that determination in a patient with known chronic pulmonary disease. If the arterial blood gas pH is less than 7.35, it is a good indication of respiratory failure. Clarify with the physician before assigning a code for the respiratory failure. Additional documentation also must be provided to support the diagnosis.

If the documentation indicates that acute respiratory failure was the reason for the admission, then it is the principal/primary diagnosis for the hospital stay.

Coding Clarification

General: Four codes are used to separately classify respiratory failure:

- Respiratory failure following shock, trauma, and surgery — 518.5
- Acute and not otherwise specified respiratory failure — 518.81
- Chronic respiratory failure — 518.83
- Acute and chronic respiratory failure — 518.84

Adult Respiratory Distress Syndrome (ARDS): Noted as another term for respiratory failure due to shock, trauma, and surgery, this condition occurs in the presence of previously normal lungs. Other terms that identify adult respiratory distress syndrome are:

- Adult hyaline membrane disease
- DeNang lung syndrome
- White lung syndrome
- Postperfusion lung
- Capillary leak Syndrome
- Trauma wet lung
- Shock lung

To report ARDS, use code 518.5 *Pulmonary insufficiency following trauma and surgery.*

Drug Overdose with Respiratory Failure: If the patient is diagnosed with a drug overdose, the poisoning code is listed first, then the respiratory failure code. It is inappropriate to use the respiratory failure as the principal/primary diagnosis based on the requirement for ventilatory support. Keep in mind that poisoning codes take precedence over the code for the resulting condition.

Respiratory Failure Associated with Nonrespiratory Conditions: Sequencing is a common problem with coding respiratory failure with nonrespiratory conditions.

The coding advice regarding the sequencing of respiratory failure has been revised and published in the AHA: Q1, 2005, 3-8. This advice supersedes previous guidelines #1 and #2 published in AHA: Q2, 1991, 3. The revision allows the sequencing of the respiratory failure to be based upon the circumstances of the admission.

If the patient is admitted with respiratory failure and another acute nonrespiratory condition or acute chronic nonrespiratory condition and both conditions are responsible for the admission and meet the definition of principal, either may be assigned as principal. Respiratory failure may be assigned as a secondary diagnosis if the respiratory failure occurs after admission.

For patients admitted with acute respiratory failure and another chronic respiratory condition, the acute respiratory failure is assigned as principal.

Chapter-specific guidelines always take precedence over general guidelines.

Coding Scenario
A 63-year-old female is admitted to the facility in acute respiratory failure. The physician's final diagnostic statement identifies that the acute respiratory failure is due to mycoplasma pneumonia.

    Code assignment: 518.81 *Acute respiratory failure* and 483 *Mycoplasma pneumoniae*

A patient is admitted following an overdose of Valium. The patient is found to be in acute respiratory failure and is placed on ventilatory support.

    Code assignment: 969.4 *Poisoning by psychotropic agents, benzodiazepine-based tranquilizers*, 305.40 *Nondependent abuse of drugs, barbiturate and similarly acting sedative or hypnotic, unspecified*, 518.81 *Acute respiratory failure*, and E853.2 *Accidental poisoning by tranquilizers, benzodiazepine-based tranquilizers*

A patient is admitted to the facility via the emergency department with severe chest pain and shortness of breath. The final diagnosis is an acute nontransmural infarction, complicated by acute respiratory failure.

    Code assignment: 410.71 *Acute myocardial infarction, subendocardial infarction* and 518.81 *Acute respiratory failure*

519 Other diseases of respiratory system

519.00		Unspecified tracheostomy complication
519.01		Infection of tracheostomy — (Use additional code to identify type of infection: 038.0-038.9, 682.1. Use additional code to identify organism: 041.00-041.9)
519.02		Mechanical complication of tracheostomy — *tracheal stenosis*
519.09		Other tracheostomy complications — *hemorrhage, fistula*
519.11		Acute bronchospasm — *bronchospasm, not otherwise specified*
	AHA: Q3, 1988, 6	

Acute bronchospasm is an abnormal contraction of the smooth muscle of the bronchi, causing narrowing and obstruction of the airway. The physiology of a bronchospasm consists of an autonomic contraction of the pulmonary muscles, often coupled with inflammation of the pleura. The bronchus becomes constricted and the mucosa inflamed, which reduces the airway's diameter and restricts breathing. When the bronchial mucosa is irritated or inflamed, it produces sticky mucus that can also plug the bronchus and further restrict airflow.

The following exposures are considered "triggers" for a bronchospastic response:

- Allergy — Inhalation or ingestion of an allergen such as animal dander, dust, certain foods, pollen, or spores
- Exercise — Overexertion or participation in exercise, usually precipitated by coughing or wheezing
- Exposures — Contact with irritants such as aerosol sprays, certain chemicals, cigarette smoke, fumes, odors, and secondary smoke from fire or other vapors
- Infection — Illness due to infection
- Stress — Emotional and psychological stress

Bronchospasm that is recurrent in nature may ultimately lead to the diagnosis of asthma.

Coding Clarification
Code 519.11 excludes acute bronchitis with bronchospasm (466.0), asthma (493.00-493.92), and bronchospasm specified as exercise induced (493.81)

Code 519.11 *Acute bronchospasm* enables reporting and monitoring of incidences and recurrences of bronchospasm in patients who have not yet been diagnosed with asthma, and/or do not meet bronchitis criteria.

Bronchospasm associated with acute bronchitis is inherent in the condition and is included in the code for acute bronchitis (466.0).

519.19	Other diseases of trachea and bronchus — *mucous plug, calcification, ulcer, stenosis*
	AHA: Q3, 2002, 18
519.2	Mediastinitis — *inflammation of the tissue between the organs behind the sternum*

Diseases of the Respiratory System

519.3 Other diseases of mediastinum, not elsewhere classified — *fibrosis, hernia, retraction*

519.4 Disorders of diaphragm — *diaphragmitis, paralysis, relation*

519.8 Other diseases of respiratory system, not elsewhere classified — *cyst of pleura*
AHA: Q4, 1989, 12

519.9 Unspecified disease of respiratory system — *unknown, but including chronic respiratory disease not otherwise specified*

520–579
Diseases of the Digestive System

This chapter classifies diseases and disorders of all of the organs along the alimentary (digestive) tract — the long, muscular tube that begins at the mouth and ends at the anus. The major digestive organs include the pharynx, esophagus, stomach, and intestines. Accessory, or secondary, organs include the salivary and parotid glands, jaw, teeth, and the supporting structures of teeth, tongue, liver, gallbladder and biliary tract, pancreas, and peritoneum.

Structures that support the digestive process from outside this continuous tube are also included in this system: gallbladder, pancreas, and liver. These organs provide secretions that are critical to food absorption and use by the body.

The digestive system is a group of organs that breaks down and changes food chemically for absorption as simple, soluble substances by blood, lymph systems, and body tissues. The digestive system begins in the mouth, continues in the pharynx and esophagus, the stomach, the small and large intestines, the rectum, and the anus.

Digestion involves mechanical and chemical processes. Mechanical actions include chewing in the mouth, churning action in the stomach, and intestinal peristaltic action. These mechanical forces move the food through the digestive tract and mix it with secretions containing enzymes, which accomplish three chemical reactions: the conversion of carbohydrates to simple sugars, the breakdown of proteins into amino acids, and the conversion of fats into fatty acids and glycerol.

The stomach churns and mixes the food with hydrochloric acid and enzymes and gradually releases materials into the upper small intestine (the duodenum) through the pyloric sphincter.

The majority of the digestive process occurs in the small intestine where most foods are hydrolysed and absorbed. The products of digestion are actively or passively transported through the wall of the small intestine and assimilated into the body. The stomach and the large intestine (colon) can also absorb water, alcohol, certain salts and crystalloids, and some drugs. Water-soluble digestive products (minerals, amino acids, and carbohydrates) are transferred into the blood system and transported to the liver. Many fats, resynthesized in the intestinal wall, are picked up by the lymphatic system and enter the blood stream through the vena caval system, bypassing the liver.

Remaining undigested matter is passed into the large intestine (the colon) where water is extracted. This solid mass (the stool) is propelled into the rectum, where it is held until excreted through the anus.

Diseases and disorders that interfere with this function are classified here, along with diseases and disorders that affect the organs of the digestive tract, although they may have no direct affect on digestion. For example, dental caries have a direct effect on digestion because they interfere with mastication, the mechanical breakdown of food by chewing. Portal hypertension does not directly affect digestion, but is included because it represents a disease of a digestive system organ. Portal hypertension would have no discernible effect on the digestive process until the disease has progressed to the point that the liver can no longer perform its function as a digestive organ.

520–529 Diseases of Oral Cavity, Salivary Glands, and Jaws

This category includes diseases and disorders of the jaw, salivary and parotid glands, teeth, gingiva and periodontium, lips, oral mucosa, and tongue.

Traumatic injuries to teeth and supporting structures may be more appropriately classified to Chapter 17 injury codes. Most Chapter 9 codes relate to disorders of the development of teeth rather than trauma.

520 Disorders of tooth development and eruption

This rubric includes disorders of tooth development and eruption in all patients regardless of age. It is one of the few categories in ICD-9-CM that classifies congenital anomalies and hereditary disturbances outside of Chapter 14 Congenital Anomalies (740-759).

520.0	Anodontia — *absence of teeth*
520.1	Supernumerary teeth — *distomolar, fourth molar, mesiodens, paramolar*
520.2	Abnormalities of size and form of teeth —*525.10 fusion, concrescence, gemination, macrodontia, microdontia, dens evaginates, dens in dente, taurodontism, tuberculum paramolar*
520.3	Mottled teeth — *dental fluorosis, enamel opacities, mottling of enamel*

Section of molar

Section of incisor

Coding Clarification
Excessive use of fluoride can cause mottled bleaching of the enamel. The problem can be particularly evident in communities with drinking water containing greater than two parts per million, which can cause dental fluorosis. The signs are whitish flecks or spots, particularly on the front teeth, or dark spots or stripes in more severe cases. While tooth-whitening products can approve appearance in most cases, discoloration of enamel can also be a structural problem that requires proper diagnosis and treatment.

520.4	Disturbances of tooth formation — *aplasia and hypoplasia of cementum, dilaceration of tooth, enamel hypoplasia, Horner's or Turners tooth, hypocalcification*
520.5	Hereditary disturbances in tooth structure, not elsewhere classified — *amelogenesis, dentinogenesis, odontogenesis, dentinal dysplasia, shell teeth*
520.6	Disturbances in tooth eruption — *embedded, impacted, obstructed, premature eruption, prenatal, premature shedding of deciduous tooth*
	AHA: Q2, 2005, 15; Q1, 2006, 18
520.7	Teething syndrome
520.8	Other specified disorders of tooth development and eruption — *not otherwise specified, pre-eruptive color change*
520.9	Unspecified disorder of tooth development and eruption

Coding Clarification
Excluded from this rubric is exfoliation of teeth, classified to 525.0-525.19.

521 Diseases of hard tissues of teeth

This rubric includes the crown, dentin, enamel, and cementum of the tooth. This rubric includes caries of the cementum, dentin, enamel, as well as infantile melanodontia and white spot lesions of the teeth.

Dental caries are a demineralization of a tooth's enamel caused by acids produced by bacteria, particularly *Streptococcus mutans*. Pit and fissure decay begins in the narrow grooves on the top of the crown and the cheek side of the back teeth and progresses rapidly. Smooth surface decay grows the slowest and begins as a white spot where bacteria are dissolving the calcium of the enamel. Root decay occurs in the cementum covering the root surface when gums have receded.

Attrition is the normal wearing away of the substance or structure of a tooth through regular use, while abrasion is wearing away of a tooth through an unnatural mechanical process. Erosion is a progressive eating away or destruction of the hard substance of a tooth by a chemical, not bacterial, process. Pathological resorption is a condition in which calcified tissue of the root is lost from the tooth through an absorption and removal process happening within the cementum and dentin, into the root canal, triggered by occlusive trauma

Diseases of the Digestive System

and disease, such as neoplastic activity. Internal resorption is an unusual form of pathological resorption that begins in the center of the tooth, with inflamed and hyperplastic pulp tissue filling the resorbed central area and showing pink through the crown of the tooth.

Variations in intraoral mechanical forces, such as chewing or grinding of the teeth, determine the continued formation of bacteria on the teeth and the plaque that can lead to dental caries. Other causes are related to feeding behaviors, such as baby bottle tooth decay in infants, in addition to craniofacial problems, neurologic abnormalities, or impaired cognitive abilities that can interfere with proper dental care.

The bacteria that cause caries are microflora that are present not only in the oral cavity but also in the gastrointestinal tract and other parts of the body, increasing the risk of many disease states and changes in health status due to oral diseases. For example, poorly controlled diabetes (characterized by hyperglycemia and increased salivary glucose) is associated with an increased risk of several dental diseases and conditions.

Diagnosis of dental caries generally involves the use of a sharp explorer, a viewing mirror, and an artificial light source, as well as the drying of tooth surfaces to improve visibility. Radiographs or fiberoptic illumination may reveal smaller caries on the hidden surfaces between adjacent teeth. Four major types of primary prevention are fluoride therapy, fissure-sealant therapy, dietary counseling, and oral-hygiene measures.

There are multiple types of cracked teeth. Treatment and outcome depend largely on the type, location, and extent of the crack. A cracked tooth is one in which a crack extends from the chewing surface of the tooth vertically toward the root but is not completely divided into two segments. Root canal therapy is often required to treat the injured pulp, and a crown is placed to hold and protect the cracked tooth. If the crack extends below the gingival tissue line, extraction is required. A split tooth is frequently the result of a crack that has progressed into fragments that can be separated. A split tooth cannot be saved intact, but a part of the tooth may be saved by endodontic treatment and a crown or other restorative process. Vertical root fractures start in the tooth's root and extent upward toward the chewing surface. These fractures are frequently discovered when the surrounding gum and bone develop infection. Treatment may involve tooth extraction or endodontic surgery in which the fractured root is removed but a portion of the tooth can be saved.

Code	Description
521.00	Unspecified dental caries
521.01	Dental caries limited to enamel — *initial caries and white spot lesion* **AHA:** Q4, 2001, 44
521.02	Dental caries extending into dentine
521.03	Dental caries extending into pulp
521.04	Arrested dental caries
521.05	Odontoclasia — *infantile melanodontia and melanodontoclasia* **AHA:** Q4, 2001, 44
521.06	Dental caries pit and fissure
521.07	Dental caries of smooth surface
521.08	Dental caries of root surface
521.09	Other dental caries
521.10	Excessive attrition (approximal wear) (occlusal wear), unspecified
521.11	Excessive attrition (approximal wear) (occlusal wear), limited to enamel
521.12	Excessive attrition (approximal wear) (occlusal wear), extending into dentine
521.13	Excessive attrition (approximal wear) (occlusal wear), extending into pulp
521.14	Excessive attrition (approximal wear) (occlusal wear), localized
521.15	Excessive attrition (approximal wear) (occlusal wear), generalized
521.20	Diseases of hard tissues of teeth, abrasion, unspecified
521.21	Diseases of hard tissues of teeth, abrasion, limited to enamel
521.22	Diseases of hard tissues of teeth, abrasion, extending into dentine
521.23	Diseases of hard tissues of teeth, abrasion, extending into pulp
521.24	Diseases of hard tissues of teeth, abrasion,, localized
521.25	Diseases of hard tissues of teeth, abrasion,, generalized
521.30	Diseases of hard tissues of teeth, erosion, unspecified
521.31	Diseases of hard tissues of teeth, erosion, limited to enamel
521.32	Diseases of hard tissues of teeth, erosion, extending into dentine
521.33	Diseases of hard tissues of teeth, erosion, extending into pulp
521.34	Diseases of hard tissues of teeth, erosion, localized
521.35	Diseases of hard tissues of teeth, erosion, generalized
521.40	Diseases of hard tissues of teeth, pathological resorption, unspecified
521.41	Diseases of hard tissues of teeth, pathological resorption, internal
521.42	Diseases of hard tissues of teeth, pathological resorption, external
521.49	Diseases of hard tissues of teeth, other pathological resorption

521.5	Hypercementosis — *excessive deposits of cementum on the root of the tooth; cementation hyperplasia*		
521.6	Ankylosis of teeth — *abnormal union of tooth to surrounding bone*		
521.7	Intrinsic posteruptive color changes — *staining due to drugs, metal, pulpal bleeding, or not otherwise specified*		
521.81	Cracked tooth		

Coding Clarification
This code excludes broken or fractured tooth due to trauma (873.63, 873.73). No code should be assigned for asymptomatic craze lines in enamel.

521.89	Other specific diseases of hard tissues of teeth — *sensitive dentin; irradiated dentin*
521.9	Unspecified disease of hard tissues of teeth

Coding Scenario
A 19-year old boy presents to his dentist for his semiannual oral exam after the recent removal of his orthodontic braces. The dentist discovers initial decay and white spots on the buccal smooth surface of his lower canines where the edge of the metal braces had been secured to the teeth for the last two years. He is advised to practice good brushing habits and informed that the initial decay will progress very slowly and not require filling for a while yet.

> Code assignment: 521.01 *Dental caries limited to enamel* and 521.07 *Dental caries of smooth surface*

522 Diseases of pulp and periapical tissues

The center of the tooth and its soft tissues are known as the pulp. It extends from the bottom of the crown to the bottom of the root and is made up of blood vessels that carry oxygen and nutrients back and forth from the heart. Nerves lining the pulp respond to heat, cold, and pressure.

An advanced bacterial infection of the pulp can, if untreated, spread to the root. If the root of the tooth dies, the toothache may stop, but the infection remains active and continues to spread and destroy tissue.

Signs and symptoms of acute apical periodontitis include swollen and red gum that may drain thick purulent material and often a throbbing pain that tends to radiate along the jaw. There is sensitivity of the teeth to hot or cold, possible fever and swollen glands of the neck, and a swollen area of the jaw in very serious cases. Biting or closing the mouth tightly also increases pain. The presence of an abscess, which is a collection of pus, requires immediate dental attention and antibiotics to control the infection, often prior to surgical intervention (e.g., root canal or, in extreme cases, an apicoectomy to drain the abscess prior to a root canal).

522.0	Pulpitis — *abscess, polyp; acute or chronic*
522.1	Necrosis of dental pulp — *death of pulp tissue; pulp gangrene*
522.2	Dental pulp degeneration — *denticles, pulp calcifications, pulp stones*
522.3	Abnormal hard tissue formation in dental pulp — *secondary or irregular dentin*
522.4	Acute apical periodontitis of pulpal origin — *severe inflammation of periodontal ligament, resulting from pulpal inflammation or necrosis*
522.5	Periapical abscess without sinus — *dental or dentoalveolar*
522.6	Chronic apical periodontitis — *persistent inflammation of periodontal ligament, from granuloma or not elsewhere specified*
522.7	Periapical abscess with sinus — *dental or alveolar process fistula*
522.8	Radicular cyst of dental pulp — *apical, periapical, radiculodental, periodontal cyst*
522.9	Other and unspecified diseases of pulp and periapical tissues — *not specified elsewhere or unknown*

Coding Clarification
Diseases of the pulp often begin with bacterial invasion of the pulp after attacking the dentin. Acute and chronic pulpitis (522.0) are conditions, often bacterial, accompanied by severe pain and acute inflammation causing pulp death and subsequent pulp extirpation or extraction. Necrosis of dental pulp (522.1) is a condition in which the pulp has been killed by acute or chronic inflammation; because the pulp is dead, pulp extirpation or tooth extraction is necessary. Periapical tissue surrounds the base of the tooth and a periapical abscess is an infection of the pulp and periapical tissue.

523 Gingival and periodontal diseases

Gingival and periodontal diseases include acute and chronic gingivitis, gingival recession, acute and chronic periodontitis, accretions on teeth, as well as other specified periodontal diseases such as gingival polyps and peripheral giant cell granuloma.

Gingivitis, or inflammation of the gums, may be either acute or chronic. Acute gingivitis has a sudden onset, is of short duration, and is painful, while chronic gingivitis has a slower onset, a longer duration, and is often painless. Gingivitis is often attributed to the presence of bacteria, but there are other types that are not primarily plaque related. Diabetes, leukemia, or other systemic diseases can aggravate plaque-associated gingivitis. Endocrine changes such as puberty or pregnancy; medications such as nifedipine, cyclosporin, and phenytoin; and malnutrition or vitamin C deficiency may also exacerbate gingivitis. If gingivitis remains untreated, progression to periodontitis is possible.

Non-plaque-induced gingivitis can be the result of certain bacterial pathogens such as *Neisseria gonorrhea*, or viral or fungal infections; mucocutaneous disorders such as lichen planus or pemphigoid; allergic reactions to restorative substances, toothpaste, or gum; or physical, chemical, or thermal trauma. Underlying factors also include genetic disorders, such as hereditary gingival fibromatosis. These gingival diseases are classified differently from plaque-associated gingivitis.

There are no symptoms in the early stages of gingivitis. Signs and symptoms of advanced gingivitis and periodontitis include blood on the tooth brush when brushing the teeth, swollen and red gums, tenderness when the gums are touched, pus around the teeth, bad taste in the mouth, and visible deposits of tartar or calculus on the teeth. Acute periodontitis describes an inflammatory disease of the bony and ligamentous supporting tissues of the teeth; however, this term is not often used in the dental community. Highly destructive types of periodontitis are named "aggressive periodontitis" with further classifications denoting localized or generalized forms. Immune deficiencies and genetic factors are believed to be potential causes for all types of aggressive periodontitis. If the condition is localized and treated, the outlook is optimistic.

The term "chronic" periodontitis signifies the progression of the disease over time without treatment and does not mean that the disease is untreatable, but patients with severe and widespread periodontitis have a high risk for tooth loss. The disease typically progresses slowly, although there may be spurts of destruction. The disease progression rate is also influenced by local factors, systemic diseases, and extrinsic factors such as smoking.

Chronic periodontitis is further classified as localized or generalized depending on the percentage of sites involved, i.e., whether greater than or less than 30 percent. Severity is determined by the amount of clinical attachment loss (CAL) and is designated as slight (1-2 mm CAL), moderate (3-4 mm CAL), or severe (> 5 mm CAL).

Diagnostic measures for detecting periodontitis include screening and recording pocket depth, which is the point where the connective tissue attaches to the tooth, testing for tooth mobility or movement, and x-rays. Treatment includes deep cleaning, scaling, and gingival curettage, oral or topical antibiotics, tissue regeneration, bone grafting, nonsteroidal anti-inflammatory drugs, bone-restoring agents, and stimulation of gum tissue growth using an enamel matrix protein derivative.

Code	Description
523.00	Acute gingivitis, plaque induced — *acute gingivitis, not otherwise specified*
523.01	Acute gingivitis, non-plaque induced
523.10	Chronic gingivitis, plaque induced — *chronic gingivitis, not otherwise specified; gingivitis, not otherwise specified*
523.11	Chronic gingivitis, non-plaque induced
523.20	Gingival recession, unspecified
523.21	Gingival recession, minimal
523.22	Gingival recession, moderate
523.23	Gingival recession, severe
523.24	Gingival recession, localized
523.25	Gingival recession, generalized
523.30	Aggressive periodontitis, unspecified
523.31	Aggressive periodontitis, localized — *periodontal abscess*
523.32	Aggressive periodontitis, generalized
523.33	Acute periodontitis
523.40	Chronic periodontitis, unspecified
523.41	Chronic periodontitis, localized
523.42	Chronic periodontitis, generalized
523.5	Periodontosis — *inflammation of the tissues that surround and support the teeth*
523.6	Accretions on teeth — *foreign material on surface of teeth, usually plaque or calculus*
523.8	Other specified periodontal diseases — *cysts, hemorrhage, occlusion, pocket, ulcer, pain, fibromatosis, lesions, giant cell granuloma*
523.9	Unspecified gingival and periodontal disease

Coding Clarification

Excluded from this category are acute necrotizing ulcerative gingivitis (101), herpetic gingivostomatitis (054.2), acute apical periodontitis (522.4), chronic apical periodontitis (522.6), periapical abscess (522.5, 522.7), and leukoplakia of gingiva (528.6).

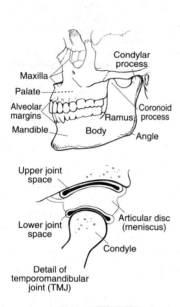

524 Dentofacial anomalies, including malocclusion

Malocclusion is an abnormal alignment of teeth and the way that the upper and lower teeth fit together (bite). It is often hereditary and may cause problems with biting and chewing but can usually be corrected with a brace on the teeth and proper orthodontic care.

Tuberosity of the jaw is seen as an elongated, raised, or protruding area on the angle of the jawbone. Sometimes the tuberosity can be raised or uneven after tooth extraction. Surgical correction of the tuberosity can be performed to correct a defect.

Dentofacial anomalies classified in this chapter may be acquired or due to congenital anomalies not classified to Chapter 14. Look in the ICD-9-CM index under both the condition and the main term "Anomaly, anomalous" to ensure proper code assignment.

Subcategory 524.0 classifies conditions affecting the size of the jaw, including hyperplasia, hypoplasia, macrogenia, and microgenia.

524.00	Unspecified major anomaly of jaw size
524.01	Maxillary hyperplasia — *overgrowth or overdevelopment of maxillary bone*
524.02	Mandibular hyperplasia — *overgrowth or overdevelopment of jaw bone*
524.03	Maxillary hypoplasia — *incomplete or underdevelopment of maxillary bone*
524.04	Mandibular hypoplasia — *incomplete or underdevelopment of jaw bone*
524.05	Macrogenia — *abnormal largeness of the chin*
524.06	Microgenia — *abnormal smallness of the chin*
524.07	Excessive tuberosity of jaw
524.09	Other specified major anomaly of jaw size — *not otherwise specified*

Subcategory 524.1 classifies inequality in the size or shape of one side of the maxilla and/or mandible compared with the other, or a difference in placement or arrangement of one of the jawbones about the craniofacial axis. These anomalies include prognathism, retrognathism, and maxillary asymmetry. Prognathism is anterior protrusion of the mandible or maxilla beyond the projection of the forehead. Retrognathism is the location of the maxilla or mandible behind the frontal plane of the forehead; it also is used as a general term meaning underdevelopment of the maxilla or mandible.

Subcategory 524.2 classifies dental arch anomalies. The dental arch is the curved structure of a line created by the buccal surfaces or the central grooves of all natural teeth and the residual ridge of missing teeth in the upper or lower jaw. Anomalies may occur as a malocclusion—an abnormal contact line between the biting and chewing tooth surfaces of the upper or lower teeth, an overbite or overlapping of upper teeth over the lower when biting down, or inadequate or excessive interarch distances—the vertical space defined between the upper and lower alveolar or residual arches, or ridges. Angle's class I is a malocclusion with correct mesiodistal relationship of the first permanent molars. Angle's class II, also called a distoclusion, is a posterior malocclusion in which the lower jaw and its first permanent molar is positioned further back than the upper. Angle's class III, also called a mesioclusion, is a protrusive malocclusion in which the lower jaw is more forward than the upper and its first permanent molar is positioned nearer to the center line of the arch than the upper. Returning the dental arch to proper positioning usually requires carefully planned orthodontic care, possibly concurrent with orthognathic surgery to reposition one or both jaws.

524.10	Unspecified anomaly of relationship of jaw to cranial base — *prognathism and retrognathism*
524.11	Maxillary asymmetry — *unequal development*
524.12	Other jaw asymmetry
524.19	Other specified anomaly of relationship of jaw to cranial base — *not otherwise specified*
524.20	Unspecified anomaly of dental arch relationship
524.21	Anomaly of dental arch relationship, malocclusion, Angle's class I

Diseases of the Digestive System

Code	Description
524.22	Anomaly of dental arch relationship, malocclusion, Angle's class II
524.23	Anomaly of dental arch relationship, malocclusion, Angle's class III
524.24	Anomaly of dental arch relationship, open anterior occlusal relationship
524.25	Anomaly of dental arch relationship, open posterior occlusal relationship
524.26	Anomaly of dental arch relationship, excessive horizontal overlap
524.27	Anomaly of dental arch relationship, reverse articulation
524.28	Anomaly of dental arch relationship, anomalies of interarch distance
524.29	Other anomalies of dental arch relationship

Subcategory 524.3 classifies anomalies of tooth position. Crowding occurs when teeth come in too close to one another have no room for the normal spacing that should be present between the teeth. Crowding also causes overlapping and displacement of adjacent teeth in various directions. Excessive spacing is the opposite problem when a tooth is too far apart from its neighboring tooth, leaving an unfilled gap between them.

Horizontal displacement may be seen as crowns and roots out of the normal line, including "tipping" in their position. Vertical displacement may present as supra-eruption of a tooth in which it continues to grow out from the gingiva when the opposing tooth is missing in the other jaw, and may require placing the missing tooth and adjusting the height of the other. Infra-eruption of a tooth occurs when has not sufficiently erupted above the gum line. Tooth rotation is the malposition of a tooth that has turned about its own longitudinal axis. The interocclusal distance in teeth is determined from the biting/chewing contact surfaces of teeth in the maxilla (upper jaw) and the mandible (lower jaw) when the lower jaw is in the normal resting position. This natural space or clearance may be either greater than normal or insufficient. These problems may require orthodontic care to move the teeth into proper position and/or the strategic removal of certain teeth.

Code	Description
524.30	Anomaly of tooth position, unspecified
524.31	Crowding of teeth
524.32	Excessive spacing of teeth
524.33	Horizontal displacement of teeth
524.34	Vertical displacement of teeth
524.35	Rotation of tooth/teeth
524.36	Insufficient interocclusal distance of teeth (ridge)
524.37	Excessive interocclusal distance of teeth
524.39	Other anomalies of tooth position
524.4	Unspecified malocclusion
524.50	Dentofacial functional abnormality, unspecified
524.51	Abnormal jaw closure
524.52	Limited mandibular range of motion
524.53	Deviation in opening and closing of the mandible
524.54	Insufficient anterior guidance
524.55	Centric occlusion maximum intercuspation discrepancy
524.56	Dentofacial functional abnormality, non-working side interference
524.57	Lack of posterior occlusal support
524.59	Other dentofacial functional abnormalities

Subcategory 524.6 classifies temporomandibular joint disorders. The temporomandibular joints (TMJ) are located just in front of the ears and attach the mandible to the skull allowing the jaw to move. Symptoms of TMJ disorders include pain in the jaw, headache, stiffness in the jaw, earaches and popping or clicking sounds when opening the mouth. Symptoms may be often be alleviated with pain-relief medications and heat/cold, and other palliative measures. Oftentimes, such TMJ problems resolve themselves over time. In some instances, surgery is required to correct the problem.

Code	Description
524.60	Unspecified temporomandibular joint disorders — *TMJ syndrome; including Costen's syndrome*
524.61	Adhesions and ankylosis (bony or fibrous) of temporomandibular joint — *a union or stiffening of the TMJ due to bony or fibrous union across the joint*
524.62	Arthralgia of temporomandibular joint — *pain of TMJ, not inflammatory in nature*
524.63	Articular disc disorder (reducing or non-reducing) of temporomandibular joint
524.64	Temporomandibular joint sounds on opening and/or closing the jaw
524.69	Other specified temporomandibular joint disorders — *not otherwise specified, snapping jaw*

Subcategory 524.7 classifies anomalies of the dental alveoli and alveolar ridge, including hyperplasia and hypoplasia. Dental alveoli are the tooth sockets of the maxilla and mandible. The alveolar ridge is the bony process of the maxilla or mandible that contains the tooth sockets. Hyperplasia of the alveoli is an overgrowth or overdevelopment of bone, and hypoplasia of the alveoli is an underdevelopment or agenesis of bone.

A vertical displacement of the alveolus and teeth includes the extrusion or extended movement of the tooth and the root cavity, or socket in the jawbone where the tooth is held, beyond the normal occlusal plane when the opposing occlusal force is missing. The occlusal plane is the hypothetical surface on which upper and lower teeth meet when biting or chewing. The plane appears as a straight line to the lateral view, even though it is actually a compound curved surface, and the planar reference points are taken from specific points within the dental arches. A structural aberration that results in canting or tipping of the occlusal plane is a deviation that may require orthopedic and/or orthodontic care to achieve the true horizontal and vertical references for the occlusal plane that are the optimal end-point of treatment for the best mandibular maxillary relationship.

524.70	Unspecified alveolar anomaly
524.71	Alveolar maxillary hyperplasia — *overgrowth or underdevelopment of alveolar tissue of the maxillary bones*
524.72	Alveolar mandibular hyperplasia — *overgrowth or underdevelopment of alveolar tissue of the mandibular bones*
524.73	Alveolar maxillary hypoplasia — *incomplete or underdevelopment of alveolar tissue of the maxillary bones*
524.74	Alveolar mandibular hypoplasia — *incomplete or underdevelopment of alveolar tissue of the mandibular bones*
524.75	Vertical displacement of alveolus and teeth
524.76	Occlusal plane deviation
524.79	Other specified alveolar anomaly — *not otherwise specified*
524.81	Anterior soft tissue impingement
524.82	Posterior soft tissue impingement
524.89	Other specified dentofacial anomalies
524.9	Unspecified dentofacial anomalies

Coding Scenario

A 24-year-old female comes to her primary care physician to complain that her jaw continually pops when she makes a movement to open or close it in such a way that she actually feels the "pop". Sometimes she also experiences mobility problems with the jaw to get it open with increased loudness it the joint sounds, especially in the morning. She hasn't had pain in the jaw at this point, however. The physician listens for the joint sounds and gives the initial diagnosis of temporomandibular joint sounds.

Code assignment: 524.64 *Temporomandibular joint sounds on opening and/or closing the jaw*

525 Other diseases and conditions of the teeth and supporting structures

Tooth loss can be caused by a variety of causes. Congenital conditions such as Papillon Lefevre syndrome, systemic conditions such as Langerhan's cell histiocytosis, loss of supporting structures, trauma, periodontal disease, and dental caries may be responsible for loosing teeth.

A bacterium that spreads into the bony tissues under the gums, supporting the teeth causes advanced gingivitis. This is called periodontitis.

Dental caries are a demineralization of a tooth's enamel caused by acids produced by bacteria. Advanced dental caries can cause decay and loss of a tooth.

Partial edentulism is the loss of one or multiple teeth and complete edentulism is the loss of all teeth. Edentulism is divided into four classes, defined by the level of difficulty or complexity in treatment for complete edentulism, and how compromised the presenting diagnostic criteria are in partial edentulism. Class IV is the most debilitating, requiring reconstructive surgery when all teeth are missing or the most severely compromised oral manifestations with poor outcome prognosis in partial edentulism. Treatment is primarily prosthodontic in nature with missing teeth or adjacent structures being restored or replaced with artificial, biocompatible substitutes.

The alveolar ridge is the line formed by the alveolar process, the root cavities or sockets of the jawbones. Edentulous ridges have lost the teeth that were once held in those sockets. Atrophy presents as a wasting and shrinking of the size of the alveolar ridge that previously held teeth. Severe atrophy may present as small, knife-like edges along the alveolar ridge and produce a sunken appearance to the mouth and lips, leaving a protruding chin, especially with anterior atrophy of the maxilla and mandible. Severe forms require oral maxillofacial surgery to reconstruct the maxilla and/or mandible. Bone grafts may be used for ridge augmentation, also possible orthopedic bone plates, a reconstruction of the vestibule of the mouth, and complete dentures.

Restorations are defined as materials or methods used to replace lost teeth or tooth structure, such as fillings, inlays, onlays, crowns, bridges, or complete or partial dentures. Dental restorative materials used include amalgam, composite resin, silicate, acrylic, synthetic, and plastic. These methods are not permanent and may suffer failure over time. They may develop recurrent cavities; become defective due to marginal breakdown; undergo corrosion or discoloration; fracture and partially or completely fall out; or the tooth structure surrounding the restoration may fracture.

Restoration problems may appear as open margins surrounding restoration sites, causing an increased potential for plaque retention and gingival inflammation; irreparable overhanging of dental restorative materials, promoting plaque accumulation and causing nondestructive subgingival flora to become destructive; fractured dental restorative material, which can allow bacterial entry, resulting in pulp and periapical disease; biologically incompatible contours, known as unacceptable morphology that can lead to development of chronic lesions and bone loss; allergies to dental restorative material; and poor aesthetics of existing restoration, producing an undesirable appearance.

525.0	Exfoliation of teeth due to systemic causes — *loss of teeth due to underlying condition*
525.10	Unspecified acquired absence of teeth — *(Code first class of edentulism: 525.40-525.44, 525.50-525.54)* **AHA:** Q4, 2001, 44; Q4, 2005, 74
525.11	Loss of teeth due to trauma— (Code first class of edentulism: 525.40-525.44, 525.50-525.54) **AHA:** Q4, 2005, 74
525.12	Loss of teeth due to periodontal disease— (Code first class of edentulism: 525.40-525.44, 525.50-525.54) **AHA:** Q4, 2005, 74
525.13	Loss of teeth due to caries— (Code first class of edentulism: 525.40-525.44, 525.50-525.54) **AHA:** Q4, 2005, 74
525.19	Other loss of teeth— (Code first class of edentulism: 525.40-525.44, 525.50-525.54) **AHA:** Q4, 2005, 74
525.20	Unspecified atrophy of edentulous alveolar ridge
525.21	Minimal atrophy of the mandible
525.22	Moderate atrophy of the mandible
525.24	Minimal atrophy of the maxilla
525.25	Moderate atrophy of the maxilla
525.26	Severe atrophy of the maxilla
525.3	Retained dental root
525.40	Complete edentulism, unspecified — (Use additional code to identify cause of edentulism: 525.10-525.19) **AHA:** Q4, 2005, 74
525.41	Complete edentulism, class I — (Use additional code to identify cause of edentulism: 525.10-525.19) **AHA:** Q4, 2005, 74
525.42	Complete edentulism, class II — (Use additional code to identify cause of edentulism: 525.10-525.19)
525.43	Complete edentulism, class III — (Use additional code to identify cause of edentulism: 525.10-525.19) **AHA:** Q4, 2005, 74
525.44	Complete edentulism, class IV — (Use additional code to identify cause of edentulism: 525.10-525.19) **AHA:** Q4, 2005, 74
525.50	Partial edentulism, unspecified — (Use additional code to identify cause of edentulism: 525.10-525.19) **AHA:** Q4, 2005, 74
525.51	Partial edentulism, class I — (Use additional code to identify cause of edentulism: 525.10-525.19) **AHA:** Q4, 2005, 74
525.52	Partial edentulism, class II — (Use additional code to identify cause of edentulism: 525.10-525.19) **AHA:** Q4, 2005, 74
525.53	Partial edentulism, class III — (Use additional code to identify cause of edentulism: 525.10-525.19) **AHA:** Q4, 2005, 74
525.54	Partial edentulism, class IV — (Use additional code to identify cause of edentulism: 525.10-525.19) **AHA:** Q4, 2005, 74

Subcategory 525.6 Unsatisfactory restoration of teeth, includes defective bridges, crowns, and fillings. It excludes unsatisfactory endodontic treatm5ent (526.61-526.69), and dental restoration status (V45.84).

525.60	Unspecified unsatisfactory restoration of tooth — *unspecified defective dental restoration*
525.61	Open restoration margins — *open margin on tooth restoration; dental restoration failure of marginal integrity*
525.62	Unrepairable overhanging of dental restorative margins — *overhang of tooth restoration*
525.63	Fractured dental restorative material without loss of material

This code excludes cracked tooth (521.81) and fractured tooth (873.63, 873.73).

525.64	Fractured dental restorative material with loss of material

This code excludes cracked tooth (521.81) and fractured tooth (873.63, 873.73).

525.65	Contour of existing restoration of tooth biologically incompatible with oral health — *unacceptable contours or morphology of existing restoration; dental restoration failure of periodontal anatomical integrity*
525.66	Allergy to existing dental restorative material — (Use additional E code to identify the specific type of allergy)
525.67	Poor aesthetics of existing restoration — *aesthetically inadequate or displeasing dental restoration*
525.69	Other unsatisfactory restoration of tooth
525.8	Other specified disorders of the teeth and supporting structures — *not otherwise specified, cicatrix, cleft, hemorrhage, lesion, or enlargement of alveolar process or tissue; loose tooth; obliteration of vestibule*
525.9	Unspecified disorder of the teeth and supporting structures — *unknown cause of pain or other symptom*

526 Diseases of the jaws

Odontogenic cysts are developmental cysts arising from the enamel organ of teeth and include about 90 percent of all jaw cysts. While it is sometimes difficult to differentiate which type of odontogenic cyst is present, some have distinguishing features.

The radicular cyst is the most common of the odontogenic cysts; associated with a nonvital tooth, it is present at the apex of the root of a tooth or teeth. Other odontogenic cysts include residual cysts associated with the removal of teeth and primordial cysts associated with undeveloped teeth. Globulomaxillary cysts are located in the anterior region of the upper jaw and dentigerous cysts form in association with an unerupted permanent tooth, although they can occasionally surround a primary tooth, due to fluid accumulation.

Dentigerous cysts are found in children and adolescents. Adults can have dentigerous cysts associated with unerupted third molars. These cysts may expand, causing displacement or resorption of adjacent teeth. In a radiograph, dentigerous cysts appear as a dark area around the crown of the tooth.

Treatment for the dentigerous cyst includes removal and microscopic examination of the cyst wall since the cyst lining may have a neoplastic change, such as ameloblastoma, squamous cell carcinoma, or mucoepidermoid carcinoma. Marsupialization is a second method of treatment that involves removing the overlying soft tissue and bone, allowing discharge of matter.

Endodontic treatment failure is related to perforations of the root canal occurring during root canal treatment, in which an opening is made into the pulp chamber. The pulp is removed, and the root canals are cleaned, enlarged, and shaped into a form that can be filled. The pulp chamber and root canals are then filled and sealed, before a crown or other restorative material is placed over the tooth.

Two of the more frequently encountered problems include penetration of the pulp chamber floor in multi-rooted teeth during access and labial perforation during access through crowned anterior teeth.

Root canal fillings ideally fill the entire obliterated pulp space and provide a seal at the surface where the cementum and dentin of the tooth's root join (dentinocemental junction). Overextension of filler or extrusion of sealer may act as chronic irritants, preventing the healing of periapical disease or causing apical breakdown in areas that were previously without pathology. Endodontic underfill is another complication of root canal treatment in which the pulp space is inadequately filled. Radiography is one of the most commonly used diagnostic measures to determine complications of root canal procedures. Depending upon its etiology, failure of endodontic treatment is most often treated in one of three ways: root canal retreatment, periradicular surgery, and extraction.

526.0	Developmental odontogenic cysts — *dentigerous, eruption, follicular, lateral development, keratocyst, primordial cyst*
526.1	Fissural cysts of jaw — *globulomaxillary, incisor canal, median anterior maxillary, medial palatal, nasopalatine*
526.2	Other cysts of jaws — *aneurysmal, hemorrhagic, traumatic*
526.3	Central giant cell (reparative) granuloma
526.4	Inflammatory conditions of jaw — *abscess, osteitis, sequestrum of jawbone, periostitis*
526.5	Alveolitis of jaw — *inflammation of alveoli or tooth socket of jaw; dry socket; alveolar osteitis*
526.61	Perforation of root canal space
526.62	Endodontic overfill
526.63	Endodontic underfill
526.69	Other periradicular pathology associated with previous endodontic treatment
526.81	Exostosis of jaw — *bony projection that develops from cartilage of jaw*
526.89	Other specified disease of the jaws — *not otherwise specified, cherubism, fibrous dysplasia, latent bone cyst, fistula, perforation, unilateral condylar hyper- or hypoplasia of mandible*
526.9	Unspecified disease of the jaws — *unknown cause of pain or other symptom*

527 Diseases of the salivary glands

The salivary glands secrete a predominantly alkaline fluid that moistens the mouth, softens food, and aids in digestion. The three major salivary glands include the submaxillary glands around the mouth under the lower jaw, the sublingual glands beneath the tongue, and the parotid glands in front of each ear. Saliva is antimicrobial and works against a host of bacteria associated with oral and systemic diseases. Large salivary mucins are antiviral as are cystatins that are active against herpes viruses. Saliva also contains histatins, anti-fungal proteins that are potent inhibitors of candida, which is normally kept in check at extremely low levels in the mouth. The sublingual glands secrete the enzyme lysozyme, which destroys bacterial invasion with methods to include degrading bacterial membranes, inhibiting the growth and metabolism of certain bacteria, and disrupting bacterial enzyme systems. The saliva of the parotid gland contains the enzyme amylase that aids in the digestion of carbohydrates. In addition to

Diseases of the Digestive System

these glands, there are hundreds of minor saliva glands in the lips, inner cheek area (buccal mucosa), and in other linings of the mouth and throat. Salivary calculi account for more than 50 percent of the major salivary gland diseases and are the most common cause of acute and chronic salivary gland infections.

Code	Description
527.0	Atrophy of salivary gland — *wasting away or death of tissue*
527.1	Hypertrophy of salivary gland — *overgrowth or over development of tissue; Mikulicz's syndrome*
527.2	Sialoadenitis — *inflammation*
527.3	Abscess of salivary gland — *pocket of pus*
527.4	Fistula of salivary gland — *abnormal sinus tract communicating between salivary gland and another site*
527.5	Sialolithiasis — *formation or presence of salivary calculus; stone, sialodocholithiasis*
527.6	Mucocele of salivary gland — *dilated salivary gland filled with accumulation of mucous*
527.7	Disturbance of salivary secretion — *hyposecretion, ptyalism, sialorrhea, xerostomia, Zagari's disease*
527.8	Other specified diseases of the salivary glands — *not otherwise specified, stenosis, stricture or obstruction of salivary duct; pneumoparotid; sialosis; obstruction of Stensen's or submaxillary duct; sialectasia*
527.9	Unspecified disease of the salivary glands — *unknown disorder*

Coding Clarification

Atrophy (527.0) in the diseases of the salivary glands is defined as a wasting away or death of tissue, while hypertrophy (527.1) is overgrowth or overdevelopment of tissue of the salivary glands. Sialoadenitis (527.2) is the inflammation of a salivary gland and sialolithiasis (527.5) is the formation or presence of a salivary calculus.

528 Diseases of the oral soft tissues, excluding lesions specific for gingiva and tongue

Stomatitis is any inflammatory condition of the oral mucosa and may include oral tissue infections or inflammatory conditions of the periodontium, dentition, or periapices. Oral mucositis is a form of stomatitis and typically presents as redness or ulcerations.

Mucosal inflammation, or mucositis, affects the tissues that line the mouth, throat, stomach, intestines, rectum, and anus. A frequent, debilitating complication of chemotherapy or radiation treatment, mucositis occurs when the epithelial cells lining the gastrointestinal tract break down, leaving the mucosal tissue susceptible to infection and ulceration. Manifestations can include ulcers in the soft tissues of mucosal surfaces throughout the body, particularly the mouth. Oral mucositis occurs in 20 percent to 40 percent of patients treated solely with chemotherapy. In patients receiving combination chemotherapy and radiation therapy, particularly those with head and neck cancer, the occurrence rate increases to up to 50 percent. Since the ability of cells to reproduce is affected by antineoplastic therapy, healing of the oral mucosa is slowed, leaving the patient more susceptible to opportunistic mouth infections. Damaged mucosa is a point of entry for bacteria and fungi, and mucositis is also associated with febrile neutropenia.

Mild cases of mucositis may respond to topical pain relief such as gels or creams. Analgesics such as acetaminophen may be helpful for relieving moderate pain, and severe pain may require stronger oral or injectable pain medications. Symptom improvement may also be obtained with allopurinol or vitamin E. Treatment of stomatitis varies, depending on the underlying cause. An infectious or systemic cause can often be treated with medication. Correction of underlying vitamin B12, iron, or folate deficiencies is indicated for chronic problems with aphthous stomatitis. Medication can also be applied to oral canker sores.

Cancrum oris, or noma, is sudden, rapidly progressive tissue destruction. The mucous membranes (e.g., gums, lining of the cheeks) become inflamed and develop ulcers. The infection spreads from the mucous membranes to the skin. The tissues in the lips and cheeks die. Rapid, painless tissue breakdown continues and this gangrenous process can destroy the soft tissue and bone. Noma can also affect the mucous membranes of the genitals, spreading to the genital skin (this is sometimes called noma pudendi). Risk factors include Kwashiorkor and other forms of severe malnutrition, poor sanitation and poor cleanliness, disorders such as measles or leukemia, and living in an underdeveloped country.

Signs and symptoms include red and tender gums and inner cheeks, ulcers that develop a foul-smelling drainage, and eventual destruction of the bones around the mouth cause deformity and loss of teeth. A physical exam shows inflamed areas of the mucous membranes, mouth ulcers, and skin ulcers, and other signs of malnutrition. Noma can be fatal if left untreated or heal over time even without treatment. However, it can cause massive tissue destruction before healing. Treatment with penicillin and improving nutrition halts progression of the disease. Skin lesions eventually heal even without treatment, but severe scarring and deformity can develop.

Keratinized tissue is made up of keratin, the main protein constituent in the epidermis, hair, and nails. Soft keratin is found in epithelial tissue. Healthy attached keratinized mucosa that presents in an even thickness on residual ridge gingiva in the edentulous patient is ideal for denture stability, because dentures rely on the residual alveolar ridge and oral mucosa for support and retention. Sometimes the keratinized epithelium present on a residual ridge is not enough or is in excess. In these cases, the amount of tissue must either be augmented or decreased before restorative measures can be carried out.

528.00		Stomatitis and mucositis, unspecified — ulcerative and vesicular, not otherwise specified
528.01		Mucositis (ulcerative) due to antineoplastic therapy — (Use additional E code to identify adverse effects of therapy, such as radiation therapy [E879.2] or antineoplastic and immunosuppressive drugs [E930.7, E933.1])
528.02		Mucositis (ulcerative) due to other drugs — (Use additional E code to identify drug)
528.09		Other stomatitis and mucositis

Coding Clarification
This subcategory excludes diphtheritic stomatitis (032.0), epizootic stomatitis (078.4), oral thrush (112.0), gingivitis (523.0-523.1), cellulitis and abscess of the mouth (528.3), and Stevens-Johnson syndrome (695.1).

528.1	Cancrum oris — gangrenous, ulcerative, inflammatory lesion of mouth
528.2	Oral aphthae — canker sore, aphthous stomatitis, periadenitis mucosa necrotica recurrens
528.3	Cellulitis and abscess of oral soft tissues — oral fistula, Ludwig's angina
528.4	Cysts of oral soft tissues — dermoid, epidermoid, Epstein's pearl, nasolabial, nasoalveolar, lymphoepithelial
528.5	Diseases of lips — abscess, cellulitis, fistula, hypertrophy; cheilitis, celiodynia, cheilosis AHA: Sept-Oct, 1986, 10
528.6	Leukoplakia of oral mucosa, including tongue — white patch on oral mucosa which cannot be attributed to a specific disease; lip, tongue, mucosa, gingiva
528.71	Minimal keratinized residual ridge mucosa
528.72	Excessive keratinized residual ridge mucosa
528.79	Other disturbances of oral epithelium, including tongue
528.8	Oral submucosal fibrosis, including of tongue
528.9	Other and unspecified diseases of the oral soft tissues — cheek/lip biting; denture sore mouth; denture stomatitis, melanoplakia; buccal lesion; fistula in soft palate; redundant uvula; melanoplakia

529 Diseases and other conditions of the tongue

Geographic tongue is described as a common and harmless condition in which one or more irregularly shaped patches appear on the tongue, in a design that may resemble a map of a country. The center area is redder than the rest of the tongue and the edges of the patch are whitish in color. The etiology is unknown, although a viral infection is assumed and it may be associated with a variety of inflammatory or allergic conditions as well. Geographic tongue often goes away without treatment, but can be treated with topical steroids such as topical Lidex gel.

529.0	Glossitis — abscess or traumatic ulceration of tongue; Riga-Fede disease
529.1	Geographic tongue — benign migratory glossitis; glossitis areata exfoliativa
529.2	Median rhomboid glossitis — asymptomatic lesion of dorsum of tongue due to Candida albicans infection
529.3	Hypertrophy of tongue papillae — black hairy tongue; coated tongue, lingua villosa nigra, hypertrophy of foliate papillae
529.4	Atrophy of tongue papillae — bald tongue, glazed tongue, Hunter's or Moeller's glossitis, glossodynia exfoliativa, smooth atrophic tongue
529.5	Plicated tongue — fissured, furrowed, scrotal
529.6	Glossodynia — painful tongue; glossopyrosis
529.8	Other specified conditions of the tongue — not otherwise specified, cicatrix, hemorrhage, paralysis, glossoncus, glossoplegia, atrophy, crenated, enlargement, hypertrophy, hemiatrophy, glossocele, glossoptosis
529.9	Unspecified condition of the tongue

530–538 Diseases of Esophagus, Stomach, and Duodenum

530 Diseases of esophagus

This category includes diseases and disorders of the esophagus, a muscular, tubular structure that serves as a conduit for the passage of food and water from the pharynx to the stomach. It functions by transporting food and fluids from the mouth to the stomach (and sometimes in the reverse direction) by a combination of gravity and peristaltic waves. The esophagus is equipped with two sphincters. The first is the pharyngeal-esophageal sphincter located at the level of the cricoid cartilage; the second is the gastroesophageal sphincter (also known as the lower esophageal sphincter) located at the level of the esophageal hiatus of the diaphragm.

Subcategory 530.0 classifies a neuromuscular disorder characterized by an absence of peristalsis, dilation of the body of the esophagus, and a conically narrowed cardioesophageal junction. The dominant symptom is dysphagia. Vigorous achalasia is a variant form characterized by recurring esophageal spasms.

Subcategory 530.1 classifies inflammation of the esophagus due to reflux, chemicals, and infection. Reflux esophagitis, sometimes referred to as peptic or regurgitant esophagitis, is the most common form of esophagitis and is caused by the reflux of acid and pepsin from the stomach into the esophagus. Normally, the gastroesophageal sphincter prevents the reflux of gastric juice into the esophagus, but a variety of conditions can compromise the sphincter's competency. Frequently, hiatal hernia is an underlying cause of sphincter incompetence. Other causes are pregnancy, certain drugs (anticholinergic agents, calcium channel blockers, beta-adrenergic agonists), scleroderma, obesity, placement of nasogastric tubes, and surgical vagotomy.

Chemical (corrosive) esophagitis is a chemical burn caused by ingestion and regurgitation of caustic liquids or solids. The caustic agent may result in sloughing of the mucous membrane, edema and inflammation of the submucosa, thrombosis of the esophageal vessels, secondary infection, perforation, and mediastinitis. Chemical esophagitis can cause severe damage and may constitute a medical emergency depending on the strength of the chemical and the length of time the chemical remains in the esophagus.

Esophagitis due to infection is relatively rare.

Signs and symptoms of esophagitis include heartburn after eating or while resting in recumbent position, chest pain sometimes masquerading as angina pectoris, regurgitation (water brash) and dysphagia due to inflammatory edema or stricture in the distal esophagus, and in patients with chemical esophagitis and a history of ingesting caustic liquids or solids, intense pain and chemical burns of the lips, buccal cavity, and tongue.

Esophagoscopy and biopsy may be performed to assess the severity of the esophagitis and rule out associated conditions such as strictures, ulcers, and carcinoma. Esophageal manometry may be performed to assess competency of the gastroesophageal sphincter. An acid perfusion test, also known as the Bernstein test, may be done to reproduce the pain associated with reflux and an acid reflux test may be performed to monitor the intraesophageal pH after instillation of hydrochloric acid into the stomach. Barium swallow and upper GI series are of limited diagnostic importance except in the most severe cases.

Therapies include alterations in diet and mealtimes, antacids, drugs to increase gastroesophageal sphincter tone such as bethanechol and metoclopramide, and avoidance of drugs known to decrease gastroesophageal sphincter pressure (anticholinergic agents, beta-adrenergic drugs). Surgical intervention includes antireflux surgery such as Nissen fundoplication, Belsey fundoplication, placement of an Angelchik ring (prosthesis) around the distal esophagus, and replacement of the esophagus with segments of stomach, jejunum, or colon in cases of severe damage.

An esophagostomy is an artificial opening from the esophagus to outside the body. Esophagostomies are performed on infants born with congenital esophageal atresia, as an interim treatment method to prepare the upper esophagus for a primary anastomosis procedure, by gradual elongation and lowered placement of the esophagostomy with traction on the distal end. Esophagostomies are also performed on patients with swallowing disorders, or dysphasia, when nonoral feedings are needed and the placement of other enteral feeding tubes is contraindicated. Patients with amyotrophic lateral sclerosis (Lou Gehrig's disease) or muscular dystrophy affecting their throat muscles and ability to eat may have an esophagostomy done to place a tube through the neck for feeding. A complication occurs when the stoma or skin surrounding it becomes infected, or when there is a malfunction occurring anywhere along the surgical opening from the esophagus to the skin surface.

530.0	Achalasia and cardiospasm — *failure of the esophagogastric sphincter to relax; aperistalsis of esophagus; megaesophagus*
530.10	Unspecified esophagitis — (Use additional E code to identify cause, if induced by chemical or drug) AHA: Q3, 2005, 17
530.11	Reflux esophagitis — (Use additional E code to identify cause, if induced by chemical or drug) — *inflammation of the lower esophagus from regurgitation of acid gastric contents* AHA: Q3, 1991, 20; Q1, 1992, 17; Q4, 1993, 27; Q4, 1995, 82

530.12	Acute esophagitis — (Use additional E code to identify cause, if induced by chemical or drug)		530.83	Esophageal leukoplakia — *white patch in the esophagus which cannot be attributed to a specific disease*
530.19	Other esophagitis — (Use additional E code to identify cause, if induced by chemical or drug) — *not otherwise specified, chemical burn, abscess, postoperative esophagitis*		530.84	Tracheoesophageal fistula — *acquired communication between trachea and esophagus*
	AHA: Q3, 1991, 20; Q1, 1992, 17; Q4, 1993, 27; Q3, 2001, 10		530.85	Barrett's esophagus
			530.86	Infection of esophagostomy
			530.87	Mechanical complication of esophagostomy

Coding Clarification

Associated conditions include perforation and bleeding, ulcer formation, secondary infection, mediastinitis, tracheoesophageal fistulas, strictures, hiatal hernia, aspiration pneumonia, and carcinoma.

Assign code 530.10 for unspecified esophagitis, 530.11 for reflux esophagitis, and 530.19 for other specified types of esophagitis.

530.2 ✓sth	Ulcer of esophagus — (Use additional E code to identify cause, if induced by chemical or drug) — *fungal, peptic, due to ingestion of aspirin, chemicals, medicine*
	AHA: Q4, 2003, 63
530.20	Ulcer of esophagus without bleeding — (Use additional E code to identify cause, if induced by chemical or drug)
530.21	Ulcer of esophagus with bleeding — (Use additional E code to identify cause, if induced by chemical or drug)
530.3	Stricture and stenosis of esophagus — *compression, obstruction*
	AHA: Q1, 1988, 13; Q2, 1997, 3; Q2, 2001, 4
530.4	Perforation of esophagus — *rupture; Boerhaave's syndrome*
530.5	Dyskinesia of esophagus — *curling, corkscrew, spasm; Barsony-Polgar or Barsony-Teschendorf syndromes*
	AHA: Nov-Dec, 1984, 19; Q1, 1988, 13
530.6	Diverticulum of esophagus, acquired — *herniated pouch or sac opening within the esophagus; epiphrenic, pharyngoesophageal, subdiaphragmatic, hypopharyngeal; esophagocele; traction, pulsion, pouch*
	AHA: Jan-Feb, 1985, 3
530.7	Gastroesophageal laceration-hemorrhage syndrome — *Mallory-Weiss syndrome*

Coding Clarification

Subcategory 530.7 classifies mucosal laceration (or vertical tear) of the esophagus or cardioesophageal junction. More commonly known as Mallory-Weiss syndrome, this condition follows prolonged or forceful vomiting.

530.81	Esophageal reflux — *regurgitation of contents of stomach into the esophagus, without inflammation*
	AHA: Q4, 1992, 27; Q1, 1995, 7; Q2, 2001, 4
530.82	Esophageal hemorrhage — *bleeding, except for varices*
	AHA: Q1, 2005, 17

530.89	Other specified disorder of the esophagus — *not otherwise specified, including cyst, deviation, erosion, fistula, pain, necrosis, relaxation, insufficiency*
530.9	Unspecified disorder of esophagus

531 Gastric ulcer
AHA: Q4, 1990, 27; Q1, 1991, 15

This rubric classifies a condition formed by discreet tissue destruction within the lumen of the stomach. The destruction is due to the action of hydrochloric (gastric) acid and pepsin on areas of gastric mucosa having a decreased resistance to ulceration.

Signs and symptoms of gastric ulcer include pain exacerbated by eating, weight loss, repeated vomiting — which is a sign of possible gastric outlet obstruction — vomiting of frank red blood or "coffee ground" material, and black and tarry stools or heme positive stools if the ulcer is bleeding.

Lab work may show hypochromic blood loss anemia. Gastric analysis shows acid pH after administration of histamine or pentagastrin with usual finding of low to normal secretion of gastric acid. An upper GI series may be performed and an upper endoscopy with biopsy may be done to determine the ulcer's benign or malignant status.

Therapies include antacids, diet modification, H2 receptor antagonist drugs such as cimetidine and ranitidine, and other therapeutic agents (sucralfate, carbenoxolone, bismuth, certain prostaglandins, tricyclic antidepressants such as doxepin). In addition, gastric irradiation may be performed to reduce acid production temporarily in patients who cannot tolerate drugs or surgery. Other therapies include distal subtotal gastrectomy, subtotal gastrectomy with wedge resection of gastric ulcer, vagotomy with drainage, and vagotomy with antrectomy.

Associated conditions include acute and/or chronic blood loss anemia and gastric outlet obstruction.

The following fifth-digit subclassification is for use with categories 531-535:
0   without mention of obstruction
1   with obstruction

531.0 ⌐5th Acute gastric ulcer with hemorrhage — (Use additional E code to identify drug, if drug induced) — *sudden, severe; prepyloric, pylorus, stomach; with bleeding*
AHA: Nov-Dec, 1984, 15; Q4, 1990, 27; Q1, 1991, 15

531.1 ⌐5th Acute gastric ulcer with perforation — (Use additional E code to identify drug, if drug induced) — *sudden, severe; prepyloric, pylorus, stomach; with leaking stomach contents*
AHA: Q4, 1990, 27; Q1, 1991, 15

531.2 ⌐5th Acute gastric ulcer with hemorrhage and perforation — (Use additional E code to identify drug, if drug induced) — *sudden, severe; prepyloric, pylorus, stomach; with bleeding and leaking stomach contents*
AHA: Q4, 1990, 27; Q1, 1991, 15

531.3 ⌐5th Acute gastric ulcer without mention of hemorrhage or perforation — (Use additional E code to identify drug, if drug induced) — *sudden, severe; prepyloric, pylorus, stomach; without bleeding or leaking stomach contents*
AHA: Q4, 1990, 27; Q1, 1991, 15

531.4 ⌐5th Chronic or unspecified gastric ulcer with hemorrhage — (Use additional E code to identify drug, if drug induced) — *persistent; prepyloric, pylorus, stomach; with bleeding*
AHA: Q4, 1990, 22; Q4, 1990, 27; Q1, 1991, 15

531.5 ⌐5th Chronic or unspecified gastric ulcer with perforation — (Use additional E code to identify drug, if drug induced) — *persistent; prepyloric, pylorus, stomach; with leaking stomach contents*
AHA: Q4, 1990, 27; Q1, 1991, 15

531.6 ⌐5th Chronic or unspecified gastric ulcer with hemorrhage and perforation — (Use additional E code to identify drug, if drug induced) — *persistent; prepyloric, pylorus, stomach; with bleeding and leaking stomach contents*
AHA: Q4, 1990, 27; Q1, 1991, 15

531.7 ⌐5th Chronic gastric ulcer without mention of hemorrhage or perforation — (Use additional E code to identify drug, if drug induced) — *persistent; prepyloric, pylorus, stomach; without bleeding or leaking stomach contents*
AHA: Q4, 1990, 27; Q1, 1991, 15

531.9 ⌐5th Gastric ulcer, unspecified as acute or chronic, without mention of hemorrhage or perforation — (Use additional E code to identify drug, if drug induced) — *unknown whether sudden or persistent; prepyloric, pylorus, stomach; unknown status of bleeding or leaking stomach contents*
AHA: Q4, 1990, 27; Q1, 1991, 15

Coding Clarification
A common factor in peptic ulcer is the presence of *Helicobacter pylori*, which is treated with bismuth salicylate and oral amoxicillin. The *H. pylori* should be reported secondarily with 041.86.

532 Duodenal ulcer
AHA: Q4, 1990, 27; Q1, 1991, 15

Duodenal ulcers are ulcers formed in the duodenum by discreet tissue destruction due to the actions of hydrochloric (gastric) acid and pepsin on areas of the mucosa having a decreased resistance to ulceration. Duodenal ulcers occur about five times more frequently than gastric ulcers. About 95 percent occur in the area of the duodenal bulb or cap.

Signs and symptoms of a duodenal ulcer include pain with cramps, burning, gnawing, heartburn, vomiting of highly acidic fluid with no retained food, deep epigastric tenderness, voluntary muscle guarding, unilateral rectus spasm over duodenal bulb, and melena and occult blood in stools in chronic ulcers. Pain diminishes by eating, but recurs two to three hours later.

Gastric analysis shows acid in all cases and a basal and maximal gastric hypersecretion of hydrochloric acid in some patients. Lab work may show hypochromic blood loss anemia. Radiographs demonstrate ulcer crater formation when the ulcer is not obscured by duodenal bulb formation. Esophagogastroduodenoscopy proves duodenal ulcer in cases not demonstrated radiographically.

Therapies include antacids, diet modification, H2 receptor antagonist drugs such as cimetidine and ranitidine, and other therapeutic agents (sucralfate, carbenoxolone, bismuth, certain prostaglandins, tricyclic antidepressants such as doxepin). Surgical interventions include subtotal gastrectomy, vagotomy, antrectomy, gastrojejunostomy, and total gastrectomy.

The following fifth-digit subclassification is for use with categories 531-535:
0   without mention of obstruction
1   with obstruction

532.0 ☑sth Acute duodenal ulcer with hemorrhage — (Use additional E code to identify drug, if drug induced) — *sudden, severe; duodenum, postpyloric; with bleeding*
AHA: Q4, 1990, 22; Q4, 1990, 27; Q1, 1991, 15

532.1 ☑sth Acute duodenal ulcer with perforation — (Use additional E code to identify drug, if drug induced) — *sudden, severe; duodenum, postpyloric; with leaking stomach contents*
AHA: Q4, 1990, 27; Q1, 1991, 15

532.2 ☑sth Acute duodenal ulcer with hemorrhage and perforation — (Use additional E code to identify drug, if drug induced) — *sudden, severe; duodenum, postpyloric; with bleeding and leaking stomach contents*
AHA: Q4, 1990, 27; Q1, 1991, 15

532.3 ☑sth Acute duodenal ulcer without mention of hemorrhage or perforation — (Use additional E code to identify drug, if drug induced) — *sudden, severe; duodenum, postpyloric; without bleeding or leaking stomach contents*
AHA: Q4, 1990, 27; Q1, 1991, 15

532.4 ☑sth Chronic or unspecified duodenal ulcer with hemorrhage — (Use additional E code to identify drug, if drug induced) — *persistent; duodenum, postpyloric; with bleeding*
AHA: Q4, 1990, 27; Q1, 1991, 15

532.5 ☑sth Chronic or unspecified duodenal ulcer with perforation — (Use additional E code to identify drug, if drug induced) — *persistent; duodenum, postpyloric; with leaking stomach contents*
AHA: Q4, 1990, 27; Q1, 1991, 15

532.6 ☑sth Chronic or unspecified duodenal ulcer with hemorrhage and perforation — (Use additional E code to identify drug, if drug induced) — *persistent; duodenum, postpyloric; with bleeding and leaking stomach contents*
AHA: Q4, 1990, 27; Q1, 1991, 15

532.7 ☑sth Chronic duodenal ulcer without mention of hemorrhage or perforation — (Use additional E code to identify drug, if drug induced) — *persistent; duodenum, postpyloric; without bleeding or leaking stomach contents*
AHA: Q4, 1990, 27; Q1, 1991, 15

532.9 ☑sth Duodenal ulcer, unspecified as acute or chronic, without mention of hemorrhage or perforation — (Use additional E code to identify drug, if drug induced) — *unknown whether sudden or persistent; duodenum, postpyloric; unknown status of bleeding or leaking stomach contents*
AHA: Q4, 1990, 27; Q1, 1991, 15

533 Peptic ulcer, site unspecified
AHA: Q4, 1990, 27; Q1, 1991, 15

This rubric classifies acute or chronic benign ulcer occurring in a portion of the digestive tract accessible to gastric secretions. Peptic ulcers result from the corrosive action of acid gastric juice on vulnerable epithelium.

This rubric includes only peptic ulcers for which no site has been specified.

The following fifth-digit subclassification is for use with categories 531-535:
0   without mention of obstruction
1   with obstruction

533.0 ☑sth Acute peptic ulcer, unspecified site, with hemorrhage — (Use additional E code to identify drug, if drug induced) — *sudden, severe; site unknown; with bleeding*
AHA: Q4, 1990, 27; Q1, 1991, 15

533.1 ☑sth Acute peptic ulcer, unspecified site, with perforation — (Use additional E code to identify drug, if drug induced) — *sudden, severe; site unknown; with leaking stomach contents*
AHA: Q4, 1990, 27; Q1, 1991, 15

533.2 ☑sth Acute peptic ulcer, unspecified site, with hemorrhage and perforation — (Use additional E code to identify drug, if drug induced) — *sudden, severe; site unknown; with bleeding and leaking stomach contents*
AHA: Q4, 1990, 27; Q1, 1991, 15

533.3 ☑sth Acute peptic ulcer, unspecified site, without mention of hemorrhage and perforation — (Use additional E code to identify drug, if drug induced) — *sudden, severe; site unknown; without bleeding or leaking stomach contents*
AHA: Q4, 1990, 27; Q1, 1991, 15

533.4 ☑sth Chronic or unspecified peptic ulcer, unspecified site, with hemorrhage — (Use additional E code to identify drug, if drug induced) — *persistent; site unknown; with bleeding*
AHA: Q4, 1990, 27; Q1, 1991, 15

533.5 ☑sth Chronic or unspecified peptic ulcer, unspecified site, with perforation — (Use additional E code to identify drug, if drug induced) — *persistent; site unknown; with leaking stomach contents*
AHA: Q4, 1990, 27; Q1, 1991, 15

533.6 ☑sth Chronic or unspecified peptic ulcer, unspecified site, with hemorrhage and perforation — (Use additional E code to identify drug, if drug induced) — *persistent; site unknown; with bleeding and leaking stomach contents*
AHA: Q4, 1990, 27; Q1, 1991, 15

533.7 ☑sth Chronic peptic ulcer, unspecified site, without mention of hemorrhage or perforation — (Use additional E code to identify drug, if drug induced) — *persistent; site unknown; without bleeding or leaking stomach contents*
AHA: Q2, 1989, 16; Q4, 1990, 27; Q1, 1991, 15

Diseases of the Digestive System

533.9 ⌐sth Peptic ulcer, unspecified site, unspecified as acute or chronic, without mention of hemorrhage or perforation — *unknown whether sudden or persistent; site unknown; unknown status of bleeding or leaking stomach contents*
AHA: Q4, 1990, 27; Q1, 1991, 15

Coding Clarification
Peptic ulcers may occur in the esophagus (subcategory 530.2), stomach (category 531), duodenum (category 532), jejunum and gastrojejunal area (category 534), and ileum (569.82).

534 Gastrojejunal ulcer
AHA: Q4, 1990, 27; Q1, 1991, 15

This rubric classifies ulcer formation at or proximal to the junction of a previous gastrojejunal anastomosis. The signs and symptoms, diagnostics, therapies, and associated conditions are virtually the same as for gastric or duodenal ulcers.

The following fifth-digit subclassification is for use with categories 531-535:
0 without mention of obstruction
1 with obstruction

534.0 ⌐sth Acute gastrojejunal ulcer with hemorrhage — *sudden, severe; jejunal, gastrocolic, gastrointestinal, marginal, stomal, anastomotic; with bleeding*
AHA: Q4, 1990, 27; Q1, 1991, 15

534.1 ⌐sth Acute gastrojejunal ulcer with perforation — *sudden, severe; jejunal, gastrocolic, gastrointestinal, marginal, stomal, anastomotic; with leaking stomach contents*
AHA: Q4, 1990, 27; Q1, 1991, 15

534.2 ⌐sth Acute gastrojejunal ulcer with hemorrhage and perforation — *sudden, severe; jejunal, gastrocolic, gastrointestinal, marginal, stomal, anastomotic; with bleeding and leaking stomach contents*
AHA: Q4, 1990, 27; Q1, 1991, 15

534.3 ⌐sth Acute gastrojejunal ulcer without mention of hemorrhage or perforation — *sudden, severe; jejunal, gastrocolic, gastrointestinal, marginal, stomal, anastomotic; without bleeding or leaking stomach contents*
AHA: Q4, 1990, 27; Q1, 1991, 15

534.4 ⌐sth Chronic or unspecified gastrojejunal ulcer with hemorrhage — *persistent; jejunal, gastrocolic, gastrointestinal, marginal, stomal, anastomotic; with bleeding*
AHA: Q4, 1990, 27; Q1, 1991, 15

534.5 ⌐sth Chronic or unspecified gastrojejunal ulcer with perforation — *persistent; jejunal, gastrocolic, gastrointestinal, marginal, stomal, anastomotic; with leaking stomach contents*
AHA: Q4, 1990, 27; Q1, 1991, 15

534.6 ⌐sth Chronic or unspecified gastrojejunal ulcer with hemorrhage and perforation — *persistent; jejunal, gastrocolic, gastrointestinal, marginal, stomal, anastomotic; with bleeding and leaking stomach contents*
AHA: Q4, 1990, 27; Q1, 1991, 15

534.7 ⌐sth Chronic gastrojejunal ulcer without mention of hemorrhage or perforation — *persistent; jejunal, gastrocolic, gastrointestinal, marginal, stomal, anastomotic; without bleeding or leaking stomach contents*
AHA: Q4, 1990, 27; Q1, 1991, 15

534.9 ⌐sth Gastrojejunal ulcer, unspecified as acute or chronic, without mention of hemorrhage or perforation — *unknown whether sudden or persistent; jejunal, gastrocolic, gastrointestinal, marginal, stomal, anastomotic; unknown status of bleeding or leaking stomach contents*
AHA: Q4, 1990, 27; Q1, 1991, 15

535 Gastritis and duodenitis
AHA: Q4, 1991, 25; Q2, 1992, 9

Gastritis is an inflammation of the lining of the stomach and duodenitis is inflammation of the duodenum. Gastritis can take on several forms, including Watermelon gastritis, which is a hemorrhagic condition that has a watermelon like appearance. Ulcers of the duodenal bulb can often be hidden between the folds. Both diseases can progress to erosion, ulceration, and bleeding. Causes, which are the same for both disorders, include alcohol, prolonged irritation from the use of nonsteroidal anti-inflammatory drugs (NSAIDs), infection with the bacteria *Helicobacter pylori*, pernicious anemia, degeneration related to age, or chronic bile reflux. Symptoms include upper abdominal pain aggravated by eating, indigestion, nausea, vomiting, and dark stools. Complications include severe loss of blood and an increased risk of gastric or duodenal cancer. Diagnosis is by a gastroscopy, an esophagogastroduodenoscopy (EGD), a complete blood count for anemia, and a positive guaiac stool. Treatment for either gastritis or duodenitis depends on the cause, such as H2 blockers and antacids to reduce HCL production, unless the cause is from anti-inflammatory medications, antibiotic therapy for conditions caused by bacterial infection, and antacids to decrease gastric acid. Other treatments include vitamin B12 for pernicious anemia and laser therapy for severe forms (e.g., watermelon gastritis).

This rubric classifies self-limiting illnesses characterized by nausea, vomiting, anorexia, epigastric pain, and some systemic symptoms. Manifestations may be variable but anorexia is a consistent feature.

The following fifth-digit subclassification is for use with categories 531-535:

0 without mention of obstruction
1 with obstruction

535.0 ⌐sth Acute gastritis — *severe inflammation of stomach*
AHA: Nov-Dec, 1986, 9; Q4, 1991, 25; Q2, 1992, 8; Q2, 1992, 9

535.1 ⌐sth Atrophic gastritis — *inflammation of the stomach with atrophy of the mucous membrane and destruction of the peptic glands*
AHA: Q4, 1991, 25; Q2, 1992, 9; Q1, 1994, 18

535.2 ⌐sth Gastric mucosal hypertrophy — *increase in size and number of cells in tissue of gastric mucosa; Menetrier's syndrome*
AHA: Q4, 1991, 25; Q2, 1992, 9

535.3 ⌐sth Alcoholic gastritis

535.4 ⌐sth Other specified gastritis — *including allergic, bile-induced, irritant, superficial, toxic*5373
AHA: Q4, 1990, 27; Q4, 1991, 25; Q2, 1992, 9

535.5 ⌐sth Unspecified gastritis and gastroduodenitis — *unknown type*
AHA: Q4, 1991, 25; Q2, 1992, 9; Q3, 2005, 17

535.6 ⌐sth Duodenitis — *inflammation of the intestine between the pylorus and the jejunum*
AHA: Q4, 1991, 25; Q2, 1992, 9; Q3, 2005, 17

536 Disorders of function of stomach

As food is eaten, it passes from the mouth through the esophagus and to the stomach. Acids in the stomach break down food, while the lower esophageal sphincter stops stomach acid from backing up into the esophagus. The contractile activity of the stomach helps to mix, grind, and evacuate small portions of chyme into the small bowel, while the rest of the chyme is mixed and ground. Anatomically, the stomach can be divided into three major regions: fundus (the most proximal), corpus, and antrum.

The term "functional" generally applies to disorders described by symptoms when no organic explanation is detected using common diagnostic procedures. Achlorhydria (536.0) is the absence of hydrochloric acid in the stomach. There are varying degrees of achlorhydria, although, the older the patient, the greater the deficiency up to a complete absence of hydrochloric acid. Symptoms frequently occur several hours after eating and include flatulence and often alternating constipation and diarrhea. Gastroparesis (536.3) is a disorder in which the stomach takes too long to empty its contents. Cause is unknown, although disruption of nerve stimulation to the intestine is a possible cause. Gastroparesis is often a complication of Type I diabetes; it occurs less often in people with Type II diabetes. Symptoms of gastroparesis are nausea, vomiting, an early feeling of fullness when eating, weight loss, abdominal bloating, and abdominal discomfort. In most cases, gastroparesis is usually a chronic condition, although treatment does help manage the condition. Risk factors include diabetes, systemic sclerosis, previous vagotomy, previous gastrectomy, visceral neuropathy, and use of anticholinergic medication.

536.0 Achlorhydria — *the absence of stomach acid, usually the result of atrophy of gastric mucosa; gastric anacidity*

536.1 Acute dilatation of stomach — *acute distention; Potain's syndrome*

536.2 Persistent vomiting — *habit, uncontrollable, Leyden's disease; not associated with pregnancy*

536.3 Gastroparesis — *a slight degree of paralysis within the muscular coat of the stomach*
AHA: Q4, 1994, 42; Q2, 2001, 4; Q2, 2004, 7

536.40 Unspecified gastrostomy complication

536.41 Infection of gastrostomy — (Use additional code to specify type of infection: 038.0-038.9, 041.00-041.9. Use additional code to identify organism: 041.00-041.9)

536.42 Mechanical complication of gastrostomy

536.49 Other gastrostomy complications — *not otherwise specified*
AHA: Q4, 1998, 42

536.8 Dyspepsia and other specified disorders of function of stomach — *hypermotility, hourglass contraction, hyperacidity, indigestion, pain, hypertonicity, Reichmann's syndrome, spasms, hypochlorhydria, hyperchlorhydria, Rossbach's disease*
AHA: Nov-Dec, 1984, 9; Q2, 1989, 16; Q2, 1993, 6

536.9 Unspecified functional disorder of stomach — *unknown disorder or disturbance*

537 Other disorders of stomach and duodenum

537.0 Acquired hypertrophic pyloric stenosis — *construction, obstruction, stricture*
AHA: Jan-Feb, 1985, 14; Q2, 2001, 4

537.1 Gastric diverticulum — *herniated pouch or sac opening within the stomach or duodenum*
AHA: Jan-Feb, 1985, 4

537.2 Chronic duodenal ileus — *persistent obstruction between the pylorus and jejunum*

537.3 Other obstruction of duodenum — *cicatrix, stenosis, stricture, volvulus*

537.4 Fistula of stomach or duodenum — *gastrocolic, gastrojejunocolic*

537.5 Gastroptosis — *downward displacement of the stomach*

537.6 Hourglass stricture or stenosis of stomach — *cascade stomach*

537.81 Pylorospasm — *spasmodic contraction of the distal aperture of the stomach*
AHA: Q4, 1991, 25

Diseases of the Digestive System

537.82	Angiodysplasia of stomach and duodenum (without mention of hemorrhage) — *vascular abnormalities of stomach and duodenum, without bleeding* AHA: Q4, 1990, 4; Q4, 1991, 25; Q3, 1996, 10
537.83	Angiodysplasia of stomach and duodenum with hemorrhage — *vascular abnormalities of stomach and duodenum, with bleeding* AHA: Q4, 1991, 25
537.84	Dieulafoy lesion (hemorrhagic) of stomach and duodenum
537.89	Other specified disorder of stomach and duodenum — *not otherwise specified, prolapse, rupture, intestinal metaplasia of gastric mucosa, lesion, necrosis, gastrolith, hypertony, obstruction, volvulus, efferent loop syndrome, passive congestion, mechanical difficulty of gastroduodenal stoma* AHA: Nov-Dec, 1984, 7; Q4, 1991, 25; Q3, 2005, 15
537.9	Unspecified disorder of stomach and duodenum
538	Gastrointestinal mucositis (ulcerative) — (Use additional E code to identify adverse effects of therapy, such as radiation therapy [E879.2] or antineoplastic and immunosuppressive drugs [E930.7, E933.1])

This code excludes mucositis of the mouth and oral soft tissue, which is reported with a code from range 528.00-528.09.

Mucosal inflammation, or mucositis, affects the tissues that line the gastrointestinal tract. A frequent, debilitating complication of chemotherapy or radiation treatment, mucositis occurs when the epithelial cells lining the GI tract break down, leaving the mucosal tissue susceptible to infection and ulceration. The chemotherapeutic drugs that cause the most severe mucositis include dactinomycin, plicamycin, methotrexate, and 5-fluorouracil. Agents such as doxorubicin, paclitaxel, and capecitabine are also often associated with gastrointestinal mucositis. Nonchemotherapeutic drugs may also cause adverse reactions that manifest as mucositis. Complications of mucositis range from mild symptoms that require little intervention to severe, sometimes fatal, problems such as malnutrition, hypovolemia, or electrolyte abnormalities. Nausea and vomiting are frequent side-effects of antineoplastic therapy; this may further complicate the mucositis.

Coding Clarification
Whether the mucositis is of oral tissue (528.01 or 528.02), gastrointestinal (538), or cervical/vagina/vulva (616.81), if due to antineoplastic therapy or to other drugs, use an additional E code to identify adverse effects of therapy or drug. If applicable, mucositis due to antineoplastic and immunosuppressive drugs or radiation therapies will be identified first, followed by the appropriate causative external causes (E code) sequenced second. Assign the appropriate additional code — E930.7 *Antineoplastic antibiotics*, E933.1 *Antineoplastic and immunosuppressive drugs*, or E879.2 for radiation therapy — as the causative agent.

540–543   Appendicitis

Appendicitis is inflammation of the vermiform appendix. It is usually initiated by obstruction of the appendiceal lumen by a fecalith, inflammation, neoplasm, or foreign body. The obstruction is followed by infection, edema, and frequently infarction of the appendiceal wall. Intraluminal tension develops rapidly and tends to cause mural necrosis and perforation.

Signs and symptoms of appendicitis include abdominal pain, usually beginning with epigastric or periumbilical pain associated with one or two episodes of vomiting. The abdominal pain may shift during the next 12 hours to the right lower quadrant (McBurney's point) where it persists as steady soreness aggravated by walking or coughing, anorexia, moderate malaise, slight to moderate fever, constipation (or occasionally diarrhea), rebound tenderness, and spasm.

Blood work may show moderate increase in white blood cells to 10,000/cu mm to 20,000/cu mm with an increase in neutrophils. Urinalysis may show a presence of microscopic hematuria and pyuria and barium enema may be used to visualize the entire appendix in uncertain cases.

Therapies include antibiotic therapy, nasogastric intubation, rehydration, and appendectomy with few exceptions.

Appendicitis is the most common nonobstetrical complication of pregnancy.

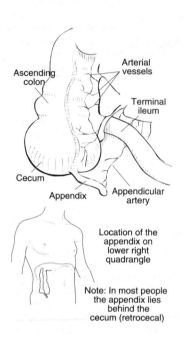

540 Acute appendicitis
AHA: Nov-Dec, 1984, 19

540.0 Acute appendicitis with generalized peritonitis — *fulminating, gangrenous, obstructive; with perforation, rupture*
AHA: Nov-Dec, 1984, 19

540.1 Acute appendicitis with peritoneal abscess — *generalized peritonitis; pocket of pus*
AHA: Nov-Dec, 1984, 19

540.9 Acute appendicitis without mention of peritonitis — *without rupture, perforation, peritonitis*
AHA: Nov-Dec, 1984, 19; Q4, 1997, 52; Q1, 2001, 15

543 Other diseases of appendix

543.0 Hyperplasia of appendix (lymphoid) — *increase in size and number of cells of appendix*

543.9 Other and unspecified diseases of appendix — *not otherwise specified, adhesion, cyst, mucocele, stercolith, fecalith, fistula, sloughing, strangulation, atrophy, intussusception, diverticulum, concretion*

550–553 *Hernia of Abdominal Cavity*

The definition of a hernia of the abdominal cavity is the protrusion of tissue, an organ, or part of an organ through an abnormal opening in the wall of the body cavity in which it is normally confined. The majority of hernias are abdominal resulting from herniation of abdominal contents through the internal or external inguinal rings, femoral rings, or defects in the abdominal wall resulting from trauma or improper healing after a surgical procedure.

550 Inguinal hernia
AHA: Nov-Dec, 1985, 12

An inguinal hernia is defined as a condition in which a loop of intestine enters the inguinal canal, a tubular passage through the lower layers of the abdominal wall. A hernia occurs when part of an organ protrudes through a weak point or tear in the thin muscular wall that holds the abdominal organs in place. A direct inguinal hernia creates a bulge in the groin area, and an indirect hernia descends into the scrotum. Inguinal hernias occur less often in women than men.

Hernias are caused by congenital (defects at birth) or age-related weaknesses in the abdominal walls. In males, they are often congenital and caused by an improper closure of the abdominal cavity. They can also be caused by an increase in pressure within the abdominal cavity due to heavy lifting, straining, violent coughing, obesity, or pregnancy.

Signs and symptoms include a protrusion in the groin area between the pubis and the top of the leg in the area known as the inguinal region of the abdomen or pain during urination or a bowel movement or when lifting a heavy object. The pain can be sharp and immediate. There may be a dull aching sensation, nausea, or constipation; these feelings typically get worse toward the end of the day or after standing for long periods of time and may disappear when lying down.

A hernia that can be pushed back into the abdominal cavity (called a reducible hernia) is not considered an immediate health threat, though it does require surgery to repair the hernia. A hernia that cannot be pushed back in (called a nonreducible hernia) may lead to dangerous complications such as the obstruction of the flow of the intestinal contents or intestinal blood supply (strangulation), leading to tissue death, and requires immediate surgery.

The following fifth-digit subclassification is for use with category 550:

0 unilateral or unspecified (not specified as recurrent)
1 unilateral or unspecified, recurrent
2 bilateral (not specified as recurrent)3bilateral, recurrent

Diseases of the Digestive System

Code	Description
550.0 ⌐sth	Inguinal hernia, with gangrene — *direct, double, indirect, oblique, sliding hernia; incarceration, irreducibility, strangulation* **AHA:** Nov-Dec, 1985, 12
550.1 ⌐sth	Inguinal hernia, with obstruction, without mention of gangrene — *direct, double, indirect, oblique, sliding hernia; incarceration, irreducibility, strangulation* **AHA:** Nov-Dec, 1985, 12
550.9 ⌐sth	Inguinal hernia, without mention of obstruction or gangrene — *direct, double, indirect, oblique, sliding hernia* **AHA:** Nov-Dec, 1985, 12

551 Other hernia of abdominal cavity, with gangrene

Code	Description
551.00	Femoral hernia with gangrene, unilateral or unspecified (not specified as recurrent)
551.01	Femoral hernia with gangrene, recurrent unilateral or unspecified
551.02	Femoral hernia with gangrene, bilateral, (not specified as recurrent)
551.03	Femoral hernia with gangrene, recurrent bilateral
551.1	Umbilical hernia with gangrene — *abnormal protrusion of the intestine at the umbilicus*
551.20	Unspecified ventral hernia with gangrene — *abnormal protrusion of tissue through the abdominal wall, cause unknown*
551.21	Incisional ventral hernia, with gangrene — *abnormal protrusion of tissue through the abdominal wall, postoperative*
551.29	Other ventral hernia with gangrene — *abnormal protrusion of tissue through the abdominal wall, not otherwise specified*
551.8	Hernia of other specified sites, with gangrene — *Gruber's, Hesselbach's Rieux's; ischiorectal, lumbar, obturator, sciatic, retroperitoneal*
551.9	Hernia of unspecified site, with gangrene — *enterocele, epiplocele, interstitial, intestinal, intraabdominal, sacroepiplocele*
553.3	Diaphragmatic hernia without mention of obstruction or gangrene — *hiatal, paraesophageal, thoracic stomach* **AHA:** Q1, 2000, 6; Q2, 2001, 6

552 Other hernia of abdominal cavity, with obstruction, but without mention of gangrene

Code	Description
552.00	Unilateral or unspecified femoral hernia with obstruction
552.01	Recurrent unilateral or unspecified femoral hernia with obstruction
552.02	Bilateral femoral hernia with obstruction
552.03	Recurrent bilateral femoral hernia with obstruction
552.1	Umbilical hernia with obstruction — *abnormal protrusion of the intestine of the umbilicus; incarcerated, irreducible, strangulated*
552.20	Unspecified ventral hernia with obstruction — *abnormal protrusion of tissue through the abdominal wall, cause unknown; incarcerated, irreducible, strangulated*
552.21	Incisional hernia with obstruction — *abnormal protrusion of tissue through the abdominal wall, postoperative; incarcerated, irreducible, strangulated* **AHA:** Q3, 2003, 11
552.29	Other ventral hernia with obstruction — *abnormal protrusion of tissue through the abdominal wall, not otherwise specified; incarcerated, irreducible, strangulated*
552.3	Diaphragmatic hernia with obstruction — *hiatal, esophageal, paraesophageal, thoracic stomach; incarcerated, irreducible, strangulated*
552.8	Hernia of other specified site, with obstruction — *other sites including Gruber's, Hesselbach's Rieux's; Treitz's, ischiorectal, lumbar, obturator, retroperitoneal; incarcerated, irreducible, strangulated* **AHA:** Q1, 2004, 10
552.9	Hernia of unspecified site, with obstruction — *unknown site*

553 Other hernia of abdominal cavity without mention of obstruction or gangrene

Subcategory 553.3 reports a protrusion of part of the stomach through the esophageal hiatus of the diaphragm. The esophageal hiatus is the opening in the diaphragm between the central tendon and the hiatus aorticus where the esophagus and the two vagus nerves pass. Clinicians recognize two different types of esophageal hiatal hernias: paraesophageal and sliding (by far the more common type of hiatal hernia).

The paraesophageal hiatal hernia is characterized by all or part of the stomach herniating into the thorax immediately adjacent and to the left of a nondisplaced gastroesophageal junction. Reflux of the gastric contents does not occur because the gastroesophageal sphincter functions normal. Although this type of hiatal hernia is usually asymptomatic, complications can include hemorrhage, incarceration, obstruction, and strangulation.

With a sliding hiatal hernia, the upper stomach, along with the cardioesophageal junction, herniates upward into the posterior mediastinum. The stomach displacement may be stationary, or it may actually slide in and out of the thorax with movement, after a large meal, or with alterations of the pressure in the abdominal and thoracic cavities. Esophageal reflux and esophagitis are characteristic and due to abnormalities in the esophageal sphincter. Sliding hiatal hernia may be complicated by development of ulcers or structure formation. Carcinoma is occasionally associated with sliding hiatal hernia.

Signs and symptoms of diaphragmatic hernia without mention of obstruction or gangrene include dysphagia, and retrosternal and epigastric burning in sliding hiatal hernia with reflux esophagitis.

Diagnostic tests include x-ray examination and fluoroscopy with or without contrast to demonstrate a protrusion of the stomach through the esophageal hiatus. Esophagoscopy and biopsy assess the severity of any esophagitis and rule out associated conditions such as strictures, polyps, ulcers, and carcinomas. Esophageal motility studies assess the competency of the esophageal sphincter and prolonged monitoring of the patient's pH in the lower esophagus establishes the presence of abnormal reflux.

Therapies include diet and antacids for esophagitis. There is no intervention for asymptomatic hiatal hernias. Surgery (for about 15 percent of patients with persistent and severe symptoms) includes Nissen fundoplication, Belsey fundoplication, and placement of a doughnut-shaped silicone prosthesis around the intraabdominal esophagus (Angelchik procedure) for uncomplicated hernias. The Collis procedure or Collis-Nissen operation, may be performed when the hernia is associated with acquired short esophagus. Other treatments include vagotomy, antrectomy, or a Roux-en-Y gastrojejunostomy when scar tissue around the gastroesophageal junction from previous surgery prevents a fundoplication.

Associated conditions include reflux esophagitis, esophageal stricture, polyps, ulcer formation with or without bleeding, carcinoma, and Saint's triad (hiatal hernia, gallbladder disease, and colon diverticulosis).

553.00	Unilateral or unspecified femoral hernia without mention of obstruction or gangrene, unilateral or unspecified
553.01	Femoral hernia without mention of obstruction or gangrene, recurrent unilateral or unspecified
553.02	Femoral hernia without mention of obstruction or gangrene, bilateral
553.03	Femoral hernia without mention of obstruction or gangrene, recurrent bilateral
553.1	Umbilical hernia without mention of obstruction or gangrene — *abnormal protrusion of the intestine at the umbilicus; paraumbilical*
553.20	Unspecified ventral hernia without mention of obstruction or gangrene — *abnormal protrusion of tissue through the abdominal wall; cause unknown* AHA: Q3, 2003, 6; Q2, 2006, 10
553.21	Incisional hernia without mention of obstruction or gangrene — *abnormal protrusion of tissue through the abdominal wall; postoperative* AHA: Q3, 2003, 6
553.29	Other ventral hernia without mention of obstruction or gangrene — *not otherwise specified; including epigastric, spigelian*
553.3	Diaphragmatic hernia without mention of obstruction or gangrene — *hiatal, paraesophageal, thoracic stomach* AHA: Q1, 2000, 6; Q2, 2001, 6
553.8	Hernia of other specified sites of abdominal cavity without mention of obstruction or gangrene — *appendix, obturator, pudendal, retroperitoneal, sciatic, lumbar, ischiatic, ischiorectal, duodenojejunal, mesenteric, mesocolon, omental*
553.9	Hernia of unspecified site of abdominal cavity without mention of obstruction or gangrene

555–558 Noninfectious Enteritis and Colitis

555 Regional enteritis

Regional enteritis is a form of inflammatory bowel disease characterized by a chronic granulomatous disease. Also known as Crohn's disease, regional enteritis most often affects the large intestines but may occur anywhere in the gastrointestinal tract (e.g., mouth, esophagus, stomach, duodenum, large intestine, appendix, and anus). The disease often results in multiple bowel resections.

Associated conditions include multiple strictures, bacterial overgrowth, and malabsorption.

555.0	Regional enteritis of small intestine — *Crohn's disease, granulomatous enteritis; duodenum, ileum, jejunum*
555.1	Regional enteritis of large intestine — *Crohn's disease, granulomatous enteritis; colon, large bowel, rectum* AHA: Q3, 1999, 8
555.2	Regional enteritis of small intestine with large intestine — *Crohn's disease, granulomatous enteritis; regional ileocolitis* AHA: Q1, 2003, 18
555.9	Regional enteritis of unspecified site AHA: Q2, 2005, 11

556 Ulcerative colitis
AHA: Q3, 1999, 8

Ulcerative colitis is a disease that causes inflammation and ulcers in the top layers of the lining of the large intestine. The inflammation usually occurs in the rectum and lower part of the colon, but it may affect the entire colon and makes the colon empty frequently, causing diarrhea. Ulcers form in places where the inflammation has killed colon cells; the ulcers bleed and produce pus and mucous.

Ulcerative colitis rarely affects the small intestine except for the lower section, called the ileum. The disease can be difficult to diagnose because its symptoms are similar to other intestinal disorders such as irritable bowel syndrome and Crohn's disease, which usually occurs in the small intestine but may occur anywhere in the GI tract.

The most common symptoms of ulcerative colitis are abdominal pain and bloody diarrhea. Patients also may experience fatigue, weight loss, and rectal bleeding.

Blood tests may be performed to check for anemia, which could indicate bleeding in the colon or rectum. Blood tests may also reveal a high white blood cell count. A stool sample indicates whether there is bleeding or infection in the colon or rectum. A colonoscopy visualizes the inside of the colon and rectum. A barium enema x-ray of the colon allows a clear view of the colon, including any ulcers or other abnormalities. Treatment for ulcerative colitis depends on the seriousness of the disease. Most people are treated with medication, although in severe cases, a patient may need surgery to remove the diseased colon.

556.0	Ulcerative (chronic) enterocolitis — *persistent inflammation of the mucous membrane of small and large intestines* **AHA:** Q3, 1999, 8
556.1	Ulcerative (chronic) ileocolitis — *persistent inflammation of the mucous membrane of ileum and colon* **AHA:** Q3, 1999, 8
556.2	Ulcerative (chronic) proctitis — *persistent inflammation of the mucous membrane of the rectum* **AHA:** Q3, 1999, 8
556.3	Ulcerative (chronic) proctosigmoiditis — *persistent inflammation of the mucous membrane of the sigmoid colon and rectum* **AHA:** Q3, 1999, 8
556.4	Pseudopolyposis of colon
556.5	Left sided ulcerative (chronic) colitis
556.6	Universal ulcerative (chronic) colitis — *persistent inflammation of the mucous membrane of the entire colon* **AHA:** Q3, 1999, 8
556.8	Other ulcerative colitis
556.9	Unspecified ulcerative colitis **AHA:** Q1, 2003, 10

557 Vascular insufficiency of intestine

Visceral ischemic syndromes are associated with atherosclerotic lesions obstructing the celiac trunk, superior mesenteric artery, and inferior mesenteric artery: embolism, mesenteric venous thrombosis, and aneurysms. Narrowing of the superior mesenteric artery often presents with intense abdominal pain that results in vomiting or loose bowel movements. Gradual occlusion of this artery causes severe pain around the navel within one hour of eating because of the increased demand for blood to the intestines for digestion. The abdomen becomes distended and the stool becomes bloody. The intestine turns gangrene because of the lack of blood being supplied to the area. Surgical intervention for embolectomy or bypass reconstruction of the obstructing lesions is usually necessary to avoid extensive intestinal necrosis or death. The major causes of small intestinal hemorrhage are infectious vascular infarctions, vascular anomalies, bleeding disorders, and tumors. Interference with blood flow to the colon is the cause of ischemic colitis (557.1), an inflammation disorder of the large intestine. Risks include a history of peripheral vascular disease, stroke, low blood pressure, congestive heart failure, diabetes, and abdominal radiation exposure. Other risk factors include previous aortic surgery with accidental damage to the artery supplying the colon.

557.0	Acute vascular insufficiency of intestine — *infarction, necrosis, hemorrhage, gangrene, thrombosis, embolism* **AHA:** Q4, 2001, 53
557.1	Chronic vascular insufficiency of intestine — *abdominal angina, ischemic colitis or enteritis, stricture, artery syndrome, vascular insufficiency, Wilkie's syndrome* **AHA:** Nov-Dec, 1984, 7; Nov-Dec, 1986, 11; Q4, 1990, 4; Q3, 1996, 9
557.9	Unspecified vascular insufficiency of intestine

558 Other noninfectious gastroenteritis and colitis

Other and unspecified noninfectious gastroenteritis and colitis include gastroenteritis and colitis that do not have an infectious or presumed infectious origin. The three most common forms are enteritis, gastroenteritis, and diarrhea, not otherwise specified.

Often, enteritis, gastroenteritis, and diarrhea, when specified as due to an underlying condition, should be classified to a different category. Infectious disease is the most frequent cause of gastritis and gastroenteritis and is classified to Chapter 1 Infectious and Parasitic Diseases (001-139).

Commonly caused by infection, diarrhea may also be caused by chronic bowel disease, malabsorption states, food poisoning, adverse reactions to medications, and dietary factors such as malnutrition and food allergy. Diarrhea also may be the result of cholestatic syndromes, pancreatic disease, metabolic disease, neurological disease, psychogenic disorders, heavy metal poisoning, laxative abuse, reflex from other viscera, and immunodeficiency disease.

558.1	Gastroenteritis and colitis due to radiation — radiation enterocolitis
558.2	Toxic gastroenteritis and colitis — (Use additional E code to identify cause)
558.3	Gastroenteritis and colitis, allergic — (Use additional code to identify type of food allergy: V15.01-V15.05)
558.9	Other and unspecified noninfectious gastroenteritis and colitis

560–569 Other Diseases of Intestines and Peritoneum

560 Intestinal obstruction without mention of hernia

This category includes functional obstruction of the intestines, usually the colon. Also known as adynamic ileus, this condition represents a neurogenic impairment of peristalsis that can lead to complete intestinal obstruction. The intraabdominal etiologies for paralytic ileus include gastrointestinal surgery (997.4), peritoneal irritations (such as intraabdominal hemorrhage, ruptured viscus, pancreatitis or peritonitis), or anoxic organic obstruction. Other etiologies include drugs with anticholinergic properties, renal colic, vertebral fractures, spinal cord injuries, uremia, severe infection, diabetic coma, and electrolyte imbalances.

Signs and symptoms of paralytic ileus include continuous mild to moderate abdominal pain, vomiting, constipation, and abdominal distention. There may be absent borborygmus, minimal to absent bowel sounds, and signs of dehydration. Lab work may show hemoconcentration and or electrolyte imbalances. Leukocytosis, anemia, or elevated serum amylase may be present depending on the initiating condition. X-ray of the abdomen shows distended gas-filled loops of bowel and may show air-fluid levels in the distended bowel.

Therapies include bed rest, restriction of oral intake, rehydration, and gastrointestinal suctioning. Surgical decompression via enterostomy or cecostomy may be performed in severe cases. Associated conditions include dehydration and other electrolyte imbalances.

When assigning 560.1, also classify any initiating diseases or disorders such as those outlined in the definition.

560.0	Intussusception — *prolapse of one section of bowel into an immediate adjacent section; invagination* AHA: Q4, 1998, 82
560.1	Paralytic ileus — *adynamic, paralysis* AHA: Jan-Feb, 1987, 13
560.2	Volvulus — *knotting, strangulation, torsion, twists*
560.30	Unspecified impaction of intestine
560.31	Gallstone ileus — *obstruction by gallstone*
560.39	Other impaction of intestine — *fecal reservoir syndrome, fecal impaction, enterolith, concretion* AHA: Q4, 1998, 38
560.81	Intestinal or peritoneal adhesions with obstruction (postoperative) (postinfection) — *abnormal joining of separate tissue in the peritoneum or intestine* AHA: Nov-Dec, 1987, 9; Q3, 1995, 6; Q4, 1995, 55
560.89	Other specified intestinal obstruction — *mural thickening causing obstruction, sympathicotonic obstruction, Ogilvie's syndrome* AHA: Q1, 1988, 6; Q2, 1997, 3
560.9	Unspecified intestinal obstruction

562 Diverticula of intestine
AHA: Jan-Feb, 1985, 1; Q4, 1991, 25

Report any associated peritonitis with an additional code (567.0-567.9). Excluded from this rubric are congenital diverticulum of the colon (751.5), diverticulum of the appendix (543.9), and Meckel's diverticulum (751.0).

Use the codes in subclassification 562.1 to report formation of a pouch or sac in the colon due to pressure from within the colon. Diverticula and diverticulosis tend to occur in higher-pressure areas, such as the sigmoid colon, and dissect along the course of nutrient vessels. They consist of a mucosal coat and serosa and usually herniate through the muscularis of the colon.

Signs and symptoms of diverticula of the colon include left lower quadrant pain, either steady or severe lasting for days; cramping, intermittent and relieved by bowel movement; and constipation (or occasionally diarrhea). Guaiac testing shows occult blood in 20 percent of patients with diverticulosis. X-ray reveals diverticula and in some cases colonic spasm and interhaustral thickening or narrowing of the colonic lumen. Endoscopic exam with or without biopsy is performed when bleeding occurs to rule out other pathology. Therapies include increased bulk and fiber in diet, anticholinergic medications to control sigmoid colon spasm, and antibiotics for diverticulitis. Surgical resection of the involved portion of bowel may be performed when there are recurrent bouts of diverticulitis or to treat complications such as hemorrhage, perforation, and abscess formation.

True diverticula contain all layers of the bowel and are rare in the colon. False diverticula consist of mucosa and submucosa that have herniated through the muscularis. For coding purposes, the terms "true" and "false" have no significance and should be treated as nonessential modifiers.

Diverticula of the colon are considered pulsion type because they are pushed out by intraluminal pressure. In the ICD-9-CM index, the term "pulsion" is an essential modifier under the main term "Diverticula, diverticulosis, diverticulum," leading to code 530.6 for diverticula of the esophagus. Do not assign this code for a pulsion diverticula when it refers to other anatomic sites such as the colon.

562.00	Diverticulosis of small intestine (without mention of hemorrhage) — (Use additional code to identify any associated peritonitis: 567.0-567.9) — *sac-like herniations of the mucosal lining; duodenum, ileum, jejunum* AHA: Jan-Feb, 1985, 1; Q4, 1991, 25
562.01	Diverticulitis of small intestine (without mention of hemorrhage) — (Use additional code to identify any associated peritonitis: 567.0-567.9) — *inflammation of sac-like herniations of mucosal lining; duodenum, ileum, jejunum* AHA: Jan-Feb, 1985, 1; Q4, 1991, 25
562.02	Diverticulosis of small intestine with hemorrhage — (Use additional code to identify any associated peritonitis: 567.0-567.9) — *sac-like herniations of the mucosal lining; duodenum, ileum, jejunum; bleeding* AHA: Jan-Feb, 1985, 1; Q4, 1991, 25
562.03	Divertulitis of small intestine with hemorrhage — (Use additional code to identify any associated peritonitis: 567.0-567.9) — *inflammation of sac-like herniations of mucosal lining; duodenum, ileum, jejunum; bleeding* AHA: Jan-Feb, 1985, 1; Q4, 1991, 25
562.10	Diverticulosis of colon (without mention of hemorrhage) — (Use additional code to identify any associated peritonitis: 567.0-567.9) — *sac-like herniations of the mucosal lining* AHA: Jan-Feb, 1985, 1; Jan-Feb, 1985, 5; Q4, 1990, 21; Q4, 1991, 25; Q3, 2002, 15; Q3, 2005, 17
562.11	Diverticulitis of colon (without mention of hemorrhage) — (Use additional code to identify any associated peritonitis: 567.0-567.9) — *inflammation of sac-like herniations of mucosal lining* AHA: Jan-Feb, 1985, 1; Jan-Feb, 1985, 5; Q4, 1991, 25; Q1, 1996, 14
562.12	Diverticulosis of colon with hemorrhage — (Use additional code to identify any associated peritonitis: 567.0-567.9) — *sac-like herniations of the mucosal lining; bleeding* AHA: Jan-Feb, 1985, 1; Q4, 1991, 25
562.13	Diverticulitis of colon with hemorrhage — (Use additional code to identify any associated peritonitis: 567.0-567.9) — *inflammation of sac-like herniations of mucosal lining; bleeding* AHA: Jan-Feb, 1985, 1; Q4, 1991, 25

564 Functional digestive disorders, not elsewhere classified

564.00	Unspecified constipation
564.01	Slow transit constipation
564.02	Outlet dysfunction constipation
564.09	Other constipation
564.1	Irritable bowel syndrome — *IBS, irritable bowel* AHA: Q1, 1988, 6
564.2	Postgastric surgery syndromes — *dumping, jejunal, postgastrectomy, postvagotomy syndromes* AHA: Q1, 1995, 11
564.3	Vomiting following gastrointestinal surgery
564.4	Other postoperative functional disorders — *diarrhea*
564.5	Functional diarrhea — *diarrhea with no detectable organic cause*
564.6	Anal spasm — *proctalgia fugax*
564.7	Megacolon, other than Hirschsprung's — *dilatation of colon; faulty bowel habit syndrome*
564.81	Neurogenic bowel
564.89	Other functional disorders of intestine — *atony of colon* AHA: Q1, 1988, 6
564.9	Unspecified functional disorder of intestine

Coding Clarification
Excluded from this rubric are functional disorders of the stomach (536.0-536.9) and digestive disorders that have been specified as psychogenic (306.4).

565 Anal fissure and fistula

The last part of the rectum (anal canal) is a section about 1.5 inche567.

s long, which ends with the anus. An anal fissure is a tear in the lining of the anus frequently caused by constipation when a dry bowel movement results in a break in the tissue. However, fissures can also occur with severe bouts of diarrhea, inflammation, injury to the anal canal during childbirth, and laxative abuse. A fissure can be painful during and following bowel movements because of the muscles that control the passage of stool and keep the anus tightly closed at other times. When those muscles expand, it stretches the fissure open. A fistula is a channel or tract that develops in the presence of inflammation and infection. The channel usually runs from the rectum to an opening in the skin around the anus. Since fistulas are infected channels, there is usually some drainage.

565.0	Anal fissure — *nontraumatic tear*
565.1	Anal fistula — *anorectal, rectum to skin*

Coding Clarification
Excluded from this rubric are traumatic fissures (863.89, 863.99), and fistulas of the rectum to internal organs. Refer to the ICD-9-CM index to classify fistulas of the rectum to internal organs.

567 Peritonitis and retroperitoneal infections
Use this rubric to report acute or chronic inflammation of the peritoneum, retroperitoneal abscesses or other infections, choleperitonitis, and sclerosing mesenteritis. These conditions may arise in response to agents such as bacteria, viruses, bile, hydrochloric acid, and chemicals such as continuous ambulatory peritoneal dialysis (CAPD) fluid. Other causative agents include parasites, fungi, and foreign bodies such as barium sulfate, used in diagnostic roentgenographic studies. Ruptured viscus and surgical procedures are two common underlying factors in secondary peritonitis. Chronic peritonitis can lead to dense, widespread abdominal adhesions.

567.0	Peritonitis in infectious diseases classified elsewhere — (Code first underlying disease) — *secondary to underlying disease*
567.1	Pneumococcal peritonitis
567.21	Peritonitis *(acute) generalized* — *male pelvic peritonitis* AHA: Q4, 2005, 74
567.22	Peritoneal abscess — *abdominopelvic, mesenteric, omental, retrocecal, subdiaphragmatic, subhepatic, subphrenic abscess* AHA: Q4, 2005, 74
567.23	Spontaneous bacterial peritonitis AHA: Q4, 2005, 74
567.29	Other suppurative peritonitis — *subphrenic peritonitis* AHA: Q4, 2005, 74
567.31	Psoas muscle abscess AHA: Q4, 2005, 74

The psoas muscle connects the lumbar vertebrae to the femur and flexes the trunk or thigh. An abscess may appear externally visible on the flank or down the anterior thigh and present with fever, flank pain, and inability to fully move the hip. The common cause of psoas abscess was previously considered to be tuberculosis. Today psoas abscess is more commonly associated with severe kidney or other infections caused by a number of organisms including staphylococcus.

567.38	Other retroperitoneal abscess AHA: Q4, 2005, 74, 77
567.39	Other retroperitoneal infections AHA: Q4, 2005, 74
567.81	Choleperitonitis — *peritonitis due to bile* AHA: Q4, 2005, 74

Choleperitonitis is infection and inflammation of the peritoneum caused by the escape of bile from its normal ducts, passages, or gallbladder due to rupture, leakage, or trauma.

567.82	Sclerosing mesenteritis — *peritoneal fat necrosis, idiopathic sclerosing mesenteric fibrosis, mesenteric lipodystrophy, mesenteric panniculitis, retractile mesenteritis* AHA: Q4, 2005, 74, 77

Sclerosing mesenteritis is a rare disease process that forms mesenteric masses or thickening, more commonly of the small bowel but also the mesocolon. The disease usually presents around age 60, with a higher predominance in men. Signs and symptoms include abdominal pain, masses, diarrhea, nausea, vomiting, and weight loss. Sclerosing mesenteritis is a combination of fat necrosis, chronic inflammation, and fibrosis occurring in the mesentery, commonly manifesting as a single mass of diffuse thickening, although additional lesions are sometimes reported. Masses are hard and gritty and may be from 1.0 to 40.0 cm. Patients may require surgical resection when bowel obstruction occurs. The numerous other terms applied to this disease process, such as mesenteric panniculitis, retractile mesenteritis, and mesenteric lipodystrophy share the same common clinical and histological features and are generally considered to be different spectrums of the single disease.

567.89	Other specified peritonitis —*chronic proliferative peritonitis, mesenteric saponification, peritonitis due to bile or urine* AHA: Q4, 2005, 74
567.9	Unspecified peritonitis AHA: Q1, 2004, 10

Coding Clarification
Excluded from this rubric are peritonitis defined as benign paroxysmal (277.3), female pelvic (614.5, 614.7), periodic familial (277.3), puerperal (670), or in cases of abortion (rubrics 634-638), appendicitis (540.0-540.1), or ectopic/molar pregnancy (639.0).

568 Other disorders of peritoneum

568.0	Peritoneal adhesions (postoperative) (postinfection) — *abdominal wall, diaphragm,*

intestine, male pelvis, mesenteric, omentum, stomach, adhesive bands
AHA: Sept-Oct, 1985, 11; Q3, 1995, 7; Q4, 1995, 55; Q3, 2003, 7, 11

568.81 Hemoperitoneum (nontraumatic) — *blood in the peritoneal cavity*
568.82 Peritoneal effusion (chronic) — *persistent escape of fluid within the peritoneal cavity*
568.89 Other specified disorder of peritoneum — *not otherwise specified, including acquired deforming, hemorrhage, rupture, degeneration, cyst, granuloma, pneumatosis*
568.9 Unspecified disorder of peritoneum

569 Other disorders of intestine

569.0 Anal and rectal polyp — *not otherwise specified*
569.1 Rectal prolapse — *procidentia; anus, rectum*
569.2 Stenosis of rectum and anus — *stricture*
569.3 Hemorrhage of rectum and anus — *bleeding*
AHA: Q3, 2005, 17
569.41 Ulcer of anus and rectum — *solitary, stercoral*
569.42 Anal or rectal pain — *proctalgia*
AHA: Q1, 1996, 13; Q1, 2003, 8
569.49 Other specified disorder of rectum and anus — *not otherwise specified, hypertrophy of anal papillae; granuloma, rupture, male proctocele/rectocele, relaxation, paralysis, cicatrix*
569.5 Abscess of intestine — *pocket of pus*
569.60 Unspecified complication of colostomy or enterostomy
569.61 Infection of colostomy or enterostomy — (Use additional code to identify organism: 041.00-041.9. Use additional code to specify type of infection: 038.0-038.9, 682.2)
569.62 Mechanical complication of colostomy and enterostomy — *malfunction*
AHA: Q4, 1995, 58; Q4, 1998, 44; Q1, 2003, 10; Q2, 2005, 11
569.69 Other complication of colostomy or enterostomy — *not otherwise specified, fistula, hernia, stenosis, prolapse*
AHA: Q4, 1995, 58; Q3, 1998, 16
569.81 Fistula of intestine, excluding rectum and anus — *abnormal communication between intestine and other internal organ or site*
AHA: Q4, 1991, 25; Q3, 1999, 8
569.82 Ulceration of intestine
569.83 Perforation of intestine — *hole through the intestinal wall*
AHA: Q4, 1991, 25
569.84 Angiodysplasia of intestine (without mention of hemorrhage) — *degenerative dilation of vasculature of intestine, without bleeding*
AHA: Q4, 1990, 4; Q4, 1990, 21; Q4, 1991, 25; Q3, 1996, 10
569.85 Angiodysplasia of intestine with hemorrhage — *degenerative dilation of vasculature of intestine, with bleeding*
AHA: Q4, 1991, 25; Q3, 1996, 9
569.86 Dieulafoy lesion (hemorrhagic) of intestine
569.89 Other specified disorder of intestines — *not otherwise specified, enteroptosis, granuloma, prolapse, acquired deformity, sacculation, Lane's, Glenard's, or Payr's disease*
AHA: Q4, 1991, 25; Q3, 1996, 9
569.9 Unspecified disorder of intestine

570–579 Other Diseases of Digestive System

570 Acute and subacute necrosis of liver
AHA: Q1, 2000, 22; Q2, 2005, 9

This valid three-digit code includes acute or subacute hepatitis, acute hepatic failure, parenchymatous degeneration, and yellow atrophy.

571 Chronic liver disease and cirrhosis

Use this rubric to report chronic liver disease and cirrhosis not due to infection. The liver is the largest gland in the body and serves many metabolic purposes including secretion of bile. Chronic alcohol use leads to three similar forms of liver disease: steatosis (fatty liver), hepatitis, and cirrhosis. The conditions have many overlapping features and each may occur without involvement of alcohol. Alcoholic cirrhosis accounts for about 60 percent of all cirrhosis cases and the risk appears to rise with the amount of alcohol consumed daily. The liver tends to shrink and become fibrotic.

Hepatitis is the inflammation of the liver, which is usually due to viral infection classified elsewhere or to toxic agents such as alcohol or drugs. Cirrhosis of the liver is a chronic, progressive disease characterized by damage to the hepatic parenchymal cells and nodular regeneration, fibrosis formation, and disturbance of the normal architecture. Two different types of cirrhosis have been described based on the amount of regenerative activity in the liver: chronic sclerosing cirrhosis in which the liver is small and hard and nodular cirrhosis in which the liver may be initially quite enlarged.

571.0 Alcoholic fatty liver
571.1 Acute alcoholic hepatitis — *severe inflammation of the liver due to alcoholic liver disease; Zieve's syndrome*
AHA: Q2, 2002, 4
571.2 Alcoholic cirrhosis of liver — *fibrosis and dysfunction of the liver due to alcoholic liver disease; Laennec's cirrhosis*
AHA: Nov-Dec, 1985, 14; Q1, 2002, 3; Q2, 2002, 4
571.3 Unspecified alcoholic liver damage
571.40 Unspecified chronic hepatitis
571.41 Chronic persistent hepatitis

571.49	Other chronic hepatitis — *not otherwise specified, Beam-Kunkel-Slater syndrome, Wadenstrom's hepatitis* **AHA:** Nov-Dec, 1985, 14; Q3, 1999, 19
571.5	Cirrhosis of liver without mention of alcohol — *fibrosis and dysfunction of the liver not due to alcohol consumption; cryptogenic, macronodular, micronodular; posthepatic, postnecrotic; Cruveilhier-Baumgarten cirrhosis*
571.6	Biliary cirrhosis — *fibrosis and dysfunction of the liver due to obstruction or infection of bile ducts; cholangitic, cholestatic*
571.8	Other chronic nonalcoholic liver disease — *not otherwise specified, fatty liver without alcohol, hardening liver, chronic yellow atrophy* **AHA:** Q2, 1996, 12
571.9	Unspecified chronic liver disease without mention of alcohol — *unknown disease of liver*

572 Liver abscess and sequelae of chronic liver disease

Hepatic coma (572.2) is characterized by slow or rapid onset of bizarre behavior, disorientation, flapping tremors of extended arms, hyperactive reflexes, and later lethargy and coma. It seems to be caused by intoxication with ammonia, a product of protein digestion that the diseased liver fails to convert into urea. Hepatic encephalopathy is a complication of advanced liver disease probably caused by cerebral toxins, including ammonia, certain amines, and fatty acids. The symptoms are similar to those of a hepatic coma.

Hepatorenal syndrome (572.4) is combined liver and kidney failure that is usually caused by serious injury to the liver associated with hemorrhage, shock, and acute renal insufficiency. Hepatic necrosis is the destruction of functional liver tissue and can lead to the clinical syndrome hepatic failure, which may be induced by hepatotoxic drugs and may lead to progressive encephalopathy and death.

572.0	Abscess of liver — *pocket of pus*
572.1	Portal pyemia — *inflammation of portal vein or its branches; phlebitis, thrombophlebitis, pylephlebitis*
572.2	Hepatic coma — *portal-systemic encephalopathy* **AHA:** Q3, 1995, 14; Q1, 2002, 3; Q2, 2005, 9
572.3	Portal hypertension — *abnormally high blood pressure in the portal vein* **AHA:** Q3, 2005, 15
572.4	Hepatorenal syndrome — *kidney failure associated with liver disease; Heyd's syndrome* **AHA:** Q3, 1993, 15
572.8	Other sequelae of chronic liver disease — *not elsewhere specified, adhesion, granuloma*

Coding Clarification
Excluded from this rubric is amebic liver abscess (006.3) and hepatorenal syndrome following delivery (674.8x).

573 Other disorders of liver
Code first underlying disease as appropriate.

573.0	Chronic passive congestion of liver — *persistent accumulation of escaped blood in liver tissue*
573.1	Hepatitis in viral diseases classified elsewhere — (Code first underlying disease: 074.8, 075, 078.5) — *secondary to underlying disease*
573.2	Hepatitis in other infectious diseases classified elsewhere — (Code first underlying disease, 084.9) — *secondary to underlying disease*
573.3	Unspecified hepatitis — (Use additional E code to identify cause)
573.4	Hepatic infarction — *area of dead liver tissue due to an interruption in circulation in that area*
573.8	Other specified disorders of liver — *hepatoptosis, hypertrophy, hemorrhage, obstruction, induration, lesion, prolapse, nontraumatic rupture*
573.9	Unspecified disorder of liver — *distention, palpable or torpid liver*

Coding Clarification
Excluded from this rubric are amyloid or lardaceous degeneration of liver (277.3), congenital cystic liver disease (751.62), glycogen infiltration of liver (271.0), hepatomegaly not otherwise specified (789.1), and portal vein obstruction (452).

574 Cholelithiasis
Use this rubric to report the presence or formation of concretions (calculi or "gallstones") in the gallbladder. The concretions contain cholesterol, calcium carbonate, or calcium bilirubinate either in pure forms or in various combinations. Many factors contribute to concretion formation, but they generally can be grouped into three categories: abnormal composition of bile, abnormal contractility of the gallbladder, and abnormal epithelial secretions. The disease is rare in children, and the rate of incidence is greater in people of native American ancestry and in women.

Choledocholithiasis is the presence or formation of concretions in any of the bile ducts. Common duct stones usually originate in the gallbladder, but may form spontaneously in the common duct following cholecystectomy. Features, in addition to those of cholecystitis, that suggest choledocholithiasis include C578.1

harcot's triad and cholangitis. Charcot's triad is a symptom complex consisting of frequently recurring attacks of severe, persistent, right upper quadrant pain lasting for hours; chills and fever associated with severe colic; and a history of jaundice chronologically associated with abdominal pain. Secondary pancreatitis, biliary cirrhosis, and hypoprothrombinemia may complicate choledocholithiasis.

Signs and symptoms of cholelithiasis include cramps or severe epigastric pain, nausea and vomiting, heartburn, eructation, flatulence, sensation of dullness in stomach, jaundice, distention of gallbladder, and pain on palpation of gallbladder. It is asymptomatic in many patients. X-rays of abdomen may show cholelithiasis, but most concretions are made up of cholesterol, which is radiolucent and cannot be visualized. Gallbladder ultrasound, HIDA scanning (a form of radionuclide excretion scan involving the intravenous injection of iminodiacetic acid), and oral cholecystography confirm the diagnosis. Lab work reveals cholesterol crystal formation in bile and granules of calcium bilirubinate in duodenal aspirate with acute cholecystitis. Lab work may reveal increased white blood cell count and serum bilirubin.

Therapies include administration of chenodeoxycholic acid for one to two years to dissolve concretions in asymptomatic patients; in asymptomatic diabetic patients, cholecystectomy is performed to avoid serious future complications. For acute cholecystitis, cholecystectomy (by open incision, laparoscopy, or endoscopically) is performed at the time of the acute cholecystitis, or electively four to six weeks after recovery in uncomplicated cases. A cholangiogram detects concretions blocking the common bile duct. If concretions are found, there is common bile duct exploration or insertion of T-tube with infusion of mono-octanoin to dissolve the stones.

Associated conditions include acute cholecystitis (including its major complications of empyema, perforations, pericholecystic abscess, bile peritonitis, and cholecystenteric fistulas), chronic cholecystitis, biliary adhesions, secondary pancreatitis, postcholecystectomy syndrome, Crohn's disease, liver damage, and obesity.

The following fifth-digit subclassification is for use with category 574:

0 without mention of obstruction

1 with obstruction

574.0 ✓5th Calculus of gallbladder with acute cholecystitis — *severe inflammation due to gallstone(s); cholelithiasis*
AHA: Q4, 1996, 32

574.1 ✓5th Calculus of gallbladder with other cholecystitis — *inflammation, persistent or unspecified, due to gallstone(s); cholelithiasis*
AHA: Q2, 1996, 13; Q4, 1996, 32,69; Q3, 1999, 9

574.2 ✓5th Calculus of gallbladder without mention of cholecystitis — *presence of gallstone(s) without inflammation*

574.3 ✓5th Calculus of bile duct with acute cholecystitis — *severe inflammation of gallbladder due to stone(s) in bile duct*

574.4 ✓5th Calculus of bile duct with other cholecystitis — *inflammation, persistent and unspecified, of gallbladder due to stone(s) in bile duct*

574.5 ✓5th Calculus of bile duct without mention of cholecystitis — *presence of bile duct stone(s) without inflammation of gallbladder*
AHA: Q3, 1994, 11

574.6 ✓5th Calculus of gallbladder and bile duct with acute cholecystitis — *presence of bile duct and gallbladder stones with severe inflammation*
AHA: Q4, 1996, 32

574.7 ✓5th Calculus of gallbladder and bile duct with other cholecystitis — *presence of bile duct and gallbladders stones, inflammation persistent and unspecified*
AHA: Q4, 1996, 32

574.8 ✓5th Calculus of gallbladder and bile duct with acute and chronic cholecystitis

574.9 ✓5th Calculus of gallbladder and bile duct without cholecystitis — *stones of gallbladder and bile duct without inflammation*
AHA: Q4, 1996, 32

575 Other disorders of gallbladder

Excluded from this rubric are cholelithiasis (rubric 574) and Hartmann's pouch of intestine (V44.3).

Acute cholecystitis is acute inflammation of the gallbladder without mention of cholelithiasis (calculi or "gallstones" of the gallbladder or bile ducts). This condition may be caused by obstruction of the cystic duct by another process (such as a malignant tumor), bile stasis ("sludge" formation, which is a precipitant of calcium bilirubinate calculi formation), or infection due to organisms such as *Escherichia coli*, *E. clostridia*, or *Salmonella typhi*.

Biliary sludge can be obstructive or non-obstructive. Assign 576.2 for bile duct obstruction due to sludge with no calculus formation. Assign 576.8 for non-obstructive biliary sludge with no calculus formation.

About 95 percent of acute cholecystitis is due to obstruction of the cystic duct by a gallstone impacted in Hartmann's pouch and classified to category 574.

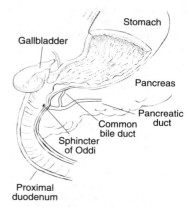

Location of the biliary tract

Use subclassification 575.1 to report cholecystitis not otherwise specified and chronic cholecystitis without mention of cholelithiasis (calculi or "gallstones" of the gallbladder or bile ducts). Chronic cholecystitis rarely occurs in the absence of lithiasis but can occur in conditions such as cholesterolosis and adenomatous hyperplasia.

575.0	Acute cholecystitis — *severe inflammation gallbladder, no stones* **AHA:** Q3, 1991, 17
575.10	Cholecystitis, unspecified — *inflammation of gallbladder of unknown type, no stones* **AHA:** Q4, 1996, 32
575.11	Chronic cholecystitis — *persistent inflammation of gallbladder, no stones* **AHA:** Q4, 1996, 32
575.12	Acute and chronic cholecystitis — *occlusion, stenosis, stricture, without stones* **AHA:** Q4, 1996, 32; Q4, 1997, 52
575.2	Obstruction of gallbladder — *occlusion, stenosis, and stricture of cystic duct or gallbladder without mention of calculus*
575.3	Hydrops of gallbladder — *abnormal collection of fluid, gallbladder* **AHA:** Q2, 1989, 13
575.4	Perforation of gallbladder — *hole in gallbladder wall*
575.5	Fistula of gallbladder — *abnormal communication between gallbladder and other tissue*
575.6	Cholesterolosis of gallbladder — *abnormal deposits of cholesterol in tissue of gallbladder* **AHA:** Q4, 1990, 17
575.8	Other specified disorder of gallbladder — *adhesions, atrophy, cyst, hypertrophy, ulcer, calcification, infarct, sepsis, torsion, Hartmann's pouch, Rokitansky-Aschoff sinuses* **AHA:** Q2, 1989, 13; Q4, 1990, 26
575.9	Unspecified disorder of gallbladder — *pain in gallbladder for unknown cause*

576 Other disorders of biliary tract

576.0	Postcholecystectomy syndrome — *jaundice or abnormal pain following cholecystectomy* **AHA:** Q1, 1988, 10
576.1	Cholangitis — *inflammation of bile duct; recurrent, secondary, chronic, primary, acute, suppurative, sclerosing* **AHA:** Q2, 1999, 13
576.2	Obstruction of bile duct — *occlusion, stenosis, stricture; Mirizzi's syndrome* **AHA:** Q2, 1999, 13; Q1, 2001, 8; Q3, 2003, 17-18
576.3	Perforation of bile duct — *hole in the wall of bile duct*
576.4	Fistula of bile duct — *abnormal communication between bile duct and other tissue*
576.5	Spasm of sphincter of Oddi — *abnormal contraction in muscle of the threshold between bile duct and duodenum*
576.8	Other specified disorders of biliary tract — *adhesions, atrophy, cyst, hypertrophy, stasis, ulcer, cicatrix, obliteration, torsion of bile duct; abscess or inflammation of hepatic duct* **AHA:** Q2, 1999, 14; Q3, 2003, 17
576.9	Unspecified disorder of biliary tract

Coding Clarification
Excluded from this rubric are disorders of the biliary tract involving the cystic duct or gallbladder (575.0-575.9).

577 Diseases of pancreas
Signs and symptoms of diseases of the pancreas include abdominal pain, weakness, dizziness, somnolence, grossly bloody or "coffee ground" vomitus, grossly bloody or black and tarry stools, and a history of bleeding diathesis. Other signs and symptoms include chronic conditions such as

Diseases of the Digestive System

diverticulosis, fall in blood pressure of more than 10 mm Hg or rise in pulse rate of more than 20 beats per minute between supine and standing positions, altered level of consciousness, pallor, diaphoresis, and peripheral vasoconstriction.

577.0	Acute pancreatitis — *severe inflammation; necrotic, acute, hemorrhagic, subacute, suppurative, infective; including Fitz's syndrome* **AHA:** Q2, 1989, 9; Q2, 1996, 13; Q2, 1998, 19; Q3, 1999, 9
577.1	Chronic pancreatitis — *persistent inflammation; infectious, interstitial, painless, recurrent, relapsing* **AHA:** Q3, 1994, 11; Q2, 1996, 13; Q1, 2001, 8
577.2	Cyst and pseudocyst of pancreas
577.8	Other specified disease of pancreas — *atrophy, calculus, cirrhosis, fibrosis, necrosis, fistula, hyperfunction, insufficiency, sclerosis, nontraumatic rupture, duct obstruction; Hadfield-Clarke or Burke's syndrome* **AHA:** Q1, 2001, 8
577.9	Unspecified disease of pancreas

Coding Clarification
Excluded from this rubric are mumps pancreatitis (072.3), islet cell tumor of pancreas (211.7), and pancreatic steatorrhea (579.4).

578 Gastrointestinal hemorrhage
AHA: Q4, 1990, 20; Q2, 1992, 9

Use this rubric to report bleeding of the stomach, ileum, jejunum, duodenum, and/or colon. The condition may be described as acute or chronic and involve a grossly bloody (visible) appearance or be detected by laboratory examination only (occult bleeding). GI bleeding is classified as either hematemesis (vomiting of blood), blood in stool which includes melena (partially digested blood showing as dark tarry stools) and hematochezia (passage of red blood in stools), and GI bleeding not specified as hematemesis or blood in stool.

Diagnostic tests may include a CBC to reveal normal hematocrit and hemoglobin for the first six hours of acute bleeding (the body can compensate for acute blood loss by vasoconstriction, delaying the intravascular fluids from entering the bloodstream). A peripheral blood smear in an acute hemorrhage longer than six hours often demonstrates normochromic and normocytic blood loss anemia. In chronic GI hemorrhage (acute exacerbation of chronic GI hemorrhage), a peripheral blood smear is characteristic of chronic blood loss showing microcytic, hypochromic anemia with marked increase in reticulocyte count. Abnormal BUN and creatinine levels suggest bleeding in the upper GI tract, and elevated liver enzymes indicate hypoperfusion of the liver following a bleeding episode. Nasogastric aspiration may be performed to confirm an upper GI bleed and an upper or lower endoscopy identifies the exact site and pathology of the bleeding. Upper GI series or barium enema locates the site when bleeding is inactive at the time of the test and a nuclear bleeding scan, such as technetium-labeled red cell scan and technetium sulfur-colloid scan, locates the site in the lower GI tract when bleeding is minimal. An angiography may be performed for both upper and lower GI bleeding and is often performed in anticipation of surgery.

Therapies include gastric lavage for upper GI bleeding confined to the stomach and medical management for lower GI bleeding unless the bleeding becomes life threatening. Therapeutic angiography using selective intra-arterial vasopressin or selective embolization of a bleeding vessel to control GI hemorrhage is also used. Use of an endoscopic laser or a heat probe induces coagulation, while surgery is directed at the etiology when bleeding is severe (e.g., gastrectomy and Billroth I reconstruction for GI bleeding due to perforated gastric ulcer or hemicolectomy for extensive diverticulosis of the colon).

Associated conditions include acute and/or chronic blood loss anemia, dehydration, gastritis, diverticulitis, neoplasms, arteriovenous malformations, chronic renal failure, diabetes mellitus, chronic obstructive lung disease, colitis, bleeding diathesis, chronic liver disease, Osler-Weber-Rendu syndrome, and valvular heart disease.

This category excludes bleeding of the anus and rectum for classification purposes. The terms "upper" and "lower" have no value as modifiers for classification of GI bleeding. GI bleeding must be assigned to code 578.9 *Hemorrhage of gastrointestinal tract, unspecified* when not further defined as hematemesis or blood in stool. Since upper GI bleeding may present not only as hematemesis but also as melena and even hematochezia in some cases, the codes are distinguished by the presentation of the GI bleeding, not the site.

Use subclassification 578.0 to report vomiting of frank red or partially digested blood. Hematemesis usually is indicative of bleeding of the upper gastrointestinal tract. Occult bleeding can be detected by analysis of vomitus or nasogastric tube aspiration. Gastric and gastroduodenal ulcers, gastritis, arteriovenous malformations, and neoplasms are the most common etiologies for hematemesis.

Certain conditions such as epistaxis may cause the patient to swallow and then vomit blood. Such vomiting of swallowed blood sometimes masquerades as hematemesis due to gastrointestinal hemorrhage.

Use subclassification 578.1 to report passage of frank red or partially digested blood in the stools which may be due to a condition in the upper or lower GI tract.

The general term "rectal bleeding" is used by clinicians to describe GI hemorrhage (classified here) or bleeding from sites within the rectum or anus classified to code 569.3. If the etiology of the rectal bleeding is a condition of the gastrointestinal tract excluding the anus and rectum, assign this code. Occult bleeding may be detected by performing a guaiac test on a stool sample. A positive guaiac test without further documentation of GI bleeding is classified to code 792.1 *Nonspecific abnormal findings in stool contents*.

578.0	Hematemesis — *vomiting blood* AHA: Q4, 1990, 20; Q2, 1992, 9; Q2, 2002, 4
578.1	Blood in stool — *melena* AHA: Q4, 1990, 20; Q2, 1992, 8; Q2, 1992, 9; Q2, 2006, 17
578.9	Unspecified, hemorrhage of gastrointestinal tract — *not otherwise specified* AHA: Nov-Dec, 1986, 9; Q4, 1990, 20; Q2, 1992, 9; Q3, 2005, 17

Coding Clarification
Excluded from this rubric are gastrointestinal hemorrhage with angiodysplasia of stomach and duodenum (537.83), angiodysplasia of intestine (537.85), diverticulitis and diverticulosis (rubric 562), gastritis and duodenitis (535.0-535.6), and duodenal, gastric, gastrojejunal, or peptic ulcer (531.00-534.91).

579 Intestinal malabsorption

The mucosal layer of the intestine is crucial for the body to prevent bacteria, antigens, and undigested food from seeping through the gastrointestinal barrier and into the systemic circulation. Intestinal malabsorption (e.g., the inadequate absorption of nutrients from the small intestine) of the mucosal layer can result in weight loss and abnormal appearing stools. An increasingly permeable mucosal layer can result in a chronically overreactive immune system that can lead to inflammatory bowel disease (IBD) and its progression. Factors affecting permeability include lesions of the small intestine, amyloidosis, the lack of digestive enzymes (e.g., lactose intolerance), and surgical operations. Blockage of the intestinal lymphatic vessels, which are important in fat absorption, also may lead to malabsorption. A comprehensive digestive stool analysis can be performed in the diagnosis of malabsorption since the test evaluates a stool sample for digestion, absorption, intestinal function, and microbial flora. A small intestine biopsy is necessary for the diagnosis of many diseases of the intestinal mucosa such as celiac sprue, abetalipoproteinemia, and Whipple's disease. Certain diseases such as Crohn's have a patchy distribution and may yield a normal biopsy if normal mucosa is sampled.

Celiac disease (also called coeliac, nontropical sprue, celiac sprue, gluten intolerant enteropathy, or gluten sensitive enteropathy) is a condition in which there is a chronic reaction to certain proteins, commonly referred to as glutens, found in some cereal grains. This reaction destroys the villi in the small intestine, with resulting malabsorption of nutrients.

The disease affects both sexes and it can begin at any age, from infancy (as soon as cereal grains are introduced) to later life (even though the individual has consumed cereal grains all along). The onset of the disease seems to require genetic predisposition and some kind of trigger, such as overexposure to wheat, a pregnancy, an operation, or a viral infection.

579.0	Celiac disease — *crisis, rickets, gluten enteropathy, nontropical spur*
579.1	Tropical sprue — *diarrhea associated with enteric infection and nutritional deficiency*
579.2	Blind loop syndrome
579.3	Other and unspecified postsurgical nonabsorption
579.4	Pancreatic steatorrhea — *passage of large amounts of fat in the feces due to absence of pancreatic juice from intestine*
579.8	Other specified intestinal malabsorption
579.9	Unspecified intestinal malabsorption AHA: Q4, 2004, 59

580–629
Diseases of the Genitourinary System

This chapter classifies diseases and disorders of the kidney, ureter, bladder, urethra, prostate, male genital organs, female and male breast, and female genital organs.

Coding Clarification
Excluded from this chapter is hypertensive renal disease, found in rubric 403. Signs and symptoms of genitourinary system disorders that may describe the emerging nature of the patient's condition are found in rubric 788, which includes codes specific to incontinence of urine, painful or frequent urination, and kidney pain. Also, some genitourinary diseases are familial linked. Family history can be found in rubrics V16-V19.

580–589 Nephritis, Nephrotic Syndrome, and Nephrosis

The kidneys are behind the parietal peritoneum at the back of the abdominal cavity. They are located on either side of the vertebral column from the level of the 12th thoracic vertebra to the 3rd lumbar vertebra. The left kidney is often slightly larger than the right, and usually slightly higher in position, presumably because of the space taken by the liver. The kidneys are encased in heavy cushions of fat, which, with the renal fasciae connective tissue, anchors them in place. The average kidney is about 11.0 centimeters by 7.0 centimeters by 3.0 centimeters and roughly oval with a medial indentation (bean-shaped). The concave notch at this indentation is called the hilum, and is where structures enter and leave the kidney. Tough, white, fibrous connective tissue encapsulates each kidney.

The outer region of the kidney is the cortex. The medulla is the inner region, consisting of about a dozen distinct triangular wedges of tissue called the renal pyramids. The papilla (points) of the pyramids face inward and jut into cuplike structures, called calyces, where urine is collected for transport via the renal pelvis out of the kidney and into the ureter. The functional units of the kidney are the nephrons. Nephrons are microscopic units that process blood and form urine by filtration, reabsorption, and secretion. There are more than one million nephrons in each kidney, which make up the bulk of the organ's tissue.

580 Acute glomerulonephritis

Acute glomerulonephritis is acute inflammation in the glomeruli of the kidneys. Also known as acute hemorrhagic glomerulonephritis and acute nephritis, this condition frequently is a late complication of pharyngitis or skin infection.

Signs and symptoms of acute glomerulonephritis include a history of infection usually streptococcal, a history of concurrent systemic vasculitis or hypersensitivity reaction, malaise, headache, anorexia, low-grade fever, mild generalized edema, and retinal hemorrhages.

In acute glomerulonephritis, urinalysis reveals hematuria (may be microscopic or grossly bloody or coffee colored) and urine sediment containing protein, hyaline and granular casts in large numbers, and erythrocyte casts. Blood work reveals elevated BUN and creatinine, rapid sedimentation rate, and mild normochromic anemia. Therapies include antibiotics to eradicate the underlying infection (e.g., streptococcal pharyngitis), symptomatic treatment to prevent overhydration and hypertension, and dietary restriction of protein and sodium. Associated conditions include hypertension, hypertensive encephalopathy, congestive heart failure, infection (e.g., streptococcal pharyngitis, skin cellulitis), and retinal hemorrhage.

When acute glomerulonephritis does not heal within one to two years, or when it progresses to chronic renal failure or chronic renal insufficiency, it is designated as chronic glomerulonephritis.

Acute glomerulonephritis with lesion of proliferative glomerulonephritis is characterized by hypercellularity of the glomeruli. The condition is due to proliferation of endothelial and/or mesangial cells and infiltration of the tissues with neutrophils and monocytes.

Acute glomerulonephritis with lesion of rapidly progressive glomerulonephritis is acute glomerulonephritis with lesion characterized by rapid deterioration of kidney function, usually a few weeks to two months. Most patients who survive this condition, which is also known as acute crescentic glomerulonephritis, develop chronic renal failure within two years.

580.0	Acute glomerulonephritis with lesion of proliferative glomerulonephritis — *acute nephritis*
580.4	Acute glomerulonephritis with lesion of rapidly progressive glomerulonephritis — *acute nephritis with lesion of necrotizing glomerulitis*
580.81	Acute glomerulonephritis with other specified pathological lesion in kidney in disease classified elsewhere — (Code first underlying disease: 002.0, 070.0-070.9, 072.79, 421.0)
580.89	Other acute glomerulonephritis with other specified pathological lesion in kidney — *acute glomerulonephritis with lesion of exudative nephritis*
580.9	Acute glomerulonephritis with unspecified pathological lesion in kidney — *hemorrhagic glomerulonephritis specified as acute*

Coding Clarification
It is rare that a patient would be assigned codes from both categories 580 and 582 during the same episode of care. Acute exacerbation of chronic glomerulonephritis is classified to chronic glomerulonephritis (582) alone when the exacerbation refers to a progressive deterioration or worsening of symptoms of chronic glomerulonephritis. When the cause of the exacerbation is known, such as an intercurrent infection (e.g., streptococcal septicemia, 038.0), report the infection along with a code from category 582.

581 Nephrotic syndrome
Nephrotic syndrome is a condition characterized by proteinuria more than 3.5 g/100 ml, hypoalbuminemia less than 3 g/100 ml, hyperlipemia (cholesterol greater than 300 mg/100 ml), and massive edema. Usually due to some form of glomerulonephritis, nephrotic syndrome may result in chronic renal failure.

Nephrotic syndrome with lesion of proliferative glomerulonephritis is nephrotic syndrome with lesion characterized by hypercellularity of the glomeruli. The condition is due to proliferating endothelial and/or mesangial cells, and infiltration of the tissues with neutrophils and monocytes as a result of acute or membranoproliferative glomerulonephritis.

Nephrotic syndrome with lesion of membranous glomerulonephritis is nephrotic syndrome with lesion characterized by insidious onset of proteinuria. It is the result of protein deposits and diffuse thickening of the capillary basement membrane of the glomeruli.

Nephrotic syndrome with lesion of membranoproliferative glomerulonephritis is nephrotic syndrome with lesion characterized by infiltration of inflammatory cells, proliferating intrinsic glomerular cells, and altered structure and function of the basement membrane of the glomeruli.

581.0	Nephrotic syndrome with lesion of proliferative glomerulonephritis
581.1	Nephrotic syndrome with lesion of membranous glomerulonephritis — *epimembranous nephritis; idiopathic membranous glomerular disease*
581.2	Nephrotic syndrome with lesion of membranoproliferative glomerulonephritis — *nephrotic syndrome with lesion of lobular glomerulonephritis; nephrotic syndrome with lesion of mesangiocapillary glomerulonephritis*
581.3	Nephrotic syndrome with lesion of minimal change glomerulonephritis — *foot process disease; lipoid necrosis; minimal change nephrotic syndrome*
581.81	Nephrotic syndrome with other specified pathological lesion in kidney in diseases classified elsewhere — (Code first underlying disease: 084.9, 250.4, 277.3, 446.0, 710.0)
581.89	Other nephrotic syndrome with specified pathological lesion in kidney — *glomerulonephritis with edema and lesion of exudative nephritis*
581.9	Nephrotic syndrome with unspecified pathological lesion in kidney — *nephritis, nephrotic NOS; nephritis with edema NOS*

582 Chronic glomerulonephritis
Chronic glomerulonephritis is a slowly progressing disease (up to 30 years in some cases) characterized by chronic inflammation of the glomeruli, which results in sclerosis, scarring, and eventual chronic renal failure. Etiologies for chronic glomerulonephritis include primary renal disorders (classified to categories 580 and 581) and systemic diseases such as Goodpasture's syndrome, systemic

lupus erythematosus, amyloidosis, and hemolytic-uremic syndrome.

Signs and symptoms of chronic glomerulonephritis include azotemia, nausea, vomiting, fatigue, malaise, pruritus, dyspnea, hematuria, and hypertension. An urinalysis reveals hematuria (may be microscopic or grossly bloody or coffee colored) and urine sediment containing protein, cylindruria (granular tube casts), and erythrocyte casts. Blood work reveals elevated BUN and creatinine, rapid sedimentation rate, and mild normochromic anemia. X-ray or renal ultrasound shows bilateral smaller kidneys and a renal biopsy identifies the underlying disease.

Therapies include antibiotics to treat any intercurrent infections, drugs such as diuretics to control hypertension, IV hydration, and fluid restriction or diuresis to correct fluid and electrolyte imbalances. There are dietary restrictions of sodium and protein and renal dialysis or renal transplant for patients with ESRD (end stage renal disease or chronic renal failure).

Associated conditions include congestive heart failure, and fluid, electrolyte, and acid-base imbalances. There may be hypertension, hypertensive encephalopathy, intercurrent infection, and underlying disease (e.g., systemic lupus erythematosus).

Chronic glomerulonephritis with lesion of proliferative glomerulonephritis is chronic glomerulonephritis with lesion characterized by hypercellularity of the glomeruli due to proliferation of endothelial and/or mesangial cells and infiltration of the tissues with neutrophils and monocytes as a result of repeated attacks of acute inflammation.

Chronic glomerulonephritis with lesion of membranous glomerulonephritis is chronic glomerulonephritis with lesion characterized by the insidious onset of proteinuria. It is the result of protein deposits and diffuse thickening of the capillary basement membrane of the glomeruli.

Chronic glomerulonephritis with lesion of membranoproliferative glomerulonephritis is chronic glomerulonephritis with lesion characterized by infiltration of inflammatory cells, proliferation of intrinsic glomerular cells, and altered structure and function of the basement membrane of the glomeruli.

Chronic glomerulonephritis with lesion of rapidly progressive glomerulonephritis is chronic glomerulonephritis with lesion characterized by rapid deterioration of kidney function, usually a few weeks to two months. Most patients with this condition, also known as chronic crescentic glomerulonephritis, develop chronic renal failure within one to two years.

582.0	Chronic glomerulonephritis with lesion of proliferative glomerulonephritis — chronic (diffuse) proliferative glomerulonephritis
582.1	Chronic glomerulonephritis with lesion of membranous glomerulonephritis — focal glomerulonephritis; segmental hyalinosis AHA: Sept-Oct, 1984, 16
582.2	Chronic glomerulonephritis with lesion of membranoproliferative glomerulonephritis — chronic endothelial glomerulonephritis; chronic mesangiocapillary glomerulonephritis
582.4	Chronic glomerulonephritis with lesion of rapidly progressive glomerulonephritis — chronic nephritis with lesion of necrotizing glomerulitis
582.81	Chronic glomerulonephritis with other specified pathological lesion in kidney in diseases classified elsewhere
582.89	Other chronic glomerulonephritis with specified pathological lesion in kidney — chronic glomerulonephritis with lesion of exudative nephritis
582.9	Chronic glomerulonephritis with unspecified pathological lesion in kidney — chronic hemorrhagic glomerulonephritis; small white kidney AHA: Q2, 2001, 12

Coding Clarification
Refer to the ICD-9-CM index under "Glomerulonephritis, due to or associated with" for a list of underlying (etiologic) conditions that can cause glomerulonephritis. The index refers you to codes in categories 580-583 in slanted brackets, indicating a manifestation code. Modify these suggested manifestation codes according to the amount of specificity in the physician's diagnostic statement. For example, for glomerulonephritis due to or associated with tuberculosis, the ICD-9-CM index lists codes 016.0x to classify the underlying disease of tuberculosis (add the appropriate fifth digit) and 583.81 for the manifestation of glomerulonephritis not specified as acute or chronic in diseases classified elsewhere. If the diagnostic statement specifies that the patient has chronic glomerulonephritis due to tuberculosis, the proper codes would be 016.0x and 582.81 for chronic glomerulonephritis in diseases classified elsewhere.

583 Nephritis and nephropathy, not specified as acute or chronic

Nephritis and nephropathy, not specific as acute or chronic, with lesion of proliferative glomerulonephritis are diseases with lesion characterized by hypercellularity of the glomeruli due to proliferating endothelial and/or mesangial cells, and infiltration of the tissues with neutrophils and monocytes as a result of acute inflammation.

Nephritis and nephropathy, not specified as acute or chronic, with lesion of membranous glomerulonephritis are diseases with lesion characterized by the insidious onset of proteinuria and unspecified nephritis or nephropathy. They are the result of protein deposits and diffuse thickening of the capillary basement membrane of the glomeruli.

Nephritis and nephropathy, not specified as acute or chronic, with lesion of membranoproliferative glomerulonephritis are diseases with lesion characterized by infiltration of inflammatory cells, proliferation of intrinsic glomerular cells, and alteration of the structure and function of the basement membrane of the glomeruli.

Nephritis and nephropathy, not specified as acute or chronic, with lesion of rapidly progressive glomerulonephritis are severe forms of glomerulonephritis with lesion characterized by rapid deterioration of kidney function, usually a few weeks to two months. Most patients with these diseases, also known as crescentic glomerulonephritis, develop chronic renal failure within one to two years.

583.0	Nephritis and nephropathy, not specified as acute or chronic, with lesion of proliferative glomerulonephritis — *proliferative nephritis NOS; proliferative nephropathy NOS*
583.1	Nephritis and nephropathy, not specified as acute or chronic, with lesion of membranous glomerulonephritis — *membranous glomerulonephritis NOS; membranous nephropathy NOS*
583.2	Nephritis and nephropathy, not specified as acute or chronic, with lesion of membranoproliferative glomerulonephritis — *membranoproliferative nephropathy NOS; nephritis NOS, with lesion of hypocomplementemic, lobular, or mesangiocapillary glomerulonephritis*
583.4	Nephritis and nephropathy, not specified as acute or chronic, with lesion of rapidly progressive glomerulonephritis — *necrotizing or rapidly progressive nephritis NOS; nephritis, unspecified, with lesion of necrotizing glomerulitis*
583.6	Nephritis and nephropathy, not specified as acute or chronic, with lesion of renal cortical necrosis — *nephritis NOS; renal cortical necrosis NOS*
583.7	Nephritis and nephropathy, not specified as acute or chronic, with lesion of renal medullary necrosis — *nephritis NOS with (renal) medullary [papillary] necrosis*
583.81	Nephritis and nephropathy, not specified as acute or chronic, with other specified pathological lesion in kidney, in diseases classified elsewhere
583.89	Other nephritis and nephropathy, not specified as acute or chronic, with specified pathological lesion in kidney — *glomerulitis with lesion of exudative nephritis; renal disease with lesion of interstitial nephritis*
583.9	Nephritis and nephropathy, not specified as acute or chronic, with unspecified pathological lesion in kidney — *glomerulitis NOS; nephritis NOS*

Coding Clarification
Refer to the ICD-9-CM index under "Glomerulonephritis, due to or associated with" for a list of underlying (etiologic) conditions that can cause glomerulonephritis. Note that the index will refer you to codes in categories 580-583 in slanted brackets, indicating a manifestation code. Modify these suggested manifestation codes according to the amount of specificity in the physician's diagnostic statement. For example, for glomerulonephritis due to or associated with tuberculosis, the ICD-9-CM index lists codes 016.0x to classify the underlying disease of tuberculosis (add the appropriate fifth digit) and 583.81 for the manifestation of glomerulonephritis not specified as acute or chronic in diseases classified elsewhere. If the diagnostic statement specifies that the patient has chronic glomerulonephritis due to tuberculosis, the proper codes would be 016.0x and 582.81 for chronic glomerulonephritis in diseases classified elsewhere.

Coding Scenario
The patient is admitted for hemodialysis. The patient is a Type I diabetic with progressive nephropathy. The physician also documents chronic renal failure in the medical history.

> Code assignment: 250.41 *Diabetes with renal manifestations*, 583.81 *Nephritis and nephropathy, not specified as acute or chronic, in diseases classified elsewhere*, and 585.9 *Chronic kidney disease, unspecified*

584 Acute renal failure
AHA: Q2, 1992, 5; Q4, 1992, 22; Q1, 1993, 18

Acute renal failure is sudden interruption of renal function following any one of a variety of conditions that insult the normal kidney. Although usually reversible with treatment, acute renal failure may progress to chronic renal insufficiency and chronic renal failure or death. Recovery from acute renal failure is marked by a conversion from an oliguric phase to a diuretic phase within a few days to six weeks.

The causes of acute renal failure are classified to prerenal, intrinsic (renal), or postrenal. Prerenal failure is due to diminished blood flow to the kidneys caused by conditions such as dehydration, shock, embolism, cardiac failure, hepatic failure, or sepsis. Intrinsic failure results from diseases and disorders of the kidneys. Acute tubular necrosis is the most common cause of renal failure, and results from conditions such as systemic lupus erythematosus, sickle cell disease, nephrotoxins, renal ischemia, acute pyelonephritis, and acute poststreptococcal glomerulonephritis. Postrenal failure is caused by bilateral obstruction of urinary outflow, as seen with ureteral calculi, blood clots, neoplasms, benign prostatic hypertrophy, and urethral strictures.

Signs and symptoms of acute renal failure include, in early stages, oliguria, sometimes anuria, azotemia, hypotension, electrolyte imbalances, fever and chills (indicating infection), anorexia, nausea, vomiting, diarrhea or constipation, uremic breath, headache, mental changes, pruritus, pallor, purpura, fluid overload, edema, and Kussmaul respirations. Blood work shows elevated BUN, serum creatinine, and potassium, decreased serum calcium, arterial pH, and bicarbonate. Urinalysis reveals urine specific gravity of approximately 1.010 (indicating isosthenuria) and sometimes protein and cellular debris. Radiology studies such as kidney ultrasound, intravenous pyelography, retrograde pyelography, and nephrotomography identify the pathology such as outflow obstruction or hydronephrosis. Therapies include dietary management and restriction of fluid intake with careful monitoring of electrolytes, and peritoneal dialysis or hemodialysis to control uremia.

584.5	Acute renal failure with lesion of tubular necrosis — *sudden onset of renal failure, compared to chronic, due to lower nephron necrosis; acute tubular necrosis* AHA: Q2, 1992, 5; Q4, 1992, 22; Q1, 1993, 18
584.6	Acute renal failure with lesion of renal cortical necrosis — *severe decline in kidney function due to destruction of kidney filtering tissue, sudden onset* AHA: Q2, 1992, 5; Q4, 1992, 22; Q1, 1993, 18
584.7	Acute renal failure with lesion of renal medullary (papillary) necrosis — *necrotizing renal papillitis* AHA: Q2, 1992, 5; Q4, 1992, 22; Q1, 1993, 18
584.8	Acute renal failure with other specified pathological lesion in kidney — *acute renal failure with pathological lesion in kidney NEC* AHA: Nov-Dec, 1985, 1; Q2, 1992, 5; Q4, 1992, 22; Q1, 1993, 18
584.9	Unspecified acute renal failure AHA: Q2, 2005, 18

Documentation Issues

Documentation in the record that may indicate the presence of renal failure could include:

- Markedly elevated values of serum creatinine or BUN, or diminished creatinine clearance.
- Clinical manifestations and laboratory findings of the degree of renal impairment primarily noted as the renal failure progresses. For example:
  - acidemia
  - anemia
  - hyperkalemia
  - hyperphosphatemia
  - hypocalcemia
  - renal osteodystrophy
  - uremic symptoms, (e.g., nausea, hemorrhagic conditions, vomiting, itching)

The above may be indicators of renal failure but confirmation and documentation from the physician must be obtained before assigning a code for renal failure from the chronic kidney disease category, 585, acute renal failure category, 584, or unspecified renal failure category, 586.

If documentation identifies kidney disease with hypertension, clarify with the physician as to whether the hypertension is malignant or accelerated. If the documentation identifies that the kidney disease and hypertension are unrelated or the cause and effect relationship cannot be established, code each separately.

When the documentation identifies kidney disease and diabetes but does not identify a cause and effect relationship, contact the physician for clarification. If the physician confirms that the kidney disease is a manifestation of the diabetes, list the diabetes code first followed by the code identifying the specific type of kidney disease.

If the diagnostic statement identifies hypertension, chronic renal failure, and diabetes, verify the cause and effect relationship of the chronic kidney disease with the physician. If the chronic kidney disease is due to the diabetes, use 250.4x and the appropriate code from category 585 as a secondary manifestation code; then code also the specific type of hypertension. However, if the physician confirms that this is hypertensive kidney disease (includes renal failure) due to diabetes, report 250.4x and a code from category 403, with a fifth digit of "1," to identify the chronic kidney disease and an additional code from 585.1-585.6 to identify the stage of the kidney disease.

When the physician documents azotemia, clarify whether or not the diagnosis of azotemia refers to the presence of acute renal failure or chronic renal failure. Unless acute or chronic renal failure is confirmed and documented by the physician, azotemia is reported with code 790.6 *Other abnormal blood chemistry.*

Coding Clarification
Excluded from this rubric are acute renal failure following labor and delivery (669.3x), posttraumatic (958.5), that complicating abortion (rubrics 634-638), or ectopic/molar pregnancy (639.3).

Acute renal failure secondary to systemic lupus erythematosus (SLE) nephritis is coded in accordance with instructional notes; first to SLE, followed by a code for the nephritis in diseases classified elsewhere with an additional code assignment for the acute renal failure.

Diabetes Mellitus: Diabetes is one of a number of the ICD-9-CM classification categories that is used as a primary code to classify both the disease and its major manifestations. Additional codes should be used to provide more specificity in defining the manifestations. When a cause and effect relationship between the renal failure and the diabetes has been established, the diabetes code 250.4x is listed first with the appropriate renal failure code listed as an additional code. Accordingly, if the diagnosis does not indicate a cause and effect relationship between the diabetes and renal failure, the code for the renal failure may be listed first.

General Guidelines: Renal failure (category 584 *Acute renal failure,* 585 *Chronic kidney disease,* and 586 *Renal failure, unspecified*) is the progression of renal insufficiency to the point at which renal function becomes further impaired and apparent clinical manifestations, such as anemia, develop. Renal insufficiency is more an abnormal laboratory assessment, while renal failure includes both the abnormal laboratory and the clinical findings.

Chronic kidney disease is caused by a number of progressive diseases such as diabetes, primary hypertension, nephrosis, nephritis, obstructive uropathy, systemic lupus erythematosus (SLE), polycystic kidney disease, and other congenital disorders. In cases of chronic renal failure that becomes irreversible, the treatment may be either dialysis or transplantation.

It is possible for acute renal failure to be only temporary; the patient's renal function may be regained after interventions such as dialysis.

Hypertensive Heart and Chronic Kidney Disease: Category 404 identifies hypertensive heart and chronic kidney disease. The fifth-digit subclassification denotes the presence or absence of heart failure and the stage of chronic kidney disease. An additional code from category 585 should be assigned to further identify the stage of chronic kidney disease. An additional code should also be assigned from range 428.0-428.43 to identify the type of heart failure, if known.

In many cases, renal failure is only seen in hypertensive heart and chronic kidney disease when the hypertension becomes malignant or accelerated. In these cases, 404.00 *Hypertensive heart and chronic kidney disease, malignant, without heart failure and with chronic kidney disease stage I through stage IV or unspecified* would be assigned together with 585.9 identifying the chronic renal failure as unspecified. Keep in mind that the code for malignant or accelerated hypertension can only be assigned if the physician documents it as such. Category 404 excludes acute renal failure, which is coded to category 584 *Acute renal failure.*

Hypertensive Chronic Kidney Disease: Category 403 identifies hypertensive chronic kidney disease. The stage of chronic kidney disease is identified with a fifth digit of 0 (stage I through stage IV, or unspecified), or 1 (stage V or end stage renal disease). An additional code should be assigned from category 585 to further denote the stage of chronic kidney disease.

In many cases, renal failure is seen in hypertensive kidney disease only when the hypertension becomes malignant or accelerated. In these cases, code 403.00 *Hypertensive chronic kidney disease, malignant, with chronic kidney disease stage I through stage IV or unspecified* would be assigned together with 585.9 identifying the chronic renal failure as unspecified. Keep in mind that the code for malignant or accelerated hypertension can be assigned only if the physician documents it as such.

Category 403 excludes acute renal failure, which is coded to category 584 *Acute renal failure.*

Tumor Lysis Syndrome: This condition occurs as a result of massive doses of chemotherapy in the bloodstream. Two codes are required to report it accurately: 584.8 *Acute renal failure with other specified pathological lesion in kidney* and E933.1 *Adverse effect in therapeutic use, antineoplastic and immunosuppressive drugs*, or a code that would identify the specific drug used in therapy.

Coding Scenario
A patient is admitted and treated for acute renal failure and essential hypertension.

> Code assignment: 584.9 *Acute renal failure, unspecified* and 401.9 *Essential hypertension, unspecified*

A patient is seen for acute renal failure that has an established hypertensive renal nephrosclerosis.

> Code assignment: 584.9 *Acute renal failure, unspecified* and 403.90 *Hypertensive chronic kidney disease, unspecified, with chronic kidney disease stage I through stage IV, or unspecified*

585 Chronic kidney disease (CKD)

AHA: Sept-Oct, 1984, 3; Nov-Dec, 1985, 15; Q4, 1989, 1; Q3, 1991, 8; Q1, 1993, 18; Q3, 1996, 9; Q2, 1998, 20; Q3, 1998, 6,7; Q4, 1998, 55; Q1, 2001, 3; Q2, 2001, 12,13; Q2, 2003, 7; Q4, 2003, 61, 111; Q1, 2004, 5; Q4, 2005, 68, 77

Chronic kidney disease is a multisystem disease due to a progressive loss of renal function. It usually develops gradually as a consequence of a wide spectrum of diseases such as primary and secondary glomerular disease, diabetes mellitus, and hereditary renal disease such as polycystic kidneys, hypertension, obstructive uropathy, chronic infection, and interstitial nephritis.

Signs and symptoms of chronic kidney disease include weakness, fatigue, peripheral edema, headaches, pallor, thirst, anorexia, weight loss, nausea, vomiting, pruritus, polyuria (early stages), oliguria (late stages), nocturia, mental changes, and may remain asymptomatic until more than 75 percent of renal function is lost. Blood work shows elevated BUN, serum creatinine, and potassium; decreased serum calcium, arterial pH, and bicarbonate; and normochromic, normocytic anemia. An urinalysis reveals urine specific gravity of approximately 1.010 (indicating isosthenuria) and sometimes protein, glucose, WBCs, RBCs, waxy and granular casts. A chest x-ray may show cardiac enlargement, interstitial edema, lung edema, and frank pulmonary congestion. Other radiology, such as x-rays of the kidney-ureter-bladder, intravenous pyelography, renal arteriography, and renal scans such as selected radionuclide studies and ultrasound may aid in diagnosis and treatment. Kidney biopsy and histological examination identify underlying pathology.

Therapies include dietary management such as protein restriction, iron and/or folate supplements, and restriction of fluid intake with careful monitoring of urine volume and electrolytes. Other therapies include transfusion of blood or blood products to treat anemia, peritoneal dialysis or hemodialysis to control uremia in patients with ESRD, and renal transplant for patients with ESRD.

Associated conditions include normochromic, normocytic anemia, electrolyte imbalances, underlying disease (e.g., diabetes mellitus, hypertension), cardiovascular complications (congestive heart failure, dysrhythmias, uremic pericarditis, pericardial effusion), respiratory complications (Kussmaul respirations due to acidosis, uremic pleuritis, uremic pneumonitis, pleural effusion), renal osteodystrophy (bone disease), and gastrointestinal complications (gastritis, pancreatitis, duodenal ulcer, uremic colitis).

Documentation Issues
When the loss of renal function is incomplete, the term "chronic renal insufficiency" is often used. When the loss of renal function is complete, the term "end-stage renal disease" or "chronic uremia" may be used. Because chronic kidney disease causes major changes in all body systems, signs and symptoms may be widespread and varied.

Documentation in the record that may indicate the presence of renal failure could include:

- Markedly elevated values of serum creatinine or BUN, or diminished creatinine clearance.
- Clinical manifestations and laboratory findings of the degree of renal impairment primarily noted as the renal failure progresses. For example:
  - acidemia
  - anemia
  - hyperkalemia
  - hyperphosphatemia
  - hypocalcemia
  - renal osteodystrophy
  - uremic symptoms, (e.g., nausea, hemorrhagic conditions, vomiting, itching)

The above may be indicators of renal failure but confirmation and documentation from the physician must be obtained before assigning acode for renal failure from the chronic kidney disease category, 585, acute renal failure category, 584, or unspecified renal failure category, 586.

If documentation identifies kidney disease with hypertension, clarify with the physician as to whether the hypertension is malignant or accelerated. If the documentation identifies that the kidney disease and hypertension are unrelated or the cause and effect relationship cannot be established, code each separately.

When the documentation identifies kidney disease and diabetes but does not identify a cause and effect relationship, contact the physician for clarification. If the physician confirms that the kidney disease is a manifestation of the diabetes, list the diabetes code first followed by the code identifying the specific type of kidney disease.

If the diagnostic statement identifies hypertension, chronic kidney disease, and diabetes, verify the cause and effect relationship of the chronic kidney disease with the physician. If the chronic kidney disease is due to the diabetes, use 250.4x and the appropriate code from 585 as a secondary manifestation code; then code also the specific type of hypertension. However, if the physician confirms that this is hypertensive kidney disease (includes renal failure) due to diabetes, report with 250.4x and a code from category 403, with a fifth digit of "1" to identify the chronic kidney disease and an additional code from 585.1-585.6 to identify the stage of the kidney disease.

585.1	Chronic kidney disease, Stage I
585.2	Chronic kidney disease, Stage II (mild)
585.3	Chronic kidney disease, Stage III (moderate)
	AHA: Q4, 2005, 69
585.4	Chronic kidney disease, Stage IV (severe)
585.5	Chronic kidney disease, Stage V
585.6	End stage renal disease
	AHA: Q4, 2005, 79
585.9	Chronic kidney disease, unspecified
	AHA: Q4, 2005, 79

Stages of CKD

At risk—(no GFR abnormalities)—When the patient is at risk for developing CKD, the patient is tested for indications of organ compromise. Treatment is directed at management of the associated underlying risk factors (diabetes, hypertension, etc.).

Stage 1 — Some kidney damage with normal or slightly increased GFR (>90) is categorized at stage 1 CKD. Evaluation and management is focused on treatment of risk factors.

Stage 2 — Mild kidney damage with a GFR value of 60–89 is categorized at stage 2 CKD. The patient is evaluated for rate of disease progression, and treatment is directed at slowing the rate of loss of function.

Stage 3 — Moderate kidney damage with a GFR value of 30–59 is categorized at stage 3 and evaluated for complications of CKD. Treatment is directed at any complications that have developed as a result of the compromise and preventing further complications from developing.

Stage 4 — Severe kidney damage and a GFR value of 15–29 is categorized at stage 4 CKD. At this stage, a nephrologist is required to manage the disease. Treatment is directed at preparing the patient for kidney replacement therapy.

Stage 5 — Severe kidney damage that has progressed to a GFR value of less than 15 is categorized at stage 5 CKD. At this stage, the nephrologist or other physician formulates the degree of kidney failure. Dialysis or transplantation is required.

End-stage renal disease (ESRD)_This stage of CKD as defined by the federal government indicates a patient is undergoing chronic treatment by dialysis or transplantation for stage 5 chronic kidney disease.

Coding Clarification

Dialysis Disequilibrium Syndrome: This condition is reported with code 276.9 *Electrolyte and fluid disorder not elsewhere classified*. Code also the underlying disease such as chronic kidney disease (585), and also report the renal dialysis status (V45.1).

General Guidelines: Renal failure (category 584 *Acute renal failure*, category 585 *Chronic kidney disease*, and 586 *Renal failure, unspecified*) is the progression of renal insufficiency to the point at which renal function becomes further impaired and apparent clinical manifestations, such as anemia, develop. Renal insufficiency is more an abnormal laboratory assessment, while renal failure includes both the abnormal laboratory and the clinical findings.

Chronic kidney disease is caused by a number of progressive diseases such as diabetes, primary hypertension, nephrosis, nephritis, obstructive uropathy, systemic lupus erythematosus (SLE), polycystic kidney disease, and other congenital disorders. In cases of chronic renal failure that becomes irreversible, the treatment may be either dialysis or transplantation.

It is possible for acute renal failure to be only temporary; the patient's renal function may be regained after interventions such as dialysis.

Infection of Dialysis Catheter: If the patient develops an infection or an inflammatory reaction due to the dialysis catheter, report with code 996.68. Additional codes should also be reported to identify the bacterial agent (e.g., *Staphylococcus aureus*, 041.11) and the stage of chronic kidney disease (585.x).

Hypertensive Chronic Kidney Disease: Code first the hypertensive chronic kidney disease (403.00-403.91) selecting the appropriate fourth digit to indicate type of hypertensive disease — malignant, benign, or unspecified. Then assign the fifth digit to indicate stage of chronic kidney disease — '0' for stages I-IV and '1' for Stage V or ESRD. In addition, assign the appropriate 585.x that describes the specific stage of CKD. Code also kidney transplant status (V42.0), if applicable. Additional codes may be reported to describe other manifestations such as uremic neuropathy (357.4) and uremic pericarditis (420.0).

Hypertensive Heart and Chronic Kidney Disease: Code first the hypertensive heart chronic kidney disease (404.00-404.94) selecting the appropriate fourth digit to indicate type of hypertensive disease — malignant, benign, or unspecified. Then assign the fifth digit to indicate the presence of heart failure and stage of CKD. In addition, assign the appropriate 585.x that describes the specific stage of CKD. Code the type of heart failure (428.0-428.9) if applicable and known. Code also kidney transplant status (V42.0), if applicable. Additional codes may be reported to describe other manifestations such as uremic neuropathy (357.4) and uremic pericarditis (420.0).

Diabetes Mellitus: Diabetes is one of a number of the ICD-9-CM classification categories that is used as a primary code to classify both the disease and its major manifestations. Additional codes should be used to provide more specificity in defining the manifestations. When a cause and effect relationship between renal failure and diabetes has been established, the diabetes code 250.4x is listed first with the appropriate renal failure code listed as an additional code. Accordingly, if the diagnosis does not indicate a cause and effect relationship between the diabetes and renal failure, the code for the specified type of renal failure may be listed first.

Coding Scenario

A patient is admitted for hemodialysis. The patient is an insulin-dependent, Type I diabetic with progressive nephropathy. The physician also documents chronic renal failure in the medical history.

> Code assignment: 250.41 *Diabetes with renal manifestations,* Type 1 583.81 *Nephritis and nephropathy, not specified as acute or chronic, in diseases classified elsewhere,* and 585.9 *Chronic kidney disease, unspecified*

A patient is diagnosed with chronic renal failure secondary to nephrosclerosis with uremia due to gout.

> Code assignment: 274.10 *Gouty nephropathy, unspecified* and 585.9 *Chronic kidney disease, unspecified*

586 Unspecified renal failure ◘
AHA: Q1, 1993, 18; Q3, 1998, 6

Documentation Issues

Documentation in the record that may indicate the presence of renal failure could include:

- Markedly elevated values of serum creatinine or BUN, or diminished creatinine clearance.
- Clinical manifestations and laboratory findings of the degree of renal impairment primarily noted as the renal failure progresses. For example:
  - acidemia
  - anemia
  - hyperkalemia
  - hyperphosphatemia
  - hypocalcemia
  - renal osteodystrophy
  - uremic symptoms, (e.g., nausea, hemorrhagic conditions, vomiting, itching)

The above may be indicators of renal failure but confirmation and documentation from the physician must be obtained before assigning the code for renal failure.

If documentation identifies renal failure with hypertension, clarify with the physician as to whether the hypertension is malignant or accelerated. If the documentation identifies that the renal failure and hypertension are unrelated, or the cause and effect relationship cannot be established, code each separately.

When the documentation identifies renal failure and diabetes but does not identify a cause and effect relationship, contact the physician for clarification. If the physician confirms that the renal failure is a manifestation of the diabetes, list the diabetes code first followed by the code identifying the specific type of renal failure.

Unless acute renal failure or chronic renal failure is confirmed and documented by the physician, azotemia is reported with code 790.6 *Other abnormal blood chemistry.*

Coding Clarification
Excluded from this rubric are renal failure following labor and delivery (669.3x), posttraumatic (958.5), that complicating abortion (rubrics 634-638) or ectopic/molar pregnancy (639.3x), extrarenal or prerenal uremia (788.9), or renal failure with any condition classifiable to 401 (403.0-403.9 with fifth-digit "1").

Diabetes Mellitus: Diabetes is one of a number of the ICD-9-CM classification categories that is used as a primary code to classify both the disease and its major manifestations. Additional codes should be used to provide more specificity in defining the manifestations. When a cause and effect relationship between the renal failure and the diabetes has been established, the diabetes code 250.4x is listed first with the appropriate renal failure code listed as an additional code. Accordingly, if the diagnosis does not indicate a cause and effect relationship between the diabetes and renal failure, the code for the renal failure may be listed first.

General Guidelines: Renal failure (category 584 *Acute renal failure*, 585 *Chronic kidney disease*, and 586 *Renal failure, unspecified*) is the progression of renal insufficiency to the point at which renal function becomes further impaired and apparent clinical manifestations, such as anemia, develop. Renal insufficiency is more an abnormal laboratory assessment, while renal failure includes both the abnormal laboratory and the clinical findings.

Chronic kidney disease is caused by a number of progressive diseases such as diabetes, primary hypertension, nephrosis, nephritis, obstructive uropathy, systemic lupus erythematosus (SLE), polycystic kidney disease, and other congenital disorders. In cases of chronic renal failure that becomes irreversible, the treatment may be either dialysis or transplantation.

Secondary Hypertension: Category 405 *Secondary hypertension* does not include renal failure, so two codes are necessary to identify cases of renal failure with secondary hypertension.

587 Unspecified renal sclerosis

Coding Clarification
Excluded from this rubric is arteriolar or arteriosclerotic nephrosclerosis (403.00-403.92).

588 Disorders resulting from impaired renal function

Secondary hyperparathyroidism results from releasing increased levels in response to deconditioning of the body to parathyroid hormone PTH due to another disease process, such as renal failure. PTH helps regulate the levels of calcium and phosphorus in the body, induces the release of calcium from bone, the amount of calcium taken from food, intestinal absorption of calcium, and the excretion of calcium in the urine. Renal osteodystrophy is caused by the kidney failing to maintain the appropriate level of calcium in the blood, which affect bone health. Nephrogenic diabetes is caused by the failure of the kidneys to absorb filtered fluids. Hypercalcemia, or increased levels of calcium in the blood, is a sign of hyperparathyroidism, when accompanied by a concurrent increase in the level of PTH hormone.

588.0	Renal osteodystrophy — *azotemic osteodystrophy; renal dwarfism; renal rickets*
588.1	Nephrogenic diabetes insipidus — *kidneys fail to resorb filtered fluids, leading to extreme thirst and frequent urination*
588.81	Secondary hyperparathyroidism (of renal origin) AHA: Q4, 2004, 58-59
588.89	Other specified disorders resulting from impaired renal function
588.9	Unspecified disorder resulting from impaired renal function — *disorder NOS due to impaired renal function*

Coding Clarification
Report 252.02 for hyperparathyroidism from non-renal causes.

589 Small kidney of unknown cause

589.0	Unilateral small kidney
589.1	Bilateral small kidneys
589.9	Unspecified small kidney — *of unknown cause*

Coding Clarification
These codes are considered nonspecific codes and should be used only when a more specific diagnosis of acquired or congenital small kidney cannot be determined.

590–599 Other Diseases of Urinary System

590 Infections of kidney

590.00 Chronic pyelonephritis without lesion of renal medullary necrosis — (Code, if applicable, any causal condition first. Use additional code to identify organism, such as E. coli, 041.4) — *chronic pyelitis, or pyonephrosis, without lesion of renal medullary necrosis use additional code to identify organism*

590.01 Chronic pyelonephritis with lesion of renal medullary necrosis — (Code, if applicable, any causal condition first. Use additional code to identify organism, such as E. coli, 041.4) — *chronic pyelitis or pyonephrosis with lesion of renal medullary necrosis use additional code to identify organism*

590.10 Acute pyelonephritis without lesion of renal medullary necrosis — (Use additional code to identify organism, such as E. coli, 041.4) — *acute pyelitis or acute pyonephrosis without lesion of renal medullary necrosis*

590.11 Acute pyelonephritis with lesion of renal medullary necrosis — (Use additional code to identify organism, such as E. coli, 041.4) — *acute pyelitis or acute pyonephrosis with lesion of renal medullary necrosis*

590.2 Renal and perinephric abscess — (Use additional code to identify organism, such as E. coli, 041.4) — *nephritic abscess; perirenal abscess*

590.3 Pyeloureteritis cystica — (Use additional code to identify organism, such as E. coli, 041.4) — *ureteritis cystica; infection of renal pelvis and ureter*

590.80 Unspecified pyelonephritis — (Use additional code to identify organism, such as E. coli, 041.4) — *pyelonephritis NOS*
AHA: Q4, 1997, 40; Q1, 1998, 10

590.81 Pyelitis or pyelonephritis in diseases classified elsewhere — (Code first underlying disease, 016.0. Use additional code to identify organism, such as E. coli, 041.4) — *in disease classified elsewhere*

590.9 Unspecified infection of kidney — (Use additional code to identify organism, such as E. coli, 041.4)

Coding Clarification
Use an additional code to identify infective agents, such as *Escherichia coli* (041.4).

591 Hydronephrosis
AHA: Q2, 1998, 9

Use this code to report dilation of the renal pelvis and calyces due to the obstruction of the flow of urine. Obstruction occurring at the ureteropelvic junction is sometimes referred to as primary hydronephrosis, and obstruction at any point distal to the ureteropelvic junction is sometimes referred to as secondary hydronephrosis.

Signs and symptoms of hydronephrosis include a history of any condition causing urinary obstruction, colicky pain in acute hydronephrosis, dull and aching flank pain in chronic hydronephrosis, and hematuria. Blood work may show azotemia (excess urea and other nitrogenous byproducts). Urinalysis may reveal red blood cells and pyuria if a concomitant urinary infection is present. Radiology, such as intravenous pyelography, cystoureterography, and kidney ultrasound, identify the site of the obstruction and confirm the diagnosis.

Therapies include cystoscopy to correct conditions such as benign prostatic hypertrophy and ureteral calculus (basket extraction of calculus or stent insertion), extracorporeal shock wave lithotripsy to break up calculi in the kidney or ureter, nephrostomy for severe obstructions, and surgery to correct conditions such as strictures, neoplasms, and congenital malformations.

Associated conditions include urinary tract infection, urinary calculus formation, benign prostatic hypertrophy or prostate cancer, urinary stricture formation, and congenital abnormalities.

Coding Clarification
Excluded from this code are congenital hydronephrosis (753.29) and hydroureter (593.5).

592 Calculus of kidney and ureter

Use this rubric to report stones of the kidney and ureter. Most stones are composed of calcium salts or magnesium/ammonium phosphate; most are idiopathic. Other stones may be composed of cystine or uric acid, and are a result of a defect in urinary acidification.

Nausea, infection, severe pain, and hematuria usually accompany kidney stones, if the stone is obstructing the flow of urine. If there is no obstruction, there may be no symptoms.

Ureteral calculi have migrated to the ureter from the kidney, and obstruction can compromise renal function. Symptoms are the same as for renal calculi.

592.0 Calculus of kidney — *renal calculus or stone; staghorn calculus*
AHA: Q1, 2000, 4

592.1 Calculus of ureter — *ureteric stone; ureterolithiasis*
AHA: Q1, 1991, 11; Q1, 1998, 10; Q2, 1998, 9

592.9 Unspecified urinary calculus — *renal or ureteral calculus NOS*
AHA: Q4, 1997, 40; Q1, 1998, 10

Coding Clarification
Excluded from this rubric is nephrocalcinosis (275.4).

593 Other disorders of kidney and ureter

The ureter is the tube leading from the kidney to the urinary bladder. It is approximately 28.0 centimeters long and is composed of three layers of tissue. The inner layer is a mucous lining. The smooth, muscular middle layer propels the urine from the kidney to the bladder by peristalsis. The outer layer is fibrous connective tissue. Each ureter leaves the kidney from the hilum, a concave notch on the middle surface, and enters the bladder through a narrow valve-like orifice that prevents backflow of urine to the kidney.

593.0 Nephroptosis — *floating kidney; mobile kidney*
593.1 Hypertrophy of kidney — *enlargement of kidney*
593.2 Acquired cyst of kidney — *peripelvic (lymphatic) cyst*
AHA: Q4, 1990, 3
593.3 Stricture or kinking of ureter — *stricture of pelviureteric junction*
AHA: Q2, 1998, 9
593.4 Other ureteric obstruction — *idiopathic retroperitoneal fibrosis; occlusion NOS of ureter*
AHA: Q2, 1997, 4
593.5 Hydroureter — *dilation of ureter due to obstructed urinary flow*
593.6 Postural proteinuria — *benign postural proteinuria; orthostatic proteinuria*
593.70 Vesicoureteral reflux, unspecified or without reflex nephropathy — *backflow of urine from bladder into ureter*
AHA: Q4, 1994, 42
593.71 Vesicoureteral reflux with reflux nephropathy, unilateral — *one-sided backflow of urine into ureter, causing renal scarring*
AHA: Q4, 1994, 42
593.72 Vesicoureteral reflux with reflux nephropathy, bilateral — *backflow of urine into ureters on both sides, causing renal scarring*
AHA: Q4, 1994, 42
593.73 Vesicoureteral reflux with reflux nephropathy, NOS — *backflow of urine into ureters, causing renal scarring*
AHA: Q4, 1994, 42
593.81 Vascular disorders of kidney — *renal artery embolism; renal artery hemorrhage; renal artery thrombosis; renal infarction*
593.82 Ureteral fistula — *intestinoureteral fistula*
593.89 Other specified disorder of kidney and ureter — *adhesions, kidney or ureter; periureteritis; ureteral polyp; ureterocele*

593.9 Unspecified disorder of kidney and ureter — *renal disease NOS; salt-losing nephritis or syndrome; Thorn's syndrome*
AHA: Q1, 1993, 17; Q4, 2005, 79

Coding Clarification
Use this code series for kidney and ureter disorders that are not further specified as acute or chronic or are lacking a stated pathology or cause with the exception that 593.9 reports only acute renal disease/insufficiency, or renal disease that is unspecified. Renal disease/insufficiency stated as chronic is excluded here and is assigned to 585.9. Also classified to this code are syndromes of low salt, salt-losing, or salt depletion not further specified, as well as salt-losing or salt-wasting nephritis, nephropathy, or renopathy not further specified.

594 Calculus of lower urinary tract

The lower urinary tract includes every part of the urinary system, except the kidneys. While the kidneys filter blood and produce urine, the remainder of the system stores and eliminates the waste liquid. The ureters carry urine from the kidneys to the bladder, the urinary bladder stores urine, and the urethra carries urine out of the body. Bladder stones are usually the result of another urologic problem such as urinary tract infection, bladder diverticulum, neurogenic bladder, or an enlarged prostate. Approximately 95 percent of all bladder stones occur in men. Bladder stones can cause irritation and damage inside the urinary tract, while chronic irritation with bladder calculi predisposes the bladder to cancer. Clinical signs include blood in the urine, frequent urination, increased thirst, abdominal distention or pain, and penile pain in males. Diagnosis is based on history; physical examination; x-rays, including x-rays taken with dye being placed into the bladder; urinalysis; and urine culture. Treatment includes drinking six to eight glasses of water each day to increase urinary output and help the stones pass. Stones that are not excreted spontaneously may be removed using a cystoscope or open surgery. Extracorporeal shock wave lithotripsy may be an alternative to surgery. Medications are rarely used to dissolve the stones.

594.0 Calculus in diverticulum of bladder — *stone in pouch of bladder wall*
594.1 Other calculus in bladder — *urinary bladder stone*
594.2 Calculus in urethra — *urinary stone in urethra*
594.8 Other lower urinary tract calculus — *suburethral urinary stone*
AHA: Jan-Feb, 1985, 16
594.9 Unspecified calculus of lower urinary tract

595 Cystitis

This rubric reports infections and inflammations of the bladder. An additional code should be reported to identify the infectious agent, as in E. coli 041.4. If the bladder inflammation or infection is due to a disease classified elsewhere, code first the underlying disease.

The urinary bladder is an expandable and collapsible bag located behind the symphysis pubis (pubic bone) and below the parietal peritoneum. This protective membrane covers only the top of the bladder. The bladder has a strong, specialized muscular layer called the detrusor muscle, a network of muscle bundles that run in all directions. The lining of the bladder is a mucous transitional epithelium that forms folds called rugae. These specialized tissue layers allow for the distension of the bladder as it fills with urine from the kidneys.

There are three openings in the floor of the bladder. The two ureters enter at the back of the bladder, guarded by the valve-like narrow regions that prevent backflow up to the kidneys. The opening into the urethra is in the front lower corner of the bladder. The bladder has two major functions: it stores urine before it leaves the body and, by means of the urethra, expels urine from the body.

Cystitis is a common complication of catheterization. When this occurs, report 996.64 *Infection and inflammatory reaction due to indwelling urinary catheter* and a cystitis code from this rubric.

595.0	Acute cystitis — (Use additional code to identify organism, such as E. coli, 041.4) — *acute infection of bladder* AHA: Q2, 1999, 15
595.1	Chronic interstitial cystitis — (Use additional code to identify organism, such as E. coli, 041.4) — *Hunner's ulcer; panmural fibrosis of bladder; submucous cystitis*
595.2	Other chronic cystitis — (Use additional code to identify organism, such as E. coli, 041.4) — *chronic cystitis NOS; subacute cystitis*
595.3	Trigonitis — (Use additional code to identify organism, such as E. coli, 041.4) — *follicular cystitis; acute or chronic trigonitis; urethrotrigonitis*
595.4	Cystitis in diseases classified elsewhere — (Code first underlying disease: 006.8, 039.8, 120.0-120.9, 122.3, 122.6. Use additional code to identify organism, such as E. coli, 041.4)
595.81	Cystitis cystica — (Use additional code to identify organism, such as E. coli, 041.4) — *bladder inflammation due to multiple cysts*
595.82	Irradiation cystitis — (Use additional code to identify organism, such as E. coli, 041.4) — *bladder inflammation due to radiation*
595.89	Other specified types of cystitis — (Use additional code to identify organism, such as E. coli, 041.4) — *bladder abscess; emphysematous cystitis*
595.9	Unspecified cystitis — (Use additional code to identify organism, such as E. coli, 041.4)

Coding Clarification

Excluded from this rubric are prostatocystitis (601.3), cystitis in diphtheria (032.84), gonococcal cystitis (098.11, 098.31), monilial cystitis (112.2), trichomonal cystitis (131.09), and tuberculous cystitis (subclassification 016.1).

596 Other disorders of bladder
AHA: March-April, 1987, 10

Subclassification 596.0 reports a condition, also known as bladder outlet obstruction or vesicourethral obstruction, that occurs mostly in males and usually as a consequence of benign prostatic hypertrophy or prostatic cancer. It also may occur in either sex due to strictures (formed following radiation therapy, cystoscopy, catheterization injury, or infection), blood clots, bladder cancer, impacted calculi, extrinsic tumors, or disease compressing the bladder neck.

Bladder neck obstruction is associated with complications such as hydronephrosis, hydroureteronephrosis, or ureteronephrosis. The obstruction also may be due to bladder thickening and hypertrophy, trabeculation, or diverticula; hypertrophy and subsequent dilatation and atony of the renal pelvis; or renal parenchymal compression and ischemic atrophy.

Use subclassification 596.5 to report functional disorders of the bladder, the musculomembranous sac that serves as a reservoir for urine received from the kidneys through the ureters and as a contractile organ actively expelling its contents into the urethra. Functional disorders prevent the bladder from performing either or both of these functions. Included are hypertonicity, low bladder compliance, paralysis, neurogenic bladder, and detrusor sphincter dyssynergia.

Hypertonicity refers to excessive muscle tonus or tension. In the bladder, it usually refers to prolonged detrusor (bladder) muscle spasms and hypersensitivity or hyperreflexia of the detrusor muscle.

Low bladder compliance refers to the relative change in bladder volume when measured against bladder (detrusor muscle) pressure. Compliance can be measured by inflow cystometry. If the cystometry demonstrates a large bladder volume with little pressure change in the bladder, the patient has a bladder of high compliance; if the cystometry reveals a tense, firm bladder with high pressure, the bladder is of low compliance.

Paralysis of the bladder is a general term meaning loss of the ability of the detrusor muscles to contract. Such paralysis may have a variety of etiologies such as trauma, drugs, disease, or other structural or functional disorders in the bladder muscle or nerves.

Neurogenic bladder is due to a nervous system lesion. Terms used to describe neurogenic bladder are spastic bladder, reflex bladder, and flaccid bladder.

Detrusor sphincter dyssynergia, also known as bladder neck dyssynergia, is a condition in which urinary outflow is obstructed because the bladder neck fails to relax or tightens when the detrusor muscle contracts during micturition. The condition is rarely observed in females.

596.0		Bladder neck obstruction — (Use additional code to identify urinary incontinence: 625.6, 788.30-788.39) — *contracture of bladder neck or other vesicoureteral orifice* **AHA:** Nov-Dec, 1986, 10; March-April, 1987, 10; Q2, 2001, 14; Q3, 2002, 28
596.1		Intestinovesical fistula — (Use additional code to identify urinary incontinence: 625.6, 788.30-788.39) — *enterovesical fistula; vesicorectal fistula* **AHA:** March-April, 1987, 10
596.2		Vesical fistula, not elsewhere classified — (Use additional code to identify urinary incontinence: 625.6, 788.30-788.39) — *urethrovesical fistula; vesicocutaneous fistula* **AHA:** March-April, 1987, 10
596.3		Diverticulum of bladder — (Use additional code to identify urinary incontinence: 625.6, 788.30-788.39) — *bladder diverticulitis* **AHA:** March-April, 1987, 10
596.4		Atony of bladder — (Use additional code to identify urinary incontinence: 625.6, 788.30-788.39) — *hypotonicity of bladder; bladder inertia* **AHA:** March-April, 1987, 10
596.51		Hypertonicity of bladder — (Use additional code to identify urinary incontinence: 625.6, 788.30-788.39) — *hyperactivity of bladder; overactivity of bladder* **AHA:** March-April, 1987, 10
596.52		Low bladder compliance — (Use additional code to identify urinary incontinence: 625.6, 788.30-788.39) — *small or sensitive bladder that requires frequent emptying* **AHA:** March-April, 1987, 10
596.53		Paralysis of bladder — (Use additional code to identify urinary incontinence: 625.6, 788.30-788.39) — *bladder unable to contract* **AHA:** March-April, 1987, 10
596.54		Neurogenic bladder, NOS — (Use additional code to identify urinary incontinence: 625.6, 788.30-788.39) — *loss of bladder control most often due to spinal nerve damage from injury or neurological disease* **AHA:** March-April, 1987, 10; Q1, 2001, 12
596.55		Detrusor sphincter dyssynergia — (Use additional code to identify urinary incontinence: 625.6, 788.30-788.39) — *loss of coordination between bladder emptying nerves and external urethral sphincter* **AHA:** March-April, 1987, 10
596.59		Other functional disorder of bladder — (Use additional code to identify urinary incontinence: 625.6, 788.30-788.39) — *detrusor instability* **AHA:** March-April, 1987, 10
596.6		Nontraumatic rupture of bladder — (Use additional code to identify urinary incontinence: 625.6, 788.30-788.39) — *spontaneous tear in bladder wall* **AHA:** March-April, 1987, 10
596.7		Hemorrhage into bladder wall — (Use additional code to identify urinary incontinence: 625.6, 788.30-788.39) — *hyperemia of bladder* **AHA:** March-April, 1987, 10
596.8		Other specified disorder of bladder — (Use additional code to identify urinary incontinence: 625.6, 788.30-788.39) — *calcified bladder; bladder hypertrophy* **AHA:** Jan-Feb, 1985, 8; March-April, 1987, 10
596.9		Unspecified disorder of bladder — (Use additional code to identify urinary incontinence: 625.6, 788.30-788.39) — *bladder disease NOS* **AHA:** Jan-Feb, 1985, 8; March-April, 1987, 10

Coding Clarification
Congenital bladder neck obstruction is excluded from this subclassification and should be reported with 753.6.

Use an additional code to report any urinary incontinence (625.6, 788.30-788.39).

Bladder Outlet Obstruction: In cases of benign prostatic hypertrophy with bladder outlet obstruction, the prostatic hypertrophy (600.00-600.01) is listed first and an additional code for the obstruction (596.0) is secondary, because the obstruction is typically a part of the condition due to the prostatic hypertrophy.

Lower Urinary Tract Symptoms (LUTS): When lower urinary tract symptoms such as incomplete bladder emptying (788.21), nocturia (788.43), straining on urination (788.65), weak urinary stream (788.62), or urinary retention (788.20), urgency

(788.63), obstruction (599.69), incontinence (788.30ñ788.39), hesitancy (788.64), or frequency (788.41) are noted with benign prostatic hypertrophy (600.00–600.01), these are reported as secondary codes.

597 Urethritis, not sexually transmitted, and urethral syndrome

- **597.0** Urethral abscess — *periurethral abscess; bulbourethral gland abscess*
- **597.80** Unspecified urethritis — *urethritis NOS*
- **597.81** Urethral syndrome NOS
- **597.89** Other urethritis — *Cowperitis (males); urethral ulcer; para-urethritis; littritis (males); adenitis, Skene's glands (females)*

Coding Clarification
Excluded from this rubric is nonspecific urethritis, so stated, reported with 099.4.

598 Urethral stricture
A urethral stricture is a narrowing of the urethra. The urethra is a small tube lined with mucous membrane that leads from the bladder to the exterior of the body. In the male, it is approximately 20.0 centimeters long and passes through the prostate gland just below the bladder, where it joins the ejaculatory ducts. The tube extends forward and down to enter the base of the penis, and travels centrally through the length of the penis to end as a urinary meatus at the tip. In the female, the urethra lies directly behind the symphysis pubis and in front of the vagina, and is only about 3.0 centimeters long.

The function of the urethra in the female is to void urine from the bladder reservoir. In the male, the urethra is part of two different systems: in addition to voiding urine, the urethra also serves as the pathway for semen (fluid containing sperm) as it is ejaculated out of the body through the penis. Urine is prevented from mixing with semen during ejaculation by the reflex closure of the sphincter muscles guarding the opening into the bladder.

- **598.00** Urethral stricture due to unspecified infection — (Use additional code to identify urinary incontinence: 625.6, 788.30-788.39) — *urethral stricture due to infection NOS*
- **598.01** Urethral stricture due to infective diseases classified elsewhere — (Code first underlying disease: 095.8, 098.2, 120.0-120.9. Use additional code to identify urinary incontinence: 625.6, 788.30-788.39)
- **598.1** Traumatic urethral stricture — (Use additional code to identify urinary incontinence: 625.6, 788.30-788.39) — *postobstetric urethral stricture*
- **598.2** Postoperative urethral stricture — (Use additional code to identify urinary incontinence: 625.6, 788.30-788.39) — *postcatheterization stricture of urethra*
  AHA: Q3, 1997, 6
- **598.8** Other specified causes of urethral stricture — (Use additional code to identify urinary incontinence: 625.6, 788.30-788.39) — *other specified cause of urethral stricture NEC*
  AHA: Nov-Dec, 1984, 9
- **598.9** Unspecified urethral stricture — (Use additional code to identify urinary incontinence: 625.6, 788.30-788.39) — *pinhole meatus; ankylurethria*

Coding Clarification
Use an additional code to identify urinary incontinence (625.6; 788.30-788.39). Code first the underlying disease, as appropriate.

599 Other disorders of urethra and urinary tract
The definition of urinary tract infection, site not specified, is a wide variety of clinical conditions characterized by a significant number of microorganisms in an unspecified part of the urinary tract. Predisposing factors for urinary tract infection include, but are not limited to, calculi or other urinary tract obstruction, foreign bodies such as stents or catheters, congenital urinary anomalies, pregnancy, diabetes mellitus, neurogenic bladder, immunosuppression (such as following renal transplant), and vesicovaginal or intestinal fistulas. Many urinary tract infections recur due to bacterial persistence or reinfection from new organisms outside the urinary tract. Women are approximately 10 times more likely to develop a urinary tract infection than men.

Signs and symptoms of urinary tract infection, site not specified, include history of recurrent urinary tract infections, burning pain on urination, polyuria, suprapubic or abdominal pain, fever, and turbid, foul-smelling, dark urine. Urinalysis shows significant bacteriuria, often accompanied by proteinuria, hematuria, and pyuria, and urine culture reveals growth of more than 100,000 colonies of a single organism. Blood work may reveal neutrophilic leukocytosis and positive blood culture, especially if the infection involves the upper urinary tract. Radiology, such as intravenous urography or pyelography, voiding cystography, and renal ultrasound, may demonstrate complicating factors such as calculi, abscess formation, hydronephrosis, and congenital anomalies. Cystoscopy and ureteral catheterization to obtain differential urine specimens localize the infection site.

Therapies include antibiotics such as ampicillin, gentamicin, tetracycline, and tobramycin. Surgery can correct complications due to urinary tract infections (such as ureteral strictures) and conditions that predispose the patient to chronic or recurrent urinary tract infections (such as ureteral calculi or congenital abnormalities).

Associated conditions include urosepsis, diabetes mellitus, pregnancy (complicated), urinary tract obstruction (e.g., calculi, fibrosis), neurogenic bladder, congenital urinary tract anomalies, benign prostatic hypertrophy, prostatitis, infected diverticula, foreign bodies, vesicovaginal and intestinal fistulas, ureteral stump following nephrectomy, papillary necrosis, and urachal cyst.

Infections of the prostate, vagina, epididymis, and testis are classified elsewhere but may be swept into the nonspecific diagnosis of urinary tract infection by some clinicians.

Urinalysis and the urine culture are the most important indicators for urinary tract infection. Urine specimens, including the so-called "clean-catch" midstream specimen, are subject to contamination during collection from microorganisms surrounding the external urethra or by improper handling and storage. Thus, the presence of three or more species of microorganisms growing in large numbers suggests contamination, except in patients who have had an indwelling catheter for a long time. Also, patients who have received antibiotic therapy for any reason prior to testing may present false negative test results.

599.0   Urinary tract infection, site not specified — (Use additional code to identify organism, such as E. coli, 041.4) — *bacteriuria; pyuria*
AHA: Q1, 1992, 13; Q2, 1995, 7; Q2, 1996, 7; Q4, 1996, 33; Q1, 1998, 5; Q2, 1999, 15; Q4, 1999, 6; Q4, 2003, 79; Q2, 2004, 13; Q3, 2005, 12

Documentation Issues

When the documentation does not identify that the cause of the infection was due to the procedure (postoperative), clarification is required from the physician before a code is assigned identifying the infection as a procedural complication. If documentation cannot be obtained specifically stating the cause and effect relationship with the procedure, code 599.0 should be assigned.

When the documentation indicates urosepsis, the physician should be contacted to clarify whether the urosepsis is intended to mean generalized sepsis (septicemia) caused by leakage of urine or toxic urine by-products into the general vascular circulation, or that the urine is contaminated by bacteria, bacterial by-products, or perhaps other toxic material but without other findings (599.0). The alphabetic index refers the coder to urinary tract infection, but this may not be what the physician meant by this term. If the information is unobtainable, it is appropriate to use the index that defaults to code 599.0 for urosepsis.

Ask the physician if the site of the infection is known, and request an addendum to the medical record if the answer is affirmative.

Coding Clarification

This subcategory excludes urinary tract infection of newborn which is reported with code 771.82.

Secondary to Noncandidal Yeast: To properly report the urinary tract infection secondary to noncandidal yeast, use two codes: 599.0 *Urinary tract infection, site not specified* and 117.9 *Other and unspecified mycoses.*

Septicemia Secondary to Urinary Tract Infection: If microorganisms or their toxins from a localized urinary infection haves entered into the patient's blood stream and developed into systemic infection, septicemia, use only a code from category 038. Code 599.0 *Urinary tract infection, site not specified* is not reported as an additional code. If the code from category 038 identifies the causative organism, it is not necessary to report a code from category 041 (e.g., pseudomonas septicemia 038.43).

Specified Organism: When the causative organism has been identified, it is reported as an additional code to the urinary tract infection (599.0). Using E. Coli as an example, a note is provided in the Tabular List, under category code 041 that states "This category is provided to be used as an additional code where it is desired to identify the bacterial agent in diseases classified elsewhere."

599.1	Urethral fistula — *urinary fistula NOS*
	AHA: Q3, 1997, 6
599.2	Urethral diverticulum — *pouch in urethral wall*
599.3	Urethral caruncle — *urethral polyp*
599.4	Urethral false passage — *passage without opening at urethral meatus*
599.5	Prolapsed urethral mucosa — *urethrocele*
599.60	Urinary obstruction, unspecified — (Use additional code to identify urinary incontinence: 625.6, 788.30-788.39) — *obstructive uropathy NOS*
	AHA: Q4, 2005, 80
599.69	Urinary obstruction, not elsewhere classified
	AHA: Q4, 2005, 80

599.7 Hematuria — *benign hematuria; essential hematuria*
AHA: Q3, 1995, 8; Q1, 2000, 5

Coding Clarification
Subcategory 599.6 excludes urinary tract obstruction due to hyperplasia of the prostate, which is coded to 600.0-600.9 with the appropriate fifth digit.

Hematuria reports a condition in which blood appears in the urine. Also known as hemuresis, hematuria may present as gross, visible blood in the urine or as RBCs visible only under microscopy (microscopic hematuria). Hematuria may be due to a urethral infection; bladder neoplasms; or radiation injury, ureteral calculus, or kidney conditions such as polycystic disease, renal artery thrombosis, or trauma. Hematuria also can be caused by systemic disorders such as hemophilia, sickle cell crisis, thrombocytopenia, anaphylactoid purpura with renal involvement, and adverse effect of anticoagulant therapy.

Often the presentation of the hematuria gives clues as to the source of the bleeding. When blood appears only during the first fraction of voided urine (initial hematuria), the source is likely the anterior urethra or prostate gland. When blood appears during the terminal fraction of voided urine (terminal hematuria), the source is likely in the posterior urethra, vesicle neck, or trigone. Blood mixed with the total urine volume (total hematuria) is from the kidneys, ureters, or bladder. Painful hematuria usually indicates infection, calculi, trauma, or foreign body in the lower urinary tract. Painless hematuria is often associated with a neoplasm or vascular disorder.

The definition of other specified disorders of urethra and urinary tract is disorders of the urethra and urinary tract not elsewhere classifiable, such as urethral hypermobility, intrinsic (urethral) sphincter deficiency, and urethral instability.

Urethral hypermobility refers to inferior and posterior motion of the urethra into the potential space of the vagina and is due to a loss of urethral supporting and backing structures of the pelvis and pelvic floor. Urethral hypermobility is associated with pathologies such as vaginal prolapse and cystoceles and is commonly seen in females with urinary stress incontinence.

Intrinsic (urethral) sphincter deficiency (ISD) is due to intrinsic sphincteric damage in which the urethra is usually well supported but there is a posterior rotation and opening of the bladder neck and posterior urethra during straining.

Urethral instability is a reflex relaxation of the urethral muscle with or without detrusor muscle contraction resulting in incontinence. This condition is commonly associated with females who have multiple sclerosis.

599.81 Urethral hypermobility — (Use additional code to identify urinary incontinence: 625.6, 788.30-788.39) — *hypermobility*

599.82 Intrinsic (urethral) sphincter deficiency (ISD) — (Use additional code to identify urinary incontinence: 625.6, 788.30-788.39) — *deficiency*
AHA: Q2, 1996, 15

599.83 Urethral instability — (Use additional code to identify urinary incontinence: 625.6, 788.30-788.39) — *instability*

599.84 Other specified disorders of urethra — (Use additional code to identify urinary incontinence: 625.6, 788.30-788.39) — *nontraumatic rupture of urethra; urethral cyst; malacoplakia of urethra*

599.89 Other specified disorders of urinary tract — (Use additional code to identify urinary incontinence: 625.6, 788.30-788.39) — *hymeno-urethral fusion; suburethral cyst*

599.9 Unspecified disorder of urethra and urinary tract

Coding Clarification
Excluded from this rubric is candidiasis of urinary tract (112.2). Use an additional code to identify the infective agent, as in *E. coli* (041.4).

Site Specificity: One of the most important aspects of coding urinary tract infections is site specificity in the medical record documentation. "UTI" is commonly used as a synonym for acute cystitis, acute pyelonephritis, and acute urethritis. Cystitis and urethritis are infections of the lower urinary tract, and pyelonephritis is an infection of the upper urinary tract. Cystitis is more often seen in females, whereas urethritis is more commonly seen in males.

If the site of the infection is known, do not use code 599.0. Code 599.0 is reserved for cases in which no attempt was made to document the site of the infection. Do not use 599.0 as an accompanying code to a specific urinary tract infection code. However, if two specific sites are named, it is correct to code them both (e.g., 595.0 *Acute cystitis* and 590.10 *Acute pyelonephritis without lesion of renal medullary necrosis*).

Remember that UTIs attributable to sexually transmitted diseases are coded to the infectious disease chapter.

Coding Scenario
A patient is seen in the clinic for painful urination and fever. A urine culture shows the bacterial agent Pseudomonas. The physician's diagnostic statement confirms a urinary tract infection due to Pseudomonas.

Code assignment: 599.0 *Urinary tract infection, site not specified* and 041.7 *Pseudomonas*

A 79-year-old male is readmitted for a urinary tract infection due to a urinary retention catheter.

Code assignment: 996.64 *Infection and inflammatory reaction due to internal prosthetic device, implant, and graft, indwelling urinary catheter* and 599.0 *Urinary tract infection, site not specified*

The patient's list of diagnoses reads acute pyelonephritis, acute cystitis, and urosepsis. After physician query, it is determined that urosepsis was not used as a synonym for septicemia.

Code assignment: Code 590.10 *Acute pyelonephritis without lesion of renal medullary necrosis* and 595.0 *Acute cystitis*

600–608 Diseases of Male Genital Organs

The male reproductive system includes the two testes that produce spermatozoa (sperm) and male hormones. A system of ducts conveys sperm to the exterior of the body. This includes the epididymis and vas deferens, the seminal vesicles (glands which contribute secretions to semen), and the external genitalia, the scrotum, and penis. The prime function of the male genital system is sexual intercourse and propagation of the species.

600 Hyperplasia of prostate
AHA: Nov-Dec, 1986, 10; Q3, 1992, 7; Q3, 1994, 12; Q4, 2000, 43; Q3, 2005, 20

This rubric classifies a condition believed to arise as fibrostromal proliferation in the periurethral glands. The etiology is unknown, but a relationship between aging and prostate enlargement is well documented. Most theories regarding the cause of benign prostatic hypertrophy focus on possible hormonal imbalances occurring in the male after age 50. The disease usually becomes symptomatic after age 60 and is due to median and/or lateral lobe (inner gland) enlargement. The outer prostate glands are pushed against the prostate capsule, resulting in a thick pseudocapsule referred to as the surgical capsule. As the enlargement continues and intracapsular pressure increases, urinary outflow is obstructed due to impingement of the urethra. Frequently, the typical signs and symptoms of benign prostatic hypertrophy are referred to as "prostatism."

Signs and symptoms of hyperplasia of the prostate include reduced urinary stream caliber and force, urinary hesitancy, feelings of incomplete voiding, nocturia, straining to initiate urination, severe urgency, suprapubic pain, bladder distention when in urinary retention, hematuria, increased urine residual, and prostate enlargement palpable with rectal exam. Urinalysis may reveal concomitant infection. Blood work may show elevated serum creatinine and BUN with prolonged obstruction. Excretory urograms reveal ureteral dilation, hydronephrosis or hydroureteronephrosis, or post voiding urinary retention. Pelvic ultrasound may be used to calculate exact amounts of residual urine. Cystoscopy shows enlargement of periurethral prostate glands and demonstrates secondary bladder wall changes such as trabeculation, vesicle calculi, acute and/or chronic inflammation due to infection, and bladder diverticula.

Therapies include sexual stimulation, prostatic massage, and catheterization for acute urine retention, which may result in a return to adequate voiding function. Other therapies include alpha-adrenergic drugs, such as terazosin and prazosin, to relax the external sphincter and prevent contractions of the prostatic capsule, prostatectomy (transurethral, retropubic, suprapubic, or peroneal) for patients with moderate to severe obstruction, and cryosurgery or transurethral balloon urethroplasty for patients who are poor surgical risks.

Code	Description
600.00	Hypertrophy (benign) of prostate without urinary obstruction and other lower urinary tract symptoms (LUTS) — (Use additional code to identify urinary incontinence: 788.30-788.39) — *benign prostatic hypertrophy* **AHA:** Q1, 2003, 6
600.01	Hypertrophy (benign) of prostate with urinary obstruction and other lower urinary tract symptoms (LUTS) — (Use additional code to identify urinary incontinence: 788.30-788.39) — *benign prostatic hypertrophy* **AHA:** Q1, 2003, 6; Q4, 2003, 64
600.10	Nodular prostate without urinary obstruction — (Use additional code to identify urinary incontinence: 788.30-788.39) — *small mass of tissue that swells, knots, or is a protuberance in the prostate*
600.11	Nodular prostate with urinary obstruction — (Use additional code to identify urinary incontinence: 788.30-788.39) — *small mass of tissue that swells, knots, or is a protuberance in the prostate, impeding the flow of urine*

Diseases of the Genitourinary System

Code	Description
600.20	Benign localized hyperplasia of prostate without urinary obstruction and other lower urinary tract symptoms (LUTS) — (Use additional code to identify urinary incontinence: 788.30-788.39) — *associated with age, enlargement caused by proliferation of grandular and stromal elements; typically starting in the fifth decade of life*
600.21	Benign localized hyperplasia of prostate with urinary obstruction and other lower urinary tract symptoms (LUTS) — (Use additional code to identify urinary incontinence: 788.30-788.39) — *associated with age, enlargement caused by proliferation of grandular and stromal elements; typically starting in the fifth decade of life, impeding the flow of urine*
600.3	Cyst of prostate — *sacs of fluid which differentiates this form from nodular or adenomatous tumors valid four digit code*
600.90	Hyperplasia of prostate, unspecified, without urinary obstruction and other lower urinary tract symptoms (LUTS) — (Use additional code to identify urinary incontinence: 788.30-788.39) — *associated with age, enlargement caused by proliferation of grandular and stromal elements; typically starting in the fifth decade of life*
600.91	Hyperplasia of prostate, unspecified, with urinary obstruction and other lower urinary tract symptoms (LUTS) — (Use additional code to identify urinary incontinence: 788.30-788.39)

Coding Clarification
Excluded from this rubric are benign neoplasm of the prostate (222.2) and malignant neoplasm of the prostate (185).

Bladder Outlet Obstruction: In cases of benign prostatic hypertrophy with bladder outlet obstruction, the prostatic hypertrophy (600.00-600.01) is listed first and an additional code for the obstruction (596.0) is secondary, because the obstruction is typically a part of the condition due to the prostatic hypertrophy.

Lower Urinary Tract Symptoms (LUTS): When lower urinary tract symptoms such as incomplete bladder emptying (788.21), nocturia (788.43), straining on urination (788.65), weak urinary stream (788.62), hesitancy (788.64), or frequency (788.41) are noted with benign prostatic hypertrophy (600.00-600.01), these are reported as secondary codes.

Coding Scenario
A 69-year-old male is admitted to the facility with urinary retention and undergoes a transurethral resection of the prostate (TURP). The final diagnosis is benign prostatic hypertrophy.

Code assignment: 600.01 *Hypertrophy (benign) of prostate, with urinary obstruction and other lower urinary tract symptoms (LUTS)* and 599.69 *Urinary obstruction, not elsewhere classified*, and 788.20 *Retention of urine, unspecified*

601 Inflammatory diseases of prostate

Code	Description
601.0	Acute prostatitis — (Use additional code to identify organism: 041.0, 041.1) — *sudden onset of inflammation of prostate*
601.1	Chronic prostatitis — (Use additional code to identify organism: 041.0, 041.1) — *persistent inflammation of prostate*
601.2	Abscess of prostate — (Use additional code to identify organism: 041.0, 041.1) — *pus pocket in wall of prostate*
601.3	Prostatocystitis — (Use additional code to identify organism: 041.0, 041.1) — *inflammation of both prostate and bladder*
601.4	Prostatitis in diseases classified elsewhere — (Code first underlying disease: 016.5, 039.8, 095.8, 116.0. Use additional code to identify organism: 041.0, 041.1)
601.8	Other specified inflammatory disease of prostate — (Use additional code to identify organism: 041.0, 041.1) — *cavitary prostatitis; granulomatous prostatitis*
601.9	Unspecified prostatitis — (Use additional code to identify organism: 041.0, 041.1) — *prostatitis NOS*

Coding Clarification
Use an additional code to identify the infective agent, such as Staphylococcus (041.1) or Streptococcus (041.0). For prostatitis in diseases classified elsewhere, code first the underlying disease. Excluded from this rubric are gonococcal prostatitis (098.12, 098.32), monilial prostatitis (112.2), and trichomonal prostatitis (131.03).

602 Other disorders of prostate

Code	Description
602.0	Calculus of prostate — *prostatic stone*
602.1	Congestion or hemorrhage of prostate — *bleeding or collection of fluid in prostate*
602.2	Atrophy of prostate — *loss of prostatic tissue*
602.3	Dysplasia of prostate — *prostatic intraepithelial neoplasia I (PIN I) and prostatic intraepithelial neoplasia II (PIN II)* AHA: Q4, 2001, 46
602.8	Other specified disorder of prostate — *prostatic fistula; prostatic infarction; periprostatic adhesions; prostatorrhea*
602.9	Unspecified disorder of prostate — *palpable prostate*

Coding Clarification
This subcategory excludes prostatic intraepithelial neoplasia III (PIN III), which is reported with code 233.4.

603 Hydrocele
Included in this rubric is a hydrocele of the spermatic cord, testis, or tunica vaginalis. The tunica vaginalis is the double-layer membrane that surrounds each testis; it consists of an outer parietal

layer and an inner visceral serous layer. In the embryo, the tunica vaginalis is an extension of the peritoneum, the membrane in the abdominal cavity. If, after it sepa-rates, the closure is not complete, fluid collects above the testes in a painless swelling called a hydrocele.

603.0	Encysted hydrocele
603.1	Infected hydrocele — (Use additional code to identify organism) — *infection in fluid-filled sac in testicular membrane*
603.8	Other specified type of hydrocele — *other specified hydrocele NEC*
603.9	Unspecified hydrocele — *hydrocele NOS*

Coding Clarification
Excluded from this rubric is a congenital hydrocele, reported with 778.6.

604 Orchitis and epididymitis

The testes are two small oval glands contained in the scrotum. The left testis is usually about 1.0 centimeter lower in the scrotal sac than the right. Both are suspended in the pouch by scrotal tissue and the spermatic cords; they are separated by a central partition. Dense, fibrous tissue, the tunica albuginea, encases each testis, enters the gland, and divides the glandular tissue into some 200 or 300 lobules. Each lobule contains coiled seminiferous tubules that produce sperm and which converge into about 20 small ducts that pass through the tunica albuginea and enter the epididymis.

The testes have two main functions: the production of sperm (spermatogenesis) and the secretion of hormones, mostly testosterone, which is responsible for the development of sexual characteristics in adolescent males and for the functioning of the male reproductive system.

Each epididymis lies along the top and back of the testis. It consists of a single, tightly coiled tube, enclosed in fibrous connective tissue casing. The epididymis tube is extremely small in diameter, but about 6.0 meters long. It forms a comma-shaped structure, with the blunt head at the top, a central body, and a tapered tail, which connects to the vas deferens.

The epididymis has three main functions, serving as one of the ducts through which the sperm pass, as a storage reservoir for maturing sperm, and as a contributor to seminal fluid.

604.0	Orchitis, epididymitis, and epididymo-orchitis, with abscess — (Use additional code to identify organism: 041.0, 041.1, 041.4) — *testicular abscess*
604.90	Unspecified orchitis and epididymitis — (Use additional code to identify organism: 041.0, 041.1, 041.4) — *orchitis and epididymitis NOS*
604.91	Orchitis and epididymitis in disease classified elsewhere — (Code first underlying disease: 032.89, 095.8, 125.0-125.9. Use additional code to identify organism: 041.0, 041.1, 041.4)
604.99	Other orchitis, epididymitis, and epididymo-orchitis, without mention of abscess — (Use additional code to identify organism: 041.0, 041.1, 041.4) — *orchitis, epididymitis and epididymo-orchitis, without mention of abscess NOS*

Coding Clarification
Use an additional code to identify the infective agent, such as *E. coli* (041.4), *Staphylococcus* (041.1), or *Streptococcus* (041.0). For orchitis and epididymitis in diseases classified elsewhere, code first the underlying disease. Excluded from this rubric are gonococcal orchitis (098.13, 098.33), mumps (072.0), tuberculous orchitis (016.5), and tuberculous epididymitis (016.4).

605 Redundant prepuce and phimosis

The prepuce is the double-layered sheath of skin covering the glans. Fused to the glans at birth by a shared membrane, the foreskin separates from the glans as the membrane dissolves. Phimosis refers to narrowness of the preputial sphincter that prevents the foreskin from being drawn back over the glans. A long foreskin, often due to redundant prepuce, may retain moisture, affecting the inner aspect of the prepuce and the glans. Balanitis, an inflammation of the glans, may develop in the devitalized tissues. Phimosis and persistent balanitis are the most common medical reasons for circumcision in the United States.

606 Male infertility
AHA: Q2, 1996, 9

A male is considered infertile when either of the two following conditions exists:

1. Inadequate sperm production: about 20 million sperm per milliliter of fluid is considered the lower limit of male fertility.

2. Abnormality in structure or motility of sperm that makes it unable to reach or penetrate the egg.

The most common male infertility factors include azoospermia (no sperm cells are produced) and oligospermia (few sperm cells are produced). Sometimes, sperm cells are malformed or they die before they can reach the egg. In some cases, a genetic disease such a cystic fibrosis or a chromosomal abnormality may be a factor.

Conditions that can cause male infertility include:

- Varicose veins in the spermatic cord since blood retained around the testes leads to an increase in temperature, which damages sperm
- Undescended testicles, which creates a higher temperature within the testes and, subsequently, impairs sperm production
- Radiation, chemotherapy, or removal of one or both testicles
- Hypothalamic or pituitary disorder
- Drug use, including alcohol, marijuana, female sex hormones, and the drugs used in chemotherapy

In addition, according to studies, the average sperm count is dropping worldwide, which may be due to both occupational and environmental exposure to chemicals that can disrupt hormone functions.

Tests for male infertility include sperm and semen analysis, physical exam for factors such as obstruction or congenital abnormality, a medical history as to the possibility of hormonal abnormality. The physical exam may indicate small, soft testicles, and hormone testing for FSH and testosterone may suggest that hormonal treatment may be beneficial. A biopsy can indicate if infection, injury, or other abnormality is interfering with the testis ability to produce sperm. Genetic testing may be performed to analyze whether azoospermia is associated with a chromosomal or DNA abnormality.

Between 30 and 50 percent of infertility in couples is attributable to the male.

606.0	Azoospermia — *Sertoli cell syndrome; Del Castillo's syndrome; infertility due to germinal cell aplasia*	
	AHA: Q2, 1996, 9	
606.1	Oligospermia — *due to germinal cell desquamation; hypospermatogenesis*	
	AHA: Q2, 1996, 9	
606.8	Infertility due to extratesticular causes — *due to drug therapy, infection, radiation*	
	AHA: Q2, 1996, 9	
606.9	Unspecified male infertility	

Coding Clarification

To report sperm count for fertility testing, see V26.21 *Fertility testing* or V26.22 *Aftercare following sterilization reversal.*

607 Disorders of penis

The penis is the organ of copulation and lies under the bladder, with the apex pointing downwards. It is composed of three cylindrical layers of tissue, which are enclosed in fibrous connective tissue, with an outer layer of skin. The smaller, lower cylinder is called the corpus spongiosum, through which the urethra passes to the external urinary meatus. The two upper and larger cylinders are the corpora cavernosa. At the end of the penis, the corpus spongiosum overlaps the ends of the corpora cavernosa, forming the bulging structure of the glans penis. Over this is a double fold of retractable skin called the prepuce, or foreskin. Surgical removal of foreskin is called circumcision.

The functions of the penis are copulation and to provide transport of semen through the urethra. Urine from the bladder is also excreted via the urethra.

Peyronie's disease is distinguished by plaque, or hard lump, that forms on the penis, due to causes unknown. The plaque develops on the upper or lower side of the penis in layers containing erectile tissue. It begins as a localized inflammation and can develop into a hardened scar.

Cases of Peyronie's disease range from mild to severe. Symptoms may develop slowly or appear overnight. Most of the time, the plaque that has hardened reduces flexibility, causing pain and forcing the penis to bend or arc during erection. The pain typically decreases over time, but the bend in the penis may remain a problem, making sexual intercourse complicated. In a small percentage of patients with the milder form of the disease, inflammation may resolve without pain or bending.

607.0	Leukoplakia of penis — *kraurosis*	
607.1	Balanoposthitis — (Use additional code to identify organism) — *balanitis*	
607.2	Other inflammatory disorders of penis — (Use additional code to identify organism) — *boil of corpus cavernosum*	
607.3	Priapism — *painful erection*	
607.81	Balanitis xerotica obliterans — *induratio penis plastica*	
607.82	Vascular disorders of penis — *embolism of corpus cavernosum; hemorrhage of corpus cavernosum*	
607.83	Edema of penis — *edema*	
607.84	Impotence of organic origin — *impotence, organic*	
	AHA: Q3, 1991, 11	
607.85	Peyronie's disease — *hardening of the corpora cavernosa of the penis, producing a fibrous chordee*	
	AHA: Q4, 2003, 64	
607.89	Other specified disorder of penis — *atrophy of corpus cavernosum; cicatrix; phagedena*	
607.9	Unspecified disorder of penis — *disorder NOS*	

Coding Clarification
Excluded from this rubric is phimosis (605) and impotence of inorganic origin (302.72).

608 Other disorders of male genital organs
608.0 Seminal vesiculitis — (Use additional code to identify organism) — *abscess of seminal vesicle; vesiculitis (seminal)*
608.1 Spermatocele — *epididymal cyst filled with sperm-containing fluid*
608.2 ⮕sth Torsion of testis

The testicle develops intra-abdominally in the abdomen and subsequently moves down into position into the scrotum. The blood supply follows along, trailing behind like a tail. Once in position in the scrotum, the testicle is encased in a sack called the tunica vaginalis. Early in life, the testicle can move around within the tunica vaginalis but progressively becomes more static as the patient continues to develop and age. This process of immobilization accounts for the increased incidence of torsion in the pediatric and young adult population.

Testicular torsion generally refers to a twisting of the testicle or spermatic cord structures that cuts off the blood supply to the testes. This is an emergent condition because of the risk of associated ischemia or testicular necrosis due to the interrupted circulation of blood and oxygen to the organ.

- Extravaginal torsion: Torsion of the spermatic cord just below the tunica vaginalis attachments that usually manifests in the neonatal period after having developed in utero. This type of torsion accounts for approximately 5 percent of all torsions. It is usually associated with high birth weight.
- Intravaginal torsion: Torsion within the tunica vaginalis also called the "bell-clapper" anomaly. It usually occurs in older children, with peak incidence occurring at approximately 13 years of age. This type of torsion accounts for roughly 16 percent of emergency room torsion encounters. Of note, the left testis is most frequently affected, with only 2 percent of cases presenting as bilateral torsions.
- The appendix testis is a small solid projection of tissue on the outer surface of the testis, which is a remnant of the embryologic mullerian duct. Torsion of this anatomical site was not previously separately classifiable. This type of torsion is often difficult to clinically differentiate from torsion of the testis.

The most common symptom associated with torsion is a sudden pain and tenderness in the scrotum or iliac fossa. The pain can present unilaterally or bilaterally, or spread into the groin, abdomen, or flank. Another term for this is "referred pain," whereby pain manifests in another site from its point of origin, or underlying cause. In these cases, an examination of the external genitalia is necessary to avoid misdiagnosis. This pain can occur when the patient is at rest or is active. Intermittent torsion is also possible, with pain symptoms that wax and wane. Other symptoms include nausea, vomiting, dysuria, swelling, and erythema. If left untreated, with progression of ischemia, the testicle is likely to become atrophic or necrotic. The degree and duration of torsion greatly influences the prognosis of whether the testes can be salvaged. In acute presentation, a delay of six to 24 hours between the onset of symptoms and surgical intervention significantly reduces the possibility of testicular salvage. Some clinical research has suggested that retention of an ischemic testicle can result in pathological changes to the remaining testis, and that a correlation may exist between the duration of torsion and abnormal semen production. This is of particular concern with the more dormant, mild-degree torsions in patients for which fertility is an issue.

Clinically, acute scrotal swelling in pediatric males usually indicates torsion of the testis until ruled out in the majority of patients. The presence of telltale signs and symptoms upon physical examination is usually sufficient to diagnose torsion. However, lab studies can assist in the diagnosis of torsion. A urinalysis or culture may help to exclude differential diagnoses of UTI or epididymitis in more quiescent or intermittent torsions. Imaging studies can also help diagnostic efforts. Doppler sonogram can confirm whether arterial blood flow is disrupted, and nuclear scans can rule out other conditions.

Urgent or emergent surgical intervention is required upon diagnosis of torsion. Manual torsion can be attempted under certain conditions but often is only temporary in nature and requires close follow-up. The potential for future definitive surgical intervention remains. In general, surgical options vary according to the age of the patient. In neonatal patients who are diagnosed with congenital torsion, an orchidopexy (anchoring) of the testes can be performed. In neonatal patients who develop spontaneous torsion, emergent surgical exploration is required to determine the appropriate corrective procedure. Postoperatively, a successful operation should yield restorative results, including a return of normal testicular appearance, positive arterial blood flow, and relief of pain. If a patient requires an orchiectomy due to necrosis, a testicular prosthesis may be elected at a later time.

608.20	Torsion of testis, unspecified
608.21	Extravaginal torsion of spermatic cord
608.22	Intravaginal torsion of spermatic cord
608.23	Torsion of appendix testis
608.24	Torsion of appendix epididymis
608.3	Atrophy of testis — *wasting of testicular tissue*
608.4	Other inflammatory disorder of male genital organs — (Use additional code to identify organism) — *scrotal boil; cellulitis of testicle*
608.81	Specified disorder of male genital organs in diseases classified elsewhere — (Code first underlying disease: 016.5, 125.0-125.9)
608.82	Hematospermia — *blood in ejaculate* AHA: Q4, 2001, 46
608.83	Specified vascular disorder of male genital organs — *testicular hematoma; hematocele, NOS, male* AHA: Q4, 2003, 110
608.84	Chylocele of tunica vaginalis — *chylocele*
608.85	Stricture of male genital organs — *stricture of vas deferens*
608.86	Edema of male genital organs — *fluid retention in male reproductive structure*
608.87	Retrograde ejaculation
608.89	Other specified disorder of male genital organs — *specified disorders NEC*
608.9	Unspecified disorder of male genital organs — *neuralgia; pain*

Coding Clarification
Use an additional code to identify the infective agent in infections and inflammatory disorders. In disorders of male genital organs in disease classified elsewhere, code first the underlying disease.

610-611 Disorders of Breast
The mammary glands are accessory organs of the female reproductive system, and are contained within the breast.

Each breast contains 15 to 20 lobes of glandular tissue consisting of smaller lobuli of alveoli (secreting cells) and ducts. The smaller ducts unite into a single milk-carrying duct for each lobe and these converge toward the nipple. The glandular tissue is contained within dense connective tissue that attaches to the pectoral muscle with suspensory ligaments, which extend from the skin to the pectoral muscle to provide support.

The nipple is located near the tip of each breast, surrounded by a circular area of pigmented and irregular surfaced skin called the areola.

The function of the mammary gland is lactation, which is the secretion of colostrum and subsequently milk for the nourishment of newborn infants. Successful lactation relies on pre- and postnatal production of hormones including progesterone, estrogen, prolactin, and oxytocin.

610 Benign mammary dysplasias
Benign mammary dysplasia, also known as chronic cystic mastitis or fibrocystic breast disease, is commonly found in normal breasts and believed to be a normal variant of tissue, and not a disease. Symptoms include a dense, irregular, and bumpy consistency in the breast tissue, especially in the outer upper quadrants and breast discomfort that is persistent or that occurs intermittently. Symptoms may range from mild to severe and typically peak just before each menstrual period and improve immediately after the menstrual period. Self-care may include restricting dietary fat and caffeine. Oral contraceptives may be prescribed because they often decrease the symptoms. Danazol, a synthetic androgen, may be used in severe cases.

610.0	Solitary cyst of breast — *cyst (solitary)*
610.1	Diffuse cystic mastopathy — *cysts scattered throughout* AHA: Q2, 2006, 10
610.2	Fibroadenosis of breast — *cystic fibroadenosis of breast; diffuse fibroadenosis*
610.3	Fibrosclerosis of breast — *fibrosclerosis*
610.4	Mammary duct ectasia — *periductal mastitis*
610.8	Other specified benign mammary dysplasias — *mazoplasia; sebaceous cyst*
610.9	Unspecified benign mammary dysplasia — *benign NOS*

611 Other disorders of breast

611.0	Inflammatory disease of breast — *acute or chronic abscess of areola; mammillary fistula; acute or subacute mastitis*
611.1	Hypertrophy of breast — *massive pubertal hypertrophy*
611.2	Fissure of nipple — *crack in nipple*
611.3	Fat necrosis of breast — *fat necrosis (segmental)*
611.4	Atrophy of breast — *wasting of breast tissue*
611.5	Galactocele
611.6	Galactorrhea not associated with childbirth — *flow of milk*
611.71	Mastodynia — *pain*
611.72	Lump or mass in breast — *lump* AHA: Q2, 2003, 4-5
611.79	Other sign and symptom in breast — *induration; inversion of nipple; thickening*
611.8	Other specified disorder of breast — *hematoma, (nontraumatic); infarction; pendulous*
611.9	Unspecified breast disorder — *disorder NOS*

614–616 Inflammatory Disease of Female Pelvic Organs

614 Inflammatory disease of ovary, fallopian tube, pelvic cellular tissue, and peritoneum

- **614.0** Acute salpingitis and oophoritis — (Use additional code to identify organism: 041.0, 041.1) — *any condition classifiable to 614.2, specified as acute or subacute*
- **614.1** Chronic salpingitis and oophoritis — (Use additional code to identify organism: 041.0, 041.1) — *hydrosalpinx; salpingitis follicularis*
- **614.2** Salpingitis and oophoritis not specified as acute, subacute, or chronic — (Use additional code to identify organism: 041.0, 041.1) — *pyosalpinx; tubo-ovarian inflammatory disease*
  AHA: Q2, 1991, 5
- **614.3** Acute parametritis and pelvic cellulitis — (Use additional code to identify organism: 041.0, 041.1) — *acute inflammatory pelvic disease*
- **614.4** Chronic or unspecified parametritis and pelvic cellulitis — (Use additional code to identify organism: 041.0, 041.1) — *chronic inflammatory pelvic disease; abscess of broad ligament; pelvic cellulitis*
- **614.5** Acute or unspecified pelvic peritonitis, female — (Use additional code to identify organism: 041.0, 041.1) — *metroperitonitis*
  AHA: Q4, 2005, 74
- **614.6** Pelvic peritoneal adhesions, female (postoperative) (postinfection) — (Use additional code to identify any associated infertility, 628.2. Use additional code to identify organism: 041.0, 041.1) — *peritubal adhesions, tubo-ovarian adhesions*
  AHA: Q3, 1994, 12; Q3, 1995, 7; Q1, 2003, 4; Q3, 2003, 6
- **614.7** Other chronic pelvic peritonitis, female — (Use additional code to identify organism: 041.0, 041.1)
- **614.8** Other specified inflammatory disease of female pelvic organs and tissues — (Use additional code to identify organism: 041.0, 041.1) — *specified inflammatory disease of female pelvic organs and tissues NEC*
- **614.9** Unspecified inflammatory disease of female pelvic organs and tissues — (Use additional code to identify organism: 041.0, 041.1)

615 Inflammatory diseases of uterus, except cervix

- **615.0** Acute inflammatory disease of uterus, except cervix — (Use additional code to identify organism: 041.0, 041.1) — *any condition classifiable to 615.9, specified as acute or subacute*
- **615.1** Chronic inflammatory disease of uterus, except cervix — (Use additional code to identify organism: 041.0, 041.1) — *any condition classifiable to 615.9, specified as chronic*
- **615.9** Unspecified inflammatory disease of uterus — (Use additional code to identify organism: 041.0, 041.1) — *endometritis; endomyometritis; perimetritis; pyometra*

616 Inflammatory disease of cervix, vagina, and vulva

- **616.0** Cervicitis and endocervicitis — (Use additional code to identify organism: 041.0, 041.1) — *cervicitis with or without mention of erosion or ectropion; Nabothian (gland) cyst of follicle*
- **616.10** Unspecified vaginitis and vulvovaginitis — (Use additional code to identify organism: 041.0, 041.1, 041.4) — *postirradiation vaginitis; vaginitis NOS*
- **616.11** Vaginitis and vulvovaginitis in diseases classified elsewhere — (Code first underlying disease, 127.4.)
- **616.2** Cyst of Bartholin's gland — (Use additional code to identify organism: 041.0, 041.1) — *fluid-filled sac within one of the paired glands*
- **616.3** Abscess of Bartholin's gland — (Use additional code to identify organism: 041.0, 041.1) — *pocket of pus within one of the paired glands*
- **616.4** Other abscess of vulva — (Use additional code to identify organism: 041.0, 041.1) — *vulvar carbuncle; vulvar boil*
- **616.50** Unspecified ulceration of vulva — (Use additional code to identify organism: 041.0, 041.1) — *ulcer NOS of vulva*
- **616.51** Ulceration of vulva in disease classified elsewhere — (Code first underlying disease: 016.7, 136.1.)
- **616.8** Other specified inflammatory disease of cervix, vagina, and vulva

The cells of the mucosal tissues are especially vulnerable to damage by chemotherapy, radiation therapy, and immune system and other diseases. Oral mucositis is the most common anatomic manifestation, but mucositis can also occur throughout the body where there are mucous membranes; through the entire digestive tract; anywhere from the esophagus to the rectum, and also at genital and respiratory sites.

Mucositis of female genital sites such as the cervix, vagina, and vulva present with signs of inflammation, redness, pseudomembrane formation, bleeding, or open sores (ulcers). Symptoms include pain and discomfort, a "raw" feeling, sticky secretions, or bleeding and swelling of mucous membranes.

The severity of mucositis ranges from mild to severe, depending on the type of treatment response to therapies, immune and hematological status, as well as other factors. Duration of illness depends upon the severity of the condition and effectiveness of treatment.

There is no single treatment or preventative measure for mucositis. Instead, treatment is often palliative in nature, or directed at specific problems such as preventing infection, ensuring adequate hygiene, controlling bleeding, and controlling pain. Oral, local, or topical or IV pain medications, irrigation, and treatment of secondary infections are commonly indicated. Corticosteroid medications are often helpful in reducing inflammation.

616.81	Mucositis (ulcerative) of cervix, vagina and vulva — (Use additional E code to identify adverse effects of therapy, such as radiation therapy [E879.2] or antineoplastic and immunosuppressive drugs [E930.7, E933.1])
616.89	Other inflammatory disease of cervix, vagina and vulva — *caruncle, ulcer, Bartholin's gland adenitis*
616.9	Unspecified inflammatory disease of cervix, vagina, and vulva — (Use additional code to identify organism: 041.0, 041.1) — *vaginal disorder NOS*

Coding Clarification
If applicable, mucositis due to antineoplastic and immunosuppressive drugs or radiation therapies will be identified first, followed by the appropriate causative external causes (E code) sequenced second. Assign the appropriate additional code — E930.7 *Antineoplastic antibiotics*, E933.1 *Antineoplastic and immunosuppressive drugs*, or E879.2 for radiation therapy — as the causative agent.

617–629 Other Disorders of Female Genital Tract

617 Endometriosis
Endometriosis is the presence of endometrial tissue (functioning endometrial glands and stoma) outside of its normal location (lining the uterine cavity). The etiology is unknown, though previous uterine surgery or heredity may be predisposing factors.

Signs and symptoms of endometriosis include acquired dysmenorrhea characterized by pain (that usually begins five to seven days before menstruation and lasts two to three days) in the lower abdomen, vagina, posterior pelvis, or back; bleeding from the vagina, rectum, or bladder depending on the site involved; dyspareunia; or cramps. A pelvic exam may locate sites of endometriosis, while laparoscopy confirms the diagnosis and stage of disease. Diagnostic radiology such as barium enema may rule out malignancy or inflammatory bowel disease.

Therapies include drugs such as progestins, danazol (a testosterone derivative), oral contraceptives, surgery ranging from local excision of endometrial tissue and preservation of the pelvic organs (for women who wish to bear children) to total abdominal hysterectomy with bilateral salpingo-oophorectomy (for older women and those with extensive disease).

Associated conditions include infertility, spontaneous abortion, and pelvic adhesions.

617.0	Endometriosis of uterus — *adenomyosis; cervical endometriosis*
	AHA: Q3, 1992, 7
617.1	Endometriosis of ovary — *chocolate cyst of ovary; endometrial cystoma of ovary*
617.2	Endometriosis of fallopian tube — *aberrant uterine mucosal tissue inflaming tissues of fallopian tube*
617.3	Endometriosis of pelvic peritoneum — *aberrant uterine mucosal tissue inflaming tissues of peritoneum*
617.4	Endometriosis of rectovaginal septum and vagina — *aberrant uterine mucosal tissue inflaming tissues behind or in vagina*
617.5	Endometriosis of intestine — *endometriosis of appendix, colon or rectum*
617.6	Endometriosis in scar of skin — *aberrant uterine mucosal tissue inflaming scar tissues*
617.8	Endometriosis of other specified sites — *endometriosis of bladder, lung, umbilicus, vulva*
617.9	Endometriosis, site unspecified — *endometriosis NOS*

618 Genital prolapse
Genital prolapse is the protrusion or projection of pelvic organs into the vagina or outside the vaginal opening caused by weakening or damaged support structures. Types of prolapse include:

- Uterine prolapse: descent of the uterus and cervix down the vaginal canal due to weak or damaged pelvic support structures
- Cystocele: tissues supporting the wall between the bladder and the vagina weaken, allowing a portion of the bladder to descend and protrude into the vagina
- Urethrocele: urethra descends and presses into the vagina
- Rectocele: tissues supporting the wall between the vagina and the rectum weaken allowing the rectum to descend and protrude into the vagina
- Enterocele: portion of intestine herniates and protrudes into the vagina
- Vaginal vault prolapse: vagina descends, usually following a hysterectomy
- A perineocele in the female is a hernia in the perineum occurring between the rectum and the vagina. In the male, it is a hernia between the rectum and prostate.

Symptoms of prolapse vary according to the organs involved and the severity of the prolapse. Those commonly reported include aching discomfort in the pelvic region, urinary and bowel problems, and dull backache.

There are a number of contributing factors that can cause genital prolapse, including pregnancy and childbirth, menopause, raised pressure in the abdomen, and genetic predisposition.

Diagnosis involves a medical history and a physical examination, including a rectal exam if a rectocele or enterocele is suspected. The woman may be asked to cough or push down during the exam to raise the pressure in the abdomen and push any prolapse downwards, making it easier to see or feel.

There is a range of treatment options available for prolapse, both non-surgical and surgical. Non-surgical approaches include reducing pressure placed on the pelvis, pessaries (e.g., device that is inserted into the upper part of the vagina to provide support to the pelvic structures), and hormonal therapy. Surgical treatment includes vaginal repair, hysterectomy and vaginal repair, vaginal vault repair, and uterine preservation surgery (i.e., partial amputation of the cervix and the shortening of supporting ligaments).

When a hysterectomy is performed without an accompanying suspension procedure, vaginal vault prolapse or a prolapse of the cervico-vaginal stump may occur in approximately 5 percent to 30 percent of cases. Alternately, suspension procedures performed at the time of hysterectomy carry a small risk of failure, resulting in an iatrogenic prolapse.

Post-hysterectomy, the portion of the cervix left in situ may collapse and descend down the vaginal vault, resulting in tears of the fascial points of attachment. This can also occur when the cervical stump is pushed out of the vaginal vault by loops of small intestine. Similar conditions include post-hysterectomy vaginal vault or cervical stump prolapse or enterocele. Historically, the cervix was removed at the time of hysterectomy to reduce the risk of cervical cancer. However, if indicated, the patient may opt to leave the cervix in place so as to either help support the vaginal vault or to preserve or improve sexual function.

Common signs and symptoms include a mass or protrusion from the vagina, with pelvic pressure, urinary incontinence, or constipation and backache. Prolapse symptoms vary according to the degree of severity of the prolapse:

- Mild: Discomfort, a sensation of dragging down in the pelvic region.
- Moderate: Increased vaginal pressure, more pronounced discomfort and pain while standing or dyspareunia.
- Severe: The pelvic organs become visible from the vagina; urinary and/or fecal incontinence, dyspareunia, constipation, dropping of the pelvic organs so far below that they become visible from the vagina.

Treatment includes both medical and surgical options. Nonsurgical (medical) options include:

- Pessary: A small device inserted vaginally to help support the pelvic organs. Most commonly used to treat mild to moderate prolapse. Surgical intervention is necessary to treat severe prolapse.
- Kegel exercises: Exercises aimed at strengthening the pelvic floor muscles. Pelvic strengthening can also assist in retention of a pessary device.
- Hormone replacement therapy (HRT): Assists in support of pelvic organs by improving the quality of pelvic tissues.

Surgical techniques vary according to the type and severity of prolapse; however, post-hysterectomy prolapse correction requires a suspension procedure. Suspension procedures anchor the cervical stump or vagina to strong ligaments in the posterior pelvic cavity. Both vaginal and laparoscopic surgical approaches are available; however, the laparoscopic approach is becoming preferred; which enables suspension sutures to be placed higher in the pelvis than with the vaginal approach, which also improves post-surgical results.

Sacro-spinus colpopexy is a type of suspension procedure increasingly performed to treat post-hysterectomy prolapse. Similar terms include hitch operation, or sacral hitch repair. For this correction, synthetic mesh is attached to the top of the cervical stump, and the mesh is anchored or sutured onto the sacral bone. This procedure is relatively new and is expected to decrease the chance of recurrence.

Sacro-colpopexy can also be performed by suturing polypropylene tape bilaterally near the coccyx bone to the site of the prolapse.

Surgical approaches can vary, but a posterior suspension can be performed least invasively via bilateral buttock incisions with the assistance of a tunneling device. Regardless of the surgical approach, these types of repairs use surgical tape to create a sort of synthetic ligament. During healing, collagen deposits around the tape, which lifts and supports the cervical stump back into position.

Diseases of the Genitourinary System

In lieu of a vaginal vault suspension procedure, total colpocleisis is an option for women with a complete prolapse, who do not wish to remain sexually active. This procedure is typically performed for elderly women of fragile health. Total colpocleisis procedure is often performed with an accompanying sling procedure to correct urinary incontinence. Under local, epidural, or spinal anesthesia, a transvaginal approach is used to close the vagina on the inside.

618.00	Prolapse of vaginal walls without mention of uterine prolapse, unspecified
618.01	Cystocele without mention of uterine prolapse, midline
618.02	Cystocele without mention of uterine prolapse, lateral
618.03	Urethrocele without mention of uterine prolapse
618.04	Rectocele without mention of uterine prolapse
618.05	Perineocele without mention of uterine prolapse
618.09	Other prolapse of vaginal walls without mention of uterine prolapse
618.1	Uterine prolapse without mention of vaginal wall prolapse — (Use additional code to identify urinary incontinence: 625.6, 788.31, 788.33-788.39) — *descensus uteri; complete uterine prolapse*
618.2	Uterovaginal prolapse, incomplete — (Use additional code to identify urinary incontinence: 625.6, 788.31, 788.33-788.39) — *downward displacement of uterus into vagina*
618.3	Uterovaginal prolapse, complete — (Use additional code to identify urinary incontinence: 625.6, 788.31, 788.33-788.39) — *downward displacement and exposure of uterus within external genitalia*
618.4	Uterovaginal prolapse, unspecified — (Use additional code to identify urinary incontinence: 625.6, 788.31, 788.33-788.39) — *uterine prolapse NOS*
618.5	Prolapse of vaginal vault after hysterectomy — (Use additional code to identify urinary incontinence: 625.6, 788.31, 788.33-788.39) — *posthysterectomy vaginal vault prolapse*
618.6	Vaginal enterocele, congenital or acquired — (Use additional code to identify urinary incontinence: 625.6, 788.31, 788.33-788.39) — *pelvic enterocele, congenital or acquired*
618.7	Genital prolapse, old laceration of muscles of pelvic floor — (Use additional code to identify urinary incontinence: 625.6, 788.31, 788.33-788.39)
618.81	Incompetence or weakening of pubocervical tissue
618.82	Incompetence or weakening of rectovaginal tissue
618.83	Pelvic muscle wasting
618.84	Cervical stump prolapse
618.89	Other specified genital prolapse
618.9	Unspecified genital prolapse — (Use additional code to identify urinary incontinence: 625.6, 788.31, 788.33-788.39) — *prolapsus*

Documentation Issues
Coders should review the record for physician documentation of urinary incontinence. If present, this condition should be reported with additional code 625.6 or with an appropriate code from subcategory 788.3.

Coding Scenario
A 37-year-old woman who gave birth one year ago is experiencing sensations of bladder fullness, or incomplete emptying after urination and urine leakage or incontinence upon changing position. Upon physical examination, the physician notes bulging in the anterior vaginal wall, some loss of normal vaginal rugae, but the lateral vaginal sulcus is intact and diagnoses her with a central defect cystocele with overflow incontinence.

Code assignment: 618.01 *Cystocele, midline* and 788.38 *Overflow incontinence*

619 Fistula involving female genital tract
A fistula is an abnormal channel or duct connecting an organ to another organ, body cavity, or the surface. Types include:

- Blind (open on one end, but connects to two structures)
- Complete (external and internal openings)
- Incomplete (tube from the skin is closed on the inside and does not connect to any internal organ or structure)

Fistulas of the female genital tract include rectovaginal, vesicovaginal, vaginoperineal, cervicovesical, ureterovaginal, urethrovesico-vaginal, and enterovaginal.

619.0	Urinary-genital tract fistula, female — *cervicovesical, ureterovaginal, urethrovesicovaginal fistula*
619.1	Digestive-genital tract fistula, female — *intestinouterine, rectovulvar, uterorectal fistula*
619.2	Genital tract-skin fistula, female — *vaginoperineal fistula*
619.8	Other specified fistula involving female genital tract — *cervical, vaginal fistula*
619.9	Unspecified fistula involving female genital tract — *genital tract fistula NOS*

620 Noninflammatory disorders of ovary, fallopian tube, and broad ligament

620.0	Follicular cyst of ovary — *cyst of graafian follicle*
620.1	Corpus luteum cyst or hematoma — *lutein cyst*
620.2	Other and unspecified ovarian cyst — *corpus albicans cyst of ovary; retention cyst NOS of ovary*
620.3	Acquired atrophy of ovary and fallopian tube — *senile involution of ovary*

620.4	Prolapse or hernia of ovary and fallopian tube — *displacement of ovary and fallopian tube; salpingocele*		621.6	Malposition of uterus — *anteversion of uterus; retroflexion of uterus*
620.5	Torsion of ovary, ovarian pedicle, or fallopian tube — *torsion of accessory tube; torsion of hydatid of Morgagni*		621.7	Chronic inversion of uterus — *uterus is turned inside out*
			621.8	Other specified disorders of uterus, not elsewhere classified — *boggy uterus; sclerotic endometrium*
620.6	Broad ligament laceration syndrome — *Masters-Allen syndrome*		621.9	Unspecified disorder of uterus — *uterine disorder NOS*
620.7	Hematoma of broad ligament — *hematocele, broad ligament*			

621 Disorders of uterus, not elsewhere classified

A uterine polyp is a growth from the endometrium. The polyp can contain endometrial, fibrous and muscular tissue. The polyp may cause pain and bleeding and may interfere with fertility. Surgical intervention may be required to treat a symptomatic polyp.

Uterine subinvolution is failure of the uterus to return to normal size after a physiological hypertrophy as in child birth or infection. Treatment may include curettage, methergine or antibiotics.

Endometrial hyperplasia is described as an abnormal overgrowth of the normal cells that line the uterus, called the endometrium. This overgrowth often causes heavy or prolonged menstrual flow (menorrhagia), bleeding after menopause, and bleeding between normal periods or at irregular intervals (metrorrhagia). Endometrial hyperplasia results from estrogen production in excess or prolonged amounts of estrogen, such as a reaction to hormone replacement therapy after menopause. The difference between simple and complex is determined by cytology studies where arborescent cell clusters are observed along with the types of branching and number of layers of stromal bundles inside the clusters.

621.0	Polyp of corpus uteri — *endometrial polyp*
621.1	Chronic subinvolution of uterus
621.2	Hypertrophy of uterus — *bulky uterus*
621.30	Endometrial hyperplasia, unspecified
621.31	Simple endometrial hyperplasia without atypia
621.32	Complex endometrial hyperplasia without atypia
621.33	Endometrial hyperplasia with atypia
621.4	Hematometra
621.5	Intrauterine synechiae — *adhesions of uterus; Asherman's syndrome*

622 Noninflammatory disorders of cervix

Cervical dysplasia is described as abnormal cells in the cervix. These cells are precancerous and could lead to invasive carcinoma. Cervical dysplasia is usually asymptomatic and is usually diagnosed by annual Pap smears from the cervix. The difference between mild and moderate dysplasia of the cervix is based on cytology studies. CIN grade I is considered mild dysplasia and CIN grade II is considered moderate dysplasia.

622.0	Erosion and ectropion of cervix — *ulcer of cervix*
622.10	Dysplasia of cervix, unspecified
622.11	Mild dysplasia of cervix
622.12	Moderate dysplasia of cervix
622.2	Leukoplakia of cervix (uteri)
622.3	Old laceration of cervix — *adhesions of cervix*
622.4	Stricture and stenosis of cervix — *atresia (acquired) of cervix; cervical contracture*
622.5	Incompetence of cervix — *cervical incompetence*
622.6	Hypertrophic elongation of cervix — *overgrowth of cervix extends downward into vagina*
622.7	Mucous polyp of cervix — *polyp NOS of cervix*
622.8	Other specified noninflammatory disorder of cervix — *senile) atrophy of cervix; fibrosis of cervix*
622.9	Unspecified noninflammatory disorder of cervix — *noninflammatory NOS*

Coding Clarification
Report 233.1 for CIN grade III or severe cervical dysplasia.

Report 795.04 for Pap smear of the cervix with low grade squamous intraepithelial lesion (LGSIL).

Report 795.05 for Pap smear of the cervix with high grade squamous intraepithelial lesion (HGSIL).

623 Noninflammatory disorders of vagina

623.0	Dysplasia of vagina — *abnormal cells*
623.1	Leukoplakia of vagina — *thickened white patches*
623.2	Stricture or atresia of vagina — *(Use additional E code to identify any external cause)*
623.3	Tight hymenal ring — *rigid hymen, acquired or congenital; tight introitus*
623.4	Old vaginal laceration — *scarring*
623.5	Leukorrhea, not specified as infective — *thick, white discharge*
623.6	Vaginal hematoma — *blood pocket*

Diseases of the Genitourinary System

623.7	Polyp of vagina — *mucosal growth*	
623.8	Other specified noninflammatory disorder of vagina	
623.9	Unspecified noninflammatory disorder of vagina — *noninflammatory disease NOS*	

624 Noninflammatory disorders of vulva and perineum

624.0	Dystrophy of vulva — *kraurosis; leukoplakia*
624.1	Atrophy of vulva — *wasting of external genitalia*
624.2	Hypertrophy of clitoris — *overgrowth of erectile body at anterior cleft of vulva*
624.3	Hypertrophy of labia — *vulvar hypertrophy NOS*
624.4	Old laceration or scarring of vulva
624.5	Hematoma of vulva — *pocket of blood in tissue*
624.6	Polyp of labia and vulva — *mucosal growth*
624.8	Other specified noninflammatory disorder of vulva and perineum — *cyst; edema; vitiligo*
	AHA: Q1, 1995, 8; Q1, 2003, 13
624.9	Unspecified noninflammatory disorder of vulva and perineum — *unspecified*

625 Pain and other symptoms associated with female genital organs

625.0	Dyspareunia — *pain during sexual intercourse*
625.1	Vaginismus — *colpospasm; vulvismus*
625.2	Mittelschmerz — *ovulation pain*
625.3	Dysmenorrhea — *painful menstruation*
	AHA: Q2, 1994, 12
625.4	Premenstrual tension syndromes — *premenstrual syndrome; menstrual migraine*
	AHA: Q4, 2003, 116
625.5	Pelvic congestion syndrome — *congestion-fibrosis syndrome*
625.6	Female stress incontinence — *involuntary escape of urine during coughing, laughing or sneezing*
625.8	Other specified symptom associated with female genital organs — *palpable uterus; perineal swelling; vicarious (nasal) menstruation*
	AHA: Nov-Dec, 1985, 16
625.9	Unspecified symptom associated with female genital organs — *pain in broad ligament, ovary, round ligament*

626 Disorders of menstruation and other abnormal bleeding from female genital tract

A woman's monthly cycle can be divided into three segments: menstruation, the follicular phase, and the luteal phase. During the middle, or follicular, segment, follicle stimulating hormone (FSH) prompts eggs in the ovary to mature and sprout a follicle, or layer of cells, which secrete estrogen. Estrogen levels then build until at their peak FSH is turned off and luteinizing hormone (LH) takes over. LH causes ovulation, the departure of the egg from the ovary. Progesterone, master hormone of the last, or luteal, stage continues development of the endometrium, the lining of the uterus. When conception does not occur, all hormone levels drop and menstruation begins. Uterine muscles contracting to squeeze out the lining may cause cramping; painful cramping is thought to be due to higher levels of prostaglandins. The egg bursting out of the ovary can cause pain on one side low in the abdomen 12 to 14 days after a period. Menstruation can begin at any time between the ages of 8 to 18; menopause generally occurs between the ages of 40 to 60.

626.0	Absence of menstruation — *amenorrhea (primary) (secondary)*
626.1	Scanty or infrequent menstruation — *hypomenorrhea; oligomenorrhea*
626.2	Excessive or frequent menstruation — *menometrorrhagia; menorrhagia; polymenorrhea*
	AHA: Q2, 1994, 12
626.3	Puberty bleeding — *pubertal menorrhagia*
626.4	Irregular menstrual cycle — *irregular periods*
626.5	Ovulation bleeding — *regular intermenstrual bleeding*
626.6	Metrorrhagia — *irregular intermenstrual bleeding*
626.7	Postcoital bleeding — *vaginal bleeding after sexual intercourse*
626.8	Other disorder of menstruation and other abnormal bleeding from female genital tract — *delayed menstruation*
626.9	Unspecified disorder of menstruation and other abnormal bleeding from female genital tract — *paramenia*

627 Menopausal and postmenopausal disorders

Menopause refers to a process occurring in a female's reproductive life. Physically, this process has four stages:

1. Premenopause refers to the cusp of menopause. Periods may be irregular, but there are no classic menopausal symptoms such as hot flashes or vaginal dryness. Irregularity can run from shorter or longer periods with bouts of amenorrhea (no period).

2. Perimenopause refers to the onset of symptoms, such as erratic periods, hot flashes, and vaginal dryness, which are indicators of a drop in estrogen. This stage lasts about four years, covering the first two years prior to the last period to the next two years following the last menstrual period. Decreased levels of estrogen affects REM sleep, which precipitates the stress, depression, and anxiety associated with menopause.

3. Menopause refers to the final menstrual period, which is marked once the female has had no periods for one year. Vaginal bleeding after more than one year of a menstrual period is considered normal.

4. Postmenopause refers to the third of a woman's life, ranging from women who have been free of menstrual periods for at least one year to women celebrating a century birthday.

Use subclassification 627.1 to report bleeding from the female reproductive tract (vulva, vagina, cervix, or endometrium) occurring one year or more after menopause.

Signs and symptoms of postmenopausal bleeding include vaginal bleeding, excess cervical mucus, and atrophy of vaginal mucosa. Lab work such as analysis of cytologic smears from the cervix and endocervical canal, blood work to assess hormone levels, and dilation and curettage (D&C) may show pathological findings in the endometrium.

Therapies include estrogen creams to correct estrogen deficiency, D&C, and hysterectomy for endometrial carcinoma.

Associated conditions include hormonal imbalances, cancer, atrophic changes of the vagina or endometrium, and adverse effects of estrogen therapy.

627.0	Premenopausal menorrhagia — *climacteric menorrhagia; preclimacteric menorrhagia*
627.1	Postmenopausal bleeding — *bleeding after onset of menopause*
627.2	Symptomatic menopausal or female climacteric states — *climacteric syndrome*
627.3	Postmenopausal atrophic vaginitis — *senile (atrophic) vaginitis*
627.4	Symptomatic states associated with artificial menopause — *postartificial menopause syndromes*
627.8	Other specified menopausal and postmenopausal disorder — *atrophic menopausal cervix; postmenopausal endometrium (atrophic)*
627.9	Unspecified menopausal and postmenopausal disorder — *menopausal disorder NOS*

Coding Clarification

To report post-menopausal status without symptoms or disorder, see V49.81 *Postmenopausal status* (age-related) (natural). Excluded from this rubric is premature menopause NOS, classifiable to 256.31.

628 Female infertility
AHA: Q1, 1995, 7; Q2, 1996, 9

This rubric classifies the inability to conceive for at least a one year period after regular intercourse in the absence of contraceptive measures. There are three basic types of infertility: functional, anatomic, and psychogenic.

Functional infertility is due to impairment of the complex hormonal interactions involved in female reproduction. Anatomic infertility can be the result of congenital malformation, scarring or adhesions due to previous infection, atrophy due to hormone deficiency, or any other condition that mechanically impairs or prevents conception. An example of psychogenic infertility is the failure to ovulate due to the stress of marital discord (codes 628.0 and 306.59).

628.0	Female infertility associated with anovulation — (Use additional code for any associated Stein-Levanthal syndrome, 256.4) — *anovulatory cycle* AHA: Q1, 1995, 7; Q2, 1996, 9
628.1	Female infertility of pituitary-hypothalamic origin — (Code first underlying disease: 253.0-253.4, 253.8)
628.2	Female infertility of tubal origin — (Use additional code for any associated peritubal adhesions, 614.6) — *tubal occlusion; tubal stenosis* AHA: Q1, 1995, 7; Q2, 1996, 9
628.3	Female infertility of uterine origin — (Use additional code for any associated tuberculous endometriosis, 016.7) — *infertility associated with congenital anomaly of uterus; nonimplantation* AHA: Q1, 1995, 7; Q2, 1996, 9
628.4	Female infertility of cervical or vaginal origin — *infertility associated with anomaly of cervical mucus, or congenital structural anomaly* AHA: Q1, 1995, 7; Q2, 1996, 9
628.8	Female infertility of other specified origin — *other specified cause* AHA: Q1, 1995, 7; Q2, 1996, 9
628.9	Female infertility of unspecified origin — *unknown cause* AHA: Q1, 1995, 7; Q2, 1996, 9

Coding Clarification

As appropriate, code first the underlying cause, as in adiposogenital dystrophy (253.8) or anterior pituitary disorder (253.0-253.4).

629 Other disorders of female genital organs

Although not practiced in this country, female circumcision or castration is practiced in other countries, from which the U.S. is receiving a number of immigrant populations. The World Health Organization has termed this as female genital mutilation, or FGM. Women who have undergone this type of mutilation present with a special set of serious problems and concerns not normally seen in relation to gynecological healthcare. Problems include difficult intercourse, childbirth, and pelvic infections. Those physicians who see a large immigrant population may have up to two thirds of their female patients present with some form of FGM.

Three levels of genital mutilation are practiced. The first type is known as clitoridectomy, with part or the entire clitoris removed. The second type involves the clitoris and the labia minora being amputated. These two types account for 85% of those who have had female castration performed. The third type is a severe form in which the clitoris is removed and most or all of the labia minora are also cut off. The labia majora are incised and made into a hood of skin to heal over the urethral and vaginal opening. After healing, another small opening is made for release of urine and menstrual blood. This third type is called infibulation. These patients require deinfibulation to permit intercourse, the deliver of a baby, or a pelvic exam. They also present with many more pelvic infections due to the interference of fluid drainage. Some women may also have had deinfibulation done to deliver a baby and then been reinfibulated. A greater risk of maternal and fetal death occurs for subsequent pregnancies.

629.0	Hematocele, female, not elsewhere classified
629.1	Hydrocele, canal of Nuck — *cyst of canal of Nuck (acquired)*
629.20	Female genital mutilation status, unspecified
	AHA: Q4, 2004, 88
629.21	Female genital mutilation, Type I status
629.22	Female genital mutilation, Type II status
	AHA: Q4, 2004, 90
629.23	Female genital mutilation, Type III status
	AHA: Q4, 2004, 90
629.29	Other female genital mutilation status — *genital cutting or mutilation Type IV, or other female genital cutting status*
629.81	Habitual aborter without current pregnancy

Habitual spontaneous abortion (or recurrent miscarriage) status can be defined as the loss of three or more consecutive pregnancies. Multiple causes can be attributed to recurrent miscarriage, such as maternal illness and hormone imbalances, polycystic ovarian syndrome, immunity disorders, uterine disease, and malfunction and lifestyle issues. However, chromosomal abnormalities and the presence of antiphospholipid antibodies are some of the most common underlying factors that precipitate encounters for genetic testing associated with recurrent spontaneous abortions.

It has been estimated that more than half of spontaneous abortions can be attributed to chromosomal abnormalities; whereby a defective sperm or ovum grows into a nonsustainable fetus. In order to diagnose the underlying genetic abnormality, a karyotype test can map out the chromosomes of the fetal tissue. Even though chromosomal abnormalities account for the majority of spontaneous abortions, only about 5 percent of abnormalities are attributed to parental genes as a role in the miscarriage. Chromosomal studies conducted via a sample of the parent's blood can explain (in genetic terms, at least) the underlying cause of the genetic malfunction. Abnormal karyotypes predispose a patient to the risk of recurrent miscarriages. Depending on the degree of risk and the patient's desire to conceive, as well as other clinical considerations, the patient may or may not be able to conceive successfully. Options for these patients may include using donor eggs or sperm, or adoption.

This code excludes habitual aborter with current pregnancy, which is reported with a code from category 646.3.

Coding of circumstances associated with habitual abortion status are as follows:

With current pregnancy, assign a code from category 634 *Spontaneous abortion*; when the pregnancy terminated in spontaneous abortion; assign a code from subcategory 646.3 *Habitual aborter*, if this factor is complicating the current pregnancy; for encounter for supervision of high-risk pregnancy assign V23.2 *Pregnancy with history of abortion*.

Without current pregnancy, assign code 629.81 *Habitual aborter without current pregnancy*; for encounter for seeking care or testing, not currently pregnant.

Assign V26.32 *Other genetic testing of female*, or V26.35 *Encounter for testing of male partner of habitual aborter*, for encounters for testing of the partners.

629.89	Other specified disorders of female genital organs
629.9	Unspecified disorder of female genital organs

Coding Scenario

A 25-year-old immigrant woman is seen by a physician with intense pelvic and vulvar pain. He suspects a severe pelvic inflammatory condition or infection and upon examination, notes that access to the introitus is severely compromised with external genitalia in a healed, but mutilated appearance. It is necessary for the artificially created covering to be surgically removed before any pelvic exam can be carried out. This is all performed at the same time under general anesthesia and a diagnosis of acute inflammatory pelvic disease is returned. The pathology report confirms the presence of group A streptococcus.

> Code assignment: 614.3 *Acute parametritis and pelvic cellulites*; 041.01 *Streptococcal infection, group A, in diseases classified elsewhere*; 629.22 *Female genital mutilation status, Type III*

630–677
Complications of Pregnancy, Childbirth, and the Puerperium

This chapter classifies diseases and disorders that occur during pregnancy, childbirth, and the six weeks immediately following childbirth.

630–633 Ectopic and Molar Pregnancy

A molar pregnancy is abnormal products of conception and an ectopic pregnancy is the implantation of normal products of conception in an anatomic location other than the uterus. Use an additional code from rubric 639 to identify any complications.

630 Hydatidiform mole OK

Hydatidiform mole is an abnormal product of conception in which the epithelial covering of the chorionic villi proliferates with dissolution and cystic cavitation of the avascular stroma of the villi. The result is a mass of cells that resembles a bunch of grapes. This condition also is called cystic or vesicular mole.

Signs and symptoms of hydatidiform mole include bleeding, usually in the first trimester, larger than expected uterus for gestational age, nausea and vomiting, preeclampsia, and passage of vesicular tissue.

Lab work positive for hydatidiform mole reveals HCG greater than 100,000 mIU/ml. Amniography reveals a honeycomb appearance of the mole; an exam of a flat plate of the abdomen fails to show fetal skeleton after 15 weeks; and an ultrasound reveals abnormalities of the fetus and gestational sac. Therapies include suction curettage to evacuate the mole before completion of 20 weeks of gestation, primary hysterectomy in patients not desiring further pregnancies, and prophylactic chemotherapy in patients whose HCG titer rises or plateaus following pregnancy.

Coding Clarification
Associated conditions include malignancy in 20 percent of all patients with hydatidiform mole pregnancies. However, these malignancies are excluded from this rubric and are reported with 236.1.

631 Other abnormal product of conception OK

Included in this rubric are carneous mole, Breus' mole, and blighted ovum.

632 Missed abortion OK
AHA: Q1, 2001, 5

ICD-9-CM defines a missed abortion as the retention of a fetus for at least four weeks after fetal demise but before completion of 22 weeks of gestation. In the United States, this period of time varies according to state law and may be as few as 19 weeks.

Signs and symptoms of missed abortion include the disappearance of normal signs of pregnancy and failure of the uterus to grow.

Diagnostic tests include a pelvic exam that may reveal brownish vaginal discharge, no fresh bleeding, and a closed cervix, though no adnexal abnormalities. Lab work may reveal negative beta HCG and a significantly low plasma fibrinogen level in midtrimester missed abortion. An ultrasound will show there is no fetal cardiac activity. Therapies include dilation and curettage or dilation and evacuation if the pregnancy has not reached the second trimester. If the pregnancy is into the second trimester, laminaria, suppositories, or amniotic injections of prostaglandin are used to induce delivery of the products of conception.

A missed abortion may occur at any time during the pregnancy before completion of 22 weeks of gestation but usually occurs during the second trimester.

Coding Clarification
Retention of abnormal products of conception is excluded from this rubric and reported with 630 or 631. Also excluded from this rubric are failed induced abortion, classified to rubric 638, and fetal death (656.4).

633 Ectopic pregnancy
AHA: Q4, 2002, 61

Tubal pregnancy is the implantation of a fertilized ovum in the fallopian tube, more often on the right than the left. This condition is more common in women who have had previous tubal disease, such as endometriosis of the fallopian tube, tubal surgeries, or infertility due to tubal disease. A tubal pregnancy may occur in any patient, though approximately 40 percent of these pregnancies occur in women between the ages of 20 and 29.

Signs and symptoms of a tubal pregnancy include mild to severe abdominal pain and occasionally nausea and vomiting before rupture. Abnormal uterine bleeding after a rupture occurs in approximately 75 percent of cases. In a tubal pregnancy, the pelvic exam shows adnexal tenderness and possible severe pain on palpation or movement of the cervix and uterus. Pregnancy tests are positive in 82.5 percent of cases. Lab work shows elevated urine urobilinogen and an ultrasound may reveal an empty uterine cavity with products of conception outside the uterus. Laparoscopy may allow direct visualization of the ectopic pregnancy as will laparotomy (performed more often when profound hemorrhage is suspected).

Therapies include laparoscopy or laparotomy to remove the ectopic pregnancy. If the patient is concerned about fertility, fimbrioplasty and salpingostomy are performed to leave the fallopian tube in place. If fertility is not an issue, the tube is removed, the tubal disease corrected, and there is lysis of adhesions in the opposite adnexa. In cases with minimal or no bleeding and without rupture, there is milking of the pregnancy from the fimbriated end of the tube.

Code	Description
633.0 ⌐sth	Abdominal pregnancy — (Use additional code from category 639 to identify any associated complications) — *intraperitoneal pregnancy* **AHA:** Q4, 2002, 61
633.00	Abdominal pregnancy without intrauterine pregnancy — (Use additional code from category 639 to identify any associated complications)
633.01	Abdominal pregnancy with intrauterine pregnancy — (Use additional code from category 639 to identify any associated complications)
633.1 ⌐sth	Tubal pregnancy — (Use additional code from category 639 to identify any associated complications) — *fallopian pregnancy; rupture of (fallopian) tube due to pregnancy* **AHA:** Q2, 1990, 27; Q4, 2002, 61
633.10	Tubal pregnancy without intrauterine pregnancy — (Use additional code from category 639 to identify any associated complications)
633.11	Tubal pregnancy with intrauterine pregnancy — (Use additional code from category 639 to identify any associated complications)
633.2 ⌐sth	Ovarian pregnancy — (Use additional code from category 639 to identify any associated complications) — *fertilized ovum implants on ovary* **AHA:** Q4, 2002, 61
633.20	Ovarian pregnancy without intrauterine pregnancy — (Use additional code from category 639 to identify any associated complications)
633.21	Ovarian pregnancy with intrauterine pregnancy — (Use additional code from category 639 to identify any associated complications)
633.8 ⌐sth	Other ectopic pregnancy — (Use additional code from category 639 to identify any associated complications) — *intraligamentous pregnancy; mesometric pregnancy* **AHA:** Q4, 2002, 61
633.80	Other ectopic pregnancy without intrauterine pregnancy — (Use additional code from category 639 to identify any associated complications)
633.81	Other ectopic pregnancy with intrauterine pregnancy — (Use additional code from category 639 to identify any associated complications)

Coding Clarification
Subclassification 633.8 reports implantation of a fertilized ovum in other specified sites such as the cervix, the uterine musculature (mesometric), or uterine cornua (horn). Signs and symptoms of other ectopic pregnancy include mild to severe abdominal pain and occasionally nausea and vomiting before rupture. Frequently after rupture, there is abnormal uterine bleeding in approximately 75 percent of cases. Therapies, depending on the implantation site, include termination using such procedures as wedge resection of the uterus, fimbrioplasty, supracervical hysterectomy, unilateral salpingo-oophorectomy, and total abdominal hysterectomy.

Code	Description
633.9 ⌐sth	Unspecified ectopic pregnancy — (Use additional code from category 639 to identify any associated complications) — *unknown* **AHA:** Q4, 2002, 61

633.90	Unspecified ectopic pregnancy without intrauterine pregnancy — (Use additional code from category 639 to identify any associated complications)
633.91	Unspecified ectopic pregnancy with intrauterine pregnancy — (Use additional code from category 639 to identify any associated complications)

Coding Scenario

A 29-year-old female is admitted for tubal pregnancy. The patient undergoes a left salpingectomy for removal of the tubal pregnancy. A pathology report confirms the diagnosis and identifies an embryonic cyst. The physician's final diagnostic statement is fallopian tube pregnancy and hydatid cyst of Morgagni.

Code assignment: 633.10 *Tubal pregnancy without intrauterine pregnancy* and 752.11 *Embryonic cyst of fallopian tube*

634–639 Other Pregnancy with Abortive Outcome

Retained Products of Conception: When the patient is admitted following a spontaneous or legally induced abortion for retained products of conception, the patient is considered to have an incomplete abortion.

Septicemia and Septic Shock Associated With Abortion: Septicemia is defined as systemic disease caused by the presence of toxins or micro-organisms in the bloodstream. It is evidenced by infection with fever or hypothermia, tachypnea, tachycardia, and impaired organ system perfusion, such as altered mental status, oliguria, and relative hypotension. Metabolic acidosis may also be present secondary to impaired organ perfusion, as evidenced by either an increased lactate level, increased anion gap, or reduced blood pH. Because it is difficult to isolate the infectious organism in blood cultures, it may still be appropriate to code the septicemia in view of the clinical data. Report with a code from categories 634-638 with the appropriate fourth digit to identify the sepsis ("0") and/or septic shock ("5"). A fifth digit is also required to identify the stage of the abortion.

634 Spontaneous abortion
AHA: Q2, 1991, 16

The definition of spontaneous abortion is complete or incomplete expulsion of the products of conception before completion of 22 weeks of gestation. Spontaneous abortions may be complete with the expulsion of the entire products of conception, or incomplete with the retention of part of the products of conception, usually the placenta.

In an incomplete abortion, the amniotic sac and fetus may be expelled without the chorion and decidua, only the embryo may be expelled, or the amniotic sac may rupture with passage of the fetus alone. Incomplete abortion requires evacuation of the remaining tissue by curettage. Fever and abdominal pain may indicate infection.

Most spontaneous abortions are associated with abnormal products of conception such as abnormal karyotype. Overall, about 10 percent are thought to have chromosomal abnormalities.

In pregnancies of about 14 weeks or less, therapies include suction, sharp curettage, or both to remove remaining conceptus. If bleeding is brisk, a 5 percent dextrose solution is administered in lactated ringers with 10 units of oxytocin per 500 ml; antibiotics are used to control infection. In pregnancies greater than 14 weeks of gestation, oxytocin is administered intravenously or prostaglandin E2 is inserted by vaginal suppository to expedite the abortion.

The following fifth-digit subclassification is used to identify stage of abortion with categories 634-637:

0 unspecified
1 incomplete
2 complete

634.0 ⌐5th	Spontaneous abortion complicated by genital tract and pelvic infection — *miscarriage complicated by salpingitis* AHA: Q2, 1991, 16
634.1 ⌐5th	Spontaneous abortion complicated by delayed or excessive hemorrhage — *miscarriage complicated by excessive bleeding* AHA: Q2, 1991, 16

Severe hemorrhage must be present for codes from 634.1 to be assigned correctly.

634.2 ⌐5th	Spontaneous abortion complicated by damage to pelvic organs or tissues — *miscarriage complicated by uterine rupture* AHA: Q2, 1991, 16
634.3 ⌐5th	Spontaneous abortion complicated by renal failure — *miscarriage complicated by renal failure* AHA: Q2, 1991, 16

Spontaneous abortion complicated by renal failure is expulsion of the products of conception before completion of 22 weeks of gestation, complicated by renal failure in the mother.

634.4 ✓sth Spontaneous abortion complicated by metabolic disorder — *miscarriage complicated by diabetes mellitus*
AHA: Q2, 1991, 16

Spontaneous abortion complicated by metabolic disorder is expulsion of the products of conception before completion of 22 weeks of gestation, complicated by metabolic disorders such as diabetes mellitus.

634.5 ✓sth Spontaneous abortion complicated by shock — *miscarriage complicated by shock*
AHA: Q2, 1991, 16

Spontaneous abortion complicated by shock is expulsion of the products of conception before completion of 22 weeks of gestation, complicated by maternal shock, which is an acute peripheral circulatory failure due to an aberration of circulatory control or loss of circulating fluid. Signs and symptoms of spontaneous abortion complicated by shock include hypotension, coldness of skin, tachycardia, anxiety, or sudden disturbance of mental equilibrium.

634.6 ✓sth Spontaneous abortion complicated by embolism — *miscarriage complicated by embolism*
AHA: Q2, 1991, 16

Spontaneous abortion complicated by embolism is expulsion of the products of conception before completion of 22 weeks of gestation, complicated by sudden blocking of an artery by a clot or foreign material in the mother.

The following fifth-digit subclassification is used to identify stage of abortion with categories 634-637:
0   unspecified
1   incomplete
2   complete

634.7 ✓sth Spontaneous abortion with other specified complications — *miscarriage complicated by other specified complication*
AHA: Q2, 1991, 16

634.8 ✓sth Spontaneous abortion with unspecified complication — *miscarriage with unspecified complication*
AHA: Q2, 1991, 16

634.9 ✓sth Spontaneous abortion without mention of complication — *miscarriage without mention of complication*
AHA: Q2, 1991, 16

Coding Clarification
Threatened Abortion: The outcome of the encounter indicates the proper code assignment. If the products of conception are expelled, the appropriate code from category 634 is assigned. A code from categories 640-648 and 651-657 may be used to identify the condition causing the abortion. If the threatened abortion does not culminate in an abortion, the appropriate code from category 640 is assigned.

Coding Scenario
A patient is admitted for a D&C following spontaneous abortion of an 18-week gestational age fetus. The pathology report reveals products of conception were removed by curettage. The patient is discharged home.

Code assignment: 634.91 *Spontaneous abortion without mention of complication, incomplete*

635 Legally induced abortion
AHA: Q2, 1994, 14

A legally induced abortion is the intentional expulsion of the products of conception from the uterus by medical professionals working within the boundaries of the law.

The following fifth-digit subclassification is used to identify stage of abortion with categories 634-637:
0   unspecified
1   incomplete
2   complete

635.0 ✓sth Legally induced abortion complicated by genital tract and pelvic infection — *therapeutic, complicated by salpingitis*
AHA: Q2, 1994, 14

635.1 ✓sth Legally induced abortion complicated by delayed or excessive hemorrhage — *therapeutic, complicated by excessive bleeding*
AHA: Q2, 1994, 14

635.2 ✓sth Legally induced abortion complicated by damage to pelvic organs or tissues — *therapeutic, complicated by uterine rupture*
AHA: Q2, 1994, 14

635.3 ✓sth Legally induced abortion complicated by renal failure — *therapeutic, complicated by renal failure*
AHA: Q2, 1994, 14

635.4 ✓sth Legally induced abortion complicated by metabolic disorder — *therapeutic, complicated by diabetes mellitus*
AHA: Q2, 1994, 14

635.5 ✓sth Legally induced abortion complicated by shock — *therapeutic, complicated by shock*
AHA: Q2, 1994, 14

635.6 ✓sth Legally induced abortion complicated by embolism — *therapeutic, complicated by embolism*
AHA: Q2, 1994, 14

635.7 ⌐sth Legally induced abortion with other specified complications — *therapeutic, with other specified complication*
AHA: Q2, 1994, 14

635.8 ⌐sth Legally induced abortion with unspecified complication — *therapeutic, with unknown complication*
AHA: Q2, 1994, 14

635.9 ⌐sth Legally induced abortion without mention of complication — *therapeutic abortion*
AHA: Q2, 1994, 14

Coding Scenario
Following a legally performed abortion, a patient is admitted for retained products of conception and septic shock. The causative organism is unknown.

Code assignment: 635.51 *Legally induced abortion complicated by shock, incomplete*

636 Illegally induced abortion
An illegally induced abortion is the intentional expulsion of the products of conception from the uterus by individuals working outside the boundaries of the law.

The following fifth-digit subclassification is used to identify stage of abortion with categories 634-637:
0 unspecified
1 incomplete
2 complete

636.0 ⌐sth Illegally induced abortion complicated by genital tract and pelvic infection — *criminal, complicated by salpingitis*

636.1 ⌐sth Illegally induced abortion complicated by delayed or excessive hemorrhage — *criminal, complicated by excessive bleeding*

636.2 ⌐sth Illegally induced abortion complicated by damage to pelvic organs or tissue — *criminal, complicated by uterine rupture*

636.3 ⌐sth Illegally induced abortion complicated by renal failure — *criminal, complicated by renal failure*

636.4 ⌐sth Illegally induced abortion complicated by metabolic disorder — *criminal, complicated by diabetes mellitus*

636.5 ⌐sth Illegally induced abortion complicated by shock — *criminal, complicated by shock*

636.6 ⌐sth Illegally induced abortion complicated by embolism — *criminal, complicated by embolism*

636.7 ⌐sth Illegally induced abortion with other specified complications — *criminal, with other specified complication*

636.8 ⌐sth Illegally induced abortion with unspecified complication — *criminal, with unknown complication*

636.9 ⌐sth Illegally induced abortion without mention of complication — *criminal abortion*

637 Legally unspecified abortion
Use this rubric when documentation does not support a choice of a legally or an illegally induced abortion.

The following fifth-digit subclassification is used to identify stage of abortion with categories 634-637:
0 unspecified
1 incomplete
2 complete

637.0 ⌐sth Legally unspecified abortion complicated by genital tract and pelvic infection — *complicated by salpingitis*

637.1 ⌐sth Legally unspecified abortion complicated by delayed or excessive hemorrhage — *complicated by excessive bleeding*

637.2 ⌐sth Legally unspecified abortion complicated by damage to pelvic organs or tissues — *complicated by uterine rupture*

637.3 ⌐sth Legally unspecified abortion complicated by renal failure — *complicated by renal failure*

637.4 ⌐sth Legally unspecified abortion complicated by metabolic disorder — *complicated by diabetes mellitus*

637.5 ⌐sth Legally unspecified abortion complicated by shock — *complicated by shock*

637.6 ⌐sth Legally unspecified abortion complicated by embolism — *complicated by embolism*

637.7 ⌐sth Legally unspecified abortion with other specified complications — *with other specified complication*

637.8 ⌐sth Legally unspecified abortion with unspecified complication — *with unknown complication*

637.9 ⌐sth Legally unspecified abortion without mention of complication — *without mention of complication*

638 Failed attempted abortion
A failed attempted abortion is the attempted, although failed, intentional expulsion of the products of conception from the uterus.

638.0 Failed attempted abortion complicated by genital tract and pelvic infection — *failed therapeutic, complicated by salpingitis*

638.1 Failed attempted abortion complicated by delayed or excessive hemorrhage — *failed therapeutic, complicated by excessive bleeding*

638.2 Failed attempted abortion complicated by damage to pelvic organs or tissues — *failed therapeutic, complicated by ruptured fallopian tube*

638.3 Failed attempted abortion complicated by renal failure — *failed therapeutic, complicated by renal failure*

638.4 Failed attempted abortion complicated by metabolic disorder — *failed therapeutic, complicated by diabetes mellitus*

638.5 Failed attempted abortion complicated by shock — *failed therapeutic, complicated by shock*

638.6 Failed attempted abortion complicated by embolism — *failed therapeutic, complicated by embolism*

638.7	Failed attempted abortion with other specified complication — *failed therapeutic, with other specified complication*
638.8	Failed attempted abortion with unspecified complication — *failed therapeutic, with unspecified complication*
638.9	Failed attempted abortion without mention of complication — *failed therapeutic, without mention of complication*

639 Complications following abortion or ectopic and molar pregnancies

This rubric reports complications that follow an abortion or an ectopic or molar pregnancy. It is used when the complication (not the abortion or the ectopic or molar pregnancy) is the reason for the current episode of care. For example, a patient is readmitted one week after treatment for a tubal pregnancy, presenting with generalized sepsis. Codes 639.0x *General tract and pelvic infection* and 038.9 *Unspecified septicemia* would be used for the second admission. Code 633.1x *Tubal pregnancy* would not be used since it pertains only to the previous episode of care.

Genital tract and pelvic infection following an abortion, especially one performed illegally, is commonly caused by both aerobic and anaerobic organisms. The infection may be localized to the products of conception or it may result in endometritis, salpingo-oophoritis, peritonitis, or septicemia.

Signs and symptoms of genital tract and pelvic infection include pain, bleeding, fever, vaginal discharge, and recent illegal abortion. Lab work shows elevated white blood count and cultures identify organisms causing infection, generally gram-negative bacilli (most commonly *Escherichia coli* and *Bacteroides fragilis*) and gram-positive cocci (particularly *enterococci* and *beta-hemolytic streptococci*). The infective agent may be reported secondarily.

639.0	Genital tract and pelvic infection following abortion or ectopic and molar pregnancies — *endometritis, salpingitis, septicemia molar pregnancies*
639.1	Delayed or excessive hemorrhage following abortion or ectopic and molar pregnancies — *secondary*
639.2	Damage to pelvic organs and tissues following abortion or ectopic and molar pregnancies — *laceration or perforation of bladder, broad ligament, periurethral tissue or uterus molar pregnancies*
639.3	Renal failure following abortion or ectopic and molar pregnancies — *secondary*
639.4	Metabolic disorders following abortion or ectopic and molar pregnancies — *secondary*
639.5	Shock following abortion or ectopic and molar pregnancies — *secondary*
639.6	Embolism following abortion or ectopic and molar pregnancies — *secondary*
639.8	Other specified complication following abortion or ectopic and molar pregnancies — *secondary*
639.9	Unspecified complication following abortion or ectopic and molar pregnancies — *secondary*

Coding Clarification
This rubric also is used when the complication cannot be identified at the fourth-digit level in code categories 634-638. For example, a patient admitted for missed abortion also develops generalized sepsis during the same episode of care. Codes 632 *Missed abortion*, 639.0, and 038.9 would be used for this admission; the infection cannot be identified at the fourth-digit level for missed abortions.

Coding Scenario
A patient is diagnosed with sepsis and shock following an abortion performed two days prior.

> Code assignment: 639.0 *Genital and pelvic infection following abortion or ectopic and molar pregnancies* and 639.5 *Shock following abortion or ectopic and molar pregnancies*

640–649 Complications Mainly Related to Pregnancy

Codes in this section describe conditions that affect the management of pregnancy, labor or delivery, and the puerperium, even if the condition was present before pregnancy.

640 Hemorrhage in early pregnancy
AHA: Q2, 1990, 11

Early pregnancy is defined as before the completion of 22 weeks gestation.

Signs and symptoms of threatened abortion include bleeding and uterine cramping without cervical dilation.

Therapies include bed rest and observation. Use the fifth-digit 0 if the episode of care is unspecified or not applicable; fifth-digit 1 when the threatened abortion is treated successfully and the patient goes on to deliver at term; and fifth-digit 3 if the threatened abortion is treated successfully without delivery.

Subclassification 640.8 reports bleeding during pregnancy that does not pose a threat of aborting the fetus. Bleeding may occur at any time during the pregnancy, although it is most prevalent during the first trimester when the risk of aborting the fetus is greater than during either the second or third trimester. The patient's pelvic exam reveals no evidence of spontaneous abortion, either complete or incomplete; CBC may indicate anemia if heavy bleeding is present; and an ultrasound is negative for placental abnormalities. Associated conditions that would be reported instead of 640.8x include placenta previa (641.1x), premature separation of placenta (641.2x), and coagulation defects in mother (641.3x).

Medical record documentation must indicate that the patient did not deliver during the current episode of care. If medical record documentation indicates that the physician was concerned about the likelihood of abortion, although there was no abortion, see 640.0x *Threatened abortion*. If medical record documentation such as ultrasound reports indicates an antepartum hemorrhagic condition affecting the placenta, see category 641 *Antepartum hemorrhage, abruptio placentae, and placenta previa* for alternative code selections.

> The following fifth-digit subclassification is for use with category 640 to denote the current episode of care.
>
> 0 unspecified as to episode of care or not applicable
>
> 1 delivered, with or without mention of antepartum condition
>
> 3 antepartum condition or complication

640.0 ⌐sth⌐ Threatened abortion — *potential abortion marked by bloody uterine discharge*
AHA: Q2, 1990, 11

640.8 ⌐sth⌐ Other specified hemorrhage in early pregnancy — *menstruation during pregnancy*
AHA: Q2, 1990, 11

640.9 ⌐sth⌐ Unspecified hemorrhage in early pregnancy — *early pregnancy hemorrhage NOS*
AHA: Q2, 1990, 11

Coding Clarification
Only the fifth-digits 0, 1, and 3 apply to the 640 rubric.

Threatened Abortion: The outcome of the encounter indicates the proper code assignment. If the products of conception are expelled, the appropriate code from category 634 is assigned. A code from categories 640-648 and 651-657 may be used to identify the condition causing the abortion. If the threatened abortion does not culminate in an abortion, the appropriate code from category 640 is assigned.

641 Antepartum hemorrhage, abruptio placentae, and placenta previa
AHA: Q2, 1990, 11

Antepartum hemorrhage, abruptio placentae, and placenta previa present with bleeding before the onset of labor (antepartum hemorrhage), premature separation of a normal placenta (abruptio placentae), and implantation of the placenta over or near the internal cervical os (placenta previa).

> The following fifth-digit subclassification is for use with category 641 to denote the current episode of care.
>
> 0 unspecified as to episode of care or not applicable
>
> 1 delivered, with or without mention of antepartum condition
>
> 3 antepartum condition or complication

641.0 ⌐sth⌐ Placenta previa without hemorrhage — *low implantation of placenta without hemorrhage*
AHA: Q2, 1990, 11

The definition of placenta previa without hemorrhage is implantation of the placenta over or near the internal os of the cervix. With total previa, the placenta completely covers the internal cervical os. Vaginal exam is contraindicated if placenta previa is suspected; ultrasound locates the exact position of the placenta. Therapies include bed rest if the patient is not near term; if the patient is at term, delivery of the fetus is usually by cesarean section.

If the fetus is not delivered during this episode of care, use the fifth digit 3 to indicate an antepartum condition.

641.1 ⌐sth⌐ Hemorrhage from placenta previa — *marginal placenta previa with hemorrhage; low lying placenta with hemorrhage*
AHA: Q2, 1990, 11

The definition of hemorrhage from placenta previa is implantation of the placenta over or near the internal os of the cervix with bleeding. With total previa, the placenta completely covers the internal cervical os. With partial previa, the placenta covers a portion of the internal cervical os.

Signs and symptoms of hemorrhage from placenta previa include sudden painless vaginal bleeding, beginning late in pregnancy, followed by painless massive bright red bleeding. Vaginal exam is contraindicated if placenta previa is suspected; ultrasound locates the exact position of the placenta. Therapies include bed rest if bleeding is minor and the patient is not near term, and if bleeding is substantial, blood transfusion and tocolytic agents are administered. If the fetus is not delivered during this episode of care, use the fifth digit 3 to indicate an antepartum condition.

Excluded from this subclassification is hemorrhage from vasa previa, reported with 663.5x.

641.2 ⌐sth⌐ Premature separation of placenta — *ablatio placentae; Couvelaire uterus; premature*

separation of normally implanted placenta; abruptio placentae
AHA: Q2, 1990, 11

Premature separation of the placenta is separation of the placenta from the site of uterine implantation before delivery of the fetus. There are two forms of placental separation: concealed, in which the hemorrhage is confined to the uterine cavity; and external, in which blood drains through the cervix. The placenta may detach either entirely or partially. Etiologies are numerous and difficult to ascertain but include advanced maternal age, multiparity, uterine distention, vascular deficiency and/or deterioration, uterine anomalies, cigarette smoking, and alcohol abuse.

Signs and symptoms of premature separation of the placenta include abdominal or back pain and visible hemorrhage, depending on the degree of separation and blood loss, irritable abdomen, and tender and often hypertonic uterus.

To avoid precipitating greater hemorrhage, pelvic exam is contraindicated until diagnosis of abruptio placentae established. CBC may show reduced platelets and anemia, depending on the degree of hemorrhage; ultrasound determines the degree of separation and viability of the fetus. Therapies include fetal monitoring to determine if the fetus is in any distress, blood transfusion if severe hemorrhage is present, delivery of the fetus if either bleeding persists or separation is total.

641.3 ⌐sth Antepartum hemorrhage associated with coagulation defects — *antepartum or intrapartum hemorrhage associated with afibrinogenemia, hyperfibrinolysis; hypofibrinogenemia*
AHA: Q2, 1990, 11

641.8 ⌐sth Other antepartum hemorrhage — *antepartum or intrapartum hemorrhage associated with trauma or uterine leiomyoma*
AHA: Q2, 1990, 11

641.9 ⌐sth Unspecified antepartum hemorrhage — *antepartum hemorrhage NOS; spots of pregnancy*
AHA: Q2, 1990, 11

642 Hypertension complicating pregnancy, childbirth, and the puerperium
AHA: Q2, 1990, 11

Hypertension complicating pregnancy, childbirth, and the puerperium may be benign, preexisting, chronic, or secondary to renal disease.

The following fifth-digit subclassification is for use with category 642 to denote the current episode of care.

0   unspecified as to episode of care or not applicable

1   delivered, with or without mention of antepartum condition

2   delivered, with mention of postpartum complication

3   antepartum condition or complication

4   postpartum condition or complication

642.0 ⌐sth Benign essential hypertension complicating pregnancy, childbirth, and the puerperium — *elevated arterial blood pressure; essential or chronic hypertension specified as complicating, or as a reason for obstetric care during pregnancy, childbirth, or the puerperium*
AHA: Q2, 1990, 11

Benign essential hypertension complicating pregnancy, childbirth, and the puerperium is blood pressure of 140/90 or greater before the onset of pregnancy or in the first trimester of pregnancy. Signs and symptoms of benign essential hypertension complicating pregnancy, childbirth, and the puerperium include a history of chronic benign hypertension. Examination reveals hypertension without other signs of preeclampsia such as proteinuria or nondependent edema. EKG may reveal left ventricular hypertrophy and lab work often shows elevated serum creatinine. A chest x-ray may reveal cardiomegaly. Therapies include antihypertensive drugs of established long-term safety for mother and fetus such as methyldopa, clonidine, and labetalol.

642.1 ⌐sth Hypertension secondary to renal disease, complicating pregnancy, childbirth, and the puerperium — *elevated arterial blood pressure due to kidney disease; hypertension secondary to renal disease*
AHA: Q2, 1990, 11

Hypertension secondary to renal disease, complicating pregnancy, childbirth, and the puerperium is preexisting renal disease that results in hypertension. Blood pressure is 140/90 or greater before the onset of pregnancy or in the first trimester of pregnancy. Signs and symptoms of hypertension secondary to renal disease, complicating pregnancy, childbirth, and the puerperium, include a history of chronic renal disease with resultant hypertension. Examination reveals hypertension, and edema. EKG may reveal left ventricular hypertrophy and lab work often shows elevated BUN and serum creatinine levels. A chest x-ray may reveal cardiomegaly. Fetal monitoring, fetal nonstress tests, and oxytocin challenge tests determine if pregnancy should be continued. Often, delivery, usually by cesarean section, is prescribed if blood pressure can no longer be controlled and the fetus has completed more than 22 weeks of gestation.

Therapies include antihypertensive drugs of established long-term safety for mother and fetus such as methyldopa, clonidine, and labetalol.

642.2 ⌐5th⌐ Other pre-existing hypertension complicating pregnancy, childbirth, and the puerperium — hypertensive heart and renal disease or malignant hypertension specified as complicating, or as a reason for obstetric care during pregnancy, childbirth, or the puerperium
AHA: Q2, 1990, 11

642.3 ⌐5th⌐ Transient hypertension of pregnancy — gestational hypertension; transient hypertension, so described, in pregnancy, childbirth, or the puerperium
AHA: Q2, 1990, 11; Q3, 1990, 4

642.4 ⌐5th⌐ Mild or unspecified pre-eclampsia — pre-eclampsia NOS or toxemia (pre-eclamptic) NOS
AHA: Q2, 1990, 11

Mild or unspecified pre-eclampsia is the development of borderline hypertension, albuminuria, and unresponsive edema between the 20th week of pregnancy and the end of the first week postpartum. Signs and symptoms of mild or unspecified pre-eclampsia include weight gain of more than two pounds in one week and nondependent edema of the hands and feet. Examination shows hypertension of 140/90 or slightly higher or rise in systolic pressure of 20 mm Hg or diastolic of 15 mm Hg, and nondependent edema of the face or hands. Lab work reveals albuminuria of 1+ or greater and rising serum creatinine. Therapies include bed rest and delivery once the fetus has reached a suitable age of gestation to be viable and antihypertensive drugs of established long-term safety for mother and fetus such as methyldopa, clonidine, and labetalol.

Excluded from 642.4x are albuminuria in pregnancy without hypertension (646.2x) and edema in pregnancy without mention of hypertension (646.1x).

642.5 ⌐5th⌐ Severe pre-eclampsia — HELLP syndrome; toxemia (pre-eclamptic), severe
AHA: Nov-Dec, 1985, 3; Q2, 1990, 11

642.6 ⌐5th⌐ Eclampsia complicating pregnancy, childbirth or the puerperium — toxemia with convulsions; eclamptic toxemia
AHA: Q2, 1990, 11

642.7 ⌐5th⌐ Pre-eclampsia or eclampsia superimposed on pre-existing hypertension — secondary
AHA: Q2, 1990, 11

642.9 ⌐5th⌐ Unspecified hypertension complicating pregnancy, childbirth, or the puerperium — childbirth, or the puerperium; hypertension NOS without mention of albuminuria or edema, complicating pregnancy, childbirth, or the puerperium
AHA: Q2, 1990, 11

Documentation Issues
The physician must clearly indicate if the patient has eclampsia, pre-eclampsia, or hypertension during pregnancy for accurate code assignment to be made.

Pre-eclampsia or eclampsia may be accompanied by pulmonary edema. An additional code indicating the pulmonary edema is only assigned when the pulmonary edema is documented as cardiogenic.

Coding Clarification
Eclampsia: This is a condition occurring during pregnancy or the immediate post-partum period noted by convulsions, coma, and edema with associated pre-eclampsia. Report with code 642.6x *Eclampsia complicating pregnancy, childbirth or the puerperium.* A fifth digit must be assigned to indicate the episode of care.

Hypertension During Pregnancy: If the medical record states hypertension with mild proteinuria, report code 642.4x *Mild or unspecified pre-eclampsia.* If the hypertension is associated with severe proteinuria, this is indicated by code 642.5x *Severe pre-eclampsia.* When the medical record documentation states transient hypertension of pregnancy or gestational hypertension, code 642.3x. These codes require the assignment of a fifth digit to indicate the episode of care.

If the patient has pre-existing hypertension that is affecting or complicating the obstetrical care, code 642.0x is assigned. This coding guideline is supported by an includes note in the tabular chapter of the ICD-9-CM manual.

Hypertension secondary to renal disease that is complicating the obstetrical care during pregnancy, childbirth, or the postpartum period is assigned to code 642.1x. This code requires the assignment of a fifth digit to indicate the episode of care.

Pre-eclampsia: This is a condition affecting women during pregnancy with one or more of the following symptoms: hypertension, proteinuria, oliguria, cerebral or visual disturbances, and pulmonary edema.

Mild pre-eclampsia is defined as hypertension associated with mild edema and proteinuria late in pregnancy. Assign code 642.4x with the appropriate fifth digit to indicate the episode of care.

Hypertension in the last trimester of pregnancy is also assigned code 642.4x.

Severe pre-eclampsia is specified as hypertension associated with either albuminuria or edema or both. Assign code 642.5x with the appropriate fifth digit indicating the episode of care. It may also be described as HELLP syndrome.

Coding Scenario
An inpatient delivers a liveborn female infant. Following the delivery, she has a blood pressure of 210/120, proteinuria, and edema. The patient suffers convulsions five hours post delivery.

> Code assignment: 642.62 *Eclampsia complicating pregnancy, childbirth or the puerperium, delivered, with mention of postpartum complication*

A patient who is 32 weeks pregnant is admitted due to severe hypertension, elevated liver function tests, and low platelet count. The diagnosis of HELLP is indicated.

> Code assignment: 642.53 *Severe pre-eclampsia, antepartum condition or complication*

A patient at 35-week gestational age is seen in her physician's office with transient elevation of blood pressure during pregnancy.

> Code assignment: 642.33 *Transient hypertension of pregnancy, antepartum condition or complication*

643 Excessive vomiting in pregnancy
AHA: Q2, 1990, 11

This category is used to describe vomiting that affects management of the pregnancy.

The following fifth-digit subclassification is for use with category 643 to denote the current episode of care.

0   unspecified as to episode of care or not applicable

1   delivered, with or without mention of antepartum condition

3   antepartum condition or complication

643.0 ⌐sth   Mild hyperemesis gravidarum — *hyperemesis gravidarum, mild or unspecified, starting before the end of the 22nd week of gestation*
AHA: Q2, 1990, 11

643.1 ⌐sth   Hyperemesis gravidarum with metabolic disturbance — *hyperemesis gravidarum starting before the end of the 22nd week of gestation, with metabolic disturbance, such as carbohydrate depletion, dehydration or electrolyte imbalance*
AHA: Q2, 1990, 11

643.2 ⌐sth   Late vomiting of pregnancy — *excessive vomiting starting after 22 completed weeks of gestation*
AHA: Q2, 1990, 11

643.8 ⌐sth   Other vomiting complicating pregnancy — (Use additional code to specify cause) — *vomiting due to organic disease or other cause, specified as complicating pregnancy, or as a reason for obstetric care during pregnancy*
AHA: Q2, 1990, 11

643.9 ⌐sth   Unspecified vomiting of pregnancy — *vomiting as a reason for care during pregnancy, length of gestation unknown*
AHA: Q2, 1990, 11

Coding Clarification
Only fifth-digits 0, 1, and 3 apply to codes in the 643 rubric.

644 Early or threatened labor
AHA: Q2, 1990, 11

Threatened labor is regular, painful uterine contractions at least twice every 10 minutes for a 30-minute period of time with effacement or dilation of the cervix occurring after completion of 22 weeks of gestation but before completion of 37 weeks. There is neither rupture of membranes nor delivery of the fetus. The contractions cease and the cervix stops dilating.

The following fifth-digit subclassification is for use with category 644 to denote the current episode of care. Valid fifth-digits are in brackets [ ] after each code, unless noted at the rubric.

0   unspecified as to episode of care or not applicable

1   delivered, with or without mention of antepartum condition

3   antepartum condition or complication

644.0 ⌐sth   Threatened premature labor — *premature labor after 22 weeks, but before 37 completed weeks of gestation*
AHA: Q2, 1990, 11

644.1 ⌐sth   Other threatened labor — *false labor after 37 completed weeks of gestation; including Braxton Hicks contractions*
AHA: Q2, 1990, 11

644.2 ⌐sth   Early onset of delivery — *onset (spontaneous) of delivery before 37 completed weeks of gestation*
AHA: Q2, 1990, 11; Q2, 1991, 16

Coding Clarification
Early onset of delivery is delivery of an infant after completion of 22 weeks of gestation but before completion of 37 weeks. Signs and symptoms of early onset of delivery include uterine contractions lasting at least 30 seconds and occurring at 10-minute intervals (at least) during a 30-minute period

of time and continued dilation and effacement of the cervix over a period of time despite medications to stop.

Therapies include hydration and sedation once the patient is admitted in premature labor, tocolysis to try to prevent progression, and, when this fails, delivery of the infant.

Only the fifth-digits 0 or 1 are valid for 644.2. The fifth-digit 0, unspecified as to episode of care or not applicable, will rarely, if ever, be assigned as the subcategory implies delivery.

Abortion with Delivery of Liveborn Fetus: An attempt to terminate pregnancy may result in the delivery of a liveborn fetus. When this occurs, ICD-9-CM code 644.2x is assigned. Hospitals also assign the appropriate code from category V27 *Outcome of delivery* to indicate the live birth.

Retained Products of Conception: When the patient is admitted following a spontaneous or legally induced abortion for retained products of conception, the patient is considered to have an incomplete abortion.

Threatened Abortion: The outcome of the encounter indicates the proper code assignment. If the products of conception are expelled, the appropriate code from category 634 is assigned. A code from categories 640-648 and 651-657 may be used to identify the condition causing the abortion. If the threatened abortion does not culminate in an abortion, the appropriate code from category 640 is assigned.

Coding Scenario
A patient is admitted for an induced abortion. Following prostaglandin suppositories and cervical dilation, a single liveborn male fetus is delivered.

> Code assignment: 644.21 *Early onset of delivery, with or without mention of antepartum condition*. Hospitals will also code V27.0 *Single liveborn*

645 Late pregnancy
AHA: Q2, 1990, 11; Q4, 1991, 26; Q4, 2000, 43

Post-term pregnancy is a normal pregnancy of more than 40 weeks, up to 42 weeks. A prolonged pregnancy is normal pregnancy that has advanced beyond 42 weeks of gestation. Postdatism may be treated by careful fetal monitoring with no intervention until there are indications the fetus is at risk. Postmaturity syndrome is a term that may be applied to both mothers and infants. In mothers, the syndrome is characterized by prolonged gestation, sometimes excessive fetal size, failing placental function, and impending fetal demise. When the term is used to describe infant pathology, it is classified to 766.2 *Post-term infant, not "heavy for dates."*

The following fifth-digit subclassification is for use with category 645 to denote the current episode of care.

0 unspecified as to episode of care or not applicable
1 delivered, with or without mention of antepartum condition
3 antepartum condition or complication

645.1 [sth] Post term pregnancy — *pregnancy over 40 completed weeks to 42 completed weeks gestation*
AHA: Q2, 1990, 11; Q4, 1991, 26; Q4, 2000, 43

645.2 [sth] Prolonged pregnancy — *pregnancy which has advanced beyond 42 completed weeks gestation*
AHA: Q2, 1990, 11; Q4, 1991, 26; Q4, 2000, 43

Coding Clarification
Only the fifth-digits 0, 1, and 3 apply to the 645 rubric.

646 Other complications of pregnancy, not elsewhere classified
AHA: Q2, 1990, 11; Q4, 1995, 59

The following fifth-digit subclassification is for use with category 646 to denote the current episode of care. Valid fifth-digits are in brackets [ ] after each code, unless noted at the rubric.

0 unspecified as to episode of care or not applicable
1 delivered, with or without mention of antepartum condition
2 delivered, with mention of postpartum complication
3 antepartum condition or complication
4 postpartum condition or complication

646.0 [sth] Papyraceous fetus — *skin of fetus resembles paper*
[0,1,3]
AHA: Q2, 1990, 11; Q4, 1995, 59

646.1 [sth] Edema or excessive weight gain in pregnancy, without mention of hypertension — *gestational edema; maternal obesity syndrome*
AHA: Q2, 1990, 11; Q4, 1995, 59

646.2 [sth] Unspecified renal disease in pregnancy, without mention of hypertension — *gestational proteinuria; albuminuria or nephropathy NOS in pregnancy or the puerperium*
AHA: Q2, 1990, 11; Q4, 1995, 59

646.3 [sth] Pregnancy complication, habitual aborter — *miscarried at least three times*
[0,1,3]
AHA: Q2, 1990, 11; Q4, 1995, 59

646.4 [sth] Peripheral neuritis in pregnancy
646.5 [sth] Asymptomatic bacteriuria in pregnancy

646.6 ⌐sth Infections of genitourinary tract in pregnancy — secondary
AHA: Q2, 1990, 11; Q4, 1995, 59; Q4, 2004, 90

646.7 ⌐sth Liver disorders in pregnancy — *icterus gravis, or necrosis of liver, or acute yellow atrophy of liver (obstetric) (true)*
[0,1,3]
AHA: Q2, 1990, 11; Q4, 1995, 59

646.8 ⌐sth Other specified complications of pregnancy — *fatigue during pregnancy; herpes gestationis; pruritic gravidarum; ptyalism in pregnancy*
AHA: Jan-Feb, 1985, 15; Q2, 1990, 11; Q4, 1995, 59; Q3, 1998, 16

646.9 ⌐sth Unspecified complication of pregnancy — *pregnancy complication NOS*
[0,1,3]
AHA: Q2, 1990, 11; Q4, 1995, 59

Coding Clarification

Additional codes should be reported to further specify the complication. Do not report 646.3x *Pregnancy complication, habitual aborter* in the case of a current abortion (rubric 634) or if the patient is not currently pregnant (629.81). Report 646.9x *Unspecified complication of pregnancy* for herpes gestationis, insufficient weight gain in pregnancy, retinitis gravidarum, ptyalism pregnancy, pruritic gravidarum, or uterine size-date discrepancy.

647 Infectious and parasitic conditions in the mother classifiable elsewhere, but complicating pregnancy, childbirth, or the puerperium
AHA: Q2, 1990, 11

Subclassification 647.0 reports a pregnancy complicated by an infection of microorganism *Treponema pallidum*, which causes venereal disease that leads to many structural and cutaneous lesions and may be transmitted to the fetus in utero.

> The following fifth-digit subclassification is for use with category 647 to denote the current episode of care. Valid fifth-digits are in brackets [ ] after each code, unless noted at the rubric.
>
> 0 unspecified as to episode of care or not applicable
> 1 delivered, with or without mention of antepartum condition
> 2 delivered, with mention of postpartum complication
> 3 antepartum condition or complication
> 4 postpartum condition or complication

647.0 ⌐sth Maternal syphilis complicating pregnancy, childbirth, or the puerperium — (Use additional code(s) to further specify complication) — secondary
AHA: Q2, 1990, 11

647.1 ⌐sth Maternal gonorrhea complicating pregnancy, childbirth, or the puerperium — (Use additional code(s) to further specify complication) — secondary
AHA: Q2, 1990, 11

647.2 ⌐sth Other maternal venereal diseases complicating pregnancy, childbirth, or the puerperium — (Use additional code(s) to further specify complication) — secondary
AHA: Q2, 1990, 11

647.3 ⌐sth Maternal tuberculosis complicating pregnancy, childbirth, or the puerperium — (Use additional code(s) to further specify complication) — secondary
AHA: Q2, 1990, 11

Subclassification 647.3 reports a pregnancy complicated by infection by mycobacterium and characterized by the formation of tubercles and caseous necrosis in the tissues.

647.4 ⌐sth Maternal malaria complicating pregnancy, childbirth, or the puerperium — (Use additional code(s) to further specify complication) — secondary
AHA: Q2, 1990, 11

Subclassification 647.4 reports a pregnancy complicated by a febrile disease caused by protozoa that are parasitic in the red blood cells. Symptoms, including fever, chills, and sweating, occur at intervals corresponding with a new generation of the parasites.

647.5 ⌐sth Maternal rubella complicating pregnancy, childbirth, or the puerperium — (Use additional code(s) to further specify complication) — secondary
AHA: Q2, 1990, 11

Subclassification 647.5 reports a pregnancy complicated by infection with a mild viral disease (German measles) known to cause birth defects.

647.6 ⌐sth Other maternal viral disease complicating pregnancy, childbirth, or the puerperium — (Use additional code(s) to further specify complication) — secondary
AHA: Jan-Feb, 1985, 15; Q2, 1990, 11

647.8 ⌐sth Other specified maternal infectious and parasitic disease complicating pregnancy, childbirth, or the puerperium — secondary
AHA: Q2, 1990, 11

647.9 ⌐sth Unspecified maternal infection or infestation complicating pregnancy, childbirth, or the puerperium — (Use additional code(s) to further specify complication) — secondary
AHA: Q2, 1990, 11

Coding Clarification

Use additional codes to further specify the complications.

648 Other current conditions in the mother classifiable elsewhere, but complicating pregnancy, childbirth, or the puerperium
AHA: Q2, 1990, 11

This rubric includes the listed conditions when complicating the pregnant state, aggravated by the pregnancy, or when it is the main reason for the obstetric care.

> The following fifth-digit subclassification is for use with category 648 to denote the current episode of care. Valid fifth-digits are in brackets [ ] after each code, unless noted at the rubric.
>
> 0 unspecified as to episode of care or not applicable
> 1 delivered, with or without mention of antepartum condition
> 2 delivered, with mention of postpartum complication
> 3 antepartum condition or complication
> 4 postpartum condition or complication

648.0 [✓-5th] Maternal diabetes mellitus complicating pregnancy, childbirth, or the puerperium — (Use additional code(s) to identify the condition) — *secondary*
AHA: Q2, 1990, 11; Q3, 1991, 5, 11

This subclassification reports pregnancy complicated by insulin- or non-insulin-dependent diabetes mellitus affecting the management and health of the mother and fetus during pregnancy. Signs and symptoms of diabetes mellitus include a history of diabetes, insulin- or non-insulin-dependent, with associated conditions such as ketoacidosis. Blood glucose may reveal hyper- or hypoglycemia during pregnancy. Urine culture and sensitivity may reveal asymptomatic urinary tract infection and markedly elevated glycosylated hemoglobin. Other lab work includes tests for electrolyte levels, BUN, and creatinine to evaluate any renal involvement. Ultrasound, fetal biophysical profiles, and other fetal tests may be performed to monitor fetal growth and detect any major congenital anomalies.

Patients with diabetes mellitus are more apt to develop pre-eclampsia or eclampsia. If medical record documentation indicates that either condition is present, assign an additional code.

This category excludes gestational diabetes (648.8x).

648.1 [✓-5th] Thyroid dysfunction complicating pregnancy, childbirth, or the puerperium — (Use additional code(s) to identify the condition) — *secondary*
AHA: Q2, 1990, 11

648.2 [✓-5th] Maternal anemia complicating pregnancy, childbirth, or the puerperium — (Use additional code(s) to identify the condition) — *secondary*
AHA: Q2, 1990, 11

Signs and symptoms of anemia include fatigue, palpitations, tachycardia, dyspnea, and pallor. In anemia, the CBC hemoglobin is 10g/100 ml. Red cells may be microcytic and hypochromic; reticulocytes and platelets may be normal or increased in number. For patients with iron deficiency anemia, lab work reveals serum iron below 30mcg/100 ml and elevated total iron binding capacity. For patients with folic acid anemia, lab work reveals low vitamin B12 levels. Therapies include iron therapy (oral, IV, or parenteral). Associated conditions include sickle cell anemia, sickle cell trait, and major and minor thalassemia. Anemia may be found in as many as 80 percent of pregnancies and is due mostly to dietary iron deficiency. Although rare, anemia also may be due to folic acid deficiency.

648.3 [✓-5th] Maternal drug dependence complicating pregnancy, childbirth, or the puerperium — (Use additional code(s) to identify the condition) — *secondary*
AHA: Q4, 1988, 8; Q2, 1990, 11; Q2, 1998, 13

648.4 [✓-5th] Maternal mental disorders complicating pregnancy, childbirth, or the puerperium — (Use additional code(s) to identify the condition) — *secondary*
AHA: Q2, 1990, 11; Q4, 1995, 63; Q2, 1998, 13

648.5 [✓-5th] Maternal congenital cardiovascular disorders complicating pregnancy, childbirth, or the puerperium — (Use additional code(s) to identify the condition) — *secondary*
AHA: Q2, 1990, 11

648.6 [✓-5th] Other maternal cardiovascular diseases complicating pregnancy, childbirth, or the puerperium — (Use additional code(s) to identify the condition) — *secondary*
AHA: Q2, 1990, 11; Q3, 1998, 11

648.7 [✓-5th] Bone and joint disorders of maternal back, pelvis, and lower limbs, complicating pregnancy, childbirth, or the puerperium — *secondary*
AHA: Q2, 1990, 11

648.8 [✓-5th] Abnormal maternal glucose tolerance, complicating pregnancy, childbirth, or the puerperium — (Use additional code(s) to identify the condition) (Use additional code, if applicable, for associated long-term (current) insulin use, V58.67) — *secondary*
AHA: Q2, 1990, 11; Q3, 1991, 5; Q4, 2004, 56

Subclassification 648.8 is reported when the patient has had abnormal glucose tolerance or gestational diabetes although a definitive diagnosis of diabetes mellitus has not been made.

648.9 [✓5th] Other current maternal conditions complicating pregnancy, childbirth, or the puerperium — (Use additional code(s) to identify the condition) — secondary
AHA: Nov-Dec, 1987, 10; Q2, 1990, 11; Q4, 2004, 88, 90

Coding Clarification
Use an additional code to describe the condition. Excluded from this rubric are conditions both known or suspected of having affected the fetus, which are reported with codes from rubric 655 *Known or suspected fetal abnormality affecting management of mother*.

This subclassification reports conditions affecting the management of the pregnancy and delivery in the absence of combination codes. This code and the appropriate code from another chapter of ICD-9-CM indicate the treatment of the condition that is affecting management of the pregnancy.

649 Other conditions or status of the mother complicating pregnancy, childbirth, or the puerperium

The following fifth-digit subclassification is for use with category 649 to denote the current episode of care. Valid fifth digits are in brackets [ ] after each code, unless noted at the rubric.

0 unspecified as to episode of care or not applicable
1 delivered, with or without mention of antepartum condition
2 delivered, with mention of postpartum complication
3 antepartum condition or complication
4 postpartum condition or complication

649.0 [✓5th] Tobacco use disorder complicating pregnancy, childbirth, or the puerperium

Women who smoke during pregnancy are at greater risk of having a miscarriage or a low-birth-weight baby. Smoking during pregnancy is attributed to be the underlying cause for 20 percent to 30 percent of all low-birth-weight babies. Additional risks to the mother include:

- Preterm birth
- Ectopic pregnancy
- Miscarriage
- Placenta previa and abruption
- Intrauterine growth restriction
- Other complications

Risks to the fetus and newborn include:

- SIDS
- Permanent physical impairment
- Childhood asthma

- Upper respiratory and ear infections
- Other health hazards

Smoking cessation should be initiated as early as possible in the pregnancy to improve the health benefits for the baby. Cessation programs are the most effective when started early in the pregnancy; however not all pharmaceutical aids are indicated for all pregnant patients. All but the heaviest of smokers are encouraged to stop smoking using nonmedical methods. Generally, nicotine replacement is considered only when nonmedical treatments fail. Clinicians must weight the risks and benefits associated with nicotine replacements and their safety and efficacy, although the potential benefits are currently thought to outweigh the risks.

649.1 [✓5th] Obesity complicating pregnancy, childbirth, or the puerperium — (Use additional code to identify the obesity)

Research has shown that obesity in pregnancy (body mass index of 30 or higher) poses significant risks to the mother and baby, such as:

- Labor and delivery complications, such as shoulder dystocia
- Thromboembolism
- Delivery of large-for-gestational-age (LGA) infants; macrosomia
- Increased need for cesarean section
- Maternal hypertension or pre-eclampsia
- Gestational diabetes
- Birth defects, especially neural tube defects

The increased rates of obesity and preterm births nationwide have led to studies to determine whether the conditions are linked. Although, so far, the findings have not directly linked the two conditions, obesity poses increased risks of maternal complications that may contribute to preterm births.

Weight-loss programs are usually not recommended during pregnancy because they could rob the fetus of the calories and nutrients it needs for normal development. Alternately, prenatal care should include testing for congenital anomalies, and breastfeeding should be encouraged post-delivery.

649.2 [✓5th] Bariatric surgery status complicating pregnancy, childbirth, or the puerperium — *gastric banding, gastric bypass, obesity surgery status*

It is recommended that patients wait for 12 to 18 months status post-surgery to become pregnant. Fertility generally increases post-surgery for those obese patients who had previously experienced infertility, because the dramatic weight loss often results in the spontaneous return of normal ovulation. However, the demands on the patient's body to adjust to the reduced size of the stomach and the absorption of nutrients is contrary to that needed for the normal growth and development of a fetus. For these reasons, patients are advised to use birth control during the rapid weight loss that follows the surgery. Once the body has adjusted to surgery and its metabolism has stabilized, pregnancy is no longer contraindicated, as it was in the past. Prenatal care with adequate nutritional support and supplementation is advised. This may involve the patient's obstetrician working as a team with her bariatric surgeon and a nutritionist.

649.3 ⌐sth   Coagulation defects complicating pregnancy, childbirth, or the puerperium — (Use additional code to identify the specific coagulation defect)

There are a number of conditions and complications that originate prior to pregnancy and complicate its course, manifest during pregnancy, or are secondary results of other complicating conditions that can alter normal coagulation in the body. Depending on the type of coagulation defect, transfusion or other management may be indicated. Because transfusions during pregnancy pose significant risks, increased monitoring of blood coagulation factors are often necessary to adequately manage the patient. Some of those conditions are as follows:

- Complicating factors such as hypertension or pre-eclampsia can result in a hypercoagulation state that can precipitate thromboemboblism.
- Disseminated intravascular coagulation (DIC) is a serious condition that can result in tissue damage and abnormal bleeding when physiological complications cause material from the inside of the womb to get into the mother's bloodstream.
- Inherited diseases such as von Willebrand disease and hemophilia put patients at a high risk of bleeding problems early in pregnancy and in the puerperium. In some cases, this can result in first trimester bleeding and miscarriage. Patients with this inherited coagulopathy have increased rates of postabortal anemia and hemorrhage. These inherited conditions often carry significant risk to the offspring, necessitating genetic testing.
- Certain medications are contraindicated in pregnancy because they can cause coagulation defects. For example, aspirin and other nonsteroidal anti-inflammatory drugs (NSAIDs) should be avoided in late pregnancy. These drugs can adversely affect maternal platelet function and increase the risk of antepartum and postpartum hemorrhage, as well as cause premature closure of the fetal ductus arteriosus, delaying labor and birth.

- Antiphospholipid syndrome (APS) is a disorder that causes a hypercoagulable state that predisposes the patient to recurrent vascular thromboses, which can result in recurrent spontaneous abortions. APS can be primary in nature or secondary to an autoimmune or rheumatic disorder. During pregnancy, management may necessitate treatment with subcutaneous heparin injection or low doses of aspirin antepartum or postpartum, although contraindicated at the time of delivery.

This subcategory excludes coagulation defects causing antepartum hemorrhage (641.3) and postpartum coagulation defects (666.3).

649.4 ⌐sth   Epilepsy complicating pregnancy, childbirth, or the puerperium — (Use additional code to specify the type of epilepsy)

Many anti-epileptic drugs pose significant risk when taken during pregnancy; however, so do epileptic seizures. For many patients, to simply stop taking their medication is ill-advised. Some recommendations for minimizing the risks to the mother include getting seizures under control and staying consistent with the lowest dosage possible of the single most effective medication, and having the medication levels regularly monitored. The greatest risks are those that the fetus will face either due to the antiepileptic medications or inherited factors. Some of these include an increased risk of:

- Malformation
- Development delay
- Hereditary epilepsy
- Infant mortality
- Neonatal internal hemorrhaging
- Low birth weight and/or prematurity

Epilepsy affects women differently. This is partly due to the hormonal effects associated with pregnancy and menstrual cycles, which are affected by epilepsy. Two specific hormones are especially important: estrogen, which increases the electrical activity of the brain, and progesterone, which has the reverse effect. The coordination of the hormonal process and seizure management with antiepileptic drugs during pregnancy pose special challenges. Fortunately, despite these challenges, approximately 90 percent of pregnant women who have epilepsy deliver healthy babies.

649.5 ⌐sth   Spotting complicating pregnancy
[0, 1, 3]

Spotting is very light bleeding that can vary in color from pink to red to brown. Some spotting is normal during pregnancy, and requires monitoring. However, it can also be a sign of a potentially serious complication or other condition necessitating prompt treatment. Therefore, it's often necessary for the obstetrician to investigate and rule out possible problems. Some of the conditions to be ruled out include:

- Miscarriage or ectopic pregnancy: Typically spotting is accompanied by abdominal pain or cramping. These conditions can be ruled out by ultrasound between seven and 11 weeks that confirm a viable fetus with a healthy heart beat. If this is the case, the chances of the pregnancy progressing to term are greater than 90 percent.
- Infection: Any infection that inflames the cervix can result in spotting, which should resolve with treatment of the infection. Some infections can pose serous risks to the fetus if left untreated.
- Placenta previa: A serious condition whereby the placenta separates from the uterus. This is a serious condition that can result in miscarriage or premature labor.
- Labor: Spotting late in pregnancy (typically after week 37) can be a sign of early labor; that the mucus plug has passed; or that the cervix is beginning to soften in preparation for labor.

This subcategory excludes antepartum hemorrhage (641.0-641.9) and hemorrhage in early pregnancy (640.0-640.9).

649.6 ⌐sth Uterine size discrepancy complicating pregnancy

Uterine size and expected date of delivery can be difficult to estimate. Ultrasonography is routinely performed to gain an accurate, objective assessment and to confirm fetal viability, development, and health. Upon routine exam, the fundal height (centimeters above the pubic symphysis) should correspond to gestational age. This is not an exact science, so if there are discrepancies between the patient's subjective estimation of last menstrual period, fundal height, and other factors, the physician will perform ultrasonography to rule out conditions such as:

- Multiple pregnancy
- Macrosomia
- Polyhydramnios or oligohydramnios
- Intrauterine growth retardation

Uterine size and date discrepancies can carry the risk of obstructed labor; requiring intervention and/or cesarean section. Repeat ultrasonography may be necessary to assess for conditions such as polyhydramnios and cephalopelvic disproportion that may develop late in pregnancy and pose labor and delivery complications.

Coding Clarification
640.0 Tobacco use: Since tobacco use is a condition classified to Chapter 5, Mental Disorders, assigning this code was done judiciously to avoid the stigma of a diagnosis from that chapter. Reporting the condition as a mental disorder seemed imprecise or misrepresentative. Since code 640.0 accurately describes tobacco use complicating pregnancy, code 305.1 is no longer assigned as a secondary diagnosis.

649.1 Obesity: This subcategory (649.1) is assigned for pre-existing obesity. Excessive weight gain during pregnancy is assigned to subcategory 646.1 *Edema or excessive weight gain in pregnancy, without mention of hypertension.*

649.20 Bariatric surgery status: This code eliminates the need to assign an additional V code identifying the status of bariatric surgery (V45.86) for a pregnancy case.

649.3 Coagulation defects: Coagulation defects that result in antepartum hemorrhage, classifiable to 641.3 *Antepartum hemorrhage associated with coagulation defects,* is excluded from this code.

649.4 Epilepsy: Code 649.4 provides a specific obstetrics code for the condition complicating pregnancy but also requires the use of an additional code to specify the type of epilepsy.

649.5 Spotting: The term "spotting" is not synonymous with hemorrhage and is not necessarily treated with the same degree of acuity or intensity. Code 649.5 *Spotting complicating pregnancy* excludes both antepartum hemorrhage (641.0-641.9) and hemorrhage in early pregnancy (640.0-640.9), which are more accurately classified elsewhere.

649.6 Uterine size date discrepancy: This code enables reporting this condition when it is either a preliminary notation of a specific condition yet to be confirmed or ruled out, versus an other type of uterine size and date discrepancy altogether.

650–659 Normal Delivery, and Other Indications for Care in Pregnancy, Labor, and Delivery

650 Normal delivery ✓
AHA: Q4, 1995, 28,59; Q3, 2000, 5; Q3, 2001, 12; Q2, 2002, 10

The definition of delivery in a completely normal case is spontaneous vaginal delivery of a single live infant after completion of 38 to 42 weeks of gestation, with cephalic presentation, without instrumentation, and with no antepartum or postpartum conditions or complications.

Documentation Issues
Examine the medical record documentation to determine if there were any conditions, early in the pregnancy, that affected management of the patient.

Coding Clarification
This category is appropriate to use if an episiotomy was performed, membranes were ruptured artificially, or the placenta was extracted manually. If forceps or vacuum extraction were used to assist delivery, see category 669 *Other complications of labor and delivery, not elsewhere classified*. Rubric 650 is for use as a single diagnosis code and is not to be used with any other code in the range 630-676. Use an additional code to indicate the outcome of delivery (V27).

Threatened Abortion: The outcome of the encounter indicates the proper code assignment. If the products of conception are expelled, the appropriate code from category 634 is assigned. A code from categories 640-648 and 651-657 may be used to identify the condition causing the abortion. If the threatened abortion does not culminate in an abortion, the appropriate code from category 640 is assigned.

651 Multiple gestation

The following fifth-digit subclassification is for use with category 651 to denote the current episode of care.

0   unspecified as to episode of care or not applicable
1   delivered, with or without mention of antepartum condition
3   antepartum condition or complication

Code		Description
651.0	✓5th	Twin pregnancy — *two fetuses*
651.1	✓5th	Triplet pregnancy — *three fetuses*
651.2	✓5th	Quadruplet pregnancy — *four fetuses*
651.3	✓5th	Twin pregnancy with fetal loss and retention of one fetus — *vanishing twin syndrome (651.33)*
651.4	✓5th	Triplet pregnancy with fetal loss and retention of one or more
651.5	✓5th	Quadruplet pregnancy with fetal loss and retention of one or more
651.6	✓5th	Other multiple pregnancy with fetal loss and retention of one or more fetus(es)
651.7	✓5th	Multiple gestation following (elective) fetal reduction — *reduction of multiple fetuses*
651.8	✓5th	Other specified multiple gestation
651.9	✓5th	Unspecified multiple gestation — *superfecundation; superfetation*

Coding Clarification
Use an additional code from rubric V27 to indicate the outcome of delivery in multiple births, identifying livebirths and stillborn births in cases of multiple births. If one or more fetus is malpositioned, also report a code from subclassification 652.6. Only the fifth-digits 0, 1, and 3 apply to the 651 rubric.

Elective Fetal Reduction: Subcategory 651.4 is intended to identify those cases of elective fetal reduction to reduce the risk to the remaining fetuses. The pregnancy is still considered high-risk even after the elective reduction. The other subcategories 651.3-651.6 allow the identification of cases of spontaneous fetal reduction during a multiple gestation pregnancy.

652 Malposition and malpresentation of fetus

The following fifth-digit subclassification is for use with category 652 to denote the current episode of care.

0   unspecified as to episode of care or not applicable
1   delivered, with or without mention of antepartum condition
3   antepartum condition or complication

Code		Description
652.0	✓5th	Unstable lie of fetus — (Code first any associated obstructed labor, 660.0) — *changing fetal position*
652.1	✓5th	Breech or other malpresentation successfully converted to cephalic presentation — (Code first any associated obstructed labor, 660.0) — *cephalic version NOS*
652.2	✓5th	Breech presentation without mention of version — (Code first any associated obstructed labor, 660.0) — *breech delivery (assisted) (spontaneous) NOS*

Breech presentation without mention of version is presentation of buttocks first without successful version. There are three forms of breech presentation: frank, in which the legs of the fetus extend over the abdomen and thorax so that the feet lie beside the face; complete, in which the fetal position is maintained so that the legs are flexed and crossed; and incomplete, in which one or both lower legs and feet are prolapsed into the vagina. Foot or knee presentations are subdivisions of incomplete breech presentation and are coded to 652.8x.

In breech presentation, the abdominal exam (four maneuvers of Leopold) identifies the fetal back on one side and the small parts on the opposite side. Lower fetal pole is less distinct, especially if engagement has occurred. Fetal heart tones are heard near the midline, slightly above and to one side of the umbilicus. If the cervix is slightly dilated and the membranes are ruptured, vaginal exam may allow palpation and identification of the presenting part; ultrasound reveals breech presentation. Delivery may be by cesarean section, breech extraction, manual assist, or spontaneous, depending on various obstetrical factors, including age and weight of the fetus and type of breech.

652.3 ✓5th   Transverse or oblique presentation of fetus — (Code first any associated obstructed labor, 660.0) — *oblique lie; transverse lie*

652.4 ✓5th   Fetal face or brow presentation of fetus — (Code first any associated obstructed labor, 660.0) — *mentum presentation*

652.5 ✓5th   High fetal head at term — (Code first any associated obstructed labor, 660.0) — *failure of head to enter pelvic brim*

652.6 ✓5th   Multiple gestation with malpresentation of one fetus or more — (Code first any associated obstructed labor, 660.0)

652.7 ✓5th   Prolapsed arm of fetus — (Code first any associated obstructed labor, 660.0) — *arm protrudes through birth canal*

652.8 ✓5th   Other specified malposition or malpresentation of fetus — (Code first any associated obstructed labor, 660.0) — *compound presentation; nuchal hitch (arm)*

652.9 ✓5th   Unspecified malposition or malpresentation of fetus — (Code first any associated obstructed labor, 660.0) — *malpresentation NOS*

Coding Clarification

Any obstructed labor (660.0x) would be sequenced first, followed by a code from this rubric to identify malposition of the fetus. Only the fifth-digits 0, 1, and 3 apply to the 652 rubric.

653   Disproportion in pregnancy, labor, and delivery

Disproportion in this rubric refers to maternal and fetal structural abnormalities or disproportions that interfere with normal delivery. Cephalopelvic disproportion is a disparity between the size of the maternal pelvis and the fetal head that precludes vaginal delivery. In fetopelvic disproportion, the presenting part of the baby is too large to fit through the mother's pelvis; labor progresses to a certain degree and then labor stops. The cervix stops dilating and delivery is by forceps, vacuum extractor, or cesarean section. When an attempt at forceps delivery proves too difficult, the obstetrician should perform a cesarean section. The fetus may be seriously injured or the infant may die if fetopelvic disproportion is encountered after the body has been delivered and the head is trapped. Prolonged labor due to cephalopelvic disproportion (CPD) is a leading cause of maternal death in the developing world. An unusually large fetus increases the likelihood of cephalopelvic disproportion requiring hospitalization for Cesarean delivery or shoulder dystocia during vaginal birth. Fetal anomalies such as hydrocephaly, encephalocele, and soft tissue tumors may obstruct labor and require fetal imaging based on vaginal or abdominal exam or when the fetus presents. Caesarean section is a way to reduce mortality resulting from obstructed labor. In addition, efforts to widen the birth canal are used to save the life of both mother and fetus, especially in third world countries where a Caesarean may increase the incidence of infection and maternal death. Perineotomy is a procedure to widen the lower portion of the birth canal, and symphysiotomy is a surgical widening at the upper level of the birth canal.

The following fifth-digit subclassification is for use with category 653 to denote the current episode of care.

0   unspecified as to episode of care or not applicable

1   delivered, with or without mention of antepartum condition

3   antepartum condition or complication

653.0 ✓5th   Major abnormality of bony pelvis, not further specified, in pregnancy — (Code first any associated obstructed labor, 660.1) — *pelvic deformity NOS*

653.1 ✓5th   Generally contracted pelvis in pregnancy — (Code first any associated obstructed labor, 660.1) — *contracted pelvis NOS*

653.2 ✓5th   Inlet contraction of pelvis in pregnancy — (Code first any associated obstructed labor, 660.1) — *inlet contraction (pelvis)*

653.3 ✓5th   Outlet contraction of pelvis in pregnancy — (Code first any associated obstructed labor, 660.1) — *outlet contraction (pelvis)*

653.4 ✓5th   Fetopelvic disproportion — (Code first any associated obstructed labor, 660.1) — *cephalopelvic disproportion NOS; disproportion of mixed maternal and fetal origin, with normally formed fetus*

Fetopelvic disproportion is a condition in which the presenting part of a normally formed fetus is too large to pass through the pelvic canal. Upon palpation of the abdomen, a large presenting part of the fetus in proportion to the mother's pelvic canal is revealed. Ultrasound determines fetal size, with therapy that includes cesarean delivery.

653.5 ✓5th   Unusually large fetus causing disproportion — (Code first any associated obstructed labor, 660.1) — *disproportion of fetal origin with normally formed fetus*

Use this subclassification to report an unusually large fetus too large to pass through the pelvic canal. Upon palpation of the abdomen, a disproportionately large fetus is revealed. Ultrasound determines fetal size. Therapies include cesarean delivery.

653.6 ✓5th   Hydrocephalic fetus causing disproportion — (Code first any associated obstructed labor,

653.7 [✓sth] 660.1) — *large head of fetus disproportionate to maternal pelvis*
Other fetal abnormality causing disproportion — (Code first any associated obstructed labor, 660.1) — *conjoined twins; fetal ascites; fetal myelomeningocele; fetal sacral teratoma*

653.8 [✓sth] Fetal disproportion of other origin — (Code first any associated obstructed labor, 660.1)

653.9 [✓sth] Unspecified fetal disproportion — (Code first any associated obstructed labor, 660.1) — *disproportion NOS*

Coding Clarification
If labor is obstructed, sequence the obstruction (660.1x) first, followed by a code from this rubric to report the disproportion. Only the fifth-digits 0, 1, and 3 apply to the 653 rubric.

654 Abnormality of organs and soft tissues of pelvis complicating pregnancy, childbirth, or the puerperium

The following fifth-digit subclassification is for use with category 654 to denote the current episode of care. Valid fifth-digts are in brackets [ ] at the end of each code, unless noted at the rubric.

0 unspecified as to episode of care or not applicable
1 delivered, with or without mention of antepartum condition
2 delivered, with mention of postpartum complication
3 antepartum condition or complication
4 postpartum condition or complication

654.0 [✓sth] Congenital abnormalities of pregnant uterus complicating pregnancy, childbirth, or the puerperium — (Code first any associated obstructed labor, 660.2) — *double uterus; uterus bicornis*

654.1 [✓sth] Tumors of body of pregnant uterus — (Code first any associated obstructed labor, 660.2) — *fibroids*

654.2 [✓sth] [0,1,3] Previous cesarean section complicating pregnancy, childbirth, or the puerperium — (Code first any associated obstructed labor, 660.2) — *scar from previous cesarean delivery*
AHA: Q1, 1992, 8

Use codes in 654.2 to report pregnancy, childbirth, or the puerperium complicated by a uterine scar caused by a previous cesarean section. Therapies include vaginal or repeat cesarean delivery.

654.3 [✓sth] Retroverted and incarcerated gravid uterus — (Code first any associated obstructed labor, 660.2) — *uterus is tilted so that it cannot rise above the sacral promontory*

654.4 [✓sth] Other abnormalities in shape or position of gravid uterus and of neighboring structures — (Code first any associated obstructed labor, 660.2) — *cystocele; pendulous abdomen; rectocele*

654.5 [✓sth] Cervical incompetence complicating pregnancy, childbirth, or the puerperium — (Code first any associated obstructed labor, 660.2) — *presence of Shirodkar suture with or without cervical incompetence*

Use codes in subclassification 654.5 to report dilation of the cervix, usually leading to second-trimester abortion. The etiology may be congenital or due to acquired causes such as previous surgical dilation, conization, breech extraction, or other trauma of delivery. Signs and symptoms of cervical incompetence include a history of previous late spontaneous abortions. A cervical exam allows passage of No. 8 Hegar dilator past the internal cervical os. Hysterosalpingostomy demonstrates a widened cervical os. Therapies include McDonald, Shirodkar, or other cerclage procedure (placement of encircling suture about the cervical os using heavy nonabsorbable suture or mercilene tape) to prevent protrusion and consequent rupture of the amniotic sac, followed by removal of the suture at 38 weeks or when labor begins.

654.6 [✓sth] Other congenital or acquired abnormality of cervix complicating pregnancy, childbirth, or the puerperium — (Code first any associated obstructed labor, 660.2) — *cicatricial cervix; cervical polyp; stenosis or stricture of cervix*

654.7 [✓sth] Congenital or acquired abnormality of vagina complicating pregnancy, childbirth, or the puerperium — (Code first any associated obstructed labor, 660.2) — *septate vagina; vaginal stenosis or stricture*

654.8 [✓sth] Congenital or acquired abnormality of vulva complicating pregnancy, childbirth, or the puerperium — (Code first any associated obstructed labor, 660.2) — *fibrosis of perineum; persistent hymen; rigid perineum*
AHA: Q1, 2003, 14

654.9 [✓sth] Other and unspecified abnormality of organs and soft tissues of pelvis complicating pregnancy, childbirth, and the puerperium — *uterine scar NEC; dystocia syndrome*

If labor is obstructed, sequence the obstruction (660.2x) first, followed by a code from this rubric to report the abnormality of organs and soft tissues of the pelvis.

655 Known or suspected fetal abnormality affecting management of mother
AHA: Q3, 1990, 4

The following fifth-digit subclassification is for use with category 655 to denote the current episode of care.

0 unspecified as to episode of care or not applicable
1 delivered, with or without mention of antepartum condition
3 antepartum condition or complication

655.0 ⌐sth Central nervous system malformation in fetus affecting management of mother — *fetal or suspected fetal; anencephaly, hydrocephalus or spina bifida (with myelomeningocele)*

655.1 ⌐sth Chromosomal abnormality in fetus affecting management of mother — *known to have damaged or mutated chromosome resulting in abnormality*

655.2 ⌐sth Hereditary disease in family possibly affecting fetus, affecting management of mother

655.3 ⌐sth Suspected damage to fetus from viral disease in mother, affecting management of mother — *maternal rubella*

655.4 ⌐sth Suspected damage to fetus from other disease in mother, affecting management of mother — *maternal alcohol addiction or maternal listerosis or maternal toxoplasmosis*

655.5 ⌐sth Suspected damage to fetus from drugs, affecting management of mother — *drug damage*

655.6 ⌐sth Suspected damage to fetus from radiation, affecting management of mother — *radiation damage*

655.7 ⌐sth Decreased fetal movements — *reduction in fetal movements*
AHA: Q4, 1997, 41

655.8 ⌐sth Other known or suspected fetal abnormality, not elsewhere classified, affecting management of mother — *suspected damage to fetus from environmental toxins or intrauterine contraceptive device*

655.9 ⌐sth Unspecified fetal abnormality affecting management of mother

Coding Clarification
Report codes in this rubric when the listed conditions in the fetus are reasons for observation or obstetrical care of the mother or for termination of the pregnancy. Only the fifth-digits 0, 1, and 3 apply to the 655 rubric.

656 Other fetal and placental problems affecting management of mother

The following fifth-digit subclassification is for use with category 656 to denote the current episode of care.

0 unspecified as to episode of care or not applicable

1 delivered, with or without mention of antepartum condition

3 antepartum condition or complication

656.0 ⌐sth Fetal-maternal hemorrhage affecting management of mother — *leakage (microscopic) of fetal blood into maternal circulation*

656.1 ⌐sth Rhesus isoimmunization affecting management of mother — *anti-D [Rh] antibodies; Rh incompatibility*

656.2 ⌐sth Isoimmunization from other and unspecified blood-group incompatibility affecting management of mother — *ABO isoimmunization*

656.3 ⌐sth Fetal distress affecting management of mother — *metabolic acidemia*
AHA: Nov-Dec, 1986, 4

The definition of fetal distress is metabolic abnormalities, notably hypoxia, and acidosis, which affect the functions of vital organs of the fetus. Fetal distress can occur at any time during pregnancy, or during or because of the stress of uterine contractions and medications. In fetal distress, the fetal heart monitor reveals acceleration or deceleration of fetal heart rate, flattened heart rate baseline, and extreme and variable deceleration of uterine tachysystole and tetanic contractions. Fetal scalp blood sampling (blood pH) reveals fetal distress. Therapies include administration of oxygen to the mother.

Coding Clarification
Fetal distress can be both a nonreassuring fetal status as well as life-threatening condition. As directed by the index, coders are to assign a code from subcategory 656.8x for reporting nonreassuring fetal distress. Subcategory 659.7 was created to capture the abnormal heart rhythm conditions that are often termed "fetal distress." Coders should only assign 656.3x, Fetal distress to cases of the most serious life-threatening situations, such as fetal metabolic acidemia. Documentation must support assignment of the 656.3x codes.

Excluded from this subclassification are abnormal fetal acid-base balance (656.8x), abnormality in fetal heart rate or rhythm (659.7x), or meconium in liquor (656.8x).

656.4 ⌐sth Intrauterine death affecting management of mother — *fetal death NOS; fetal death after completion of 22 weeks' gestation; missed delivery*

656.5 ⌐sth Poor fetal growth affecting management of mother — *"light for dates"; "placental insufficiency"; "small for dates"*

656.6 ⌐sth Excessive fetal growth affecting management of mother — *"large for dates"*

656.7 ⌐sth Other placental conditions affecting management of mother — *abnormal placenta; placental infarct*

656.8 ⌐sth Other specified fetal and placental problems affecting management of mother — *abnormal acid-base balance; intrauterine abscess; lithopedion*

656.9 ⌐sth Unspecified fetal and placental problem affecting management of mother

Coding Clarification
Report codes in this rubric when the listed conditions in the fetus are a reason for observation or obstetrical care of the mother or for termination of

the pregnancy. Only the fifth-digits 0, 1, and 3 apply to the 656 rubric.

657 Polyhydramnios

Polyhydramnios is excess amniotic fluid surrounding the fetus and can occur when the fetus fails to swallow and absorb amniotic fluid in excess of normal amounts due to, among other causes, gastrointestinal obstruction and neurological problems. Decreases or excessive amounts of amniotic fluid may be associated with abnormalities in the fetus. This condition is discovered at or before delivery and is evaluated during the infant's hospital stay. Documenting polyhydramnios may include:

- History of the pregnancy
- History of past pregnancies and the health of children delivered
- Other family history

If there is a concern regarding polyhydramnios, the amount of amniotic fluid can be estimated using ultrasound. The amount of fluid that is normal changes with gestational age; however, polyhydramnios is typically defined as a total fluid volume of greater than 24.0 centimeters.

> The following fifth-digit subclassification is for use with category 657 to denote the current episode of care.
> 0 unspecified as to episode of care or not applicable
> 1 delivered, with or without mention of antepartum condition
> 3 antepartum condition or complication

657.0 ⌐5th⌐ Polyhydramnios — *excessive amniotic fluid*
AHA: Q4, 1991, 26

Coding Clarification
This code requires a fifth-digit. Assign a 0 for fourth-digit placement with this code, and then assign the appropriate fifth-digit. Only the fifth-digits 0, 1, and 3 apply to the 657 rubric.

658 Other problems associated with amniotic cavity and membranes

> The following fifth-digit subclassification is for use with category 658 to denote the current episode of care.
> 0 unspecified as to episode of care or not applicable
> 1 delivered, with or without mention of antepartum condition
> 3 antepartum condition or complication

658.0 ⌐5th⌐ Oligohydramnios — *presence of abnormally low amount of amniotic fluid*
658.1 ⌐5th⌐ Premature rupture of membranes in pregnancy — *rupture of amniotic sac less than 24 hours prior to onset of labor*
658.2 ⌐5th⌐ Delayed delivery after spontaneous or unspecified rupture of membranes — *prolonged rupture of membranes NOS; rupture of amniotic sac 24 hours or more prior to the onset of labor*
658.3 ⌐5th⌐ Delayed delivery after artificial rupture of membranes
658.4 ⌐5th⌐ Infection of amniotic cavity — *amnionitis; membranitis; chorioamnionitis*
658.8 ⌐5th⌐ Other problems associated with amniotic cavity and membranes — *amnion nodosum; amniotic cyst; infarct of amnion; cyst of chorion*

Coding Clarification
Amniotic fluid embolism (673.1x) is excluded from this rubric. Only the fifth-digits 0, 1, and 3 apply to the 658 rubric.

659 Other indications for care or intervention related to labor and delivery, not elsewhere classified

An "elderly" pregnant woman will be 35 years of age or older at expected date of delivery. A primigravida is pregnancy with a first child, while a multigravida is pregnancy with a second or greater pregnancy.

> The following fifth-digit subclassification is for use with category 659 to denote the current episode of care.
> 0 unspecified as to episode of care or not applicable
> 1 delivered, with or without mention of antepartum condition
> 3 antepartum condition or complication

659.0 ⌐5th⌐ Failed mechanical induction of labor — *failure of induction of labor by surgical or other instrumental methods*
659.1 ⌐5th⌐ Failed medical or unspecified induction of labor — *failed induction NOS; failure of induction of labor by medical methods, such as oxytocic drugs*
659.2 ⌐5th⌐ Maternal pyrexia during labor, unspecified — *fever while the patient is in labor*
659.3 ⌐5th⌐ Generalized infection during labor — *septicemia during labor*
659.4 ⌐5th⌐ Grand multiparity, with current pregnancy — *birth to six or more children previously*
659.5 ⌐5th⌐ Elderly primigravida — *beyond the age norm for a first pregnancy*
AHA: Q3, 2001, 12
659.6 ⌐5th⌐ Elderly multigravida — *age at delivery at least 35, and has experienced at least one pregnancy previously*
AHA: Q3, 2001, 12
659.7 ⌐5th⌐ Abnormality in fetal heart rate or rhythm — *depressed fetal heart tones, including brachycardia, tachycardia*
AHA: Q4, 1998, 48
659.8 ⌐5th⌐ Other specified indications for care or intervention related to labor and delivery — *age less than 16 years at expected date of delivery*
AHA: Q3, 2001, 12

659.9 ⌐sth Unspecified indication for care or intervention related to labor and delivery

Coding Clarification
Supervision only of the pregnancy of an elderly primigravida is reported with V23.81; supervision of an elderly multigravida with V23.82. Only the fifth-digits 0, 1, and 3 apply to the 659 rubric.

660–669 Complications Occurring Mainly in the Course of Labor and Delivery

660 Obstructed labor
AHA: Q3, 1995, 10

Labor is described in stages. The latent phase lasts from several hours to as long as three days with uterine contractions and passage of the mucus plug. During the first stage, the contractions come at intervals and may be accompanied by mild pain. The cervix dilates until its opening is large enough to allow the passage of the infant and by the end of the first stage, the amniotic sac breaks. The first stage can last many hours in obstructed labor, where the baby is unusually large or badly angled. Obstructed labor may be due to anatomical abnormalities, prematurity, and unusual orientation of the child in the uterus, such as breech presentation (e.g., head last in the birth canal) and transverse presentation (e.g., sideways position in the birth canal). Obstructed labor is a leading cause of maternal and fetal death.

The following fifth-digit subclassification is for use with category 660 to denote the current episode of care.

0 unspecified as to episode of care or not applicable
1 delivered, with or without mention of antepartum condition
3 antepartum condition or complication

660.0 ⌐sth Obstruction caused by malposition of fetus at onset of labor — (Use additional code from 652.0-652.9 to identify condition) — *secondary*
AHA: Q3, 1995, 10

660.1 ⌐sth Obstruction by bony pelvis during labor and delivery — (Use additional code from 653.0-653.9 to identify condition) — *secondary*
AHA: Q3, 1995, 10

660.2 ⌐sth Obstruction by abnormal pelvic soft tissues during labor and delivery — (Use additional code from 654.0-654.9 to identify condition) — *secondary*
AHA: Q3, 1995, 10

660.3 ⌐sth Deep transverse arrest and persistent occipitoposterior position during labor and delivery

660.4 ⌐sth Shoulder (girdle) dystocia during labor and delivery — *impacted shoulders*
AHA: Q3, 1995, 10

660.5 ⌐sth Locked twins — *one twin is in breech position, the other high in head position, rendering vaginal delivery impossible*
AHA: Q3, 1995, 10

660.6 ⌐sth Unspecified failed trial of labor — *failed trial of labor*
AHA: Q3, 1995, 10

660.7 ⌐sth Unspecified failed forceps or vacuum extractor — *application of ventouse or forceps*
AHA: Q3, 1995, 10

660.8 ⌐sth Other causes of obstructed labor — *(Use additional code to identify condition) — other specified causes of obstructed labor NEC*
AHA: Q3, 1995, 10; Q4, 2004, 88

660.9 ⌐sth Unspecified obstructed labor — *dystocia NOS or fetal dystocia NOS or maternal dystocia NOS*
AHA: Q3, 1995, 10

Coding Clarification
Additional codes may be required to report the cause of the obstruction and should be sequenced secondarily to the code from this rubric. Only the fifth-digits 0, 1, and 3 apply to the 660 rubric.

661 Abnormality of forces of labor
Labor is diagnosed when there is regular uterine activity in association with cervical dilatation or effacement. Labor can be obstructed due to weak uterine muscle contractions and other problems during the stages of labor. Uterine inertia, or poor contraction strength, is a common reason for prolonged latent phase. Uterine inertia can be primary (e.g., when few contractions are initiated or do not start) or secondary (e.g., the slowing down of labor). Slow progress at the end of the first stage may be due to cephalopelvic disproportion, malposition, or poor contraction strength. An oxytocin infusion helps overcome malposition or poor contraction strength. In the third stage, the uterus may be prevented from contracting effectively by fragments of placenta that remain in the uterus after delivery or by benign growths of uterine muscle within the uterine wall; however, in most cases, the uterine muscle simply fails to contract adequately.

The following fifth-digit subclassification is for use with category 661 to denote the current episode of care.

0 unspecified as to episode of care or not applicable
1 delivered, with or without mention of antepartum condition
3 antepartum condition or complication

661.0 ⌐sth Primary uterine inertia — *weakness of uterus during first stage of labor; including failure of*

661.1 [✓sth] cervical dilation; hypotonic uterine dysfunction, primary
Secondary uterine inertia — *weakness of uterus in second stage of labor; including arrested active phase of labor; hypotonic uterine dysfunction, secondary*

661.2 [✓sth] Other and unspecified uterine inertia — *desultory labor; irregular labor; slow slope active phase of labor*

661.3 [✓sth] Precipitate labor — *rapid labor and delivery*

Precipitate labor is cervical dilation of 5.0 centimeters or more per hour for primigravidas and 10.0 centimeters or more per hour for multigravidas. Usually, precipitate labor is the result of extraordinarily forceful uterine contractions or low birth canal resistance.

661.4 [✓sth] Hypertonic, incoordinate, or prolonged uterine contractions — *cervical spasm; dyscoordinate labor; hourglass contraction of uterus; retraction ring (Band's) (pathological); uterine spasm*

661.9 [✓sth] Unspecified abnormality of labor

Coding Clarification
Only the fifth-digits 0, 1, and 3 apply to the 661 rubric.

662 Long labor
Labor is described in stages. During the first stage, the cervix dilates until its opening is large enough to allow the passage of the infant. The first stage can last many hours in obstructed labor, where the baby is unusually large or badly angled. The second stage begins with the complete dilation and effacement of the cervix and ends at the birth. During the third stage of labor, which occurs within the first hour of birth, placental material is expelled through the birth canal. Labor averages about 13 hours for first deliveries and about eight hours for subsequent deliveries. Dystocia, or difficult labor, includes labor that fails to progress, prolonged labor, or difficult childbirth. Dysfunctional labors due to cephalopelvic disproportion (CPD) occur when the baby is too large to pass safely through the mother's pelvis.

The following fifth-digit subclassification is for use with category 662 to denote the current episode of care.

0 unspecified as to episode of care or not applicable
1 delivered, with or without mention of antepartum condition
3 antepartum condition or complication

662.0 [✓sth] Prolonged first stage of labor
662.1 [✓sth] Unspecified prolonged labor — *unknown stage*
662.2 [✓sth] Prolonged second stage of labor
662.3 [✓sth] Delayed delivery of second twin, triplet, etc

Coding Clarification
Only the fifth-digits 0, 1, and 3 apply to the 662 rubric.

663 Umbilical cord complications during labor and delivery
This rubric covers umbilical complications at birth, which include:

- Occult prolapse — occurs with intact membranes when the cord is expelled before the presenting part or is trapped in front of a shoulder.

- Overt prolapse — occurs with ruptured membranes when the cord is in front of the presenting part. It most commonly occurs spontaneously with breech presentation but also occurs with vertex presentation, particularly when membranes are ruptured and the presenting part is not engaged. Treatment is immediate delivery and the practitioner must hold the presenting part up off the prolapsed cord to prevent further, prolonged compression. The cord is kept in the vagina to prevent drying.

- Vasa previa — the umbilical cord is the presenting part, a dangerous condition since the umbilical vessels can become pinched off or rupture as they are compressed between the fetus and the walls of the birth canal.

The following fifth-digit subclassification is for use with category 663 to denote the current episode of care.

0 unspecified as to episode of care or not applicable
1 delivered, with or without mention of antepartum condition
3 antepartum condition or complication

663.0 [✓sth] Prolapse of cord, complicating labor and delivery — *presentation of cord; an emergent situation*

663.1 [✓sth] Cord around neck, with compression, complicating labor and delivery — *cord tightly around neck*

663.2 [✓sth] Other and unspecified cord entanglement, with compression, complicating labor and delivery — *entanglement of cords of twins in mono-amniotic sac; knot in cord (with compression)*

663.3 [✓sth] Other and unspecified cord entanglement, without mention of compression, complicating labor and delivery

663.4 [✓sth] Short cord complicating labor and delivery — *lacks appropriate amount of slack, increasing risk of placental abruption*

663.5 [✓sth] Vasa previa complicating labor and delivery — *umbilical cord is presenting part*

663.6 [✓sth] Vascular lesions of cord complicating labor and delivery — *bruising; hematoma; thrombosis of vessels*

663.8 [✓sth] Other umbilical cord complications during labor and delivery — *velamentous insertion of umbilical cord; ruptured umbilical cord*

663.9 ⌐sth Unspecified umbilical cord complication during labor and delivery

Coding Clarification
Only the fifth-digits 0, 1, and 3 apply to the 663 rubric.

A loose nuchal cord that is reduced without incident may be reported on the mother's record even though there is no effect on the treatment of the mother. Report any cord compression that affects the baby on the baby's record.

664 Trauma to perineum and vulva during delivery
AHA: Nov-Dec, 1984, 10; Q1, 1992, 11

This category includes a laceration, rupture, or a tear of the perineum and vulva during delivery due to damage from instruments such as forceps or from an extension of an episiotomy.

The following fifth-digit subclassification is for use with category 664 to denote the current episode of care.

0 unspecified as to episode of care or not applicable
1 delivered, with or without mention of antepartum condition
4 postpartum condition or complication

664.0 ⌐sth First-degree perineal laceration during delivery — *perineal laceration, rupture or tear involving fourchette, hymen, labia, skin, vagina or vulva*
AHA: Nov-Dec, 1984, 10; Q1, 1992, 11

664.1 ⌐sth Second-degree perineal laceration during delivery — *perineal laceration, rupture or tear (following episiotomy) involving pelvic floor, perineal muscles, or vaginal muscles*
AHA: Nov-Dec, 1984, 10; Q1, 1992, 11

664.2 ⌐sth Third-degree perineal laceration during delivery — *perineal laceration, rupture or tear (following episiotomy) involving anal sphincter, rectovaginal septum or sphincter, NOS*
AHA: Nov-Dec, 1984, 10; Q1, 1992, 11

664.3 ⌐sth Fourth-degree perineal laceration during delivery — *secondary*
AHA: Nov-Dec, 1984, 10; Q1, 1992, 11

664.4 ⌐sth Unspecified perineal laceration during delivery — *central laceration*
AHA: Nov-Dec, 1984, 10; Q1, 1992, 8; Q1, 1992, 11

664.5 ⌐sth Vulvar and perineal hematoma during delivery
664.8 ⌐sth Other specified trauma to perineum and vulva during delivery
664.9 ⌐sth Unspecified trauma to perineum and vulva during delivery

Coding Clarification
Only the fifth-digits 0, 1, and 3 apply to the 664 rubric.

665 Other obstetrical trauma

The following fifth-digit subclassification is for use with category 665 to denote the current episode of care. Valid fifth-digts are in brackets [ ] at the end of each code, unless noted at the rubric.

0 unspecified as to episode of care or not applicable
1 delivered, with or without mention of antepartum condition
2 delivered, with mention of postpartum complication
3 antepartum condition or complication
4 postpartum condition or complication

665.0 ⌐sth Rupture of uterus before onset of labor
[0,1,3]

665.1 ⌐sth Rupture of uterus during and after labor — *rupture of uterus NOS*
[0,1]

665.2 ⌐sth Obstetrical inversion of uterus — *failure of placenta to separate from uterus, facilitating the turning of the uterus inside out*
[0,2,4]

665.3 ⌐sth Obstetrical laceration of cervix
[0,1,4]

665.4 ⌐sth High vaginal laceration during and after labor — *laceration of vaginal wall or sulcus without mention of perineal laceration*
[0,1,4]

665.5 ⌐sth Other obstetrical injury to pelvic organs — *injury to bladder or urethra*
[0,1,4]
AHA: March-April, 1987, 10

665.6 ⌐sth Obstetrical damage to pelvic joints and ligaments — *avulsion of inner symphyseal cartilage; damage to coccyx; separation of symphysis pubis*
[0,1,4]
AHA: Nov-Dec, 1984, 12

665.7 ⌐sth Obstetrical pelvic hematoma — *hematoma of vagina*
[0,1,2,4]

665.8 ⌐sth Other specified obstetrical trauma
[0,4]

665.9 ⌐sth Unspecified obstetrical trauma — *obstetrical trauma NOS*
[0,4]

666 Postpartum hemorrhage
AHA: Q1, 1988, 14

Postpartum hemorrhage is vaginal bleeding in excess of 500 ml during the third stage of labor, in the immediate postpartum period, or after the first 24 hours following delivery. Therapies include manual exploration of the uterine cavity for retained placenta and curettage of the uterine cavity.

Postpartum hemorrhage due to etiologies other than a retained placenta or membranes is classified elsewhere. Other etiologies for postpartum hemorrhage include lacerations of the cervix, vagina, or perineum, rupture of the uterus, a hypotonic myometrium due to general anesthesia, and overdistension of the uterus due to an abnormally large fetus or multiple gestation.

The following fifth-digit subclassification is for use with category 666 to denote the current episode of care.

0   unspecified as to episode of care or not applicable
2   delivered, with mention of postpartum complication
4   postpartum condition or complication

666.0 ⌐sth Third-stage postpartum hemorrhage — *hemorrhage associated with retained, trapped, or adherent placenta; retained placenta NOS*
AHA: Q1, 1988, 14

666.1 ⌐sth Other immediate postpartum hemorrhage — *atony of uterus with hemorrhage; hemorrhage within the first 24 hours following delivery of placenta; postpartum hemorrhage (atonic) NOS*
AHA: Q1, 1988, 14

666.2 ⌐sth Delayed and secondary postpartum hemorrhage — *hemorrhage after the first 24 hours following delivery; hemorrhage associated with retained portions of placenta or membranes; postpartum hemorrhage specified as delayed or secondary; retained products of conception NOS*
AHA: Q1, 1988, 14

666.3 ⌐sth Postpartum coagulation defects — *postpartum afibrinogenemia or fibrinolysis*
AHA: Q1, 1988, 14

Coding Clarification
Postpartum hemorrhage may be associated with a retained, trapped, or adherent placenta (666.0x). It also may occur within the first 24 hours following delivery of the fetus but not be associated with a retained portion of the placenta and/or membranes (code 666.1x). Delayed or secondary postpartum hemorrhage refers to hemorrhage occurring after the first 24 hours after delivery of the fetus and usually is associated with a retained portion of the placenta and/or membranes (666.2x). Code 666.3x includes postpartum coagulation defects, as seen in hypofibrinogenemia or thrombocytonia. Only the fifth-digits 0, 2, and 4 apply to the 666 rubric.

Uterine atony without hemorrhage is not included in category 666; rather, it is reported with a code from subcategory 669.8.

667 Retained placenta or membranes, without hemorrhage
AHA: Q1, 1988, 14

The placenta is normally delivered within 30 minutes of the birth. If the placenta does not deliver spontaneously, the practitioner will administer an analgesic and reach into the uterus to retrieve the placenta. If the placenta delivers spontaneously, the practitioner will check the placenta for completeness. If the placenta is not complete, the practitioner will examine the uterus and try to remove the residual pieces. In some cases, the uterus will be suctioned or scraped to remove residual tissues. If retained placenta is left untreated, there is a high risk of maternal death. However, manual removal of the placenta is an invasive procedure with its own serious complications of hemorrhage, infection, or genital tract trauma. Noninvasive techniques include injecting saline solution and oxytocin into the umbilical vein. This code reports the diagnosis without hemorrhage.

The following fifth-digit subclassification is for use with category 667 to denote the current episode of care.

0   unspecified as to episode of care or not applicable
2   delivered, with mention of postpartum complication
4   postpartum condition or complication

667.0 ⌐sth Retained placenta without hemorrhage — *placenta accreta, retained placenta NOS, or retained placenta, total, no hemorrhage*
AHA: Q1, 1988, 14

667.1 ⌐sth Retained portions of placenta or membranes, without hemorrhage — *retained products of conception, following delivery, without hemorrhage*
AHA: Q1, 1988, 14

Coding Clarification
Only the fifth-digits 0, 2, and 4 apply to the 667 rubric.

668 Complications of the administration of anesthetic or other sedation in labor and delivery
This rubric includes complications arising from the administration of a general or local anesthetic, analgesic, or other sedation in labor or delivery.

The following fifth-digit subclassification is for use with category 668 to denote the current episode of care.

0   unspecified as to episode of care or not applicable
1   delivered, with or without mention of antepartum condition
2   delivered, with mention of postpartum complication
3   antepartum condition or complication
4   postpartum condition or complication

668.0 ⌐sth Pulmonary complications of the administration of anesthesia or other sedation in labor and delivery — (Use additional code(s) to further specify complication) — *pressure collapse of lung or inhalation or aspiration of stomach contents or secretions following anesthesia or other sedation; Use additional code to further specify complication*

668.1 ⌐sth Cardiac complications of the administration of anesthesia or other sedation in labor and delivery — (Use additional code(s) to further specify complication)

668.2 ⌐sth Central nervous system complications of the administration of anesthesia or other sedation in labor and delivery — *cerebral anoxia following anesthesia or other sedation; Use additional code to further specify complication*

668.8 ⌐sth Other complications of the administration of anesthesia or other sedation in labor and delivery — (Use additional code(s) to further specify complication) — *other specified complications of anesthesia or other sedation use additional code to further specify complication*
AHA: Q2, 1999, 9

668.9 ⌐sth Unspecified complication of the administration of anesthesia or other sedation in labor and delivery — (Use additional code(s) to further specify complication) — *anesthesia complication NOS, obstetric use additional code to further specify complication*

Coding Clarification
Additional codes may be required to further identify the specific complications. This rubric excludes a reaction to a spinal or lumbar puncture or a spinal headache (349.0).

669 Other complications of labor and delivery, not elsewhere classified

The following fifth-digit subclassification is for use with category 669 to denote the current episode of care. Valid fifth-digts are in brackets [ ] at the end of each code, unless noted at the rubric.

0   unspecified as to episode of care or not applicable
1   delivered, with or without mention of antepartum condition
2   delivered, with mention of postpartum complication
3   antepartum condition or complication
4   postpartum condition or complication

669.0 ⌐sth Maternal distress — *metabolic disturbance*
669.1 ⌐sth Shock during or following labor and delivery — *obstetric shock*
669.2 ⌐sth Maternal hypotension syndrome — *low arterial blood pressure in the mother*
669.3 ⌐sth [0,2,4] Acute renal failure following labor and delivery
669.4 ⌐sth Other complications of obstetrical surgery and procedures — *cardiac arrest or failure following cesarean or other obstetrical surgery or procedure, including delivery NOS*
669.5 ⌐sth [0,1] Forceps or vacuum extractor delivery without mention of indication — *delivery by ventouse*
669.6 ⌐sth [0,1] Breech extraction, without mention of indication
669.7 ⌐sth [0,1] Cesarean delivery, without mention of indication
669.8 ⌐sth Other complications of labor and delivery
669.9 ⌐sth Unspecified complication of labor and delivery — *sudden death during childbirth*

670–677 Complications of the Puerperium

Categories 671 and 673-676 include the listed conditions even if they occur during pregnancy or childbirth.

670 Major puerperal infection
Puerperal infection refers to bacterial infection following childbirth. The bacteria are normally found in the mother's genital tract, but may be introduced from the woman's intestine and skin or from the practitioner. The genital tract, particularly the uterus, is the most commonly infected site and in a major episode, the infection can spread to other parts of the body. The primary symptom is a fever between birth and 10 days postpartum. Endometritis is the most prominent of these infections and can occur if the uterus has retained a piece of the placenta.

The following fifth-digit subclassifications are for use with category 670 to denote the current episode of care.

0   unspecified as to episode of care or not applicable
2   delivered, with mention of postpartum complication
4   postpartum condition or complication

670.0 ⌐sth Major puerperal infection — *infection and inflammation in the days following childbirth; puerperal endometritis, fever, pelvic cellulitis or sepsis*
AHA: Q2, 1991, 7; Q4, 1991, 26

Coding Clarification
Select the appropriate fifth-digit subclassification for this code and use a 0 as the fourth-digit.

This rubric excludes infection following abortion (639.0), minor genital tract infection following delivery (646.6x), puerperal pyrexia (672), and urinary tract infection following delivery (646.6x). Only the fifth-digits 0, 2, and 4 apply to the 670 rubric.

671 Venous complications in pregnancy and the puerperium

The following fifth-digit subclassifications are for use with category 671 to denote the current episode of care.

0   unspecified as to episode of care or not applicable
1   delivered, with or without mention of antepartum condition
2   delivered, with mention of postpartum complication
3   antepartum condition or complication
4   postpartum condition or complication

Complications of Pregnancy, Childbirth, and the Puerperium

671.0 ⌐5th Varicose veins of legs in pregnancy and the puerperium — *distended tortuous veins of the lower extremities associated with pregnancy*

671.1 ⌐5th Varicose veins of vulva and perineum in pregnancy and the puerperium — *distended tortuous veins on the external female genitalia and perineum associated with pregnancy*

671.2 ⌐5th Superficial thrombophlebitis in pregnancy and the puerperium — *inflammation and blood clot of superficial vein following childbirth; thrombophlebitis (superficial)*

671.3 ⌐5th Deep phlebothrombosis, antepartum — *inflammation and blood clot of deep vein in pregnant patient; deep-vein thrombosis, antepartum*
[0,1,3]

671.4 ⌐5th Deep phlebothrombosis, postpartum — *inflammation and blood clot of deep vein in pregnant patient; deep-vein thrombosis, postpartum*
[0,2,4]

671.5 ⌐5th Other phlebitis and thrombosis in pregnancy and the puerperium — *cerebral venous thrombosis; thrombosis of intracranial venous sinus*

671.8 ⌐5th Other venous complications in pregnancy and the puerperium — *hemorrhoids*

671.9 ⌐5th Unspecified venous complication in pregnancy and the puerperium — *phlebitis NOS; thrombosis NOS*

672 Pyrexia of unknown origin during the puerperium

Select the appropriate fifth-digit subclassification for this code, and use a 0 as the fourth-digit.

The following fifth-digit subclassifications are for use with category 672 to denote the current episode of care.

0 unspecified as to episode of care or not applicable
2 delivered, with mention of postpartum complication
4 postpartum condition or complication

672.0 ⌐5th Pyrexia of unknown origin during the puerperium — *postpartum fever NOS; puerperal fever NOS; puerperal pyrexia NOS*
AHA: Q4, 1991, 26

673 Obstetrical pulmonary embolism

This rubric reports pulmonary emboli in pregnancy, childbirth, or the puerperium, or specified as puerperal.

The following fifth-digit subclassifications are for use with category 673 to denote the current episode of care.

0 unspecified as to episode of care or not applicable
1 delivered, with or without mention of antepartum condition
2 delivered, with mention of postpartum complication
3 antepartum condition or complication
4 postpartum condition or complication

673.0 ⌐5th Obstetrical air embolism — *bubble of air blocking artery in the lung, associated with pregnancy*

673.1 ⌐5th Amniotic fluid embolism — *bubble of amniotic fluid blocking artery in mother's lung*

673.2 ⌐5th Obstetrical blood-clot embolism — *puerperal pulmonary embolism NOS*
AHA: Q1, 2005, 6

673.3 ⌐5th Obstetrical pyemic and septic embolism — *blockage of the artery in the lung, associated with infection in pregnancy*

673.8 ⌐5th Other obstetrical pulmonary embolism — *fat embolism*

Coding Clarification
Excluded are emboli following abortion (639.6).

674 Other and unspecified complications of the puerperium, not elsewhere classified

The following fifth-digit subclassifications are for use with category 674 to denote the current episode of care. Valid fifth-digts are in brackets [ ] at the end of each code, unless noted at the rubric.

0 unspecified as to episode of care or not applicable
1 delivered, with or without mention of antepartum condition
2 delivered, with mention of postpartum complication
3 antepartum condition or complication
4 postpartum condition or complication

674.0 ⌐5th Cerebrovascular disorders in the puerperium — *secondary*

674.1 ⌐5th Disruption of cesarean wound — *dehiscence or disruption of uterine wound*
[0,2,4]

674.2 ⌐5th Disruption of obstetrical perineal wound — *breakdown of perineum; secondary perineal tear; disruption of episiotomy wound*
[0,2,4]

674.3 ⌐5th Other complications of obstetrical surgical wounds — *hematoma, hemorrhage or infection of cesarean or perineal wound*
[0,2,4]
AHA: Q2, 1991, 7

674.4 ⌐5th Placental polyp
[0,2,4]

674.5 ⌐5th Peripartum cardiomyopathy

674.8 ⌐5th Other complications of the puerperium — *hepatorenal syndrome, following delivery; subinvolution of the uterus; puerperal cardiac thrombosis*
[0,2,4]
AHA: Q3, 1998, 16

674.9 ⌐5th Unspecified complications of the puerperium — *sudden death of unknown cause during the puerperium*
[0,2,4]

675 Infection of the breast and nipple associated with childbirth

Included in this rubric are the listed conditions as they occur during childbirth, pregnancy, or in the puerperium.

The following fifth-digit subclassifications are for use with category 675 to denote the current episode of care.

0 unspecified as to episode of care or not applicable
1 delivered, with or without mention of antepartum condition
2 delivered, with mention of postpartum complication
3 antepartum condition or complication
4 postpartum condition or complication

675.0 ✓sth Infection of nipple associated with childbirth — *abscess of the nipple*
675.1 ✓sth Abscess of breast associated with childbirth — *mammary abscess; purulent abscess*
675.2 ✓sth Nonpurulent mastitis associated with childbirth — *lymphangitis of breast; interstitial mastitis*
675.8 ✓sth Other specified infection of the breast and nipple associated with childbirth
675.9 ✓sth Unspecified infection of the breast and nipple associated with childbirth

676 Other disorders of the breast associated with childbirth and disorders of lactation

Included in this rubric are the listed conditions as they occur during childbirth, pregnancy, or in the puerperium.

The following fifth-digit subclassifications are for use with category 676 to denote the current episode of care.

0 unspecified as to episode of care or not applicable
1 delivered, with or without mention of antepartum condition
2 delivered, with mention of postpartum complication
3 antepartum condition or complication
4 postpartum condition or complication

676.0 ✓sth Retracted nipple associated with childbirth — *drawing back of the projected surface of the mammary gland*
676.1 ✓sth Cracked nipple associated with childbirth — *fissure of nipple*
676.2 ✓sth Engorgement of breasts associated with childbirth — *abnormally high accumulation of milk in the breast ducts*
676.3 ✓sth Other and unspecified disorder of breast associated with childbirth — *absence of milk secretion by the breast*
676.4 ✓sth Failure of lactation — *agalactia*

676.5 ✓sth Suppressed lactation
676.6 ✓sth Galactorrhea — *Chiari-Frommel syndrome*
676.8 ✓sth Other disorders of lactation — *galactocele*
676.9 ✓sth Unspecified disorder of lactation

677 Late effect of complication of pregnancy, childbirth, and the puerperium OK
AHA: Q4, 1994, 42; Q1, 1997, 9

Documentation Issues
Documentation must clearly indicate that the condition is a result of a complication that initially developed during the pregnancy, delivery, or the postpartum period to substantiate a late effect code selection.

Coding Clarification
Code first any sequelae. This category is to be used to indicate conditions in 632-648.9x and 651-676.9x as the cause of the late effect classifiable elsewhere. The "late effects" include conditions specified as such, or as sequelae, which may occur at any time after the puerperium.

Etiology: A late effect of pregnancy, childbirth, and the puerperium is a condition identified as being caused by or the sequel of a complication initially arising during this period (e.g., conditions classified to categories 632-648.9x and 651-676.9x). It does not include those conditions treated during the pregnancy, delivery, and postpartum period.

To report the late effect of complication of pregnancy, childbirth, and the puerperium, use code 677. This code does not require a fourth or fifth digit. Code also any sequelae of the complication.

Coding Scenario
A patient who is six months post-delivery of an infant is seen for rectal dilation. She has scarring secondary to a third degree laceration resulting from delivery.

Code assignment: 677 *Late effect of complication of pregnancy, childbirth, and the puerperium* and 569.2 *Stenosis of rectum and anus*

680–709

Diseases of the Skin and Subcutaneous Tissue

This chapter classifies diseases and disorders of the epidermis, dermis, subcutaneous tissue, nails, sebaceous glands, sweat glands, and hair and hair follicles.

680–686 Infections of Skin and Subcutaneous Tissue

This range of codes classifies infections of the skin and subcutaneous tissue into diseases and disorders such as boils, carbuncles, furuncles, cellulitis, abscess, lymphadenitis, local infections, and pilonidal cysts. When assigning a code from categories 680-686, also assign a code (as a secondary code) to identify the infective organism, such as staphylococcus (code 041.1).

680 Carbuncle and furuncle

Carbuncles and furuncles are infections caused by either aerobic or anaerobic bacterial organisms. A carbuncle is a collection of pus contained in a cavity or sac. A furuncle is a painful nodule formed by circumscribed inflammation of the skin and subcutaneous tissue that encloses a central core.

Signs and symptoms of carbuncles and furuncles include pain, fluctuating or fixed mass, fever, chills, and malaise with furuncle in active stage. A gram stain and culture (if open wound or pus is present) may be performed to identify the infective organism. Therapies include antimicrobials (penicillin).

680.0	Carbuncle and furuncle of face — *single boil or cluster of boils on sites including ear, nose, temple*
680.1	Carbuncle and furuncle of neck — *single boil or cluster of boils, neck*
680.2	Carbuncle and furuncle of trunk — *back, breast, chest, flank, groin, perineum, umbilicus, abdominal wall*
680.3	Carbuncle and furuncle of upper arm and forearm — *arm, axilla, shoulder*
680.4	Carbuncle and furuncle of hand — *finger, thumb, wrist*
680.5	Carbuncle and furuncle of buttock — *anus, gluteal region*
680.6	Carbuncle and furuncle of leg, except foot — *ankle, knee, thigh, hip*
680.7	Carbuncle and furuncle of foot — *heel, toe*
680.8	Carbuncle and furuncle of other specified sites — *head except face; scalp*
680.9	Carbuncle and furuncle of unspecified site — *unknown site*

Coding Clarification
Use an additional code to identify the infective organism, typically streptococcus or staphylococcus. Use the appropriate fourth digit to indicate the anatomic location of the furuncle or carbuncle. Excluded from this rubric are carbuncles of the eye, lacrimal apparatus, and orbit, classified to rubrics in the nervous system chapter of ICD-9-CM, and those of the genital system, classified to the chapter on diseases of the genitourinary system.

Excluded from this range are certain infections of the skin classified to Chapter 1 Parasitic and Infectious Diseases of ICD-9-CM, including erysipelas (035), erysipeloid of Rosenbach (027.1), herpes (rubrics 053 and 054), molluscum contagiosum (078.0), and viral warts (078.1).

681 Cellulitis and abscess of finger and toe
AHA: Jan-Feb, 1987, 12; Q2, 1991, 5

Cellulitis and abscess of the finger and toe are infections often caused by group A streptococci or *Staphylococcus aureus* but may be caused by other organisms. Cellulitis is an infection of the dermis and subcutaneous tissues. An abscess is a collection of pus resulting from an acute or chronic localized infection associated with tissue destruction.

Signs and symptoms of cellulitis and abscess of the finger and toe include erythema, warmth, edema, and pain.

Lab work reveals elevated sedimentation rate and mild leukocytosis with left shift. A gram stain and culture of the lesion identify the infective organism. Therapies include antimicrobials (penicillin or cephalosporin). Associated conditions include surgical wounds, cutaneous ulcers of the skin, and diabetes mellitus.

Code	Description
681.00	Unspecified cellulitis and abscess of finger — (Use additional code to identify organism) — *sudden, severe inflammation of finger not otherwise specified* AHA: Jan-Feb, 1987, 12; Q2, 1991, 5
681.01	Felon — (Use additional code to identify organism) — *cellulitis in fleshy tip of finger; Whitlow* AHA: Jan-Feb, 1987, 12; Q2, 1991, 5
681.02	Onychia and paronychia of finger — (Use additional code to identify organism) — *in or around fingernail; panaritium, perionychia* AHA: Jan-Feb, 1987, 12; Q2, 1991, 5
681.10	Unspecified cellulitis and abscess of toe — (Use additional code to identify organism) — *sudden, severe inflammation of toe not otherwise specified* AHA: Jan-Feb, 1987, 12; Q2, 1991, 5; Q1, 2005, 14
681.11	Onychia and paronychia of toe — (Use additional code to identify organism) — *in or around toenail; panaritium, perionychia* AHA: Jan-Feb, 1987, 12; Q2, 1991, 5
681.9	Cellulitis and abscess of unspecified digit — (Use additional code to identify organism)

Documentation Issues
If the documentation has an unclear diagnostic statement as to the site or type of injury, it will be necessary to obtain clarification from the physician to make an accurate code selection.

When the documentation identifies cellulitis following the repair of a laceration, clarification should be made with the physician whether the cellulitis is a postoperative infection or solely a complicated wound infection. Do not assume that the wound is the problem and the origin of the infection rather than the surgical procedure.

Coding Clarification
Use an additional code to identify the infective organism, typically streptococcus or staphylococcus. When cellulitis occurs with a chronic skin ulcer (category 707), code both conditions.

Cellulitis Associated with Pregnancy or Delivery: There are times when a patient will develop pelvic cellulitis after delivery or following an abortion. In these instances, only codes indicating the puerperal infection (codes from chapter 11) are indicated. The cellulitis is not coded separately.

Cellulitis Secondary to Superficial Injury: When cellulitis is the result of a superficial injury, burn, or frostbite, two codes are required: one for the cellulitis and one describing the injury.

Gangrenous Cellulitis: If the documentation indicates that gangrenous cellulitis is present, code 785.4 is assigned in addition to the injury or ulcer code and not a code from categories 681-682.

Open Wound with Cellulitus: When cellulitis is associated with an open wound, the code for a complicated open wound is assigned followed by the code for cellulitis when the patient is being seen primarily for treatment of the open wound. However, if the patient is being seen primarily for treatment of the cellulitis and the open wound is minor and does not require specific treatment, the appropriate code for cellulitis is indicated followed by an additional code identifying the complicated open wound.

Postoperative Cellulitis: Cellulitis resulting from a postoperative wound infection requires two codes: 998.59 *Other postoperative infection* and the appropriate code from categories 681 and 682 identifying the cellulitis.

Skin Ulcers and Cellulitus: A frequent complication of chronic skin ulcers is cellulitis. Since the codes identifying chronic skin ulcers (707.0-707.9) do not include any mention of cellulitis, two codes are necessary. Code both the chronic skin ulcer and the cellulitis.

Coding Scenario
A patient is being treated for a gangrenous abscess of the big toe of the right foot.

> Code assignment: 785.4 *Gangrene* and 681.10 *Unspecified cellulitis and abscess of toe*

682 Other cellulitis and abscess
AHA: Sept-Oct, 1985, 10; Jan-Feb, 1987, 12; Q2, 1991, 5

Cellulitis and abscess are infections caused by streptococci, staphylococci, or other organisms. Cellulitis is an infection of the dermis and subcutaneous tissues, more severe in patients with lower resistance to infection (e.g., diabetics). An abscess is a collection of pus resulting from an acute or chronic localized infection associated with tissue destruction.

Signs and symptoms of other cellulitis and abscess include edema, warmth, redness, pain, and interference with function. A gram stain and culture of the lesion identify the infective organism. Blood work usually reveals negative cultures, while

Diseases of the Skin and Subcutaneous Tissue

serological testing, specifically measurement of anti-DNAse B, confirms streptococcal etiology. Therapies include antimicrobials (penicillin).

682.0   Cellulitis and abscess of face — (Use additional code to identify organism) — *cheek, chin, forehead, nose, temple, submandibular region*
AHA: Sept-Oct, 1985, 10; Jan-Feb, 1987, 12; Q2, 1991, 5

682.1   Cellulitis and abscess of neck — (Use additional code to identify organism) — *sudden severe suppurative inflammation and edema in muscle or subcutaneous tissue*
AHA: Sept-Oct, 1985, 10; Jan-Feb, 1987, 12; Q2, 1991, 5

682.2   Cellulitis and abscess of trunk — (Use additional code to identify organism)

682.3   Cellulitis and abscess of upper arm and forearm — (Use additional code to identify organism) — *axilla, shoulder*
AHA: Sept-Oct, 1985, 10; Jan-Feb, 1987, 12; Q2, 1991, 5; Q2, 2003, 7

682.4   Cellulitis and abscess of hand, except fingers and thumb — (Use additional code to identify organism) — *wrist*
AHA: Sept-Oct, 1985, 10; Jan-Feb, 1987, 12; Q2, 1991, 5

682.5   Cellulitis and abscess of buttock — (Use additional code to identify organism) — *gluteal region*
AHA: Sept-Oct, 1985, 10; Jan-Feb, 1987, 12; Q2, 1991, 5

682.6   Cellulitis and abscess of leg, except foot — (Use additional code to identify organism) — *ankle, knee, thigh, hip*
AHA: Sept-Oct, 1985, 10; Jan-Feb, 1987, 12; Q2, 1991, 5; Q4, 2003, 108; Q3, 2004, 5

682.7   Cellulitis and abscess of foot, except toes — (Use additional code to identify organism) — *heel*
AHA: Sept-Oct, 1985, 10; Jan-Feb, 1987, 12; Q2, 1991, 5

682.8   Cellulitis and abscess of other specified site — (Use additional code to identify organism) — *scalp, pterygopalatine fossa, head, except face*
AHA: Sept-Oct, 1985, 10; Jan-Feb, 1987, 12; Q2, 1991, 5

682.9   Cellulitis and abscess of unspecified site — (Use additional code to identify organism) — *unknown site*
AHA: Sept-Oct, 1985, 10; Jan-Feb, 1987, 12; Q2, 1991, 5

Documentation Issues
If the documentation has an unclear diagnostic statement as to the site or type of injury, it will be necessary to obtain clarification from the physician to make an accurate code selection.

When the documentation identifies cellulitis following the repair of a laceration, clarification should be made with the physician whether the cellulitis is a postoperative infection or solely a complicated wound infection. Do not assume that the wound is the problem and the origin of the infection rather than the surgical procedure.

Coding Clarification
Use an additional code to identify the infective organism, typically streptococcus. Abscess and lymphangitis are included in this code category. Sequencing should follow the guidelines for selection of the principal diagnosis. When cellulitis or abscess occurs with chronic skin ulcer (category 707), code both conditions.

Cellulitis Associated with Pregnancy or Delivery: There are times when a patient will develop pelvic cellulitis after delivery or following an abortion. In these instances, only codes indicating the puerperal infection (codes from chapter 11) are indicated. The cellulitis is not coded separately.

Cellulitis Secondary to Superficial Injury: When cellulitis is the result of a superficial injury, burn, or frostbite, two codes are required: one for the cellulitis and one describing the injury.

Gangrenous Cellulitis: If the documentation indicates that gangrenous cellulitis is present, code 785.4 is assigned in addition to the injury or ulcer code and not a code from categories 681-682.

Open Wound with Cellulitus: When cellulitis is associated with an open wound, the code for a complicated open wound is assigned followed by the code for cellulitis when the patient is being seen primarily for treatment of the open wound. However, if the patient is being seen primarily for treatment of the cellulitis and the open wound is minor and does not require specific treatment, the appropriate code for cellulitis is indicated followed by an additional code identifying the complicated open wound.

Postoperative Cellulitis: Cellulitis resulting from a postoperative wound infection requires two codes: 998.59 *Other postoperative infection* and the appropriate code from categories 681 and 682 identifying the cellulitis.

Septic Leukocytoclastic Vasculitis: Two codes are required to report this condition: 446.29 *Other specified hypersensitivity angiitis* and a code from category 682 *Other cellulitis and abscess*.

Skin Ulcers and Cellulitus: A frequent complication of chronic skin ulcers is cellulitis. Since the codes identifying chronic skin ulcers (707.0-707.9) do not include any mention of cellulitis, two codes are necessary. Code both the chronic skin ulcer and the cellulitis.

Coding Scenario
An 8-year-old male is seen in the physician's office with cellulitis of the left forearm. The patient's mother states that there was an insect bite in the area and believes the skin infection resulted from scratching the bite.

>Code assignment: 682.3 *Other cellulitis and abscess of upper arm and forearm* and 913.5 *Superficial injury of elbow, forearm, and wrist, insect bite, nonvenomous, infected*

A patient has an open wound of the left upper leg with the development of cellulitis.

>Code assignment: 682.6 *Other cellulitis and abscess of leg, except foot* and 890.1 *Open wound of hip and thigh, complicated*

A patient had a coronary bypass graft 10 days ago and is admitted today with cellulitis of the incision site.

>Code assignment: 998.5 *Postoperative infection* and 682.2 *Cellulitis and abscess of trunk*

683 Acute lymphadenitis ▣
Acute lymphadenitis is sudden, severe inflammation of the lymph nodes. The infection may be due to streptococci, staphylococci, or other organisms. Therapies include antimicrobials (penicillin).

Coding Clarification
Use an additional code to identify the infective organism, typically streptococcus. Abscess and acute lymphangitis are included in this code category. Chronic or subacute, mesenteric, and unspecified lymphadenitis are excluded. Sequencing should follow the guidelines for selection of the principal diagnosis. When cellulitis or abscess associated with acute lymphadenitis occurs with a chronic skin ulcer (category 707), code both conditions.

684 Impetigo ▣
Impetigo is a superficial skin infection. There are two types of impetigo: bullous and vesicular. With bullous impetigo, fragile bullae form rapidly, break early, and heal centrally, leaving crusted erosions. Vesicular impetigo originates as small vesicles or pustules that break, exposing a red, moist base, and secrete a honey-yellow to white-brown crust. Usually caused by streptococci, staphylococci, or both, impetigo occurs most frequently after a minor skin injury such as a cut, scrape, or insect bite but infrequently may also develop on healthy skin.

Signs and symptoms of impetigo include skin lesions, itching, and mild pain. Blood work reveals elevated sedimentation rate. A gram stain and culture of the lesion identify the infective organism, and antistreptolysin-O (ASO) titers detect streptococcal infection. Therapies include triple antibiotic ointment (bacitracin, Polysporin, and neomycin applied three times daily).

Coding Clarification
Excluded from this rubric is impetigo herpetiformis, reported with 694.3.

685 Pilonidal cyst
A pilonidal cyst is a hair-containing cyst or sinus located at the sacrococcygeal area, which often has a sinus that opens at a postanal dimple.

Signs and symptoms of pilonidal cyst include edema, warmth, redness, pain, and interference with function. A gram stain and culture of the lesion identify the infective organism. Blood work usually identifies negative culture. Therapies include incision and drainage or circumferential excision. Use the appropriate fourth digit to indicate the presence or absence of an abscess.

685.0	Pilonidal cyst with abscess — *cyst and abscess in sacrococcygeal tissue, including sinus or fistula*
685.1	Pilonidal cyst without mention of abscess — *cyst in sacrococcygeal tissue, including sinus or fistula*

686 Other local infection of skin and subcutaneous tissue
This rubric classifies other local infections of the skin and subcutaneous tissue including pyoderma, pyogenic granuloma, granuloma, or dermatitis due to a pus-forming organism such as those classified to rubric 041. Therapies include antibiotics and incision and drainage of larger lesions.

686.00	Unspecified pyoderma — *dermatitis unknown*
686.01	Pyoderma gangrenosum — *persistent, debilitating dermatitis with boggy blue-red ulcers* AHA: Q4, 1997, 42
686.09	Other pyoderma — *not elsewhere classified*
686.1	Pyogenic granuloma of skin and subcutaneous tissue — *septic, suppurative, telangiectaticum*
686.8	Other specified local infections of skin and subcutaneous tissue — *dermatitis vegetans; Andrew's pustular bacteride; Brandt's syndrome; Danbold-Closs syndrome; Spiegler-Fendt sarcoid*
686.9	Unspecified local infection of skin and subcutaneous tissue — *skin infection or fistula, unknown*

690–698 Other Inflammatory Conditions of Skin and Subcutaneous Tissue

Excluded from this range of codes is panniculitis, classified to 739.30-739.39.

690 Erythematosquamous dermatosis

Erythematosquamous dermatosis is an inflammatory, scaly condition of the skin predominantly affecting the scalp and face.

Signs and symptoms of erythematosquamous dermatosis include dandruff, itching, dry skin, and crusted scalp lesion ("cradle cap") in infants. Therapies include hydrocortisone cream for facial lesions and dandruff shampoo for scalp and other hairy areas.

690.10	Unspecified seborrheic dermatitis — *not otherwise specified* AHA: Q4, 1995, 58	
690.11	Seborrhea capitis — *exclusive to scalp; cradle cap* AHA: Q4, 1995, 58	
690.12	Seborrheic infantile dermatitis — *itchy and scaly inflammation of skin in infants* AHA: Q4, 1995, 58	
690.18	Other seborrheic dermatitis — *not otherwise specified, including Unna's disease* AHA: Q4, 1995, 58	
690.8	Other erythematosquamous dermatosis — *parakeratosis*	

Coding Clarification

Excluded from this rubric are eczematous dermatitis of the eyelid (373.31), parakeratosis variegata (696.2), psoriasis (rubric 696), and seborrheic keratosis (702).

691 Atopic dermatitis and related conditions

691.0	Diaper or napkin rash — *psoriasiform napkin eruption; ammonia dermatitis*
691.8	Other atopic dermatitis and related conditions — *atopic dermatitis; Besnier's prurigo; atopic neurodermatitis; prurigo-asthma syndrome; intrinsic eczema*

692 Contact dermatitis and other eczema

This rubric classifies rash as a result of a substance that comes in contact with the skin. Initially, the rash is limited to the site of contact but may spread.

Signs and symptoms of contact dermatitis and other eczema include transient redness to severe swelling, itching, and vesiculation. Therapies include identification and elimination of the offending agent, topical corticosteroid gel in less acute situations, emollient, and other protective ointment for dry dermatitis.

692.0	Contact dermatitis and other eczema due to detergents — *allergic reaction*
692.1	Contact dermatitis and other eczema due to oils and greases — *allergic reaction*
692.2	Contact dermatitis and other eczema due to solvents — *chlorocompound, cyclohexane, ester, glycol, hydrocarbon, ketone groups*
692.3	Contact dermatitis and other eczema due to drugs and medicines in contact with skin — (Use additional E code to identify drug) — *arnica, fungicides, iodine, keratolytics, mercurials, neomycin, pediculocides, phenols, scabicides; dermatitis medicamentosa*
692.4	Contact dermatitis and other eczema due to other chemical products — *acids, adhesive plaster, alkalis, caustics, dichromate, insecticide, nylon, plastic, rubber* AHA: Q2, 1989, 16
692.5	Contact dermatitis and other eczema due to food in contact with skin — *cereals, fish, flour, fruit, meat, milk*
692.6	Contact dermatitis and other eczema due to plants (except food) — *lacquer tree; poison ivy, oak, sumac; primrose; ragweed*

Subcategory 692.7 reports photodamage to the skin. Photodamage is a serious medical condition that has been identified with an increased risk of premalignant skin lesions, such as actinic keratosis, and skin malignancies such as basal cell carcinoma and melanoma.

692.70	Unspecified dermatitis due to sun
692.71	Contact dermatitis and other eczema due to sunburn — *first degree and sunburn NOS* AHA: Q4, 2001, 47

Interestingly, no differentiation is made between first, second, and third degree sunburn in ICD-9-CM.

Do not use a sunburn code to report a burn received in a tanning booth. Instead, report that burn with 692.82.

692.72	Acute dermatitis due to solar radiation — (Use additional E code to identify drug, if drug-induced) — *Berlogue dermatitis, photoallergic response, phototoxic response, polymorphus light eruption*

Use subclassification 692.72 to report acute contact photosensitive reaction due to solar radiation. Contact photosensitive reaction is categorized as photoallergic or phototoxic. Sunburn is excluded from this code, see 692.71 and 692.76-692.77.

Photoallergic contact dermatitis is an allergic dermatitis caused by a photosensitizing substance plus sunlight in a sensitized person. The clinical presentation is similar to allergic contact dermatitis except that sunlight must be present to induce the reaction. If the photosensitizer acts internally, it is photodrug dermatitis; if it acts externally, it is a photocontact dermatitis. Some examples of oral photodrug dermatitis photosensitizers are diuretics such as Diuril, hypoglycemics such as Orinase, and phenothiazine such as Thorazine. Examples of topical photocontact dermatitis photosensitizers are antimicrobials such as bithionol and antihistamines such as Benadryl. Report an E code secondarily to identify the drug if the dermatitis is drug-induced.

Phototoxic contact dermatitis is a nonimmunologic reaction that occurs two to six hours after the skin has been exposed to a photosensitizing agent and solar radiation. The clinical presentation is similar to sunburn. Some examples of phototoxic dermatitis are phototoxic tar dermatitis (dermatitis associated with coal tar, creosote, or pitch), phytophotodermatitis, dermatitis bullosa striata pratensis (grass or meadow dermatitis), and berloque (perfume) dermatitis.

| 692.73 | Actinic reticuloid and actinic granuloma — *skin growths the result of persistent inflammation of the skin as a reaction to solar rays* |

Use subclassification 692.73 to report a severe and chronic form of photosensitivity (actinic reticuloid) and skin lesion (actinic granuloma). Usually affecting males between the ages of 45 and 70, actinic reticuloid requires complete avoidance of sunlight and other forms of ultraviolet radiation since it is resistant to treatment with sunscreens and steroids.

Actinic granuloma begins as papules and nodules. These lesions grow very slowly and eventually become annular. Persistent for years, actinic granuloma is believed to be due to defective repair of connective tissue damaged by sun and heat.

| 692.74 | Other chronic dermatitis due to solar radiation — *solar elastosis, chronic solar skin damage* |

Use subclassification 692.74 to report other specified and unspecified forms of chronic dermatitis due to solar radiation. Included are conditions such as actinic cheilitis, actinic solar elastosis, Favre-Racouchot syndrome, "sailor's skin," and "farmer's skin."

692.75	Disseminated superficial actinic porokeratosis (DSAP)
692.76	Sunburn of second degree
692.77	Sunburn of third degree
692.79	Other dermatitis due to solar radiation — *hydroa aestivale; photodermatitis, photosensitiveness*
692.81	Dermatitis due to cosmetics

| 692.82 | Dermatitis due to other radiation — *infrared lights, ultraviolet lights, tanning beds, x-rays* |

AHA: Q3, 2000, 5; Q4, 2001, 47

Coding Clarification
Use subclassification 692.82 to report dermatitis due to forms of radiation other than solar radiation, such as x-rays, radiation from tanning beds, infrared rays, ionizing radiation, ultraviolet light (excluding sunlight), and gamma rays.

| 692.83 | Dermatitis due to metals — *jewelry* |

Use subclassification 692.83 to report dermatitis due to exposure to or contact with metals or metallic salts. Nickel, the chromates, and mercury are the most common causes of metal dermatitis in the United States. Other metals associated with dermatitis are rhodium, platinum, cobalt, tungsten, cadmium, beryllium, vanadium, and zinc. Metals and metal salts can occur in soap and detergents, cosmetics, hair dyes, and tattoos.

| 692.84 | Contact dermatitis and other eczema due to animal (cat) (dog) dander |

Contact dermatitis is an allergic reaction of the skin characterized by a rash or hives. This is usually an immune reaction to a protein found in animal dander. This may be a result of direct contact with an animal or contact with fabric containing the animal dander.

| 692.89 | Contact dermatitis and other eczema due to other specified agent — *not elsewhere specified, including dermatitis due to weather, dyes, preservatives, blister beetle dermatitis, enema rash, caterpillar dermatitis* |
| 692.9 | Contact dermatitis and other eczema, due to unspecified cause |

Coding Clarification
Use the appropriate fourth digit to indicate the causative agent. An E code from the table of drugs and chemicals should be reported secondarily to report an adverse effect from a drug or chemical.

Excluded from this rubric are allergy NOS (995.3), contact dermatitis of the eyelids (373.32), dermatitis due to a substance taken internally (rubric 693), eczema of the external ear (380.22), perioral dermatitis (695.3), urticarial reactions (708.0-708.9, 995.1), and seborrheic keratosis (702.11-702.19).

693 Dermatitis due to substances taken internally
Use this rubric to report dermatitis due to the ingestion of drugs, chemicals, foodstuffs, or other substances. The condition usually manifests with an abrupt onset of diffuse, symmetric erythematous eruptions. The cause may be an allergic reaction,

adverse effect, drug interaction, idiosyncratic reaction, or some other cause.

693.0   Dermatitis due to drugs and medicines taken internally — (Use additional E code to identify drug) — *dermatitis medicamentosa not otherwise specified*

The definition of dermatitis due to drugs and medicines taken internally is systemic erythematous inflammation of the skin, also known as dermatitis medicamentosa or drug eruption. The condition may mimic inflammatory skin conditions such as eczema, toxic erythema, and erythroderma. Onset may be sudden (e.g., urticaria or angioedema after penicillin) or delayed.

Signs and symptoms of dermatitis due to drugs and medicines taken internally include mild rash to toxic epidermal microlysis, malaise, fever, arthralgia, and headache. Therapies include cessation of the offending drug; lubricant for dry, itching, maculopapular eruption; and corticosteroid for the existing rash.

ICD-9-CM coding rules regarding poisonings and adverse effects must be followed using the table of drugs and chemicals.

693.1   Dermatitis due to food taken internally — *infested food*
693.8   Dermatitis due to other specified substances taken internally — *not specified elsewhere*
693.9   Dermatitis due to unspecified substance taken internally

Coding Clarification
Excluded from this rubric are adverse effect NOS of drugs and medicines (995.2), allergy NOS (995.3), contact dermatitis (rubric 692), and urticarial reactions (708.0-708.9, 995.1).

694 Bullous dermatoses
Use this rubric to report cutaneous lesions of bullous dermatoses. The primary lesion in many diseases, bullae are large blisters that form at some level of the skin.

694.0   Dermatitis herpetiformis — *dermatosis herpetiformis; Duhring's disease, Brocq-Duhring disease; hydroa herpetiformis*
694.1   Subcorneal pustular dermatosis — *Sneddon-Wilkinson disease*
694.2   Juvenile dermatitis herpetiformis — *juvenile pemphigoid*
694.3   Impetigo herpetiformis — *rare dermatosis of third trimester with multiply symptoms*
694.4   Pemphigus — *erythematosus, foliaceus, vegetans, vulgaris; Senear-Usher syndrome*
694.5   Pemphigoid — *bullous, herpes circinatus bullosus, senile dermatitis herpetiformis*

The definition of pemphigoid is chronic, benign eruption, including benign pemphigus and bullous pemphigoid. Pemphigoid is seen chiefly in the elderly and in individuals with autoimmune disease. Signs and symptoms of pemphigoid include tense bullae on normal or reddened skin. Immunofluorescence studies confirm the diagnosis. Therapies include prednisone.

694.60   Benign mucous membrane pemphigoid without mention of ocular involvement — *cicatricial pemphigoid, mucosynechial atrophic bullous dermatitis*
694.61   Benign mucous membrane pemphigoid with ocular involvement — *cicatricial pemphigoid, mucosynechial atrophic bullous dermatitis*
694.8   Other specified bullous dermatosis — *not specified elsewhere*
694.9   Unspecified bullous dermatosis

695 Erythematous conditions
Erythema has many causes, including an immunologic reaction triggered by circulating immune complexes, drugs (penicillin, barbiturates, sulfonamides), and infection (herpes simplex, Mycoplasma pneumoniae). Etiology is unknown in many of the erythematous conditions. Treatments include painkillers and ice packs to ease the pain of nodules and medical attention directed toward the underlying disease.

Papules, plaques, and bulls eye (target) lesions are diagnostic of erythema multiforme (695.1). On mucous membranes, it begins as blisters and progresses to ulcers. A more advanced form, Stevens-Johnson syndrome, can be fatal.

Recurring mouth and genital ulcers, and inflammation of the uvea are characteristic of Behcet's syndrome (695.2), which can also affect the retina, brain, joints, skin, and bowels.

Rosacea (695.3) is a hereditary, chronic disorder characterized by groups of arterioles, capillaries, and venules that become dilated, resulting in small papules and pustules, especially around the nose, forehead, cheekbones, and chin. Patients with progressive rosacea may be seen by an ophthalmologist to detect early subclinical complications.

Red plaques with an expanding inflammatory border and hypopigmented atrophic scarring is characteristic of discoid lupus erythematosus (695.4), which is not usually associated with systemic manifestations. Lesions are commonly in areas exposed to sunlight such as the face, ears, neck, and scalp.

695.0 Toxic erythema — *erythema venenatum*
Use subcategory 695.0 to report erythematous eruptions of a wide anatomic area caused by bacterial or other toxins or administration of medications in toxic dosages.

695.1 Erythema multiforme — *toxic epidermal necrolysis, erythema iris; herpes iris; syndromes: Lyell's; Stevens-Johnson, Baader', Flessinger-Rendu, Klauder's*

695.2 Erythema nodosum — *painful inflammation of tissue of lower extremities usually caused by a hypersensitivity reaction, and sometimes seen as a manifestation of disease, as in sarcoidosis*

695.3 Rosacea — *erythematosa acne; rhinophyma; perioral dermatitis; rosacea acne*

695.4 Lupus erythematosus — *discoid lupus erythematosus, not disseminated*

Coding Clarification
Use subcategory 695.4 to report lupus erythematosus, a chronic disease that causes inflammation of the connective tissue of the skin only. Occurring worldwide, this disease affects nine times as many women as men, usually those of childbearing age, and can lead to scarring and permanent disfigurement.

Signs and symptoms of lupus erythematosus include erythematous, round scaling papules usually on malar prominences, the bridge of the nose, scalp, and external auditory canals. Thickened areas of skin may later scar.

Lab work reveals leukopenia, positive LE cells test in only 10 percent of patients. A skin biopsy shows immunoglobulins or complement components. Therapies include reduced exposure to sunlight, topical corticosteroid for lesions, and antimalarials (Plaquenil).

This subcategory includes discoid lupus erythematosus but excludes lupus vulgaris NOS (017.0) and systemic lupus erythematosus (710.0).

695.81 Ritter's disease — *generalized staph syndrome causing exfoliation and raw skin in infants*

695.89 Other specified erythematous condition — *erythema intertrigo; pityriasis rubra; dermatitis epidemica; syndromes: Savill's; Sweet's, Wilson-Brocq, Bury's, Leiner's*
AHA: Sept-Oct, 1986, 10

695.9 Unspecified erythematous condition

696 Psoriasis and similar disorders
Use this category to report a common skin disease characterized by patches of inflamed, red skin, covered by silvery scales and sometimes accompanied by painful swelling and stiffness of the joints (arthritis). With psoriasis, new cells are produced 10 times faster than normal, but the rate at which old cells are shed is unchanged. Consequently, the stratum corneum becomes thickened with flaky, immature skin cells. Occurring predominantly over the elbows, knees, scalp, and trunk, psoriasis tends to run in families, affects men and women equally, and usually appears between the ages of 10 and 30.

Therapies include moderate exposure to sunlight or phototherapy and the use of an emollient for mild cases, ointment containing coal tar or anthralin for moderate cases, and topical corticosteroids and oral methotrexate for severe cases.

696.0 Psoriatic arthropathy — *psoriasis associated with joint disease*

696.1 Other psoriasis and similar disorders — *acrodermatitis continua, dermatitis repens, Willan-Plumbe syndrome*

696.2 Parapsoriasis — *parakeratosis variegata; parapsoriasis lichenoides chronica; pityriasis lichenoides et varioliformis; Brocq's parapsoriasis; Mucah-Haberman syndrome; Wise's disease*

696.3 Pityriasis rosea — *pityriasis circinata (et maculata)*

696.4 Pityriasis rubra pilaris — *Devergie's disease, lichen ruber acuminatus*

696.5 Other and unspecified pityriasis — *not otherwise specified*

696.8 Other psoriasis and similar disorders — *not otherwise specified*

697 Lichen
This rubric describes papular skin diseases characterized by small lesions set close together. A biopsy is performed to make the diagnosis of the particular form of the disease and treatments include topical corticosteroids to reduce itching and induce regression of the lesions. Hyperpigmented areas may persist after the lesions have resolved. An example from this rubric is lichen sclerosus, which is a skin disorder that affects the vulva. The cause is unknown and, similar to other diseases in this rubric, the condition resembles the appearance of lichens (mixture of fungi and algae) found in nature.

697.0 Lichen planus — *planopilaris, ruber planus*
Use subcategory 697.0 to report an inflammatory cutaneous and mucous membrane condition characterized by pruritic, violaceous, and flattop papules with fine white streaks and symmetric distribution. Signs and symptoms of lichen planus include chronic papules, acute lesions of the skin and mucous membranes, and severe itching. Histopathology of the skin lesion confirms the diagnosis. Therapies include topical, intralesional, and systemic steroids, antihistamines, psoralens

plus long-wave ultraviolet light, and oral griseofulvin.

697.1	Lichen nitidus — *Pinkus' disease*
697.8	Other lichen, not elsewhere classified — *ruber moniliforme, striata*
697.9	Unspecified lichen

Coding Clarification
Excluded from this rubric are obtusus corneus (698.3), congenital pilaris (757.39), ruber acuminatus (696.4), sclerosus of atrophicus (701.9), scrofulosus (017.0), simplex chronicus (698.3), congenital spinulosus (757.39), and urticatus (698.2).

698 Pruritus and related conditions

Use this rubric to report conditions characterized by an intense itching and/or burning sensation of the skin. Most cases of generalized pruritus are due to dry skin but may be due to a variety of dermatologic or systemic conditions. Therapies include elimination of soaps or detergents, cessation of all but necessary medications, the application of moisturizers while the skin is wet, tranquilizers in severe cases, and topical or systemic corticosteroids as well as antihistamines and antiserotonin drugs.

Pruritus (itching) may be related to a wide variety of conditions classifiable elsewhere, such as scabies, atopic dermatitis, sunburn, uremia, and contact dermatitis. In most cases, the pruritus is an integral part of the disease and is not reported separately. Excluded from this rubric is pruritus that is psychogenic in nature (306.3).

698.0	Pruritus ani — *intense anal itch*
698.1	Pruritus of genital organs — *intense genital itch*
698.2	Prurigo — *lichen urticatus; Hebra's prurigo; urticaria papulosa; mitis prurigo; prurigo simplex*
698.3	Lichenification and lichen simplex chronicus — *neurodermatitis; prurigo nodularis; Brocq's lichen simplex chronicus; Hyde's or Vidal's disease*
698.4	Dermatitis factitia (artefacta) — (Use additional code to identify any associated mental disorder) — *dermatitis ficta, neurotic excoriation*
698.8	Other specified pruritic conditions — *not classified elsewhere, including hiemalis, senilis, winter itch*
698.9	Unspecified pruritic disorder

700–709 Other Diseases of Skin and Subcutaneous Tissue

Excluded from this range of codes are conditions confined to the eyelids (373.0–374.9) and congenital conditions of the hair, skin, and nails (759.0–759.9).

700 Corns and callosities

Calluses and corns are knobs of hyperkeratotic tissue caused by pressure or friction, most commonly seen in the bony prominences of the feet or hands. Benign conditions, they can cause pain that requires treatment by a podiatrist or physician.

701 Other hypertrophic and atrophic conditions of skin

701.0	Circumscribed scleroderma — *Addison's keloid, morphea, localized dermatosclerosis, von Zambusch's disease, lichen sclerosus et atrophicus*
701.1	Acquired keratoderma — *elastosis perforans serpiginosa; acquired ichthyosis, acquired keratoderma palmaris et plantaris; keratosis blennorrhagica*
	AHA: Q4, 1994, 48
701.2	Acquired acanthosis nigricans — *keratosis nigricans*
701.3	Striae atrophicae — *atrophic skin spots; striae disease; senile degenerative atrophy; atrophy blanche of Milian*
701.4	Keloid scar — *hypertrophic scar, cheloid*

Keloid scars are tumors consisting of actively growing hypertrophic cutaneous scar tissue. They occur as a result of trauma or irritation such as burns, incisions, vaccinations, insect bites, and other stimuli. Ulcerated keloids are prone to carcinomatous transformation, but the majority behave as benign neoplasms. Dark-skinned races are particularly susceptible to keloid formation. Hypertrophic scars are similar to keloids except they lack the characteristic tumor formation of keloids and do not grow beyond the margins of the original injury.

Signs and symptoms of keloid scar include a history of surgery or skin trauma, overreactive visible scar formation, itching, and burning. A skin biopsy may be performed to determine the histopathology. Therapies include surgical or laser excision, z-plasty when the scar crosses a flexion surface, cryotherapy (freezing with liquid nitrogen), radiation therapy, and injection of corticosteroid such as Kenalog-10.

In many cases, keloids and hypertrophic scars are residuals of previous trauma or surgery. If the etiology of the keloid or hypertrophic scar is known and described as a late effect, assign a secondary code describing the late effect. For example, if the diagnosis were residual keloid due to a previously treated burn of the hand, codes 701.4 and 906.6 would be assigned.

| 701.5 | Other abnormal granulation tissue — *excessive granulation* |
| 701.8 | Other specified hypertrophic and atrophic condition of skin — *atrophia cutis senilis, cutis* |

laxa senilis, acantholysis, pachydermatitis, Pick-Herxheimer or Gougerot-Carteaud syndrome, elastosis senilis, folliculitis ulerythematosa reticulata, confluent and reticulate papillomatosis

701.9 Unspecified hypertrophic and atrophic condition of skin — *skin tag, atrophoderma, pendulous abdomen, redundant skin, or unknown*

Coding Clarification
Excluded form this rubric are dermatomyositis (710.0), hereditary edema of the legs (757.0), and scleroderma (generalized) (710.3).

702 Other dermatoses

702.0 Actinic keratosis — *sharply outlined warty growth usually caused by sun damage to skin*
AHA: Q1, 1992, 18

Use subcategory 702.0 to report precancerous warty lesions due to the cumulative effect of overexposure to sunlight. These lesions also are known as solar or senile keratosis, keratoderma, keratoma, acanthosis verrucosa, verruca senilis, and plana senilis. Therapies include cryotherapy (freezing with liquid nitrogen) and 5-Fluorouracil.

Use subcategory 702.1 to report superficial noninvasive tumors (usually multiple) originating in the epidermis. Characterized by numerous yellow or brown sharply marginated, oval, raised lesions, these tumors also are known as seborrheic warts or verrucae. They occur commonly in middle-aged or older patients. Therapies include shaving the lesions.

702.11 Inflamed seborrheic keratosis — *warty growth of basaloid sells not otherwise specified*
AHA: Q4, 1994, 48
702.19 Other seborrheic keratosis
702.8 Other specified dermatoses — *acanthotic nevus, cutaneous horn, sebaceous nevus, or not otherwise specified*

Coding Clarification
Excluded from this rubric is carcinoma in situ (232.0-232.9).

703 Diseases of nail

Nails are hard, keratinized cells of epidermis that consist of a nail body, a free edge, and a nail root. Vascular tissue gives the visible nail body its pink color, except at the whitish lunula where the vascular tissue does not show through. The nail groove is between the nail fold and the nail bed, which is the epidermis beneath the nail. The cuticle, or eponychium, is a narrow band of epidermis that adheres to the nail wall. The thickened stratum corneum below the free edges is referred to as the hyponychium. The nail matrix, at the proximal end of the nail bed, promotes nail growth, which occurs when superficial cells of the matrix transform into nail cells. In the process, the harder layer is pushed forward over the stratum germinativum. The average growth rate for fingernails is about 1.0 millimeter per week; growth is slower for the toenails. Onychomycosis (703.8) is an infection of the nail or nail bed caused by pathogenic fungi.

An ingrowing nail is a painful condition, usually of the big toe, in which one or both edges of the nail press into the adjacent skin, leading to infection and inflammation. Common causes include poor personal hygiene, tight-fitting shoes, and incorrect nail cutting. Therapies include soaking, antibiotics to control infection, and removal of the nail edge. Excluded from this subclassification is nail infection, reported with 681.9.

703.0 Ingrowing nail — *unguis incarnatus; with infection*
703.8 Other specified disease of nail — *dystrophia unguium, hypertrophy, leukonychia, onychauxis, onycholysis, acquired polyunguia; subungual hemorrhage; horn of nail; Beau's lines; acquired anonychia; koilonychia, acquired pachyonychia, or not otherwise specified*
703.9 Unspecified disease of nail

Coding Clarification
Excluded from this rubric are congenital anomalies of the nail (757.5) and onychia and paronychia (681.02, 681.11).

704 Diseases of hair and hair follicles

The primary function of hair is protection (i.e., eyebrows and eyelashes protect the eyes from foreign objects). Hair follicles (downgrowths into the dermis) develop during the third and fourth months of fetal life and by the sixth month the follicles produce lanugo, which is shed from the trunk prior to birth. Several months after birth, a coarser hair, vellus, develops and the remaining lanugo is shed from the eyebrows, eyelids, and scalp and replaced by terminal hairs. Terminal hairs also develop in the axillary and pubic regions and on the face at puberty.

The hair shaft, which projects above the surface of the skin, is made up of the inner medulla, which consists of cells containing eleidin and air spaces; the cortex, which contains pigment granules in dark hair but mostly are in white hair; and the cuticle, the outermost layer of the shaft. The root is the portion below the surface that penetrates into the dermis and, like the shaft, consists of a medulla, cortex, and cuticle. The color of hair is due primarily to melanin.

Diseases of the Skin and Subcutaneous Tissue

704.00	Unspecified alopecia — *loss of hair, type unknown*	
704.01	Alopecia areata — *patchy loss of hair; usually temporary*	
704.02	Telogen effluvium — *temporary excessive hair loss due to stressor like childbirth, surgery, weight loss*	
704.09	Other alopecia — *folliculitis decalvans; oligotrichia, Quinquaud's disease, tinea decalvans, pseudopelade*	
704.1	Hirsutism — *excessive hair growth; acquired lanuginosa, polytrichia*	
704.2	Abnormalities of the hair — *atrophic hair, clastothrix, fragilitas crinium, trichorrhexis nodosa*	
704.3	Variations in hair color — *canities, premature gray, heterochromia, acquired poliosis circumscripta*	
704.8	Other specified disease of hair and hair follicles — *ingrown hair, folliculitis, perifolliculitis, sycosis, Bockhart's impetigo, mentagra*	
704.9	Unspecified disease of hair and hair follicles	

Coding Clarification
Excluded from this rubric are congenital anomalies (757.4).

705 Disorders of sweat glands

A sweat, or sudoriferous, gland is a type of exocrine gland that eliminates perspiration to cool the skin. The sweat glands are a simple cuboidal or columnar epithelium with pale-staining cells. The base of the sweat glands has a row of myoepithelial cells wrapped around the outside of the gland. Eccrine sweat glands are found in skin throughout the body, particularly on the forehead, scalp, axillae, palms, and soles and produce watery and neutral or slightly acidic sweat. Apocrine sweat glands are in the axilla, areola, and circumanal region and begin to function in puberty and produce viscid milky secretions in response to external stimuli. Apocrine glands accumulate secretory products at the outer margin of the cell and that portion pinches off to form the secretion; the remaining part of the cell repairs itself and repeats the process.

705.0	Anhidrosis — *diminished sweating; hypohidrosis, oligohidrosis*	
705.1	Prickly heat — *heat rash, sudamina, miliaria rubra, sweat retention syndrome*	
705.21	Primary focal hyperhidrosis **AHA:** Q4, 2004, 91	
705.22	Secondary focal hyperhidrosis **AHA:** Q4, 2004, 91	
705.81	Dyshidrosis — *usually affecting hands and feet; cheiropompholyx, pompholyx*	
705.82	Fox-Fordyce disease — *rare eruption of follicular papules of axillae, nipples, pubic region*	
705.83	Hidradenitis — *inflammation of sweat gland; Pollitzer's disease, hidradenitis suppurativa*	

Hyperhidrosis is the clinical disorder of excessive sweating, beyond what the body requires to maintain thermal control. This condition may be generalized, often called secondary hyperhidrosis, occurring with another associated condition such as metabolic or endocrine disorder, malignancies, drugs, substance abuse, toxins, infections, cardiovascular disorders, or respiratory failure.

Primary hyperhidrosis occurs in the absence of any underlying or causative condition, and is almost always focal, confined to one or more specific areas of the body, like the axilla, the soles of the feet, the palms, or the face. Secondary hyperhidrosis may also occur as focal, however, when it is caused by a local condition or treatment, such as radiation therapy to a specific tumor location, or spinal disease or injury. Hyperhidrosis is first treated by a trial of topical medication applications with surgery as a final step.

Use subclassification 705.83 to report inflammation of the apocrine sweat glands occurring in the axillae, anogenital regions, nipples, and under the female breast. The condition may produce chronic abscesses or sinus tract formation. In most cases, hidradenitis is caused by the obstruction of the apocrine sweat pores due to the application of underarm deodorants, irritant depilatories, or other topical ointments or creams. Signs and symptoms of hidradenitis include large painful abscesses resulting from double comedones and extensive deep dermal inflammation, weight loss, fever, malaise, local pain, and tenderness. A gram stain and culture of the lesion identify the infective organism. Therapies include antimicrobials (penicillin), surgical excision, and plastic repair of the affected area in chronic conditions.

Sequence an additional code secondarily to identify the infective organism, typically streptococcus or staphylococcus.

705.89	Other specified disorder of sweat glands — *not otherwise specified, including bromhidrosis, chromhidrosis, abscess, cyst, granulosis rubra nasi, urhidrosis, osmidrosis, hematidrosis*
705.9	Unspecified disorder of sweat glands

Coding Clarification
Report 780.8 for generalized hyperhidrosis.

Coding Scenario
A 17-year-old male comes to his primary care physician complaining of sweating under the arms and on his palms. He says his shirts seem to be

continually wet, and his hands may drip with sweat, but this occurs only during waking hours and seems to stop when he is asleep. It is now interfering with daily activities as he cannot maintain a proper grip on the ball during sports and his embarrassing underarms are causing him social anxieties. The physician diagnoses him with focal primary hyperhidrosis and informs him of treatment choices such as topical and systemic agents, iontophoresis, and botox injections to be considered before surgical sweat gland resection

> Code assignment: 705.21 *Primary focal hyperhidrosis*

706 Diseases of sebaceous glands

A sebaceous gland is one of several types of glands located in the skin and occurs most commonly in association with hair follicles (i.e., on the face and scalp and in the genital area). These glands produce sebum, a thick, slightly oily secretion that conditions the skin, which empties into the hair follicle.

Acne (706.0, 706.1) is an inflammatory skin condition characterized by superficial skin eruptions that occur when sebaceous glands within the hair follicles become plugged, because secretion occurs faster than the oil and skin cells can exit the follicle. If the plug ruptures the wall of the follicle, the oil, dead skin cells, and bacteria found on the surface of the skin can enter to form the infected pustules (e.g., pimples). The condition usually begins at puberty and affects 75 percent of all teenagers to some extent, probably due to hormonal changes that stimulate the sebaceous glands. Sebaceous hyperplasia (706.8) describes sebaceous glands enlarged by a central hair follicle that can appear on the forehead or cheeks as small yellow bumps up to 3.0 millimeters in diameter.

706.0	Acne varioliformis — *frontalis, necrotica*
706.1	Other acne — *conglobata, cystic, pustular, vulgaris, comedo, blackhead*
706.2	Sebaceous cyst — *atheroma, keratin cyst, infected steatoma, wen*

Coding Clarification

A sebaceous cyst is a slowly developing, benign cystic tumor of the skin containing follicular, keratinous, and sebaceous material. Frequently found on the scalp, ears, face, back, or scrotum, sebaceous cysts may grow very large and become infected by bacteria. An exam reveals a firm, globular, movable, and nontender tumor. Therapies include incision and expression of contents for small lesions (milium); for larger lesions, surgical excision of the cyst walls.

706.3	Seborrhea — *excessive production of sebum*

Coding Clarification
Excluded from this subclassification are dermatitis (690.10) and keratosis (702.11-702.19).

706.8	Other specified disease of sebaceous glands — *asteatosis cutis, xerosis cutis*
706.9	Unspecified disease of sebaceous glands

707 Chronic ulcer of skin
AHA: Q4, 2004, 92

Use this rubric to report a chronic defect of the skin, deeper than erosion or excoriation, extending at least into the dermal layer. Chronic ulcers usually are due to chronic inflammation, ischemia, or both.

707.00	Decubitus ulcer, unspecified site
	AHA: Q1, 2004, 14
707.01	Decubitus ulcer, elbow
707.02	Decubitus ulcer, upper back
707.03	Decubitus ulcer, lower back
	AHA: Q1, 2005, 16
707.04	Decubitus ulcer, hip
707.05	Decubitus ulcer, buttock
707.06	Decubitus ulcer, ankle
707.07	Decubitus ulcer, heel
	AHA: Q1, 2005, 16
707.09	Decubitus ulcer, other site

Documentation Issues
Documentation may identify synonymous terms for decubitus ulcers such as bed sores, plaster ulcer, pressure sore, or ulcer.

There are six stages to a decubitus ulcer that may be documented but have no effect on code selection. Code selection is based on the location of the decubitus ulcer.

Coding Clarification
Use subclassification 707.0x to report a condition, also known as a bedsore or pressure sore, that affects superficial tissues and may also deepen to affect muscle and bone. Usually occurring over a bony prominence at the sacrum, hip, heel, shoulder, or elbow, decubitus ulcers develop in patients who are bedridden, unconscious, or immobile, for example, stroke or spinal cord injury victims. Intrinsic loss of pain and pressure sensations, disuse atrophy, malnutrition, anemia, and infection play roles in the formation of decubitus ulcers. Herpes simplex virus is suspected in immunocompromised patients. In early stages, the condition is reversible, but left untended, a decubitus ulcer can become extensively infected, necrotic, and, ultimately, irreversible.

Diseases of the Skin and Subcutaneous Tissue

Signs and symptoms of decubitus ulcer include: in the first stage, deep pink, red, or mottled skin that is warm, firm, or stretched tightly across the area; in the second stage, blistering, cracking, or abrasion of the skin; in the third stage, a crater-like sore with involvement of underlying structures, and exposure of fat; in the fourth stage, necrosis extended through skin and fat to the muscle; in the fifth stage, advanced fat and muscle necrosis; and in the sixth stage, bone destruction and osteomyelitis.

Therapies include a high protein, well-balanced diet, application of absorbable gelatin sponges (Gelfoam), a change in the patient's position every two hours, and the use of egg-crate mattresses and protective padding (sheepskin). Other therapies include stimulation of the affected area by gentle massage to facilitate circulation (thus healing), debridement (excisional, chemical, and whirlpool), or deeper surgery with closure or skin grafting for advanced stages.

Recurrent Decubitus Ulcer with Failed Graft: A recurrent decubitus ulcer that has had multiple failed grafts is reported with 996.52 *Mechanical complication of device, implant or graft* and a code from the 707.0 subcategory.

Residual Pressure Sore with Recurrent Ischial Sinus: This condition is classified as a decubitus ulcer. The formation of the ischial sinus in the decubitus ulcer is an integral component of the disease progression and no additional code is assigned.

Coding Scenario
A patient has had multiple grafting procedures for treatment of an extensive decubitus ulcer of the buttock. The patient is being readmitted for failure of the skin graft.

   Code assignment: 996.52 *Mechanical complication of device, implant, or graft* and 707.05 *Decubitus ulcer, buttock*

An elderly patient is transferred from an extended care facility for treatment of a decubitus ulcer of the heel. The physician also identifies the patient as a Type I diabetic with related progressive peripheral vascular disease.

   Code assignment: 707.07 *Decubitus ulcer, heel,* 250.71 *Diabetes with peripheral circulatory disorders, Type I, not stated as uncontrolled,* and 443.81 *Peripheral angiopathy in diseases classified elsewhere*

707.10		Ulcer of lower limb, unspecified — *unknown site, not calf*
		AHA: Q4, 1999, 15; Q4, 2000, 44; Q4, 2002, 43; Q3, 2004, 5
707.11		Ulcer of thigh — *between hip and knee*
		AHA: Q4, 1999, 15; Q4, 2000, 44
707.12		Ulcer of calf
707.13		Ulcer of ankle
707.14		Ulcer of heel and midfoot — *plantar surface of midfoot*
		AHA: Q4, 1999, 15; Q4, 2000, 44
707.15		Ulcer of other part of foot — *toes*
		AHA: Q4, 1999, 15; Q4, 2000, 44
707.19		Ulcer of other part of lower limb — *not otherwise specified*
		AHA: Q4, 1999, 15; Q4, 2000, 44
707.8		Chronic ulcer of other specified site — *groin, hand, neck, perineum, sacrum, scalp, submental*
707.9		Chronic ulcer of unspecified site — *unknown skin site*

Coding Clarification
Code, if applicable, any causal condition first, as in atherosclerosis with ulceration (440.23), chronic venous hypertension with ulcer (459.31), chronic venous hypertension with ulcer and inflammation (459.33), postphlebitic syndrome with ulcer (459.11), postphlebitic syndrome with ulcer and inflammation (459.13), and diabetes (250.80-250.83). Codes are chosen according to ulcer site. In some cases, multiple codes may be required.

708 Urticaria

Use this rubric to report eruption of itching edema of the skin (hives). Often due to hypersensitivity to a drug, food, or insect stings or bites, urticaria also may be due to such stimuli as physical exercise, heat, cold, sunlight, anxiety, and tension. Most episodes are acute and self-limiting over a period of one to two weeks.

Signs and symptoms of urticaria include pruritus, wheals that may remain small or may enlarge, rings of erythema, and edema. Therapies include cessation of nonessential medication or other causative factors, oral antihistamine (Benadryl, Atarax, and Periactin), and prednisone in more severe cases (associated with angioedema).

708.0	Allergic urticaria — *allergic hives*
708.1	Idiopathic urticaria — *hives of unknown cause*
708.2	Urticaria due to cold and heat — *hives due to heat or cold*
708.3	Dermatographic urticaria — *hives raised as a result of scratching*
708.4	Vibratory urticaria — *hives as a response to vibration*
708.5	Cholinergic urticaria

708.8	Other specified urticaria — *nettle rash, recurrent periodic rash, chronic hives*
708.9	Unspecified urticaria — *hives of unknown cause*

Coding Clarification
Excluded from this rubric are angioneurotic edema (995.1), Quincke's edema (995.1), hereditary angioedema (277.6), giant urticaria (995.1), papulosa urticaria (698.2), and urticaria pigmentosa (757.33).

709 Other disorders of skin and subcutaneous tissue

709.00	Dyschromia, unspecified — *variation of skin pigmentation of unknown cause*
709.01	Vitiligo
709.09	Other dyschromia — *Civatte's poikiloderma, classic piebaldism, café au lait spots, xanthosis, Sutton's or Schamberg's disease, liver spots*
709.1	Vascular disorder of skin — *angioma serpiginosum, purpura annularis telangiectodes, Gougerot-Blum syndrome, Majocchi's disease*
709.2	Scar condition and fibrosis of skin — *adherent scar, cicatrix, disfigurement* **AHA:** Nov-Dec, 1984, 19
709.3	Degenerative skin disorder — *calcinosis circumscripta or cutis, colloid milium, Miescher-Leder syndrome, Wagner's disease, skin deposits*
709.4	Foreign body granuloma of skin and subcutaneous tissue
709.8	Other specified disorder of skin — *epithelial hyperplasia, menstrual dermatosis, vesicular eruption, dermatosis papulosa nigra, macules, papules, sclerosing lipogranuloma* **AHA:** Nov-Dec, 1987, 6
709.9	Unspecified disorder of skin and subcutaneous tissue

710–739

Diseases of the Musculoskeletal System and Connective Tissue

This chapter classifies diseases and disorders of the bones, muscles, cartilage, fascia, ligaments, synovia, tendons, and bursa.

Connective tissue disorders classified to Chapter 13 are those primarily affecting the musculoskeletal system. Injuries and certain congenital disorders of the musculoskeletal system are classified elsewhere.

Many codes for the manifestation of musculoskeletal diseases due to specified infections and other diseases and disorders classified elsewhere are included in this chapter. Also included are many codes describing the residuals of previous diseases, disorders, and injuries classified as late effects. These codes often can be identified by the term "acquired" in the description.

710–719 Arthropathies and Related Disorders

Excluded from this section are disorders of the spine (720.0-724.9).

710 Diffuse diseases of connective tissue

This rubric reports a group of diseases in which the primary lesion appears to be damage to collagen, a protein that is the major component of connective tissue. Collagen (rheumatoid) diseases, attributed largely to disorders of the immune complex mechanism, include myositis, sclerosis, dermal atrophy, arthritis, vasculitis, nephritis, carditis, subcutaneous nodules, polyserositis, and lupus erythematosus. Many of these conditions, such as polyarteritis nodosa (a connective tissue disease that is a form of vasculitis), are classified to other chapters.

Category 710 includes diffuse diseases of connective tissues; most are collagen diseases whose effects are not mainly confined to a single body system. For proper code assignment, follow the ICD-9-CM index carefully and read the includes and excludes notes pertaining to this category. Also excluded are those diffuse diseases affecting mainly the cardiovascular system, as in polyarteritis and other allied conditions (446.0-446.7).

710.0 Systemic lupus erythematosus — (Use additional code to identify manifestation: 424.91, 581.81, 582.81, 583.81) — *disseminated, Libman-Sacks disease, L.E. cell phenomenon*
AHA: Q2, 1997, 8; Q2, 2003, 7-8

Use subclassification 710.0 to report an inflammatory autoimmune disorder that may affect multiple organ systems. The disease is usually chronic, and the clinical course is mild to fulminating. Clinical exacerbations and remissions of manifestations involving the skin, serosal surfaces, central nervous system, kidneys, and blood cells are characteristic. Arthralgia, symmetrical arthritis, and inflammatory muscle involvement are common musculoskeletal features of acute systemic lupus erythematosus. The disease is most prevalent in women, particularly black women, of childbearing age.

No single etiology for the disease has been discovered, but initiation and expression of the disease has been associated with hormonal influences, genetic factors, loss of tolerance to autoantigens, and certain viruses and drugs. The hands and wrist are two sites commonly affected by lupus arthritis.

Signs and symptoms of systemic lupus erythematosus include fever, anorexia, malaise, weight loss, and skin lesions identical to chronic discoid lupus erythematosus, redness and edema affecting the nose and cheeks revealing a classic butterfly rash, photosensitivity and other ocular manifestations, and joint symptoms with or without acute synovitis. Lab work may show mild normochromic, normocytic anemia, or occasionally autoimmune hemolytic anemia. Lab work also may reveal leukopenia, lymphopenia, and thrombocytopenia. Therapies include limited, symptomatic intervention, such as topical sunscreens for photosensitivity, in mild, benign forms of the disease, in addition to nonsteroidal antiinflammatory medications to control fever, joint complaints, and serositis, as well as antimalarial drugs (chloroquine, hydroxychloroquine) and topical corticosteroids for skin manifestations. Systemic corticosteroids are prescribed for more severe manifestations involving the heart and kidneys. Immunosuppressive agents (such as cyclophosphamide, chlorambucil, and azathioprine) may be prescribed in cases resistant to corticosteroids.

Associated conditions include endocarditis, renal failure due to proliferative glomerulonephritis, nephritis or nephritis syndrome, Raynaud's phenomenon, anemia, pleurisy and pleural effusion, bronchopneumonia, restrictive lung diseases, vasculitis (with resulting ileus and peritonitis), and Hashimoto's thyroiditis.

The physician should document a causal relationship between SLE and the associated condition(s). If the causal relationship exists, sequence the SLE first followed by an additional code for the condition. If a causal relationship does not exist, sequencing would depend on the circumstances of admission, and SLE may be listed as an additional code.

Excluded from this code is lupus erythematosus (discoid) not otherwise specified (695.4).

710.1 Systemic sclerosis — (Use additional code to identify manifestation: 359.6, 517.2) — *acrosclerosis, CREST or Weissenbach-Thibierge syndrome, scleroderma, progressive systemic sclerosis*
AHA: Q1, 1988, 6

Use 710.1 to report widespread small vessel obliteration and fibrotic thickening of the skin and multiple organs, including the alimentary tract, kidneys, lungs, muscles, joints, nerves, and heart. When localized to the face and extremities (with Raynaud's phenomena), it is called acrosclerosis. A distinct form of systemic sclerosis is CREST syndrome, which stands for subcutaneous Calcinosis, Raynaud's phenomenon, Esophageal motility dysfunction, Sclerodactyly, and Telangiectasia.

Associated conditions include Raynaud's phenomena, subcutaneous calcinosis (nodular deposition of calcium salts in the subcutaneous tissues or muscles), ulcers and infection of the finger tips, telangiectasia, malabsorption syndrome, and carpal tunnel syndrome.

Excluded from this code is circumscribed scleroderma (701.0).

710.2 Sicca syndrome — *keratoconjunctivitis sicca, including Sjögren's disease*

Use 710.2 to report Sjögren's syndrome resulting from lymphocytic infiltration of lacrimal and salivary glands. An idiopathic, autoimmune disorder, Sjögren's syndrome is characterized by xerostomia (dry mouth), keratoconjunctivitis sicca (dry eyes), and parotid gland enlargement. Primary Sjögren's syndrome presents a wide variety of clinical manifestations due to a wider involvement of the exocrine glands. The organs involved may include the skin, lung, GI tract, kidney, muscles, nerves, spleen, and thyroid. Secondary Sjögren's syndrome is limited to symptoms of the lacrimal and salivary glands.

Lab work may reveal a higher frequency of human lymphocytic antigen HLA-DR3 in primary Sjögren's syndrome and of HLA-DR4 in secondary Sjögren's syndrome.

Associated conditions include rheumatoid arthritis and other collagen diseases.

710.3 Dermatomyositis — *poikilodermatomyositis, polymyositis with skin involvement, Petges-Cléjat or Unverricht-Wagner syndromes*

Use 710.3 to report nonsuppurative inflammation of the skin, subcutaneous tissues, and muscles with necrosis of muscle fibers. The disease complex is differentiated from polymyositis by the presence of a characteristic rash of edema and erythema and a heliotrope discoloration particularly around the eyes.

Physical exam reveals prominent proximal muscle weakness. Lab work shows elevated muscle enzymes. Electromyograph (EMG) reveals myopathic patterns and muscle biopsy reveals inflammatory infiltrates.

Associated conditions include malignancy of visceral organs in adults.

710.4 Polymyositis — *chronic, progressive, inflammatory symmetrical weakness of limb girdles, with pain*

Use 710.4 to report a condition identical to dermatomyositis without the characteristic skin lesions.

710.5 Eosinophilia myalgia syndrome — (Use additional E code to identify drug, if drug-induced) — *toxic oil syndrome*
AHA: Q4, 1992, 21

Use 710.5 to report a multisystem inflammatory and fibrosing illness associated with ingestion of L-tryptophan, an oral nutritional substance of amino acids. It includes toxic oil syndrome and eosinophilic fasciitis.

Signs and symptoms of eosinophilia myalgia syndrome include a history of over-the-counter use of nutritional supplements containing L-tryptophan, muscle and joint pain, weakness, swelling of the arms and legs, fever, and rash. Blood work shows increased circulating eosinophils.

Associated conditions include pneumonia, cardiac arrhythmia, pulmonary hypertension (cor pulmonale), and polyneuropathy.

710.8 Other specified diffuse disease of connective tissue — *not elsewhere classified*
AHA: March-April, 1987, 12

Subcategory 710.8 includes carpal tunnel osteolysis syndrome.

710.9 Unspecified diffuse connective tissue disease — *unknown collagen disease*

Coding Clarification

Category 710 includes diffuse diseases of connective tissues; most are collagen diseases whose effects are not mainly confined to a single body system. For proper code assignment, follow the ICD-9-CM index read the includes and excludes notes pertaining to this category. Also excluded are those diffuse diseases affecting mainly the cardiovascular system, as in polyarteritis and other allied conditions (446.0-446.7).

711 Arthropathy associated with infections
AHA: Q1, 1992, 17

This rubric includes infections of the articular joints of bones, and must be differentiated from infections of the bones classifiable to category 730.

Direct microbial contamination may cause a primary infection of the articular joints. The routes of infection include open fractures, surgical procedures, diagnostic needle aspirations, and therapeutic drug injections.

The following fifth-digit subclassification is for use with categories 711-712, 715-716, 718-719, and 730. Valid fifth-digits are in brackets [ ] at the end of each code.

0 site unspecified
1 shoulder region (acromioclavicular joint, clavicle, glenohumeral joint, scapula, sternoclavicular joint)
2 upper arm (elbow joint, humerus)
3 forearm (radius, ulna, wrist joint)
4 hand (carpus, metacarpus, phalanges)
5 pelvic regions and thigh (buttock, femur, hip joint)
6 lower leg (fibula, knee joint, patella, tibia)
7 ankle and foot (ankle joint, metatarsus, phalanges, tarsus, other joints in foot)
8 other specified sites (head, neck, ribs, skull, trunk, vertebral column)
9 multiple sites

711.0 ⌐sth Pyogenic arthritis — (Use additional code to identify infectious organism: 041.0-041.8) — *due to infectious organism, including staph, strep, H. influenzae, E. coli, pneumococcus*
AHA: Q1, 1991, 15; Q1, 1992, 16; Q1, 1992, 17

Use codes in subcategory 711.0 to report an acute, destructive bacterial process in a joint following infection, usually occurring as acute monoarticular (single joint) arthritis. The knee and large joints are most often involved.

Signs and symptoms of pyogenic arthritis include fever, joint pain, decreased range of motion, and swelling and redness over the affected joint. Gross examination of aspirated synovial (joint) fluid confirms the presence of pus (pyarthrosis); a gram stain and culture may detect microorganisms and crystals; an examination with polarizing microscope reveals crystals. Therapies include removal of inflammatory material by aspiration or incision and drainage, antibiotic therapy that may be prolonged, and resting the joint in a stable position.

Associated conditions include systemic or localized infections, intravenous drug abuse, recent trauma or surgery, pyogenic arthropathy, septicemia, and osteomyelitis.

Not all pyogenic joint infections are classifiable to subcategory 711.0. Before assigning code 711.0, carefully review the entries in the ICD-9-CM index under the terms "Arthritis, arthritic," "due to or associated with," and the includes note under subcategory 711.4 for any bacterial organism not specifically referenced under category 041. List a code from category 041 as a secondary code to identify the specific organism responsible for the arthritis or arthropathy.

711.1 ⌐sth Arthropathy associated with Reiter's disease and nonspecific urethritis — (Code first underlying disease: 099.3, 099.4) — *arthritis, arthropathy, polyarthritis, polyarthropathy code first underlying disease as: 099.4, 099.3*
AHA: Q1, 1992, 17

Use codes in subcategory 711.1 to report seronegative reactive arthritis. Occurring predominantly in the lower extremities, it is triggered by urethritis, cervicitis, or dysenteric infections. The syndrome consists of a triad of nonspecific (nongonococcal or simple) urethritis, conjunctivitis (or sometimes uveitis), and arthritis, and sometimes appears with mucocutaneous lesions. There is a close correlation between this disease and the presence of the histocompatibility antigen HLA-B27.

These manifestation codes include arthropathy with Reiter's disease and nonspecific urethritis. ICD-9-CM classifies etiology first, then manifestation, to remain compatible with the dual classification concept used in the international version of ICD-9.

711.2 ⌐sth Arthropathy in Behcet's syndrome — (Code first underlying disease, 136.1) — *arthritis, arthropathy, polyarthritis, polyarthropathy code first underlying disease 136.1*
AHA: Q1, 1992, 17

Use codes in subcategory 711.2 to report a multisystem disorder of unknown etiology named after the Turkish dermatologist who first described it. Recurrent oral and genital ulcers, uveitis, seronegative arthritis, and central nervous system abnormalities characterize the syndrome. The arthritic component involves large and small joints with a nonspecific, self-limiting synovitis and, in more than two-thirds of the patients, commonly affects the knees and ankles. The arthritic changes resemble those of rheumatoid arthritis but are milder and lead only to shallow erosions of the articular cartilage in the more severe cases. Therapies include immunomodulating drugs and corticosteroids.

Associated conditions include cranial nerve palsies, encephalitis, mental disturbances, spinal cord lesions, convulsions, and, although rarely, death.

These manifestation codes include arthropathy associated with Behcet's syndrome (136.1). ICD-9-CM classifies etiology first, then manifestation, to remain compatible with the dual classification concept used in the international version of ICD-9.

711.3 ⌐sth Postdysenteric arthropathy — (Code first underlying disease: 002.0-002.9, 008.0-009.5) — *secondary to gastrointestinal infection*
AHA: Q1, 1992, 17

Use codes in subcategory 711.3 to report rare enteropathic arthropathies due to a wide range of specific dysentery-causing organisms, Shigella, and typhoid fever.

These manifestation codes include postdysenteric arthropathy, and are distinguished from subcategory 713.1 by an infectious or parasitic etiology for the enteropathic arthritis. ICD-9-CM classifies etiology first, then manifestation, to remain compatible with the dual classification concept used in the international version of ICD-9.

Excluded from this subclassification is salmonella arthritis (003.23).

711.4 ⌐sth Arthropathy associated with other bacterial diseases — (Code first underlying disease, such as: diseases classifiable to 010-040 (except 036.82), 090-099 (except 098.50)) — *secondary*
AHA: Q1, 1992, 17

Use codes in subcategory 711.4 to report arthropathy due to a wide variety of bacteria, excluding the pyogenic organisms identified under subcategory 711.0 and bacterial arthropathies classified elsewhere.

These manifestation codes include arthropathy associated with other bacterial diseases. ICD-9-CM classifies etiology first, then manifestation, to remain compatible with the dual classification concept used in the international version of ICD-9.

Excluded from this rubric are gonococcal arthritis (098.50) and meningococcal arthritis (036.82).

711.5 ⌐sth Arthropathy associated with other viral diseases — (Code first underlying disease, such as: diseases classifiable to 045-049, 050-079 (except 056.71), 480, 487) — *secondary*
AHA: Q1, 1992, 17

Use codes in subcategory 711.5 to report arthropathy associated with a wide variety of other viral diseases including rubella, mumps, infectious mononucleosis, lymphogranuloma venereum, variola, and many others.

These manifestation codes include arthropathy associated with other viral diseases. Arthropathy associated with viral hepatitis should also be classified here. ICD-9-CM classifies etiology first, then manifestation, to remain compatible with the dual classification concept used in the international version of ICD-9.

Excluded from this subclassification is arthropathy due to rubella (056.7).

711.6 ✎5th Arthropathy associated with mycoses — (Code first underlying disease: 110.0-118) — *secondary*
AHA: Q1, 1992, 17

Use codes in subcategory 711.6 to report arthropathy due to mycoses. Mycoses are diseases caused by fungi. A variety of fungal organisms may lodge in the synovium and create suppurative or granulomatous lesions. The synovium usually is the primary site of joint involvement, but secondary infection can spread from the marrow cavity to the subchondral bone and then into the articular tissues.

These manifestation codes includes arthropathy associated with mycoses. ICD-9-CM classifies etiology first, then manifestation, to remain compatible with the dual classification concept used in the international version of ICD-9.

711.7 ✎5th Arthropathy associated with helminthiasis — (Code first underlying disease: 125.0-125.9) — *secondary*
AHA: Q1, 1992, 17

Use codes in subcategory 711.7 to report arthropathy due to parasitic infection of helminths (worms), hydatid cysts, or helminth larvae.

These manifestation codes include arthropathies associated with helminthiases. ICD-9-CM classifies etiology first, then manifestation, to remain compatible with the dual classification concept used in the international version of ICD-9.

711.8 ✎5th Arthropathy associated with other infectious and parasitic diseases — (Code first underlying disease, such as: diseases classifiable to 080-088, 100-104, 130-136) — *secondary*
AHA: Q3, 1990, 14; Q4, 1991, 15; Q1, 1992, 17

The manifestation codes in subcategory 711.8 include arthropathy associated with other infectious and parasitic diseases. ICD-9-CM classifies etiology first, then manifestation, to remain compatible with the dual classification concept used in the international version of ICD-9.

Excluded from this subclassification is arthropathy associated with sarcoidosis (713.7).

711.9 ✎5th Unspecified infective arthritis — *infective agent unknown*
AHA: Q1, 1992, 17

Coding Clarification

Direct microbial infections resulting from surgical, diagnostic, and therapeutic procedures are classified to categories 996-999.

Excluded from this rubric is rheumatic fever (390).

Most of the arthropathies classified here are due to indirect (secondary) infections, and require a second code to identify the infectious organism or the underlying disease.

Arthritis as a Late Effect: As mentioned earlier, arthritis can be a late effect or a residual of a disease process or injury.

In most circumstances, the residual condition or nature of the late effect is coded first, followed by the late effect code for the cause of the residual condition, except when instructed otherwise by the alphabetic index of the ICD-9-CM manual.

Arthritis Associated with Other Diseases: Arthritis can be a manifestation or symptom of other diseases or conditions. For example:

Arthritis due to Lyme Disease: A common manifestation of Lyme disease is joint pain (arthralgia) and arthritis. These symptoms occur early in the disease process and each should be separately coded.

In instances when the patient has both Lyme disease and the clinical manifestation of arthritis, code 088.81 is assigned as well as the code indicating arthritis associated with other parasitic diseases (711.8x).

Multiple Coding: There are times when arthritis will require multiple codes. In these instances, the alphabetic index of the ICD-9-CM manual will identify a code for both the etiology and the manifestation following the subentry term, with the second code italicized and in slanted brackets. Both codes should be assigned and in the sequence that the patient presents.

Type of Arthritis: The term arthritis is used by medical personnel to describe more than 100 various forms of rheumatic disease. Arthritis can affect multiple body systems and/or sites including joints, muscles, connective tissues, skin, and internal organs. The most widespread forms of arthritis are osteoarthritis and rheumatoid arthritis. This disease can also be the sequelae of other disease processes or caused by infectious organisms.

Osteoarthritis: The most common form of arthritis is osteoarthritis (OA). Physicians often call this form of arthritis by various terms including degenerative joint disease (DJD), osteoarthrosis, degenerative arthritis, and hypertrophic arthritis.

Osteoarthritis noted as generalized is a chronic noninflammatory arthritis that affects multiple sites, commonly of older patients, marked by degeneration of articular cartilage and enlargement of bone, and pain and stiffness occurring with any type of activity but subsiding when the patient rests. This form should be reported with subcategory code 715.0x. Only three of the 10 fifth digits available for osteoarthritis may be used with this subcategory: 0, 4, and 9.

There are two categories of localized osteoarthritis: primary and secondary.

- Primary osteoarthritis is also known as idiopathic or polyarticular degenerative arthritis. Primarily this form affects joints of the spine, knee, hip, and small joints of the hands and feet.
- Secondary osteoarthritis, also known as monarticular arthritis, is due to an illness or injury and affects the joint of one area. Possible causes include, but are not limited to, infectious, metabolic, endocrine, or neuropathic diseases; diseases that alter the normal function and structure of the cartilage (e.g., Paget's disease, gout, chondrocalcinosis, etc.); and acute or chronic injuries or trauma.

Rheumatoid Arthritis: Rheumatoid arthritis is a disease of the autoimmune system that can affect the entire body. This disease can occur during childhood (called juvenile rheumatoid arthritis) or adulthood. Single or multiple sites may be affected.

Pyogenic Arthritis: This form of arthritis is due to an acute inflammation of the synovial membranes with purulent effusion into the joint caused by a bacterial infection. It may also be referred to in the medical record documentation as suppurative arthritis or suppurative synovitis. It may progress and become chronic resulting in sinus formation, osteomyelitis, and joint deformity.

When reporting pyogenic arthritis, use subcategory code 711.0 with the appropriate fifth digit to identify the specific site. An additional code indicating the infectious organism is assigned if it is known.

Pyogenic arthritis can also affect other tissues and organs. When this occurs, the code for the condition responsible for the encounter is assigned as well as a code for the pyogenic arthritis (711.0x).

Gout: This is an acute recurrent arthritis in which excessive uric acid in the blood is deposited in the peripheral joints. It may be chronic, which can cause progressive debilitation. However, all hyperuricemia is not gout, and all hyperuricemia does not progress to gout.

Coding Scenario
A patient with recently diagnosed Lyme disease is seen in the office for follow-up. She is now complaining of joint pain and swelling of the knees. The physician states that arthritis due to the Lyme disease is now present.

> Code assignment: 088.81 *Lyme disease* and 711.86 *Arthropathy associated with other infectious and parasitic diseases, lower leg (fibula, knee joint, patella, tibia)*

A patient who was treated five years ago for Lyme disease is now seen in the office for residual arthritic pain. After examination, the physician's diagnostic statement indicates that the patient has arthritis secondary to Lyme disease. The medical record identifies that the patient is cured of Lyme disease, but still has the residual arthritis of multiple sites from the disease.

> Code assignment: 139.8 *Late effect of other and unspecified infectious and parasitic diseases* and 711.89 *Arthropathy associated with other infectious and parasitic diseases, multiple sites*

712 Crystal arthropathies

Use this rubric to report chondrocalcinosis, arthritis, and synovitis, as well as pseudogout and calcium pyrophosphate dehydrate deposition (CPDD) disease. The presence, and not the chemical composition, of crystals (apatite and hydroxyapatite, calcium pyrophosphate, calcium and dicalcium phosphate, calcium oxalate, and lipid crystals) acts as irritants. The mechanisms of initial precipitation are unknown, but predisposing conditions such as degradation of the cartilage matrix may be involved. Once the crystals have accumulated, they are taken up by phagocytic cells, initiating the inflammatory sequence. This in turn causes additional damage to the affected tissues.

The term chondrocalcinosis refers to calcification of articular cartilage. Articular chondrocalcinosis also is known as pseudogout since the disease is characterized by calcified deposits in the cartilage, but is free of the urate crystals found in gout. Aspiration and examination of synovial fluid allows precise diagnosis. Therapies include aspiration of the acutely inflamed joint; drugs such as corticosteroid injections; nonsteroidal, anti-inflammatory drugs; and intravenous colchicine.

> The following fifth-digit subclassification is for use with categories 711-712, 715-716, 718-719, and 730. Valid fifth-digits are in brackets [ ] at the end of each code.
>
> 0   site unspecified

1 shoulder region (acromioclavicular joint, clavicle, glenohumeral joint, scapula, sternoclavicular joint)
2 upper arm (elbow joint, humerus)
3 forearm (radius, ulna, wrist joint)
4 hand (carpus, metacarpus, phalanges)
5 pelvic regions and thigh (buttock, femur, hip joint)
6 lower leg (fibula, knee joint, patella, tibia)
7 ankle and foot (ankle joint, metatarsus, phalanges, tarsus, other joints in foot)
8 other specified sites (head, neck, ribs, skull, trunk, vertebral column)
9 multiple sites

712.1 [✓5th] Chondrocalcinosis due to dicalcium phosphate crystals — (Code first underlying disease, 275.4) — *crystal-induced arthritis*

The manifestation codes in subcategory 712.1 include chondrocalcinosis due to dicalcium phosphate crystals. ICD-9-CM classifies etiology first, then manifestation, to remain compatible with the dual classification concept used in the international version of ICD-9.

712.2 [✓5th] Chondrocalcinosis due to pyrophosphate crystals — (Code first underlying disease, 275.4) — *crystal-induced arthritis*

Use codes in subcategory 712.2 to report chondrocalcinosis due to pyrophosphate crystals, which is a calcium pyrophosphate dehydrate deposition (CPPD) disease and type II crystal deposition disease.

The manifestation codes include chondrocalcinosis due to pyrophosphate crystals. ICD-9-CM classifies etiology first, then manifestation, to remain compatible with the dual classification concept used in the international version of ICD-9.

712.3 [✓5th] Chondrocalcinosis, cause unspecified — (Code first underlying disease, 275.4)

Codes in subcategory 712.3 include chondrocalcinosis due to unspecified cause. ICD-9-CM classifies etiology first, then manifestation, to remain compatible with the dual classification concept used in the international version of ICD-9.

712.8 [✓5th] Other specified crystal arthropathies

Use codes in subcategory 712.8 to report other specified crystal arthropathies due to lipid crystals, apatite and hydroxyapatite, calcium oxalate, calcium phosphate, and other identifiable crystals not elsewhere classifiable.

712.9 [✓5th] Unspecified crystal arthropathy — *crystal-induced arthritis, type unknown*

Coding Clarification
This category includes crystal (mineral) deposition arthropathies with the exception of gouty arthropathy, which is classified to code 274.0. Crystal deposition disease type I refers to gouty arthropathy due to uric acid crystals and should be classified to subcategory 274.0; type II crystal deposition disease includes the disorders classified to subcategory 712.2.

713 Arthropathy associated with other disorders classified elsewhere
This rubric includes manifestation codes used to classify arthropathy associated with other disorders classified elsewhere. ICD-9-CM classifies etiology first, then manifestation, to remain compatible with the dual classification concept used in the international version of ICD-9.

713.0 Arthropathy associated with other endocrine and metabolic disorders — (Code first underlying disease: 243-244.9, 252.0, 253.0, 270.2, 272.0-272.9, 275.0, 279.00-279.09) — *secondary*

713.1 Arthropathy associated with gastrointestinal conditions other than infections — (Code first underlying disease: 555.0-555.9, 556.0-556.9) — *secondary*

713.2 Arthropathy associated with hematological disorders — (Code first underlying disease: 202.3, 203.0, 204.0-208.9, 282.4-282.7, 286.0-286.2) — *secondary*

713.3 Arthropathy associated with dermatological disorders — (Code first underlying disease: 695.1, 695.2) — *secondary*

713.4 Arthropathy associated with respiratory disorders — (Code first underlying disease, such as: diseases classifiable to 490-519) — *secondary*

713.5 Arthropathy associated with neurological disorders — (Code first underlying disease: 094.0, 250.6, 336.0) — *secondary*

713.6 Arthropathy associated with hypersensitivity reaction — (Code first underlying disease: 287.0, 999.5) — *secondary*

713.7 Other general diseases with articular involvement — (Code first underlying disease: 135, 277.3x) — *secondary*
AHA: Q2, 1997, 12

713.8 Arthropathy associated with other conditions classifiable elsewhere — (Code first underlying disease) — *secondary*

Coding Clarification
Whenever the physician's diagnostic statement specifies etiology for the patient's arthropathy, a code from category 713 should be used as a secondary code. For example, the diagnosis "arthropathy due to hemochromatosis" is assigned codes 275.0 and 713.0, and the diagnosis "arthropathic multiple myeloma of the hip" is

assigned codes 203.0x and 713.2. In the first case, the cause and effect relationship is stated; in the second, the relationship is implied. The term "associated with" in the code title indicates that both parts of the title may be in the physician's diagnostic statement. The word "as" in the notation *"code first underlying disease as"* under each subcategory indicates an incomplete list of etiologies.

Coding Scenario
A patient develops arthritis of multiple joints as a result of her ulcerative colitis.

> Code assignment: 556.9 *Ulcerative colitis, unspecified* and 713.1 *Arthropathy associated with gastrointestinal conditions other than infectious*

714   Rheumatoid arthritis and other inflammatory polyarthropathies
AHA: Q2, 1995, 3

714.0   Rheumatoid arthritis — (Use additional code to identify manifestation: 357.1, 359.6) — *chronic rheumatic polyarthritis*
AHA: Q1, 1990, 5; Q2, 1995, 3; Q2, 2006, 20

Rheumatoid arthritis is a chronic, systemic inflammatory disease of unknown etiology, characterized by a variable but prolonged course with exacerbations and remissions of joint pains and swelling. In early stages, the disease attacks the joints of the hands and feet. As the disease progresses, more joints become involved. Also known as primary progressive arthritis and proliferative arthritis, the disease often leads to progressive deformities, which may develop rapidly and cause permanent disability.

Clinical manifestations of rheumatoid arthritis are highly variable, particularly in the mode of onset, distribution, degree of severity, and rate of progression. Joint disease is the major manifestation; systemic involvement (spleen, liver, eyes, etc.) is rare.

Signs and symptoms of rheumatoid arthritis include articular inflammation, malaise, weight loss, paresthesia, Raynaud's phenomenon, periarticular pain and stiffness, symmetrical joint swelling and stiffness, warmth, and tenderness (most severe in the morning, somewhat subsiding during the day).

Lab work includes a complete blood count (CBC) to reveal anemia, elevated white blood cell count (WBC), and elevated erythrocyte sedimentation rate (ESR). Various serological tests may be used to detect rheumatoid factor, but false positive and false negative results are not unusual; typically, tests show elevated gamma globulins IgM and IgC during both acute and chronic phases. X-rays of affected joints early in the disease reveal evidence of periarticular soft tissue swelling and joint effusion. As the disease progresses, x-rays show regional osteoporosis, osteolysis of subchondral bone, narrowing of cartilage spaces, and, in the late stages, subluxation, dislocation, and ankylosis.

Therapies include medical treatment directed toward pain relief and reduction of inflammation with a wide variety of drugs including gold salts, corticosteroids, and nonsteroidal antiinflammatory drugs for preservation of function and prevention of deformities. Physical and occupational therapy and splinting of joints are other therapies, as well as surgery such as arthrodesis, synovectomy, tendon grafts and transplantations, arthroplasty, capsulectomy, and capsulotomy.

Associated conditions include nonspecific pericarditis and pleuritis, pulmonary fibrosis, secondary amyloidosis, leukopenia, arteritis, and adverse effect of medications used to treat rheumatoid arthritis.

714.1   Felty's syndrome — *rheumatoid arthritis with splenoadenomegaly and leukopenia*
AHA: Q2, 1995, 3

The definition of Felty's syndrome is the association of rheumatoid arthritis with splenomegaly and leukopenia. Mild anemia and thrombocytopenia may accompany the variable severe neutropenia, and skin and pulmonary infections are frequent complications.

714.2   Other rheumatoid arthritis with visceral or systemic involvement — *rheumatoid carditis*
AHA: Q2, 1995, 3

Other rheumatoid arthritis with visceral or systemic involvement occurs in the connective tissue components of the cardiovascular, reticuloendothelial, digestive, and respiratory system.

714.3 ⌐sth   Juvenile chronic polyarthritis

Juvenile chronic polyarthritis is a rheumatoid-like disorder occurring in children (onset prior to age 17), involving one or more joints. Juvenile rheumatoid arthritis has a much more favorable prognosis than adult-onset disease.

The disease process for juvenile rheumatoid arthritis and polyarthritis is different genetically and immunologically from rheumatoid arthritis in adults, but the condition is still classified to subcategory 714.3 with the appropriate fifth digit, depending on the clinical presentation.

714.30	Polyarticular juvenile rheumatoid arthritis, chronic or unspecified — *number of joints affected unspecified, Still's disease*

AHA: Q2, 1995, 3

Polyarticular juvenile rheumatoid arthritis, chronic or unspecified, is systemic juvenile arthritis or polyarthritis, also known as Still's disease, that interferes with growth and development.

714.31	Polyarticular juvenile rheumatoid arthritis, acute — *affecting many joints*

AHA: Q2, 1995, 3

Polyarticular juvenile rheumatoid arthritis, acute, is systemic juvenile arthritis or polyarthritis, also known as Still's disease, described as acute. Typically, the acute phase includes high fever, erythematous rash, anemia, generalized lymphadenopathy, and, in some cases, hepatosplenomegaly, iridocyclitis, and pericarditis.

714.32	Pauciarticular juvenile rheumatoid arthritis — *affecting only a few joints*

AHA: Q2, 1995, 3

Pauciarticular juvenile rheumatoid arthritis is a disease, also known as oligoarticular juvenile arthritis, affecting a small number of joints, usually two to five. It is associated with chronic iridocyclitis in 25 to 30 percent of patients and can lead to blindness.

714.33	Monoarticular juvenile rheumatoid arthritis — *affecting one joint*

AHA: Q2, 1995, 3

Monoarticular juvenile rheumatoid arthritis is juvenile arthritis limited to one joint.

Pauciarticular juvenile arthritis may be used to describe monoarticular juvenile arthritis. In such cases, verify the diagnosis with the physician to ensure proper code assignment.

714.4	Chronic postrheumatic arthropathy — *chronic rheumatoid nodular fibrositis, Jaccoud's syndrome*

AHA: Q2, 1995, 3

The definition of chronic postrheumatic arthropathy is a form of arthropathy of the hands and feet caused by repeated attacks of rheumatic arthritis. Also called Jaccoud's syndrome, this disease is characterized by flexion deformities, particularly of the metacarpophalangeal joints, and is associated with pronounced ulnar deviation of the fingers. Chronic rheumatoid nodular fibrositis is a variation of this disease characterized by the presence of subcutaneous nodules in the region of the previously involved joints.

714.81	Rheumatoid lung — *Caplan's syndrome, diffuse interstitial rheumatoid lung disease, fibrosing alveolitis*

AHA: Q2, 1995, 3

Rheumatoid lung is diseases of the lung associated with rheumatoid arthritis, including Hamman-Rich syndrome (when associated with rheumatoid arthritis) and Caplan's syndrome, a syndrome of rheumatoid pneumoconiosis seen in patients with concomitant coal worker's pneumoconiosis.

714.89	Other specified inflammatory polyarthropathies — *not otherwise specified*

AHA: Q2, 1995, 3

714.9	Unspecified inflammatory polyarthropathy

Documentation Issues

The physician should clearly indicate the type of arthritis and the sites affected by the condition for appropriate code selection to be made.

When pyogenic arthritis is documented and the infectious organism has not been identified, contact the physician for clarification as an additional code should be used to identify the infectious organism.

If conditions that are integral to the disease process of the arthritis are mentioned in the final diagnostic statement, they should not be assigned as additional codes (e.g., pain, joint swelling).

Coding Scenario

A 10-year-old patient in seen in the rheumatology clinic complaining of joint pain and swelling with early morning fatigue. After a comprehensive evaluation, it is determined that she is in the early stages of juvenile rheumatoid arthritis.

> Code assignment: 714.30 *Polyarticular juvenile rheumatoid arthritis, chronic or unspecified*

715 Osteoarthrosis and allied disorders

Osteoarthrosis and allied disorders are degenerative, rather than inflammatory, diseases of one or more joints. Also known as osteoarthritis and degenerative joint disease, osteoarthrosis is most conspicuous in the large joints and initiated by local deterioration of the articular cartilage. It progressively destroys the cartilage, remodels the subchondral bone, and causes a secondary inflammation of the synovial membrane.

Signs and symptoms of osteoarthrosis and allied disorders include pain in the affected joints, muscle spasm, crepitation, and atrophy of surrounding muscles without evidence of inflammation.

Lab work is usually of little value, although examination of synovial fluid may demonstrate increased mucin content. X-rays of affected joints readily show narrowing of articular space, subchondral sclerosis and cysts, osteophyte formation, and joint remodeling.

Therapies include pain and weight management, reduction of secondary inflammation of the synovial membrane, and physical and occupational therapy to help the patient maintain joint function and prevent or correct joint deformities. Surgery such as osteotomy near the joint improves biomechanics and soft tissue operations such as release of muscle contractions and neurectomy may help relieve intractable pain. For osteoarthritis of the hip, therapy includes hip preserving surgery (excision of osteophytes, curettage and bone grafting of acetabular cysts, proximal femoral osteotomy and muscle release) or hip reconstruction (cup arthroplasty, total hip replacement, femoral head replacement, and arthrodesis).

Assignment of the fourth digit to codes in this category is based on whether the disease is generalized or localized and whether it is primary or secondary.

The following fifth-digit subclassification is for use with categories 711-712, 715-716, 718-719, and 730. Valid fifth-digits are in brackets [ ] beneath each code.

0   site unspecified
1   shoulder region (acromioclavicular joint, clavicle, glenohumeral joint, scapula, sternoclavicular joint)
2   upper arm (elbow joint, humerus)
3   forearm (radius, ulna, wrist joint)
4   hand (carpus, metacarpus, phalanges)
5   pelvic regions and thigh (buttock, femur, hip joint)
6   lower leg (fibula, knee joint, patella, tibia)
7   ankle and foot (ankle joint, metatarsus, phalanges, tarsus, other joints in foot)
8   other specified sites (head, neck, ribs, skull, trunk, vertebral column)
9   multiple sites

715.0 ✓sth   Osteoarthrosis, generalized — *degenerative*
[0,4,9]   *joint disease, multiple joints; primary generalized hypertrophic osteoarthrosis*

Generalized disease is osteoarthrosis involving many joints without any known preexisting abnormality. Localized osteoarthrosis is disease confined to a limited number of sites, generally one or two of the larger weight-bearing joints, such as the hip or knee.

715.1 ✓sth   Osteoarthrosis, localized, primary —
[0-8]   *idiopathic localized osteoarthropathy*

Primary osteoarthrosis is idiopathic or due to some constitutional or genetic factor.

715.2 ✓sth   Osteoarthrosis, localized, secondary —
[0-8]   *coxae malum senilis*

Secondary osteoarthrosis is due to some identifiable initiating factor. These factors include obesity, trauma, congenital malformations, superimposition of fibrosis and scarring from previous inflammatory disease or infection, foreign bodies, malalignment of joints, metabolic or circulatory bone diseases, and iatrogenic factors such as osteoarthrosis caused by continuous pressure on the joint surfaces during orthopedic treatment of congenital deformities. Secondary osteoarthroses should be paired with a second code describing the causative injury, disorder, or disease.

715.3 ✓sth   Osteoarthrosis, localized, not specified
[0-8]   whether primary or secondary — *Otto's pelvis*
AHA: Q2, 2004, 15; Q3, 2004, 12

715.8 ✓sth   Osteoarthrosis involving or with mention of
[0, 9]   more than one site, but not specified as generalized

715.9 ✓sth   Osteoarthrosis, unspecified whether
[0-8]   generalized or localized

Documentation Issues
The physician should clearly indicate the type of arthritis and the sites affected by the condition for appropriate code selection to be made.

When pyogenic arthritis is documented and the infectious organism has not been identified, contact the physician for clarification as an additional code should be used to identify the infectious organism.

If conditions that are integral to the disease process of the arthritis are mentioned in the final diagnostic statement, they should not be assigned as additional codes (e.g., pain, joint swelling).

Coding Clarification
Type of Arthritis: The term arthritis is used by medical personnel to describe more than 100 various forms of rheumatic disease. Arthritis can affect multiple body systems and/or sites including joints, muscles, connective tissues, skin, and internal organs. The most widespread forms of arthritis are osteoarthritis and rheumatoid arthritis. This disease can also be the sequelae of other disease processes or caused by infectious organisms.

Osteoarthritis: The most common form of arthritis is osteoarthritis (OA). Physicians often call this form of arthritis by various terms including degenerative joint disease (DJD), osteoarthrosis, degenerative arthritis, and hypertrophic arthritis.

Osteoarthritis noted as generalized is a chronic noninflammatory arthritis that affects multiple sites, commonly of older patients, marked by degeneration of articular cartilage and enlargement of bone, and pain and stiffness occurring with any type of activity but subsiding when the patient rests. This form should be reported with subcategory code 715.0x. Only three of the 10 fifth digits available for osteoarthritis may be used with this subcategory: 0, 4, and 9.

Coding Scenario
A patient is seen in the office for a follow-up examination of her osteoarthritis in the right knee.

> Code assignment: 715.96 *Osteoarthritis, unspecified whether generalized or localized, lower leg (fibula, knee joint, patella, tibia)*

716 Other and unspecified arthropathies
AHA: Q2, 1995, 3

The following fifth-digit subclassification is for use with categories 711-712, 715-716, 718-719, and 730. Valid fifth-digits are in brackets [ ] beneath each code.

0 site unspecified
1 shoulder region (acromioclavicular joint, clavicle, glenohumeral joint, scapula, sternoclavicular joint)
2 upper arm (elbow joint, humerus)
3 forearm (radius, ulna, wrist joint)
4 hand (carpus, metacarpus, phalanges)
5 pelvic regions and thigh (buttock, femur, hip joint)
6 lower leg (fibula, knee joint, patella, tibia)
7 ankle and foot (ankle joint, metatarsus, phalanges, tarsus, other joints in foot)
8 other specified sites (head, neck, ribs, skull, trunk, vertebral column)
9 multiple sites

716.0 ✓5th   Kaschin-Beck disease — *endemic*
[0-9]   *polyarthritis*
                 AHA: Q2, 1995, 3

716.1 ✓5th   Traumatic arthropathy — *following injury*
[0-9]   **AHA:** Q2, 1995, 3

716.2 ✓5th   Allergic arthritis — *immunological reaction*
[0-9]   *following exposure to antigen*
                 AHA: Q2, 1995, 3

Allergic arthritis is associated with a hypersensitive state acquired through exposure to an allergen.

Loosening of orthopedic implants (including prostheses and other devices) due to an allergic or inflammatory reaction to chromium, cobalt, or nickel in the implant is classified as a postoperative complication. In such cases, use code 996.66 or 996.67 to classify the postoperative complication, followed by 716.2x to further describe the nature of the complication.

Excluded from this subclassification is arthritis associated with Henoch-Schonlein purpura or serum sickness (713.6).

716.3 ✓5th   Climacteric arthritis — *menopausal*
[0-9]   **AHA:** Q2, 1995, 3

716.4 ✓5th   Transient arthropathy
[0-9]

716.5 ✓5th   Unspecified polyarthropathy or polyarthritis
[0-9]

716.6 ✓5th   Unspecified monoarthritis — *unknown type*
[0-8]   **AHA:** Q2, 1995, 3

716.8 ✓5th   Other specified arthropathy — *not*
[0-9]   *otherwise specified, including due to old epiphyseal slip, villous arthritis*
                 AHA: Q2, 1995, 3

716.9 ✓5th   Unspecified arthropathy
[0-9]

Coding Scenario
A patient with a previous fracture of the left wrist is diagnosed with osteoarthritis due to the fracture.

> Code assignment: 716.13 *Traumatic arthropathy, forearm (radius, ulna, wrist joint)* and 905.2 *Late effect of fracture of upper extremities*

717 Internal derangement of knee
This rubric includes degenerative disorders of the articular cartilage or meniscus of the knee, as well as the late effects of acute trauma to the knee classifiable to category 836.

717.0   Old bucket handle tear of medial meniscus — *old bucket handle tear of unspecified cartilage*

717.1   Derangement of anterior horn of medial meniscus

717.2   Derangement of posterior horn of medial meniscus

717.3   Other and unspecified derangement of medial meniscus — *degeneration of internal semilunar cartilage*

Code 717.3 includes tears of the medial cartilage, or the meniscus, of the knee that may be described as radial, peripheral, horizontal cleavage type, flap, and complex tears.

717.40   Unspecified derangement of lateral meniscus
717.41   Bucket handle tear of lateral meniscus
717.42   Derangement of anterior horn of lateral meniscus
717.43   Derangement of posterior horn of lateral meniscus
717.49   Other derangement of lateral meniscus — *not otherwise specified*

Code 717.49 includes tears of the lateral meniscus of the knee that may be described as radial, peripheral, horizontal cleavage type, flap, and complex tears.

717.5 Derangement of meniscus, not elsewhere classified — *congenital discoid meniscus, cyst of semilunar cartilage*

Code 717.5 includes other forms of meniscal derangements, such as cysts of any meniscus and congenital discoid lateral or medial meniscus.

717.6 Loose body in knee — *joint mice, rice bodies*

Loose body in knee is joint mice, rice bodies, and debris described as cartilaginous (cartilage only, radiolucent on x-rays), osseous (bony), osteocartilaginous, and fibrous. Osteochondritis dissecans is commonly the cause; other causes include synovial chondromatosis, osteophytes, fractured articular surfaces, and damaged menisci.

717.7 Chondromalacia of patella — *degeneration or softening of articular cartilage of patella*
AHA: Nov-Dec, 1984, 9; March-April, 1985, 14

717.81 Old disruption of lateral collateral ligament
717.82 Old disruption of medial collateral ligament
717.83 Old disruption of anterior cruciate ligament
717.84 Old disruption of posterior cruciate ligament
717.85 Old disruption of other ligament of knee — *capsular ligament*
717.89 Other internal derangement of knee — *not otherwise specified, calcification, derangement of ligament, slipped patella, intraligamentous cyst, Haglund-Lawen-Frund syndrome, Budinger-Lawen-Ludloff-Lawen disease*

Code 717.89 includes old disruptions of the arcuate complex, medial capsule, lateral capsule, and popliteus.

717.9 Unspecified internal derangement of knee

Coding Clarification
This rubric excludes acute derangement of the knee and current injury (836.0-836.6), ankylosis (718.5x), contracture (718.4x), deformity (736.4-736.6), and recurrent dislocation (718.3x).

718 Other derangement of joint

The following fifth-digit subclassification is for use with categories 711-712, 715-716, 718-719, and 730. Valid fifth-digits are in brackets [ ] beneath each code.

0 site unspecified
1 shoulder region (acromioclavicular joint, clavicle, glenohumeral joint, scapula, sternoclavicular joint)
2 upper arm (elbow joint, humerus)
3 forearm (radius, ulna, wrist joint)
4 hand (carpus, metacarpus, phalanges)
5 pelvic regions and thigh (buttock, femur, hip joint)
6 lower leg (fibula, knee joint, patella, tibia)
7 ankle and foot (ankle joint, metatarsus, phalanges, tarsus, other joints in foot)
8 other specified sites (head, neck, ribs, skull, trunk, vertebral column)
9 multiple sites

718.0 Articular cartilage disorder — *meniscus old rupture, old tear*
[0-5, 7-9]
718.1 Loose body in joint — *joint mice*
[0-5, 7-9]

Loose body in joint is joint mice, rice bodies, and debris described as cartilaginous, osseous (bony), osteocartilaginous, or fibrous in joints other than the knee.

718.2 Pathological dislocation — *spontaneous; not recurrent and not from injury*
[0-9]

Pathological dislocation is dislocation of an articular joint due to a disease process (e.g., poliomyelitis), rather than trauma.

Code 718.2 should be accompanied by a second ICD-9-CM code identifying the specific pathology (etiology of the pathological dislocation).

718.3 Recurrent dislocation of joint — *occurring again and again*
[0-9]
AHA: Nov-Dec, 1987, 7

Recurrent dislocation of a joint is chronic, subsequent, additional, and repeated dislocations or subluxations of a joint due to trauma.

718.4 Contracture of joint — *strong resistance to stretch*
[0-9]
AHA: Q4, 1998, 40

Contracture of a joint is a disorder characterized by restriction of joint motion due to contraction of the muscles that articulate the joint. The condition may be due to tonic spasm, fibrosis, loss of musculature equilibrium, or disuse atrophy.

718.5 Ankylosis of joint — *immobility*
[0-9]
718.6 Unspecified intrapelvic protrusion of acetabulum — *protrusio acetabuli, cause unknown*
[0, 5]
718.7 Developmental dislocation of joint
[0-9]

Excluded from this subclassification are congenital dislocation of joint (754.0-755.8) and traumatic dislocation of joint (830-839).

718.8 Other joint derangement, not elsewhere classified — *flail joint, instability of joint*
[0-9]

The codes in this subclassification may be used as an additional code to classify instability of a joint secondary to removal of a prosthesis. Use code 909.3

when the instability is described as a late effect of the prosthesis removal.

718.9 [5th] Unspecified derangement of joint —
[0-5, 7-9] *unknown cause*

719 Other and unspecified disorders of joint

The following fifth-digit subclassification is for use with codes 719.0-719.6 and 719.8-719.9. Valid fifth-digits are in brackets [ ] beneath each code.

0   site unspecified
1   shoulder region (acromioclavicular joint, clavicle, glenohumeral joint, scapula, sternoclavicular joint)
2   upper arm (elbow joint, humerus)
3   forearm (radius, ulna, wrist joint)
4   hand (carpus, metacarpus, phalanges)
5   pelvic regions and thigh (buttock, femur, hip joint)
6   lower leg (fibula, knee joint, patella, tibia)
7   ankle and foot (ankle joint, metatarsus, phalanges, tarsus, other joints in foot)
8   other specified sites (head, neck, ribs, skull, trunk, vertebral column)
9   multiple sites

719.0 [5th] Effusion of joint — *hydrarthrosis, swelling*
[0-9]   *of joint*

Effusion of joint is the escape of fluid from blood vessels or lymphatics into joint spaces. Hemorrhagic effusion is from blood. Hydrarthrosis is the accumulation of watery fluid in a joint. Effusion indicates synovial irritation due to disease or trauma (excluding current injury).

Therapies include aspiration of a tense effusion.

719.1 [5th] Hemarthrosis — *blood in the joint*
[0-9]

Hemarthrosis is the presence of gross blood in the joint spaces, excluding that due to current injury or hemophilia.

719.2 [5th] Villonodular synovitis
[0-9]

Villonodular synovitis is a form of inflammation involving the synovial membranes of joints. There are two types of villonodular synovitis: pigmented and nonpigmented.

Therapies include steroidal and nonsteroidal medication to reduce inflammation and synovectomy when nonoperative therapy fails.

Villonodular synovitis may be a form of benign neoplasm of the connective tissue of the synovium, or be representative of granulomatous disease. The term "villonodular synovitis" is sometimes used to describe conditions such as xanthofibroma, giant cell tumor of tendon sheath, and benign synovioma, which are classified elsewhere.

719.3 [5th] Palindromic rheumatism — *Hench-*
[0-9]   *Rosenberg syndrome, intermittent hydrarthrosis*

Palindromic rheumatism is sudden and recurring attacks of moderate to severe joint pain and swelling. The etiology is unknown but the condition has been associated with irritants and allergic reactions.

719.4 [5th] Pain in joint — *arthralgia*
[0-9]

719.5 [5th] Stiffness of joint, not elsewhere classified
[0-9]

719.6 [5th] Other symptoms referable to joint — *joint*
[0-9]   *crepitus, snapping hip*
                     AHA: Q1, 1994, 15

719.7 Difficulty in walking — *disorders of joints*
            AHA: Q2, 2004, 18; Q2, 2004, 15

719.8 [5th] Other specified disorders of joint — *not*
[0-9]   *otherwise specified, including calcification, fistula*

719.9 [5th] Unspecified disorder of joint
[0-9]

Coding Clarification
Subcategory 719.7 describes disorders of the joints and should not be used to describe problems with ambulation after hip replacement surgery. For post-hip replacement gait problems, assign 781.2. No fifth digit is required for code 719.7. This is a valid four-digit code.

720–724   Dorsopathies

720 Ankylosing spondylitis and other inflammatory spondylopathies

Ankylosing spondylitis is a form of chronic inflammation of the spine and the sacroiliac joints. Chronic inflammation in these areas causes pain and stiffness in and around the spine and can lead to a complete fusion of the vertebrae, a process called ankylosis. Ankylosis causes total loss of mobility of the spine and it is a systemic rheumatic disease, causing inflammation in joints away from the spine, as well as inflammation in organs such as the eyes, heart, lungs, and kidneys. The disease is more common in males. In women, joints away from the spine are more frequently affected. Although ankylosing spondylitis can occur at any age, onset usually falls in the second and third decades; the cause is believed to be genetic. Common symptoms include back pain and stiffness over a period of weeks or months and lasting longer than three months, and early morning stiffness improved by warm shower or light exercise. Diagnosis depends on the history of symptoms, physical examination, and x-ray findings. X-rays are taken of the sacroiliac joints to note changes in tissues caused by inflammation, although tissue changes do not always appear on x-rays in the early stages of the disease. There is no cure and treatment consists of medicines to alleviate the pain and stiffness (i.e., non-steroidal anti-inflammatory drugs), daily exercises that incorporate stretching and strengthening, and good posture habits.

Ankylosing spondylitis shares many features with other arthritic conditions, such as psoriatic arthritis, reactive arthritis, arthritis associated with Crohn's disease, and ulcerative colitis. The conditions are collectively referred to as spondyloarthropathies.

720.0	Ankylosing spondylitis — *arthritis primarily of the sacroiliac joints and to varying degree, the rest of the spine and peripheral joints, with no new bone formation; Marie-Strumpell spondylitis*

Ankylosing spondylitis is a chronic, progressive inflammatory disease of unknown etiology involving primarily the small apophyseal and costovertebral joints of the spine and sacroiliac. This disease also is known as Marie-Strumpell or Bekhterev disease.

720.1	Spinal enthesopathy — *Romanus lesion; disorder of peripheral ligamentous or muscular attachments of spine*
720.2	Sacroiliitis, not elsewhere classified — *pain and inflammation within the joint or the junction of sacrum and hip*
720.81	Inflammatory spondylopathies in diseases classified elsewhere — (Code first underlying disease, 015.0) — *secondary to underlying disease*
720.89	Other inflammatory spondylopathies — *not otherwise specified*
720.9	Unspecified inflammatory spondylopathy — *unknown type*

721 Spondylosis and allied disorders
AHA: Q2, 1989, 14

Spondylosis and allied disorders are degenerative, rather than inflammatory conditions. Myelopathy is a qualifying term describing diseases and disturbances of the spinal cord. Paresthesia, loss of sensation, and loss of sphincter control are among the most common forms of myelopathy.

721.0	Cervical spondylosis without myelopathy — *cervical or cervicodorsal; in the neck* AHA: Q2, 1989, 14
721.1	Cervical spondylosis with myelopathy — *spondylogenic compression of cervical spinal cord; vertebral artery compression or anterior spinal artery compression syndromes* AHA: Q2, 1989, 14
721.2	Thoracic spondylosis without myelopathy — *upper back, T1-T12* AHA: Q2, 1989, 14
721.3	Lumbosacral spondylosis without myelopathy — *lower back, L1-L5* AHA: Q2, 1989, 14; Q4, 2002, 107
721.41	Spondylosis with myelopathy, thoracic region — *upper back, T1-T12* AHA: Q2, 1989, 14
721.42	Spondylosis with myelopathy, lumbar region — *lower back, L1-L5* AHA: Q2, 1989, 14
721.5	Kissing spine — *Baastrup's, Michotte's syndromes* AHA: Q2, 1989, 14
721.6	Ankylosing vertebral hyperostosis — *hypertrophy or exostosis causing immobility* AHA: Q2, 1989, 14
721.7	Traumatic spondylopathy — *Kummell's disease* AHA: Q2, 1989, 14
721.8	Other allied disorders of spine — *not otherwise specified, arthritis of coccyx* AHA: Q2, 1989, 14
721.90	Spondylosis of unspecified site without mention of myelopathy — *unknown cause, but without compression of spinal cord* AHA: Q2, 1989, 14
721.91	Spondylosis of unspecified site with myelopathy — *unknown cause, but with compression of spinal cord* AHA: Q2, 1989, 14

Coding Clarification
Assignment of a fourth digit to codes in this category is based on the presence or absence of myelopathy. For coding purposes, myelopathy includes any symptomatic impingement, compression, disruption, or disturbance of the spinal cord or blood supply of the spinal cord due to spondylosis.

Neurogenic Bladder: Many conditions may result in neurogenic bladder including cauda equina syndrome, injury to the spine and spinal cord, spondylitis, neoplasms, fractures, and congenital defects. When the neurogenic bladder is not due to a spinal condition, it is classified to one of the bladder dysfunction categories.

Spondylosis: This is a compression of any or all of the nerve roots of the cauda equina and causes a variety of sensory and motor deficits. Spondylosis with myelopathy indicates deficits due to nerve compression and would include neurogenic bladder. However, it is appropriate to code lumbar or sacral spondylosis with neurogenic bladder by reporting both codes 721.42 and 344.61.

Diseases of the Musculoskeletal System and Connective Tissue

Pain or neuritis is a symptom of spondylosis and therefore does not need to be coded in addition to a code from categories 721-722.

722 Intervertebral disc disorders
AHA: Q1, 1988, 10

An intervertebral disk is the flexible plate that connects any two adjacent vertebrae in the spine; they cushion the spinal cord from the impact produced by the body's movements. Each disk is composed of a gelatinous material in the center, called the nucleus pulposus, surrounded by rings of a fibrous tissue. With age, these disks can degenerate and dry out, and the fibers holding them in place can tear. Eventually, the disk torn from the tissue can rupture the fibrocartilaginous material, which releases the nucleus pulposus. Pressure may force the nucleus pulposus outward, placing pressure on the spinal cord and causing pain. Disk herniation most commonly affects the lumbar region between the fifth lumbar vertebra and the first sacral vertebra. However, disk herniation also occurs in the cervical spine. Muscle weakness or bladder and bowel function interference because of the pressure on a nerve root often requires a diskectomy.

722.0 Displacement of cervical intervertebral disc without myelopathy — *neuritis or radiculitis due to displacement or rupture of cervical intervertebral disc; neck, C1-C7; without compression of spinal cord*
AHA: Q1, 1988, 10

722.10 Displacement of lumbar intervertebral disc without myelopathy — *lumbago, neuritis, radiculitis, or sciatica due to displacement of intervertebral disc; lower back, L1-L5; without compression of spinal cord*
AHA: Q1, 1988, 10; Q4, 2002, 107; Q1, 2003, 7; Q3, 2003, 12

722.11 Displacement of thoracic intervertebral disc without myelopathy — *lumbago, neuritis, radiculitis, or sciatica due to displacement of intervertebral disc; upper back, T1-T12; without compression of spinal cord*
AHA: Q1, 1988, 10

722.2 Displacement of intervertebral disc, site unspecified, without myelopathy — *lumbago, neuritis, radiculitis, or sciatica due to displacement of intervertebral disc; unknown site in spine; without compression of spinal cord*
AHA: Q1, 1988, 10

722.3 Schmorl's nodes

Schmorl's nodes describe the prolapse of the nucleus pulposus into an adjoining vertebra, as seen on x-rays of the spine.

722.30 Schmorl's nodes, unspecified region — *nodule caused by prolapse of disk pulp into adjacent vertebra, unknown site in spine*
AHA: Q1, 1988, 10

722.31 Schmorl's nodes, thoracic region — *nodule caused by prolapse of disk pulp into adjacent vertebra, upper back, T1-T12*
AHA: Q1, 1988, 10

722.32 Schmorl's nodes, lumbar region — *nodule caused by prolapse of disk pulp into adjacent vertebra, lower back, L1-L5*
AHA: Q1, 1988, 10

722.39 Schmorl's nodes, other spinal region — *nodule caused by prolapse of disk pulp into adjacent vertebra, cervical, C1-C7, or not otherwise specified*
AHA: Q1, 1988, 10

722.4 Degeneration of cervical intervertebral disc — *cervicothoracic intervertebral disc*
AHA: Q1, 1988, 10

722.51 Degeneration of thoracic or thoracolumbar intervertebral disc

722.52 Degeneration of lumbar or lumbosacral intervertebral disc
AHA: Q4, 2004, 133; Q2, 2006, 18

722.6 Degeneration of intervertebral disc, site unspecified — *unknown site*
AHA: Q1, 1988, 10

722.70 Intervertebral disc disorder with myelopathy, unspecified region — *with compression on spine, unknown site in spine*
AHA: Q1, 1988, 10

722.71 Intervertebral cervical disc disorder with myelopathy, cervical region — *with compression on spine, in neck, C1-C7*
AHA: Q1, 1988, 10

722.72 Intervertebral thoracic disc disorder with myelopathy, thoracic region — *with compression on spine, upper back, T1-T12*
AHA: Q1, 1988, 10

722.73 Intervertebral lumbar disc disorder with myelopathy, lumbar region — *with compression on spine, lower back, L1-L5*
AHA: Q1, 1988, 10

722.8 Postlaminectomy syndrome

Postlaminectomy syndrome is a complex of symptoms following laminectomy surgery. It includes conditions and syndromes described as postfusion, postmicrosurgery, and postchemonucleolysis.

722.80 Postlaminectomy syndrome, unspecified region — *unknown site on spine*
AHA: Jan-Feb, 1987, 7; Q1, 1988, 10

722.81 Postlaminectomy syndrome, cervical region — *neck, C1-C7*
AHA: Jan-Feb, 1987, 7; Q1, 1988, 10

722.82	Postlaminectomy syndrome, thoracic region — *upper back, T1-T12*	
	AHA: Jan-Feb, 1987, 7; Q1, 1988, 10	
722.83	Postlaminectomy syndrome, lumbar region — *lower back, L1-L5*	
	AHA: Jan-Feb, 1987, 7; Q1, 1988, 10; Q2, 1997, 15	
722.90	Other and unspecified disc disorder of unspecified region — *calcification, discitis, unknown site on spine*	
	AHA: Nov-Dec, 1984, 19; Q1, 1988, 10	
722.91	Other and unspecified disc disorder of cervical region — *calcification, discitis, neck, C1-C7*	
	AHA: Q1, 1988, 10	
722.92	Other and unspecified disc disorder of thoracic region — *calcification, discitis, upper back, T1-T12*	
	AHA: Q1, 1988, 10	
722.93	Other and unspecified disc disorder of lumbar region — *calcification, discitis, lower back, L1-L5*	
	AHA: Q1, 1988, 10	

Coding Clarification

Herniated Disc: When sciatica is the result of a slipped or degenerative intervertebral disc, the sciatica is a symptom of the disc disease and does not need to be coded separately. For lateral disc herniation, assign an appropriate code from the 722.0-722.2 subcategories.

Intervertebral Disc Space Infection: An intervertebral disc space infection is a condition also known as discitis and is classified to category 722.

Neurogenic Bladder: Many conditions may result in neurogenic bladder including cauda equina syndrome, injury to the spine and spinal cord, spondylitis, neoplasms, fractures, and congenital defects. When the neurogenic bladder is not due to a spinal condition, it is classified to one of the bladder dysfunction categories.

Posterior midline disk prolapse: A compression of the nerve roots at the level of L2-3 may result in acute cauda equina syndrome. In these instances, code 722.73 should be reported as well as code 344.61 to indicate both the prolapsed disc and the cauda equina syndrome with neurogenic bladder.

Postoperative Back Pain: A patient who has post-laminectomy lumbar back pain with no herniated disc or other condition causing this pain should be classified to code 722.83 *Postlaminectomy syndrome, lumbar region*. However, if after diagnostic testing it is determined that there is a condition present, such as a herniated disc that is causing that pain, then code the causative condition.

Spinal Stenosis: There are two forms of spinal stenosis: degeneration of the intervertebral disc (arthritic) and congenital. Degenerative spinal stenosis is classified to category 722. Congenital spinal stenosis is classified to categories 723-724.

Spondylosis: Pain or neuritis is a symptom of spondylosis and therefore does not need to be coded in addition to a code from categories 721-722.

Coding Scenario

A patient is seen with herniation of the L3-L4. The medical record indicates that no myelopathy is present.

Code assignment: 722.10 *Displacement of lumbar intervertebral disc without myelopathy*

A 69-year-old female is seen with acute mid-back pain. It is determined by x-ray that she has degenerative disc disease of the thoracic spine.

Code assignment: 722.51 *Degeneration of thoracic or thoracolumbar intervertebral disc*

A 54-year-old male is seen by his neurologist 10 weeks post laminectomy. He is complaining of back pain radiating down the right leg. An MRI reveals no further herniation. The physician indicates in the medical record that the patient has postlaminectomy syndrome.

Code assignment: 722.83 *Postlaminectomy syndrome, lumbar region*

723 Other disorders of cervical region
AHA: Q2, 1989, 14; Q3, 1994, 14

723.0	Spinal stenosis in cervical region — *stricture in neck region, C1-C7*	
	AHA: Q2, 1989, 14; Q3, 1994, 14; Q4, 2003, 101	
723.1	Cervicalgia — *pain in neck region,*	
	AHA: Q2, 1989, 14; Q3, 1994, 14	
723.2	Cervicocranial syndrome — *Barre-Lieou, craniovertebral, or posterior cervical sympathetic syndromes*	
	AHA: Q2, 1989, 14; Q3, 1994, 14	
723.3	Cervicobrachial syndrome (diffuse)	
723.4	Brachial neuritis or radiculitis nos — *radicular syndrome of upper limbs*	
	AHA: Q2, 1989, 14; Q3, 1994, 14	
723.5	Torticollis, unspecified — *contracture of neck*	
	AHA: Q2, 1989, 14; Q3, 1994, 14; Q1, 1995, 7; Q2, 2001, 21	
723.6	Panniculitis specified as affecting neck — *cutaneous nodules caused by subcutaneous inflammatory reaction*	
	AHA: Q2, 1989, 14; Q3, 1994, 14	
723.7	Ossification of posterior longitudinal ligament in cervical region	

723.8	Other syndromes affecting cervical region — not otherwise specified, including, video display tube syndrome, occipital neuralgia, Klippel's disease	
	AHA: Q2, 1989, 14; Q3, 1994, 14; Q1, 2000, 7	

Code 723.8 includes cervical instability syndromes, including C1-2 rotary instability syndrome.

723.9	Unspecified musculoskeletal disorders and symptoms referable to neck	

Documentation Issues
To ensure correct code assignment of a herniated disc, the physician should include in the documentation the presence or absence of myelopathy.

Spinal stenosis that is not documented as being degenerative or congenital is classified to categories 723-724; however, it is advisable to ask for clarification from the physician before assigning a nonspecific code. The physician should document the type of spinal stenosis, such as degenerative or congenital, in the medical record.

Coding Clarification
Spinal Stenosis: There are two forms of spinal stenosis: degeneration of the intervertebral disc (arthritic) and congenital. Degenerative spinal stenosis is classified to category 722. Congenital spinal stenosis is classified to categories 723-724.

Misnomer: Occipital neuralgia is actually a neuropathy. The condition is characterized by pain in the occiput and suboccipital region, involving nerve entrapment or impingement. It may be a consequence of injury, arthritis, trauma, compression of the occipital nerves, or tumors of the second and third cervical dorsal roots. Treatment depends on symptoms if the cause of the neuralgia is unknown. If the cause is known, treatment is directed to it. Some treatments include anticonvulsants for atypical facial pain, tricyclic antidepressants for pain similar to tic douloureux, local nerve blocks, injections of local anesthetics, and steroids.

Coding Scenario
A 24-year-old female presents with throbbing pain in the back of the head, toward the base of the skull. Her history is negative for any head trauma. After workup, the diagnosis is documented to be occipital neuralgia.

Code assignment: Code 723.8 *Other syndromes affecting cervical region*

A 48-year-old male is seen in the emergency department with numbness over the base of the skull. His history is negative for any head trauma and is currently being treated for arthritis. The diagnosis is documented as occipital neuralgia. There is no documentation found in the medical record that would warrant reporting the arthritis as the underlying condition.

Code assignment: 723.8 *Other syndromes affecting cervical region*

724	**Other and unspecified disorders of back**	
	AHA: Q2, 1989, 14	
724.00	Spinal stenosis, unspecified region other than cervical — *stricture, unknown site in spine*	
	AHA: Q2, 1989, 14	
724.01	Spinal stenosis of thoracic region — *stricture, upper back, T1-T12*	
	AHA: Q2, 1989, 14	
724.02	Spinal stenosis of lumbar region — *stricture, lower back, L1-L5*	
	AHA: Q2, 1989, 14; Q4, 1999, 13	
724.09	Spinal stenosis, other region other than cervical — *stricture, other site, cervical site excluded*	
	AHA: Q2, 1989, 14	
724.1	Pain in thoracic spine — *upper back, T1-T12*	
	AHA: Q2, 1989, 14	
724.2	Lumbago — *lower back, L1-L5*	
	AHA: Nov-Dec, 1985, 12; Q2, 1989, 14	
724.3	Sciatica — *neuralgia of sciatic nerve*	
	AHA: Q2, 1989, 12; Q2, 1989, 14	
724.4	Thoracic or lumbosacral neuritis or radiculitis, unspecified — *vertebral bodies impingement syndrome, radicular syndrome of lower limbs*	
	AHA: Q2, 1989, 14; Q2, 1999, 3	
724.5	Unspecified backache — *specifics unknown*	
	AHA: Q2, 1989, 14	
724.5	Unspecified backache — *specifics unknown*	
	AHA: Q2, 1989, 14	
724.6	Disorders of sacrum — *ankylosis, instability, or Thiele syndrome*	
	AHA: Q2, 1989, 14	
724.70	Unspecified disorder of coccyx	
724.71	Hypermobility of coccyx	
724.79	Other disorder of coccyx — *pain, coccygodynia*	
	AHA: Q2, 1989, 14	
724.8	Other symptoms referable to back — *ossification of posterior longitudinal ligament, sacral panniculitis, muscle spasm, stiffness in back*	
	AHA: Q2, 1989, 14	
724.9	Other unspecified back disorder	

Documentation Issues
To ensure correct code assignment of a herniated disc, the physician should include in the documentation the presence or absence of myelopathy.

Spinal stenosis that is not documented as being degenerative or congenital is classified to categories 723-724; however, it is advisable to ask for clarification from the physician before assigning a nonspecific code. The physician should document the type of spinal stenosis, such as degenerative or congenital, in the medical record.

Coding Clarification
Spinal Stenosis: There are two forms of spinal stenosis: degeneration of the intervertebral disc (arthritic) and congenital. Degenerative spinal stenosis is classified to category 722. Congenital spinal stenosis is classified to categories 723-724.

725–729 Rheumatism, Excluding the Back

725 Polymyalgia rheumatica OK
Polymyalgia rheumatica is a self-limiting disease of the elderly which often develops abruptly with joint and muscle pain and stiffness of the pelvis and shoulder girdle in association with fever, malaise, fatigue, weight loss, and anemia. The disease bears a close relationship with giant cell arteritis, and the two conditions often occur concomitantly.

726 Peripheral enthesopathies and allied syndromes
Peripheral enthesopathies and allied syndromes are disorders of peripheral ligamentous or muscular attachments. The term "enthesopathy" is an obscure medical term meaning disease of the ligamentous or muscular attachments of a joint.

726.0   Adhesive capsulitis of shoulder
Adhesive capsulitis of the shoulder is frozen shoulder syndrome, characterized by development of diffuse capsulitis of the glenohumeral joint with subsequent adherence of the inflamed capsule to the humeral head. Contracture due to the shrunken, adherent capsule prevents motion in the glenohumeral joint; that is, the joint is "frozen" in one position. The capsulitis may be caused by a variety of intrinsic and extrinsic disorders such as bicipital tendinitis, calcific supraspinatus tendinitis, basal pleurisy, and subphrenic inflammation.

Therapies include arthroscopic lavage, distension, and instillation of cortisone.

726.1 5th   Rotator cuff syndrome of shoulder and allied disorders
Rotator cuff syndrome of the shoulder and allied disorders are disorders of the ligamentous or muscular attachments of the shoulder joint and allied syndromes of the rotator cuff. The rotator cuff is a musculotendinous structure that blends with the joint capsule and is attached to the humerus. The supraspinatus is the major muscle that contributes to the formation of the rotator cuff.

726.10   Unspecified disorders of bursae and tendons in shoulder region — *rotator cuff or supraspinatus syndromes*
AHA: Q2, 2001, 11

726.11   Calcifying tendinitis of shoulder — *hardening and inflammation of tendons due to calcium deposits*

726.12   Bicipital tenosynovitis — *inflammation of the tendon and tendon sheath surrounding the long head of the biceps*

726.19   Other specified disorders of rotator cuff syndrome of shoulder and allied disorders — *not otherwise specified, including painful arc syndrome*

726.2   Other affections of shoulder region, not elsewhere classified — *periarthritis, scapulohumeral fibrositis, Duplay's or shoulder impingement syndromes*

726.30   Unspecified enthesopathy of elbow — *disorder of the attachment of muscle or tendon to bone, site unknown*

726.31   Medial epicondylitis of elbow — *disorder of the attachment of muscle or tendon to bone*

726.32   Lateral epicondylitis of elbow — *disorder of the attachment of muscle or tendon to bone, tennis/ golfer's elbow*

726.33   Olecranon bursitis — *inflammation of bursa; elbow*

Olecranon bursitis is inflammation of the olecranon bursa. There are two olecranon bursae: one lies deep to the triceps tendon and the other between the skin and olecranon process. The latter is more commonly inflamed.

726.39   Other enthesopathy of elbow region — *not otherwise specified*

726.4   Enthesopathy of wrist and carpus — *disorder of the attachment of muscle or tendon to bone, bursitis, periarthritis*

726.5   Enthesopathy of hip region — *disorder of the attachment of muscle or tendon to bone, bursitis, periarthritis; gluteal, trochanteric, or psoas tendinitis, iliac crest spur*

Enthesopathy of the hip region is a complex of conditions such as iliotibial band syndrome of the hip, trochanteric bursitis, subgluteal bursitis, iliopectineal bursitis, trochanteric tendinitis (with calcification), psoas and tibiopsoas tendinitis, iliac crest spur, and snapping hip syndrome.

726.60   Unspecified enthesopathy of knee — *disorder of the attachment of muscle or tendon to bone, bursitis, periarthritis, site unknown*

726.61   Pes anserinus tendinitis or bursitis — *inflammation of the combined insertion of*

	tendinous expansions of satirise, gracilis, and semitendinosus muscles
726.62	Tibial collateral ligament bursitis — *Pellegrini-Stieda syndrome*
726.63	Fibular collateral ligament bursitis — *inflammation of bursa*
726.64	Patellar tendinitis — *inflammation of patellar tendon*
726.65	Prepatellar bursitis — *inflammation of bursa* AHA: Q2, 2006, 15
726.69	Other enthesopathy of knee — *infrapatellar, subpatellar*

Code 726.69 includes iliotibial band syndrome of the knee, infrapatellar bursitis, subpatellar bursitis, medial gastrocnemius bursitis, and semimembranosus bursitis.

726.70	Unspecified enthesopathy of ankle and tarsus — *disorder of the attachment of muscle or tendon to bone, site unknown*
726.71	Achilles bursitis or tendinitis — *Albert's disease*
726.72	Tibialis tendinitis — *anterior or posterior*
726.73	Calcaneal spur
726.79	Other enthesopathy of ankle and tarsus — *not otherwise specified, peroneal tendinitis*

Subclassification 726.79 includes peroneal tendinitis, "pump bump" and tendinitis of the flexor hallucis longus, flexor digitorum longus, extensor hallucis longus, and extensor digitorum longus.

726.8	Other peripheral enthesopathies — *not otherwise specified*
726.90	Enthesopathy of unspecified site — *unknown site*
726.91	Exostosis of unspecified site — *bone spur NOS* AHA: Q2, 2001, 15

727 Other disorders of synovium, tendon, and bursa

727.0 Synovitis and tenosynovitis

Synovitis is inflammation of a synovial membrane, especially the synovium that lines articular joints. In a normal synovial joint, the smooth and reciprocally shaped cartilaginous opposing surfaces permit a fluid, frictionless, and painless articulation. Irregularities, disease, and damage to the articular surfaces lead to progressive degenerative changes resulting in pain and limitation of movement. The joint capsule is particularly sensitive to stretching and increased fluid pressure.

Tenosynovitis is the inflammation of a tendon and its synovial sheath. It is also known as tendosynovitis, tendovaginitis, tenontothecitis, tenontolemmitis, and vaginal or tendinous synovitis. At the site of friction, the tendon is enveloped by a sheath consisting of a visceral and parietal layer of synovial membrane and is lubricated by a synovial-like fluid containing hyaluronate. The synovial sheath is in turn covered by a dense, fibrous tissue sheath. Irregularities, disease, and damage to the tendon's attachment to the articular joints may lead to progressive degenerative changes with resultant limitation of movement and pain. The synovial membranes of tendon sheaths and bursae are capable of the same inflammatory reactions to abnormal conditions as the synovial membranes of joints.

727.00	Unspecified synovitis and tenosynovitis — synovitis NOS, tenosynovitis NOS
727.01	Synovitis and tenosynovitis in diseases classified elsewhere — (Code first underlying disease: 015.0-015.9) — secondary to an underlying disease
727.02	Giant cell tumor of tendon sheath
727.03	Trigger finger (acquired)
727.04	Radial styloid tenosynovitis — de Quervain's disease
727.05	Other tenosynovitis of hand and wrist — not otherwise specified
727.06	Tenosynovitis of foot and ankle
727.09	Other synovitis and tenosynovitis — buttock, elbow, hip, knee
727.1	Bunion — enlargement of the first metatarsal head caused by inflammation of bursa, frequently resulting in lateral displacement of the great toe

A bunion is a localized friction-type bursitis located at either the medial or dorsal aspect of the first metatarsophalangeal joint. Bunions of the medial aspect are usually associated with hallux valgus.

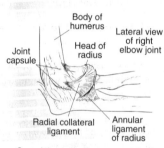

Synovial membranes are contained within the joint capsule

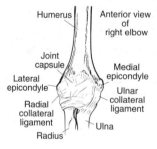

727.2	Specific bursitides often of occupational origin — chronic crepitant synovitis of wrist, miner's elbow or knee

Specific bursitides often of occupational origin is friction-type bursitis of various sites excluding bunions. Examples of these bursitides are "housemaid's knee," "student's elbow," and "weaver's bottom."

Ganglia can be found on either the dorsal or volar aspect

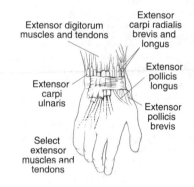

Select extensor muscles and tendons

727.3	Other bursitis disorders — not otherwise specified
727.4 ⌐sth	Ganglion and cyst of synovium, tendon, and bursa

Ganglion and cyst of synovium, tendon, and bursa are thin-walled cystic lesions of unknown etiology containing thick, clear, mucinous fluid, possibly due to mucoid degeneration. Arising in relation to periarticular tissues, joint capsules, and tendon sheaths, ganglia are limited to the hands and feet and are most common in the dorsum of the wrist.

727.40	Unspecified synovial cyst — round, cystic swelling of unspecified synovial site AHA: Q2, 1997, 6
727.41	Ganglion of joint — round, cystic swelling
727.42	Ganglion of tendon sheath — round, cystic swelling
727.43	Unspecified ganglion — round, cystic swelling of unspecified site
727.49	Other ganglion and cyst of synovium, tendon, and bursa — round cystic swelling of bursa
727.50	Unspecified rupture of synovium — nontraumatic, unknown site

727.51	Synovial cyst of popliteal space — *Baker's cyst of knee*			

Synovial cyst of the popliteal space is Baker's cysts, sometimes called popliteal cysts. In children, Baker's cysts are common but usually are asymptomatic and regress spontaneously. In adults, Baker's cysts, in conjunction with synovial effusion due to rheumatoid arthritis or degenerative joint disease, may produce significant impairment. When a Baker's cyst interferes with normal knee function, surgical exploration and excision of the cyst is indicated.

Baker's cysts are classified under subcategory 727.5 for rupture of synovium because the cysts usually communicate with the knee joint through a long and tortuous duct, allowing the cyst to become distended by any synovial effusion and possibly extend down as far as the mid calf.

727.59   Other rupture of synovium — *other*

Rupture of tendon, nontraumatic, is a rupture due to pathology rather than trauma or injury. A normal tendon seldom ruptures even with strenuous activity, but if it has become damaged by disease (e.g., secondary to tenosynovitis) or degenerated due to the fraying caused by friction (e.g., due to bony erosion), it may rupture even with normal activity. Degeneration occurs in rheumatic arthritis, lupus erythematosus, hyperparathyroidism, and systemic steroid use, or when steroids are injected directly into a tendon.

Therapies include reconstructive surgery to repair or replace the abnormal part of the ruptured tendon.

727.60	Nontraumatic rupture of unspecified tendon — *unknown tendon*
727.61	Complete rupture of rotator cuff
727.62	Nontraumatic rupture of tendons of biceps (long head)
727.63	Nontraumatic rupture of extensor tendons of hand and wrist

Subclassification 727.63 includes the extensor pollicis longus, extensor pollicis brevis, extensor digitorum communis, extensor indicis, and the abductor pollicis longus tendons.

727.64	Nontraumatic rupture of flexor tendons of hand and wrist

Subclassification 727.64 includes the flexor digitorum superficialis, flexor digitorum profundus, and the flexor pollicis longus tendons.

727.65	Nontraumatic rupture of quadriceps tendon
727.66	Nontraumatic rupture of patellar tendon
727.67	Nontraumatic rupture of Achilles tendon
727.68	Nontraumatic rupture of other tendons of foot and ankle — *not otherwise specified*
727.69	Nontraumatic rupture of other tendon — *not otherwise specified*
727.81	Contracture of tendon (sheath) — *acquired short Achilles tendon*
727.82	Calcium deposits in tendon and bursa — *calcification or calcific tendonitis, not otherwise specified*
727.83	Plica syndrome — *plica knee* **AHA:** Q4, 2000, 44
727.89	Other disorders of synovium, tendon, and bursa — *abscess, hemorrhage, union of bursa or tendon, pseudobursa* **AHA:** Q2, 1989, 15
727.9	Unspecified disorder of synovium, tendon, and bursa — *specifics unknown, including sloughing tendon, slipped tendon, degeneration of synovial membrane, tenophyte*

728 Disorders of muscle, ligament, and fascia

Muscle is an organ composed of one of three types of muscle tissue (skeletal, cardiac, or smooth) that is specialized for contraction to produce voluntary or involuntary movements. Ligament is dense, regularly arranged connective tissue that attaches bone to bone. The fascia is thin connective tissue covering, or separating, the muscles and internal organs of the body. It varies in thickness, density, elasticity, and composition. Fascia, muscles, and ligaments are normally exposed to stress throughout life. Damage occurs when the muscle or connective tissue is exposed to higher-than-usual stress levels, such as sudden excessive stress, or the result of repetitive stress. Whether damaged by repetitive overuse or by acute injury, treatment includes a brief period of relative rest, with length depending on the extent of injury, followed by gradual movement and activity.

728.0	Infective myositis — *purulent, suppurative*

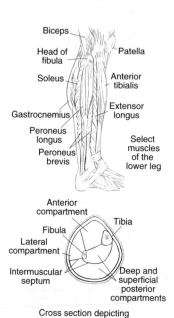

Cross section depicting compartments of lower leg

Infective myositis is inflammation of the voluntary muscles due to infection. It is usually secondary to osteomyelitis or a penetrating wound, but hematogenous infection can occur in debilitated patients or patients with suppressed immunity.

Signs and symptoms of infective myositis include marked swelling and pain, usually confined to shoulder girdle and arms, but may affect any part of the body.

Code	Description
728.10	Unspecified calcification and ossification — *massive calcification*
728.11	Progressive myositis ossificans — *Munchmeyer's syndrome*
728.12	Traumatic myositis ossificans — *myositis ossificans (circumscripta)*
728.13	Postoperative heterotopic calcification — *occurring at the site of surgery*
728.19	Other muscular calcification and ossification — *not otherwise specified, including polymyositis ossificans*
728.2	Muscular wasting and disuse atrophy, not elsewhere classified — *hemiatrophy of leg, myofibrosis*
728.3	Other specific muscle disorders — *arthrogryposis, immobility syndrome*
728.4	Laxity of ligament — *looseness or relaxation*
728.5	Hypermobility syndrome
728.6	Contracture of palmar fascia — *Dupuytren's contracture*
728.71	Plantar fascial fibromatosis — *plantar fascia syndrome, contracture, traumatic fasciitis*
728.79	Other fibromatoses of muscle, ligament, and fascia — *not otherwise specified, Garrod's or knuckle pads, nodular fasciitis, subcutaneous or proliferative pseudosarcomatous fibromatosis*
728.81	Interstitial myositis
728.82	Foreign body granuloma of muscle — *talc granuloma of muscle*
728.83	Rupture of muscle, nontraumatic
728.84	Diastasis of muscle — *diastasis recti*
728.85	Spasm of muscle
728.86	Necrotizing fasciitis — (Use additional code to identify infectious organism, 041.00-041.89, 785.4, if applicable)
728.87	Muscle weakness (generalized)— *weariness and fatigue of muscles* AHA: Q4, 2003, 66; Q1, 2005, 13
728.88	Rhabdomyolysis — *muscle breakdown or dissolution of muscle, related to myoglobin in the urine; may be due to extreme and prolonged physical exertion* AHA: Q4, 2003, 66
728.89	Other disorder of muscle, ligament, and fascia — (Use additional E code to identify drug, if drug-induced) — *not otherwise specified, thecal abscess; cicatrix of muscle; calcification, contraction or cyst of ligament; contraction, eosinophilic, hernia of fascia* AHA: Q2, 2001, 14,15; Q3, 2002, 28
728.9	Unspecified disorder of muscle, ligament, and fascia

Coding Clarification
Report 618.83 for pelvic muscle wasting and disuse atrophy.

Muscle Weakness: Code assignment of 728.87 *Muscle weakness (generalized)* must be distinguished from code 780.79 *Generalized weakness*. Generalized muscle weakness is a result of musculoskeletal disorders, neuromuscular disease, nerve damage due to trauma or degenerative disease, or psychological and metabolic disorders. Generalized weakness is an ill-defined condition of lethargy, malaise, and tiredness.

729 Other disorders of soft tissues

Code	Description
729.0	Rheumatism, unspecified and fibrositis — *specifics unknown*
729.1	Unspecified myalgia and myositis — *unspecified generalized musculoskeletal pain, stiffness and easy fatigability*
729.2	Unspecified neuralgia, neuritis, and radiculitis — *pain along an inflamed nerve, with inflammation of the root of the associated spinal nerve, site unspecified*

Panniculitis, unspecified, is inflammation of subcutaneous fat. The term often is used solely to refer to an inflammation of the panniculus adiposa of the abdominal wall. Miscellaneous forms of panniculitis include those resulting from trauma, insulin injections, pancreatitis, allergic reactions, insect toxins, angiitis, idiopathic cold agglutinins, and sclerosing lipogranulomas.

Many variations of panniculitis, such as erythema nodosum (tuberculous and nontuberculous) and erythema pernio, are classified elsewhere. When coding panniculitis, obtain as much specific information as possible and follow the ICD-9-CM index carefully.

729.30	Panniculitis, unspecified site — *Weber-Christian disease*
729.31	Hypertrophy of fat pad, knee — *infrapatellar fat pad*
729.39	Panniculitis of other sites — *not otherwise specified*
729.4	Unspecified fasciitis — *inflammation of the fibrous tissue that acts to compartmentalize muscle*
	AHA: Q2, 1994, 13
729.5	Pain in soft tissues of limb — *not otherwise specified*
729.6	Residual foreign body in soft tissue

Subcategory 729.7 reports nontraumatic compartment syndrome. Muscle groups in the arms and legs are separated by fascia, or thick layers of tissue. Inside each layer of fascia is a compartment, a limited space containing muscle tissue, nerves, and blood vessels. Fascia do not expand; therefore any swelling within a compartment will result in increased pressure. This in turn constricts the muscles, blood vessels, and nerves. Sufficiently high pressure will block blood flow to the compartment, potentially leading to permanent injury to the muscle and nerves. If the pressure persists, the limb may become necrotic and require amputation.

Nontraumatic compartment syndrome can have numerous underlying causes. Most often occurring in the lower leg or forearm, compartment syndrome may also occur in other sites such as the hand, foot, thigh, upper arm, abdomen, or buttock. Repetitive activities such as running or other forms of vigorous exercise or sports can result in a form of compartment syndrome known as exertional compartment syndrome. Other underlying causes can include seizures, nephrotic syndrome, or everyday exercise activities such as horseback riding or stationary bicycle use.

The characteristic symptom of compartment syndrome is severe pain that is unresponsive to elevation or analgesics. In advanced cases, there may be decreased sensation, weakness, and pallor of the skin. Definitive diagnosis is accomplished by measuring compartmental pressure. A needle attached to a pressure meter is inserted directly into the compartment. Diagnosis is confirmed when the compartment pressure is greater than 45 mmHg or when the pressure is within 30 mmHg of the diastolic blood pressure. If chronic compartment syndrome is suspected, this test must be performed immediately following the activity that causes pain.

Treatment for compartment syndrome may initially consist of rest, ice, and elevation. However, depending upon acuity or chronicity of the condition, emergent or elective fasciotomy (surgical release) is often required. Fascial incisions are made in order to relieve the pressure buildup. The wounds are often left open and covered with a sterile bandage for 48 to 72 hours, after which they are closed during a second surgery. Skin grafts may be necessary for wound closure.

Prognosis for compartment syndrome depends largely on the underlying cause. If the condition is diagnosed and treated promptly, there is an excellent chance of recovery of the muscles and nerves within the compartment. However, delayed diagnosis can result in permanent nerve injury and loss of muscle function; this can occur after 12 to 24 hours of compression. In the most severe cases, amputation may be required.

729.71	Nontraumatic compartment syndrome of upper extremity — *arm, forearm, shoulder, wrist, hand and fingers*
729.72	Nontraumatic compartment syndrome of lower extremity — *hip, buttock, thigh, leg, foot and toes*
729.73	Nontraumatic compartment syndrome of abdomen
729.79	Nontraumatic compartment syndrome of other sites

Coding Clarification

Exertional compartment syndrome is a nontraumatic compartment syndrome due to repetitive motion/impact seen in legs of runners, feet of ballet dancers, and arms of tennis players.

For traumatic compartment syndrome or compartment syndrome not otherwise specified, see subcategory 958.9.

729.81	Swelling of limb
729.82	Cramp of limb
729.89	Other musculoskeletal symptoms referable to limbs
729.9	Other and unspecified disorders of soft tissue — *not otherwise specified, polyalgia, nontraumatic compartment or Profichet's syndrome*

Coding Clarification

Traumatic compartment syndrome not otherwise specified is assumed to be traumatic and is classified to subcategory 958.9. An exclusion note under code 729.7 directs the coder to subcategory 958.9 for the correct classification of compartment syndrome not otherwise specified, or due to trauma.

730–739 Osteopathies, Chondropathies, and Acquired Musculoskeletal Deformities

730 Osteomyelitis, periostitis, and other infections involving bone
AHA: Q4, 1997, 43

Osteomyelitis, periostitis, and other infections involving bone is a broad spectrum of bone infections. Osteomyelitis is an inflammation of bone and bone marrow. The condition is commonly due to a pathogen such as bacteria, virus, protozoa, or fungus. Periostitis is an inflammation of the periosteum, the thick fibrous membrane covering all of the surfaces of bones except at the articular cartilage. The combination of osteomyelitis and periostitis is periosteomyelitis.

The pathogenesis of osteomyelitis, periostitis, and periosteomyelitis follows three general routes of infection. Hematogenous osteomyelitis (acute) is a form of osteomyelitis common to children where blood-borne organisms settle in the metaphyseal vascular bed of the rapidly developing long bones. Osteomyelitis may develop as an extension of a contiguous infection, particularly infections involving ischemic, diabetic, or neurotrophic ulcers. The third route of infection is by direct inoculation of pathogens through an open wound created by injury or a surgical procedure.

Signs and symptoms of osteomyelitis, periostitis, and other infections involving bone include pain and unwillingness to move the affected area and, occasionally, malaise, fever, chills, and anorexia. Sometimes the site of infection closest to the surface may be detected by palpation.

Lab work includes aspiration with a large bore needle for gram stain and a culture to confirm the diagnosis and reveal the pathogenic agent. Blood cultures may be positive in patients with acute hematogenous osteomyelitis. Bone scans such as scintigraphy are useful, although other factors may cause false positive results and false negative results are possible with acute hematogenous osteomyelitis.

Therapies include long-term antibiotic therapy and surgery to incise and drain the involved area and remove necrotic debris in severe acute cases. Other surgery includes sequestrectomy, excision of multiple sinus tracts, craterization, saucerization, partial excision of bone, and bone grafting for chronic osteomyelitis.

Associated conditions include skin ulcers of various types, septicemia, diabetes, tuberculosis, poliomyelitis, neuropathy, septic arthritis, and trauma (such as compound fractures).

Osteomyelitis may result from direct inoculation from a traumatic or surgical wound. In these cases, follow the Department of Health and Human Services (DHHS) definitions regarding principal and other diagnoses code sequencing and ICD-9-CM coding rules regarding late effects and complications of surgical and medical care where applicable.

The following fifth-digit subclassification is for use with categories 711-712, 715-716, 718-719, and 730. Valid fifth-digits are in brackets [ ] beneath each code.

0   site unspecified
1   shoulder region (acromioclavicular joint, clavicle, glenohumeral joint, scapula, sternoclavicular joint)
2   upper arm (elbow joint, humerus)
3   forearm (radius, ulna, wrist joint)
4   hand (carpus, metacarpus, phalanges)
5   pelvic regions and thigh (buttock, femur, hip joint)
6   lower leg (fibula, knee joint, patella, tibia)
7   ankle and foot (ankle joint, metatarsus, phalanges, tarsus, other joints in foot)
8   other specified sites (head, neck, ribs, skull, trunk, vertebral column)
9   multiple sites

730.0 Acute osteomyelitis — (Use additional code to identify organism, 041.1, also use additional code to identify major osseous defect (731.1) if applicable.) — *abscess of any bone except accessory sinus, jaw, or mastoid*
[0-9]
AHA: Q4, 1997, 43; Q1, 2004, 14

Acute osteomyelitis is diseases including periostitis and periosteomyelitis in acute and subacute forms. Clinically, patients fall into two groups: those who respond to intravenous antibiotics and those who require surgical intervention.

730.1 Chronic osteomyelitis — (Use additional code to identify organism, 041.1, also use additional code to identify major osseous defect (731.1) if applicable.) — *Brodie's abscess, Busquet's disease, sequestrum, sclerosing osteomyelitis of Garre*
[0-9]
AHA: Q4, 1997, 43

Chronic osteomyelitis is persistent, recurring infection of bone and/or draining sinuses, often regarded as controllable but incurable.

730.2 [0-9]	5th	Unspecified osteomyelitis — (Use additional code to identify organism, 041.1, also use additional code to identify major osseous defect (731.1) if applicable.) — *osteitis or osteomyelitis of unknown origin, with or without periostitis* **AHA:** Q4, 1997, 43
730.3 [0-9]	5th	Periostitis without mention of osteomyelitis — (Use additional code to identify organism, 041.1) — *abscess without mention of osteomyelitis* **AHA:** Q4, 1997, 43
730.7 [0-9]	5th	Osteopathy resulting from poliomyelitis — (Code first underlying disease: 045.0-045.9. Use additional code to identify organism) — *secondary to polio* **AHA:** Q4, 1997, 43
730.8 [0-9]	5th	Other infections involving bone in diseases classified elsewhere — (Code first underlying disease: 002.0, 015.0-015.9. Use additional code to identify organism) — *secondary to underlying disease* **AHA:** Q3, 1991, 10; Q2, 1997, 16; Q4, 1997, 43
730.9 [0-9]	5th	Unspecified infection of bone — (Use additional code to identify organism, 041.1)

731 Osteitis deformans and osteopathies associated with other disorders classified elsewhere

Osteitis deformans and osteopathies associated with other disorders classified elsewhere include the disseminated bone disorder known as Paget's disease. Characterized by slow and progressive enlargement and deformity of multiple bones, Paget's disease is associated with unexplained acceleration of both deposition and resorption of bone. During the early (osteolytic) phase of the disease, resorption exceeds deposition, and the bone, although enlarged, becomes sponge-like, weakened, and deformed. The second (osteosclerotic) phase is marked by deposition exceeding resorption resulting in the bones becoming thick and dense. The disease sometimes is associated with an invariably fatal form of malignant osteogenic sarcoma as a result of hyperactive osteoblast activity. Etiology is unknown, but there is some evidence that it may be triggered by a "slow virus" that affects primarily the osteoclasts.

731.0	Osteitis deformans without mention of bone tumor — *Paget's disease of bone*
731.1	Osteitis deformans in diseases classified elsewhere — (Code first underlying disease: 170.0-170.9) — *secondary to underlying disease*
731.2	Hypertrophic pulmonary osteoarthropathy — *Bamberger-Marie disease, Minkowski's, Pierre Marie-Bamberger, or thoracogenous rheumatic syndromes*
731.3	Major osseous defects — (Code first the underlying disease, if known: 170.0-170.9, 730.00-730.29, 733.00-733.09, 733.40-733.49, 996.45)

Major osseous defects are conditions that occur as a result of extensive bone loss. Underlying causes for osseous defects are varied. They may or may not be associated with previous joint replacement, and may include osteomyelitis, osteoporosis, pathological fractures, trauma, or benign or malignant neoplasms. One of the most common causes, however, is periprosthetic osteolysis from a previous joint replacement.

The repair of major osseous defects is a primary concern in many types of bone surgeries, including primary or revision arthroplasty procedures. Following revision total joint replacement procedures, one of the most important variables in ascertaining the complexity, resource intensity, recovery times, and patient outcomes is the extent of bone loss that has taken place around the prosthesis. If bone loss is minimal, the majority of these procedures can be carried out with standard implants. Resource utilization, recovery times, and patient outcomes are consistent with those associated with initial hip and knee replacement. Conversely, when bone loss is extensive, bony defect reconstruction often necessitates specialized implants, the use of cadaver (allograft) bone, extended hospitalization and recovery times, and less-than-optimal patient outcomes. Although more commonly occurring with hip replacements, major osseous defects affect knee replacements as well.

Other methods of osseous defect repair may include autogenous, allogenic, xenogenic, or synthetic bone grafts. Demineralized bone matrix or bone morphogenic protein (BMP) is often used to fill osseous defects in nonunion repair and repair of certain vertebral fractures.

731.8	Other bone involvement in diseases classified elsewhere — (Code first underlying disease. Use additional code to specify bone condition) — *secondary to underlying disease* **AHA:** Q2, 1997, 16; Q4, 1997, 43; Q1, 2004, 14

Coding Clarification
Code 731.3 *Major osseous defects*, may be reported secondary to the causal condition or independently.

In cases of joint prosthesis failure, code 731.3 should be reported in addition to the mechanical complication code 996.45 *Peri-prosthetic osteolysis*. However, this is not an etiology/manifestation mandatory dual coding situation.

732 Osteochondropathies

Osteochondropathies are self-limiting disorders of unknown etiology that mostly affect children (juvenile osteochondrosis) 3 to 10 years of age. Four phases in the pathogenesis of the disease have been identified: necrosis, revascularization with bone deposition and resorption, bone healing, and bone deformity. The fourth phase often is associated with degenerative arthropathy and is subject to ICD-9-CM coding rules regarding late effects, where applicable.

732.0	Juvenile osteochondrosis of spine — *marginal or vertebral epiphysis of Scheuermann or spine; vertebral epiphysitis*
732.1	Juvenile osteochondrosis of hip and pelvis — *acetabulum, head of femur, iliac crest, symphysis pubis; coxa plana, ischiopubic synchondrosis of van Neck, Wadenstrom's disease, pseudocoxalgia*
732.2	Nontraumatic slipped upper femoral epiphysis — *slipped upper femoral epiphysis, not otherwise specified*
732.3	Juvenile osteochondrosis of upper extremity — *capitulum of humerus if Panner, carpal lunate of Kienbock, head of humerus of Haas, heads of metacarpals of Mauclaire, lower ulna of Burns, radial head of Brailsford*
732.4	Juvenile osteochondrosis of lower extremity, excluding foot — *primary patellar center of Köhler, proximal tibia of Blount, secondary patellar center of Sinding-Larsen, tibial tubercle of Osgood-Schlatter; tibia vara, Blount-Barber or Erlacher-Blount syndromes*
732.5	Juvenile osteochondrosis of foot — *astragalus of Diaz, calcaneum of Sever, second metatarsal of Freiberg, fifth metatarsal of Iselin, os tibiale externum of Haglund, tarsal navicular of Köhler, calcaneal apophysitis, epiphysitis os calcis, Mouchet's disease*
732.6	Other juvenile osteochondrosis — *apophysitis, epiphysitis, osteochondritis, osteochondrosis of site not otherwise specified*
732.7	Osteochondritis dissecans

Osteochondritis dissecans is a form of osteochondropathy in which the convex surfaces of certain pressure epiphyses are susceptible to avascular necrosis. When a small tangential segment of subchondral bone becomes separated or "dissected" from the remaining portion of the epiphysis by reactive fibrous and granulation tissue, it is designated an osteochondritis or osteochondrosis dissecans.

732.8	Other specified forms of osteochondropathy — *adult osteochondrosis of spine*
732.9	Unspecified osteochondropathy — *apophysitis, epiphysitis, osteochondritis, osteochondrosis, not specified as adult or juvenile, of site not otherwise specified*

Coding Clarification

Many osteochondroses are identified by their eponyms (e.g., Kienbock's disease of the carpal lunate) and can be found under the main terms "Disease," "Osteochondrosis," and "Syndrome" in the ICD-9-CM index.

733 Other disorders of bone and cartilage

Osteoporosis is generalized bone disease characterized by decreased osteoblastic formation of matrix combined with increased osteoclastic resorption of bone, resulting in a marked decrease in bone mass. Osteoporosis often presents with osteopenia, which is a decrease in bone mineralization. Osteoporosis is classified into two major groups: primary and secondary. Primary osteoporosis implies that the condition is a fundamental disease entity and may be further broken down into involutional disease (e.g., juvenile). Secondary osteoporosis attributes the condition to an underlying clinical disease, medical condition, or medication.

Signs and symptoms of osteoporosis include chronic and intermittent back pain (due to vertebral microfractures), skeletal remodeling such as dorsal kyphosis, or loss of height.

Lab work usually shows normal results although metabolic studies may reveal a negative calcium balance. Radiographs and bone scans determine the extent and severity of osteoporosis and osteopenia and may reveal fresh or old evidence of pathological fractures. Quantitative computed tomography (CT) and single and dual energy x-ray absorptiometry (DEXA) measure bone density, and bone biopsy occasionally is done for histological studies.

Therapies include medical management such as dietary manipulation, calcitonin, diphosphonate's, vitamin D, calcium and sodium fluoride, and estrogen therapy following menopause.

Associated conditions include pathological fractures; in the case of secondary osteoporosis, a wide range of underlying factors such as anemia, hormone-related disorders, hepatic disease, starvation and anorexia, small intestine disease, mastocytosis, hemochromatosis, acromegaly, and conditions resulting from gastrectomy and treatment with anticonvulsants may be involved.

Diseases of the Musculoskeletal System and Connective Tissue

733.00	Unspecified osteoporosis — *wedging of vertebra not otherwise specified* **AHA:** Q2, 1998, 12; Q3, 2001, 19
733.01	Senile osteoporosis — *bone mass reduction, usually without abnormality of mineral or organic content, in postmenopausal women*
733.02	Idiopathic osteoporosis — *bone mass reduction, usually without abnormality of mineral or organic content, not the result of disease or trauma*
733.03	Disuse osteoporosis
733.09	Other osteoporosis — (Use additional E code to identify drug) — *not otherwise specified, including drug-induced osteoporosis, Preiser's disease* **AHA:** Q4, 2003, 108

Coding Clarification
In subcategory 733.0, use an additional code to identify major osseous defect (731.3) if applicable.

Subcategory 733.1 reports pathological fractures.

A pathological fracture occurs at a site weakened by preexisting disease. These fractures are often differentiated from traumatic fractures by clinically assessing the magnitude of the trauma or stress causing the fracture. A relatively minor trauma or stress can cause a pathological fracture in bones diseased by osteoporosis and other metabolic bone disease, disseminated bone disorders, inflammatory bone diseases, Paget's disease, neoplasms, or any other condition that can compromise bone strength and integrity.

733.10	Pathologic fracture, unspecified site — *spontaneous fracture, site unknown* **AHA:** Nov-Dec, 1985, 16; Nov-Dec, 1986, 10; Q4, 1993, 25
733.11	Pathologic fracture of humerus — *spontaneous fracture* **AHA:** Nov-Dec, 1985, 16; Nov-Dec, 1986, 10; Q4, 1993, 25
733.12	Pathologic fracture of distal radius and ulna — *spontaneous fracture* **AHA:** Nov-Dec, 1985, 16; Nov-Dec, 1986, 10; Q4, 1993, 25
733.13	Pathologic fracture of vertebrae — *spontaneous fracture* **AHA:** Nov-Dec, 1985, 16; Nov-Dec, 1986, 10; Q4, 1993, 25; Q3, 1999, 5
733.14	Pathologic fracture of neck of femur — *spontaneous fracture* **AHA:** Nov-Dec, 1985, 16; Nov-Dec, 1986, 10; Q4, 1993, 25; Q1, 1996, 16; Q1, 2001, 1
733.15	Pathologic fracture of other specified part of femur — *spontaneous fracture* **AHA:** Nov-Dec, 1985, 16; Nov-Dec, 1986, 10; Q4, 1993, 25; Q2, 1998, 12
733.16	Pathologic fracture of tibia or fibula — *spontaneous fracture* **AHA:** Nov-Dec, 1985, 16; Nov-Dec, 1986, 10; Q4, 1993, 25
733.19	Pathologic fracture of other specified site — *spontaneous fracture, site not otherwise specified* **AHA:** Nov-Dec, 1985, 16; Nov-Dec, 1986, 10; Q4, 1993, 25

Excluded from this subclassification is stress fracture (733.93-733.95).

When a fracture is due to a minor injury, the physician must determine if the injury was sufficient to cause the fracture or if the fracture is pathologic. Documentation must support the code selection of a pathological fracture (733.1x).

733.20	Unspecified cyst of bone (localized) — *unknown site*
733.21	Solitary bone cyst — *unicameral bone cyst*
733.22	Aneurysmal bone cyst
733.29	Other cyst of bone — *not otherwise specified, fibrous dysplasia*
733.3	Hyperostosis of skull — *formation of new, abnormal bone on the inner aspect of cranial bones; leontiasis ossium, Buchem's, Morel-Moore, and Morgagni-Stewart-Morel syndromes*

Aseptic necrosis of bone is infarction of bone tissue due to noninfectious etiologies such as fractures (avascular necrosis due to fracture), ischemic disorders, and immunosuppressive agents such as corticosteroids following renal transplants. It leads to degenerative joint disease or nonunion of fracture.

Osteonecrosis can be used to describe a wide variety of disorders, both infectious and noninfectious, resulting in bone infarction.

Some conditions falling under the general category of osteonecrosis are due to infectious etiologies and should be classified elsewhere. For example, osteonecrosis associated with acute staphylococcal osteomyelitis is classified to subcategories 730.0x and 041.1. Osteonecrosis unspecified as to infectious or noninfectious etiology is classified to subcategory 730.1x. When reporting a code from subcategory 733.4, an additional code should also be assigned to identify major osseous defect (731.3) if applicable.

733.40	Aseptic necrosis of bone, site unspecified — *death of bone tissue not due to infection, unknown site*
733.41	Aseptic necrosis of head of humerus — *death of bone tissue not due to infection*
733.42	Aseptic necrosis of head and neck of femur — *death of bone tissue not due to infection*
733.43	Aseptic necrosis of medial femoral condyle — *death of bone tissue not due to infection*

733.44	Aseptic necrosis of talus — *death of bone tissue not due to infection*	
733.49	Aseptic necrosis of other bone site — *death of bone tissue not due to infection, site not otherwise specified*	
733.5	Osteitis condensans — *piriform sclerosis of ilium*	
733.6	Tietze's disease — *painful swell and inflammation of unknown origin of rib cartilage; costochondral junction syndrome, costochondritis*	
733.7	Algoneurodystrophy — *disuse atrophy of bone, Sudeck's atrophy*	
733.81	Malunion of fracture — *broken bone heals in misalignment* **AHA:** Q2, 1994, 5	
733.82	Nonunion of fracture — *broken bone fails to heal* **AHA:** Nov-Dec, 1984, 18; Q2, 1994, 5	
733.90	Disorder of bone and cartilage, unspecified — *specifics unknown*	
733.91	Arrest of bone development or growth — *Harris lines, epiphyseal arrest*	
733.92	Chondromalacia — *localized, except patella, systemic, tibial plateau*	
733.93	Stress fracture of tibia or fibula — *stress reaction of tibia or fibular* **AHA:** Q4, 2001, 48	
733.94	Stress fracture of the metatarsals — *stress reaction of metatarsals* **AHA:** Q4, 2001, 48	
733.95	Stress fracture of other bone — *stress reaction of other bone* **AHA:** Q4, 2001, 48	
733.99	Other disorders of bone and cartilage — *not otherwise specified, diaphysitis, hypertrophy of bone, relapsing polychondritis, Bruck's disease, slipped rib, xiphoiditis, ossification of cartilage* **AHA:** Jan-Feb, 1987, 14	

Coding Clarification
Nature of Pathological Fractures: A pathological fracture is a spontaneous fracture that occurs without external injury or by a minor or slight injury to a weakened bone. Bone density may become weakened by a number of conditions including but not limited to bone cysts, bone tumors, hyperparathyroidism, nutritional maladies, congenital anomalies, osteoporosis, Paget's disease, or osteomyelitis.

Because a fracture must either be traumatic (due to an injury) or pathological (due to weakened bone), a code from categories 800-829 must never accompany a code from category 733.

Report 380.03 for chondritis of pinna.

Coding Scenario
A 92-year-old female patient is seen complaining of pain of her left leg and back. She denies any traumatic injury. Upon x-ray examination, the physician determines that the patient has a pathological compression fracture of the L-3 vertebral body.

Code assignment: 733.13 *Pathologic fracture of vertebrae*

734 Flat foot OK
Flat feet have a low arch and leave a nearly complete imprint; there is only a slight inward curve where the arch should be. The stretching or tearing of the posterior tibial tendon, which supports the arch and helps lift the heel off the ground, can lead to an adult acquired flatfoot deformity. Causes include trauma, overuse, and medical conditions such as obesity, diabetes, previous surgery, and steroid injections. The condition progresses from pain, swelling, and weakness of the tendon to a rigid flattening of the foot and ankle pain. Treatment depends on the stage of progression at the time of examination. Early stages can be treated non-surgically by rest and anti-inflammatory drugs. Orthotics and minor tendon surgery can help in advanced states, while later stages may require reconstructive surgery to stabilize the foot and ankle.

735 Acquired deformities of toe
735.0	Hallux valgus (acquired) — *deformity in which the great toe angles toward other toes of that foot*	
735.1	Hallux varus (acquired) — *deformity in which the great toe angles away from other toes of that foot*	
735.2	Hallux rigidus — *limited motion of great toe due to painful flexion; also called hallux rigidus*	
735.3	Hallux malleus — *hammer toe of big toe*	
735.4	Other hammer toe (acquired) — *hammer toe, other than big toe*	
735.5	Claw toe (acquired) — *contracture of toe*	
735.8	Other acquired deformity of toe — *hypertrophic, overriding, overlapping, or pigeon toe*	
735.9	Unspecified acquired deformity of toe	

736 Other acquired deformities of limbs
736.00	Unspecified deformity of forearm, excluding fingers	
736.01	Cubitus valgus (acquired) — *deformity in which the forearm angles away from the body*	
736.02	Cubitus varus (acquired) — *deformity in which the forearm angles toward the body*	
736.03	Valgus deformity of wrist (acquired) — *deformity in which the wrist angles away from the body*	
736.04	Varus deformity of wrist (acquired) — *deformity in which the wrist angles toward the body*	

Diseases of the Musculoskeletal System and Connective Tissue

736.05	Wrist drop (acquired) — *paralysis or injury of extensor muscles of hand and fingers causing flexion of wrist*		736.79	Other acquired deformity of ankle and foot — *not otherwise specified, pronation of ankle or foot, varus talipes, valgus talipes*

Wrist drop is a condition in which the wrist remains flexed downward and is unable to be extended. It is often caused by injury to the radial nerve of the forearm or paralysis of the muscles in the hand and wrist.

736.06	Claw hand (acquired) — *contracture of hand*

A claw hand is characterized by curved or bent fingers, making the hand appear claw-like. Claw hand can be something that a child is born with (congenital) or can develop as a consequence of disorders (acquired).

736.07	Club hand, acquired
736.09	Other acquired deformities of forearm, excluding fingers — *not otherwise specified, intrinsic swan neck hand*
736.1	Mallet finger — *constant flexion of distal joint*
736.20	Unspecified deformity of finger
736.21	Boutonniere deformity — *fixed flexion of proximal interphalangeal joint and hyperextension of distal interphalangeal joint*
736.22	Swan-neck deformity
736.29	Other acquired deformity of finger — *not otherwise specified, shallow acetabulum, acquired short ip, wandering acetabulum*
	AHA: Q2, 1989, 13; Q2, 2005, 7
736.30	Unspecified acquired deformity of hip
736.31	Coxa valga (acquired) — *angle formed by the head and neck of the femur and axis of the shaft is increased*
736.32	Coxa vara (acquired) — *angle formed by the head and neck of the femur and axis of the shaft is decreased*
736.39	Other acquired deformities of hip — *not otherwise specified*
	AHA: Q2, 1991, 18
736.41	Genu valgum (acquired) — *"knock-knee;" knees close together, ankles far apart*
736.42	Genu varum (acquired) — *"bowleg," knees far apart, ankles close together*
736.5	Genu recurvatum (acquired) — *"back-knee," hyperextension of knee*
736.6	Other acquired deformities of knee — *not otherwise specified*
736.70	Unspecified deformity of ankle and foot, acquired
736.71	Acquired equinovarus deformity — *clubfoot*
736.72	Equinus deformity of foot, acquired — *tip-toe walking deformity*
736.73	Cavus deformity of foot, acquired — *abnormally high arch*
736.74	Claw foot, acquired — *contracture deformity*
736.75	Cavovarus deformity of foot, acquired
736.76	Other acquired calcaneus deformity — *not otherwise specified*
736.79	Other acquired deformity of ankle and foot — *not otherwise specified, pronation of ankle or foot, varus talipes, valgus talipes*
736.81	Unequal leg length (acquired)
736.89	Other acquired deformity of other parts of limb — *not otherwise specified, including angulation or torsion of tibia; bowing of femur, fibula, tibia, winged scapula*
736.9	Acquired deformity of limb, site unspecified

737 Curvature of spine

Curvature of the spine is a deformity of the spine when it is not in straight alignment or with proper convexity. Kyphosis is an abnormal increase in the thoracic convexity as viewed from the side. Lordosis is the anterior convexity of the cervical and lumbar spine as viewed from the side.

737.0	Adolescent postural kyphosis — *acquired abnormal convex curve of spine*
737.10	Kyphosis (acquired) (postural)
737.11	Kyphosis due to radiation
737.12	Kyphosis, postlaminectomy
737.19	Other kyphosis (acquired) — *not otherwise specified*
737.20	Lordosis (acquired) (postural) — *not due to disease or injury*
737.21	Lordosis, postlaminectomy
737.22	Other postsurgical lordosis
737.29	Other lordosis (acquired)

Scoliosis is lateral curvature of the spine and kyphoscoliosis is a lateral curvature of the spine with extensive flexion. Scoliosis may be described as structural or nonstructural depending on whether the condition is reversible. Etiologies for nonstructural scoliosis include poor posture, pain, muscle spasms, and uneven limb lengths.

Specific etiologies for osteopathic scoliosis include fractures and dislocations of the spine, rickets, osteomalacia, and thoracogenic conditions such as unilateral pulmonary disease, or deformities caused by unilateral surgical procedures. Neuropathic scoliosis etiologies include acquired conditions such as poliomyelitis, paraplegia, syringomyelia, and Friedreich's ataxia.

737.30	Scoliosis (and kyphoscoliosis), idiopathic — *not due to disease or injury*
	AHA: Q3, 2003, 19
737.31	Resolving infantile idiopathic scoliosis
737.32	Progressive infantile idiopathic scoliosis
737.33	Scoliosis due to radiation
737.34	Thoracogenic scoliosis
737.39	Other kyphoscoliosis and scoliosis — *not otherwise specified*
	AHA: Q2, 2002, 16
737.40	Unspecified curvature of spine associated with other condition — (Code first associated condition: 015.0, 138, 237.7, 252.0, 277.5,

	356.1, 731.0, 733.00-733.09) — *unknown type, secondary to underlying disease*
737.41	Kyphosis associated with other condition — (Code first associated condition: 015.0, 138, 237.7, 252.0, 277.5, 356.1, 731.0, 733.00-733.09) — *abnormal convex curve of the spine as seen in profile, secondary to underlying disease*
737.42	Lordosis associated with other condition — (Code first associated condition: 015.0, 138, 237.7, 252.0, 277.5, 356.1, 731.0, 733.00-733.09) — *abnormal concave curve of the spine as seen in profile*
737.43	Scoliosis associated with other condition — (Code first associated condition: 015.0, 138, 237.7, 252.0, 277.5, 356.1, 731.0, 733.00-733.09) — *abnormal lateral curve of the spine*
737.8	Other curvatures of spine associated with other conditions — *not otherwise specified*
737.9	Unspecified curvature of spine associated with other condition

ICD-9-CM coding rules for late effects are applicable for osteopathic and neuropathic etiologies when scoliosis represents the residual of the etiology. Etiologies for myopathic scoliosis are all congenital scolioses classified in ICD-9-CM Chapter 14 Congenital Anomalies (740-759).

738 Other acquired musculoskeletal deformity

Other acquired musculoskeletal deformity is a noncongenital deformity due to a variety of conditions such as degenerative disease; a late effect of fracture, dislocation, or other soft tissue injury or infection; or pathological weakness of a musculoligamentous structure.

Deformities due to acute injury or illness are classified only to the acute injury or illness to which they pertain; an "acquired deformity" of the nasal septum due to acute fracture of the septum requires one code only (802.0).

738.0	Acquired deformity of nose — *overdevelopment of nasal bones*

Other acquired deformity of the head includes deformities of the zygoma and zygomatic arch. The zygoma is the long slender process of the temporal and malar bones on each side of the skull. The bridge formed by the articulation of the temporal and malar processes is the zygomatic arch to which the masseter muscle, which moves the lower jaw (mandible), is attached.

738.10	Unspecified acquired deformity of head
738.11	Zygomatic hyperplasia — *overgrowth*
738.12	Zygomatic hypoplasia — *undergrowth*
738.19	Other specified acquired deformity of head — *not otherwise specified* **AHA:** Q2, 2003, 13; Q1, 2006, 6
738.2	Acquired deformity of neck
738.3	Acquired deformity of chest and rib — *thorax, chest, rib, xiphoid process, pectus carinatum, pectus excavatum*
738.4	Acquired spondylolisthesis

Acquired spondylolisthesis is forward slipping of one vertebral body (with the remainder of the spinal column above it) in relation to the vertebral segment immediately below, not due to congenital deformity or fracture. Acquired spondylolisthesis may be secondary to degenerative disk disease, a late effect of fracture, or due to spondylolysis (not qualified as congenital) or pathological weakness of bone.

The subterm "traumatic" listed in the ICD-9-CM index under the main term "Spondylolisthesis" refers to spondylolisthesis due to birth or intrauterine trauma, rather than as a late effect of trauma occurring any time after birth. Traumatic spondylolisthesis is considered a congenital anomaly and is classified to code 756.12. Spondylolisthesis due to acute trauma is classified as a current injury and coded as an acute fracture of the vertebra. Spondylolisthesis as a late effect of trauma, such as a prior fracture of the vertebra, is classified as acquired using the appropriate ICD-9-CM code for late effect (e.g., 905.1).

738.5	Other acquired deformity of back or spine
738.6	Acquired deformity of pelvis — *pelvic obliquity*
738.7	Cauliflower ear
738.8	Acquired musculoskeletal deformity of other specified site — *not otherwise specified, clavicle* **AHA:** Q2, 2001, 15
738.9	Acquired musculoskeletal deformity of unspecified site

739 Nonallopathic lesions, not elsewhere classified

739.0	Nonallopathic lesion of head region, not elsewhere classified — *occipitocervical*
739.1	Nonallopathic lesion of cervical region, not elsewhere classified — *cervicothoracic*
739.2	Nonallopathic lesion of thoracic region, not elsewhere classified — *thoracolumbar*
739.3	Nonallopathic lesion of lumbar region, not elsewhere classified — *lumbosacral*
739.4	Nonallopathic lesion of sacral region, not elsewhere classified — *sacrococcygeal, sacroiliac*
739.5	Nonallopathic lesion of pelvic region, not elsewhere classified — *hip, pubic*
739.6	Nonallopathic lesion of lower extremities, not elsewhere classified — *thigh, knee, calf, foot*
739.7	Nonallopathic lesion of upper extremities, not elsewhere classified — *forearm, wrist, hand, upper arm*
739.8	Nonallopathic lesion of rib cage, not elsewhere classified
739.9	Nonallopathic lesion of abdomen and other sites, not elsewhere classified

740-759

Congenital Anomalies

Congenital anomalies may be the result of genetic factors (chromosomes), teratogens (agents causing physical defects in the embryo), or both. The anomalies may be apparent at birth or hidden and identified sometime after birth. Whatever the cause, congenital anomalies can be attributed to nearly 50 percent of deaths to full-term newborn infants.

Codes in chapter 14 are classified according to a principal or defining defect rather than to the cause (chromosome abnormalities are the exception). Regardless of the origin, dysmorphology — clinical structural abnormality — is generally the primary indication of a congenital anomaly and, in many cases, a syndrome may be classified according to a single anatomic anomaly rather than a complex of symptoms. For example, Apert's syndrome is classified to 755.55 *Acrocephalosyndactyly*. Rubric 755 classifies reduction deformities of the lower limb, and abnormal bony fusion in the feet is a single anatomic anomaly of the multi-complex syndrome that can include fusion in the hands and facial anomalies.

Coding Clarification
ICD-9-CM does not differentiate between abnormalities that are intrinsic — related to the fetus — or extrinsic — as a result of intrauterine problems, although a note in ICD-9-CM prior to rubric 754 *Certain congenital musculoskeletal deformities* identifies codes as specific to extrinsic factors. However, ICD-9-CM does make a distinction in the classification of an anomaly as compared to a deformity. An anomaly is a malformation caused by abnormal fetal development, as in transposition of great vessels or spina bifida. A deformity is an alteration in structure caused by an extrinsic force, as in intrauterine compression. The force may cause a disruption in a normal fetal structure, including congenital amputations from amniotic bands.

In some cases, two codes are necessary to describe the condition. For example, the condition thalidomide phocomelia (thalidomide influence on the developing fetus during the perinatal period) requires two codes: 755.23 *Longitudinal deficiency, combined, involving humerus, radius, and ulna (complete or incomplete)* and 760.79 *Noxious influences affecting fetus via placenta or milk*.

There is no clear methodology between what is classified to chapter 14 and a congenital anomaly classified to another chapter in ICD-9-CM. For example, oligohydramnios, a condition caused by a complication of pregnancy, is classified to chapter 15 Certain Conditions Originating in the Perinatal Period (760-779). Retinoblastoma, a tumor arising in the fetal retina and diagnosed after birth, is reported with 190.5 *Malignant neoplasm of the retina* from chapter 2 Neoplasms. The congenital absence of clotting factors is reported with codes in the rubric 286 *Coagulation defects*.

740 Anencephalus and similar anomalies
Anencephalus is a usually fatal brain defect of the newborn caused by a closure of the neural groove early in the first trimester of pregnancy. It can present in several forms:

- The cranial vault may be absent
- The cerebral hemispheres are missing or exist as masses attached to the base of the skull
- The brain is abnormally shaped

Anencephalus is identified in the patient record as acrania, partial or total absence of the skull; amyelencephalus, the absence of the brain and spinal cord; hemianencephaly, absence of half the brain; and hemicephaly, absence of one of the brain hemispheres.

740.0	Anencephalus — *anencephalus; acrania; amyelencephalus; hemicephaly; hemiencephaly*
740.1	Craniorachischisis — *craniorachischisis; Antley-Bixler syndrome*
740.2	Iniencephaly — *Iniencephaly; protrusion of brain into cord space*

Congenital Structural Defects of Cranium and Spinal Cord

Condition	Anotomy Displaced	Nature of Defect	Structural Defect Location
Craniorhachischisis	C + B	Fissure	Skull and V ertebral column
Encephalocystocele	B	Hernia of brain, filled with CSF	Skull
Holoprosencephaly	B	Forebrain defect	Brain
Hydroencephalocele	B	Brain protrudes in a sac	Skull
Hydromeningocele	M	Meninges protrude, filled with CSF	Vertebral column
Iniencephaly	B	brain protrudes into cord space	Skull
Meningoencephalocele	B + M	Brain and meninges protrude	Skull
Micrencephaly	B	abnormally small brain	Brain
Microgyria	B	abnormally small convolutions of brain	Brain
Myelomeningocele	C + M	Meninges and cord protrude	Vertebral column
Hydrocephalus	B	CSF volume too great	Brain (CSF circulation)
Syringomyelocele	C	Hernia cavity communicates with cord	Cord
Myelocystocele	C	Cord substance protrudes	Cord
Myelocele	C	Cord protrudes	Vertebral column
B= Brain		C= Skull	M= Meninges

741 Spina bifida

AHA: Q3, 1994, 7

Citing the location of the lesion is mandatory when coding spina bifida; the unspecified fifth digit should be avoided. The presence or absence of hydrocephalus is a second axis in the rubric, while spina bifida occulta is excluded from this rubric and is reported with 756.17.

Spina bifida, a defect in the vertebral column, presents in conjunction with several anomalies or it may occur as a solitary anomaly. Prognosis depends both on the number and severity of anomalies and on the size and location of the vertebral defect. Paralysis at the level below the defect is always present when the cord or spinal nerve roots are involved. Defects at the lumbosacral level can cause bladder and rectal problems. The child will often have orthopedic problems such as kyphosis or clubfoot. Death is usually ascribed to shunt complications, including infection and renal failure.

The circulation of the cerebrospinal fluid (CSF) is impeded, causing additional fluid pressure on the brain, in hydrocephalus, a condition that may be categorized as either communicating or non-communicating. In communicating hydrocephalus, there is no obstruction.

Type II is the most serious of the four types of malformations found in Arnold-Chiari or Chiari disease and the only type assigned to this subcategory. In this variation, the inferior poles of the cerebellum and the medulla protrude through the foramen magnum into the spinal canal. It is typically associated with other anomalies such as polymicrogyria, meningomyelocele, and hydrocephalus.

Subclassification 741.9 includes:

- Spinal hydromeningocele: fluid-filled sac composed of meninges protruding through the vertebral column defect
- Hydromyelocele: sac filled with CSF protruding through the wall of the spinal cord
- Meningocele: sac of meninges protruding through the skull or vertebral column
- Meningomyelocele: sac of meninges and cord protruding through the spinal column
- Myelocele: protrusion of the cord through the vertebral column
- Myelocystocele: protrusion of cord substance through the spinal canal
- Rachischisis: complete fissure in the vertebral column
- Syringomyelocele: saclike protrusion of the cord that remains in communication with the central canal of the cord

The following fifth-digit subclassification is for use with category 741:

0   unspecified region
1   cervical region
2   dorsal (thoracic) region
3   lumbar region

741.0	⌐5th	Spina bifida with hydrocephalus
741.9	⌐5th	Spina bifida without mention of hydrocephalus

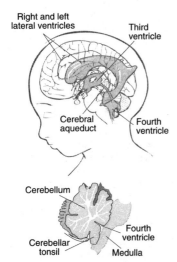

Detail of section through brain stem showing part of cerebellum herniating into the brain stem (Chiari malformation)

742 Other congenital anomalies of nervous system

742.0   Encephalocele

An encephalocele is a neural herniation of brain parenchyma and meninges that protrudes through a cranial defect. Encephalocele is also known as cranium bifidum with encephalocele, hydrencephalocele, and hydrencephalomeningocele. Lesions occur in the occipital region or anywhere in the cranial vault.

742.1   Microcephalus

In microcephalus, the head circumference is more than two standard deviations below the mean for age, sex, race, and gestation. Anomalous development, such as a chromosomal disorder or maternal phenylketonuria, during the first seven months of gestation causes primary microcephaly. Secondary microcephaly results from an insult, such as infection, trauma, anoxia, or metabolic disorders, during the last two months of gestation or during the perinatal period.

742.2	Congenital reduction deformities of brain
742.3	Congenital hydrocephalus
	AHA: Q4, 2005, 83

Ventricular enlargement, abundant cerebral spinal fluid, and, in most cases, increasing pressure are present in congenital hydrocephalus. In addition, the foramen of Magendie and the foramen of Luschka may be undeveloped, resulting in the obstruction of fluid through the aqueduct of Sylvius, which carries the cerebrospinal fluid between the midbrain and the fourth ventricle. An obstruction of the fourth ventricle outlet, as seen in Dandy-Walker syndrome (741.0 with spina bifida) describes noncommunicating hydrocephalus. Other conditions that may present include arachnoiditis and lesions such as neoplasms, cysts, and hematomas. In addition, the obstruction may be secondary to exudate, hemorrhage, or parasites.

Communicating hydrocephalus may be due to adhesions of the basilar cisterns or surface subarachnoid space following infection or hemorrhage, post developmental adhesions, vitamin A deficiency, developmental failure or erythrocyte obstruction of the arachnoid villi, or Arnold Chiari malformation (741.0).

Cerebral cysts, macroencephaly, (synonym for megalencephaly) an abnormally large head, large convolutions of the cerebrum, ulegyria, — abnormal convolutions of the cerebrum due to scarring — and porencephaly — a cerebral cyst with an opening into a ventricle — are abnormalities that may progress to hydrocephalus. These conditions are reported with 742.4.

742.4	Other specified congenital anomalies of brain
742.51	Diastematomyelia

Diastematomyelia reports a longitudinal fissure in the spinal cord that results in gait disturbance, muscular atrophy, and lack of sphincter control.

742.53   Hydromyelia

Hydromyelia reports a dilated spinal canal. It is a synonym for hydrorrhachis.

Amyelia is the absence of a spinal cord, whereas atelomyelia is an incompletely developed cord. Myelodysplasia and myelatelia are synonymous terms describing a defective spinal cord.

742.59	Other specified congenital anomaly of spinal cord
742.8	Other specified congenital anomalies of nervous system

Marcus-Gunn syndrome, also known as jaw-winking syndrome, is characterized by the onset of rapid eyelid movement, producing a winking effect, when the jaw moves. The cause is unknown.

Riley-Day syndrome, or familial dysautonomia, is primarily found in families of European-Jewish extraction. Poor sucking ability, sweating while eating, hypotonia, and insensitivity to pain characterize the condition.

742.9 Unspecified congenital anomaly of brain, spinal cord, and nervous system

Coding Clarification
Acquired hydrocephalus (331.3-331.4) is excluded from this rubric, as is hydrocephalus due to congenital toxoplasmosis (771.2). This rubric also excludes congenital central alveolar hypoventilation syndrome, which is coded to 327.25

Side view schematic of eye

743 Congenital anomalies of eye
Any structure or organ of the body is subject to a failure or deviation in development. Congenital anomalies of the eye are classified according to the specific site affected and the type of defect. They include:

- Anophthalmos: absence of an eye
- Cryptophthalmos: uninterrupted extension of an eyelid across the eyeball
- Microphthalmos: abnormally small eye

743.00	Unspecified clinical anophthalmos
743.03	Cystic eyeball, congenital
743.06	Cryptophthalmos
743.10	Unspecified microphthalmos
743.11	Simple microphthalmos

743.12 Microphthalmos associated with other anomalies of eye and adnexa

Physicians assess microphthalmos according to levels of debility. Pure microphthalmos, a condition of a small eye with a tendency to angle-closing glaucoma, is reported with 743.12 if the condition causes vision complications. Simple microphthalmos (743.11) is a small eye, which is essentially normal in functionality.

Buphthalmos is congenital glaucoma. In affected infants, a defect in the iridocorneal angle, an outlet in the anterior chamber of the eye, impedes aqueous circulation.

Glaucoma is an elevated pressure in the aqueous humor. Undetected, glaucoma can lead to nerve damage and blindness. Surgery, directed toward restoring the natural circulation of the aqueous, can prevent loss of sight. A genetic abnormality or an inflammation of the eye prior to birth can cause congenital glaucoma.

743.20	Unspecified buphthalmos
743.21	Simple buphthalmos
743.22	Buphthalmos associated with other ocular anomaly

Excluded from these subclassifications are glaucoma of childhood (365.14) and traumatic glaucoma due to birth injury (767.8).

Cataracts are milky or opaque areas on the lens of the eye that translate into milky or opaque disturbances in the field of vision. Infection during development, genetic error, or metabolites residing within the lens may be the cause. Other anomalies of the lens include aphakia, or congenital absence of the lens, and anomalies of shape including spherophakia (sphere shaped) or microphakia (small lens). An ectopic lens is a displaced lens.

A coloboma describes a part absent from an ophthalmological structure, due usually to a chromosomal defect, which presents as a fissure of the iris, the ciliary body, or the choroid (thus the common name "keyhole pupil"). It is typically associated with CHARGE syndrome (C=coloboma; H=heart; A=atresia of choanae, R=retarded growth and development, G=genital hypoplasia, E=ear anomalies). Coloboma may increase the risk of iridial tearing and often includes iris and choroid flaws.

743.30	Unspecified congenital cataract
743.31	Congenital capsular and subcapsular cataract
743.32	Congenital cortical and zonular cataract
743.33	Congenital nuclear cataract
743.34	Congenital total and subtotal cataract
743.35	Congenital aphakia
743.36	Congenital anomalies of lens shape

Congenital Anomalies

743.37	Congenital ectopic lens
743.39	Other congenital cataract and lens anomalies

Excluded from these subclassifications are cataracts that are associated with syndromes congenital in nature although not present at birth, as in craniofacial dysotosis (756.0). These cataracts are reported with 366.44.

743.41	Congenital anomaly of corneal size and shape
743.42	Congenital corneal opacity, interfering with vision
743.43	Other congenital corneal opacity
743.44	Specified congenital anomaly of anterior chamber, chamber angle, and related structures
743.45	Aniridia

Aniridia, the incomplete formation of the iris, results in vision loss. Typically, aniridia is bilateral and gives the appearance of black irises though it is the pupil — and not the iris — which is dark. An autosomal-dominant or autosomal-recessive gene can be a cause and, if so determined, the child may have other health or developmental problems.

743.46	Other specified congenital anomaly of iris and ciliary body

Anisocoria, or unequal pupils, is a common condition. In corectopia, the pupil is asymmetrically placed in the iris. Children with iris colobomata should be checked for fissure of the optic nerve and of the fundus.

743.47	Specified congenital anomaly of sclera
743.48	Multiple and combined congenital anomalies of anterior segment of eye
743.49	Other congenital anomaly of anterior segment of eye
743.51	Vitreous anomaly, congenital
743.52	Fundus coloboma
743.53	Congenital chorioretinal degeneration
743.54	Congenital folds and cysts of posterior segment of eye
743.55	Congenital macular change
743.56	Other congenital retinal changes
743.57	Specified congenital anomalies of optic disc
743.58	Congenital vascular anomalies of posterior segment of eye
743.59	Other congenital anomalies of posterior segment of eye
743.61	Congenital ptosis of eyelid

A severe case of ptosis is treated immediately after birth since it can disrupt visual development. In less severe cases, treatment is delayed until the child reaches 3 to 5 years of age.

743.62	Congenital deformity of eyelid

Ablepharon, the congenital absence of an eyelid, seldom appears as a solitary variant, which is typical of agenesis anomalies.

An accessory eyelid is an additional eyelid.

Entropion is inversion of the lower eyelid, whereas ectropion is the eversion of the lower eyelid. Both conditions require surgical correction since rubbing caused by the displacement often scars the cornea.

743.63	Other specified congenital anomaly of eyelid
743.64	Specified congenital anomaly of lacrimal gland
743.65	Specified congenital anomaly of lacrimal passages

The lacrimal glands produce the tears that moisten the eyes to keep them healthy. Tears are produced at each blink and pumped down and across the eye. Any excess tears drain through the tear duct and into the nose, which explains why noses run when crying. Excess tears can also create problems. Surgery may be required to open ducts obstructed by pus in an infection resulting from stagnant tears.

743.66	Specified congenital anomaly of orbit
743.69	Other congenital anomalies of eyelids, lacrimal system, and orbit
743.8	Other specified congenital anomalies of eye
743.9	Unspecified congenital anomaly of eye

Coding Clarification
Assign code 377.43 for congenital hyperplasia of the optic nerve.

744 Congenital anomalies of ear, face, and neck

Codes in this rubric are classified according to site and the impairment associated with the anomaly. The most significant codes in this rubric are those reporting hearing impairments, classified to subcategory 744.0. Congenital deafness, without mention of cause, is excluded from this rubric and is reported with codes from the series 389.0-389.9.

744.00	Unspecified congenital anomaly of ear causing impairment of hearing
744.01	Congenital absence of external ear causing impairment of hearing
744.02	Other congenital anomaly of external ear causing impairment of hearing
744.03	Congenital anomaly of middle ear, except ossicles, causing impairment of hearing
744.04	Congenital anomalies of ear ossicles
744.05	Congenital anomalies of inner ear
744.09	Other congenital anomalies of ear causing impairment of hearing
744.1	Congenital anomalies of accessory auricle
744.21	Congenital absence of ear lobe
744.22	Macrotia
744.23	Microtia

Microtia, external auditory canal atresia, and ossicular fusion often occur together. Auricle atresia is associated with craniofacial syndromes such as Treacher-Collins and Nager syndromes, but may occur in solitary.

744.24	Specified congenital anomaly of Eustachian tube
744.29	Other congenital anomaly of ear

Large and protruding ears, called Bat ear, can be surgically modified. Polyotia is the presence of an accessory auricle. Pointed ear, Stahl's ear, and Spoke ear describe ears pointed at the top. Darwin's tubercle, a prominence on the upper posterior of the superior ridge of the auricle; is a vestigial remnant of a folded ear.

744.3	Unspecified congenital anomaly of ear

Branchial cleft relates to embryonic development of the external auricle, the external auditory meatus, and the tympanic membrane. A sinus is a blind ending tract. A fistula is an open-ended tract.

744.41	Congenital branchial cleft sinus or fistula
744.42	Congenital branchial cleft cyst
744.43	Congenital cervical auricle
744.46	Congenital preauricular sinus or fistula
744.47	Congenital preauricular cyst
744.49	Other congenital branchial cleft cyst or fistula; preauricular sinus
744.5	Congenital webbing of neck

Pterygium colli is a webbed effect produced by an anomalous band of fascia extending from the mastoid process to the clavicle.

744.81	Macrocheilia
744.82	Microcheilia

Microcheilia is an abnormally small lip.

744.83	Macrostomia
744.84	Microstomia

Microstomia is an abnormally small mouth.

744.89	Other specified congenital anomaly of face and neck
744.9	Unspecified congenital anomaly of face and neck

745–747 Congenital Anomalies of the Cardiovascular System

One percent of all births has a cardiac anomaly. The evaluation of an infant or child with a cardiac anomaly must determine the anomalous pattern of vascularity, cardiac enlargement, whether cyanosis is present, or a combination of the possible irregularities. An anomalous vascular pattern indicates abnormal circulation. An anomalous vascularity is characterized as a transposition or transposition complex anomaly. The term transposition refers to the normal anterior-to-posterior relationships of the vessels. An enlarged heart requires an evaluation of the chambers to determine the extent of the anomaly. Cyanosis is the most common variant, followed by volume load disorders.

745 Bulbus cordis anomalies and anomalies of cardiac septal closure

Bulbus cordis relates to embryological development of the fetal heart. Persistent truncus arteriosus is the failure of the aorticopulmonary trunk to divide at the correct developmental stage. There are four classifications and an infant born with the condition presents as cyanotic and tachypneic, and may be struggling with congestive heart failure due to the effects of the abnormally increased pulmonary artery blood flow. The infant may require the Rastelli procedure, which involves separating the pulmonary artery from the primitive truncus to create a right ventricle-to-pulmonary artery conduit.

745.0	Bulbus cordis anomalies and anomalies of cardiac septal closure, common truncus
745.10	Complete transposition of great vessels
745.11	Transposition of great vessels, double outlet right ventricle

Double outlet right ventricle is a cyanotic congenital heart disease, affecting more males than females, and presents within the first 24 hours after birth. The infant is often cyanotic and tachypneic, and congestive heart failure is probable. Survival depends on the existence of a ventricular septal defect, an atrial septal defect, or a patent ductus arteriosus, which allow communication between the pulmonary and systemic circulations. Many of the operative procedures work with the anomalous anatomy to achieve operational pulmonary and systemic circulations. For example, the Jatene operation creates a corrective arterial switch.

In Taussig-Bing syndrome, the aorta is in the right ventricle, the pulmonary artery is located in both ventricles, and a ventricular septal defect is present. The child is often cyanotic due to the oxygen insufficiency resulting from the anomalies.

745.12	Corrected transposition of great vessels

Report 745.12 to identify a newborn with a transposition syndrome subsequently corrected since this transposition often involves sequelae.

745.19	Other transposition of great vessels
745.2	Tetralogy of Fallot

The tetralogy of Fallot represents 8 percent of all congenital heart diseases. The anomaly, which presents by 6 months, is a cyanotic and transposition syndrome. A right aortic arch, abnormal origin of coronary arteries, a left superior vena cava, and an enlarged bronchial artery are characteristic. Palliative repairs are performed in the

Congenital Anomalies

early years, with definitive repair reserved until 5 to 7 years of age, using the Blalock-Taussig, Pohl's, or Waterston-Cooley operations. This code excludes Fallot's triad, which is reported with 746.09.

745.3 Bulbus cordis anomalies and anomalies of cardiac septal closure, common ventricle

A common ventricle anomaly occurs when a single ventricle arises from the absence of a ventricular septum. Typically, there is transposition of the great vessels, cardiomegaly, cyanosis, congestive heart failure, and mixed pulmonary and system circulation.

745.4 Ventricular septal defect

Ventricular septal defects (VSD) may appear as solitary anomalies or present as part of a syndrome, such as Holt-Roan syndrome, trisomy 13, 18, and 21, and tetralogy of Fallot. A VSD may involve both the membranous and muscular portions of the ventricles. Approximately 80 percent involve the membranous septum. Within two to three months of birth, the infant presents with congestive heart failure. Treatment includes patching the VSD, pulmonary artery banding, and medical therapy. Common atrioventricular canal type anomalies (745.69) and single ventricle anomalies (745.3) are excluded from this code.

Eisenmenger's syndrome is a progressive cyanotic condition characterized by a VSD, pulmonary hypertension, and combined pulmonary and systemic circulations. A small, asymptomatic VSD is a primary characteristic of Roger's disease, also reported with 745.4.

745.5 Ostium secundum type atrial septal defect

Ostium secundum accounts for 90 percent of all atrial septal defects (ASD). Treatment depends on the age of the patient at evaluation and usually involves applying a patch to the ASD. An ASD left untreated can cause right heart failure, atrial fibrillation later in life, and the increased risk of blood clots leading to a stroke.

Lutembacher's syndrome, reported with 745.5, is an ASD in conjunction with mitral rheumatic stenosis. A patent foramen ovale, also reported with 745.5, is treated when other heart defects are present. The foramen ovale normally closes shortly after birth.

There are three classifications of cushion defects: complete, partial, and intermediate. A complete defect presents with congestive heart failure and all types demonstrate ostium primum. A partial defect is the most common. About 40 percent of cushion anomalies are associated with trisomy-21 (Down's syndrome), which is separately reported with 758.0.

745.60	Unspecified type congenital endocardial cushion defect
745.61	Ostium primum defect
745.69	Other congenital endocardial cushion defect
745.7	Cor biloculare

Cor biloculare describes a heart lacking both an atrial and a ventricular septum. A two-chambered heart severely compromises the newborn and few born with the condition live to the first year.

745.8	Other bulbus cordis anomalies and anomalies of cardiac septal closure
745.9	Unspecified congenital defect of septal closure

746 Other congenital anomalies of heart

Endocardial fibroelastosis is excluded from this rubric and is reported with 425.3.

746.00	Unspecified congenital pulmonary valve anomaly
746.01	Congenital atresia of pulmonary valve

Absence of the pulmonary valve is associated with hypoplastic right heart structures. An infant becomes critically ill when the foramen ovale and PDA close and result in impaired pulmonary circulation. A shunt may be placed between the aorta and the pulmonary artery or a pulmonary artery may be implanted to correct the problem.

746.02 Congenital stenosis of pulmonary valve
AHA: Q1, 2004, 16

A ventricle may become enlarged to compensate for the slow down of blood circulation due to a narrowed valve. Severe stenosis, reported with 746.02, requires surgical repair and lifelong antibiotic prophylaxis.

746.09 Other congenital anomalies of pulmonary valve

Other pulmonary insufficiencies are managed medically. The trilogy or triad of Fallot involves pulmonary stenosis, ASD, and right ventricular hypertrophy.

746.1	Congenital tricuspid atresia and stenosis
746.2	Ebstein's anomaly

In Ebstein's anomaly, the tricuspid valve is displaced downward, which can lead to fatigue palpitations and dyspnea. A portion of the RV is atrialized (i.e., thinned and dysplastic). Dilated tricuspid annulus and a dilated RA are present. Of the four classifications, "D" is the most severe, manifesting with nearly total atrialization of the RV and other cardiac anomalies such as ASD and Wolff-Parkinson-White syndrome.

746.3	Congenital stenosis of aortic valve
746.4	Congenital insufficiency of aortic valve

Thickened and stiffened valves may cause the stenosis or it may be due to the valve having only one or two cusps. If severe, the stenosis produces fatigue, dizziness, and fainting.

746.5   Congenital mitral stenosis
Fusion of the commissures of the valve causes mitral stenosis. The valves are not calcific and the treatment is a commissurotomy.

746.6   Congenital mitral insufficiency
Mitral insufficiency is regurgitation or back flow into the RA leading to decreased systemic flow. The condition overworks the heart in its efforts to pump blood to the body's periphery.

746.7   Hypoplastic left heart syndrome
Hypoplastic left heart syndrome accounts for 10 percent of all heart defects. The LV is tiny and symptoms include stenosis or atresia of the aortic and mitral valves and coarctation of the aorta. The condition can be critical and treatments include heart transplant and palliative reconstruction. If a transplant is necessary, large amounts of donor aorta must be used in the reconstruction of the aorta. If reconstruction is the selected treatment, it is performed in stages (i.e., the Norwood procedure is performed immediately, followed by the Glenn procedure three to six months later, and the Fontan reconstructive procedure at 18 to 24 months of age).

746.81   Congenital subaortic stenosis
In subaortic stenosis, the LV works hard to push the blood past the coarctation of the aorta, a condition that leads to cardiomegaly and congestive heart failure. A mild condition requires no surgery unless, over time, the stenosis worsens and leads to severe tachycardia, tachypnea, and eventually into congestive heart failure. Other milder complications include fatigue, chest pain, and fainting.

746.82   Cor triatriatum
In cor triatriatum, a small extra chamber above the LA receives the blood from the pulmonary vein. This extra chamber hampers the force of the blood entering the LA and, as a result, congestive heart failure may result.

746.83   Congenital infundibular pulmonic stenosis
Infundibular pulmonic stenosis is a narrowing of the outflow tract of the right ventricle below the pulmonary valve within the infundibulum. The condition is due to a fibrous diaphragm or to a long, narrow fibromuscular channel.

746.84   Congenital obstructive anomalies of heart, not elsewhere classified
Uhl's disease is a RV spongiform dysplasia, characteristically with paper-thin ventricle walls.

746.85   Congenital coronary artery anomaly
Anomalous Left Coronary Artery Originating from Pulmonary Artery (ALCAPA) is a serious condition and, if left untreated, only about 20 percent of children survive beyond adolescence. A single coronary artery is inadequate for perfusion and infarctions leave the heart dependent on collateral circulation to perfuse the left ventricle. Surgery establishes a two-coronary artery system through revascularization.

746.86   Congenital heart block
Congenital heart block appears as both a sole congenital variant and as part of a syndrome of congenital anomalies. An isolated variant may be associated with autoimmune diseases in the mother. In these situations, the infants are born with neonatal lupus syndrome, which disappears after 6 months of age. The heart block does not disappear. Whatever the origin of the disorder, diminished cardiac output progresses to congestive heart failure. The infant is surgically treated with pacemaker implantation.

746.87   Congenital malposition of heart and cardiac apex
There are four types of dextrocardia:

1. Dextroposition: extrinsic factor causes the heart to shift to the right, leading to hypoplastic right lung, a partial anomaly of the pulmonary venous connection to the inferior vena cava, and right-sided pulmonary collaterals.

2. Dextroversion: abnormal rotation of the cardiac loops in embryological development leads to atrioventricular or ventriculoatrial discordance, or a single ventricle, which may be part of Cantrell syndrome: omphalocele or other midline defect, lower sternal defect, anterior inferior diaphragmatic defect, parietal pericardial defect, and left ventricular diverticulum.

3. Ventriculoatrial situs inversus: associated with tetralogy of Fallot, and Kartagener's syndrome. Excluded from 746.87 is dextrocardia with complete transposition of viscera, which is reported with 759.3.

4. Levocardia: includes four variants: 1) situs solitus with normal heart, 2) levoposition (heart shifts left in the mediastinum due to dysgenesis of the left lung), 3) levoversion of situs inversus, atrioventricular and ventriculoatrial discordance, 4) situs ambiguous.

Dextrocardia and levocardia are both reported with 746.87 in ICD-9-CM.

Ectopic cordis is a serious anomaly in which the sternum is split and the heart protrudes (most common form) or the heart is displaced to the abdomen or neck. A newborn with the condition generally dies within a few days of birth in nearly 100 percent of cases. Ectopic cordis is reported with 746.87.

746.89 Other specified congenital anomaly of heart

In diverticulum of the left ventricle, the diverticulum protrudes into the epigastrium. It may or may not be an isolated anomaly.

Brugada syndrome is a combination of right bundle branch block, ST elevation, and arrhythmic right ventricular dysplasia (ARVD), which results in abnormal left ventricular electrophysiology and sudden death. The condition runs in families and is treated by implantation of an automatic cardioverter-defibrillator.

746.9 Unspecified congenital anomaly of heart

The ductus arteriosus is the natural shunt that bypasses lung circulation in the prenatal phase

Aortic ring syndrome

747 Other congenital anomalies of circulatory system

747.0 Patent ductus arteriosus

Other terms for patent ductus arteriosus (PDA) are persistent ductus arteriosus or patent ductus Botallo. The incidence is greater in females and it is one of the most common cardiovascular anomalies. The ductus arteriosus is patent during fetal life for breathing through the umbilical cord and, in most infants, closes within a few weeks of birth. A patent ductus arteriosus allows the lungs to be bypassed until birth, shunting right ventricular blood to the aorta. The condition presents two ways: if the infant is premature, the patency typically closes once the infant reaches the appropriate developmental stage. If the infant is term, with persistent patency, the infant will experience elevated left heart pressures and increased pulmonary circulation, putting undue strain on the left heart and pulmonary vasculature, leading to pulmonary vascular disease and congestive heart failure. There is an increased risk of bacterial endocarditis. PDAs are surgically corrected, no matter their size, due to probable complications.

747.10 Coarctation of aorta (preductal) (postductal)

Coarctation refers to a pinching of the aortic arch, forcing the left heart to pump past the obstruction, which leads to enlargement, increased blood pressure in arteries behind the obstruction, decreased pressure in arteries post obstruction, and congestive heart failure. In post obstruction, the aorta may enlarge to increase the risk of dilation, aneurysm, rupture, and stroke. Patients with coarctation are at lifelong risk for bacterial endocarditis and for myocardial infarction. The obstruction is resected as soon as possible after birth and the same procedure may need to be repeated in adulthood. The congestive failure subsides after corrective surgery, although there may be persistent pulmonary hypertension.

747.11 Congenital interruption of aortic arch
747.20 Unspecified congenital anomaly of aorta
747.21 Congenital anomaly of aortic arch

An anomalous arch in double aortic arch encircles the trachea or the esophagus, leading to tracheal compression and subsequent proclivity to repeated respiratory infections. The anomalous arch may be patent and always causes difficulty because of its position.

747.22 Congenital atresia and stenosis of aorta

Aortic stenosis is a progressive condition that rarely produces symptoms in the young. Progressive elevated resistance to the pumping action of the left ventricle leads to increased LV pressure and hypertrophy. Hypertrophy weakens the heart and is prodromal to heart failure. The thicker and stiffer the ventricle walls, the weaker the pumping action. The two most common forms of aortic stenosis are valvular obstruction resulting from a defect in the valve, and subaortic obstruction, found in the Left Ventricular Outlet Tract. The condition may be an isolated phenomenon or appear in conjunction with VSD, PDA, and coarctation of the aorta.

747.29   Other congenital anomaly of aorta

Aneurysms of the sinus of Valsalva may not be apparent until adulthood. If rupture occurs, the patient is subject to congestive heart failure and sudden death. Typically, the rupture occurs in either the right or left coronary sinus leading to an acute right-to-left shunt.

747.3   Congenital anomalies of pulmonary artery
          AHA: Q1, 2004, 16

Agenesis of the pulmonary artery is rare, occurring on the left more than on the right, and is usually a benign variation. When symptomatic, it results in frequent respiratory tract infections with bronchiectasis.

747.40   Congenital anomaly of great veins unspecified
747.41   Total congenital anomalous pulmonary venous connection

Total anomalous pulmonary venous return (TAPVR) allows oxygenated blood to drain into the right atrium (normally the recipient of deoxygenated blood). ASD often accompanies the condition. It is treated by severing the pulmonary return to the RA and creating a return to the LA.

747.42   Partial congenital anomalous pulmonary venous connection

Partial anomalous pulmonary venous return (PAPVR) is rarely clinically significant unless associated with sinus venosus ASD, which elevates it to significant importance.

747.49   Other congenital anomalies of great veins

In Scimitar syndrome, one lobe of the left lung is hypoplastic leading to a right shift by the heart. PAPVR is usually present, the thoracic aorta or the celiac axis supplies blood to the aorta, and there are diaphragmatic and thoracic defects.

Persistent left superior vena cava (LSVC), the most common thoracic venous anomaly, is a remnant of a structure normally disappearing during embryological development and, if a solitary variant, is seldom symptomatic or significant.

747.5   Congenital absence or hypoplasia of umbilical artery
747.60   Congenital anomaly of the peripheral vascular system, unspecified site
747.61   Congenital gastrointestinal vessel anomaly
747.62   Congenital renal vessel anomaly
747.63   Congenital upper limb vessel anomaly
747.64   Congenital lower limb vessel anomaly
747.69   Congenital anomaly of other specified site of peripheral vascular system
747.81   Congenital anomaly of cerebrovascular system
747.82   Congenital spinal vessel anomaly
747.83   Persistent fetal circulation

747.89   Other specified congenital anomaly of circulatory system
747.9   Unspecified congenital anomaly of circulatory system

Select arteries of the head

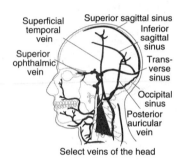

Select veins of the head

Documentation Issues

Documentation must be clear and concise for accurate code selection. The physician must identify the specific vessel involved in the arteriovenous malformation for the most appropriate code to be assigned.

Coding Clarification

Cardiac Outflow Tract Obstruction: This congenital anomaly should be reported with code 747.3 *Congenital anomalies of pulmonary artery.* Included in this code are other anomalies such as atresia, agenesis, stenosis, coarctation, and hypoplasia of the pulmonary artery as well as pulmonary arteriovenous aneurysms.

Spinal Arteriovenous Malformation: Spinal A-V malformations are anomalous communications between a vein and an artery that are congenital in nature. Congenital A-V malformations are caused by persistent embryonic vessels that fail to differentiate into veins and arteries. Spinal dural A-V malformations are the most common type in adults. These lesions develop progressive sensory motor

Congenital Anomalies

symptoms ranging from painful paraparesis to acute quadriplegia. Report with code 747.82 *Congenital spinal vessel anomaly.*

Coding Scenario
A patient is admitted for a resection of a spinal dural arteriovenous malformation.

> Code assignment: 747.82 *Congenital spinal vessel anomaly*

A patient is diagnosed with right outflow tract obstruction.

> Code assignment: 747.3 *Congenital anomalies of pulmonary artery*

748   Congenital anomalies of respiratory system

748.0	Congenital choanal atresia
748.1	Other congenital anomaly of nose
748.2	Congenital web of larynx
748.3	Other congenital anomaly of larynx, trachea, and bronchus
748.4	Congenital cystic lung
748.5	Congenital agenesis, hypoplasia, and dysplasia of lung
748.60	Unspecified congenital anomaly of lung
748.61	Congenital bronchiectasis
748.69	Other congenital anomaly of lung
748.8	Other specified congenital anomaly of respiratory system
748.9	Unspecified congenital anomaly of respiratory system

Coding Clarification
Excluded from this rubric is congenital defect of the diaphragm, which is reported with 756.6 and congenital central alveolar hypoventilation syndrome, which is reported with 327.25.

749   Cleft palate and cleft lip

Cleft palate is the fourth most common birth defect and the most common facial birth defect, affecting approximately one out of every 700 infants. While it is associated with multiple defect syndromes, it is typically associated with a cleft lip, occurring in the first few weeks of fetal development, and is multi-factorial in cause. A cleft palate is repaired at 6 to 12 months of age and may require follow up surgery at a later age. If the cleft involves the gum line, an alveolar bone graft is used in the restorative surgery.

749.00	Unspecified cleft palate
749.01	Unilateral cleft palate, complete
749.02	Unilateral cleft palate, incomplete
749.03	Bilateral cleft palate, complete
749.04	Bilateral cleft palate, incomplete
749.10	Unspecified cleft lip
749.11	Unilateral cleft lip, complete
749.12	Unilateral cleft lip, incomplete
749.13	Bilateral cleft lip, complete
749.14	Bilateral cleft lip, incomplete
749.20	Unspecified cleft palate with cleft lip
749.21	Unilateral cleft palate with cleft lip, complete
749.22	Unilateral cleft palate with cleft lip, incomplete
749.23	Bilateral cleft palate with cleft lip, complete
749.24	Bilateral cleft palate with cleft lip, incomplete
749.25	Other combinations of cleft palate with cleft lip

750   Other congenital anomalies of upper alimentary tract

750.0	Tongue tie
750.10	Congenital anomaly of tongue, unspecified
750.11	Aglossia

Aglossia is absence of the tongue. It is seen in Hanhart syndrome, a condition marked by absent tongue and serious anomalies of the limbs.

750.12	Congenital adhesions of tongue
750.13	Congenital fissure of tongue

Bifid tongue occurs when the tongue buds fail to develop normally. It is seen most often in South America.

750.15	Macroglossia

Macroglossia is an abnormally large tongue.

750.16	Microglossia

Microglossia is an abnormally small tongue.

750.19	Other congenital anomaly of tongue
750.21	Congenital absence of salivary gland
750.22	Congenital accessory salivary gland
750.23	Congenital atresia, salivary duct
750.24	Congenital fistula of salivary gland
750.25	Congenital fistula of lip
750.26	Other specified congenital anomalies of mouth
750.27	Congenital diverticulum of pharynx

A pharyngeal pouch is an abnormal pocket in the wall of the pharynx, causing difficulty in swallowing.

750.29	Other specified congenital anomaly of pharynx
753.3	Other specified congenital anomalies of kidney

A tracheoesophageal fistula, which is an abnormal opening between the trachea and the esophagus, must be repaired immediately after birth. In esophageal atresia, the esophagus ends in a blind pouch. Even though the esophagus ends in a blind pouch, it is essential that newborns are able to suck and swallow. Surgical intervention temporarily diverts the esophagus to an opening in the neck, while the infant's nutrition is maintained by IV feedings.

Esophageal stenosis is an abnormally narrowed lumen of the esophagus associated with vomiting and dysphagia.

750.4	Other specified congenital anomaly of esophagus
750.5	Congenital hypertrophic pyloric stenosis

Hypertrophic pyloric stenosis is the most common cause of surgery in the young infant, excluding hernia surgery. In this condition, the outlet to the intestines becomes blocked, leading to projectile vomiting, electrolyte imbalances, and dehydration. The condition is often diagnosed between 2 and 4 weeks of age. Pyloromyotomy may be delayed until an electrolyte disturbance or dehydration is corrected.

750.6 Congenital hiatus hernia

A hiatal hernia is an upward displacement of the stomach through the esophageal hiatus into the mediastinal cavity, leading to esophageal reflux disease. It is always corrected.

750.7 Other specified congenital anomalies of stomach

Cardiospasm is the failure of the cardiac sphincter to relax, leading to aperistalsis. In hourglass stomach, fibrous bands pinch in the stomach, giving it an hourglass appearance. When the stomach is transposed, it lies on the right side of the abdomen. Megalogastria is an abnormally large stomach and microgastria is an abnormally small stomach.

750.8 Other specified congenital anomalies of upper alimentary tract
750.9 Unspecified congenital anomaly of upper alimentary tract

Coding Clarification
This rubric excludes congenital dentofacial anomalies classified to 524.0-524.9.

The diverticulum pouch is often found about 50 cm from the ileocecal junction

751 Other congenital anomalies of digestive system

751.0 Meckel's diverticulum
AHA: Q1, 2004, 10

Meckel's diverticulum is a sacculation of the distal ileum caused by failure of the vitelline duct to atrophy. It is the most frequently occurring digestive malformation and usually presents with massive dark red rectal bleeding which is often painless to the child. Strangulation or intussusception can occur.

751.1 Congenital atresia and stenosis of small intestine

Atresia of the small intestine usually affects the ileum and is associated with trisomy-21 (Down syndrome) if it appears in the duodenum. It is diagnosed in utero through ultrasound or shortly after birth and treated with resection and primary anastomosis.

751.2 Congenital atresia and stenosis of large intestine, rectum, and anal canal

Imperforate anus is diagnosed on birth. The infant is given a diverting colostomy and corrective surgery is performed later.

751.3 Hirschsprung's disease and other congenital functional disorders of colon

Hirschsprung's disease is a massive distention of the colon with associated inability to defecate due to lack of innervation of the affected portion of the colon. It has familial associations and is more commonly seen in males. The condition is often diagnosed about 48 hours after birth, as the infant is unable to pass meconium, and treatment is immediate to prevent the onset of enterocolitis.

751.4 Congenital anomalies of intestinal fixation

Volvulus is a potential symptom of malrotation of the intestine, leading to strangulation and intestinal infarction through choking off the mesenteric artery.

751.5 Other congenital anomalies of intestine

Dolichocolon is an abnormally long colon.

A persistent cloaca is the third level of a developmental anomaly involving the persistence of a urogenital sinus. In this condition, there is a single orifice behind the clitoris and agenesis of the anus and vagina. Treatment is delayed until the child is at least 1 year of age. A colostomy is performed after birth as a temporary measure and the infant is catheterized intermittently until corrective surgery is performed.

751.60 Unspecified congenital anomaly of gallbladder, bile ducts, and liver
751.61 Congenital biliary atresia

Biliary atresia is the lack of patency of the extrahepatic ducts thought to be an obliterative process rather than a developmental anomaly. It is a serious condition, which may lead to cirrhosis of the liver. Approximately 10 percent of the cases are associated with multiple malformations, the most common being polysplenia (multiple right-sided spleens, a midline liver, a pre-duodenal portal vein, and cardiac malformations).

| 751.62 | Congenital cystic disease of liver |

Congenital polycystic disease of the liver involves the formation of numerous cysts that block the drainage of bile.

| 751.69 | Other congenital anomaly of gallbladder, bile ducts, and liver |

When the liver or gallbladder is characterized as floating, the organ is displaced and moveable.

| 751.7 | Congenital anomalies of pancreas |

If the pancreas either does not develop (agenesis) or is extremely underdeveloped (hypoplasia), intrauterine growth is retarded due to lack of the insulin, which would normally be secreted by the pancreas.

| 751.8 | Other specified congenital anomalies of digestive system |
| 751.9 | Unspecified congenital anomaly of digestive system |

752 Congenital anomalies of genital organs

| 752.0 | Congenital anomalies of ovaries |

Ovarian agenesis is associated with low set ears, a high palate, mental retardation, and edema of the extremities. The genitalia may be ambiguous. Without the estrogen produced by the ovaries, breast development and menarche do not occur.

A streak ovary contains streaks of fibrous stroma where germ cells should reside. Germ cells are absent.

752.10	Unspecified congenital anomaly of fallopian tubes and broad ligaments
752.11	Embryonic cyst of fallopian tubes and broad ligaments
752.19	Other congenital anomaly of fallopian tubes and broad ligaments
752.2	Congenital doubling of uterus

A didelphic uterus is associated with a septate vagina. It has two cervices and two small uteri. An expectant mother with a didelphic uterus may have a difficult time bringing a child to term.

| 752.3 | Other congenital anomaly of uterus |

A bicornuate uterus has two uterine cavities correctable by surgery.

A unicornuate uterus has only one lateral half and usually only one fallopian tube. This condition is associated with a high rate of miscarriage.

| 752.40 | Unspecified congenital anomaly of cervix, vagina, and external female genitalia |
| 752.41 | Embryonic cyst of cervix, vagina, and external female genitalia— *Gartner's duct cyst* |

A Gartner's duct cyst is a benign tumor-like cyst of the vagina that develops from the embryonic remnants of the Gartner's duct part of the mesonephros that develops into the reproductive organs.

| 752.42 | Imperforate hymen |
| 752.49 | Other congenital anomaly of cervix, vagina, and external female genitalia |

Synechia vulvae are fused labia minora. There is a tiny opening that permits the flow of urine from the urethra.

| 752.51 | Undescended testis |

In true cryptorchism, the testis is concealed within the abdominal cavity. In incomplete cryptorchism, the testis has partially descended within the inguinal canal and arrested. Both conditions are associated with low birth weight, with incidence increasing as birth weights decrease. Cryptorchism must be corrected through orchiopexy by age 2 or sterility will result.

| 752.52 | Retractile testis |

A retractile testis can be manipulated into the scrotum without strain.

| 752.61 | Hypospadias |

In hypospadias, the urethral meatus lies on the ventral portion of the penile shaft. Corrective surgery should be performed by 8 to 12 months of age.

| 752.62 | Epispadias |

Epispadias is rare, with the urethral meatus on the dorsal portion of the penile shaft. The penis curves upward.

| 752.63 | Congenital chordee |

Chordee is the downward bowing of the penis and is associated with hypospadias, although it may occur as a solitary variant.

| 752.64 | Micropenis |

Micropenis, a form of ambiguous genitalia, is caused by a lack of endocrine output during fetal life, specifically lack of testosterone. Typically the penis, though small, is normal in function. Testosterone shots administered in infancy allow the penis to obtain normal size.

| 752.65 | Hidden penis |
| 752.69 | Other penile anomalies |

Penile agenesis is so rare that it occurs in one out of 30 million births. The scrotum is usually normal, though the testicles are undescended.

Penile duplication presents as a bifid penis with two corpora cavernosa and two hemialgias and may range from the glans only to duplication of the entire urogenital tract.

In torsion of the penis, the rotation is typically to the left.

752.7 Indeterminate sex and pseudohermaphroditism

Indeterminate sex, pseudohermaphroditism, and intersex are interchangeable terms. This category excludes all forms of this condition but gonadal dysgenesis. As in other forms of the condition, in hermaphroditism due to gonadal dysgenesis, the external genitalia do not match the genetic makeup of the individual. The fetus begins as a female and, if the chromosome pattern is XY, develops as a boy. For reasons unrelated to the other causes of the condition, gonadal development is subpart, leading to the birth of an infant of ambiguous sex.

752.81	Scrotal transposition
752.89	Other specified anomalies of genital organs
752.9	Unspecified congenital anomaly of genital organs

Documentation Issues
If the documentation identifies congenital chordee with hypospadias, both should be coded separately. Congenital chordee (752.63) is commonly noted as an associated condition with hypospadias (752.61). This rubric excludes testicular feminization syndrome, coded to 259.5.

Coding Clarification
Excluded from this rubric are syndromes associated with anomalies in the number and form of chromosomes (758.0-758.9) and testicular feminization syndrome (257.8).

Epispadias: This condition is a partial or complete dorsal fusion anomaly of the urethra. It may appear in both male and female patients, but is typically seen in males. As a male defect it is marked by the urethral opening on the dorsal surface of the penis; in females it appears as a slit in the upper wall of the urethra. Classically this condition is seen in patients with exstrophy of the bladder. Report with code 752.62 *Epispadias*.

Hydatid Cyst of Morgagni: In female patients, this condition would be reported with code 752.11 *Embryonic cyst of fallopian tubes and broad ligaments*. If identified in a male patient, report with code 752.89 *Other specified anomalies of genital organs*.

Hypospadias: A male developmental defect characterized by an abnormal opening of the urethra on the ventral surface of the penis or on the perineum; it is also a rare defect in the vagina of females. Report with code 752.61 *Hypospadias*.

Micropenis or Microphallus: This condition is due to the developmental failure of the penis caused by either failure of testosterone to stimulate the tissues or failure of the tissues to respond to testosterone stimulation. Report with code 752.64 *Micropenis*.

Coding Scenario
A 16-month-old boy is admitted for surgical repair of hypospadias and congenital chordee.

Code assignment: 752.63 *Congenital chordee* and 752.61 *Hypospadias*

A 29-year-old female is admitted for tubal pregnancy. The patient undergoes a left salpingectomy for removal of the tubal pregnancy. A pathology report confirms the diagnosis and identifies an embryonic cyst. The physician's final diagnostic statement is fallopian tube pregnancy and hydatid cyst of Morgagni.

Code assignment: 633.10 *Tubal pregnancy* and 752.11 *Embryonic cyst of fallopian tubes and broad ligaments*

753 Congenital anomalies of urinary system

753.0 Congenital renal agenesis and dysgenesis
Renal agenesis can be either bilateral or unilateral. When bilateral, the condition is terminal due to its affect on other organs. In bilateral agenesis of the kidneys, the fetus lives in an environment of oligohydramnios, which prevents normal development of the lungs. (The lungs are dependent on a moist environment for normal development.)

753.10	Unspecified congenital cystic kidney disease
753.11	Congenital single renal cyst

There is evidence that a single congenital renal cyst is a marker for polycystic kidney disease.

753.12	Congenital polycystic kidney, unspecified type
753.13	Congenital polycystic kidney, autosomal dominant

Polycystic kidney disease, autosomal-dominant, is a progressive disease of adult onset characterized by bilateral cysts. The kidneys are enlarged and their function is impaired.

753.14	Congenital polycystic kidney, autosomal recessive

Polycystic kidney disease, autosomal-recessive, has early childhood onset. There are multiple cysts in the kidneys and liver, leading to failure of both organs.

753.15	Congenital renal dysplasia
753.16	Congenital medullary cystic kidney

Medullary cystic kidney is a disease of the renal tubules leading to proteinuria and renal failure.

753.17	Congenital medullary sponge kidney

A medullary sponge kidney demonstrates dilation of the tubules. It may be symptomatic if calcinosis develops in the tubules, leading to renal insufficiency.

753.19	Other specified congenital cystic kidney disease
753.20	Unspecified obstructive defect of renal pelvis and ureter
753.21	Congenital obstruction of ureteropelvic junction

Congenital obstruction of the ureteropelvic junction is the most common urinary tract anomaly. Its appearance is associated with other anomalies of the urinary tract such as horseshoe kidney, ectopic kidney, multicystic, and dysplastic kidney. The condition may be diagnosed antenatally and is corrected within the first few months of life. A pyeloplasty promotes normal growth and development of urinary tract structures.

753.22	Congenital obstruction of ureterovesical junction

Obstruction of the ureterovesical junction often occurs with ureteropelvic obstruction.

753.23	Congenital ureterocele
753.29	Other obstructive defect of renal pelvis and ureter
753.3	Other specified congenital anomalies of kidney

Horseshoe and discoid kidneys are the products of fusion anomalies. A discoid kidney is fused medially at both poles, while a horseshoe kidney is fused at the lower poles. Horseshoe kidney may be associated with Wilms' tumor and anomalies of a number of body systems. An ectopic kidney is on the opposite side of its ureter.

753.4	Other specified congenital anomalies of ureter

Duplication occurs most frequently among ureteral anomalies.

753.5	Exstrophy of urinary bladder

Exstrophy of the bladder is the absence of part of the lower abdominal wall and part of the anterior bladder wall, allowing the posterior bladder wall to protrude. The bladder must be closed immediately after birth, a first stage of complex reconstructive surgeries.

753.6	Congenital atresia and stenosis of urethra and bladder neck

Urethral atresia is successfully treated antenatally by placement of a vesicoamniotic shunt.

753.7	Congenital anomalies of urachus

A urachal cyst presents as an extraperitoneal mass near the umbilicus. It may become infected or rupture, possibly causing peritonitis if it drains into the peritoneum rather than through the umbilicus.

753.8	Other specified congenital anomaly of bladder and urethra

Congenital diverticulum of the bladder, also known as Hutch diverticulum, occurs where the ureter enters the bladder and may cause obstruction and deviation. The diverticulum threatens the competence of the ureterovesical valve, leading to vesicoureteral reflux.

Female hypospadias presents the urinary meatus fairly near its normal position; however, it is associated with other anomalies of the urinary-genital tract.

753.9	Unspecified congenital anomaly of urinary system

754 Certain congenital musculoskeletal deformities

Defects in this rubric are limited by ICD-9-CM notes to those defects caused by extrinsic factors (e.g., intrauterine problems including malposition and pressure).

754.0	Congenital musculoskeletal deformities of skull, face, and jaw

Dolichocephaly is a skull that is long in relation to the anterior/posterior axis. Plagiocephaly is a lopsided and twisted skull. Potter's facies is a facial appearance characterized by deep folds under the eyes. The folds are caused by oligohydramnios related to agenesis of the kidneys.

754.1	Congenital musculoskeletal deformity of sternocleidomastoid muscle

Sternocleidomastoid torticollis is apparent after birth. Because there are other non-muscular causes of congenital torticollis, the pediatrician must ascertain the cause. If it is muscular, the child should be checked for hip dysplasia, as it is frequently associated with muscular torticollis. Treatment involves daily stretching for the first year of life. If torticollis persists, surgery is necessary to correct the asymmetrical tilt to the face.

754.2	Congenital musculoskeletal deformity of spine

Congenital scoliosis, an anterior/posterior plane vertebral malformation, may appear in three variants. It can be an isolated deformity or be associated with other multi-system deformities. Approximately 20 percent of the cases include genitourinary malformations, while another 20 percent show coexistent cord defects.

Lordosis is an exaggerated inward curve in the low back.

Dislocation and subluxation of the hip occur in conjunction with ligamentous laxity of the hip joint capsules. Females are affected nine times out of 10 and there is a 30 to 50 percent incidence among breech births. Osteoarthritis, gait abnormalities, pains, and unequal leg length may result if left untreated.

754.30	Congenital dislocation of hip, unilateral
754.31	Congenital dislocation of hip, bilateral
754.32	Congenital subluxation of hip, unilateral
754.33	Congenital subluxation of hip, bilateral
754.35	Congenital dislocation of one hip with subluxation of other hip

Bowing of the long bones can occur alone or as part of a series of anomalies, of which osteogenesis imperfecta is the most known.

754.40	Congenital genu recurvatum
754.41	Congenital dislocation of knee (with genu recurvatum)
754.42	Congenital bowing of femur
754.43	Congenital bowing of tibia and fibula
754.44	Congenital bowing of unspecified long bones of leg
754.50	Congenital talipes varus

In talipes varus, the foot rotates outward, promoting walking on the outside of the sole.

Foot is plantar flexed
Tarsal bones are inverted

The congenital deformity known as clubfoot is usually bilateral. The bones and soft tissues may be normal in shape but are locked in a tortured position.

Cavus deformity

| 754.51 | Congenital talipes equinovarus |

Also known as clubfoot, talipes equinovarus is a condition in which the sole points straight back. As is the case with the other foot deformities, talipes equinovarus arises from improper alignment of the baby in utero.

| 754.52 | Congenital metatarsus primus varus |

Metatarsus primus varus is a deformity of the cuneiform bone.

| 754.53 | Congenital metatarsus varus |

Metatarsus varus is a toeing-in deformity.

| 754.59 | Other congenital varus deformity of feet |

Talipes calcaneovarus has the foot pointing out and down.

| 754.60 | Congenital talipes valgus |

Talipes valgus is a deformity in which the foot toes in, promoting walking on the inside of the soles.

| 754.61 | Congenital pes planus |

Congenital flat foot is a more severe problem than acquired flat foot.

| 754.62 | Talipes calcaneovalgus |

Talipes calcaneovalgus, in which the foot toes out, is the most common foot deformity.

| 754.69 | Other congenital valgus deformity of feet |

Talipes equinovalgus is a form of clubfoot in which the heel points outward.

| 754.70 | Unspecified talipes |
| 754.71 | Talipes cavus |

In talipes cavus, there is muscle imbalance and weakness due to many causes. The forefoot is adducted and the heel is valgus.

| 754.79 | Other congenital deformity of feet |

Pectus excavatum produces a deep indentation in the chest at the level of the breastbone. It may be a solitary phenomenon, but has a strong association with Marfan's syndrome and cardiac anomalies. More males than females are affected by the condition. Pectus carinatum, which causes the chest to curve outward like a pigeon's breast, is associated with other anomalies and is primarily a cosmetic problem.

754.81	Pectus excavatum
754.82	Pectus carinatum
754.89	Other specified nonteratogenic anomalies

755 Other congenital anomalies of limbs

Intrinsic and extrinsic factors may cause the anomalies reported by this rubric. Intrinsic factors include errors of fetal development. Extrinsic factors are the result of intrauterine problems including malposition and pressure and comprise only 2 percent of all congenital anomalies.

Polydactyly may be genetic, solitary, or part of numerous syndromes. The supernumerary digits may be rudimentary or normally formed.

Congenital Anomalies

Syndactyly of digits (webbing)
Image at right depicts a case involving fusion of bone and nail

Supernumerary digit

Code	Description
755.00	Polydactyly, unspecified digits
755.01	Polydactyly of fingers
755.02	Polydactyly of toes

Syndactyly is genetically linked and may appear in conjunction with other syndromes. When the webbing is confined to the skin, surgery is generally performed at 6 months of age to enhance normal digit development. The corrective operation involves splitting the webbing and applying skin grafts. When all five bones are fused, the situation is more complex and surgery rarely is able to provide optimal function.

Code	Description
755.10	Syndactyly of multiple and unspecified sites
755.11	Syndactyly of fingers without fusion of bone
755.12	Syndactyly of fingers with fusion of bone
755.13	Syndactyly of toes without fusion of bone
755.14	Syndactyly of toes with fusion of bone
755.20	Congenital unspecified reduction deformity of upper limb

Ectromelia is hypoplasia of the long bones in the upper limb. In hemimelia, a part of the bone of the upper limb is missing.

Code	Description
755.21	Congenital transverse deficiency of upper limb

Amelia is the congenital absence of the upper limb.

Congenital amputation of any limb may be due to constriction by fibrous amniotic bands or to teratogenic factors.

Code	Description
755.22	Congenital longitudinal deficiency of upper limb, not elsewhere classified

In complete phocomelia, the hands are attached to the trunk. In incomplete phocomelia, there may be a rudimentary long bone.

Code	Description
755.23	Congenital longitudinal deficiency, combined, involving humerus, radius, and ulna (complete or incomplete)
755.24	Congenital longitudinal deficiency, humeral, complete or partial (with or without distal deficiencies, incomplete)

Proximal phocomelia means the absence of a humerus.

Code	Description
755.25	Congenital longitudinal deficiency, radioulnar, complete or partial (with or without distal deficiencies, incomplete)
755.26	Congenital longitudinal deficiency, radial, complete or partial (with or without distal deficiencies, incomplete)
755.27	Congenital longitudinal deficiency, ulnar, complete or partial (with or without distal deficiencies, incomplete)
755.28	Congenital longitudinal deficiency, carpals or metacarpals, complete or partial (with or without incomplete phalangeal deficiency)
755.29	Congenital longitudinal deficiency, phalanges, complete or partial
755.30	Congenital unspecified reduction deformity of lower limb

Ectromelia is hypoplasia of the long bones in the lower limb. In hemimelia, a part of the bone of the lower limb is missing.

Code	Description
755.31	Congenital transverse deficiency of lower limb

Amelia is the congenital absence of one or more lower limbs.

Code	Description
755.32	Congenital longitudinal deficiency of lower limb, not elsewhere classified
755.33	Congenital longitudinal deficiency, combined, involving femur, tibia, and fibula (complete or incomplete)

Complete phocomelia of the lower limb means the direct attachment of the feet to the trunk.

Code	Description
755.34	Congenital longitudinal deficiency, femoral, complete or partial (with or without distal deficiencies, incomplete)

Proximal phocomelia of the lower limb means the absence of a femur.

Code	Description
755.35	Congenital longitudinal deficiency, tibiofibular, complete or partial (with or without distal deficiencies, incomplete)
755.36	Congenital longitudinal deficiency, tibia, complete or partial (with or without distal deficiencies, incomplete)
755.37	Congenital longitudinal deficiency, fibular, complete or partial (with or without distal deficiencies, incomplete)
755.38	Congenital longitudinal deficiency, tarsals or metatarsals, complete or partial (with or without incomplete phalangeal deficiency)

Code	Description
755.39	Congenital longitudinal deficiency, phalanges, complete or partial
755.4	Congenital reduction deformities, unspecified limb
755.50	Unspecified congenital anomaly of upper limb
755.51	Congenital deformity of clavicle
755.52	Congenital elevation of scapula

Sprengel's deformity connotes a hypoplastic and elevated scapula. Often, the hypoplastic trapezius, deltoid, or rhomboid is absent. The result may be torticollis, scoliosis, or limb length discrepancy.

Code	Description
755.53	Radioulnar synostosis

The forearm is permanently pronated in radioulnar synostosis. Most cases do not require surgery.

Code	Description
755.54	Madelung's deformity

Madelung's deformity is a dysplasia of the radius involving an exaggerated radial inclination, a short forearm, dorsal dislocation of the ulnar head, and a "V" shaped proximal carpal row. The condition may arise from an abnormal fibrous band tethering the sigmoid notch of the radius proximally to the ulna.

Code	Description
755.55	Acrocephalosyndactyly

Apert's syndrome involves premature fusing of the cranial sutures, asymmetrical facies, webbed hands, and progressive calcification and fusion of the bones of the hands, feet, and cervical spine.

Code	Description
755.56	Accessory carpal bones
755.57	Macrodactylia (fingers)
755.58	Congenital cleft hand

Lobster-claw hand, a rare disorder, affects the phalanges of the middle finger. The corresponding metacarpal may be absent and the hand is separated into medial and lateral sections by a deep cleft.

Code	Description
755.59	Other congenital anomaly of upper limb, including shoulder girdle

Cleidocranial dysostosis, or Scheutthauer-Marie-Sainton syndrome, is a genetic disease most often characterized by the absence or hypoplastic development of the collarbone.

In cubitus valgus, the forearm deviates away from the midline on extension. In cubitus varus, the forearm deviates inward when extended.

The angle between the long axes of the neck and shaft of the femur is 120-125 degrees in the normal individual. In coxa valga, this angle is increased to approximately 140 degrees, creating extreme adduction with the possibility of a superior dislocation in the immature hip. In coxa vara, this angle is abnormally decreased, creating an extreme abduction. Coxa vara is much more common than coxa valga.

Code	Description
755.60	Unspecified congenital anomaly of lower limb
755.61	Congenital coxa valga
755.62	Congenital coxa vara
755.63	Other congenital deformity of hip (joint)
755.64	Congenital deformity of knee (joint)

Genu valgum (knock-knee) is a normal part of development that may require surgical intervention if it persists beyond 10 or 12 years of age and if there are more than three inches between the ankles.

Code	Description
755.65	Macrodactylia of toes
755.66	Other congenital anomaly of toes

The correction of hallux valgus is postponed until skeletal maturity.

Code	Description
755.67	Congenital anomalies of foot, not elsewhere classified

"Coalition" and "bar" refer to an abnormal union of bones that are normally separated.

Code	Description
755.69	Other congenital anomaly of lower limb, including pelvic girdle
755.8	Other specified congenital anomalies of unspecified limb

Larsen's syndrome is a genetic, multi-system disorder that presents with multiple dislocations and other bony irregularities, as well as cylindrical fingers and unusual facies. Other symptoms include mental retardation, short stature, and cardiac abnormalities.

Code	Description
755.9	Unspecified congenital anomaly of unspecified limb

756 Other congenital musculoskeletal anomalies

Code	Description
756.0	Congenital anomalies of skull and face bones

Acrocephaly is a pointed vault of the skull.

Craniosynostosis is an abnormal fusing of the cranial sutures. In the newborn, the cranial sutures are open, serving two desired outcomes: normal delivery with a malleable head and the ability of the skull to grow to accommodate the growing brain. The sagittal suture is the most frequently occurring site of synostosis and is the least likely to be associated with genetics. Any bilateral craniosynostosis is a flag for a possible genetic relationship.

Corrective surgery is performed primarily for cosmetic reasons, although in some cases, the facial bones are affected or the brain does not have enough room and the surgery is justified for both cosmetic and medical reasons.

Oxycephaly describes a cone-shaped head.

Platybasia is an upward thrust of the odontoid bone through the foramen magnum, causing pressure on the midbrain.

Trigonocephaly is a triangular-shaped head.

Crouzon's disease combines craniosynostosis, exophthalmos, hypoplastic midface, flat sphenoids, and a large mandible. Genetic and spontaneous causes are split 50 percent. Asymmetrical exophthalmos and the large jaw are correctable.

Hypertelorism is an abnormal distance between the eyes.

First arch syndrome refers to the developmental stage of the first arch, and involves numerous craniofacial anomalies.

Oculo-auricle-vertebral (OAV) syndrome is synonymous with Goldenhar's syndrome and is non-hereditary.

Greig's syndrome is a hereditary disease involving multiple deformities of the hands and feet, macrocephaly, hypertelorism, mild mental retardation, and a broad, flat nose.

Hallman Streiff syndrome is an oculo-mandibula-facial syndrome inclusive of short stature and congenital cataracts.

Treacher-Collins, synonymous with Franceschetti's syndrome, is genetically driven and involves an eye slant, lip coloboma, micrognathia, microtia, hypoplastic zygomatic arches, and macrostomia.

756.10	Congenital anomaly of spine, unspecified
756.11	Congenital spondylolysis, lumbosacral region

Spondylolysis is a defect in the vertebra, usually L5, filled with fibrous tissue containing nerve endings that are painful due to compression.

756.12	Congenital spondylolisthesis

Spondylolisthesis is the slipping forward of one vertebra over another, often L5, and is usually associated with a spinal defect such as spina bifida occulta. Females are more often affected.

756.13	Congenital absence of vertebra
756.14	Hemivertebra

A hemivertebra, a condition that can promote scoliosis, is treated with fusion and bone graft to render it equal in height.

756.15	Congenital fusion of spine (vertebra)

Bertolotti's syndrome involves sacralization of the L4-L5 vertebrae. An L5 transverse process forms a pseudoarthrosis with the ala of S1, increasing the tilt of the vertebra and enhancing the possibility of scoliosis.

756.16	Klippel-Feil syndrome

A short neck caused by the fusion of existing cervical vertebrae and the absence of at least one cervical vertebra characterize Klippel-Feil syndrome, also known as brevicollis. It has a high rate of associated malformations or syndromes and affects females.

756.17	Spina bifida occulta

Spina bifida occulta is fairly benign in adults if not causing apparent problems during childhood. The disorder is vertebral, as in spina bifida aperta; however, skin covers the defect in the occulta form. In severe forms, which accounts for about 2 percent of the occulta cases, the condition is called spinal dysraphism to distinguish it from its benign presentation.

756.19	Other congenital anomaly of spine
756.2	Cervical rib

A cervical rib is a supernumerary rib in the cervical region, which can lead to thoracic outlet syndrome.

756.3	Other congenital anomaly of ribs and sternum
756.4	Chondrodystrophy

Chondrodystrophy, a defect of the cartilage growth mechanism, is the primary cause of short limb dwarfism, a condition characterized by decreased length of the long bones, although the diameter is not affected. The condition is hereditary. Dyschondroplasia typically affects unilateral joints and involves knobby fingers and genu valgus.

Jeune's syndrome is an asphyxiating thoracic dystrophy.

Maffucci's syndrome, another term for Kast's syndrome, is a non-hereditary dyschondroplasia and involves soft tissue hemangiomata, cyst-like bone lesions, and multiple phleboliths. The hemangiomata can enhance dysplastia.

756.50	Unspecified congenital osteodystrophy
756.51	Osteogenesis imperfecta

Osteogenesis imperfecta is a hereditary collagen disorder that produces very brittle bones. Type 1 is the most common and mildest form, with the affected person's stature being normal or near normal. Multiple fractures may occur prior to puberty, decreasing later in life. Type II is the most severe, causing death at or soon after birth. Types III and IV are treated with intramedullary rods inserted into the long bones.

756.52	Osteopetrosis

Osteopetrosis produces an overgrowth of bone that spills into the marrow and obliterates the marrow of the bones below the head and the foramina. The loss of marrow leads to anemia and heptad-splenomegaly. Osteopetrosis can lead to sight and hearing impairments because the nerves cannot emerge through their foramina in the skull.

756.53	Osteopoikilosis

Osteopoikilosis, a rare genetic disorder, manifests in multiple areas of increased bone density, although the disorder is often asymptomatic. It is associated with other disorders such as dwarfism or scleroderma.

756.54	Polyostotic fibrous dysplasia of bone
756.55	Chondroectodermal dysplasia

Chondroectodermal dysplasia is characterized by abnormal development of hair, skin, teeth, and cartilage. Polydactyly and heart anomalies are also present.

756.56	Multiple epiphyseal dysplasia
756.59	Other congenital osteodystrophy

McCune-Albright syndrome, which usually affects females, involves bone disease with enhanced potential for fractures, leg deformities, endocrine disease, and skin changes. There is wide variability in the degree of severity.

756.6	Congenital anomaly of diaphragm
756.70	Unspecified congenital anomaly of abdominal wall
756.71	Prune belly syndrome

Prune belly syndrome, also known as Eagle-Barrett disease, manifests in the absence of the lower rectus abdominus and the medial portions of the oblique muscles. There are urinary tract anomalies. About 95 percent of infants affected are males and 50 percent of all affected newborns are stillborn or die within two years of birth.

756.79	Other congenital anomalies of abdominal wall

An omphalocele is a defect in the abdominal wall involving the umbilicus. Large omphaloceles contain parts of the intestines that are reduced over time. The condition may be associated with a syndrome or may appear as a solitary variant.

756.81	Congenital absence of muscle and tendon
756.82	Accessory muscle
756.83	Ehlers-Danlos syndrome

Ehlers-Danlos syndrome, a genetic collagen disorder, causes hyperelasticity of the skin, hypermobility of the joints, and fragility of blood vessels. Wound healing is impaired.

756.89	Other specified congenital anomaly of muscle, tendon, fascia, and connective tissue

Use this code for amyotrophia congenita, congenital shortening of tendon, Ayala's disease, Bakwin-Krida syndrome, elongated ligamentum patellae, Fong's syndrome, HOOD syndrome, Krabbe's syndrome, Oestreicher-Turner syndrome, popliteal web syndrome, Pyle-Cohn disease, Schwartz- (Jambul) syndrome, Touraine's syndrome, congenital trigger finger, Turner-Kieser syndrome, and Waardenburg's syndrome.

756.9	Other and unspecified congenital anomaly of musculoskeletal system

Documentation Issues

Because it is not unusual for multiple anomalies to be present, the physician should clearly indicate in the medical record documentation those anomalies that are related vs. those that do not appear to be due to a disease process.

Coding Clarification

Craniosynostosis: This is the premature closure of one or more of the cranial sutures. This premature closure is usually incomplete and affects one suture. It can result in abnormalities of the cranial contour. This condition is classified to code 756.0.

Nager Syndrome: This is a congenital disorder that is also known as preaxial acrofacial dysostosis. In addition to anomalies of the face, patients with this condition may also have cleft palate, hypoplastic or aplastic thumb, hip dislocation, reduced stature, and mild mental retardation.

Code 756.0 is assigned to indicate the congenital anomalies of the skull and face. If any other features of the disease are present that do not appear to be indicated by using this code, those anomalies should be coded separately.

757 Congenital anomalies of the integument

757.0	Hereditary edema of legs

Congenital lymphedema is a disorder of the lymph drainage system affecting the legs. Infection is a constant threat. Garments that avoid compression and the use of gradient pumps are the common treatments.

757.1	Ichthyosis congenita

Ichthyosis congenita refers to scaly skin as a result of an excessive production of skin cells.

Sjögren-Larsson syndrome manifests with dry, scaly skin, as well as mental retardation, speech abnormalities, and spasticity. Retinal degeneration is characteristic in about 50 percent of all cases.

757.2	Dermatoglyphic anomalies
757.31	Congenital ectodermal dysplasia

Congenital ectodermal dysplasia, or hidrotic ED, is an inherited disorder primarily affecting the French. The nails are thick and there is thick skin on the palms and soles, and dark skin on the elbows and knees.

757.32	Congenital vascular hamartomas

Port wine stain, or nevus flammeus, is a hemangioma that is red and flat at birth, which thickens over time.

Congenital Anomalies

757.33 Congenital pigmentary anomaly of skin
Urticaria pigmentosa is a self-limiting rash that tends to disappear after puberty.

757.39 Other specified congenital anomaly of skin
Congenital pachydermatocele, or cutis pendula, causes the skin to hang in wrinkled folds.

757.4 Specified congenital anomalies of hair
Congenital alopecia is the failure of hair to grow or develop.

757.5 Specified congenital anomalies of nails
Anonychia is the absence of one or more fingernails.

757.6 Specified congenital anomalies of breast
757.8 Other specified congenital anomalies of the integument
757.9 Unspecified congenital anomaly of the integument

758 Chromosomal anomalies

Chromosomes are divided into two types: autosomes and sex-linked. Of the 23 pairs, only one pair, the 23rd, is related to sex and is distributed as XX in girls and XY in boys. The other 22 pairs are called autosomes. The conditions in the 758 category involve anomalies in either the sex chromosome or autosome arrangements.

758.0 Down's syndrome
Down's syndrome is the result of an extra chromosome (trisomy) on the 21st pair of chromosomes. Characteristics include hypertrophy, hearing loss due to the angle of the ear canals, developmental delay, delay in language acquisition, and heart defects.

758.1 Patau's syndrome
Patau's syndrome is also a trisomic condition involving the 13th pair of autosomes. The brain's failure to divide into lobes is a primary characteristic that can affect the senses of sight, smell, and hearing. Lip and palate (typically cleft) anomalies may be present.

758.2 Edwards' syndrome
Edwards' syndrome, a trisomic autosome 18, involves delays in growth, the respiratory system, craniofacial malformations, skeletal defects, and webbing. Mental retardation is another characteristic.

758.31 Cri-du-chat syndrome
Cri-du-chat syndrome, also called cat cry syndrome, results from a deletion of the short arm of the fifth chromosome and may vary from a tiny deletion of one band to the entire small arm. Incidence makes it one of the most common autosomal deletions with variability between 1 in 20,000-50,000 births.

Children with cri-du-chat present with an abnormally small head (microcephaly), with accompanying small jaw and chin (micrognathia), low set ears, wide set eyes (hypertelorism), and profound or severe mental retardation and psychomotor problems. The identifying characteristic diagnosed in infants is the unusual, high-pitched, cat cry.

758.32 Velo-cardio-facial syndrome
Velo-cardio-facial syndrome (VCFS) refers to the palate, the heart, and the face, where the most common, identifying signs and symptoms of this syndrome are manifested, although not in every child with VCFS. These characteristic problems include: cleft palate, heart defects, and an elongated face with almond-shaped eyes, a wide nose, and small ears. VCFS is caused by deletion of genes on a specific part of the 22nd chromosome. There is still great variation in the presentation of this disease—up to 30 different problems have been related to it, including feeding problems, weak immune systems, weak musculature, hypothyroidism, short stature, and scoliosis. It affects about 130,000 individuals in the U.S., occurring in approximately 5-8% of all those born with a cleft palate, around 1 in 700 live births.

758.39 Autosomal deletion syndromes, other autosomal deletions
Microdeletions, such as Miller-Dieker and Smith-Magenis syndromes are included under 758.33 other microdeletions. Miller-Dieker syndrome is seen when there is a deletion from the short arm of chromosome 17, sometimes in combination with duplication of the long arm. Also known as agyria (lack of sulci and gyri) and lissencephaly (smooth surface of the brain), it causes death in infancy or early childhood with an array or problems from the multiple developmental defects and abnormalities of the brain that it produces: retarded mental, speech, and motor development, neurological complications, and multiple abnormalities affecting the kidneys, heart, gastrointestinal tract, and other organs.

Smith-Magenis syndrome is also due to a deletion in a certain area of chromosome 17 that results in craniofacial changes, speech delay, hoarse voice, hearing loss in many, and behavioral problems, such as self-destructive head banging, wrist biting, and tearing at nails.

758.4 Balanced autosomal translocation in normal individual
758.5 Other conditions due to autosomal anomalies
758.6 Gonadal dysgenesis

Turner's syndrome, also known as XO syndrome, affects females. It is sex chromosome linked, occurring once every 2,500 births. Characteristics include short stature, ovarian dysgenesis, and associated heart, kidney, and thyroid disorders. Growth hormone and estrogen are used to treat the symptoms.

758.7   Klinefelter's syndrome
Klinefelter's syndrome affects only males, and involves an additional X chromosome, creating a pattern of XXY instead of XY. The condition is divided in mosaic and non-mosaic patients (mosaic implies that not all cells are affected). Characteristics include delayed language development. Injections of testosterone can counter the physical anomalies of the syndrome. Associated disorders are asthma, hypostatic leg ulcers, thrombophlebitis, and osteoporosis. Male breast cancer presents a risk 20 times that of the non-Klinefelter male and there is also an increased incidence of mediastinal germ cell cancer.

A variant of Klinefelter syndrome produces two sets of abnormal sex chromosomes, for an XX YY arrangement. Another variant is XXXXY.

758.81   Other conditions due to sex chromosome anomalies
758.89   Other conditions due to chromosome anomalies
MELAS syndrome is a mitochondrial myopathy that can lead to stroke-like episodes and encephalomyopathy. Patients are increasingly fatigued in this progressive disease.

758.9   Conditions due to anomaly of unspecified chromosome

759   Other and unspecified congenital anomalies
759.0   Congenital anomalies of spleen
Asplenia is a serious condition associated with congenital heart anomalies.

759.1   Congenital anomalies of adrenal gland
Use code 759.1 to report adrenal hypoplasia, or an absent, accessory, or aberrant adrenal gland. Excluded from this code are congenital disorders of steroid metabolism (255.2) and adrenogenital disorders (255.2).

759.2   Congenital anomalies of other endocrine glands
A thyroglossal duct cyst is a fluid-filled connective duct extending from the tongue base to the thyroid. The thyroglossal duct generally disappears during fetal development. This code reports thyroglossal duct cyst, absent parathyroid gland, accessory thyroid gland, or persistent thyroglossal or thyrolingual duct. Excluded from this code are congenital goiter (246.1) and congenital hypothyroidism (243).

759.3   Situs inversus
Situs inversus, or Kartagener's syndrome, is a condition in which the abdominal and/or thoracic organs are in reverse position.

759.4   Conjoined twins
Conjoined twins are born from a single ovum and a shared single placenta. They are always identical. The incidence is one in every 50,000 to 80,000 births, with the highest incidence in Africa and India. The twins can be joined at various sites, the most common being the thoracopagus arrangement of sharing a heart, joined at the chest, followed by omphalopagus, an anterior union at the midtrunk. Most conjoined twins miscarry or are stillborn.

759.5   Tuberous sclerosis
Tuberous sclerosis promotes benign tumors in the vital organs as well as in the eyes and skin, and affects both sexes. This condition can cause epileptic seizures and developmental delays and may be referred to as Bourneville's disease, Epiloia, Bourneville-Pringle syndrome, or Pringle's disease.

759.6   Other congenital hamartoses, not elsewhere classified
Von Hippel-Lindau syndrome involves abnormal growth of the blood vessels leading to hemangiomata and hemangioblastomata. They tend to grow in the retina, brain, cord, and adrenals. Predisposing the affected individuals to kidney cancer, it appears in the fourth decade.

Also use this code to report Jahnke's syndrome, Peutz-Jeghers syndrome, Sturge-Weber (-Dimitri) syndrome, Kalischer's syndrome, Krabbe's cutaneocerebral angioma syndrome, Lawford's syndrome, Milles' syndrome, Shimmer's syndrome, Sturge-Kalischer-Weber syndrome, and Weber-Dimitri syndrome.

759.7   Multiple congenital anomalies, so described
759.81   Prader-Willi syndrome
Prader-Willi syndrome is characterized by several conditions, including hypotonia, hypogonadism, hyperphagia, cognitive impairments, behavioral difficulties, and morbid obesity. The hypothalamus dysfunction leads to the disordered appetite (hyperphagia), which in turn causes the morbid obesity. The disorder is considered to be a deletion error in the genes.

759.82   Marfan's syndrome
Marfan syndrome is a connective tissue disorder, affecting the long limbs, fingers, and toes. Arm span often exceeds height. The face is narrow and sharply

featured and the chest may be excavatum or carinatum. The lens may be displaced, causing myopia. Other symptoms include loose joints, weakened aorta and cardiac valves, decreased lung elasticity, and scoliosis.

759.83   Fragile X syndrome

Fragile X syndrome occurs in males and females and involves mental retardation that is often more profound in males.

759.89   Other specified multiple congenital anomalies, so described
              AHA: Q2, 2004, 12; Q2, 2005, 17

This code can be reported to describe congenital malformation syndromes affecting multiple systems, not elsewhere classified, including Alport's syndrome, bird-headed dwarf (Seckel's syndrome), Brachmann-de Lange syndrome, Brachymorphism with ectopic lentis (Marchesani -(Weil) syndrome, Craniocarpotarsal dystrophy (Freeman-Sheldon syndrome), whistling-face syndrome, microencephaly, and dwarfism (Cockayne's syndrome). Other conditions reported with this code include Noonan's syndrome, Orodigitofacial dysotosis (Bardet-Biedl) syndrome, Papillon-Lege and Psaume syndrome, Rubinstein-Taybi's syndrome, Smith-Lemli Opitz syndrome, Synophthalmus, and a congenital thoracogastroschisis, umbilical fistula, or cyst.

Laurence-Moon-Biedl syndrome, reported with this code, involves obesity, mental retardation, polydactyly or syndactyly, renal disease, retinitis pigmentosa, genital hypoplasia, and, in males, hypogonadism.

Startle disease (also Kok disease, familial startle disease), reported with this code and 333.99 for abnormal movement disorders, is characterized by exaggerated and persistent startle reactions to stimuli.

759.9   Unspecified congenital anomaly

760–779
Certain Conditions Originating in the Perinatal Peroid

This chapter classifies conditions that begin during the perinatal period even if death or morbidity occur later. The perinatal period is defined as the period of time occurring before, birth through the first 28 days following birth. These codes are used to classify causes of morbidity and mortality that began in the fetus or newborn and should never be used on the mother's coding profile. Codes in this chapter may be used throughout the life of the patient, no matter the patient's age, if the condition is still present. Additional codes can be used to further specify the newborn's condition.

760–763 Maternal Causes of Perinatal Morbidity and Mortality

Use these codes to report fetal or newborn conditions caused by systemic, metabolic, or infectious diseases of the mother. Maternal diseases that can affect the health or life of the fetus or newborn include hypertension, renal disease, urinary or respiratory tract infections, and circulatory diseases (pulmonary embolism, thrombophlebitis). Categories 760-763 also include fetal or newborn conditions caused by maternal nutritional disorders; maternal injury, surgery, or death; maternal ingestion of drugs, chemicals, or alcohol; and maternal complications of labor, delivery, or both.

These codes are reserved for use on the newborn coding profile as a secondary diagnosis to follow a code from rubrics V30-V39 for liveborn infants. They also may be used as a principal diagnosis for a newborn that has been transferred or readmitted for a condition classifiable to codes 760-763. Assign a code from these categories only when there is evidence documented in the chart that the maternal condition has in fact affected the fetus or newborn.

760 Fetus or newborn affected by maternal conditions which may be unrelated to present pregnancy
AHA: Nov-Dec, 1984, 11; Q2, 1989, 14; Q3, 1990, 5; Q2, 1992, 12; Q1, 1994, 8

760.0 Fetus or newborn affected by maternal hypertensive disorders — *fetus or newborn affected by maternal hypertension*
AHA: Nov-Dec, 1984, 11; Q2, 1989, 14; Q3, 1990, 5; Q2, 1992, 12; Q1, 1994, 8

Use code 760.0 to report a fetal or newborn condition caused by maternal hypertension. The hypertension may be benign or malignant, preexisting, transient or gestational, chronic, or secondary (such as that due to renal artery stenosis). The incidence of maternal hypertension varies from 0.5 to 4 percent depending on the race and age of the mother, and averages 2.5 percent. The fetus or infant of a mother with hypertension has a 25 to 30 percent risk of prematurity and a 10 to 15 percent chance of being small for gestation age (SGA).

Therapies include resuscitation at birth for anoxia. Associated conditions include prematurity, alveolar conditions, respiratory distress syndrome, inadequate or erratic brain perfusion, acute tubular necrosis, necrotizing enterocolitis, hypotension, blood pressure peaks, hypovolemia, SGA, hypermagnesemia, thrombocytopenia, and neutropenia.

Use code 760.0 for the fetus or newborn when the maternal conditions have been classified to rubric 642.

760.1 Fetus or newborn affected by maternal renal and urinary tract diseases — *fetus or newborn affected by renal and urinary tract diseases*
AHA: Nov-Dec, 1984, 11; Q2, 1989, 14; Q3, 1990, 5; Q2, 1992, 12; Q1, 1994, 8

Use code 760.1 for the fetus or newborn when the maternal conditions have been classified to rubrics 580-599.

760.2 Fetus or newborn affected by maternal infections — *fetus or newborn affected by maternal infectious disease, but fetus not manifesting that disease*
AHA: Nov-Dec, 1984, 11; Q2, 1989, 14; Q3, 1990, 5; Q2, 1992, 12; Q1, 1994, 8

Use code 760.2 for the fetus or newborn when the maternal infectious disease has been classified to 001-136 and 487, but the fetus or newborn is not manifesting the disease. Excluded from this subcategory are congenital infectious diseases (771.0-771.8) and maternal genital tract and other localized infection (780.8).

760.3 Fetus or newborn affected by other chronic maternal circulatory and respiratory diseases — *fetus or newborn affected by chronic maternal circulatory and respiratory diseases*
AHA: Nov-Dec, 1984, 11; Q2, 1989, 14; Q3, 1990, 5; Q2, 1992, 12; Q1, 1994, 8

Use code 760.3 for the fetus or newborn when the maternal conditions are classifiable to 390-459, 490-519, or 745-748.

760.4 Fetus or newborn affected by maternal nutritional disorders — *fetus or newborn affected by nutritional disorders*
AHA: Nov-Dec, 1984, 11; Q2, 1989, 14; Q3, 1990, 5; Q2, 1992, 12; Q1, 1994, 8

Use code 760.4 for the fetus or newborn when the maternal disorders are classifiable to 260-269. Excluded from this code is fetal malnutrition (764.10-764.29).

760.5 Fetus or newborn affected by maternal injury — *fetus or newborn affected by maternal injury*
AHA: Nov-Dec, 1984, 11; Q2, 1989, 14; Q3, 1990, 5; Q2, 1992, 12; Q1, 1994, 8

Use code 760.5 for the fetus or newborn when the maternal disorders are classifiable to 800-995.

760.6 Fetus or newborn affected by surgical operation on mother

Excluded from code 760.6 are cesarean section for present delivery (763.4); damage to placenta from amniocentesis, cesarean section, or surgical induction (762.1); or previous surgery to uterus or pelvic organs (763.89).

760.70 Noxious influences affecting fetus or newborn via placenta or breast milk, unspecified noxious substance — *fetus or newborn affected by drug NEC*
AHA: Nov-Dec, 1984, 11; Q2, 1989, 14; Q3, 1990, 5; Q3, 1991, 21; Q2, 1992, 12; Q1, 1994, 8

Use code 760.70 when the fetal or newborn condition is caused by maternal ingestion of drugs or chemicals. This includes drugs taken for therapeutic purposes during pregnancy (but excludes drugs taken during labor and delivery, classified to code 763.5), drugs taken before pregnancy is known, and exposure to chemicals through the maternal work place while the fetus is in utero. Most drugs ingested during pregnancy, including their metabolites, cross the placenta and reach the fetus. Therefore, many substances have the potential for affecting the fetus. The specific effects on the fetus or newborn depend on the type of noxious substance.

Associated conditions include limb defects, skeletal and facial anomalies, mental retardation, chromosomal abnormalities, cardiac defects, and central nervous system defects.

760.71 Noxious influences affecting fetus or newborn via placenta or breast milk, alcohol — *fetal alcohol syndrome*
AHA: Nov-Dec, 1984, 11; Q2, 1989, 14; Q3, 1990, 5; Q3, 1991, 21; Q2, 1992, 12; Q1, 1994, 8

Use code 760.71 to report a fetal or newborn condition caused by maternal ingestion of alcohol during pregnancy. This code includes fetal alcohol syndrome (FAS), a condition diagnosed in patients born to chronic alcoholics who drank heavily during pregnancy. Lesser alcohol abuse results in a decreased severity of the manifestations of FAS. It is not known how much alcohol can be consumed safely.

Signs and symptoms of alcohol abuse include jitteriness, diaphoresis, and convulsions; with acute intoxication, stupor or coma, confusion, lethargy, and poor reflex responses; with fetal alcohol syndrome, pre- and postnatal growth retardation, short palpebral fissures, midfacial hypoplasia, low unparallel ears, flattened nasal bridge, and abnormal palmar creases. Toxicology tests of blood or urine reveal the presence of alcohol. Associated conditions include cardiac defects, joint contractures, and mental retardation.

This code is used to report the effects of alcohol on the fetus or newborn, including alcohol withdrawal syndrome. Note that some newborns may suffer from both fetal alcohol syndrome and alcohol withdrawal syndrome, or fetal alcohol syndrome and acute alcohol intoxication.

Certain Conditions Originating in the Perinatal Period

760.72 Noxious influences affecting fetus or newborn via placenta or breast milk, narcotics

Use code 760.72 to report fetal or newborn conditions caused by maternal ingestion of narcotics during pregnancy. Narcotics include opium, heroin, morphine, codeine, papaverine, and their many synthetics such as Demerol and methadone.

Signs and symptoms of narcotics abuse include drowsiness and "nodding," small or pinpoint pupils, urinary retention, shallow irregular respirations or apnea, and, in severe cases, hypotension, hypothermia, and pulmonary edema. Toxicology tests of blood or urine reveal the presence of narcotics. Therapies include drugs such as naloxone (Narcan).

This subclassification is used to report the effects of narcotics on the fetus or newborn. It excludes drug withdrawal syndrome, which is classified to code 779.5. Note that some newborns may suffer from both drug withdrawal syndrome and other physiopathological effects of narcotics in the perinatal period such as acute intoxication; both conditions should be coded.

760.73 Noxious influences affecting fetus or newborn via placenta or breast milk, hallucinogenic agents

Use code 760.73 to report the fetal or newborn condition caused by maternal ingestion of hallucinogenic agents during pregnancy. Hallucinogenic agents include lysergide (LSD), mescaline, psilocybin, sodium thiopental (STP), marijuana, phencyclidine (PCP), tetrahydrocannabinol (THC), and hashish.

Signs and symptoms of using hallucinogenic agents include dilated pupils, restlessness, hyperreflexia, easy distractibility, and tachycardia. Toxicology tests of blood or urine reveal the presence of hallucinogenics. Therapies include drugs such as diazepam and ammonium chloride.

This subclassification is used to report the effects of hallucinogens on the fetus or newborn. It excludes drug withdrawal syndrome, which is classified to code 779.5. Medical literature indicates that, of all hallucinogens, only chronic marijuana abuse has been associated with drug withdrawal symptoms.

760.74 Noxious influences affecting fetus or newborn via placenta or breast milk, anti-infectives — *fetus affected by antibiotics or antifungals via placenta or breast milk*
AHA: Nov-Dec, 1984, 11; Q2, 1989, 14; Q3, 1990, 5; Q3, 1991, 21; Q2, 1992, 12; Q1, 1994, 8

Use code 760.74 to report a fetal or newborn condition caused by maternal ingestion of anti-infectives, such as antibiotics and antifungals, during pregnancy. Antibiotics that have been associated with birth defects include sulfonamides, metronidazole, and tetracycline as well as antibiotics that inhibit deoxyribonucleic acid (DNA) or ribonucleic acid (RNA) synthesis such as actinomycin D, mitomycin C, adenine arabinoside, and idoxuridine.

Associated conditions include nerve damage, inhibition of bone growth, discoloration of teeth due to demineralization of enamel, and connective tissue defects.

760.75 Noxious influences affecting fetus or newborn via placenta or breast milk, cocaine

The physician should document the specific effects of the mother's cocaine use on the newborn, that is, if the newborn exhibited manifestations or mortality, tested positive for cocaine, or is experiencing drug withdrawal syndrome.

Cocaine Addiction in Newborns: Two scenarios may present in newborns who are born to cocaine-addicted mothers. The newborn may exhibit no manifestations of the drug but test positive for cocaine. In this instance, code 760.75 *Cocaine affecting fetus or newborn via placenta or breast milk* is reported. However, the infant may experience drug withdrawal. In these instances, code 779.5 *Drug withdrawal syndrome in newborn* is reported.

Newborn Delivered by Cocaine Abuser/Dependent: When a newborn is affected by the mother's use of cocaine, specified as a cause of mortality or morbidity, or when the infant has a positive drug screen, assign code 760.75.

If the infant does not exhibit an associated complication or test positive for cocaine in a drug screen, code 760.75 is not assigned.

Signs and symptoms of cocaine use include hyperactivity, hyperthermia, tachycardia, dilated pupils, and, in severe cases, convulsions, coma, and circulatory collapse. Toxicology tests of blood or urine reveal the presence of cocaine.

Therapies include drugs such as diazepam or chlorpromazine.

Associated conditions include infant drug withdrawal, renal system anomalies, central nervous system anomalies, and sudden infant death syndrome (SIDS).

760.76	Noxious influences affecting fetus or newborn via placenta or breast milk, diethylstilbestrol [DES]
760.77	Noxious influences affecting fetus or newborn via placenta or breast milk, anticonvulsants — carbamazepine, phenobarbital, phenytoin, valproic acid AHA: Q4, 2005, 82

Many antiseizure medications are a teratogen, an agent that causes physical defects in the developing fetus when exposed in utero. In many cases, the mother must take medications during pregnancy to prevent other medical conditions from occurring that present hazards to the baby.

760.78	Noxious influences affecting fetus or newborn via placenta or breast milk, antimetabolic agents — methotrexate, retinoic acid, statins AHA: Q4, 2005, 83
760.79	Noxious influences affecting fetus or newborn via placenta or breast milk, other — fetus or newborn affected by immune sera, medicinal agents NEC, or toxic substance NEC AHA: Nov-Dec, 1984, 11; Q2, 1989, 14; Q3, 1990, 5; Q3, 1991, 21; Q2, 1992, 12; Q1, 1994, 8

These codes may be used regardless of the patient's age. For example, it is not uncommon for the daughters of women who ingested diethylstilbestrol (DES) during pregnancy to develop ovarian cancer from exposure to the drug through the placenta while in utero.

In addition, these codes may be used when the fetus or newborn shows signs and symptoms of acute intoxication of the noxious influence.

Excluded from these subclassifications are anesthetic and analgesic drugs administered during labor and delivery (763.5) and drug withdrawal syndrome in newborn (779.5).

760.8	Other specified maternal conditions affecting fetus or newborn — genital tract and other localized infection affecting fetus or newborn, but fetus or newborn manifesting that disease AHA: Nov-Dec, 1984, 11; Q2, 1989, 14; Q3, 1990, 5; Q2, 1992, 12; Q1, 1994, 8
760.9	Unspecified maternal condition affecting fetus or newborn

Coding Clarification
Excluded from this rubric is maternal endocrine and metabolic disorders affecting fetus or newborn (775.0-775.9).

Coding Scenario
A newborn male is delivered in the hospital to a mother who has a past history of cocaine abuse. The newborn has no manifestations from the drug abuse; however, the infant tests positive for cocaine.

Code assignment: V30.00 *Single liveborn, born in hospital, delivered without mention of cesarean delivery* and 760.75 *Cocaine affecting fetus or newborn via placenta or breast milk*

761 Fetus or newborn affected by maternal complications of pregnancy
AHA: Q2, 1989, 14; Q3, 1990, 5

761.0	Fetus or newborn affected by incompetent cervix of mother
761.1	Fetus or newborn affected by premature rupture of membranes of mother
761.2	Fetus or newborn affected by oligohydramnios

Coding Clarification
Associated conditions include Potter's syndrome, fetal urinary tract obstruction, intrauterine growth retardation, amniotic band syndrome, fetal compression, and fetal demise.

Use code 761.2 *Fetus or newborn affected by oligohydramnios* to report a fetus or newborn affected by the presence of less than 300 ml of amniotic fluid at term.

761.3	Fetus or newborn affected by polyhydramnios — hydramnios (acute) (chronic) AHA: Q2, 1989, 14; Q3, 1990, 5

Coding Clarification
Polyhydramnios is often associated with maternal diabetes; however, the cause is unknown in approximately a third of all cases.

Associated conditions include esophageal atresia, anencephaly, spinal bifida, and isoimmunization.

Use code 761.3 to report a fetus or newborn affected by the presence of an excessive amount of amniotic fluid during pregnancy.

761.4	Fetus or newborn affected by ectopic pregnancy of mother — abdominal, intraperitoneal, and tubal AHA: Q2, 1989, 14; Q3, 1990, 5

Coding Clarification
This condition frequently occurs when the mother has some type of infertility. The most frequent site of ectopic pregnancy is within the fallopian tube. It is rare for the fetus to complete the weeks of gestation necessary to be viable.

Use code 761.4 to report a fetus or newborn affected by implantation of the fertilized ovum in an area other than the uterus, for example, the cervix, uterine tube, ovary, or abdominal or pelvic cavity.

761.5	Fetus or newborn affected by multiple pregnancy of mother — *triplet, twin births* **AHA:** Q2, 1989, 14; Q3, 1990, 5
761.6	Fetus or newborn affected by maternal death
761.7	Fetus or newborn affected by malpresentation before labor — *breech presentation, external version, oblique lie, transverse lie, unstable lie* **AHA:** Q2, 1989, 14; Q3, 1990, 5
761.8	Fetus or newborn affected by other specified maternal complications of pregnancy — *spontaneous abortion, fetus* **AHA:** Q2, 1989, 14; Q3, 1990, 5
761.9	Fetus or newborn affected by unspecified maternal complication of pregnancy

762 Fetus or newborn affected by complications of placenta, cord, and membranes
AHA: Q2, 1989, 14; Q3, 1990, 5; Q1, 1994, 8

762.0   Fetus or newborn affected by placenta previa

Use code 762.0 to report a fetus or newborn affected by the implantation of the placenta over or near the internal os of the cervix. There are two forms of placental previa: total, in which the placenta completely covers the internal cervical os; and partial, in which the placenta covers a portion of the internal cervical os. Placenta previa often results in a fetus being delivered prior to term.

Associated conditions include prematurity, alveolar conditions, respiratory distress syndrome, inadequate or erratic brain perfusion, hypotension, blood pressure peaks, infections including meningitis and sepsis, and SGA.

762.1	Fetus or newborn affected by other forms of placental separation and hemorrhage — *abruptio placentae; antepartum hemorrhage; damage to placenta from amniocentesis; cesarean section or surgical induction; blood loss; premature separation of placenta; rupture of marginal sinus* **AHA:** Q2, 1989, 14; Q3, 1990, 5; Q1, 1994, 8
762.2	Fetus or newborn affected by other forms of other and unspecified morphological and functional abnormalities of placenta — *dysfunction, infarction, insufficiency; yellow vernix syndrome* **AHA:** Q2, 1989, 14; Q3, 1990, 5; Q1, 1994, 8
762.3	Fetus or newborn affected by placental transfusion syndromes — (Use additional code to indicate resultant condition in fetus or newborn: 772.0, 776.4) — *placental and cord abnormality resulting in twin-to-twin or other transplacental transfusion* **AHA:** Q2, 1989, 14; Q3, 1990, 5; Q1, 1994, 8
762.4	Fetus or newborn affected by prolapsed cord — *cord presentation* **AHA:** Q2, 1989, 14; Q3, 1990, 5; Q1, 1994, 8
762.5	Fetus or newborn affected by other compression of umbilical cord — *cord around neck; entanglement; knot, torsion* **AHA:** Q2, 1989, 14; Q3, 1990, 5; Q1, 1994, 8; Q2, 2003, 9
762.6	Fetus or newborn affected by other and unspecified conditions of umbilical cord — *short cord, thrombosis, varices, velamentous insertion, vasa previa* **AHA:** Q2, 1989, 14; Q3, 1990, 5; Q1, 1994, 8
762.7	Fetus or newborn affected by chorioamnionitis — *amnionitis, membranitis, placentitis* **AHA:** Q2, 1989, 14; Q3, 1990, 5; Q1, 1994, 8
762.8	Fetus or newborn affected by other specified abnormalities of chorion and amnion — *not elsewhere classified* **AHA:** Q2, 1989, 14; Q3, 1990, 5; Q1, 1994, 8
762.9	Fetus or newborn affected by unspecified abnormality of chorion and amnion

Coding Clarification
Report the cord compression or entanglement as a secondary diagnosis on the baby's record only if the cord compression affected the baby. Loose nuchal cord reduction without incident may be reported on the mother's record.

763 Fetus or newborn affected by other complications of labor and delivery
AHA: Q2, 1989, 14; Q3, 1990, 5; Q1, 1994, 8

763.0	Fetus or newborn affected by breech delivery and extraction
763.1	Fetus or newborn affected by other malpresentation, malposition, and disproportion during labor and delivery — *abnormality of bony pelvis, contracted pelvis, persistent occipitoposterior position, shoulder presentation, transverse lie* **AHA:** Q2, 1989, 14; Q3, 1990, 5; Q1, 1994, 8
763.2	Fetus or newborn affected by forceps delivery — *fetus or newborn affected by forceps extraction* **AHA:** Q2, 1989, 14; Q3, 1990, 5; Q1, 1994, 8
763.3	Fetus or newborn affected by delivery by vacuum extractor
763.4	Fetus or newborn affected by cesarean delivery
763.5	Fetus or newborn affected by maternal anesthesia and analgesia — *reactions and intoxications from maternal opiates and tranquilizers during labor and delivery* **AHA:** Q2, 1989, 14; Q3, 1990, 5; Q1, 1994, 8
763.6	Fetus or newborn affected by precipitate delivery — *rapid second stage* **AHA:** Q2, 1989, 14; Q3, 1990, 5; Q1, 1994, 8
763.7	Fetus or newborn affected by abnormal uterine contractions — *fetus or newborn affected by contraction ring, hypertonic labor, hypotonic uterine dysfunction, uterine inertia or dysfunction* **AHA:** Q2, 1989, 14; Q3, 1990, 5; Q1, 1994, 8

763.81	Abnormality in fetal heart rate or rhythm before the onset of labor	
763.82	Abnormality in fetal heart rate or rhythm during labor	
763.83	Abnormality in fetal heart rate or rhythm, unspecified as to time of onset	
763.84	Meconium passage during delivery AHA: Q4, 2005, 83	

Meconium consists of the baby's first fecal material. Nearly 20 percent of infants pass meconium. Twenty to 30 percent of those will inhale meconium while still in utero or with their first breath. Depending on the amount aspirated and the viscosity, the baby's lungs can become blocked, initiating an inflammatory response and causing lung problems of differing severity. Often the baby passes meconium without incident. Not all infants who pass meconium will aspirate it, nor will they develop meconium aspiration syndrome.

763.89	Other specified complications of labor and delivery affecting fetus or newborn — *fetus or newborn affected by abnormality of maternal soft tissues, destructive operation on live fetus to facilitate delivery, induction of labor (medical), previous surgery to uterus or pelvic organs* AHA: Q2, 1989, 14; Q3, 1990, 5; Q1, 1994, 8; Q4, 1998, 46
763.9	Unspecified complication of labor and delivery affecting fetus or newborn

764–779 Other Conditions Originating in the Perinatal Period

764 Slow fetal growth and fetal malnutrition
AHA: Q2, 1989, 15; Q2, 1991, 19; Q1, 1994, 8; Q4, 2002, 63; Q3, 2004, 4

This category reports conditions in which the fetus is considerably below the normal weight of offspring of the same gestational age. Malnutrition in a fetus may be due to defective assimilation or utilization of foods or to a maternal diet that is unbalanced or insufficient. Other factors that may cause an infant to be light for dates are genetic disorders, drugs, small maternal stature, placenta previa, multiple pregnancies, hypertension, anemia, and renal disease.

This condition may be described with such terms as "small for gestational age," "low birth weight," or "intrauterine growth retardation" (IUGR).

Associated conditions include genetic disorders such as Down's syndrome, Edwards' syndrome, autosomal trisomy, and Turner syndrome.

The following fifth-digit subclassification is for use with categories 764-765 to denote birthweight:

0 unspecified
1 less than 500 grams (less than 1.1 lbs)
2 500-749 grams (1.11 to 1.67 lbs)
3 750-999 grams (1.68 to 2.23 lbs)
4 1000-1249 grams (2.24 to 2.78 lbs)
5 1250-1499 grams (2.79 to 3.34 lbs)
6 1500-1749 grams (3.35 to 3.9 lbs)
7 1750-1999 grams (3.91 to 4.5 lbs)
8 2000-2499 grams (4.51 to 5.59 lbs)
9 2500 grams or more (5.6 lbs and over)

764.0 ✓5th	"Light-for-dates" without mention of fetal malnutrition — *infants underweight for gestational age; "small for dates"* AHA: Q2, 1989, 15; Q2, 1991, 19; Q1, 1994, 8; Q4, 2002, 63
764.1 ✓5th	"Light-for-dates" with signs of fetal malnutrition — *infants "light-for-dates;" infant showing signs of fetal malnutrition, such as dry peeling skin and loss of subcutaneous tissue; intrauterine malnutrition* AHA: Q2, 1989, 15; Q2, 1991, 19; Q1, 1994, 8; Q4, 2002, 63
764.2 ✓5th	Fetal malnutrition without mention of "light-for-dates" — *infants, not underweight for gestational age, showing signs of fetal malnutrition, such as dry peeling skin and loss of subcutaneous tissue; intrauterine malnutrition* AHA: Q2, 1989, 15; Q2, 1991, 19; Q1, 1994, 8; Q4, 2002, 63
764.9 ✓5th	Unspecified fetal growth retardation — *intrauterine growth retardation; undeveloped fetus or newborn* AHA: Q2, 1989, 15; Q2, 1991, 19; Q1, 1994, 8; Q4, 2002, 63

765 Disorders relating to short gestation and unspecified low birthweight
AHA: Q2, 1989, 15; Q2, 1991, 19; Q1, 1994, 8; Q1, 1997, 6

Use this category to report short gestation and low birthweight disorders in a viable infant.

Associated conditions include alveolar conditions, respiratory distress syndrome, inadequate or erratic brain perfusion, hypotension, blood pressure peaks, infections including meningitis and sepsis, and SGA.

The following fifth-digit subclassification is for use with categories 764-765 to denote birthweight:

0 unspecified
1 less than 500 grams (less than 1.1 lbs)
2 500-749 grams (1.11 to 1.67 lbs)
3 750-999 grams (1.68 to 2.23 lbs)

4	1000-1249 grams (2.24 to 2.78 lbs)	
5	1250-1499 grams (2.79 to 3.34 lbs)	
6	1500-1749 grams (3.35 to 3.9 lbs)	
7	1750-1999 grams (3.91 to 4.5 lbs)	
8	2000-2499 grams (4.51 to 5.59 lbs)	
9	2500 grams or more (5.6 lbs and over)	

765.0 ✔sth Extreme fetal immaturity — (Use additional code for weeks of gestation: 765.20-765.29) — usually implies a birthweight of less than 1000 grams
AHA: Q2, 1989, 15; Q2, 1991, 19; Q1, 1994, 8; Q1, 1997, 6; Q4, 2002, 63; Q3, 2004, 4

765.1 ✔sth Other preterm infants — (Use additional code for weeks of gestation: 765.20-765.29) — usually implies a birthweight of 1000 to 2499 grams
AHA: Q2, 1989, 15; Q2, 1991, 19; Q1, 1994, 8; Q1, 1997, 6; Q4, 2002, 63; Q3, 2004, 4

765.20	Unspecified weeks of gestation
765.21	Less than 24 completed weeks of gestation
765.22	24 completed weeks of gestation
765.23	25-26 completed weeks of gestation
765.24	27-28 completed weeks of gestation
765.25	29-30 completed weeks of gestation
765.26	31-32 completed weeks of gestation
765.27	33-34 completed weeks of gestation
765.28	35-36 completed weeks of gestation
765.29	37 or more completed weeks of gestation

Coding Clarification
Weeks of gestation should be reported only for preterm infants, infants with extreme immaturity, and/or infants with slow fetal growth and malnutrition. Do not assign weeks of gestation codes for all newborns.

766 Disorders relating to long gestation and high birthweight

Category 766 reports disorders in a viable infant born after 42 weeks of gestation and/or described as "heavy," "large-for-dates," or greater than 4,500 grams birthweight.

766.0 Exceptionally large baby relating to long gestation — *implies a birthweight of 4500 grams or more*

Use code 766.0 to report an infant weighing over the 90th percentile for gestational age. Approximately 1 to 3 percent of neonates in the United States are considered large for gestational age. A baby may be exceptionally large when the mother has a large frame, is obese, or has diabetes. Associated conditions include hypoxia during labor and birth trauma.

766.1 Other "heavy-for-dates" infants not related to gestation period — *fetus or infant "heavy-" or "large-for-dates," regardless of period of gestation*

766.21 Post-term infant — *over 40 completed weeks to 42 completed weeks*
AHA: Q2, 2006, 12

766.22 Prolonged gestation of infant — *beyond 42 completed weeks of gestation, postmaturity*
AHA: Q2, 2006, 12

767 Birth trauma

The definition of birth trauma is injury to the fetus or newborn during delivery. Such injury may be due to breech presentation or forceps delivery.

767.0 Subdural and cerebral hemorrhage, birth trauma — (Use additional code to identify cause) — *due to birth trauma or to intrapartum anoxia or hypoxia; including subdural hematoma (localized), tentorial tear; secondary code to identify cause*

Subdural and cerebral hemorrhage is hemorrhage in or around the brain.

Signs and symptoms of subdural and cerebral hemorrhage include seizures, abnormally large head, diminished tone and/or resistance of skeletal muscles, retinal hemorrhage, positive transillumination of skull, or poor Moro's response (reaction to sudden loud noises).

Lab work reveals red blood cells in cerebral spinal fluid. A computed tomography (CT) scan of the head confirms the diagnosis.

Therapies include fluid removal by daily subdural taps.

Associated conditions include hypoxia while in utero, anoxia while in utero, and prematurity.

Excluded from this subcategory is intraventricular hemorrhage (772.10-772.14).

767.11 Birth trauma, Epicranial subaponeurotic hemorrhage (massive)

Epicranial subaponeurotic hemorrhage is the rupture of the emissary veins, connections between the dural sinuses and scalp veins. Blood accumulates in the space between the epicranial aponeurosis of the scalp and the periosteum, typically caused by vacuum extraction during delivery. The aponeurosis is a structure that connects the frontal and occipital bellies of the occipitofrontalis muscle and epicranial.

767.19 Birth trauma, Other injuries to scalp

Injuries to the scalp include caput succedaneum, subgaleal hemorrhage, and cephalhematoma. Caput succedaneum, edema of the presenting portion of the scalp, usually is a mild trauma resulting from the pressure of the fetal scalp against the uterine cervix during labor and delivery. Subgaleal hemorrhage is a greater trauma manifested by a boggy feeling over the entire scalp, and cephalhematoma is hemorrhage of the periosteum of the skull.

767.2	Fracture of clavicle, birth trauma
767.3	Other injuries to skeleton, birth trauma — *fracture of long bones, skull*
767.4	Injury to spine and spinal cord, birth trauma — *dislocation, fracture, laceration, rupture*
767.5	Facial nerve injury, birth trauma — *facial palsy, Bell's paralysis of newborn*
767.6	Injury to brachial plexus, birth trauma — *brachial, Erb (-Duchenne), and Klumpke (-Déjérine) paralysis or palsy*

Use code 767.6 to report injury of the brachial plexus nerve during delivery. Damage of this nerve can affect the muscles of the arm and shoulder.

767.7	Other cranial and peripheral nerve injuries, birth trauma — *phrenic nerve paralysis*
767.8	Other specified birth trauma — *eye damage; hematoma or liver (subcapsular), testes, vulva; rupture of liver, spleen; scalpel wound; traumatic glaucoma; hematoma of sternocleidomastoid; ruptured stomach due to injury at birth; ruptured viscera; torticollis due to birth injury*
767.9	Unspecified birth trauma — *birth injury NOS*

768 Intrauterine hypoxia and birth asphyxia
AHA: Q4, 1992, 20

Use codes in category 768 to report reduction of oxygen resulting in impending or actual cessation of life. The condition may be brought on by events such as acute blood loss, aspiration of meconium, or a tight nuchal cord.

Signs and symptoms of intrauterine hypoxia and birth asphyxia include low Apgar score, pale or cyanotic color, poor or absent respirations, and poor reflexes and muscle tone. Fetal monitor shows irregular heart rhythm. Blood gases show hypercapnia and hypoxia. Therapies include endotracheal intubation and ventilation, and IV fluids with glucose.

Associated conditions include hypoglycemia, respiratory or metabolic acidosis, coma and seizures due to anoxic brain damage, fluid retention and hyponatremia due to acute tubular necrosis, sepsis, and bowel disorders, such as necrotizing enterocolitis.

Neonatal encephalopathy is defined clinically based on a variety of factors, including abnormalities in consciousness, tone and reflexes, feeding, respirations, or seizures. These factors may result from many conditions, which may or may not result in permanent neurologic impairment, and poor outcomes may occur secondary to events occurring before or after delivery.

Hypoxic-ischemic encephalopathy (HIE) is only one form of neonatal encephalopathy and is defined as neonatal encephalopathy with intrapartum hypoxia and the lack of any other abnormality. Over 75 percent of neonatal encephalopathy cases have no clinical signs of intrapartum hypoxia. Per the ACOG/AAP report, evidence suggests that true HIE occurs in only one to two of every 10,000 births.

HIE is an acquired condition distinguished by clinical and laboratory evidence of acute brain injury due to asphyxia. Many factors can produce neurologic symptoms in the immediate newborn period that resemble those of HIE. These include prepartum and postpartum ischemia and hypoxemia, prenatal strokes, intrauterine infections, cerebral malformations, genetic factors, metabolic or autoimmune disease, and maternal drug use. The clinical features of neonatal HIE are often nonspecific; therefore, thorough examination of historical, physical-neurologic, and laboratory data are necessary for diagnosis.

Diagnostic tools include laboratory studies of blood and cerebrospinal fluids, electroencephalogram, evoked potential testing, technetium scanning, intracranial pressure (ICP) monitoring, and radiographic studies including cranial CT, ultrasonography of the head, MRI, and magnetic resonance spectroscopy.

Following the diagnosis of HIE, treatment is essentially supportive and symptomatic. Respiratory support is often necessary. Common comorbidities such as seizures and hypocalcemia require appropriate treatment. Patients with motor, speech, or cognitive disabilities require close follow-up, serial testing, and various therapy modalities, including occupational, physical, and speech therapy.

768.0	Fetal death from asphyxia or anoxia before onset of labor or at unspecified time — (Use only when associated with newborn morbidity classifiable elsewhere) — *secondary* AHA: Q4, 1992, 20
768.1	Fetal death from asphyxia or anoxia during labor — (Use only when associated with newborn morbidity classifiable elsewhere) — *secondary* AHA: Q4, 1992, 20

Certain Conditions Originating in the Perinatal Peroid

768.2 Fetal distress before onset of labor, in liveborn infant — (Use only when associated with newborn morbidity classifiable elsewhere) — *secondary; fetal metabolic acidemia first noted during labor, in liveborn infant*
AHA: Q4, 1992, 20

Use code 768.2 to report hypoxia and acidosis affecting the functions of vital organs, such as the heart and lungs, of a fetus to the point of temporary injury, permanent injury, or death.

768.3 Fetal distress first noted during labor, in liveborn infant — (Use only when associated with newborn morbidity classifiable elsewhere)

768.4 Fetal distress, unspecified as to time of onset, in liveborn infant — (Use only when associated with newborn morbidity classifiable elsewhere) — *secondary, fetal metabolic acidemia unknown as to time of onset, in liveborn infant*
AHA: Nov-Dec, 1986, 10; Q4, 1992, 20

768.5 Severe birth asphyxia — (Use only when associated with newborn morbidity classifiable elsewhere) — *secondary; birth asphyxia with neurologic involvement*
AHA: Nov-Dec, 1986, 3; Q4, 1992, 20

768.6 Mild or moderate birth asphyxia — (Use only when associated with newborn morbidity classifiable elsewhere) — *secondary;*
AHA: Nov-Dec, 1986, 3; Q4, 1992, 20

768.7 Hypoxic-ischemic encephalopathy — *HIE*

768.9 Unspecified birth asphyxia in liveborn infant — (Use only when associated with newborn morbidity classifiable elsewhere) — *anoxia NOS, asphyxia NOS, hypoxia NOS*
AHA: Q4, 1992, 20

Documentation Issues

HIE is a well-defined condition that is established by the physician and should be documented in the medical record. Assign code 768.7 *Hypoxic-ischemic encephalopathy* when the documentation and diagnosis indicate ischemic injury of the brain due to prenatal or perinatal asphyxia. Severe birth asphyxia (768.5) may result in neurologic manifestations. Asphyxia is defined as pathological changes due to lack of oxygen and is not a diagnosis of acute ischemic injury of the brain.

769 Respiratory distress syndrome in newborn
AHA: Nov-Dec, 1986, 6; Q1, 1989, 10

Use code 769 to report insufficient lung maturity of the fetus or newborn resulting in severe hypoxemia and multiple organ failure or death if left untreated. Also known as hyaline membrane disease and respiratory distress syndrome of the premature infant, this condition occurs primarily in premature infants (before completion of 37 weeks of gestation) or infants whose mothers are diabetic. It also may develop in infants whose mothers have toxemia or hypertension.

Signs and symptoms of respiratory distress syndrome include rapid labored respirations, substernal retractions, nasal alae flaring and "grunting" retractions, and low Apgar scores. Chest x-ray shows diffuse pulmonary atelectasis with overdistended alveolar ducts; blood gases show hypoxia. Therapies include IV fluids and electrolytes, oxygen therapy via nasal prongs, facemask, nasopharyngeal tube and endotracheal tube, and ventilation (CPAP, IPPV, and PEEP).

Associated conditions include respiratory or metabolic acidosis, hypoxemia, multiple organ failure, and atelectasis.

This category includes Type I respiratory distress syndrome or distress of the newborn. Type II respiratory distress syndrome or distress of the newborn is reported with 770.6, as is transient tachypnea of newborn.

770 Other respiratory conditions of fetus and newborn

770.0 Congenital pneumonia — *infective pneumonia acquired prenatally*
AHA: Q1, 2005, 10

770.10 Fetal and newborn aspiration, unspecified — *aspiration of contents of birth canal NOS;*
AHA: Q4, 2005, 83

Meconium consists of the baby's first fecal material. In a distressed state, the baby's intestinal activity increases, relaxing the anal sphincter, and passing the first bowel movement. Fetal distress during labor is a common cause of meconium aspiration. Nearly 20 percent of infants pass meconium. Twenty to 30 percent of those will inhale meconium while still in utero or with their first breath. Depending on the amount aspirated, the viscosity, and how deeply inhaled, the baby's lungs can become blocked, initiating an inflammatory response and causing severe lung problems. Aspiration does not necessarily develop into respiratory problems or meconium aspiration syndrome, which is generally defined as the presence of meconium below the vocal cords, causing respiratory problems, occurring in approximately 4 percent of deliveries with meconium staining.

Signs and symptoms of meconium aspiration include dark green streaks or colored stains in the amniotic fluid or coating the newborn; low Apgar score; rapid, labored, or suspended breathing; cyanosis; or limpness.

Code	Description
770.11	Meconium aspiration without respiratory symptoms — *meconium aspiration NOS* **AHA:** Q4, 2005, 83
770.12	Meconium aspiration with respiratory symptoms — *(Use additional code to identify any secondary pulmonary hypertension, 416.8, if applicable)* — *pneumonia or pneumonitis from meconium aspiration, meconium aspiration syndrome NOS, presence of meconium below the vocal cords* **AHA:** Q4, 2005, 83
770.13	Aspiration of clear amniotic fluid without respiratory symptoms **AHA:** Q4, 2005, 83
770.14	Aspiration of clear amniotic fluid with respiratory symptoms — *(Use additional code to identify any secondary pulmonary hypertension, 416.8, if applicable)* — *pneumonia or pneumonitis from clear amniotic fluid aspiration* **AHA:** Q4, 2005, 83

Aspiration of amniotic fluid and other birth canal contents can occur without the presence of meconium.

Code	Description
770.15	Aspiration of blood without respiratory symptoms **AHA:** Q4, 2005, 83
770.16	Aspiration of blood with respiratory symptoms — *(Use additional code to identify any secondary pulmonary hypertension, 416.8, if applicable)* — *pneumonia or pneumonitis from blood aspiration* **AHA:** Q4, 2005, 83
770.17	Other fetal and newborn aspiration without respiratory symptoms **AHA:** Q4, 2005, 83
770.18	Other fetal and newborn aspiration with respiratory symptoms — *(Use additional code to identify any secondary pulmonary* **AHA:** Q4, 2005, 83
770.2	Interstitial emphysema and related conditions of newborn — *pneumomediastinum, pneumopericardia, and pneumothorax originating in the perinatal period*
770.3	Pulmonary hemorrhage of fetus or newborn — *hemorrhage of alveolar, intraalveolar, and massive pulmonary originating in the perinatal period*
770.4	Primary atelectasis of newborn — *pulmonary immaturity NOS*
770.5	Other and unspecified atelectasis of newborn — *atelectasis NOS, partial, and secondary originating in the perinatal period; pulmonary collapse*
770.6	Transitory tachypnea of newborn — *idiopathic tachypnea, wet lung syndrome* **AHA:** Nov-Dec, 1986, 6; Q1, 1989, 10; Q3, 1993, 7; Q1, 1994, 12; Q4, 1995, 4
770.7	Chronic respiratory disease arising in the perinatal period — *bronchopulmonary dysplasia, interstitial pulmonary fibrosis of prematurity, Wilson-Mikity syndrome, bubbly lung syndrome* **AHA:** Nov-Dec, 1986, 11; Q2, 1991, 19
770.81	Primary apnea of newborn — *apneic spells NOS, essential and sleep apnea of newborn* **AHA:** Q2, 1996, 10; Q2, 1998, 10; Q4, 2002, 65
770.82	Other apnea of newborn — *obstructive apnea of newborn* **AHA:** Q2, 1996, 10; Q2, 1998, 10; Q4, 2002, 65
770.83	Cyanotic attacks of newborn
770.84	Respiratory failure of newborn — *excluding respiratory distress syndrome (769)* **AHA:** Q2, 1996, 10; Q2, 1998, 10; Q4, 2002, 65
770.85	Aspiration of postnatal stomach contents without respiratory symptoms **AHA:** Q4, 2005, 83
770.86	Aspiration of postnatal stomach contents with respiratory symptoms — *(Use additional code to identify any secondary pulmonary hypertension, 416.8, if applicable)* — *pneumonia or pneumonitis from postnatal stomach contents aspiration* **AHA:** Q4, 2005, 83
770.87	Respiratory arrest of newborn

Apnea is the absence of spontaneous breathing from any cause. Prolonged apnea is also known as respiratory arrest and is a life-threatening condition that requires immediate medical intervention. Respiratory arrest in newborns is often a result of prematurity, although other contributing factors may include congenital abnormalities, birth injury, or genetic factors. Treatment often consists of endotracheal intubation and mechanical ventilation, CPAP, or ECMO (extracorporeal membrane oxygenation).

Code	Description
770.88	Hypoxemia of newborn — *hypoxia of newborn, not otherwise specified*

Hypoxemia (insufficient oxygen in the blood) and hypoxia (insufficient oxygen in the tissues) are other complications frequently seen in prematurity. Because of structural immaturity of the lungs and deficiencies in surfactant, a substance produced in the lungs that reduces the surface tension in the small airways and alveoli, premature infants are more susceptible to these conditions. Treatment may include supplemental oxygen or administration of a pulmonary vasodilator, such as tolazoline.

Code	Description
770.89	Other respiratory problems of newborn after birth
770.9	Unspecified respiratory condition of fetus and newborn

Coding Clarification

This rubric excludes codes for meconium passage during delivery (763.84) and meconium staining (779.84).

Subcategory 770.1 classifies conditions involving aspiration together. The new codes identify a range of possible occurrences and whether respiratory function or complications have developed as a result. Other and unspecified options are available to report unspecified or not elsewhere classifiable aspiration situations that require intervention. An instructional note throughout this code category prompts the coder to assign a separate code if secondary pulmonary hypertension (416.8) occurs as a complication of the aspiration.

Coding Scenario
A healthy 41-week post-term female infant is delivered with Apgar scores of 8 at 2 minutes, and 9 at 5 minutes. Meconium staining is noted in the amniotic fluid coating the infant. Routine direct laryngoscopy revealed no meconium in the respiratory tract. The baby is cleaned and taken to her mother.

> Code assignment: V30.00 *Single liveborn, born in hospital, delivered without mention of cesarean delivery,* 766.2 *Post-term infant,* and 779.84 *Meconium staining*

771 Infections specific to the perinatal period
AHA: Nov-Dec, 1985, 4

771.0	Congenital rubella — *congenital rubella pneumonitis*
	AHA: Nov-Dec, 1985, 4

Use code 771.0 to report a fetal infection of the virus rubella while in utero. Maternal rubella infection that occurs within a month before conception and through the second trimester is associated with newborn disease.

Signs and symptoms of congenital rubella include hepatosplenomegaly, "blueberry muffin" skin, and purpuric lesions. Lab work, such as immunofluorescence or enzyme immunoassays, reveals elevated antirubella IgM or IgG titers. Therapies include management of complications.

Associated conditions include hemolytic and hypoplastic anemia, pneumonia, meningoencephalitis, glaucoma and cataracts, thrombocytopenia, cardiac deformities such as patent ductus arteriosus, and other birth defects such as microcephaly and mental retardation.

771.1	Congenital cytomegalovirus infection — *congenital cytomegalic inclusion disease*
	AHA: Nov-Dec, 1985, 4

Code 771.1 reports fetal infection with cytomegalovirus (CMV), a member of the herpes virus family, while in utero.

This subcategory includes only congenital CMV infections; that is, those acquired up until the moment of birth, including passage through the birth canal. Noncongenital CMV infections of the newborn — for example, those acquired through breast milk, in the nursery or home, or through postnatal blood transfusion — are classified elsewhere.

771.2	Other congenital infection specific to the perinatal period — *herpes simplex, listeriosis, malaria, toxoplasmosis, tuberculosis* **AHA:** Nov-Dec, 1985, 4
771.3	Tetanus neonatorum — *tetanus omphalitis* **AHA:** Nov-Dec, 1985, 4
771.4	Omphalitis of the newborn — *infection of naval cord and umbilical stump* **AHA:** Nov-Dec, 1985, 4
771.5	Neonatal infective mastitis
771.6	Neonatal conjunctivitis and dacryocystitis — *ophthalmia neonatorum NOS* **AHA:** Nov-Dec, 1985, 4
771.7	Neonatal Candida infection — *neonatal moniliasis, thrush in newborn* **AHA:** Nov-Dec, 1985, 4
771.81	Septicemia (sepsis) of newborn — (Use additional code to identify organism)
771.82	Urinary tract infection of newborn — (Use additional code to identify organism)
771.83	Bacteremia of newborn — (Use additional code to identify organism)
771.89	Other infections specific to the perinatal period — (Use additional code to identify organism) — *intra-amniotic infection of fetus NOS, infection of newborn NOS* **AHA:** Nov-Dec, 1985, 4; Q4, 2002, 66

Coding Clarification
Newborn Sepsis: Code 771.81 *Septicemia [sepsis] of newborn*, should be assigned a secondary code from category 041 *Bacterial infections in conditions classified elsewhere and of unspecified site*, to identify the organism. A code from subcategory 995.9 *Systemic inflammatory response syndrome (SIRS)*, is not necessary on a newborn record. In addition, a code from category 038 *Septicemia*, should not be used on a newborn record.

Excluded from this rubric are congenital pneumonia (770.0), congenital syphilis (090.0-090.9), maternal infectious disease as a cause of mortality or morbidity in fetus or newborn, but fetus or newborn not manifesting the disease (760.2), ophthalmia neonatorum due to gonococcus (098.40), and other infections not specifically classified to this category.

772 Fetal and neonatal hemorrhage

Blood loss in this rubric is classified according to the site of hemorrhage. Typically, in fetal and neonatal hemorrhage, the infant will be hypotensive and pale. Hypovolemic shock should be corrected immediately.

772.0	Fetal blood loss — *fetal blood loss from cut end of co-twin's cord, placenta, ruptured cord, and vasa previa; exsanguination; hemorrhage into co-twin, mother's circulation*
772.10	Intraventricular hemorrhage, unspecified grade
772.11	Intraventricular hemorrhage, Grade I — *includes bleeding into germinal matrix* **AHA:** Q4, 1988, 8; Q3, 1992, 8; Q4, 2001, 49
772.12	Intraventricular hemorrhage, Grade II — *includes bleeding into ventricle* **AHA:** Q4, 1988, 8; Q3, 1992, 8; Q4, 2001, 49
772.13	Intraventricular hemorrhage, Grade III — *includes bleeding with enlargement of ventricle* **AHA:** Q4, 1988, 8; Q3, 1992, 8; Q4, 2001, 49; Q4, 2001, 51
772.14	Intraventricular hemorrhage, Grade IV — *includes bleeding into cerebral cortex* **AHA:** Q4, 1988, 8; Q3, 1992, 8; Q4, 2001, 49
772.2	Fetal and neonatal subarachnoid hemorrhage of newborn — *from any perinatal cause*
772.3	Umbilical hemorrhage after birth — *slipped umbilical ligature*
772.4	Fetal and neonatal gastrointestinal hemorrhage
772.5	Fetal and neonatal adrenal hemorrhage
772.6	Fetal and neonatal cutaneous hemorrhage — *bruising, ecchymoses, petechiae, superficial hematoma in fetus or newborn*
772.8	Other specified hemorrhage of fetus or newborn — *hemopericardium, homothorax of newborn*
772.9	Unspecified hemorrhage of newborn

Coding Clarification
Excluded from this rubric are hematological disorders of the fetus and newborn (776.0-776.9).

773 Hemolytic disease of fetus or newborn, due to isoimmunization

In isoimmunization, the mother develops antibodies against an antigen derived from a genetically dissimilar fetus.

773.0	Hemolytic disease due to Rh isoimmunization of fetus or newborn — *premature destruction of red blood cells due to incompatibility of Rh fetal-maternal blood grouping and positive Coombs test; including anemia, erythroblastosis, hemolytic disease, jaundice due to Rh antibodies, isoimmunization, and maternal/fetal incompatibility; Rh hemolytic disease, Rh isoimmunization*

Code 773.0 reports incompatibility that occurs when an Rh-negative mother carries an Rh-positive fetus. Antibodies cross the placenta into the fetus and lead to hemolysis of the fetal blood.

Signs and symptoms of hemolytic disease due to Rh isoimmunization include scalp edema, cardiomegaly, hepatomegaly, splenomegaly, pale skin, and severe generalized edema.

Associated conditions include erythroblastosis fetalis, hydrops fetalis, ascites, polyhydramnios, pleural effusion, heart failure, anemia, and asphyxia during delivery due to an enlarged liver.

773.1	Hemolytic disease due to abo isoimmunization of fetus or newborn — *ABO hemolytic disease, ABO isoimmunization; anemia, erythroblastosis, hemolytic disease, jaundice due to ABO antibodies, isoimmunization, maternal/fetal incompatibility* **AHA:** Q3, 1992, 8

Use code 773.1 to report incompatibility that occurs when a mother with blood type O carries a fetus with blood type A or B. Antibodies cross the placenta into the fetus and cause hemolysis of the fetal blood.

Signs and symptoms of hemolytic disease due to ABO isoimmunization include scalp edema, cardiomegaly, hepatomegaly, splenomegaly, pale skin, and severe generalized edema.

Associated conditions include erythroblastosis fetalis, hydrops fetalis, ascites, polyhydramnios, pleural effusion, heart failure, anemia, and asphyxia during delivery due to an enlarged liver.

773.2	Hemolytic disease due to other and unspecified isoimmunization of fetus or newborn — *erythroblastosis NOS, hemolytic disease NOS, jaundice or anemia due to unknown blood-group incompatibility* **AHA:** Q1, 1994, 13
773.3	Hydrops fetalis due to isoimmunization — (Use additional code to identify type of isoimmunization: 773.0-773.2) — *secondary to identify type of isoimmunization*

Use code 773.3 to report gross edema of the entire body of the fetus with associated anemia due to mother-fetus blood incompatibility. The condition has a high mortality rate, especially in premature infants. Blood work reveals mother-fetus Rh and ABO incompatibility. Therapies include exchange blood transfusions, resuscitation and mechanical ventilation at birth, and thoracentesis.

Associated conditions include erythroblastosis fetalis, respiratory failure, pleural effusion, alloimmune hemolytic anemia, high output cardiac failure, and hypoproteinemia.

773.4	Kernicterus due to isoimmunization of fetus or newborn — (Use additional code to identify type of isoimmunization: 773.0-773.2) — *secondary to identify type of isoimmunization*

Kernicterus is a significantly large accumulation of bilirubin in the brain that may result in brain damage because of an incompatibility of fetal and maternal blood.

Signs and symptoms of kernicterus due to isoimmunization include jaundice, high fever, seizures, blunted Moro reflex, opisthotonic posturing, incomplete flexion of extremities, vomiting, and high-pitched cry. Therapies include phototherapy and exchange blood transfusions.

Associated conditions include mental retardation and hemolytic disease.

773.5	Late anemia due to isoimmunization of fetus or newborn

Documentation Issues
Abnormal Bilirubin: When a laboratory result indicates an elevation of the bilirubin, but the medical record lacks evidence that the infant was treated, these abnormal findings should not be coded. The physician can be queried to determine if jaundice was present.

Coding Clarification
Due to Blood-group Incompatibility: When the documentation specifies that the infant has jaundice due to blood-group incompatibility, code 773.1 *Hemolytic disease due to ABO isoimmunization* should be reported. Do not use codes 774.2 or 774.6 as additional codes because code 773.1 already includes jaundice.

Preterm Jaundice: This condition is a form of jaundice identified in an infant born before the completion of 36 weeks gestation. When the medical record documentation indicates this condition, code 774.2 *Neonatal jaundice associated with preterm delivery* should be reported.

Positive Coombs Test in a Newborn: If the physician documents the lab results, then assign the code for nonspecific findings on examination of blood. A definitive diagnosis of hemolytic disease in a newborn is based upon several criteria, only one of which is positive Coombs. Do not code based on abnormal lab results.

774 Other perinatal jaundice
Jaundice is also known as hyperbilirubinemia, which refers to the excess of bilirubin. The excess bilirubin may be caused by an overproduction of bilirubin, an impaired ability to secrete bilirubin, or a mixture of both causes.

774.0	Perinatal jaundice from hereditary hemolytic anemias — (Code first underlying disease: 282.0-282.9) — *secondary to underlying disease*
774.1	Perinatal jaundice from other excessive hemolysis — (Use additional code to identify cause) — *secondary to identify cause; including jaundice from bruising, drugs or toxins transmitted from mother, infection, polycythemia, swallowed maternal blood*
774.2	Neonatal jaundice associated with preterm delivery — *hyperbilirubinemia of prematurity; jaundice due to delayed conjugation associated with preterm delivery* **AHA:** Q3, 1991, 21
774.30	Neonatal jaundice due to delayed conjugation, cause unspecified — *Lucey-Driscoll syndrome*
774.31	Neonatal jaundice due to delayed conjugation in diseases classified elsewhere — (Code first underlying disease: 243, 277.4) — *secondary to underlying disease*
774.39	Other neonatal jaundice due to delayed conjugation from other causes — *jaundice due to delayed conjugation from causes such as breast milk inhibitors and delayed development of conjugating system*
774.4	Perinatal jaundice due to hepatocellular damage — *fetal or neonatal hepatitis, giant cell hepatitis, inspissated bile syndrome*
774.5	Perinatal jaundice from other causes — (Code first underlying cause: 271.1, 277.00-277.09, 751.61) — *Code first underlying cause, as: 271.1, 277.00-277.09, 751.61*
774.6	Unspecified fetal and neonatal jaundice — *icterus neonatorum, neonatal hyperbilirubinemia (transient), physiologic jaundice NOS* **AHA:** Q2, 1989, 15; Q1, 1994, 13
774.7	Kernicterus of fetus or newborn not due to isoimmunization — *bilirubin encephalopathy, kernicterus of newborn NOS*

Documentation Issues
When a laboratory result indicates an elevation of the bilirubin, but the medical record lacks evidence that the infant was treated, these abnormal findings should not be coded. The physician can be queried to determine if jaundice was present.

Coding Clarification
Use code 774.7 to report a significantly large accumulation of bilirubin in the brain that may result in brain damage not due to a fetal/maternal blood incompatibility (ABO incompatibility). The condition may be caused by a large influx of red blood cells through the umbilicus at the time of delivery.

Signs and symptoms of kernicterus not due to isoimmunization include jaundice, high fever, seizures, blunted Moro reflex, opisthotonic posturing, incomplete flexion of the extremities, vomiting, and high-pitched cry. Therapies include phototherapy and exchange blood transfusions. Associated conditions include mental retardation.

Due to Blood-group Incompatibility: When the documentation specifies that the infant has jaundice due to blood-group incompatibility, code 773.1 *Hemolytic disease due to ABO isoimmunization* should be reported. Do not use codes 774.2 or 774.6 as additional codes; code 773.1 already includes jaundice.

Preterm Jaundice: This condition is a form of jaundice identified in an infant born before the completion of 36 weeks gestation. When the medical record documentation indicates this condition, code 774.2 *Neonatal jaundice associated with preterm delivery* should be reported.

Coding Scenario
A 35-week-gestational age male is delivered via cesarean delivery. The physician indicates that the infant has preterm jaundice.

> Code assignment: V30.01 *Single liveborn, born in hospital, delivered by cesarean delivery* and 774.2 *Neonatal jaundice associated with preterm delivery*

775 Endocrine and metabolic disturbances specific to the fetus and newborn

This rubric includes transitory endocrine and metabolic disturbances caused by the infant's response to maternal endocrine and metabolic factors, the infant's removal from them, or the infant's adjustment to extrauterine existence.

775.0	Syndrome of "infant of diabetic mother" — maternal diabetes mellitus affecting fetus or newborn (with hypoglycemia)
	AHA: Q3, 1991, 5; Q1, 2004, 7-8

This code reports a syndrome with manifestations including macrosomia, birth asphyxia, hypoglycemia, cardiorespiratory disorders, and congenital malformations.

Signs and symptoms of syndrome of "infant of a diabetic mother" include large size (macrosomia), obesity, listlessness, limpness, poor feeding, and red florid complexion due to excessive amount of blood.

775.1	Neonatal diabetes mellitus — *diabetes mellitus syndrome in newborn*
	AHA: Q3, 1991, 6
775.2	Neonatal myasthenia gravis
775.3	Neonatal thyrotoxicosis — *hyperthyroidism (transient)*
775.4	Hypocalcemia and hypomagnesemia of newborn — *cow's mile hypocalcemia, hypocalcemic tetany, hypoparathyroidism, phosphate-loading hypocalcemia*
775.5	Other transitory neonatal electrolyte disturbances — *dehydration*
	AHA: Q1, 2005, 9
775.6	Neonatal hypoglycemia
775.7	Late metabolic acidosis of newborn

Subcategory 775.8 reports other neonatal endocrine and metabolic disturbances. Neonatal acidosis and other forms of endocrine and metabolic disturbances are frequently associated with prematurity. Acidosis may be respiratory, with an elevated $PaCO_2$; metabolic, with a normal $PaCO_2$ but a negative base excess; or a combination of both. It may also be associated with hypoxemia, hypotension or poor tissue perfusion, anemia, infection or sepsis, or respiratory distress. Determination of a newborn's acid-base status may be made by arterial blood gas (ABG) or capillary blood gas. Treatment for respiratory acidosis involves ventilation management, while that for metabolic acidosis is often directed at the underlying cause.

775.81	Other acidosis of newborn — *acidemia; mixed metabolic and respiratory acidosis*
775.89	Other neonatal endocrine and metabolic disturbances — *transitory amino-acid metabolic disturbances*
775.9	Unspecified endocrine and metabolic disturbances specific to the fetus and newborn

Coding Clarification
An infant born to a diabetic mother that presents with one or more symptoms is considered to have the "syndrome." It is not necessary for the infant to exhibit multiple symptoms to be coded as such.

An asymptomatic infant born to a diabetic mother may be assigned a code indicating a family history of certain other conditions.

Large stature in a child with no definitive underlying cause, such as endocrine disorders, should be assigned 783.9. The physician must document that the large stature is abnormal and of clinical significance.

Fetal distress (768.2-768.4) is fetal metabolic acidemia due to hypoxia or asphyxia before or during labor and delivery. Fetal distress NOS is assigned code 768.4. These code assignments are intended to identify metabolic acidemia due to insufficient oxygenation before and during labor and delivery. Subcategory 775.8 describes mixed metabolic and respiratory acidosis of the newborn, not related directly to labor and delivery.

776 Hematological disorders of fetus and newborn

776.0	Hemorrhagic disease of newborn — *diathesis, vitamin K deficiency, Minot's disease*
776.1	Transient neonatal thrombocytopenia — *due to exchange transfusion, idiopathic maternal thrombocytopenia, isoimmunization*
776.2	Disseminated intravascular coagulation in newborn
776.3	Other transient neonatal disorders of coagulation — *transient coagulation defect, newborn*
776.4	Polycythemia neonatorum — *plethora; polycythemia due to donor twin transfusion, maternal-fetal transfusion*
776.5	Congenital anemia — *anemia following fetal blood loss*
776.6	Anemia of neonatal prematurity

Use code 776.6 to report anemia in a viable infant born before completing 37 weeks of gestation in which the number of erythrocytes per cu mm and the quantity of hemoglobin are reduced. The hemoglobin nadir for premature infants is 6.5-9.0 g/100 ml as opposed to 9.5-11.0 g/100 ml for term infants. The extent of the anemia is directly related to the birth weight.

Signs and symptoms of anemia of prematurity include tachycardia, tachypnea, poor feeding, apnea, and dyspnea. Lab work shows abnormally low hemoglobin. Therapies include packed red blood cells, particularly when blood removed for testing exceeds 10 percent of estimated volume, and iron supplement.

Associated conditions include alveolar conditions, respiratory distress syndrome, inadequate or erratic brain perfusion, hypotension, blood pressure peaks, and infections including meningitis and sepsis.

776.7	Transient neonatal neutropenia — *isoimmune and maternal transfer neutropenia*
776.8	Other specified transient hematological disorders of fetus or newborn — *other specified*
776.9	Unspecified hematological disorder specific to fetus or newborn

777 Perinatal disorders of digestive system

777.1	Fetal and newborn meconium obstruction — *congenital fecaliths, meconium ileus NOS, meconium plug syndrome, delayed passage of meconium*

Meconium obstruction is obstruction of the digestive tract due to the fetal tar-like meconium.

Signs and symptoms of meconium obstruction include no stools for the first 24 to 48 hours of life, abdominal distention, symptoms of distal intestinal obstruction and incomplete obstruction, and vomiting. Radiology tests, such as a contrast enema, locate the obstruction. Therapies include contrast enema (therapeutic) and saline enemas.

This subcategory includes meconium plug syndrome but excludes meconium ileus (277.01).

777.2	Neonatal intestinal obstruction due to inspissated milk
777.3	Neonatal hematemesis and melena due to swallowed maternal blood — *swallowed blood syndrome in newborn*
777.4	Transitory ileus of newborn
777.5	Necrotizing enterocolitis in fetus or newborn — *pseudomembranous enterocolitis in newborn*
777.6	Perinatal intestinal perforation — *meconium peritonitis*
777.8	Other specified perinatal disorder of digestive system — *other specified*
777.9	Unspecified perinatal disorder of digestive system

Excluded from this rubric is intestinal obstruction classifiable to 560.0-560.9.

778 Conditions involving the integument and temperature regulation of fetus and newborn

778.0	Hydrops fetalis not due to isoimmunization — *idiopathic hydrops*

Use this code to report gross edema of the entire body of the fetus with associated anemia. Nonimmune fetal hydrops can be caused by a wide variety of diseases and disorders involving many different body systems. The infant mortality rate is very high, particularly with premature infants. Therapies include vigorous resuscitation including mechanical ventilation at birth, thoracentesis for pleural effusion, and diuresis. Associated conditions include erythroblastosis fetalis, anemia, hypoproteinemia, respiratory failure, and pleural effusion.

Most diagnostic studies, such as fetal ultrasounds and maternal blood examination, are performed in utero and are not reported in the newborn's chart.

Excluded from this subclassification is hydrops fetalis due to isoimmunization (773.3).

778.1	Sclerema neonatorum — *subcutaneous fat necrosis, Underwood's disease*
778.2	Cold injury syndrome of newborn
778.3	Other hypothermia of newborn
778.4	Other disturbance of temperature regulation of newborn — *dehydration fever, environmentally-induced pyrexia, hyperthermia, transitory fever*
778.5	Other and unspecified edema of newborn — *edema neonatorum*
778.6	Congenital hydrocele — *congenital hydrocele of tunica vaginalis*

Use code 778.6 to report a collection of fluid in the tunica vaginalis of the testicle or along the spermatic cord, or a serous dilation of a cervical duct of an infant. Almost all neonatal hydroceles are communicating and close spontaneously.

Therapies include surgery to repair persistent hydrocele (lasting more than one year) by inguinal incision and ligation of sac.

778.7	Breast engorgement in newborn — *noninfective mastitis*
778.8	Other specified condition involving the integument of fetus and newborn — *urticaria neonatorum*
778.9	Unspecified condition involving the integument and temperature regulation of fetus and newborn

779 Other and ill-defined conditions originating in the perinatal period

779.0	Convulsions in newborn — *fits and seizures in newborn* **AHA:** Nov-Dec, 1994, 11
779.1	Other and unspecified cerebral irritability in newborn — *other and unknown*
779.2	Cerebral depression, coma, and other abnormal cerebral signs in fetus or newborn — *CNS dysfunction in newborn NOS*
779.3	Feeding problems in newborn — *regurgitation, slow feeding, and vomiting in newborn* **AHA:** Q2, 1989, 15
779.4	Drug reactions and intoxications specific to newborn — *Gray syndrome from chloramphenicol administration in newborn*

Use code 779.4 to report toxic conditions and adverse drug reactions in neonates, especially premature infants, caused by the body's immature detoxification and excretion mechanisms. Gray syndrome, or gray baby syndrome, is a condition caused by an infant's inability to efficiently conjugate and eliminate the antibiotic chloramphenicol.

779.5	Drug withdrawal syndrome in newborn — *drug withdrawal syndrome in infant of dependent mother* **AHA:** Q3, 1994, 6

Code 799.5 reports a syndrome in newborns adversely affected by mothers who are addicted to, or frequent abusers of, drugs. Narcotics, cocaine, and coca plant derivatives are the most frequently abused drugs capable of causing withdrawal symptoms in the newborn, but barbiturates, other tranquilizers, amphetamines, other stimulants, and other addictive substances can cause the syndrome.

Signs and symptoms of drug withdrawal syndrome in the newborn include irritability, tremulousness, tachypnea, vomiting or diarrhea, fever, and convulsions. Toxicology tests of blood or urine identify the drug. Therapies include close monitoring for seizure activity or arrhythmias, detoxification tailored for the drug of dependence, drugs such as phenytoin sodium (Dilantin) or phenobarbital for seizures, and exchange transfusions in emergencies.

Associated conditions include fetal alcohol syndrome, dehydration, hypocalcemia, and seizures.

779.6	Termination of pregnancy (fetus) — *fetal death due to induced abortion and termination of pregnancy*
779.7	Periventricular leukomalacia
779.81	Neonatal bradycardia
779.82	Neonatal tachycardia
779.83	Delayed separation of umbilical cord
779.84	Meconium staining **AHA:** Q4, 2005, 83, 88
779.85	Cardiac arrest of newborn

Cardiac arrest is defined as the cessation of cardiac mechanical activity, manifested by the inability to detect a central pulse, unresponsiveness, and apnea. Newborn cardiac arrest can be caused by multiple factors, including the use of beta-adrenergic antagonists for the control of high blood pressure in the mother, trauma, and congenital abnormalities. Revised neonatal resuscitation guidelines have recently been published by the American Heart Association, which apply to resuscitation for neonates undergoing the transition from intrauterine to extrauterine life and also to those who have completed this transition but require resuscitation during the first few days to months following birth.

779.89	Other specified conditions originating in the perinatal period — *(Use additional code to specify condition) — atheromatosis of colon, toxemia, uremia, Harlequin color change syndrome, hypertonicity of infancy, papyraceous fetus, strophulus* **AHA:** Q1, 1994, 15; Q4, 2002, 67; Q1, 2005, 9; Q2, 2005, 15; Q1, 2006, 18
779.9	Unspecified condition originating in the perinatal period — *congenital debility NOS, stillbirth NEC*

Coding Clarification
Cocaine Addiction in Newborns: Two scenarios may present in newborns who are born to cocaine-addicted mothers. The newborn may exhibit no manifestations of the drug but test positive for cocaine. In this instance, code 760.75 *Cocaine affecting fetus or newborn via placenta or breast milk* is reported. However, the infant may experience drug withdrawal. In these instances, code 779.5 *Drug withdrawal syndrome in newborn* is reported.

Meconium staining is found as dark green colored streaks or greenish tint in the amniotic fluid. When the baby has passed meconium before birth and been exposed to meconium in the amniotic fluid for a long time, it may be born with discolored, yellowish skin. Staining in the otherwise clear amniotic fluid or of the baby's skin is a sign that meconium aspiration may have occurred, but staining may be noted in the absence of other symptoms. Meconium aspiration must be determined by exam. Code 779.84 does not include meconium passage during delivery, which is coded to 763.84, or meconium aspiration, which is coded to 770.11 or 770.12.

Coding Scenario
A mother addicted to cocaine comes to the hospital and delivers a newborn that is in drug withdrawal.

Code assignment: V30.00 *Single liveborn, born in hospital, delivered without mention of cesarean delivery* and 779.5 *Drug withdrawal syndrome in newborn*

A healthy 41-week post-term female infant is delivered with Apgar scores of 8 at two minutes, and 9 at five minutes. Meconium staining is noted in the amniotic fluid coating the infant. Routine direct laryngoscopy revealed no meconium in the respiratory tract. The baby is cleaned and taken to her mother.

Code assignment: V30.00 *Single liveborn, born in hospital, delivered without mention of cesarean delivery*, 766.21 *Post-term infant*, and 779.84 *Meconium staining*

780–799

Symptoms, Signs, and Ill-Defined Conditions

This chapter includes symptoms, signs, and abnormal results of laboratory or other investigative procedures, as well as ill-defined conditions for which there are no other, more specific diagnoses classifiable elsewhere.

In general, codes from this chapter are used to report symptoms, signs, and ill-defined conditions that point with equal suspicion to two or more diagnoses or represent important problems in medical care that may affect management of the patient. In addition, this chapter provides codes to classify abnormal findings that are reported without a corresponding definitive diagnosis. Codes for such findings can be located in the alphabetic index under such terms as "Abnormal, abnormality, abnormalities," "Decrease, decreased," "Elevation," and "Findings, abnormal, without diagnosis."

Codes from this chapter also are used to report symptoms and signs that existed on initial encounter but proved to be transient and without a specified cause. Also included are provisional diagnoses for patients who fail to return for further investigation, cases referred elsewhere for further investigation before being diagnosed, and cases in which a more definitive diagnosis was not available for other reasons.

Do not assign a code from categories 780-799 when the symptoms, signs, and abnormal findings pertain to a definitive diagnosis. For example, a patient with acute appendicitis would not need additional codes for abdominal pain (rubric 789) and abdominal rigidity (789.4). These signs and symptoms are integral to acute appendicitis and add no value to the patient's coding profile when assigned as secondary codes.

However, you may use a code from this chapter to report symptoms, signs, and abnormal findings that pertain to a particular clinical diagnosis if they represent important problems in medical care. Such problems may be useful to record because they may affect length of stay or level of nursing care and/or monitoring. Such problems also may require additional diagnostic or clinical evaluation or may affect treatment plans. In these cases, list the definitive condition as the principal diagnosis and the symptoms secondarily.

List as a secondary diagnosis any symptoms, signs, and abnormal findings that are not integral to the principal diagnosis but provide important clinical information. For example, a patient with benign prostatic hypertrophy (rubric 600) admitted in acute urinary retention might have acute urinary retention listed as a secondary diagnosis (788.2). Acute urinary retention is not integral to the disease process for benign prostatic hypertrophy, but is an indication for catheterization or surgery. Acute urinary retention can be viewed as an "important medical problem" when the medical record documentation shows the need for clinical evaluation or diagnostic procedures to rule out pathology other than benign prostatic hypertrophy as the etiology. Therapeutic treatment (e.g., catheterization prior to surgery) includes increased nursing care and/or monitoring such as catheter care or extended length of hospital stay.

List as the principal diagnosis any symptoms, signs, and abnormal findings that, after study, cannot be attributed to a definitive diagnosis classifiable to another ICD-9-CM chapter. Also, list as the principal diagnosis any symptom, sign, or abnormal finding that points to contrasting or comparative diagnoses (e.g., it points with equal suspicion to two or more diagnoses). List the contrasting or comparative diagnoses as secondary.

780–789 Symptoms

The definition of a symptom is a subjective observation reported to the physician by the patient but not confirmed by the physician. These observations depart from the structure, function, or sensation that the patient normally experiences.

780 General symptoms
AHA: March-April, 1985, 3; Q2, 1990, 3; Q2, 1990, 5; Q2, 1990, 15; Q1, 1991, 12

These subclassifications report impaired consciousness due to dysfunction of the cerebral hemispheres, the upper brainstem, or both. These codes include coma, transient alteration of awareness, persistent vegetative state, and other alterations such as drowsiness, semicoma, somnolence, stupor, or suppressed or impaired awareness or unconsciousness.

Coma is a state of profound stupor or unconsciousness from which the patient cannot be aroused by external stimuli. The etiology may be trauma, intracranial neoplasm, infection and toxic reaction to infection, poisoning and adverse effects of drugs and chemicals, hypertensive and atherosclerotic cerebrovascular disease, or thrombosis.

Transient alteration of awareness refers to symptoms of staring or transient loss of awareness. This condition has been associated with migraines, epileptic seizures, transient ischemic attacks, or psychological disorders, but in many cases the etiology is unknown.

Lab work may identify the cause based on blood work (hematocrit, respiratory gases, WBC, BUN), urinalysis (sugar, acetone, albumin, sedatives), and levels of glucose, sodium, potassium, bicarbonate, chloride, alcohol, and bromide. A gastric lavage reveals suspected poisoning. A lumbar puncture (if infection is suspected as the etiology) and culture identify the presence of white blood cells and the infective organism.

Therapies depend on etiology and may include, if the cause is unknown, temperature, pulse, respirations and blood pressure checked at frequent intervals, and glucose infusion.

Associated conditions include epidural/subdural hematoma, cerebral infarct or hemorrhage, brain tumor or abscess, brain stem infarction, tumor, hemorrhage, trauma, concussion, cerebral lacerations or contusion, cardiac arrhythmia, shock, epilepsy, infection, subarachnoid hemorrhage, catatonia, hypoglycemia, and diabetic acidosis.

780.01 Coma — *persistent unconsciousness*
AHA: March-April, 1985, 3; Q2, 1990, 3; Q2, 1990, 5; Q2, 1990, 15; Q1, 1991, 12; Q4, 1992, 20; Q3, 1996, 16

780.02 Transient alteration of awareness — *alternating states of consciousness and unconsciousness*
AHA: March-April, 1985, 3; Q2, 1990, 3; Q2, 1990, 5; Q2, 1990, 15; Q1, 1991, 12; Q4, 1992, 20

780.03 Persistent vegetative state — *awake without consciousness*
AHA: March-April, 1985, 3; Q2, 1990, 3; Q2, 1990, 5; Q2, 1990, 15; Q1, 1991, 12; Q4, 1992, 20

780.09 Other alteration of consciousness — *not specified elsewhere, including drowsiness, semicoma, somnolence, stupor*
AHA: March-April, 1985, 3; Q2, 1990, 3; Q2, 1990, 5; Q2, 1990, 15; Q1, 1991, 12; Q4, 1992, 20

780.1 Hallucinations — *auditory, visual, gustatory, olfactory, tactile*
AHA: March-April, 1985, 3; Q2, 1990, 3; Q2, 1990, 5; Q2, 1990, 15; Q1, 1991, 12

Use code 780.1 to report sensory perception of an object or event without corresponding external stimuli. Hallucinations generally take one of five forms, as follows:

- Auditory (perception of nonexistent voices or sounds)
- Visual (perception of nonexistent people, places, or other visual stimuli such as flashes of light)
- Olfactory (perception of nonexistent odors)
- Tactile (perception of nonexistent contact stimuli such as crawling insects on skin)
- Gustatory (perception of unpleasant tastes)

Hallucinations may be due to drugs or toxic substances or due to chronic conditions such as schizophrenia, depression, bipolar affective disorders, and organic brain syndromes.

780.2 Syncope and collapse — *blackout, fainting, Gower's syndrome*
AHA: March-April, 1985, 3; Nov-Dec, 1985, 12; Q2, 1990, 3; Q2, 1990, 5; Q2, 1990, 15; Q1, 1991, 12; Q3, 1995, 14; Q3, 2000, 12; Q1, 2002, 6

Signs and symptoms of syncope and collapse include motionlessness, paleness, diaphoresis, weak pulse, and shallow breathing. Physical exam reveals hypotension and postural changes in heart rate and blood pressure. Lab work may show elevated fasting blood sugar (confirming hyperglycemia) and elevated cardiac serum isoenzyme (identifying acute myocardial infarction). Hematocrit may detect anemia. An electrocardiogram (EKG) may suggest

Symptoms, Signs, and Ill-Defined Conditions

arrhythmia, conduction abnormality, ventricular hypertrophy, or myocardial infarction. A computed tomography (CT) scan of the head and brain confirms focal neurological deficit or intracranial process. Therapies depend on the etiology.

Associated conditions include seizure disorder, arrhythmias, hypovolemia, myocardial infarction, drug toxicity, and transient ischemic attack.

If the cause of the syncope is not documented, verify with the physician as to whether the cause has been established. If so, be sure the medical record is updated to support code selection. For example, if syncope is due to bradycardia, then bradycardia should be documented for accurate reporting.

Definition: Syncope is a transient loss of consciousness due to inadequate blood flow to the brain. The patient experiences generalized weakness, an inability to continue standing, and loss of consciousness. It can last anywhere from a few seconds to as long as 30 minutes. Any form of syncope is reported with code 780.2 if no specific disease process can be identified as causing the condition.

Neurocardiogenic Syncope: This type of syncope is also known as vasodepressor or vasovagal syncope. It is a condition that results from a drop in blood pressure due to failure of peripheral resistance with concomitant reduced venous return. It may also be due to slowing of the heart, emotional stress, pain, acute loss of blood, or assuming an upright position after having been supine for a prolonged period. It is not uncommon for patients who have just donated blood to experience this form of syncope.

Reaction or Hypersensitivity to Medications: When this occurs, code first the syncope (780.2) followed by an E-code to identify the type of medication.

Convulsions are a series of jerking movements of the face, trunk, or extremities, with involuntary contracture of voluntary muscles. Etiology is an acute focal or generalized disturbance in cerebral function. A small focus of diseased tissue in the cerebrum discharges abnormally in response to certain endogenous or exogenous stimuli. Spread of the discharge to other portions of the cerebrum results in convulsive activity and loss of consciousness. Codes in this subclassification are selected based on whether the convulsions are febrile in origin.

Associated conditions include hyperpyrexia (acute infection, heat stroke), central nervous system infections (meningitis, encephalitis, brain abscess), cerebral trauma (skull fracture, birth injury), cerebral edema (hypertensive encephalopathy, eclampsia), metabolic disturbances (hypoglycemia, hypoparathyroidism), and cerebral hypoxia (Adams-Stokes syndrome, anesthesia).

Complex (also atypical or complicated) febrile seizures can be defined as focal or prolonged seizures associated with fever that are either prolonged (greater than 15 minutes) or recur within 24 hours of initial onset. Although not limited exclusively to the pediatric population, complex febrile seizures most commonly occur in children between 6 months and 5 years old.

For parents and caregivers, witnessing a child experience a complex febrile seizure can be frightening. Seizures usually begin with contraction or spasms of muscles. A distinctive cry or moan may result from the force of these spasms. The patient also may fall, vomit, or urinate as he or she loses voluntary control of their muscles. The child may cease breathing until the muscles begin to periodically relax and contract again, which results in rhythmic jerking movements. A complex febrile seizure may last 15 minutes or longer.

Febrile seizures are thought to be triggered by the sudden stimulation of many brain cells at once. Both the severity of fever and the onset or rapidity of rise in temperature may be factors in initiating seizure. Fevers over 103 degrees Fahrenheit pose the greatest risk for seizure. These seizures often occur within the first 24 hours of an illness or infection, such as an upper respiratory infection or otitis media. However, complex febrile seizures may indicate a more serious problem, such as meningitis, abscess, or encephalitis. Also, fever as a reaction to DTP or MMR vaccines have been an underlying cause of febrile seizures in some patients. For these reasons, lumbar puncture may be performed to rule out more serious underlying causes. Febrile seizures may run in families, especially if underlying neurologic problems or a history of epilepsy is also present.

Children with febrile seizures should be taken to the emergency department for evaluation and treatment. However, initial response to complex febrile seizures by parents or caregivers should include moving the patient to a safe location, loosening clothing and positioning the patient on their side if possible in order to reduce the risk of chocking on saliva or vomit. Secondarily, the fever will need to be brought down as soon as possible, initially with cool compresses. Nothing should be given by mouth until the seizures have ceased and the patient is awake and responsive. At that time, normal doses of ibuprofen or acetaminophen can be given. As a preventive measure, acetaminophen or ibuprofen should be given at the first sign of a fever, along with adequate hydration to keep the fever from progressing. However, with complex and prolonged seizure, it is necessary to obtain emergency medical treatment. Diagnostic neurological testing may be indicated when seizures are complex or atypical, if the child is neurologically abnormal on exam, or if in the presence of multiple febrile seizures. Anticonvulsant medications can be given (usually rectally), but are rarely used for young pediatric patients, as the risks usually outweigh the benefits.

Codes in subcategory 780.3 classify convulsive disorders and seizures that are ill-defined, as well as sudden, acute symptomatic manifestations of other conditions. Excluded from this subclassification is neonatal convulsion (779.0). Classify convulsive or seizure disorders described as irreversible, intractable, recurrent, repetitive, chronic, or requiring maintenance with phenobarbital or Dilantin for control to rubric 345 *Epilepsy.*

780.31	Febrile convulsions — *pyrexial seizure* AHA: March-April, 1985, 3; Nov-Dec, 1987, 12; Q2, 1990, 3; Q2, 1990, 5; Q2, 1990, 15; Q1, 1991, 12; Q4, 1992, 23; Q1, 1993, 24; Q3, 1994, 9; Q1, 1997, 12; Q2, 1997, 8; Q4, 1997, 45
780.32	Complex febrile convulsions — *febrile seizures described as atypical, complex, or complicated*

This code excludes status epilepticus (345.3).

780.39	Other convulsions — *not originating with fever* AHA: March-April, 1985, 3; Nov-Dec, 1987, 12; Q2, 1990, 3; Q2, 1990, 5; Q2, 1990, 15; Q1, 1991, 12; Q4, 1992, 23; Q1, 1993, 24; Q3, 1994, 9; Q1, 1997, 12; Q2, 1997, 8; Q4, 1998, 39; Q2, 1999, 17; Q1, 2003, 7; Q4, 2004, 51

In cases where repeated admissions for seizures have occurred during the first three years after birth, verify with the physician if the patient's diagnosis of "convulsions" or "seizures" should be classified as infantile spasms, code 345.6x. If the physician does not verify that the condition is infantile spasms, and no underlying pathology is found, use code 780.39 for convulsions of unknown etiology.

When the documentation indicates the diagnosis of posttraumatic seizure disorder only, clarify with the physician if the seizure disorder is to be coded seizure (780.39) or as epilepsy (345.9x).

Benign Shuddering Attacks: This movement disorder noted in young children is not coded as an epileptic or convulsive condition. It is a nonepileptic disorder that may occur as frequently as several times a day, but typically decreases in frequency as the child ages. Use code 333.93 to classify this condition.

Drug Withdrawal: Patients may experience convulsions as a result of inappropriate use of drugs and medications.

Code 780.39 should be used to identify the physical disturbance of convulsions due to drug withdrawal. Code 292.0 would also be used to identify the drug withdrawal. Assign an additional code for the associated drug dependence (304).

If a patient experiences convulsions as a result of discontinuing a medication, use code V58.69 *Long-term (current) drug use,* in addition to the code for the convulsions. If the convulsions are a result of the patient not taking a medication as prescribed, code V15.81 *Noncompliance with medical treatment* should be identified as an additional diagnosis.

Febrile Convulsions: This is the most common seizure disorder of children; 40 percent of first time seizures are febrile. Treatment includes temperature control with acetaminophen and control of the seizures with diazepam or Ativan suppositories. This condition is identified with code 780.31 *Febrile convulsions.*

Neurocysticercosis: This condition is caused by an infestation of the larval form of the parasite Taenia solium. Brain involvement of the parasite can result in epilepsy, increased intracranial pressure, and other neurologic conditions. Two codes should be indicated: 123.1 to identify the parasitic infection and code 780.3x indicating the convulsions.

Newborn Convulsions: Convulsions of a newborn are serious and can be caused by such conditions as hypoglycemia, hypocalcemia, sepsis, or central nervous system damage. If no etiology has been determined during the newborn stay, report with code 779.0 *Convulsions in newborn.*

Code 780.3x is assigned only when repeated admissions have occurred following birth and the etiology of the convulsions is unknown.

780.4	Dizziness and giddiness — *light-headedness, vertigo not otherwise specified* AHA: March-April, 1985, 3; Q2, 1990, 3; Q2, 1990, 5; Q2, 1990, 15; Q1, 1991, 12; Q2, 1991, 17; Q2, 1997, 9; Q3, 2000, 12; Q2, 2003, 11

Symptoms, Signs, and Ill-Defined Conditions

Use code 780.4 to report the illusion of movement or a feeling of unsteadiness or light-headedness.

Associated conditions include brain stem ischemia, head trauma, multiple sclerosis, posterior fossa tumor, acoustic neuroma, labyrinthitis, Meniére's disease, vestibular neuritis, herpes zoster, and toxic levels of drugs.

Subcategory 780.5 provides codes for unspecified sleep disorders that remain a general symptom without a specifically identified sleep disorder diagnosis. Excluded from this subcategory are sleep disturbances that are alcohol or drug induced (291.82, 292.85), not organic in nature (307.40-307.49), or specified organic sleep disorders including circadian rhythm sleep disorders (327.30-327.39), organic hypersomnia (327.10-327.19), organic insomnia (327.00-327.09), organic sleep apnea (327.20-327.29), organic sleep related movement disorders (327.51-327.59), and parasomnias (327.40-327.49).

780.50 Unspecified sleep disturbance
AHA: Q4, 2005, 59

780.51 Insomnia with sleep apnea — *cessation of breathing causes sleeplessness*
AHA: March-April, 1985, 3; Q2, 1990, 3; Q2, 1990, 5; Q2, 1990, 15; Q1, 1991, 12; Q4, 2005, 59

780.52 Insomnia, unspecified — *sleeplessness not associated with apnea*
AHA: March-April, 1985, 3; Q2, 1990, 3; Q2, 1990, 5; Q2, 1990, 15; Q1, 1991, 12; Q4, 2005, 59

780.53 Unspecified hypersomnia with sleep apnea — *cessation of breathing causes excessive sleepiness*
AHA: March-April, 1985, 3; Nov-Dec, 1985, 4; Q2, 1990, 3; Q2, 1990, 5; Q2, 1990, 15; Q1, 1991, 12; Q1, 1993, 28; Q4, 2005, 59

780.54 Hypersomnia, unspecified — *sleepiness not associated with apnea*
AHA: March-April, 1985, 3; Q2, 1990, 3; Q2, 1990, 5; Q2, 1990, 15; Q1, 1991, 12; Q4, 2005, 59

780.55 Disruptions of 24-hour sleep-wake cycle, unspecified
AHA: March-April, 1985, 3; Q2, 1990, 3; Q2, 1990, 5; Q2, 1990, 15; Q1, 1991, 12; Q4, 2005, 59

780.56 Dysfunctions associated with sleep stages or arousal from sleep
AHA: Q4, 2005, 59

780.57 Unspecified sleep apnea
AHA: March-April, 1985, 3; Q2, 1990, 3; Q2, 1990, 5; Q2, 1990, 15; Q1, 1991, 12; Q1, 1993, 28; Q1, 1997, 5; Q1, 2001, 6; Q4, 2005, 59

Unspecified sleep apnea involves the abnormal cessation of breathing during sleep not otherwise classified. Sleep apnea is due to a failure of the ventilatory signals from the brain as seen in diseases of the central nervous system or an obstruction of the upper airway as seen in massive obesity or tonsillar hypertrophy. A combination of the two may also occur. Specified forms of organic sleep apnea are coded within subcategory 327.2.

People with untreated sleep apnea stop breathing repeatedly during their sleep, sometimes hundreds of times during the night and often for a minute or longer, according to the American Sleep Apnea Association. Sleep apnea affects more than 12 million Americans, according to the National Institutes of Health. Males are more prone to sleep apnea than females. Risk of sleep apnea increases for those overweight and older than 40 years of age, although sleep apnea can strike anyone at any age.

Untreated sleep apnea can cause high blood pressure and other cardiovascular disease, memory problems, weight gain, impotency, and headaches. Several treatment options exist, and research into additional options continues.

780.58 Sleep related movement disorder, unspecified
AHA: Q4, 2004, 95; Q4, 2005, 59

Sleep related movement disorder, also known as nocturnal myoclonus, is characterized by involuntary movement during sleep. This can range from slight movement to small continuous movements of the ankle or toes to wild flailing of the legs and arms. The patient may initially present with poor sleep or daytime sleepiness. The disorder is characterized by repetitive, involuntary movement during the night. The cause of this disorder is not known. Sleep studies are required for definitive diagnosis. Currently there is no cure, but medication may alleviate the symptoms.

780.59 Other sleep disturbances
AHA: Q4, 2005, 59

780.6 Fever — *pyrexia, PUO, FUO, chills with fever*
AHA: March-April, 1985, 3; Q2, 1990, 3; Q2, 1990, 5; Q2, 1990, 15; Q1, 1991, 12; Q2, 1991, 8; Q4, 1999, 26; Q3, 2000, 13; Q3, 2005, 16

Fever is an abnormal elevation of body temperature (at least 38.3 C or 101 F) for a minimum of three weeks without the etiology being determined despite exhaustive investigation. Fever that is ill-defined or unspecified also is classified here.

Therapies depend on the etiology, but include cooling blankets, cold compresses, antibiotics, and antipyretics (aspirin, acetaminophen). Associated conditions include infections, connective tissue disorders, and occult neoplasm (leukemia, lymphoma).

Excluded from this subcategory is fatigue during combat (308.0-308.9), heat (992.6), and pregnancy (646.8x); and fatigue or malaise related to neurasthenia (300.5) and senile asthenia (797).

780.71 Chronic fatigue syndrome — *severe, prolonged fatigue impairing daily function, without proven physical or psychological cause*
AHA: March-April, 1985, 3; March-April, 1987, 8; Q4, 1988, 12; Q2, 1990, 3; Q2, 1990, 5; Q2, 1990, 15; Q1, 1991, 12; Q4, 1998, 48

Chronic fatigue syndrome (CFS) also is known as myalgic encephalomyelitis, postviral fatigue syndrome, and chronic fatigue and immune dysfunction syndrome. It is marked by unrelenting exhaustion, muscle pain, cognitive disorders that patients call "brain fog," and a profound weakness that does not go away with a few good nights of sleep. There is no known cause. CFS may begin after a bout with a cold, bronchitis, hepatitis, or an intestinal bug. For some, it follows a bout of infectious mononucleosis or during a period of high stress. Unlike flu symptoms, CFS symptoms, such as a chronic headache, muscle and joint aches, and fatigue, either hang on or come and go frequently for more than six months. Some patients are bedridden; others can work or attend school at least part time, since any exertion typically worsens symptoms.

CFS is diagnosed two to four times more often in females than males and it is estimated that as many as 500,000 people in the United States have a CFS-like condition. There is no effective treatment for CFS. However, nonsteroidal anti-inflammatory drugs, such as ibuprofen, reduce body aches or fever, and nonsedative antihistamines relieve any prominent allergic symptoms, such as a runny nose.

780.79 Other malaise and fatigue — *asthenia, postviral syndrome, Stiller's asthenia, neurasthenia, albionarc*
AHA: March-April, 1985, 3; March-April, 1987, 8; Q4, 1988, 12; Q2, 1990, 3; Q2, 1990, 5; Q2, 1990, 15; Q1, 1991, 12; Q4, 1999, 26; Q1, 2000, 6; Q4, 2004, 78

780.8 Generalized hyperhidrosis — *night sweats, diaphoresis, excessive sweating*
AHA: March-April, 1985, 3; Q2, 1990, 3; Q2, 1990, 5; Q2, 1990, 15; Q1, 1991, 12

Report 705.21 for primary focal hyperhidrosis.
Report 705.22 for secondary focal hyperhidrosis.
Report 333.94 for restless legs syndrome.

780.91 Fussy infant (baby)

780.92 Excessive crying of infant (baby)
780.93 Memory loss
780.94 Early satiety
780.95 Excessive crying of child, adolescent, or adult
AHA: Q4, 2005, 89

780.96 Generalized pain — *pain, not otherwise specified*

True to the nature of generalized pain, it is a condition that is difficult to define. Often, "generalized pain" is a term used to describe pain that a patient experiences that cannot be attributed to a specific anatomic site or type or has overlapping or multiple characteristics. Usually, the term is applied before establishing an underlying cause or more specific diagnosis. Generalized pain can vary in nature as stabbing, tingling, dull or cramping, or it may exhibit one or more of these features. Mainly, the generalized term refers to pain of multiple anatomic sites or all-over "aching." Sometimes, this pain is a symptom of chronic conditions such as fibromyalgia and polymyalgia rheumatica, late effects of other illnesses such as poliomyelitis, infections such as Lyme disease, or referred pain from a quiescent injury or disease process. Treatment can be as difficult as defining the pain; effective treatment is based on obtaining an underlying diagnosis and addressing the root cause.

There is a massive variety of pain medications on the market, many of which pose a risk of dependence. Herbal remedies are available, but also pose a certain degree of risk in the absence of addressing the root cause. Interventions such as neurostimulation and neuroablation are effective when indicated. Nonmedicinal therapies run the gamut from biofeedback and electromagnetic therapy to physical therapy but, again, therapies are most effective when the cause of the pain in known. Prior to diagnosis, depression and personality disorders should be ruled out.

780.97 Altered mental status — *change in mental status*

Significant changes in mental status can occur without the patient's losing consciousness. These changes can also be described as disorientation or confusion, and often include various degrees of cognitive impairment. Some of the conditions that can cause mental status changes include:

- Alcohol or drug intoxication
- Low blood sugar
- Head trauma, head injury or concussion
- Fluid and electrolyte imbalance
- Nutritional deficiencies, such as niacin or vitamin B12

- Fever
- Sudden drop in body temperature (hypothermia)
- Hypoxia due to chronic lung disease
- Adverse effects of medications
- Infections
- Neoplasm
- Sleep deprivation
- Seizures
- Mental illness

Endocrine, neurological, psychiatric, and renal disorders can all manifest or progress with mental status changes as a sentinel sign or symptom. A change in mental status is most often noticed by family or caregivers, with the patient themselves either unaware or reluctant to seek care. Depending on the age and general health of the patient, there are a wide variety of potential underlying causes of this symptom. In pediatric populations, neurological disorders, trauma, shock, metabolic disorders, poisoning or CNS infections are most common. In the elderly, mental status changes are common effects of medication, electrolyte imbalances, or infection.

Upon examination, the physician will seek to obtain a baseline status upon which to assess future changes. Examination includes assessment of orientation, affect and mood, language, memory, judgment and insight, as well as abnormal thought content, level of consciousness and perception abnormalities. Diagnostic tests such as MRI, blood and urine lab tests, and EEG may be indicated, depending upon the patient's history and clinical presentation. Accuracy of diagnosis is imperative, since treatment depends on correcting underlying cause.

Altered mental status is reportable when it cannot be attributed to an underlying cause, or if there is no other diagnosis or condition for which mental status changes are an integral part of the disease process. This code should be used when altered mental status requires further investigation or no underlying cause is yet known.

Coding Clarification

Altered mental status due to a known condition should be coded to that condition. This code excludes altered level of consciousness, which should be reported with a code from range 780.01-780.09, and delirium not otherwise specified (780.09).

When reporting complex febrile convulsions (780.32), assign a code for the condition responsible for the fever, if known. Sequencing of codes will depend on the circumstances of the encounter/admission.

Code 780.96 *Generalized pain* should not be reported if an underlying cause or more specific site is identified that is classifiable elsewhere.

780.99 Other general symptoms — *chill(s) NOS, hypothermia not associated with environmental temperature*
AHA: March-April, 1985, 3; Nov-Dec, 1985, 12; Q2, 1990, 3; Q2, 1990, 5; Q2, 1990, 15; Q1, 1991, 12; Q3, 1993, 11; Q4, 1999, 10; Q4, 2002, 67; Q4, 2003, 103

Coding Scenario

A 72-year-old female is seen with complaints of transient dizziness. She must sit down immediately when experiencing this symptom. She states that she may have lost consciousness for a few seconds but is unsure. The physician documents syncope and will order further diagnostic testing if the patient experiences recurrence of the symptoms.

Code assignment: 780.2 *Syncope and collapse*

A patient is seen in the physician's office complaining of persistent fainting spells upon rising in the morning. She notes no other symptoms. The physician documents neurocardiogenic syncope and recommends further testing.

Code assignment: 780.2 *Syncope and collapse*

A 5-year-old male is seen in the emergency department. His mother states that he suffered a seizure. Upon examination the child is found to have otitis media and a temperature of 104.2. The physician documents the diagnosis as febrile convulsions and acute nonsuppurative otitis media.

Code assignment: 780.31 *Febrile convulsions (simple) unspecified* and 381.00 *Acute nonsuppurative otitis media, unspecified*

A 2-year-old female is admitted via the emergency department for recurrent convulsions. The physician's final diagnostic statement states recurrent convulsions.

Code assignment: 780.39 *Other convulsions*

781 Symptoms involving nervous and musculoskeletal systems
AHA: March-April, 1985, 3; Q2, 1990, 3; Q2, 1990, 5; Q2, 1990, 15; Q1, 1991, 12

781.0 Abnormal involuntary movements — *spasms, tremors, head movements, fasciculations; not otherwise specified*
AHA: March-April, 1985, 3; Q2, 1990, 3; Q2, 1990, 5; Q2, 1990, 15; Q1, 1991, 12

781.1 Disturbances of sensation of smell and taste — *anosmia, parageusia, parosmia*
AHA: March-April, 1985, 3; Q2, 1990, 3; Q2, 1990, 5; Q2, 1990, 15; Q1, 1991, 12

781.2 Abnormality of gait — *ataxic, paralytic, spastic, staggering*
AHA: March-April, 1985, 3; Q2, 1990, 3; Q2, 1990, 5; Q2, 1990, 15; Q1, 1991, 12; Q2, 2004, 15; Q2, 2005, 6

781.3 Lack of coordination — *muscular incoordination, ataxia not otherwise specified*
AHA: March-April, 1985, 3; Q2, 1990, 3; Q2, 1990, 5; Q2, 1990, 15; Q1, 1991, 12; Q3, 1997, 12; Q4, 2004, 51

781.4 Transient paralysis of limb — *transient monoplegia*
AHA: March-April, 1985, 3; Q2, 1990, 3; Q2, 1990, 5; Q2, 1990, 15; Q1, 1991, 12

781.5 Clubbing of fingers — *enlargement of soft tissues of distal fingers*
AHA: March-April, 1985, 3; Q2, 1990, 3; Q2, 1990, 5; Q2, 1990, 15; Q1, 1991, 12

781.6 Meningismus — *irritation of lining of brain or spinal cord; Dupre's syndrome, meningism*
AHA: March-April, 1985, 3; Jan Feb, 1987, 7; Q2, 1990, 3; Q2, 1990, 5; Q2, 1990, 15; Q1, 1991, 12; Q3, 2000, 13

781.7 Tetany — *extremity muscle spasms; carpopedal spasm, magnesium deficiency syndrome*
AHA: March-April, 1985, 3; Q2, 1990, 3; Q2, 1990, 5; Q2, 1990, 15; Q1, 1991, 12

Tetany is a type of cramp that causes the muscles of the hands and feet to cramp rhythmically, as well as spasms of the larynx with difficulty in breathing, nausea, vomiting, convulsions, and considerable pain. The disorder stems from a mineral imbalance, such as a lack of calcium, potassium, or magnesium, or an acid or alkaline condition of the body.

Associated conditions include poorly controlled hypoparathyroidism, hypophosphatemia, osteomalacia, renal disorders, or malabsorption syndromes. Treatment is directed at restoring metabolic balance, as by intravenous administration of calcium in cases of hypocalcemia (calcium deficiency).

781.8 Neurological neglect syndrome — *asomatognosia, hemi-akinesia, hemi-spatial neglect, sensory neglect, visuospatial neglect*
AHA: March-April, 1985, 3; Q2, 1990, 3; Q2, 1990, 5; Q2, 1990, 15; Q1, 1991, 12; Q4, 1994, 37

781.91 Loss of height — *not due to osteoporosis*
AHA: March-April, 1985, 3; Q2, 1990, 3; Q2, 1990, 5; Q2, 1990, 15; Q1, 1991, 12; Q4, 2000, 45

781.92 Abnormal posture
781.93 Ocular torticollis
781.94 Facial weakness — *facial droop*
AHA: Q4, 2003, 72

781.99 Other symptoms involving nervous and musculoskeletal systems — *acragnosis, acroagnosis, acute catatonia, floppy infant syndrome, growing pains; not otherwise specified*
AHA: March-April, 1985, 3; Q2, 1990, 3; Q2, 1990, 5; Q2, 1990, 15; Q1, 1991, 12; Q4, 2000, 45

Excluded from this rubric are depression not otherwise specified (311); pain in the limb (729.5); and disorders relating to the back (724.0-724.9), hearing (388.0-389.9), joint (718.0-719.9), limb (729.0-729.9), neck (723.0-723.9), or vision (368.0-369.9).

782 Symptoms involving skin and other integumentary tissue
AHA: March-April, 1985, 3; Q2, 1990, 3; Q2, 1990, 5; Q2, 1990, 15; Q1, 1991, 12

782.0 Disturbance of skin sensation — *anesthesia, burning, prickling, numbness, tingling, hyperesthesia, hypoesthesia, paresthesia, Berger's paresthesia, pseudohemianesthesia*
AHA: March-April, 1985, 3; Q2, 1990, 3; Q2, 1990, 5; Q2, 1990, 15; Q1, 1991, 12

782.1 Rash and other nonspecific skin eruption — *exanthem*
AHA: March-April, 1985, 3; Q2, 1990, 3; Q2, 1990, 5; Q2, 1990, 15; Q1, 1991, 12

782.2 Localized superficial swelling, mass, or lump — *subcutaneous nodules*
AHA: March-April, 1985, 3; Q2, 1990, 3; Q2, 1990, 5; Q2, 1990, 15; Q1, 1991, 12

782.3 Edema — *fluid in soft tissue; localized, anasarca, dropsy, Secretan's syndrome*
AHA: March-April, 1985, 3; Q2, 1990, 3; Q2, 1990, 5; Q2, 1990, 15; Q1, 1991, 12; Q2, 2000, 18

Edema is the accumulation of excessive amounts of fluid (water and sodium) in the intercellular tissue spaces of the body. Edema results when the balance of the lymphatic system, which normally transports excess interstitial fluid back to the intravascular space, is compromised. Pitting edema is a type of edema that retains for a time the indentation produced by pressure that forces fluid into the underlying tissues. Nonpitting edema is a type of edema that leaves no indentation when pressure is applied because fluid has coagulated in the tissues. Edema may occur at any site of the body, indicating different causes.

Excluded from this code are ascites (789.5), edema of newborn (778.5), edema of pregnancy (642.0x-642.9x, 646.1x), fluid retention (276.6), hydrops fetalis (773.3, 778.0), hydrothorax (511.8), and nutritional edema (260, 262).

782.4 Jaundice, unspecified, not of newborn — bilirubin causing yellow cast to skin; cholemia, icterus
AHA: March-April, 1985, 3; Q2, 1990, 3; Q2, 1990, 5; Q2, 1990, 15; Q1, 1991, 12

Use this code to report yellow discoloration of the skin and/or mucous membranes due to excessive levels of bilirubin in the blood. Pruritus, dark urine, and clay-colored stools commonly accompany jaundice. Etiologies for jaundice include congestive heart failure, carcinoma of the papilla of Vater or pancreas, cholecystitis and cholelithiasis, Kaye or Byler cholestasis, Laennec's or primary cirrhosis of the liver, liver abscess, hepatitis, acute or chronic pancreatitis, Dubin-Johnson syndrome, hemolytic anemia, glucose-6-phosphate dehydrogenase (G6PD) deficiency, and drug-induced hepatic insult. Lab work may include urine and fecal urobilinogen, serum bilirubin, liver enzyme tests, serum cholesterol, prothrombin, and complete blood count (CBC). Liver biopsy may rule out hepatic etiology.

Therapies depend on the etiology, such as cholecystectomy for jaundice due to cholecystitis; dietary management, including increased carbohydrates, decreased proteins, and fewer high-fat foods; frequent skin cleansing; and topical antipruritic medications for pruritus.

Jaundice in newborn (774.0-774.7) and jaundice due to isoimmunization (773.0-773.2, 773.4) are excluded from this code.

782.5 Cyanosis — deficient oxygen in blood, causing blue cast to skin
AHA: March-April, 1985, 3; Q2, 1990, 3; Q2, 1990, 5; Q2, 1990, 15; Q1, 1991, 12

Cyanosis in newborn (770.83) is excluded from this code.

782.61 Pallor — pale skin
AHA: March-April, 1985, 3; Q2, 1990, 3; Q2, 1990, 5; Q2, 1990, 15; Q1, 1991, 12

782.62 Flushing — ruddy skin, excessive blushing
AHA: March-April, 1985, 3; Q2, 1990, 3; Q2, 1990, 5; Q2, 1990, 15; Q1, 1991, 12

782.7 Spontaneous ecchymoses — hemorrhagic spots with the appearance of freckles; petechiae
AHA: March-April, 1985, 3; Q2, 1990, 3; Q2, 1990, 5; Q2, 1990, 15; Q1, 1991, 12

Ecchymoses is defined as a purplish, flat bruise that occurs when blood leaks out into the top layers of skin; the bruise is not raised but may be irregular in shape. Spontaneous ecchymoses is often a symptom of a coagulation disorder. Sometimes diagnostic tests are necessary to determine the diagnosis, such as serologic tests, biopsies, culture plus antimicrobial sensitivity, dermatrophy, and test media-ring worm.

782.8 Changes in skin texture — induration, thickening, scabs, scales
AHA: March-April, 1985, 3; Q2, 1990, 3; Q2, 1990, 5; Q2, 1990, 15; Q1, 1991, 12

782.9 Other symptoms involving skin and integumentary tissues — not otherwise specified
AHA: March-April, 1985, 3; Q2, 1990, 3; Q2, 1990, 5; Q2, 1990, 15; Q1, 1991, 12

Symptoms relating to possible breast disorders (611.71-611.79) are excluded from this rubric.

783 Symptoms concerning nutrition, metabolism, and development
AHA: March-April, 1985, 3; Q2, 1990, 3; Q2, 1990, 5; Q2, 1990, 15; Q1, 1991, 12

783.0 Anorexia — loss of appetite
AHA: March-April, 1985, 3; Q2, 1990, 3; Q2, 1990, 5; Q2, 1990, 15; Q1, 1991, 12

This code reports loss of appetite. This is a common symptom of gastrointestinal (GI) and endocrine disorders as well as psychological disturbances. Investigation of organ-specific pathology (function studies of thyroid, liver, kidney, upper GI, gallbladder), barium enema, and blood work allow assessment of nutritional status.

Associated conditions include hypopituitarism, hypothyroidism, ketoacidosis, appendicitis, cirrhosis, Crohn's disease, gastritis, hepatitis, chronic renal failure, pernicious anemia, alcoholism, anorexia nervosa, and cancer.

This subcategory does not include anorexia nervosa. Anorexia nervosa is a psychophysiological condition classified to 307.1. Also excluded is loss of appetite with a nonorganic origin (307.59).

Polyphagia refers to eating to the point of being focused only on eating (or excessive eating) before feeling full. This can be a symptom of various disorders. It can be intermittent or persistent and depending on the cause, it may or may not result in weight gain. Common causes include anxiety, premenstrual syndrome, bulimia, diabetes mellitus, gestational diabetes, Graves' disease, hyperthyroidism, hypoglycemia, and drugs such as corticosteroids, cyproheptadine, and tricyclic antidepressants.

783.1	Abnormal weight gain
783.21	Loss of weight — (Use additional code to identify Body Mass Index (BMI) if known, V85.0)
	AHA: Q4, 2005, 96
783.22	Underweight — (Use additional code to identify Body Mass Index (BMI) if known, V85.0)
	AHA: Q4, 2005, 96
783.3	Feeding difficulties and mismanagement — *typically in elderly, infants*
	AHA: March-April, 1985, 3; Q2, 1990, 3; Q2, 1990, 5; Q2, 1990, 15; Q1, 1991, 12; Q3, 1997, 12
783.40	Lack of normal physiological development, unspecified — *inadequate development, lack of development in childhood*
	AHA: March-April, 1985, 3; Q2, 1990, 3; Q2, 1990, 5; Q2, 1990, 15; Q1, 1991, 12; Q3, 1997, 4; Q4, 2000, 45
783.41	Failure to thrive — *failure to gain weight in childhood*
	AHA: March-April, 1985, 3; Q2, 1990, 3; Q2, 1990, 5; Q2, 1990, 15; Q1, 1991, 12; Q3, 1997, 4; Q4, 2000, 45; Q1, 2003, 12
783.42	Delayed milestones — *late walker, late talker*
	AHA: March-April, 1985, 3; Q2, 1990, 3; Q2, 1990, 5; Q2, 1990, 15; Q1, 1991, 12; Q3, 1997, 4; Q4, 2000, 45
783.43	Short stature — *growth failure, physical retardation in childhood*
	AHA: March-April, 1985, 3; Q2, 1990, 3; Q2, 1990, 5; Q2, 1990, 15; Q1, 1991, 12; Q3, 1997, 4; Q4, 2000, 45
783.5	Polydipsia
783.6	Polyphagia

Excluded from this subcategory are eating disorders of nonorganic origin (307.50-307.59) and dehydration.

783.7	Adult failure to thrive
783.9	Other symptoms concerning nutrition, metabolism, and development
	AHA: Q2, 2004, 3

784 Symptoms involving head and neck
AHA: March-April, 1985, 3; Q2, 1990, 3; Q2, 1990, 5; Q2, 1990, 15; Q1, 1991, 12

784.0	Headache
	AHA: Q2, 2006, 17

Use code 784.0 to report pain in the cranial vaults, orbits, or nape of neck. About 90 percent of all headaches are benign. The basic etiologies of the headache are muscle contraction (tension headache), vascular (migraine or cluster headache), or a combination.

Excluded from this subcategory are atypical face pain (350.2), migraine (346.0x-346.9x), and tension headache (307.81).

784.1	Throat pain
784.2	Swelling, mass, or lump in head and neck
784.3	Aphasia
	AHA: Q4, 2004, 78

Aphasia is impaired expression or comprehension of written or spoken language due to disease or injury of one or more of the brain's language centers: Broca's area, Wernicke's area, or arcuate fasciculus. Broca's area controls the muscle for speech (expressive aphasia). Wernicke's area controls the auditory and visual comprehension for speech (receptive aphasia). The arcuate fasciculus aids in control of the content of speech and enables repetition.

Associated conditions include Alzheimer's disease, brain tumor, cerebrovascular accident, encephalitis, head trauma, and heroin overdose.

784.40	Unspecified voice disturbance
784.41	Aphonia — *loss of voice*
	AHA: March-April, 1985, 3; Q2, 1990, 3, Q2, 1990, 5; Q2, 1990, 15; Q1, 1991, 12
784.49	Other voice disturbance — *change, hoarseness, hypernasality, dysphonia, plicae dysphonia ventricularis, rhinolalia, trachyphonia; not otherwise specified*
	AHA: March-April, 1985, 3; Q2, 1990, 3; Q2, 1990, 5; Q2, 1990, 15; Q1, 1991, 12
784.5	Other speech disturbance — *dysarthria, dysphasia, slurred speech*
	AHA: March-April, 1985, 3; Q2, 1990, 3; Q2, 1990, 5; Q2, 1990, 15; Q1, 1991, 12
784.60	Symbolic dysfunction, unspecified — *unknown variety*
	AHA: March-April, 1985, 3; Q2, 1990, 3; Q2, 1990, 5; Q2, 1990, 15; Q1, 1991, 12
784.61	Alexia and dyslexia — *organic inability or difficulty in reading*
	AHA: March-April, 1985, 3; Q2, 1990, 3; Q2, 1990, 5; Q2, 1990, 15; Q1, 1991, 12
784.69	Other symbolic dysfunction — *acalculia, agnosia, Bianchi's or Gerstmann's syndrome, palilalia, agraphia, apraxia*
	AHA: March-April, 1985, 3; Q2, 1990, 3; Q2, 1990, 5; Q2, 1990, 15; Q1, 1991, 12

Symptoms, Signs, and Ill-Defined Conditions

784.7 Epistaxis — *nosebleed*
AHA: March-April, 1985, 3; Q2, 1990, 3; Q2, 1990, 5; Q2, 1990, 15; Q1, 1991, 12; Q3, 2004, 7

Use code 784.7 to report nosebleed. Typically occurring unilaterally, epistaxis may be spontaneous or induced from the front or back of the nose. The majority of nosebleeds occur within the anterior-inferior nasal septum (Kiesselbach's plexus), but they also can occur at the point where the inferior turbinates meet the nasopharynx. In nonsevere cases, a complete blood count may reveal acute blood loss anemia, prothrombin, and activated partial thromboplastin time measurements. Therapies include application of external pressure, insertion of cotton treated with vasoconstrictor and local anesthetic, and humidified oxygen. In severe cases, therapies may include IV hydration, pinching in of the nares to control bleeding in the absence of nasal fracture, and anterior or posterior nasal packing if other measures prove ineffective in controlling bleeding.

Associated conditions include maxillofacial injury, nasal fracture, nasal tumors, orbital floor fracture, acute sinusitis, hypertension, cirrhosis, hepatitis, renal failure, skull fracture, aplastic and acute blood loss anemia, coagulation disorders, hereditary hemorrhagic telangiectasia (Rendu-Osler-Weber disease), leukemia, polycythemia vera, systemic lupus erythematosus, infectious mononucleosis, influenza, and anticoagulant use (adverse effect).

784.8 Hemorrhage from throat — *bleeding*
AHA: March-April, 1985, 3; Q2, 1990, 3; Q2, 1990, 5; Q2, 1990, 15; Q1, 1991, 12

784.91 Postnasal drip
AHA: March-April, 1985, 3; Q2, 1990, 3; Q2, 1990, 5; Q2, 1990, 15; Q1, 1991, 12

Postnasal drip (PND) is the symptom of excess fluid or mucous dripping down the back of the throat. Patients with postnasal drip may complain of:

- Constantly clearing of the throat
- Excessive swallowing
- Sore throat
- Nasal or sinus congestion
- Chronic cough
- Bad breath and a sour taste in mouth
- White or yellow coating on the tongue

Some common causes of postnasal drip include:

- Viral infections; common cold or the flu
- Illness such as otitis media or bronchitis
- Head injury
- Small objects in the nostril (especially in children)
- Sinusitis
- Allergic rhinitis
- Inhaled irritants
- Food allergies or a sensitivity to dairy products

If clinicians assume the patient has a cold, they can misdiagnose the condition and prescribe antibiotics (which are ineffective against viruses). However, this can actually aggravate post-nasal drip in the absence of infection because the antibiotics have a negative effect on beneficial bacterial, causing a secondary anaerobic bacterial imbalance. Chronic PND can cause irritation and inflammation of the sinus and result in bleeding (epistaxis) and polyp formation.

Some patients can be effectively treated for PND with antihistamines, decongestants, or a combination of both. Steroidal nasal sprays and intranasal ipratropium bromide (Atrovent) are indicated for certain types of rhinitis. Over-the-counter nasal sprays can relieve symptoms temporarily, but they carry risks with chronic use. Antibiotics can help if there is a bacterial infection present; otherwise they are either ineffective or can disrupt the natural bacterial balance and make the condition worse. Diagnostic tests such as a sinus x-ray or CT scan may be indicated in certain cases. Alternative medicine treatments are also available in the form of herbal and homeopathic remedies, and irrigation with devices such as a neti pot (as used in Ayurveda; natural Indian medicine). In cases of PND due to food allergy or sensitivity, dietary modification is necessary.

784.99 Other symptoms involving head and neck — *halitosis, choking sensation, mouth breathing, sneezing*
AHA: March-April, 1985, 3; Q2, 1990, 3; Q2, 1990, 5; Q2, 1990, 15; Q1, 1991, 12

785 Symptoms involving cardiovascular system
AHA: March-April, 1985, 3; Q2, 1990, 3; Q2, 1990, 5; Q2, 1990, 15; Q1, 1991, 12

785.0 Unspecified tachycardia — *rapid heart beat*
AHA: March-April, 1985, 3; Q2, 1990, 3; Q2, 1990, 5; Q2, 1990, 15; Q1, 1991, 12; Q2, 2003, 11

This code reports a heart rate greater than 100 beats per minute caused by the heart making an effort to deliver more oxygen to the body tissues by increasing the rate at which blood passes through the vessels. Usually, the patient will complain of palpitations or racing of the heart. Tachycardia may be the result of excitement, exercise, pain, or fever as well as caffeine and tobacco. However, it may be an early sign of a life-threatening disorder such as cardiogenic or septic shock.

Associated conditions include neurogenic shock, adult respiratory distress syndrome, chronic obstructive pulmonary disease, pneumothorax, pulmonary embolism, cardiac dysrhythmia, cardiogenic shock, congestive heart failure, hypertensive crisis, myocardial infarction, thyrotoxicosis, anemia, diabetic ketoacidosis, hyponatremia, anaphylactic shock, and septic shock.

Excluded from this subcategory is paroxysmal tachycardia (427.0-427.2) and neonatal tachycardia (779.82).

785.1	Palpitations — *awareness of heart beat* **AHA:** March-April, 1985, 3; Q2, 1990, 3; Q2, 1990, 5; Q2, 1990, 15; Q1, 1991, 12
785.2	Undiagnosed cardiac murmurs — *mitral or systolic click syndrome, heart murmur not otherwise specified* **AHA:** March-April, 1985, 3; Q2, 1990, 3; Q2, 1990, 5; Q2, 1990, 15; Q1, 1991, 12; Q4, 1992, 16
785.3	Other abnormal heart sounds — *cardiac dullness, friction fremitus, precardial friction* **AHA:** March-April, 1985, 3; Q2, 1990, 3; Q2, 1990, 5; Q2, 1990, 15; Q1, 1991, 12
785.4	Gangrene — (Code first any associated underlying condition:250.7, 443.0) — *phagedena, spreading cutaneous gangrene, gangrenous cellulitis* **AHA:** March-April, 1985, 3; March-April, 1986, 12; Q2, 1990, 3; Q2, 1990, 5; Q2, 1990, 15; Q3, 1990, 15; Q1, 1991, 12; Q3, 1991, 12; Q1, 2004, 14

Gangrene is the death of tissue due to loss of vascular supply. Gangrene may be wet (bacterial infection with cellulitis) or dry (affected area is dry and shriveled).

Associated conditions include diabetes with microangiopathy, ischemia due to atherosclerosis or embolism, and Raynaud's phenomenon. Code first any associated underlying disease.

This subcategory excludes gas gangrene due to tissue invasion by *Clostridium perfringens* or other clostridia (classified to code 040.0) and gangrene to a variety of specific sites. Refer to the ICD-9-CM index under "Gangrene, gangrenous" for specific code assignments since some specific types of gangrene are classified to other chapters.

Use codes in this subclassification to report a condition in which the blood flow to peripheral tissues and perfusion are inadequate to sustain life due to insufficient cardiac output or maladapted distribution of peripheral blood flow. The principal deficiency is a reduction in perfusion of vital tissues resulting in inadequate oxygen delivery. This facilitates aerobic metabolism, which results in anaerobic respiration. The result is increased production and accumulation of lactic acid (metabolic acidosis) with compensatory hyperventilation and respiratory alkalosis. Eventually, the homeostatic mechanisms that serve to maintain acid-base balance fail, leading to cell death and subsequent organ failure.

Cardiogenic shock is shock resulting from decreased cardiac output in heart disease. Associated conditions include disturbance of heart rate or rhythm, acute myocardial infarction, valvular heart disease, cardiomyopathy, hypoxemia secondary to pulmonary or neurologic disease, tension pneumothorax, pericardial tamponade, massive pulmonary embolism, prosthetic valve malfunction, and mixed acid-base balance disorder.

Shock due to anesthetic (995.4), anaphylactic shock (995.0), electric shock (994.8), shock following abortion (639.5), shock from lightning (994.0), shock following an obstetrical procedure (669.1), postoperative shock (998.0), or traumatic shock (958.4) are excluded from this classification.

785.50	Unspecified shock — *unknown cause* **AHA:** March-April, 1985, 3; Q2, 1990, 3; Q2, 1990, 5; Q2, 1990, 15; Q1, 1991, 12; Q2, 1996, 10
785.51	Cardiogenic shock — *failure of peripheral circulation due to heart insufficiency* **AHA:** March-April, 1985, 3; Q2, 1990, 3; Q2, 1990, 5; Q2, 1990, 15; Q1, 1991, 12; Q3, 2005, 14
785.52	Septic shock — (Code first systemic inflammatory response syndrome due to infectious process with organ dysfunction, 995.92; code first systemic inflammatory response syndrome due to noninfectious process with organ dysfunction, 995.94) — *severe sepsis with shock, severe septic infection in the blood stream or other tissue causing organ dysfunction* **AHA:** Q4, 2003, 73, 79; Q2, 2005, 18, 19
785.59	Other shock without mention of trauma — *hypervolemic, septic shock; not otherwise specified* **AHA:** March-April, 1985, 3; Q2, 1990, 3; Q2, 1990, 5; Q2, 1990, 15; Q1, 1991, 12; Q2, 2000, 3

Symptoms, Signs, and Ill-Defined Conditions

785.6 Enlargement of lymph nodes — *lymphadenopathy, swollen glands*
AHA: March-April, 1985, 3; Q2, 1990, 3; Q2, 1990, 5; Q2, 1990, 15; Q1, 1991, 12

785.9 Other symptoms involving cardiovascular system — *strong pulse, weak pulse, bruit; not otherwise specified*
AHA: March-April, 1985, 3; Q2, 1990, 3; Q2, 1990, 5; Q2, 1990, 15; Q1, 1991, 12

Coding Clarification
Excluded from this rubric is heart failure, not otherwise specified (428.9).

Septic shock is a form of organ dysfunction associated with systemic inflammatory response syndrome (SIRS) and cannot occur in the absence of severe sepsis. Septic shock can also be stated as severe sepsis with shock. Severe sepsis usually follows systemic infection along the continuum of illness severity. The infective organism is sequenced first, followed by the respective code provided for SIRS due to an infectious (995.92) process with acute organ dysfunction (severe sepsis), then the code for septic shock, 785.52, and any additional codes identifying specific acute organ failure. Severe sepsis with shock involves persistent hypotension with a systolic blood pressure < 90 mmHg, or a 40 mmHg drop in previous blood pressure, with no response to adequate fluid resuscitation. Reduced myocardial performance is an inherent characteristic in this condition; therefore, heart failure is inclusive in 785.52 and should not be listed separately.

Coding Scenario
A 74-year old male patient presents with nausea, persistent fever, hyperventilation, and prostration. Physical examination gives a respiratory rate of 30 breaths/min, temperature of 101 degrees F, pulse is 102, BP 80/55. Initial blood cultures indicate the presence of *streptococcus pyogenes*. The patient is placed on Fortaz, 2 gm IV every eight hours. The physician documents severe sepsis with shock due to streptococcal infection.

Code assignment: 038.0 *Streptococcal septicemia*, 995.92 *Severe sepsis*, and 785.52 *Septic shock*

786 Symptoms involving respiratory system and other chest symptoms
AHA: March-April, 1985, 3; Q2, 1990, 3; Q2, 1990, 5; Q2, 1990, 15; Q1, 1991, 12

786.00 Unspecified respiratory abnormality
786.01 Hyperventilation — *rapid breathing*
AHA: March-April, 1985, 3; Q2, 1990, 3; Q2, 1990, 5; Q2, 1990, 15; Q1, 1991, 12

786.02 Orthopnea — *difficult respiration except when patient is upright*
AHA: March-April, 1985, 3; Q2, 1990, 3; Q2, 1990, 5; Q2, 1990, 15; Q1, 1991, 12

786.03 Apnea — *momentary cessation in breathing*
AHA: March-April, 1985, 3; Q2, 1990, 3; Q2, 1990, 5; Q2, 1990, 15; Q1, 1991, 12; Q4, 1998, 50

This subclassification excludes sleep apnea (780.51, 780.53, and 780.57) and apnea of newborn (770.81, 770.82).

786.04 Cheyne-Stokes respiration
Cheyne-Stokes respiration is defined as an abnormal breathing pattern that is first shallow and infrequent and then increases gradually to abnormally deep and rapid, before fading away completely for about five to 30 seconds, before the next cycle of shallow breathing begins. Cheyne-Stokes respiration is often accompanied by changes in the level of consciousness; it most commonly occurs in seriously ill patients with brain or heart disorders. It may occur during sleep.

Therapies include treating the associated heart or brain disorder and prescribing the drug aminophylline.

786.05 Shortness of breath
786.06 Tachypnea — *quick, shallow breathing*
AHA: March-April, 1985, 3; Q2, 1990, 3; Q2, 1990, 5; Q2, 1990, 15; Q1, 1991, 12; Q4, 1998, 50

786.07 Wheezing — *whistling noises during breathing*
AHA: March-April, 1985, 3; Q2, 1990, 3; Q2, 1990, 5; Q2, 1990, 15; Q1, 1991, 12; Q4, 1998, 50

786.09 Other dyspnea and respiratory abnormalities — *snoring, yawning, paroxysmal dyspnea, respiratory distress; not otherwise specified*
AHA: March-April, 1985, 3; Q1, 1990, 9; Q2, 1990, 3; Q2, 1990, 5; Q2, 1990, 15; Q1, 1991, 12; Q1, 1997, 7; Q2, 1998, 10; Q4, 2005, 90

This subclassification excludes respiratory distress of newborn (770.89) and respiratory failure of newborn (770.84).

786.1 Stridor — *harsh sound associated with respiration in patients with airway obstruction*
AHA: March-April, 1985, 3; Q2, 1990, 3; Q2, 1990, 5; Q2, 1990, 15; Q1, 1991, 12

786.2 Cough
786.3 Hemoptysis — *cough with hemorrhage*
AHA: March-April, 1985, 3; Q2, 1990, 3; Q2, 1990, 5; Q2, 1990, 15; Q4, 1990, 26; Q1, 1991, 12; Q2, 2006, 17

Hemoptysis is coughing up or spitting out of blood or bloody sputum from the lungs or tracheobronchial tree. Expectoration of 200 ml of blood in a single episode suggests severe bleeding. Expectoration of 400 ml in three hours, or more than 600 ml in 16 hours, is life threatening. Bleeding into the respiratory tract by bronchial or pulmonary vessels causes hemoptysis, which reflects changes in the vascular walls and blood-clotting mechanisms. Lab work, including complete count, sputum culture and smear, and coagulation studies, may reveal anemia or infection. Chest x-ray, pulmonary arteriography, or lung scan may rule out disease such as carcinoma, tuberculosis, and pneumonia. Bronchoscopy (with biopsy), in severe hemoptysis, locates bleeding site. Therapies include placement of the patient in Trendelenburg position to promote drainage of blood from the lungs and cough suppressants to prevent blood from spreading throughout the lungs.

Associated conditions include chronic bronchitis, bronchogenic carcinoma, bronchiectasis, laryngeal cancer, bronchial adenoma, lung abscess, pneumonia (Klebsiella, pneumococcal), pulmonary arteriovenous fistula, pulmonary contusion, pulmonary edema, pulmonary embolism with infarction, pulmonary hypertension (primary), pulmonary tuberculosis and silicosis, tracheal trauma, ruptured aortic aneurysm, Wegener's granulomatosis, systemic lupus erythematosus, and coagulation disorder.

786.4   Abnormal sputum — *in color, amount, odor, quantity*
AHA: March-April, 1985, 3; Q2, 1990, 3; Q2, 1990, 5; Q2, 1990, 15; Q1, 1991, 12

786.50   Unspecified chest pain — *unknown cause*
AHA: March-April, 1985, 3; Q2, 1990, 3; Q2, 1990, 5; Q2, 1990, 15; Q1, 1991, 12; Q4, 1999, 25; Q1, 2002, 4; Q1, 2003, 6; Q2, 2006, 7

Use code 786.50 to report localized discomfort occurring in the chest. Among possible etiologies are acute myocardial infarction, angina, chest trauma, and peptic ulcer disease. Studies vary depending on the suspected etiology (e.g., electrocardiogram (EKG) for acute myocardial infarction, chest x-ray for chest trauma). Therapies include analgesics for pain control.

786.51   Precordial pain — *chest pain near heart*
AHA: March-April, 1985, 3; Q2, 1990, 3; Q2, 1990, 5; Q2, 1990, 15; Q1, 1991, 12

786.52   Painful respiration — *pleurodynia, Prinzmetal-Massumi syndrome, pleuritic pain*
AHA: Nov-Dec, 1984, 17; March-April, 1985, 3; Q2, 1990, 3; Q2, 1990, 5; Q2, 1990, 15; Q1, 1991, 12

Use this code to report a form of chest pain due to painful inhalation, expiration, or both. It may be due to pain in the chest wall (rib cage and sternum), pleura, or accessory muscles of respiration.

786.59   Other chest pain — *not otherwise specified, including discomfort, pressure, tightness in chest*
AHA: March-April, 1985, 3; Q2, 1990, 3; Q2, 1990, 5; Q2, 1990, 15; Q1, 1991, 12; Q1, 2002, 6

786.6   Swelling, mass, or lump in chest

786.7   Abnormal chest sounds — *rales, tympany, friction sounds, abnormal percussion*
AHA: March-April, 1985, 3; Q2, 1990, 3; Q2, 1990, 5; Q2, 1990, 15; Q1, 1991, 12

786.8   Hiccough — *singultus, spastic diaphragm*
AHA: March-April, 1985, 3; Q2, 1990, 3; Q2, 1990, 5; Q2, 1990, 15; Q1, 1991, 12

A hiccough, or hiccups, is defined as repetitive, involuntary, spasmodic contractions of the diaphragm. Hiccups are a symptom, not a disease. Hiccups involve the diaphragm (large, thin muscle that separates the chest from the abdomen) and phrenic nerve (nerve that connects the diaphragm to the brain). Almost everybody gets hiccups, even a fetus in a mother's womb.

Hiccups are caused by an irritation of nerves from the brain that control breathing muscles, especially the diaphragm. Causes are numerous for prolonged or recurrent hiccup episodes and include diseases of the pleura, pneumonia, uremia, alcoholism, use of certain prescription or non-prescription drugs, pregnancy, and disorders of the stomach, esophagus, bowel, or pancreas. There is no known prevention for hiccups, though prolonged episodes may require surgery to cut the phrenic nerve.

786.9   Other symptoms involving respiratory system and chest — *breath-holding spell*
AHA: March-April, 1985, 3; Q2, 1990, 3; Q2, 1990, 5; Q2, 1990, 15; Q1, 1991, 12

787 Symptoms involving digestive system
AHA: March-April, 1985, 3; Q2, 1990, 3; Q2, 1990, 5; Q2, 1990, 15; Q1, 1991, 12

Often, nausea and vomiting are symptoms of metabolic or microbial toxins or reactions to drugs, radiation, or motion (i.e., seasickness). Therapies depend on the etiology and include antiemetics (Inapsine, Reglan, Compazine, and Norzine).

Excluded from this subclassification are hematemesis not otherwise specified (578.0), excessive vomiting in pregnancy (643.0x-643.9x), regurgitation of food in newborn (779.3), habitual vomiting (536.2), psychogenic vomiting not otherwise

Symptoms, Signs, and Ill-Defined Conditions

specified (307.54), and constipation (564.00-564.09).

787.01	Nausea with vomiting
787.02	Nausea alone
787.03	Vomiting alone
787.1	Heartburn — *pyrosis, waterbrash* AHA: March-April, 1985, 3; Q2, 1990, 3; Q2, 1990, 5; Q2, 1990, 15; Q1, 1991, 12; Q2, 2001, 6
787.2	Dysphagia — *difficulty in swallowing, cricopharyngeal syndrome* AHA: March-April, 1985, 3; Q2, 1990, 3; Q2, 1990, 5; Q2, 1990, 15; Q1, 1991, 12; Q2, 2001, 4; Q4, 2003, 103, 109

Dysphagia is difficulty in swallowing. Pre-esophageal dysphagia is difficulty in emptying material from the oral pharynx into the esophagus. Esophageal dysphagia is difficulty in passing food down the esophagus. The most common symptom of esophageal disorders, dysphagia is classified as phase 1, 2, or 3. Phase 1, transfer phase, typically results from a neuromuscular disorder. Phase 2, transport phase, usually indicates spasm or carcinoma. Phase 3, entrance phase, results from lower esophageal narrowing by diverticula, esophagitis, and other disorders. Endoscopy with biopsy visualizes any gross pathology and provides specimens. Esophageal manometry measures esophageal pressure of upper and lower sphincters and detects abnormal contractions and peristalsis. Esophageal acidity test (usually performed with manometry) or acid perfusion test (Bernstein test) detects gastric acid reflux.

Associated conditions include amyotrophic lateral sclerosis, myasthenia gravis, Parkinson's disease, oral cavity tumor, carcinoma (laryngeal, esophageal, gastric), pharyngitis (chronic), airway obstruction, progressive systemic sclerosis, achalasia, and dysphagia lusoria. Associated esophageal conditions include esophageal compression (external), esophageal diverticulum, esophageal leiomyoma, esophageal obstruction by foreign body, esophagitis (corrosive, monilial, reflux), and lower esophageal ring. Other associated conditions include mediastinitis, Plummer-Vinson syndrome, systemic lupus erythematosus, hypocalcemia, syphilis, botulism, lead poisoning, and tetanus.

787.3	Flatulence, eructation, and gas pain — *bloating, tympanites, abdominal distension* AHA: March-April, 1985, 3; Q2, 1990, 3; Q2, 1990, 5; Q2, 1990, 15; Q1, 1991, 12
787.4	Visible peristalsis — *hyperperistalsis* AHA: March-April, 1985, 3; Q2, 1990, 3; Q2, 1990, 5; Q2, 1990, 15; Q1, 1991, 12
787.5	Abnormal bowel sounds — *absent or hyperactive* AHA: March-April, 1985, 3; Q2, 1990, 3; Q2, 1990, 5; Q2, 1990, 15; Q1, 1991, 12
787.6	Incontinence of feces — *encopresis, incontinence of sphincter ani* AHA: March-April, 1985, 3; Q2, 1990, 3; Q2, 1990, 5; Q2, 1990, 15; Q1, 1991, 12; Q1, 1997, 9
787.7	Abnormal feces — *bulky stools* AHA: March-April, 1985, 3; Q2, 1990, 3; Q2, 1990, 5; Q2, 1990, 15; Q1, 1991, 12
787.91	Diarrhea — *loose, copious stools* AHA: March-April, 1985, 3; Q2, 1990, 3; Q2, 1990, 5; Q2, 1990, 15; Q1, 1991, 12; Q4, 1995, 54
787.99	Other symptoms involving digestive system — *tenesmus, swelling, neuralgia, change in bowel habits* AHA: March-April, 1985, 3; Q2, 1990, 3; Q2, 1990, 5; Q2, 1990, 15; Q1, 1991, 12

788 Symptoms involving urinary system
AHA: March-April, 1985, 3; Q2, 1990, 3; Q2, 1990, 5; Q2, 1990, 15; Q1, 1991, 12

Signs and symptoms of retention of urine include distended abdomen, pain, and urgency. Therapies include catheterization and surgery, such as transurethral resection of the prostate in males. Associated conditions include benign prostatic hypertrophy, neurogenic bladder, carcinoma of the prostate, urethral stricture, and urinary tract infection.

Inability to void is a common sequela to pelvic and perineal surgery or surgery performed under spinal anesthesia. The condition is not necessarily a postoperative complication. Documentation should support the condition as a medical management problem and not solely reflect prophylactic measures such as bladder catheterization.

788.0	Renal colic — *kidney or ureter* AHA: March-April, 1985, 3; Q2, 1990, 3; Q2, 1990, 5; Q2, 1990, 15; Q1, 1991, 12; Q3, 2004, 8
788.1	Dysuria — *painful urination, strangury* AHA: March-April, 1985, 3; Q2, 1990, 3; Q2, 1990, 5; Q2, 1990, 15; Q1, 1991, 12
788.20	Unspecified retention of urine — *unknown type* AHA: March-April, 1985, 3; Q2, 1990, 3; Q2, 1990, 5; Q2, 1990, 15; Q1, 1991, 12; Q3, 1996, 10; Q1, 2003, 6; Q3, 2003, 12-13; Q2, 2004, 18
788.21	Incomplete bladder emptying
788.29	Other specified retention of urine — *not otherwise specified* AHA: March-April, 1985, 3; Q2, 1990, 3; Q2, 1990, 5; Q2, 1990, 15; Q1, 1991, 12

Signs and symptoms of urinary incontinence include stress, urge, overflow or total incontinence; intermittent leakage resulting from sudden physical strain; dribble resulting from urinary retention; inability to suppress the sudden urge to urinate; and continuous leakage. Cystoscopy with biopsy visualizes any gross pathology and provides specimens. Cystometry tests bladder compliance, capacity, and residual volume. Therapies include bladder retraining and surgery such as creation of urinary diversion.

Associated conditions include cerebrovascular accident, diabetic neuropathy, Guillain-Barré syndrome, multiple sclerosis, spinal cord injury, benign prostatic hypertrophy, bladder calculi, bladder cancer, prostatic cancer, chronic prostatitis, and urethral stricture.

788.3 ⇨sth	Urinary incontinence — (Code, if applicable, any causal condition first: 618.0-618.9, 753.23)	
	AHA: March-April, 1985, 3; Q2, 1990, 3; Q2, 1990, 5; Q2, 1990, 15; Q1, 1991, 12; Q4, 1992, 22	
788.30	Unspecified urinary incontinence — *unknown type of enuresis, bladder neck syndrome*	
788.31	Urge incontinence — *inability to control flow upon urge*	
788.32	Stress incontinence, male — *inability to control flow upon pressure*	
788.33	Mixed incontinence urge and stress (male)(female) — *urge and stress*	
788.34	Incontinence without sensory awareness — *no sensory warning*	
788.35	Post-void dribbling — *inability to control flow after urination*	
788.36	Nocturnal enuresis — *bed-wetting*	
788.37	Continuous leakage — *constant flow*	
788.38	Overflow incontinence	
788.39	Other urinary incontinence — *not otherwise specified*	
788.41	Urinary frequency — *frequent micturition*	
788.42	Polyuria — *copious micturition*	
788.43	Nocturia — *frequent nighttime micturition*	
788.5	Oliguria and anuria — *deficient secretion or suppression of urine*	
788.61	Splitting of urinary stream — *intermittent urinary stream*	
788.62	Slowing of urinary stream — *weak stream*	
788.63	Urgency of urination	
788.64	Urinary hesitancy	
788.65	Straining on urination	

Both urinary hesitancy and straining on urination are considered lower urinary tract symptoms (LUTS). LUTS are commonly associated with various types of obstructive uropathies. However, these symptoms can herald a variety of other possible etiologies depending on other clinical factors. In both sexes, LUTS may be further divided into the following categories of symptoms:

- Obstructive: Reduced force, hesitancy, straining, nocturia
- Irritative: Often associated with infection) dysuria, frequency, urgency
- Bladder storage: Daytime frequency, nocturia, urgency, incontinence
- Bladder sensation: Increase, reduction or absence of sensation
- Urinary voiding: Weak stream, spraying, intermittent, hesitancy, straining, dribbling
- Posturination: Incomplete emptying, dribbling
- Genital and lower urinary tract pain: Pelvic, bladder, urethral, vaginal, scrotal, perineal

These symptoms, or any combination of them, are considered along with the patient's clinical presentation to determine the underlying cause, which is used to determine the best intervention and course of treatment.

In male patients, LUTS including both urinary hesitancy and straining on urination are common symptoms associated with an enlarged prostate, bladder outlet obstruction (BOO), calculi, and other obstructive or functional uropathies.

In female patients, LUTS can be due to conditions such as:

- Hormonal changes; reduction or loss of estrogen
- Neuromuscular disease
- Obstructive pelvic mass
- Inverted uterus
- Cystocele
- Urethral diverticulum

788.69	Other abnormality of urination — *not otherwise specified*	
788.7	Urethral discharge — *penile discharge, urethrorrhea*	
788.8	Extravasation of urine — *escape of urine into adjacent tissues*	
788.9	Other symptoms involving urinary system — *not otherwise specified, including extrarenal uremia, tenesmus*	
	AHA: Q1, 2005, 12	

Excluded from this rubric are hematuria (599.7), nonspecific findings on examination of the urine (791.0-791.9), small kidney of unknown cause (589.0-589.9), and uremia not otherwise specified (586).

Coding Clarification
Urinary hesitancy and straining upon urination are included in the clinical term lower urinary tract

Symptoms, Signs, and Ill-Defined Conditions

symptoms (LUTS), for which there is no single unique code. Each urinary symptom would be coded separately in category 788 *Symptoms involving urinary system*, in lieu of a causal diagnosis.

Included in the 600 *Benign prostate hyperplasia* code category are specific code titles and instructional notes that direct the coder to code lower urinary tract symptoms (LUTS) in addition to BPH, when appropriate, even though the underlying cause is known.

Code, if applicable, any causal condition first, such as congenital ureterocele (753.23) and hyperplasia of prostate (600.0-600.9) with fifth-digit 1.

Excluded from this subclassification are urinary incontinence of nonorganic origin (307.6) and female stress incontinence (625.6).

789 Other symptoms involving abdomen and pelvis
AHA: March-April, 1985, 3; Q2, 1990, 3; Q2, 1990, 5; Q2, 1990, 15; Q1, 1991, 12

The following fifth-digit subclassification is to be used for codes 789.0, 789.3, 789.4, and 789.6:

0 unspecified site
1 right upper quadrant
2 left upper quadrant
3 right lower quadrant
4 left lower quadrant
5 periumbilic
6 epigastric
7 generalized
9 other specified site or multiple sites

789.0 ⌐5th⌐ Abdominal pain — *cramps, colic*
AHA: March-April, 1985, 3; Q2, 1990, 3; Q2, 1990, 2; Q2, 1990, 15; Q1, 1991, 12; Q1, 1995, 3

Use this subclassification to report localized pain or discomfort affecting the abdominal area. It may be due to drug use, the effect of toxins, or disorders of the gastrointestinal, reproductive, genitourinary, musculoskeletal, or vascular system. Blood work shows hematocrit, WBC, and differential and platelet counts. Urinalysis may identify urinary tract infection or kidney disease. Other lab work may reveal elevated liver enzymes (in hepatic disease), elevated serum bilirubin (in hepatobiliary disease), elevated serum amylase (in pancreatitis), or bacteria and parasites in stool culture (in acute diarrhea). Abdominal x-ray (supine and upright or decubitus and flat) may reveal intestinal disease or obstruction, while an ultrasound may identify aneurysms. Intravenous pyelogram (IVP) may identify renal disease or ureteral obstruction, while a sigmoidoscopy reveals condition of sigmoid colon and rectum. Associated conditions include peritonitis, perforated peptic ulcer, gallbladder disease, appendicitis, colitis, pancreatitis, lymphadenitis, pelvic inflammatory disease, intestinal obstruction, ruptured liver or spleen, ovarian cyst, ectopic pregnancy, endometriosis, pneumonia, myocardial ischemia, leukemia, nephritis, uremia, herpes zoster, and ureteral obstruction.

789.1 Hepatomegaly — *enlarged liver*
AHA: March-April, 1985, 3; Q2, 1990, 3; Q2, 1990, 5; Q2, 1990, 15; Q1, 1991, 12

789.2 Splenomegaly — *enlarged spleen*
AHA: March-April, 1985, 3; Q2, 1990, 3; Q2, 1990, 5; Q2, 1990, 15; Q1, 1991, 12

789.3 ⌐5th⌐ Abdominal or pelvic swelling, mass, or lump — *diffuse or generalized swelling or mass*
AHA: March-April, 1985, 3; Q2, 1990, 3; Q2, 1990, 5; Q2, 1990, 15; Q1, 1991, 12

789.4 ⌐5th⌐ Abdominal rigidity — *inflexibility, turgidity*
AHA: March-April, 1985, 3; Q2, 1990, 3; Q2, 1990, 5; Q2, 1990, 15; Q1, 1991, 12

789.5 Ascites — *fluid in peritoneal cavity*
AHA: March-April, 1985, 3; Q4, 1989, 11; Q2, 1990, 3; Q2, 1990, 5; Q2, 1990, 15; Q1, 1991, 12; Q2, 2005, 8

Ascites is accumulation of serous fluid in the peritoneal cavity. Signs and symptoms of ascites include abdominal discomfort, distention, dyspnea, and a flat or an inverted umbilicus. Abdominal percussion transmits fluid wave and reveals shifting dullness. Paracentesis to remove fluid (typically 50 ml to 100 ml) may reveal the following:

- High WBC (more than 300 cells/ml to 500 cells/ml suggests infection)
- Sanguineous fluid (indicative of neoplasm or tuberculosis)
- Milky or chylous fluid (common with lymphoma)
- Concentrations of protein (less than 3 g/100 ml suggests liver disease or systemic disorder)

Therapies include bed rest, sodium restriction (20 mEq/day to 40 mEq/day), spironolactone such as Aldactone (100 mg/day to 300 mg/day, orally), monitoring of body weight and urinary sodium, and peritoneal-jugular shunting.

Associated conditions include chronic or subacute liver disease (most commonly cirrhosis from alcoholism), chronic active hepatitis, severe alcoholic hepatitis without cirrhosis, hepatic vein obstruction, systemic disease (heart failure, nephrotic syndrome), carcinomatosis, and tubercular peritonitis.

If the physician documents malignant ascites, assign code 197.6 instead.

789.6 ⌐sth Abdominal tenderness — *rebound tenderness*
AHA: March-April, 1985, 3; Q2, 1990, 3; Q2, 1990, 5; Q2, 1990, 15; Q1, 1991, 12

789.9 Other symptoms involving abdomen and pelvis — *umbilical bleeding or discharge; not otherwise specified*
AHA: March-April, 1985, 3; Q2, 1990, 3; Q2, 1990, 5; Q2, 1990, 15; Q1, 1991, 12

790–796 Nonspecific Abnormal Findings

790 Nonspecific findings on examination of blood
AHA: Q2, 1990, 16

790.01 Precipitous drop in hematocrit — *drop in red blood cell count*
AHA: Q4, 2000, 46

790.09 Other abnormality of red blood cells — *morphology, volume, anisocytosis, poikilocytosis; not otherwise specified*
AHA: Q4, 2000, 46

790.1 Elevated sedimentation rate — *sed rate*

790.21 Impaired fasting glucose — *elevated fasting glucose*

790.22 Impaired glucose tolerance test (oral) — *a metabolic test that measures carbohydrate tolerance; which includes the measurement of active insulin, a test on the liver based on the ability and power to absorb and store large quantities of glucose; elevated glucose tolerance test*

790.29 Nonspecific findings, Other abnormal glucose — *abnormal non-fasting glucose, pre-diabetes*

790.3 Excessive blood level of alcohol — *indicative of alcohol consumption*
AHA: Sept-Oct, 1986, 3

790.4 Nonspecific elevation of levels of transaminase or lactic acid dehydrogenase (LDH) — *a marker for hemolysis, pulmonary embolism, liver malignancy*

790.5 Other nonspecific abnormal serum enzyme levels — *acid phosphatase, alkaline phosphate, amylase, lipase*

790.6 Other abnormal blood chemistry — *cobalt, copper, iron, lithium, magnesium, mineral, zinc*
AHA: Q4, 1988, 1

Use code 790.6 to report an abnormal finding on blood chemistry tests for which there is no corresponding diagnosis, such as copper, iron, lithium, and magnesium.

790.7 Bacteremia — (Use additional code to identify organism) — *bacteria in the blood*
AHA: Q3, 1988, 12; Q4, 1993, 29; Q2, 2003, 7

Use code 790.7 to report the presence of live bacteria circulating in the bloodstream. Bacteremia frequently results from surgical procedures (e.g., incision and drainage of an abscess or dental extractions). It also may result from colonization of indwelling urinary catheters or other invasive apparatus. Therapies include antibiotics.

Associated conditions include abscessed teeth, urinary tract infection, and infected medical device.

The term "bacteremia" is sometimes used ambiguously by clinicians to mean septicemia, which is bacteremia with clinical signs and symptoms of systemic infection and classified to rubric 038. To ensure proper classification, verify with the physician any reports of bacteremia with signs and symptoms of systemic infection such as fever, chills, prostration, nausea and vomiting, diarrhea, metastatic abscesses, and skin eruptions.

Bacteremia of newborn (771.83) is excluded from this code.

790.8 Unspecified viremia — *virus in the blood*
AHA: Q4, 1988, 10

790.91 Abnormal arterial blood gases

790.92 Abnormal coagulation profile — *bleeding time, coagulation time, PTT, PT*
AHA: Q4, 1993, 29

790.93 Elevated prostate specific antigen [PSA]

790.94 Euthyroid sick syndrome

790.95 Other nonspecific findings on examination of blood, elevated C-reactive protein (CRP)

The presence of inflammation in an arterial wall has been found to contribute to plaque rupture and artery obstruction, thereby also contributing to heart attacks and strokes, even when the patient has none of the other classic risk factors involved in atherosclerosis. Elevated C-reactive protein (CRP) found in blood as this is a marker for inflammation occurring anywhere in the body. This level can vary from day to day and tends to increase with aging, low levels of physical activity, diabetes, depression, and even sleep disorders.

C-reactive protein is recognized as a risk factor in cardiovascular disease and is becoming more and more a risk assessment factor of heart disease and stroke along with cholesterol screening. This means that patients screened for this may come from several different patient groupings, including those with hypothyroidism and/or progressive thyroid failure, premature atherosclerosis, those undergoing

Symptoms, Signs, and III-Defined Conditions

peritoneal dialysis, middle aged men and women with and without other risk factors, and those with periodontal disease. Patients presenting with periodontal disease, especially, are at risk for cardiovascular problems. The inflammation from periodontal disease allows oral bacteria to enter the bloodstream, and causes the liver to produce proteins, such as CRP, that inflame arteries and promote blood clot formation.

790.99 Other nonspecific findings on examination of blood — *not otherwise specified, including proteinemia*
AHA: Q4, 1993, 29; Q2, 2003, 14

Excluded from this rubric are abnormalities of platelets (287.0-287.9), thrombocytes (287.0-287.9), or white blood cells (288.0-288.9).

791 Nonspecific findings on examination of urine
AHA: Q2, 1990, 16

791.0 Proteinuria — *protein in urine; albuminuria, Bence-Jones proteinuria*
AHA: Q3, 1991, 8

Proteinuria is defined as urinary protein excretion of greater than 150 mg per day. The types of proteinuria can be classified as glomerular, tubular, or overflow. Glomerular disease is the most common cause, resulting in urinary loss of albumin and immunoglobulins. Tubular proteinuria occurs when tubulointerstitial disease prevents the proximal tubule from reabsorbing low-molecular-weight proteins. Tubular diseases include hypertensive nephrosclerosis and tubulointerstitial nephropathy caused by nonsteroidal anti-inflammatory drugs. In overflow proteinuria, low-molecular-weight proteins inhibit the reabsorption of filtered proteins.

Lab tests include a quantitative measurement of protein excretion, which can be done with a 24-hour urine specimen or the urine protein-to-creatinine ratio (UPr/Cr). Dipstick analysis is used in most outpatient settings to semiquantitatively measure the urine protein concentration. The sulfosalicylic acid (SSA) turbidity test qualitatively screens for proteinuria.

Therapy depends on urine to protein concentration. Proteinuria of more than two g per 24 hours (moderate to heavy) requires aggressive work-up. If the creatinine clearance is normal and if there is a clear diagnosis such as diabetes or uncompensated congestive heart failure, the underlying medical condition can be treated with close follow-up of proteinuria and renal function (creatinine clearance). Benign causes include fever, intense activity or exercise, dehydration, emotional stress, and acute illness. More serious causes include glomerulonephritis and multiple myeloma. Common secondary causes are diabetic nephropathy, amyloidosis, and systemic lupus erythematosus.

This subcategory excludes postural proteinuria (593.6) and proteinuria arising during pregnancy or the puerperium (642.0x-642.9x, 646.2x).

791.1	Chyluria — *excess lymphatic fluid in urine*
791.2	Hemoglobinuria — *blood in urine seen in a lab exam*
791.3	Myoglobinuria — *myoglobin in the urine*
791.4	Biliuria — *bile pigments in the urine*
791.5	Glycosuria — *sugar in the urine*
791.6	Acetonuria — *acetone in the urine; ketonuria*
791.7	Other cells and casts in urine — *not otherwise specified*
791.9	Other nonspecific finding on examination of urine — *crystalluria, melanuria, cocciurea, uricosuria, elevated 18-ketosteroids, catecholamines, indoleacetic acid, or VMA*
AHA: Q1, 2005, 12

Excluded from this rubric are hematuria (599.7), specific findings indicating abnormality of amino-acid transport and metabolism (270.0-270.9), and specific findings indicating abnormality of carbohydrate transport and metabolism (271.0-271.9).

792 Nonspecific abnormal findings in other body substances
AHA: Q2, 1990, 16

792.0	Nonspecific abnormal finding in cerebrospinal fluid
792.1	Nonspecific abnormal finding in stool contents — *mucus, pus, fat, abnormal color, occult stool*
AHA: Q2, 1992, 9
792.2	Nonspecific abnormal finding in semen — *abnormal spermatozoa*
792.3	Nonspecific abnormal finding in amniotic fluid — *fluid surround fetus*
AHA: Nov-Dec, 1986, 4
792.4	Nonspecific abnormal finding in saliva
792.5	Cloudy (hemodialysis) (peritoneal) dialysis affluent
792.9	Other nonspecific abnormal finding in body substances — *peritoneal, pleural, synovial, vaginal or other fluid, not elsewhere specified*

A nonspecific abnormal finding in chromosomal analysis (795.2) is excluded from the rubric.

793 Nonspecific abnormal findings on radiological and other examination of body structure
AHA: Q2, 1990, 16

This rubric includes nonspecific abnormal findings in thermography, ultrasound (echogram), and x-ray.

Coders' Desk Reference for Diagnoses

793.0	Nonspecific abnormal findings on radiological and other examination of skull and head — *upon x-ray, ultrasound, thermography*
793.1	Nonspecific abnormal findings on radiological and other examination of lung field — *coin lesion or shadow upon x-ray, ultrasound, thermography*
793.2	Nonspecific abnormal findings on radiological and other examination of other intrathoracic organs — *heart shadow, mediastinal shift upon x-ray, ultrasound, thermography*
793.3	Nonspecific abnormal findings on radiological and other examination of biliary tract — *nonvisualization of gallbladder upon x-ray, ultrasound, thermography*
793.4	Nonspecific abnormal findings on radiological and other examination of gastrointestinal tract — *upon x-ray, ultrasound, thermography*
793.5	Nonspecific abnormal findings on radiological and other examination of genitourinary organs — *filling defect of bladder, kidney or ureter upon x-ray, ultrasound, thermography* **AHA:** Q4, 2000, 46
793.6	Nonspecific abnormal findings on radiological and other examination of abdominal area, including retroperitoneum — *upon x-ray, ultrasound, thermography*
793.7	Nonspecific abnormal findings on radiological and other examination of musculoskeletal system — *upon x-ray, ultrasound, thermography*
793.80	Unspecified abnormal mammogram
793.81	Mammographic microcalcification
793.89	Other abnormal findings on radiological examination of breast
793.91	Image test inconclusive due to excess body fat — (Use additional code to identify Body Mass Index (BMI) if known)

Radiologists have reported that the prevalence of obesity in the patient population has resulted in an increased occurrence of inconclusive imaging test results due to excessive body fat. Unsatisfactory imaging can negatively impact the ability to appropriately diagnose and treat an illness, trauma, or other condition.

Unsatisfactory imaging due to excessive body fat can seriously impede the efficacy of imaging technologies to appropriately diagnose and treat an illness, trauma, or other condition. X-rays, CT scans, ultrasound, and magnetic resonance imaging equipment require accommodation by the patient; the patient has to be able to fit into or onto the examining table or machine. The patient's size or large body habitus (LBH) may preclude proper positioning. If the equipment can accommodate the patient, imaging may still be unsuccessful or unsatisfactory due to decreased visualization through the fatty tissues of the body. The x-ray or other imaging beam of light cannot penetrate the layers of fat to obtain a crisp image of its target

internal organ or structure. When this occurs, it can be difficult or impossible to get a clear picture of the organs or any abnormality. Fatty tissue can obscure conditions such as diseased organs, obstructions, vascular compromise, abnormal tissues or tumors, and problems with fetal growth and development.

793.99	Other nonspecific abnormal findings on radiological and other examinations of body structure — *abnormal placental finding; abnormal radiological findings in skin and subcutaneous tissue*

Abnormal results of function studies and radioisotope scans (794.0-794.9) are excluded from the rubric.

794 Nonspecific abnormal results of function studies
AHA: Q2, 1990, 16

This rubric includes nonspecific abnormal findings in radioisotope scans, uptake studies, and scintiphotography.

794.00	Unspecified abnormal function study of brain and central nervous system
794.01	Nonspecific abnormal echoencephalogram
794.02	Nonspecific abnormal electroencephalogram (EEG)
794.09	Other nonspecific abnormal result of function study of brain and central nervous system — *brain scan; not otherwise specified*
794.10	Nonspecific abnormal response to unspecified nerve stimulation
794.11	Nonspecific abnormal retinal function studies — *ERG*
794.12	Nonspecific abnormal electro-oculogram (EOG)
794.13	Nonspecific abnormal visually evoked potential — *VEP*
794.14	Nonspecific abnormal oculomotor studies
794.15	Nonspecific abnormal auditory function studies **AHA:** Q1, 2004, 15-16
794.16	Nonspecific abnormal vestibular function studies
794.17	Nonspecific abnormal electromyogram (EMG)
794.19	Other nonspecific abnormal result of function study of peripheral nervous system and special senses
794.2	Nonspecific abnormal results of pulmonary system function study — *lung scan, ventilatory capacity, vital capacity*
794.30	Nonspecific abnormal unspecified cardiovascular function study
794.31	Nonspecific abnormal electrocardiogram (ecg) (ekg) — *Q-T interval prolongations, Romano-Ward syndrome* **AHA:** Q4, 2005, 72

Code 794.31 excludes long QT syndrome, which is coded to 426.82.

794.39	Other nonspecific abnormal cardiovascular system function study — *ballistocardiogram, phonocardiogram, vectorcardiogram*

Symptoms, Signs, and Ill-Defined Conditions

794.4	Nonspecific abnormal results of kidney function study — *renal function test*
794.5	Nonspecific abnormal results of thyroid function study — *thyroid scan, thyroid uptake*
794.6	Nonspecific abnormal results of other endocrine function study — *pituitary, thymus, adrenal, hypothalamus*
794.7	Nonspecific abnormal results of basal metabolism function study — *BMR*
794.8	Nonspecific abnormal results of liver function study — *liver scan*
794.9	Nonspecific abnormal results of other specified function study — *bladder, pancreas, placenta, spleen*

795 Other and nonspecific abnormal cytological, histological, immunological and DNA test findings
AHA: Q2, 1990, 16

795.0 🔖sth Abnormal Papanicolaou smear of cervix and cervical HPV — *Pap smear*
AHA: Q4, 2002, 69

Women who have abnormal results of a Pap smear test returned have some kind of atypical cellular changes occurring in the cervix uteri. These changes include abnormal glandular cell changes, and high and low grade squamous intraepithelial lesions. Positive results for a DNA test to detect the presence of the human papilloma virus can be very effective in helping doctors determine which patients who have had an abnormal smear result have cancer or precancer and need immediate attention. High risk types of this virus are the cause of most cervical cancers and can now be detected with certain DNA tests. Those patients who test positive are carefully followed for cervical cancer.

The histological and immunological cell changes reported with the Bethesda system are determined by cytology studies of the cell samples taken in smear tests. Dysplasias are more definitive results returned from biopsy samples of the cervical tissue taken during colposcopy exams and not Pap smears. Colposcopy with biopsy is the next step in diagnosing abnormal smear results in high-risk patients. Pap smears are screening tests and the actual changes occurring in the cells could be more or less severe. A Pap smear that results in a low grade squamous intraepithelial lesion usually indicates there is mild dysplasia, CIN I and koilo cytotic atypia. A Pap smear result of high grade squamous intraepithelial lesion usually indicates there is a moderate dysplasia. Dysplasias can progress to cancerous conditions that may require treatments such as removal or destruction of cervical tissue, cervicectomy, or even hysterectomy.

Excluded from this subcategory (795.0) are carcinoma of cervix (233.1), cervical intraepithelial neoplasia I (622.11), cervical intraepithelial neoplasia II (622.12), cervical intraepithelial neoplasia III (233.1), dysplasia (histologically confirmed) of cervix NOS (622.10), mild dysplasia (histologically confirmed) (622.12), severe dysplasia (histologically confirmed) (233.1).

795.00	Abnormal glandular Papanicolaou smear of cervix
795.01	Papanicolaou smear of cervix with atypical squamous cells of undetermined significance (ASC-US) AHA: Q2, 2006, 3
795.02	Papanicolaou smear of cervix with atypical squamous cells cannot exclude high grade squamous intraepithelial lesion (ASC-H)
795.03	Papanicolaou smear of cervix with low grade squamous intraepithelial lesion (LGSIL)
795.04	Papanicolaou smear of cervix with high grade squamous intraepithelial lesion (HGSIL)
795.05	Cervical high risk human papillomavirus (HPV) DNA test positive
795.06	Papanicolaou smear of cervix with cytologic evidence of malignancy
795.08	Nonspecific abnormal papanicolaou smear of cervix, unsatisfactory smear AHA: Q2, 2006, 4
795.09	Other abnormal Papanicolaou smear of cervix and cervical HPV — *cervical low risk human papillomavirus (HPV) DNA positive*
795.1	Nonspecific abnormal Papanicolaou smear of other site — *Pap smear other than cervical*
795.2	Nonspecific abnormal findings on chromosomal analysis — *abnormal karyotype*
795.3 🔖sth	Nonspecific positive culture findings — *nose, sputum, throat, wound*
795.31	Nonspecific positive findings for anthrax
795.39	Other nonspecific positive culture findings
795.4	Other nonspecific abnormal histological findings
795.5	Nonspecific reaction to tuberculin skin test without active tuberculosis — *Mantoux test, PPD positive, positive TB skin test*
795.6	False positive serological test for syphilis — *Wassermann reaction*

Subcategory 795.7 reports other nonspecific immunological findings. Excluded from this subcategory is elevated prostate-specific antigen, which is reported with code 790.93. Also excluded are abnormal tumor markers and elevated tumor-associated antigens, both of which are reported with codes from range 795.81-795.89.

| 795.71 | Nonspecific serologic evidence of human immunodeficiency virus (HIV) — (This code is only to be used when a test finding is reported as nonspecific. Asymptomatic positive findings are coded to V08. If any HIV infection symptom or condition is present, see code 042. Negative |

findings are not coded.) — *nonspecific findings only*
AHA: July-Aug, 1987, 24; Q2, 1992, 11; Q1, 1993, 21, 22; Q2, 1993, 6; Q2, 2004, 11

When the medical record documentation indicates "possible," "probable," or "questionable" AIDS, not confirmed, without manifestations, the record should be returned to the physician for further clarification. Physicians also need to be aware that unacceptable terminology and abbreviations in the medical record should not be used. These terms only cause confusion in code selection.

Positive Newborn Testing: If a newborn has a positive ELISA or Western Blot test for HIV, the correct code to use is 795.71 *Nonspecific serologic evidence of human immunodeficiency virus [HIV]*. These tests may reflect the antibodies of the mother and not the baby. If the mother is positive for HIV, the antibody may cross the placenta to the newborn. The antibodies may be carried up to 18 months producing a false-positive result. These false-positive results during the newborn's first 18 months are due to the mother's antibodies carried by the newborn. The baby may later lose those antibodies, indicating that he/she was actually never infected.

795.79	Other and unspecified nonspecific immunological findings — *raised antibody titer, raised immunoglobulin level*

AHA: Q2, 1993, 6

Excluded from this rubric are nonspecific abnormalities of red blood cells (790.01 790.09).

Coding Scenario
A 39-year-old female presents to her OB/GYN physician for a colposcopy and biopsy. Her recent Pap smear returned with a diagnosis of atypical high grade squamous intraepithelial lesion (HGSIL) identified. He performs a colposcopy and biopsy. Her visit is recorded as high grade squamous intraepithelial lesion (HGSIL).

Coding assignment: 795.04 *Papanicolaou smear of cervix with high grade squamous intraepithelial lesion (HGSIL)*

Subcategory 795.8 reports abnormal tumor markers, including elevations in tumor-associated antigens and tumor-specific antigens.

Caregivers regularly evaluate elevated levels of tumor markers and antigens to help diagnose and follow up on certain types of cancer. Over the past decade, a greater understanding of the role of immunity mechanisms has improved the ability to diagnose certain neoplasms and diseases earlier than previously possible. This identification is made possible by the isolation and measurement of tumor associated antigens (TAA), tumor-specific antigens (TSA), and other tumor markers or cancer-identifying cells and biological substances. Tumor-associated antigens (TAA) are closely associated with the presence of tumor cells, and tumor-specific antigens (TSA) are unique identifiers of tumor cells. The presence of TSA is especially beneficial in diagnosing and following many types of cancer. There are many different types of TAA and TSA tests, many of which are specific to certain cancers, such as tests for elevated prostate-specific antigens (PSA) for prostate cancer, alpha-fetoprotein for hepatocellular cancer, and CA-19 for gastrointestinal and pancreatic cancer.

The term "tumor markers" describes the presence of certain molecules (including antigens, hormones and proteins) occurring in blood or tissue that are associated with the cancer. Identification and measurement of tumor markers helps clinical management by:

• Providing a screening mechanism for a healthy population or a high-risk population for the presence of cancer

• Assisting in the diagnosis of cancer or of a specific type of cancer

• Providing a measurement to evaluate the prognosis in a patient

• Providing a means of monitoring the course in a patient in remission or during surgery, radiation, or chemotherapy

Elevated carcinoembryonic antigen (CEA) levels in the blood are used to help diagnose certain benign and malignant neoplasms, and other diseases. CEA tests are primarily used to monitor patients with colorectal and advanced breast cancer; however, elevated CEA levels can also be present in other types of cancer such pancreatic, gastric, and lung. Other diseases in which it can be detected include cirrhosis, inflammatory bowel disease, chronic lung disease, and pancreatitis. CEA tests are not a substitute for a pathological diagnosis. For example, studies have found elevated CEA levels in approximately 19 percent of smokers and in 3 percent of a healthy control population.

795.81	Elevated carcinoembryonic antigen (CEA)
795.82	Elevated cancer antigen 125 (CA 125)
795.89	Other abnormal tumor markers

Coding Clarification
Subcategory 795.8 includes elevated tumor-associated antigens (TAA) and tumor-specific

antigens (TSA). It excludes elevated prostate-specific antigen (PSA), which is reported with code 790.93.

796 Other nonspecific abnormal findings
AHA: Q2, 1990, 16

796.0	Nonspecific abnormal toxicological findings — *heavy metals or drugs in blood, urine or other tissue* **AHA:** Q1, 1997, 16
796.1	Abnormal reflex
796.2	Elevated blood pressure reading without diagnosis of hypertension — *no formal diagnosis of hypertension; incidental finding* **AHA:** July-Aug, 1984, 12; Q3, 1990, 4; Q2, 2003, 11
796.3	Nonspecific low blood pressure reading
796.4	Other abnormal clinical finding
796.5	Abnormal finding on antenatal screening
796.6	Nonspecific abnormal findings on neonatal screening

This code represents a status determination or laboratory findings result and not an actual presenting diagnosis. It denotes simply that some condition for which the infant was screened during normal newborn testing, came back with positive results that the infant may possibly have an abnormal condition for which the infant will need to be tested more extensively so a specific determination or an actual diagnosis can be made.

796.9	Other nonspecific abnormal finding — *not elsewhere specified*

Refer to the ICD-9-CM Index before assigning a code from this rubric to ensure a more specific code cannot be found.

When the documentation identifies a postoperative hypertension, the physician needs to document whether it was caused by inadequate control of pain or patient agitation, and if the hypertension was merely an elevation in blood pressure without mention of hypertension (796.2) or a benign hypertension (401.1).

Elevated Blood Pressure: Also known as transient hypertension, this condition is an elevated blood pressure reading without a diagnosis of hypertension and may be characteristic of older age groups or due to emotional stress. For these cases, report code 796.2 *Elevated blood pressure reading without diagnosis of hypertension.*

Coding Scenario
A patient is seen for blood pressure checks three times a week due to transient elevated blood pressure readings.

Code assignment: 796.2 *Elevated blood pressure reading without diagnosis of hypertension*

797–799 Ill-Defined and Unknown Causes of Morbidity and Mortality

797 Senility without mention of psychosis
Senility is triggered by mental decline and its cause is related to the neurons of the nervous system. With age, some shrinkage of the brain occurs due to the loss of neurons throughout life. The shrinkage is often insignificant, but in roughly 10 percent of the elderly, the brain atrophy is severe and senility results. The five major symptoms of senility are forgetfulness, irritability, poor judgment, disorientation, and general intellectual decline. The first signs are lapses in recent memory and an inability to grasp new information. As the illness progresses, abstract thinking is impaired, judgment becomes poor, and verbal communication becomes difficult. In time, the person is unable to perform ordinary activities and becomes completely dependent on others for physical needs. Diagnosis includes personal history, physical exam, and neurological testing. In many patients, the condition is one that mimics senility and is due to causes such as toxic drug reactions or high blood pressure. There is no cure for senility and the standard management is to delay the progression of symptoms.

Senile psychoses (290.0-290.9) are excluded from this category.

798 Sudden death, cause unknown

798.0	Sudden infant death syndrome — *crib death, SIDS*

Sudden infant death syndrome (SIDS) is defined as the sudden death of an infant younger than 1 year of age that remains unexplained after a thorough case investigation, including performance of a complete autopsy, examination of the death scene, and review of the clinical history.

According to the National SIDS Resource Center, most researchers now believe that babies who die of SIDS are born with one or more conditions that make them especially vulnerable to stresses that occur in the normal life of an infant, including both internal and external influences. Maternal risk factors include cigarette smoking during pregnancy, maternal age under 20 years, poor prenatal care, low weight gain, anemia, use of illegal drugs, and a history of sexually transmitted disease or urinary tract infection.

Most deaths from SIDS occur by the end of the sixth month, with the greatest number occurring between two and four months of age. A SIDS death occurs quickly and is often associated with sleep, with no signs of suffering. More deaths are reported in the fall and winter (in both the Northern and Southern Hemispheres) and there is a 60 to 40 percent male-to-female ratio. A death is diagnosed as SIDS only after all other alternatives have been eliminated: SIDS is a diagnosis of exclusion and includes investigations of the autopsy, death scene, and a review of the victim and family case history.

798.1	Instantaneous death
798.2	Death occurring in less than 24 hours from onset of symptoms, not otherwise explained — *without sign of disease or trauma*
798.9	Unattended death — *found dead*

799 Other ill-defined and unknown causes of morbidity and mortality

799.01	Asphyxia — *lack of oxygen* AHA: Q4, 2005, 90
799.02	Hypoxemia AHA: Q4, 2005, 90; Q2, 2006, 24-25

Asphyxia is a condition caused by the inadequate intake of oxygen. Hypoxemia is defined as below normal oxygen content in the arterial blood that impairs tissue perfusion. Hypoxia is a reduction in the supply of oxygen reaching tissues and low oxygen levels in the blood from reduced oxygen intake during inspiration. Adequate tissue perfusion by the blood may still be present with hypoxia, however. These codes exclude asphyxia and hypoxemia due to hypercapnia (786.09), which is an excess of carbon dioxide in the blood, although hypercapnia can occur with asphyxia.

Therapies depend on the etiology (e.g., removal of foreign body obstructing the trachea or electrical defibrillation for cardiopulmonary arrest) and may include closed cardiac massage if a heart beat and carotid pulse are absent, and the placement of the patient in Trendelenburg position to promote drainage of water from the lungs (fresh water victim).

Other therapies include mechanical ventilation, intensive respiratory therapy, IV administration of sodium bicarbonate, inhalation or injection of beta-agonists (epinephrine, Isuprel, Alupent, Brethine) to reduce bronchospasm, and administration of corticosteroids and antibiotics.

799.1	Respiratory arrest — *cardiorespiratory failure*

Use code 799.1 to report a cessation of breathing, identified as primary, secondary, or complete. Primary respiratory arrest may be due to airway obstruction, decreased respiratory drive, or respiratory muscle weakness. Secondary respiratory arrest may be a result of cardiac arrest. Therapies include cardiopulmonary resuscitation, intubation, and ventilation.

This code excludes respiratory distress of newborn (770.89) and respiratory failure of newborn (770.84).

799.2	Nervousness
799.3	Unspecified debility — *specifics unknown*
799.4	Cachexia — (Code first underlying condition, if known) — *wasting disease; general ill health and poor nutrition* AHA: Q3, 1990, 17

The protein-wasting syndrome called cachexia most commonly occurs with lung, pancreatic, stomach, bowel, and prostate cancers, and rarely with breast cancer. It also affects people with AIDS, uncontrolled rheumatoid arthritis, severe infections, chronic lung and bowel disease, and heart failure. The cause is usually related to liver metastasis with resulting pain and loss of appetite. Sometimes the cause is mechanical, such as when a tumor grows into the stomach or blocks the intestine.

Undiagnosed and untreated cachexia is life threatening. It can decrease the effectiveness of cancer treatments such as chemotherapy and radiation therapy, and magnify their side effects.

799.81	Decreased libido — *drop off in sexual desire* AHA: Q4, 2003, 75
799.89	Other ill-defined conditions
799.9	Other unknown and unspecified cause of morbidity or mortality — *unknown cause of morbidity or mortality* AHA: Q1, 1990, 20; Q1, 1998, 4

800–999
Injury and Poisoning

800–829 Fractures

A fracture is a break in a bone resulting from two possible causes: the direct or indirect application of undue force against the bone and pathological changes resulting in spontaneous fractures. This chapter includes only those fractures that have arisen as a result of an injury. It excludes malunions and nonunions of fractured bones.

The clinician always determines whether a fracture is open or closed; this is one of the first determinations that should be made.

Closed fractures are contained beneath the skin, while open or compound fractures connote an associated open wound.

Terms that typically describe closed fractures include:

- Comminuted — a splintering of the fractured bone
- Depressed — a portion of the skull broken and driven inward from a forceful blow
- Fissured — a fracture that does not split the bone
- Greenstick — occurs in children; the bone is somewhat bent and partially broken
- Impacted — one fractured bone end wedged into another
- Linear — straight line
- Simple — intact ligaments and skin
- Slipped epiphysis — separation of the growing end of the bone (epiphysis) from the shaft of the bone that occurs in children and young adults who still have active epiphyses
- Spiral — resembles a helix

Open fractures have a distinctive vocabulary. They are always compound, with a wound leading to the fracture or the broken bone ends protruding through the skin. There is a very high risk of infection with open fractures since the tissues are exposed to contaminants. Also, there may be missiles or foreign bodies embedded in the tissues that must be removed during surgery. Puncture wounds may be present.

Both open and closed fractures may earn the descriptive term of "complicated." A complicated fracture is one in which a bone fragment has injured an internal organ. For example, the ribs may injure the lungs, liver, and spleen, depending on the nature and direction of the force causing the fracture.

800 Fracture of vault of skull
AHA: Sept-Oct, 1985, 3; Q2, 1989, 15; Q2, 1990, 7; Q3, 1990, 5; Q3, 1990, 13; Q4, 1990, 26; Q4, 1996, 36

The vault of the skull is composed of three bones: the frontal bone and two parietal bones. Fractures of the vault may be accompanied by cerebral contusion or laceration; subarachnoid, subdural, or extradural hemorrhage; or an unspecified cause of hemorrhage.

Cerebral contusions and lacerations constitute severe injury. One of the great problems associated with head trauma is that the brain sustains a double blow — the initial blow that causes the brain to travel to the opposite side of the skull, smiting the interior skull with significant force. This second blow is called contrecoup. Such force applied to the brain causes swelling and increased intracranial pressure that is very dangerous. Serious head trauma has a high mortality rate, nearly 50 percent. In addition to edema, a second complication is hemorrhage resulting from laceration of blood vessels. If the fracture is open, the brain is exposed to bacteria, compounding the danger.

Major trauma to the forebrain with no injury to the brainstem may result in survival of the patient in a chronic vegetative state for several years.

Patients who have survived severe head trauma often deal with posttraumatic epilepsy for many years.

The following fifth-digit subclassification is for use with the appropriate codes in categories 800, 801, 803, and 804:
0   unspecified state of consciousness
1   with no loss of consciousness
2   with brief [less than one hour] loss of consciousness
3   with moderate [1-24 hours] loss of consciousness
4   with prolonged [more than 24 hours] loss of consciousness and return to pre-existing conscious level
5   with prolonged [more than 24 hours] loss of consciousness, without return to pre-existing conscious level
6   with loss of consciousness of unspecified duration
9   with concussion, unspecified

800.0 ✓5th   Closed fracture of vault of skull without mention of intracranial injury
800.1 ✓5th   Closed fracture of vault of skull with cerebral laceration and contusion
800.2 ✓5th   Closed fracture of vault of skull with subarachnoid, subdural, and extradural hemorrhage
800.3 ✓5th   Closed fracture of vault of skull with other and unspecified intracranial hemorrhage
800.4 ✓5th   Closed fracture of vault of skull with intercranial injury of other and unspecified nature
800.5 ✓5th   Open fracture of vault of skull without mention of intracranial injury
800.6 ✓5th   Open fracture of vault of skull with cerebral laceration and contusion
800.7 ✓5th   Open fracture of vault of skull with subarachnoid, subdural, and extradural hemorrhage
800.8 ✓5th   Open fracture of vault of skull with other and unspecified intracranial hemorrhage
800.9 ✓5th   Open fracture of vault of skull with intracranial injury of other and unspecified nature

801 Fracture of base of skull
AHA: Sept-Oct, 1985, 3; Q2, 1989, 15; Q2, 1990, 7; Q3, 1990, 5; Q3, 1990, 13; Q4, 1990, 26; Q4, 1996, 36

Included in the description for the base of the skull are the following bones:

- Occiput — bone at the base of the skull; contains the foramen magnum, the opening in the bone that allows the spinal cord to join the brain.
- Orbital roof — the orbit has a roof and a floor. The roof is considered part of the skull base, an exception is the frontal bone that forms part of the roof of the orbit as part of the skull vault.
- Sphenoid bone — large bone containing the sphenoid sinus, forming part of the back of the orbit.
- Temporal bones (2) — adjoin the parietal, sphenoid, and occipital bones.

- Cranial fossae — anterior, middle, and posterior — The three fossae form the floor of the cranial cavity (on the superior aspect of the base of the skull) and provide a surface to support the various lobes of the brain. The frontal lobes rest on the anterior fossa, the temporal lobes on the middle fossa, and the pons and medulla oblongata are contained within the posterior fossa, with the cerebellum expanding over the medulla oblongata.

The following fifth-digit subclassification is for use with the appropriate codes in categories 800, 801, 803, and 804:
0   unspecified state of consciousness
1   with no loss of consciousness
2   with brief [less than one hour] loss of consciousness
3   with moderate [1-24 hours] loss of consciousness
4   with prolonged [more than 24 hours] loss of consciousness and return to pre-existing conscious level
5   with prolonged [more than 24 hours] loss of consciousness, without return to pre-existing conscious level
6   with loss of consciousness of unspecified duration
9   with concussion, unspecified

801.0 ✓5th   Closed fracture of base of skull without mention of intracranial injury
801.1 ✓5th   Closed fracture of base of skull with cerebral laceration and contusion
801.2 ✓5th   Closed fracture of base of skull with subarachnoid, subdural, and extradural hemorrhage
801.3 ✓5th   Closed fracture of base of skull with other and unspecified intracranial hemorrhage
801.4 ✓5th   Closed fracture of base of skull with intracranial injury of other and unspecified nature
801.5 ✓5th   Open fracture of base of skull without mention of intracranial injury
801.6 ✓5th   Open fracture of base of skull with cerebral laceration and contusion
801.7 ✓5th   Open fracture of base of skull with subarachnoid, subdural, and extradural hemorrhage
801.8 ✓5th   Open fracture of base of skull with other and unspecified intracranial hemorrhage
801.9 ✓5th   Open fracture of base of skull with intracranial injury of other and unspecified nature

802 Fracture of face bones
AHA: Sept-Oct, 1985, 3; Q2, 1989, 15; Q2, 1990, 7; Q3, 1990, 5; Q3, 1990, 13; Q4, 1990, 26; Q4, 1996, 36

The facial bones comprise the following bones:

- Nasal bone — adjoins the frontal bone to form the superior aspect of the nose
- Mandible — lower jawbone
- Maxilla — upper jawbone
- Zygomatic bones — two bones of the cheek

Injury and Poisoning

- Lacrimal bones — two bones of the tear ducts
- Vomer — inferior and interior support for nasal conchae
- Orbital plate — two bones in the area of the eye
- Palate — the roof of the mouth

The orbit is one of the most complex bony structures in the skull. The frontal, mandible, lacrimal, orbital plate, zygomatic, and sphenoid bones fit together to form support and protection for the eyeball.

The following fifth-digit subclassification is for use with the appropriate codes in categories 800, 801, 803, and 804:

0   unspecified state of consciousness
1   with no loss of consciousness
2   with brief [less than one hour] loss of consciousness
3   with moderate [1-24 hours] loss of consciousness
4   with prolonged [more than 24 hours] loss of consciousness and return to pre-existing conscious level
5   with prolonged [more than 24 hours] loss of consciousness, without return to pre-existing conscious level
6   with loss of consciousness of unspecified duration
9   with concussion, unspecified

Code	Description
802.0	Nasal bones, closed fracture
802.1	Nasal bones, open fracture
802.2 ⌐sth	Mandible, closed fracture
802.3 ⌐sth	Mandible, open fracture
802.4	Malar and maxillary bones, closed fracture
802.5	Malar and maxillary bones, open fracture
802.6	Orbital floor (blow-out), closed fracture
802.7	Orbital floor (blow-out), open fracture
802.8	Other facial bones, closed fracture
802.9	Other facial bones, open fracture

803   Other and unqualified skull fractures
AHA: Sept-Oct, 1985, 3; Q2, 1989, 15; Q2, 1990, 7; Q3, 1990, 5; Q3, 1990, 13; Q4, 1990, 26; Q4, 1996, 36

Use these codes when the record lacks specific information regarding the trauma to the head.

The following fifth-digit subclassification is for use with the appropriate codes in categories 800, 801, 803, and 804:

0   unspecified state of consciousness
1   with no loss of consciousness
2   with brief [less than one hour] loss of consciousness
3   with moderate [1-24 hours] loss of consciousness
4   with prolonged [more than 24 hours] loss of consciousness and return to pre-existing conscious level
5   with prolonged [more than 24 hours] loss of consciousness, without return to pre-existing conscious level
6   with loss of consciousness of unspecified duration
9   with concussion, unspecified

Code	Description
803.0 ⌐sth	Other closed skull fracture without mention of intracranial injury
803.1 ⌐sth	Other closed skull fracture with cerebral laceration and contusion
803.2 ⌐sth	Other closed skull fracture with subarachnoid, subdural, and extradural hemorrhage
803.3 ⌐sth	Closed skull fracture with other and unspecified intracranial hemorrhage
803.4 ⌐sth	Other closed skull fracture with intracranial injury of other and unspecified nature
803.5 ⌐sth	Other open skull fracture without mention of intracranial injury
803.6 ⌐sth	Other open skull fracture with cerebral laceration and contusion
803.7 ⌐sth	Other open skull fracture with subarachnoid, subdural, and extradural hemorrhage
803.8 ⌐sth	Other open skull fracture with other and unspecified intracranial hemorrhage
803.9 ⌐sth	Other open skull fracture with intracranial injury of other and unspecified nature

804   Multiple fractures involving skull or face with other bones
AHA: Sept-Oct, 1985, 3; Q2, 1989, 15; Q2, 1990, 7; Q3, 1990, 5; Q3, 1990, 13; Q4, 1990, 26; Q4, 1996, 36

This category is used when bones of the skull or face are fractured, together with bones in other parts of the body. If there is more specific information about the nature of the various fractures, code more specifically.

The following fifth-digit subclassification is for use with the appropriate codes in categories 800, 801, 803, and 804:
- 0 unspecified state of consciousness
- 1 with no loss of consciousness
- 2 with brief [less than one hour] loss of consciousness
- 3 with moderate [1-24 hours] loss of consciousness
- 4 with prolonged [more than 24 hours] loss of consciousness and return to pre-existing conscious level
- 5 with prolonged [more than 24 hours] loss of consciousness, without return to pre-existing conscious level
- 6 with loss of consciousness of unspecified duration
- 9 with concussion, unspecified

804.0 ✓5th Closed fractures involving skull or face with other bones, without mention of intracranial injury

804.1 ✓5th Closed fractures involving skull or face with other bones, with cerebral laceration and contusion
AHA: Q1, 2006, 6

804.2 ✓5th Closed fractures involving skull or face with other bones with subarachnoid, subdural, and extradural hemorrhage

804.3 ✓5th Closed fractures involving skull or face with other bones, with other and unspecified intracranial hemorrhage

804.4 ✓5th Closed fractures involving skull or face with other bones, with intracranial injury of other and unspecified nature

804.5 ✓5th Open fractures involving skull or face with other bones, without mention of intracranial injury

804.6 ✓5th Open fractures involving skull or face with other bones, with cerebral laceration and contusion

804.7 ✓5th Open fractures involving skull or face with other bones with subarachnoid, subdural, and extradural hemorrhage

804.8 ✓5th Open fractures involving skull or face with other bones, with other and unspecified intracranial hemorrhage

804.9 ✓5th Open fractures involving skull or face with other bones, with intracranial injury of other and unspecified nature

805-809 Fracture of Neck and Trunk

805 Fracture of vertebral column without mention of spinal cord injury
AHA: Sept-Oct, 1985, 3; Q2, 1989, 15; Q2, 1990, 7; Q3, 1990, 5; Q3, 1990, 13; Q4, 1990, 26

The vertebral column forms a protective shield around the spinal column, much as the cranium protects the brain. It allows movement through articulation of the cervical, thoracic, and lumbar vertebrae (sacral vertebrae are fused). Each vertebra has a body and a neural arch, which encase the spinal cord. Each vertebra has several prominent aspects called processes for the attachment of muscles, tendons, and other soft tissues.

The two transverse processes of the cervical vertebrae have a small foramen, the foramen transversarium, through which the vertebral artery and vein and a plexus of sympathetic nerves travel. The first cervical vertebra is called the atlas and supports the globe of the head; it has no vertebral body; instead, the part of the vertebra that would have been the body is fused with the second cervical vertebra to form an osseous pivot around which the head turns. The second cervical vertebra is called the axis.

The thoracic (dorsal) vertebrae accept the heads of the ribs. The lumbar vertebrae are the largest of the moveable vertebrae, or true vertebrae.

Below the thoracic vertebrae are the five lumbar vertebrae, which are larger than the thoracic and cervical vertebrae and support a great amount of weight.

The sacrum consists of five large vertebrae that are fused in the adult. The female sacrum is shorter and wider than the male sacrum.

The composition of the coccyx varies from three to five fused segments, though the typical configuration is four.

The spinal cord, protected by the vertebral column, shares the three meningeal layers, the dura, arachnoid, and pia maters with the brain. It is described anatomically in relation to the vertebrae at each level, but the cord is not identical to the column. In addition to nerve tracts to the brain, enclosed within the column, the spinal nerves exit the column to innervate specific muscle groups bilaterally, according to their level on the vertebral column. The part of the cord that extends below the lumbar level resembled a horse's tail to early anatomists, hence its name — cauda equina.

Similar to the brain, the cord has both gray and white matter. Hemorrhage into the gray matter is known as hematomyelia; its symptoms, which are often permanent, include muscle wasting, diminished tendon reflexes, and muscle weakness. Spinal concussion, the same contrecoup action described in the brain, can result in loss of cord function after a very severe blow or jarring.

Injury and Poisoning

The following fifth-digit subclassification is for use with codes 805.0-805.1:

0   cervical vertebra, unspecified level
1   first cervical vertebra
2   second cervical vertebra
3   third cervical vertebra
4   fourth cervical vertebra
5   fifth cervical vertebra
6   sixth cervical vertebra
7   seventh cervical vertebra
8   multiple cervical vertebra

805.0 ⌐sth	Closed fracture of cervical vertebra without mention of spinal cord injury	
805.1 ⌐sth	Open fracture of cervical vertebra without mention of spinal cord injury	
805.2	Closed fracture of dorsal (thoracic) vertebra without mention of spinal cord injury	
805.3	Open fracture of dorsal (thoracic) vertebra without mention of spinal cord injury	
805.4	Closed fracture of lumbar vertebra without mention of spinal cord injury	
805.5	Open fracture of lumbar vertebra without mention of spinal cord injury	
805.6	Closed fracture of sacrum and coccyx without mention of spinal cord injury	
805.7	Open fracture of sacrum and coccyx without mention of spinal cord injury	
805.8	Closed fracture of unspecified part of vertebral column without mention of spinal cord injury	
805.9	Open fracture of unspecified part of vertebral column without mention of spinal cord injury	

806 Fracture of vertebral column with spinal cord injury

AHA: Sept-Oct, 1985, 3; Q2, 1989, 15; Q2, 1990, 7; Q3, 1990, 5; Q3, 1990, 13; Q4, 1990, 26

A transverse cord injury will cause immediate total paralysis and sensory loss below the level of the injury. It is sometimes referred to as a complete injury. An incomplete lesion will result in partial motor and sensory loss. Depending on the site of injury, outcomes vary, ranging from respiratory paralysis (injury above C5 level); quadriplegia, which is paralysis of four limbs (C4-C5); and paralysis of the legs and partial paralysis of the arms, with abduction and flexion of the arms as movement potentials (C5-C6). C6-C7 allows shoulder movement and elbow flexion, though the lower limbs are paralyzed. Complete loss of bowel and bladder control is associated with injury to the third, fourth, and fifth sacral nerve roots or to the juncture at L1. Posterior cord syndrome is an incomplete injury resulting in motor paralysis and loss of posterior spinal column sensory function.

Paralysis to both legs and the lower portion of the body is termed paraplegia.

The documentation in the medical record should be clear for coding these injuries as either complete or incomplete. Resort to "unspecified" only if the physician fails to make the distinction.

806.00	Closed fracture of C1-C4 level with unspecified spinal cord injury
806.01	Closed fracture of C1-C4 level with complete lesion of cord
806.02	Closed fracture of C1-C4 level with anterior cord syndrome
806.03	Closed fracture of C1-C4 level with central cord syndrome
806.04	Closed fracture of C1-C4 level with other specified spinal cord injury
806.05	Closed fracture of C5-C7 level with unspecified spinal cord injury
806.06	Closed fracture of C5-C7 level with complete lesion of cord
806.07	Closed fracture of C5-C7 level with anterior cord syndrome
806.08	Closed fracture of C5-C7 level with central cord syndrome
806.09	Closed fracture of C5-C7 level with other specified spinal cord injury
806.10	Open fracture of C1-C4 level with unspecified spinal cord injury
806.11	Open fracture of C1-C4 level with complete lesion of cord
806.12	Open fracture of C1-C4 level with anterior cord syndrome
806.13	Open fracture of C1-C4 level with central cord syndrome
806.14	Open fracture of C1-C4 level with other specified spinal cord injury
806.15	Open fracture of C5-C7 level with unspecified spinal cord injury
806.16	Open fracture of C5-C7 level with complete lesion of cord
806.17	Open fracture of C5-C7 level with anterior cord syndrome
806.18	Open fracture of C5-C7 level with central cord syndrome
806.19	Open fracture of C5-C7 level with other specified spinal cord injury
806.20	Closed fracture of T1-T6 level with unspecified spinal cord injury
806.21	Closed fracture of T1-T6 level with complete lesion of cord
806.22	Closed fracture of T1-T6 level with anterior cord syndrome
806.23	Closed fracture of T1-T6 level with central cord syndrome
806.24	Closed fracture of T1-T6 level with other specified spinal cord injury
806.25	Closed fracture of T7-T12 level with unspecified spinal cord injury
806.26	Closed fracture of T7-T12 level with complete lesion of cord

Code	Description
806.27	Closed fracture of T7-T12 level with anterior cord syndrome
806.28	Closed fracture of T7-T12 level with central cord syndrome
806.29	Closed fracture of T7-T12 level with other specified spinal cord injury
806.30	Open fracture of T1-T6 level with unspecified spinal cord injury
806.31	Open fracture of T1-T6 level with complete lesion of cord
806.32	Open fracture of T1-T6 level with anterior cord syndrome
806.33	Open fracture of T1-T6 level with central cord syndrome
806.34	Open fracture of T1-T6 level with other specified spinal cord injury
806.35	Open fracture of T7-T12 level with unspecified spinal cord injury
806.36	Open fracture of T7-T12 level with complete lesion of cord
806.37	Open fracture of T7-T12 level with anterior cord syndrome
806.38	Open fracture of T7-T12 level with central cord syndrome
806.39	Open fracture of T7-T12 level with other specified spinal cord injury
806.4	Closed fracture of lumbar spine with spinal cord injury
806.5	Open fracture of lumbar spine with spinal cord injury
806.60	Closed fracture of sacrum and coccyx with unspecified spinal cord injury
806.61	Closed fracture of sacrum and coccyx with complete cauda equina lesion
806.62	Closed fracture of sacrum and coccyx with other cauda equina injury
806.69	Closed fracture of sacrum and coccyx with other spinal cord injury
806.70	Open fracture of sacrum and coccyx with unspecified spinal cord injury
806.71	Open fracture of sacrum and coccyx with complete cauda equina lesion
806.72	Open fracture of sacrum and coccyx with other cauda equina injury
806.79	Open fracture of sacrum and coccyx with other spinal cord injury
806.8	Closed fracture of unspecified vertebra with spinal cord injury
806.9	Open fracture of unspecified vertebra with spinal cord injury

807 Fracture of rib(s), sternum, larynx, and trachea

AHA: Sept-Oct, 1985, 3; Q2, 1989, 15; Q2, 1990, 7; Q3, 1990, 5; Q3, 1990, 13; Q4, 1990, 26

Twelve pairs of ribs form the thoracic cage, which protects the critical organs in the thorax and abdomen. The true ribs are the first eight ribs and the false ribs are the last four ribs. The floating ribs are the last two of the false ribs.

All of the ribs, except the floating ribs, are connected to the sternum (the breastbone) with costal cartilage.

Flail chest is one of the most dangerous thoracic injuries, resulting from an injury causing at least four fractured ribs in two locations, and pulmonary contusion, leading to hypoventilation. In flail chest, the movement of the chest is paradoxical (opposite of the natural ventilatory movement). On inhalation, the chest contracts and on expiration the chest expands. Generally, thoracic injuries carry a high mortality risk, with death attributed to hypoxemia, hypovolemia, or myocardial failure.

Fractures of the scapula, the sternum, or the first rib are indicative of applied forces.

When coding rib fractures, review the documentation to capture multiple fractures. In inpatient reimbursement, some payment algorithms are constructed according to the number of ribs fractured, making complete capture of all injuries important in all cases.

The following fifth-digit subclassification is for use with codes 807.0-807.1:

0	rib(s), unspecified
1	one rib
2	two ribs
3	three ribs
4	four ribs
5	five ribs
6	six ribs
7	seven ribs
8	eight or more ribs
9	multiple ribs, unspecified

Code	Description
807.0 ↙5th	Closed fracture of rib(s)
807.1 ↙5th	Open fracture of rib(s)
807.2	Closed fracture of sternum
807.3	Open fracture of sternum
807.4	Flail chest
807.5	Closed fracture of larynx and trachea
807.6	Open fracture of larynx and trachea

808 Fracture of pelvis

AHA: Sept-Oct, 1985, 3; Q2, 1989, 15; Q2, 1990, 7; Q3, 1990, 5; Q3, 1990, 13; Q4, 1990, 26

The pelvis includes the ilium, the ischium, the pubis, and the sacrum, which form a bony circle to protect the pelvic contents, provide stability for the vertebral column, (sacrum) and provide an appropriate surface for femoral articulation for ambulation.

The innominate bone, or hipbone, refers to the three bones making up the hipbone: the pubis, ilium, and ischium. The acetabulum is the socket for the femoral head and is found anterior to the rings of the ischium on the lateral inferior surface of the ilium. When the acetabulum is fractured, the head of the femur functions as a hammer, striking against its socket with undue force.

Note that the term hip fracture, which is often used to describe a fracture of the acetabulum, excludes the femur. A fracture of the shaft of the femur, or of the head of the femur, is anatomically distinct from a disruption of the socket of the femoral head.

Pelvic fractures in an individual age 55 and older are associated with a 9.5 percent mortality rate within one year. In fractures of the pelvic ring (circle), the mortality risk to the patient is quite immediate, due to the hemorrhagic capability of cancellous bone. While the issue of application of external fixation may be debated, all agree that the disruption must be stabilized as soon as possible to ensure a positive outcome.

808.0	Closed fracture of acetabulum
808.1	Open fracture of acetabulum
808.2	Closed fracture of pubis
808.3	Open fracture of pubis
808.41	Closed fracture of ilium
808.42	Closed fracture of ischium
808.43	Multiple closed pelvic fractures with disruption of pelvic circle
808.49	Closed fracture of other specified part of pelvis
808.51	Open fracture of ilium
808.52	Open fracture of ischium
808.53	Multiple open pelvic fractures with disruption of pelvic circle
808.59	Open fracture of other specified part of pelvis
808.8	Unspecified closed fracture of pelvis
808.9	Unspecified open fracture of pelvis

809 Ill-defined fractures of bones of trunk
AHA: Sept-Oct, 1985, 3; Q2, 1989, 15; Q2, 1990, 7; Q3, 1990, 5; Q3, 1990, 13; Q4, 1990, 26

Although this category includes a number of excludes notes, an example is a combination of rib and pelvic fractures, poorly defined in documentation.

809.0	Fracture of bones of trunk, closed
809.1	Fracture of bones of trunk, open

810–819 Fracture of Upper Limb

810 Fracture of clavicle
AHA: Sept-Oct, 1985, 3; Q2, 1989, 15; Q2, 1990, 7; Q3, 1990, 5; Q3, 1990, 13; Q4, 1990, 26

The clavicle, or collarbone, has a shaft and articulating ends — the sternal and acromial ends. The acromial end articulates with the scapula, the shoulder bone.

The following fifth-digit subclassification is for use with category 810:

0   unspecified part
1   sternal end of clavicle
2   shaft of clavicle
3   acromial end of clavicle

810.0	5th	Closed fracture of clavicle
810.1	5th	Open fracture of clavicle

811 Fracture of scapula
AHA: Sept-Oct, 1985, 3; Q2, 1989, 15; Q2, 1990, 7; Q3, 1990, 5; Q3, 1990, 13; Q4, 1990, 26

The scapula articulates with the clavicle and the humerus, the long bone in the upper arm. Its socket, the glenoid fossa, receives the humoral head. The coracoid process superior to the glenoid fossa provides a surface for attachments of muscles and tendons.

The following fifth-digit subclassification is for use with category 811:

0   unspecified part
1   acromial process
2   coracoid process
3   glenoid cavity and neck of scapula
9   other

811.0	5th	Closed fracture of scapula
811.1	5th	Open fracture of scapula

812 Fracture of humerus
AHA: Sept-Oct, 1985, 3; Q2, 1989, 15; Q2, 1990, 7; Q3, 1990, 5; Q3, 1990, 13; Q4, 1990, 26

In addition to possession of an anatomical neck, the humerus includes a surgical neck, described as that portion of the anatomical neck most likely to fracture.

812.00	Closed fracture of unspecified part of upper end of humerus
812.01	Closed fracture of surgical neck of humerus
812.02	Closed fracture of anatomical neck of humerus
812.03	Closed fracture of greater tuberosity of humerus
812.09	Other closed fractures of upper end of humerus

Code	Description
812.10	Open fracture of unspecified part of upper end of humerus
812.11	Open fracture of surgical neck of humerus
812.12	Open fracture of anatomical neck of humerus
812.13	Open fracture of greater tuberosity of humerus
812.19	Other open fracture of upper end of humerus
812.20	Closed fracture of unspecified part of humerus
812.21	Closed fracture of shaft of humerus
	AHA: Q4, 2005, 129
812.30	Open fracture of unspecified part of humerus
812.31	Open fracture of shaft of humerus
812.40	Closed fracture of unspecified part of lower end of humerus
812.41	Closed fracture of supracondylar humerus
812.42	Closed fracture of lateral condyle of humerus
812.43	Closed fracture of medial condyle of humerus
812.44	Closed fracture of unspecified condyle(s) of humerus
812.49	Other closed fracture of lower end of humerus
812.50	Open fracture of unspecified part of lower end of humerus
812.51	Open fracture of supracondylar humerus
812.52	Open fracture of lateral condyle of humerus
812.53	Open fracture of medial condyle of humerus
812.54	Open fracture of unspecified condyle(s) of humerus
812.59	Other open fracture of lower end of humerus

813 Fracture of radius and ulna
AHA: Sept-Oct, 1985, 3; Q2, 1989, 15; Q2, 1990, 7; Q3, 1990, 5; Q3, 1990, 13; Q4, 1990, 26

The radius and ulna operate in tandem, with a hinge-like motion for bending and capabilities for pronation and supination for the hand and wrist. In the anatomical position, the hands are supinated. In the pronated position, the palms are down.

Monteggia's fracture is a common fracture at the proximal end of the ulna, combined with dislocation of the radial head. In a child, closed reduction may suffice, though adults require open reduction and internal fixation (ORIF). Reduction is the repositioning of a bone into proper alignment. Dislocations, which are the disruption of the joint, are also reduced.

Another common fracture is Colles' fracture, which is a transverse fracture of the distal radius, displacing the hand. This injury typically occurs when an individual puts out a hand to break a fall.

Code	Description
813.00	Unspecified fracture of radius and ulna, upper end of forearm, closed
813.01	Closed fracture of olecranon process of ulna
813.02	Closed fracture of coronoid process of ulna
813.03	Closed Monteggia's fracture
813.04	Other and unspecified closed fractures of proximal end of ulna (alone)
813.05	Closed fracture of head of radius
813.06	Closed fracture of neck of radius
813.07	Other and unspecified closed fractures of proximal end of radius (alone)
813.08	Closed fracture of radius with ulna, upper end (any part)
813.10	Unspecified open fracture of upper end of forearm
813.11	Open fracture of olecranon process of ulna
813.12	Open fracture of coronoid process of ulna
813.13	Open Monteggia's fracture
813.14	Other and unspecified open fractures of proximal end of ulna (alone)
813.15	Open fracture of head of radius
813.16	Open fracture of neck of radius
813.17	Other and unspecified open fractures of proximal end of radius (alone)
813.18	Open fracture of radius with ulna, upper end (any part)
813.20	Unspecified closed fracture of shaft of radius or ulna
813.21	Closed fracture of shaft of radius (alone)
813.22	Closed fracture of shaft of ulna (alone)
813.23	Closed fracture of shaft of radius with ulna
813.30	Unspecified open fracture of shaft of radius or ulna
813.31	Open fracture of shaft of radius (alone)
813.32	Open fracture of shaft of ulna (alone)
813.33	Open fracture of shaft of radius with ulna
813.40	Unspecified closed fracture of lower end of forearm
813.41	Closed Colles' fracture
813.42	Other closed fractures of distal end of radius (alone)
813.43	Closed fracture of distal end of ulna (alone)
813.44	Closed fracture of lower end of radius with ulna
813.45	Torus fracture of lower end of radius
813.50	Unspecified open fracture of lower end of forearm
813.51	Open Colles' fracture
813.52	Other open fractures of distal end of radius (alone)
813.53	Open fracture of distal end of ulna (alone)
813.54	Open fracture of lower end of radius with ulna
813.80	Closed fracture of unspecified part of forearm
813.81	Closed fracture of unspecified part of radius (alone)
813.82	Closed fracture of unspecified part of ulna (alone)
813.83	Closed fracture of unspecified part of radius with ulna
813.90	Open fracture of unspecified part of forearm
813.91	Open fracture of unspecified part of radius (alone)
813.92	Open fracture of unspecified part of ulna (alone)
813.93	Open fracture of unspecified part of radius with ulna

Coding Scenario
A patient is seen in the emergency department (ED) after falling from a tree. He complains of pain in the right wrist. After x-ray examination, it is determined

that the patient has a greenstick break of the upper end of the right radius.

> Code assignment: 813.00 *Unspecified fracture of radius and ulna, upper end of forearm, closed*

A 64-year-old female involved in an automobile accident is seen in the ED. The physician documents that there is a compound fracture of the shaft of the right femur and a fracture of the left shaft of the ulna and radius.

> Code assignment: 821.11 *Fracture of other and unspecified parts of femur, shaft or unspecified part, open, shaft* and 813.23 *Fracture of radius and ulna, shaft, closed, radius with ulna*

814 Fracture of carpal bone(s)
AHA: Sept-Oct, 1985, 3; Q2, 1989, 15; Q2, 1990, 7; Q3, 1990, 5; Q3, 1990, 13; Q4, 1990, 26

The eight carpal bones are functionally linked to the placement of each bone and its articulation with various partners.

Two rows of bones, with the scaphoid bone common to each row, act as a bridge to provide stability. The first row (proximal) is comprised of the scaphoid, lunate, pisiform, and triquetrum. The second row (distal) is comprised of the scaphoid, trapezium, trapezoid, capitate, and hamate.

Fractures of the distal radius and ulna are typically referred to as wrist fractures. They articulate with the proximal carpals, though, technically, they are the bones of the forearm. The carpals, which form the wrist, are considered part of the hand.

Carpal fractures usually occur as a result of extreme dorsiflexion or extension of the wrist and require significant force to happen at all.

814.00	Unspecified closed fracture of carpal bone
814.01	Closed fracture of navicular (scaphoid) bone of wrist
814.02	Closed fracture of lunate (semilunar) bone of wrist
814.03	Closed fracture of triquetral (cuneiform) bone of wrist
814.04	Closed fracture of pisiform bone of wrist
814.05	Closed fracture of trapezium bone (larger multangular) of wrist
814.06	Closed fracture of trapezoid bone (smaller multangular) of wrist
814.07	Closed fracture of capitate bone (os magnum) of wrist
814.08	Closed fracture of hamate (unciform) bone of wrist
814.09	Closed fracture of other bone of wrist
814.10	Unspecified open fracture of carpal bone
814.11	Open fracture of navicular (scaphoid) bone of wrist
814.12	Open fracture of lunate (semilunar) bone of wrist
814.13	Open fracture of triquetral (cuneiform) bone of wrist
814.14	Open fracture of pisiform bone of wrist
814.15	Open fracture of trapezium bone (larger multangular) of wrist
814.16	Open fracture of trapezoid bone (smaller multangular) of wrist
814.17	Open fracture of capitate bone (os magnum) of wrist
814.18	Open fracture of hamate (unciform) bone of wrist
814.19	Open fracture of other bone of wrist

815 Fracture of metacarpal bone(s)
AHA: Sept-Oct, 1985, 3; Q2, 1989, 15; Q2, 1990, 7; Q3, 1990, 5; Q3, 1990, 13; Q4, 1990, 26

The metacarpals are the bones of the hand distal to the carpals and proximal to the phalanges (fingers). The fingers have three joints: the section next to the metacarpals is the proximal phalanx, the midsection is the middle phalanx, and the farthest section is the distal phalanx. The numbering convention selects the thumb as the first metacarpal and the medial finger (pinkie) as the fifth finger.

The anatomy of each phalanx is described in terms of base, body, and head. The base is the end portion closest to the head of the body, the body is the midsection of the bone, and the head is the distal end of the bone. The distal phalanx has an additional descriptor, a tuberosity. Two sesamoid bones are located close to the distal joint of the first metacarpal (thumb).

Because they project and perform many functions, the metacarpals and phalanges account for 10 percent of all fractures, of which 50 percent are work-related.

> The following fifth-digit subclassification is for use with category 815:
> 0   metacarpal bone(s), site unspecified
> 1   base of thumb [first] metacarpal
> 2   base of other metacarpal bone(s)
> 3   shaft of metacarpal bone(s)
> 4   neck of metacarpal bone(s)
> 9   multiple sites of metacarpus

815.0	✓5th	Closed fracture of metacarpal bones
815.1	✓5th	Open fracture of metacarpal bones

816 Fracture of one or more phalanges of hand
AHA: Sept-Oct, 1985, 3; Q2, 1989, 15; Q2, 1990, 7; Q3, 1990, 5; Q3, 1990, 13; Q4, 1990, 26

816.00	Closed fracture of unspecified phalanx or phalanges of hand

816.01	Closed fracture of middle or proximal phalanx or phalanges of hand
816.02	Closed fracture of distal phalanx or phalanges of hand
816.03	Closed fracture of multiple sites of phalanx or phalanges of hand
816.10	Open fracture of phalanx or phalanges of hand, unspecified
816.11	Open fracture of middle or proximal phalanx or phalanges of hand
816.12	Open fracture of distal phalanx or phalanges of hand
816.13	Open fractures of multiple sites of phalanx or phalanges of hand

817 Multiple fractures of hand bones
AHA: Sept-Oct, 1985, 3; Q2, 1989, 15; Q2, 1990, 7; Q3, 1990, 5; Q3, 1990, 13; Q4, 1990, 26

Use these categories only if the documentation is extremely sketchy.

817.0	Multiple closed fractures of hand bones
817.1	Multiple open fractures of hand bones

818 Ill-defined fractures of upper limb
AHA: Sept-Oct, 1985, 3; Q2, 1989, 15; Q2, 1990, 7; Q3, 1990, 5; Q3, 1990, 13; Q4, 1990, 26

818.0	Ill-defined closed fractures of upper limb
818.1	Ill-defined open fractures of upper limb

819 Multiple fractures involving both upper limbs, and upper limb with rib(s) and sternum
AHA: Sept-Oct, 1985, 3; Q2, 1989, 15; Q2, 1990, 7; Q3, 1990, 5; Q3, 1990, 13; Q4, 1990, 26

819.0	Multiple closed fractures involving both upper limbs, and upper limb with rib(s) and sternum
819.1	Multiple open fractures involving both upper limbs, and upper limb with rib(s) and sternum

820–829 Fracture of Lower Limb

820 Fracture of neck of femur
AHA: Sept-Oct, 1985, 3; Q2, 1989, 15; Q2, 1990, 7; Q3, 1990, 5; Q3, 1990, 13; Q4, 1990, 26

The proximal femur bears the brunt of accidents leading to fractures, compared to the other bones used for locomotion. Lower extremity fractures in children may suggest child abuse.

Fractures of the femoral shaft are relatively uncommon, while fractures of the neck are among the most frequent. Femoral neck fractures are classified in ICD-9-CM as transcervical, or pertrochanteric, with subdivisions. Radiologists often use the terminology intracapsular and extracapsular. A subcapital or intracapsular fracture of the femoral neck has the highest risk of avascular necrosis, which occurs when a severe injury disrupts the blood supply to the bone. This fracture also is inherently more unstable after surgery than an intertrochanteric fracture since the weakest part of the bone is now supporting the point of greatest stress.

If a clinician reports a proximal femur fracture as opposed to an intertrochanteric, the radiology report will state that the fracture is intertrochanteric. This coded information is crucial to achieve an accurate evaluation of patient outcomes and utilization data.

Preferred treatments for the various fractures include the following:

- Shaft fracture — intramedullary nailing; promotes fast weight-bearing capability
- Transcervical fracture — hemiarthroplasty or total hip replacement
- Intertrochanteric fracture — fixation with sliding implant

820.00	Closed fracture of unspecified intracapsular section of neck of femur
820.01	Closed fracture of epiphysis (separation) (upper) of neck of femur
820.02	Closed fracture of midcervical section of femur
820.03	Closed fracture of base of neck of femur
820.09	Other closed transcervical fracture of femur
820.10	Open fracture of unspecified intracapsular section of neck of femur
820.11	Open fracture of epiphysis (separation) (upper) of neck of femur
820.12	Open fracture of midcervical section of femur
820.13	Open fracture of base of neck of femur
820.19	Other open transcervical fracture of femur
820.20	Closed fracture of unspecified trochanteric section of femur
820.21	Closed fracture of intertrochanteric section of femur
820.22	Closed fracture of subtrochanteric section of femur
820.30	Open fracture of unspecified trochanteric section of femur
820.31	Open fracture of intertrochanteric section of femur
820.32	Open fracture of subtrochanteric section of femur
820.8	Closed fracture of unspecified part of neck of femur
820.9	Open fracture of unspecified part of neck of femur

821 Fracture of other and unspecified parts of femur
AHA: Sept-Oct, 1985, 3; Q2, 1989, 15; Q2, 1990, 7; Q3, 1990, 5; Q3, 1990, 13; Q4, 1990, 26

In children and adolescents, whose skeletons are still immature, distal epiphyseal fracture, presenting as valgus instability, results in a significant number of injuries. These fractures occur in normal play and sports activity, and are easy to overlook if the evaluation seems to point to a ligamentous sprain, rather than a physeal fracture.

821.00	Closed fracture of unspecified part of femur
821.01	Closed fracture of shaft of femur
821.10	Open fracture of unspecified part of femur
821.11	Open fracture of shaft of femur
821.20	Closed fracture of unspecified part of lower end of femur
821.21	Closed fracture of femoral condyle
821.22	Closed fracture of lower epiphysis of femur
821.23	Closed supracondylar fracture of femur
821.29	Other closed fracture of lower end of femur
821.30	Open fracture of unspecified part of lower end of femur
821.31	Open fracture of femoral condyle
821.32	Open fracture of lower epiphysis of femur
821.33	Open supracondylar fracture of femur
821.39	Other open fracture of lower end of femur

822 Fracture of patella
AHA: Sept-Oct, 1985, 3; Q2, 1989, 15; Q2, 1990, 7; Q3, 1990, 5; Q3, 1990, 13; Q4, 1990, 26

The anatomy of the knee joint and associated muscles, tendons, and ligaments predispose the occurrence of patellar fractures in conjunction with sprains or ruptures of the ligaments. Typically, injuries are due to direct application of force or twisting. A severely injured knee remains prone to re-injury, instability, or arthritis.

822.0	Closed fracture of patella
822.1	Open fracture of patella

823 Fracture of tibia and fibula
AHA: Sept-Oct, 1985, 3; Q2, 1989, 15; Q2, 1990, 7; Q3, 1990, 5; Q3, 1990, 13; Q4, 1990, 26

The malleolus is the distal end of both the tibia and the fibula and is classified to the ankle in ICD-9-CM. The lateral malleolus is part of the fibula and the medial malleolus is part of the tibia. This category is for fractures of the upper end and shaft of the tibia and fibula, or unspecified parts.

The following fifth-digit subclassification is for use with category 823:
- 0 tibia alone
- 1 fibula alone
- 2 fibula with tibia

823.0 ⌐sth	Closed fracture of upper end of tibia and fibula
823.1 ⌐sth	Open fracture of upper end of tibia and fibula
823.2 ⌐sth	Closed fracture of shaft of tibia and fibula
823.3 ⌐sth	Open fracture of shaft of tibia and fibula
823.4 ⌐sth	Torus fracture of tibia and fibula
823.8 ⌐sth	Closed fracture of unspecified part of tibia and fibula
823.9 ⌐sth	Open fracture of unspecified part of tibia and fibula

824 Fracture of ankle
AHA: Sept-Oct, 1985, 3; Q2, 1989, 15; Q2, 1990, 7; Q3, 1990, 5; Q3, 1990, 13; Q4, 1990, 26

A bimalleolar fracture is a fracture of both the lateral and medial aspects of the malleolus. Pott's fracture is any fracture of the malleolus. Dupuytren's fracture is a fracture dislocation of the ankle with the talus downwardly displaced. The talus is one of the major ankle (tarsal) bones. A trimalleolar fracture involves a fracture of the medial malleolus and the fibula with a fracture of the posterior lip of the tibia's articulating surface.

Open reduction and internal fixation is the method of treatment for bimalleolar and trimalleolar fractures.

824.0	Closed fracture of medial malleolus
	AHA: Q1, 2004, 9
824.1	Open fracture of medial malleolus
824.2	Closed fracture of lateral malleolus
824.3	Open fracture of lateral malleolus
824.4	Closed bimalleolar fracture
824.5	Open bimalleolar fracture
824.6	Closed trimalleolar fracture
824.7	Open trimalleolar fracture
824.8	Unspecified closed fracture of ankle
824.9	Unspecified open fracture of ankle

825 Fracture of one or more tarsal and metatarsal bones
AHA: Sept-Oct, 1985, 3; Q2, 1989, 15; Q2, 1990, 7; Q3, 1990, 5; Q3, 1990, 13; Q4, 1990, 26

The tarsal bones are the heel bone (calcaneus, os calcis), talus (astragalus), navicular (scaphoid), cuboid, and the lateral, medial, and intermediate cuneiform bones. The metatarsals are the five long bones of the foot extending from the tarsal bones to the phalanges, or toes.

825.0	Closed fracture of calcaneus
825.1	Open fracture of calcaneus
825.20	Closed fracture of unspecified bone(s) of foot (except toes)
825.21	Closed fracture of astragalus
825.22	Closed fracture of navicular (scaphoid) bone of foot
825.23	Closed fracture of cuboid bone
825.24	Closed fracture of cuneiform bone of foot
825.25	Closed fracture of metatarsal bone(s)
825.29	Other closed fracture of tarsal and metatarsal bones
825.30	Open fracture of unspecified bone(s) of foot (except toes)
825.31	Open fracture of astragalus
825.32	Open fracture of navicular (scaphoid) bone of foot
825.33	Open fracture of cuboid bone
825.34	Open fracture of cuneiform bone of foot,

825.35	Open fracture of metatarsal bone(s)	
825.39	Other open fractures of tarsal and metatarsal bones	

826 Fracture of one or more phalanges of foot
AHA: Sept-Oct, 1985, 3; Q2, 1989, 15; Q2, 1990, 7; Q3, 1990, 5; Q3, 1990, 13; Q4, 1990, 26

826.0	Closed fracture of one or more phalanges of foot
826.1	Open fracture of one or more phalanges of foot

827 Other, multiple, and ill-defined fractures of lower limb
AHA: Sept-Oct, 1985, 3; Q2, 1989, 15; Q2, 1990, 7; Q3, 1990, 5; Q3, 1990, 13; Q4, 1990, 26

Use these categories only if the documentation is extremely sketchy.

827.0	Other, multiple and ill-defined closed fractures of lower limb
827.1	Other, multiple and ill-defined open fractures of lower limb

828 Multiple fractures involving both lower limbs, lower with upper limb, and lower limb(s) with rib(s) and sternum
AHA: Sept-Oct, 1985, 3; Q2, 1989, 15; Q2, 1990, 7; Q3, 1990, 5; Q3, 1990, 13; Q4, 1990, 26

828.0	Multiple closed fractures involving both lower limbs, lower with upper limb, and lower limb(s) with rib(s) and sternum
828.1	Multiple fractures involving both lower limbs, lower with upper limb, and lower limb(s) with rib(s) and sternum, open

829 Fracture of unspecified bones
AHA: Sept-Oct, 1985, 3; Q2, 1989, 15; Q2, 1990, 7; Q3, 1990, 5; Q3, 1990, 13; Q4, 1990, 26

829.0	Closed fracture of unspecified bone
829.1	Open fracture of unspecified bone

830–839 Dislocation

Luxation is the term used to describe a complete dislocation, one that has separated the articulating surfaces of the joint. An incomplete dislocation, or subluxation, is one in which the joint surfaces maintain some articulation. A simple dislocation has not penetrated to make a communicating wound. An uncomplicated dislocation is not associated with other important injuries. Open dislocations are subject to infection. They are always compound. Reduction of a dislocation is by manipulation, open or closed. They should be performed immediately, although this does not ensure a good result. Avascular necrosis, traumatic arthritis, and ectopic ossification are considered threats to complete recovery.

Some dislocations are described as anterior and posterior or lateral and medial, which describe the location of the displaced bone in relation to its proper placement. For example, if the bone lies in front of its joint, the dislocation is considered to be anterior.

Dislocation of the acromioclavicular joint ranges in severity according to the degree of damage to the acromioclavicular and coracoclavicular ligaments.

Pubic symphysis and sacroiliac dislocations result from high-energy impact and are associated with other severe pelvic injuries. Regardless of the severity of injuries, a hip dislocation must be reduced first to contain blood loss and to minimize permanent damage to the pelvic structures.

The sternoclavicular joint may sustain anterior or posterior dislocations. While an anterior dislocation is simply remedied, a posterior dislocation poses a grave risk to the patient because of potential risk to critical internal thoracic organs.

Dislocation of the patella is typically lateral. The choice of open or closed reduction depends on the degree of disruption of the nearby ligaments and tendons. Intraarticular dislocations of the patella usually require open reduction. Other dislocations of the knee are serious, requiring immediate surgery to offset the risk of vascular complications.

The ankle is seldom dislocated without an accompanying fracture and is easily reduced.

830 Dislocation of jaw
AHA: Q3, 1990, 12

830.0	Closed dislocation of jaw
830.1	Open dislocation of jaw

831 Dislocation of shoulder
AHA: Q3, 1990, 12

The following fifth-digit subclassification is for use with category 831:

0	shoulder, unspecified
1	anterior dislocation of humerus
2	posterior dislocation of humerus
3	inferior dislocation of humerus
4	acromioclavicular (joint)
9	other

831.0 ✓5th	Closed dislocation of shoulder, unspecified
831.1 ✓5th	Open dislocation of shoulder

832 Dislocation of elbow
AHA: Q3, 1990, 12

The following fifth-digit subclassification is for use with category 832:
- 0 elbow, unspecified
- 1 anterior dislocation of elbow
- 2 posterior dislocation of elbow
- 3 medial dislocation of elbow
- 4 lateral dislocation of elbow
- 9 other

832.0 ⌐sth Closed dislocation of elbow
832.1 ⌐sth Open dislocation of elbow

833 Dislocation of wrist
AHA: Q3, 1990, 12

The following fifth-digit subclassification is for use with category 833:
- 0 wrist, unspecified part
- 1 radioulnar (joint), distal
- 2 radiocarpal (joint)
- 3 midcarpal (joint)
- 4 carpometacarpal (joint)
- 5 metacarpal (bone), proximal end
- 9 other

833.0 ⌐sth Closed dislocation of wrist
833.1 ⌐sth Open dislocation of wrist

834 Dislocation of finger
AHA: Q3, 1990, 12

The following fifth-digit subclassification is for use with category 834:
- 0 finger, unspecified part
- 1 metacarpophalangeal (joint)
- 2 interphalangeal (joint), hand

834.0 ⌐sth Closed dislocation of finger
834.1 ⌐sth Open dislocation of finger

835 Dislocation of hip
AHA: Q3, 1990, 12

The following fifth-digit subclassification is for use with category 835:
- 0 dislocation of hip, unspecified
- 1 posterior dislocation
- 2 obturator dislocation
- 3 other anterior dislocation

835.0 ⌐sth Closed dislocation of hip
835.1 ⌐sth Open dislocation of hip

836 Dislocation of knee
AHA: Q3, 1990, 12

Code	Description
836.0	Tear of medial cartilage or meniscus of knee, current
836.1	Tear of lateral cartilage or meniscus of knee, current
836.2	Other tear of cartilage or meniscus of knee, current
836.3	Closed dislocation of patella
836.4	Open dislocation of patella
836.50	Closed dislocation of knee, unspecified part
836.51	Closed anterior dislocation of tibia, proximal end
836.52	Closed posterior dislocation of tibia, proximal end
836.53	Closed medial dislocation of tibia, proximal end
836.54	Closed lateral dislocation of tibia, proximal end
836.59	Other closed dislocation of knee
836.60	Open dislocation of knee unspecified part
836.61	Open anterior dislocation of tibia, proximal end
836.62	Open posterior dislocation of tibia, proximal end
836.63	Open medial dislocation of tibia, proximal end
836.64	Open lateral dislocation of tibia, proximal end
836.69	Other open dislocation of knee

837 Dislocation of ankle
AHA: Q3, 1990, 12

Code	Description
837.0	Closed dislocation of ankle
837.1	Open dislocation of ankle

838 Dislocation of foot
AHA: Q3, 1990, 12

The following fifth-digit subclassification is for use with category 838:
- 0 foot, unspecified
- 1 tarsal (bone), joint unspecified
- 2 midtarsal (joint)
- 3 tarsometatarsal (joint)
- 4 metatarsal (bone), joint unspecified
- 5 metatarsophalangeal (joint)
- 6 interphalangeal (joint), foot
- 9 other

838.0 ⌐sth Closed dislocation of foot
838.1 ⌐sth Open dislocation of foot

839 Other, multiple, and ill-defined dislocations
AHA: Q3, 1990, 12

Code	Description
839.00	Closed dislocation, unspecified cervical vertebra
839.01	Closed dislocation, first cervical vertebra
839.02	Closed dislocation, second cervical vertebra
839.03	Closed dislocation, third cervical vertebra
839.04	Closed dislocation, fourth cervical vertebra
839.05	Closed dislocation, fifth cervical vertebra
839.06	Closed dislocation, sixth cervical vertebra
839.07	Closed dislocation, seventh cervical vertebra
839.08	Closed dislocation, multiple cervical vertebrae
839.10	Open dislocation, unspecified cervical vertebra

839.11	Open dislocation, first cervical vertebra	
839.12	Open dislocation, second cervical vertebra	
839.13	Open dislocation, third cervical vertebra	
839.14	Open dislocation, fourth cervical vertebra	
839.15	Open dislocation, fifth cervical vertebra	
839.16	Open dislocation, sixth cervical vertebra	
839.17	Open dislocation, seventh cervical vertebra	
839.18	Open dislocation, multiple cervical vertebrae	
839.20	Closed dislocation, lumbar vertebra	
839.21	Closed dislocation, thoracic vertebra	
839.30	Open dislocation, lumbar vertebra	
839.31	Open dislocation, thoracic vertebra	
839.40	Closed dislocation, vertebra, unspecified site	
839.41	Closed dislocation, coccyx	
839.42	Closed dislocation, sacrum	
839.49	Closed dislocation, other vertebra	
839.50	Open dislocation, vertebra, unspecified site	
839.51	Open dislocation, coccyx	
839.52	Open dislocation, sacrum	
839.59	Open dislocation, other vertebra	
839.61	Closed dislocation, sternum	
839.69	Closed dislocation, other location	
839.71	Open dislocation, sternum	
839.79	Open dislocation, other location	
839.8	Closed dislocation, multiple and ill-defined sites	
839.9	Open dislocation, multiple and ill-defined sites	

840–848 Sprains and Strains of Joints and Adjacent Muscles

A sprain is not identical to a strain and should not be used as a synonym. A sprain is an injury to the ligaments, tough fibrous tissues that bind bones together at joints. A strain is an injury to the muscles or tendons that bind muscles together and does not occur at the joint.

Sprains and strains are graded. A Type I sprain denotes minor ligamentous injury; Type II is an incomplete ligamentous injury; and Type III describes a complete disruption of the ligament. The more ligaments involved in the sprain, the more serious the injury. A Type III strain involves the complete tearing of muscle and separation from its tendon. Both sprains and strains manifest with swelling, pain, and difficulty in using and are best treated according to the RICE therapy — Rest of the affected part, Ice, Compression, and Elevation.

Areas commonly sprained include the ankle, groin, knee, and neck. Ankle sprains seldom require surgery. If the patient suffers repeated injury to the weakened ankle, surgery may be performed. If two or more ligaments are involved in a knee sprain, it is serious and likely to require corrective surgery. A mild sprain may heal in two to six weeks, while a severe sprain may require eight weeks to 10 months to heal.

Whiplash is the sudden and forceful extension and flexion of the neck and can cause death if the movement of the neck injures the brain stem. Arms and shoulders can be affected to the point of paralysis. Whiplash accounts for 10 percent of all long-term disabilities.

Sports Injuries. Acute athletic injuries are those that develop suddenly and last six months or less. Some acute injuries require time to heal, sometimes longer than six months. These include injuries to the musculoskeletal system, especially to the knees and ankles, such as bone fractures, sprains, and muscle strains, and typically result from twisting, tearing, or from lateral force, such as the blows to the side of the knee. Severe acute injuries, such as those to the head or spinal cord, usually result from accidents or extreme overexertion. Chronic athletic injuries include aches and pain of unknown origin, tendonitis, and stress fractures, which are common in athletes who consistently overuse muscles for extended periods. Diagnosis includes visual exam and manipulation of injured joints in concert with more complex procedures, such as arthroscopy for an internal exam of the joints. Common diagnostic imaging techniques include x-rays, computed tomography, ultrasound, and magnetic resonance imaging. Treatments range from cryotherapy and immobilization for simple sprains and strains to surgical procedures for fractures and tears in ligaments or tendons. Rest, physical therapy, and massage are integral to the healing of most injuries. Drugs and corticosteroids can be used to lessen pain and inflammation.

840 Sprains and strains of shoulder and upper arm

840.0	Acromioclavicular (joint) (ligament) sprain and strain
840.1	Coracoclavicular (ligament) sprain and strain
840.2	Coracohumeral (ligament) sprain and strain
840.3	Infraspinatus (muscle) (tendon) sprain and strain
840.4	Rotator cuff (capsule) sprain and strain
840.5	Subscapularis (muscle) sprain and strain
840.6	Supraspinatus (muscle) (tendon) sprain and strain
840.7	Superior glenoid labrum lesions (SLAP)
840.8	Sprain and strain of other specified sites of shoulder and upper arm
840.9	Sprain and strain of unspecified site of shoulder and upper arm

841 Sprains and strains of elbow and forearm

841.0	Radial collateral ligament sprain and strain

Injury and Poisoning

841.1	Ulnar collateral ligament sprain and strain		846.2	Sprain and strain of sacrospinatus (ligament)
841.2	Radiohumeral (joint) sprain and strain		846.3	Sprain and strain of sacrotuberous (ligament)
841.3	Ulnohumeral (joint) sprain and strain		846.8	Other specified sites of sacroiliac region sprain and strain
841.8	Sprain and strain of other specified sites of elbow and forearm		846.9	Unspecified site of sacroiliac region sprain and strain
841.9	Sprain and strain of unspecified site of elbow and forearm			

842 Sprains and strains of wrist and hand

842.00	Sprain and strain of unspecified site of wrist
842.01	Sprain and strain of carpal (joint) of wrist
842.02	Sprain and strain of radiocarpal (joint) (ligament) of wrist
842.09	Other wrist sprain and strain
842.10	Sprain and strain of unspecified site of hand
842.11	Sprain and strain of carpometacarpal (joint) of hand
842.12	Sprain and strain of metacarpophalangeal (joint) of hand
842.13	Sprain and strain of interphalangeal (joint) of hand
842.19	Other hand sprain and strain

843 Sprains and strains of hip and thigh

843.0	Iliofemoral (ligament) sprain and strain
843.1	Ischiocapsular (ligament) sprain and strain
843.8	Sprain and strain of other specified sites of hip and thigh
843.9	Sprain and strain of unspecified site of hip and thigh

844 Sprains and strains of knee and leg

844.0	Sprain and strain of lateral collateral ligament of knee
844.1	Sprain and strain of medial collateral ligament of knee
844.2	Sprain and strain of cruciate ligament of knee
844.3	Sprain and strain of tibiofibular (joint) (ligament) superior, of knee
844.8	Sprain and strain of other specified sites of knee and leg
844.9	Sprain and strain of unspecified site of knee and leg

845 Sprains and strains of ankle and foot

845.00	Unspecified site of ankle sprain and strain
845.01	Sprain and strain of deltoid (ligament) of ankle
845.02	Sprain and strain of calcaneofibular (ligament)
845.03	Sprain and strain of tibiofibular (ligament) AHA: Q1, 2004, 9
845.09	Other ankle sprain and strain
845.10	Sprain and strain of unspecified site of foot
845.11	Sprain and strain of tarsometatarsal (joint) (ligament)
845.12	Sprain and strain of metatarsophalangeal (joint)
845.13	Sprain and strain of interphalangeal (joint), of toe
845.19	Other foot sprain and strain

846 Sprains and strains of sacroiliac region

846.0	Sprain and strain of lumbosacral (joint) (ligament)
846.1	Sprain and strain of sacroiliac (ligament)

847 Sprains and strains of other and unspecified parts of back

847.0	Neck sprain and strain
847.1	Thoracic sprain and strain
847.2	Lumbar sprain and strain
847.3	Sprain and strain of sacrum
847.4	Sprain and strain of coccyx
847.9	Sprain and strain of unspecified site of back

848 Other and ill-defined sprains and strains

848.0	Sprain and strain of septal cartilage of nose
848.1	Sprain and strain of jaw
848.2	Sprain and strain of thyroid region
848.3	Sprain and strain of ribs
848.40	Sprain and strain of sternum, unspecified part
848.41	Sprain and strain of sternoclavicular (joint) (ligament)
848.42	Sprain and strain of chondrosternal (joint)
848.49	Other sprain and strains of sternum
848.5	Pelvic sprain and strains
848.8	Other specified sites of sprains and strains
848.9	Unspecified site of sprain and strain

850–854 Intracranial Injury, Excluding Those with Skull Fracture

850 Concussion
AHA: Q4, 1990, 24; Q1, 1993, 22; Q2, 1996, 6

850.0	Concussion with no loss of consciousness
850.11	Concussion, with loss of consciousness of 30 minutes or less
850.12	Concussion, with loss of consciousness 31 to 59 minutes
850.2	Concussion with moderate (1-24 hours) loss of consciousness
850.3	Concussion with prolonged (more than 24 hours) loss of consciousness and return to pre-existing conscious level
850.4	Concussion with prolonged (more than 24 hours) loss of consciousness, without return to pre-existing conscious level
850.5	Concussion with loss of consciousness of unspecified duration
850.9	Unspecified concussion

Documentation Issues

When coding concussions, the physician must document if the patient has a loss of consciousness; if the loss of consciousness was brief, moderate, or prolonged; and if the patient returned to the previous level of consciousness.

If the concussion is accompanied by cerebral laceration and contusion, the physician should also indicate the site of the laceration and if an open wound is present in addition to the above findings.

When the patient is treated for the symptoms of a concussion within 24 to 48 hours and the diagnosis is identified as "postconcussion syndrome," verify with the physician if the concussion is still in the current stage and should be reported with a code from category 850, rather than as postconcussion syndrome, code 310.2.

Coding Clarification
Also refer to category 800.

Concussion with Cerebral Laceration: Only one code is necessary to indicate a concussion with cerebral laceration. When the documentation states that this condition is present, assign a code from category 851 with a fourth digit indicating the site of the laceration and a fifth digit to identify loss of consciousness and the duration.

Postconcussion syndrome is a term used to describe the symptoms following a concussion, including headache, dizziness, anxiety, fatigue, problems concentrating, and depression. This condition is indicated with code 310.2.

Suspected Concussion: A physician may suspect that a patient has a concussion but may not have confirmed the suspicion. When coding inpatients, the appropriate code from category 850 should be reported.

When coding outpatients, rule-out and suspected conditions cannot be coded. Therefore, the appropriate code indicating the symptoms the patient is having (i.e., headache, dizziness, etc.) should be reported.

851 Cerebral laceration and contusion
AHA: Q4, 1990, 24; Q1, 1993, 22; Q4, 1996, 36

The following fifth-digit subclassification is for use with categories 851-854:

0   unspecified state of consciousness
1   with no loss of consciousness
2   with brief [less than one hour] loss of consciousness
3   with moderate [1-24 hours] loss of consciousness
4   with prolonged [more than 24 hours] loss of consciousness and return to pre-existing conscious level
5   with prolonged [more than 24 hours] loss of consciousness, without return to pre-existing conscious level

Use fifth-digit five to designate when a patient is unconscious and dies before regaining consciousness, regardless of the duration of the loss of consciousness

6   with loss of consciousness of unspecified duration
9   with concussion, unspecified

851.0 ✓5th   Cortex (cerebral) contusion without mention of open intracranial wound
851.1 ✓5th   Cortex (cerebral) contusion with open intracranial wound
851.2 ✓5th   Cortex (cerebral) laceration without mention of open intracranial wound
851.3 ✓5th   Cortex (cerebral) laceration with open intracranial wound
851.4 ✓5th   Cerebellar or brain stem contusion without mention of open intracranial wound
851.5 ✓5th   Cerebellar or brain stem contusion with open intracranial wound
851.6 ✓5th   Cerebellar or brain stem laceration without mention of open intracranial wound
851.7 ✓5th   Cerebellar or brain stem laceration with open intracranial wound
851.8 ✓5th   Other and unspecified cerebral laceration and contusion, without mention of open intracranial wound
851.9 ✓5th   Other and unspecified cerebral laceration and contusion, with open intracranial wound

852 Subarachnoid, subdural, and extradural hemorrhage, following injury
AHA: Q1, 1993, 22

The following fifth-digit subclassification is for use with categories 851-854:
- 0 unspecified state of consciousness
- 1 with no loss of consciousness
- 2 with brief [less than one hour] loss of consciousness
- 3 with moderate [1-24 hours] loss of consciousness
- 4 with prolonged [more than 24 hours] loss of consciousness and return to pre-existing conscious level
- 5 with prolonged [more than 24 hours] loss of consciousness, without return to pre-existing conscious level

  Use fifth-digit five to designate when a patient is unconscious and dies before regaining consciousness, regardless of the duration of the loss of consciousness
- 6 with loss of consciousness of unspecified duration
- 9 with concussion, unspecified

852.0 [✓5th] Subarachnoid hemorrhage following injury without mention of open intracranial wound
852.1 [✓5th] Subarachnoid hemorrhage following injury, with open intracranial wound
852.2 [✓5th] Subdural hemorrhage following injury without mention of open intracranial wound
852.3 [✓5th] Subdural hemorrhage following injury, with open intracranial wound
852.4 [✓5th] Extradural hemorrhage following injury without mention of open intracranial wound
852.5 [✓5th] Extradural hemorrhage following injury with open intracranial wound

853 Other and unspecified intracranial hemorrhage following injury
AHA: Q1, 1993, 22

The following fifth-digit subclassification is for use with categories 851-854:
- 0 unspecified state of consciousness
- 1 with no loss of consciousness
- 2 with brief [less than one hour] loss of consciousness
- 3 with moderate [1-24 hours] loss of consciousness
- 4 with prolonged [more than 24 hours] loss of consciousness and return to pre-existing conscious level
- 5 with prolonged [more than 24 hours] loss of consciousness, without return to pre-existing conscious level

  Use fifth-digit five to designate when a patient is unconscious and dies before regaining consciousness, regardless of the duration of the loss of consciousness
- 6 with loss of consciousness of unspecified duration
- 9 with concussion, unspecified

853.0 [✓5th] Other and unspecified intracranial hemorrhage following injury, without mention of open intracranial wound
853.1 [✓5th] Other and unspecified intracranial hemorrhage following injury with open intracranial wound

854 Intracranial injury of other and unspecified nature
AHA: Q2, 1992, 6; Q1, 1993, 22; Q1, 1999, 10

The following fifth-digit subclassification is for use with categories 851-854:
- 0 unspecified state of consciousness
- 1 with no loss of consciousness
- 2 with brief [less than one hour] loss of consciousness
- 3 with moderate [1-24 hours] loss of consciousness
- 4 with prolonged [more than 24 hours] loss of consciousness and return to pre-existing conscious level
- 5 with prolonged [more than 24 hours] loss of consciousness, without return to pre-existing conscious level

  Use fifth-digit five to designate when a patient is unconscious and dies before regaining consciousness, regardless of the duration of the loss of consciousness
- 6 with loss of consciousness of unspecified duration
- 9 with concussion, unspecified

854.0 [✓5th] Intracranial injury of other and unspecified nature without mention of open intracranial wound
AHA: Q2, 2005, 6
854.1 [✓5th] Intracranial injury of other and unspecified nature with open intracranial wound

860–869 *Internal Injury of Thorax, Abdomen, and Pelvis*

Internal injuries can result from a blast, blunt trauma, crushing, puncture, rupture, concussion of internal organs, laceration, and hematoma.

Blast injuries result from explosive force capable of generating shock waves that damage the body. The force can emanate from a bomb, a gas leak, or any other explosion. Blast injuries are graded as primary, secondary, tertiary, and miscellaneous. A primary blast injury affects air-filled organs such as the lungs, ears, and bowel. If the tympanic membrane is ruptured, the physician automatically assumes serious organ damage. Secondary injury results from injuries associated with flying objects. Tertiary injuries may result from striking objects while airborne. Morbidity and mortality are greatest if the explosion occurs within a confined space or under water.

The most common fatality associated with blast injury results from injury to the pulmonary system, which can result in pulmonary contusion, air embolism, free radical injury and thrombosis, lipo-oxygenation, and disseminated intravascular coagulation (DIS).

Blunt trauma has two traumatic components: compression and deceleration forces. Compression causes trauma such as rupture of the bowel, which is often a marker for more serious solid organ damage. Deceleration causes stretching and shearing injuries. A common deceleration injury is a hepatic tear along the ligamentum teres. Blunt trauma refers to abdominal injuries. In adults, automobile accidents are to blame for 66 percent of all blunt trauma injuries.

Crush injuries involve smashing, fractures, bleeding, and bruising.

A hematoma is blood that has escaped from the vascular vessels and is free in the tissues (extravascular).

860 Traumatic pneumothorax and hemothorax
AHA: Q2, 1993, 4

Pneumothorax is free gas in the pleural space with lung collapse on the affected side. The medical record may state that a hemothorax is traumatic when arising from a medical procedure, but category 860 for traumatic hemothorax is not to be assigned for the condition arising from the delivery of medical care (998.11).

When hemothorax presents, the clinician suspects further damage to the lungs and heart. An evaluation must assess the integrity of the great vessels (aorta, vena cava, pulmonary artery, and pulmonary vein), as lacerations to these vessels increase mortality risks.

860.0	Traumatic pneumothorax without mention of open wound into thorax
860.1	Traumatic pneumothorax with open wound into thorax
860.2	Traumatic hemothorax without mention of open wound into thorax
860.3	Traumatic hemothorax with open wound into thorax
860.4	Traumatic pneumohemothorax without mention of open wound into thorax
860.5	Traumatic pneumohemothorax with open wound into thorax

861 Injury to heart and lung

861.00	Unspecified injury to heart without mention of open wound into thorax
861.01	Heart contusion without mention of open wound into thorax
861.02	Heart laceration without penetration of heart chambers or mention of open wound into thorax
861.03	Heart laceration with penetration of heart chambers, without mention of open wound into thorax
861.10	Unspecified injury to heart with open wound into thorax
861.11	Heart contusion with open wound into thorax
861.12	Heart laceration without penetration of heart chambers, with open wound into thorax
861.13	Heart laceration with penetration of heart chambers and open wound into thorax
861.20	Unspecified lung injury without mention of open wound into thorax
861.21	Lung contusion without mention of open wound into thorax
861.22	Lung laceration without mention of open wound into thorax
861.30	Unspecified lung injury with open wound into thorax
861.30	Unspecified lung injury with open wound into thorax
861.31	Lung contusion with open wound into thorax
861.32	Lung laceration with open wound into thorax

862 Injury to other and unspecified intrathoracic organs

862.0	Diaphragm injury without mention of open wound into cavity
862.1	Diaphragm injury with open wound into cavity
862.21	Bronchus injury without mention of open wound into cavity
862.22	Esophagus injury without mention of open wound into cavity
862.29	Injury to other specified intrathoracic organs without mention of open wound into cavity
862.31	Bronchus injury with open wound into cavity
862.32	Esophagus injury with open wound into cavity
862.39	Injury to other specified intrathoracic organs with open wound into cavity
862.8	Injury to multiple and unspecified intrathoracic organs without mention of open wound into cavity
862.9	Injury to multiple and unspecified intrathoracic organs with open wound into cavity

863 Gastrointestinal tract injury

863.0	Stomach injury without mention of open wound into cavity
863.1	Stomach injury with open wound into cavity
863.20	Small intestine injury, unspecified site, without mention of open wound into cavity
863.21	Duodenum injury without mention of open wound into cavity

863.29	Other injury to small intestine without mention of open wound into cavity		863.92	Pancreas body injury with open wound into cavity
863.30	Small intestine injury, unspecified site, with open wound into cavity		863.93	Pancreas tail injury with open wound into cavity
863.31	Duodenum injury with open wound into cavity		863.94	Pancreas injury, multiple and unspecified sites, with open wound into cavity
863.39	Other injury to small intestine with open wound into cavity		863.95	Appendix injury with open wound into cavity
863.40	Colon injury unspecified site, without mention of open wound into cavity		863.99	Injury to other and unspecified gastrointestinal sites with open wound into cavity

863.41 Ascending (right) colon injury without mention of open wound into cavity
863.42 Transverse colon injury without mention of open wound into cavity
863.43 Descending (left) colon injury without mention of open wound into cavity
863.44 Sigmoid colon injury without mention of open wound into cavity
863.45 Rectum injury without mention of open wound into cavity
863.46 Injury to multiple sites in colon and rectum without mention of open wound into cavity
863.49 Other colon and rectum injury, without mention of open wound into cavity
863.50 Colon injury, unspecified site, with open wound into cavity
863.51 Ascending (right) colon injury with open wound into cavity
863.52 Transverse colon injury with open wound into cavity
863.53 Descending (left) colon injury with open wound into cavity
863.54 Sigmoid colon injury with open wound into cavity
863.55 Rectum injury with open wound into cavity
863.56 Injury to multiple sites in colon and rectum with open wound into cavity
863.59 Other injury to colon and rectum with open wound into cavity
863.80 Gastrointestinal tract injury, unspecified site, without mention of open wound into cavity
863.81 Pancreas head injury without mention of open wound into cavity
863.82 Pancreas body injury without mention of open wound into cavity
863.83 Pancreas tail injury without mention of open wound into cavity
863.84 Pancreas injury, multiple and unspecified sites, without mention of open wound into cavity
863.85 Appendix injury without mention of open wound into cavity
863.89 Injury to other and unspecified gastrointestinal sites without mention of open wound into cavity
863.90 Gastrointestinal tract injury, unspecified site, with open wound into cavity
863.91 Pancreas head injury with open wound into cavity

864 Injury to liver

The liver is protected by the fibrous membrane Glisson's capsule. Not all liver injuries need surgical repair. If the patient is stable hemodynamically and has no other intra-abdominal injury that requires surgery, nursing may allow for non-operative management of the injury.

The following fifth-digit subclassification is for use with category 864:

0 unspecified injury
1 hematoma and contusion
2 laceration, minor
3 laceration, moderate
4 laceration, major
5 laceration, unspecified
9 other

864.0 ✓5th Liver injury without mention of open wound into cavity
864.1 ✓5th Liver injury with open wound into cavity

865 Injury to spleen

Similar to the liver, the spleen is covered by a thick fibrous membrane, the capsule, which plays a part in grading the severity of splenic injuries.

The following fifth-digit subclassification is for use with category 865:

0 unspecified injury
1 hematoma with rupture of capsule
2 capsular tears, without major disruption of parenchyma
3 laceration extending into parenchyma
4 massive parenchymal disruption
9 other

865.0 ✓5th Spleen injury without mention of open wound into cavity
865.1 ✓5th Spleen injury with open wound into cavity

866 Injury to kidney

The kidney's capsule protects the kidney parenchyma and is part of the injury grading system for the kidney.

The following fifth-digit subclassification is for use with category 866:

0 unspecified injury
1 hematoma without rupture of capsule
2 laceration
3 complete disruption of kidney parenchyma

866.0 ⌐sth Kidney injury without mention of open wound into cavity
866.1 ⌐sth Kidney injury with open wound into cavity

867 Injury to pelvic organs
Pelvic organs include the bladder, urethra, ureters, uterus, and other specified organs, including the fallopian tubes, ovaries, prostate, seminal vesicles, and vas deferens.

867.0	Bladder and urethra injury without mention of open wound into cavity
867.1	Bladder and urethra injury with open wound into cavity
867.2	Ureter injury without mention of open wound into cavity
867.3	Ureter injury with open wound into cavity
867.4	Uterus injury without mention of open wound into cavity
867.5	Uterus injury with open wound into cavity
867.6	Injury to other specified pelvic organs without mention of open wound into cavity
867.7	Injury to other specified pelvic organs with open wound into cavity
867.8	Injury to unspecified pelvic organ without mention of open wound into cavity
867.9	Injury to unspecified pelvic organ with open wound into cavity

868 Injury to other intra-abdominal organs
The peritoneum is a serous membrane lining the abdominal cavity and reflected over the viscera, the internal organs. The portion covering the viscera is called the omentum (apron). The retroperitoneum lies behind the viscera and outside the cavity. The kidneys are in the retroperitoneum.

The following fifth-digit subclassification is for use with category 868:

0 unspecified intra-abdominal organ
1 adrenal gland
2 bile duct and gallbladder
3 peritoneum
4 retroperitoneum
9 other and multiple intra-abdominal organs

868.0 ⌐sth Injury to other intra-abdominal organs without mention of open wound into cavity
868.1 ⌐sth Injury to other intra-abdominal organs with open wound into cavity

869 Internal injury to unspecified or ill-defined organs
Use these categories only if the documentation is extremely sketchy.

869.0	Internal injury to unspecified or ill-defined organs without mention of open wound into cavity
869.1	Internal injury to unspecified or ill-defined organs with open wound into cavity

870–879 Open Wound of Head, Neck, and Trunk

A traumatic amputation and an avulsion are essentially the same. Amputation is typically reserved to describe limb injuries and avulsion describes injuries such as the tearing or ripping of fingernails or a portion of an organ, though it can be used in reference to loss of limbs.

When using the term "complicated," described in the fourth-digit of codes 870-897, it includes wounds that have delayed healing, foreign body, infection, or wounds with delayed treatment.

870 Open wound of ocular adnexa
AHA: Q4, 2001, 52

The ocular adnexa are the eyelids, the lacrimal apparatus, the orbit, and the periocular area.

870.0	Laceration of skin of eyelid and periocular area
870.1	Laceration of eyelid, full-thickness, not involving lacrimal passages
870.2	Laceration of eyelid involving lacrimal passages
870.3	Penetrating wound of orbit, without mention of foreign body
870.4	Penetrating wound of orbit with foreign body
870.8	Other specified open wound of ocular adnexa
870.9	Unspecified open wound of ocular adnexa

871 Open wound of eyeball
AHA: Q4, 2001, 52

871.0	Ocular laceration without prolapse of intraocular tissue
871.1	Ocular laceration with prolapse or exposure of intraocular tissue
871.2	Rupture of eye with partial loss of intraocular tissue
871.3	Avulsion of eye
871.4	Unspecified laceration of eye
871.5	Penetration of eyeball with magnetic foreign body
871.6	Penetration of eyeball with (nonmagnetic) foreign body
871.7	Unspecified ocular penetration
871.9	Unspecified open wound of eyeball

Injury and Poisoning

872 Open wound of ear
AHA: Q4, 2001, 52

The auricle, or pinna, is another term for the external ear. The ossicles (tiny bones) refer to the three bones facilitating hearing — the malleus, incus, and stapes.

Code	Description
872.00	Open wound of external ear, unspecified site, without mention of complication
872.01	Open wound of auricle, without mention of complication
872.02	Open wound of auditory canal, without mention of complication
872.10	Open wound of external ear, unspecified site, complicated — (Use additional code to identify infection)
872.11	Open wound of auricle, complicated — (Use additional code to identify infection)
872.12	Open wound of auditory canal, complicated — (Use additional code to identify infection)
872.61	Open wound of ear drum, without mention of complication
872.62	Open wound of ossicles, without mention of complication
872.63	Open wound of Eustachian tube, without mention of complication
872.64	Open wound of cochlea, without mention of complication
872.69	Open wound of other and multiple sites, without mention of complication
872.71	Open wound of ear drum, complicated — (Use additional code to identify infection)
872.72	Open wound of ossicles, complicated — (Use additional code to identify infection)
872.73	Open wound of Eustachian tube, complicated — (Use additional code to identify infection)
872.74	Open wound of cochlea, complicated — (Use additional code to identify infection)
872.79	Open wound of other and multiple sites, complicated — (Use additional code to identify infection)
872.8	Open wound of ear, part unspecified, without mention of complication
872.9	Open wound of ear, part unspecified, complicated — (Use additional code to identify infection)

Coding Clarification

The term "complicated" describes wounds that have delayed healing, foreign body, infection, or wounds with delayed treatment.

873 Other open wound of head
AHA: Q4, 2001, 52

Code	Description
873.0	Open wound of scalp, without mention of complication
873.1	Open wound of scalp, complicated — (Use additional code to identify infection)
873.20	Open wound of nose, unspecified site, without mention of complication
873.21	Open wound of nasal septum, without mention of complication
873.22	Open wound of nasal cavity, without mention of complication
873.23	Open wound of nasal sinus, without mention of complication
873.29	Open wound of nose, multiple sites, without mention of complication
873.30	Open wound of nose, unspecified site, complicated — (Use additional code to identify infection)
873.31	Open wound of nasal septum, complicated — (Use additional code to identify infection)
873.32	Open wound of nasal cavity, complicated — (Use additional code to identify infection)
873.33	Open wound of nasal sinus, complicated — (Use additional code to identify infection)
873.39	Open wound of nose, multiple sites, complicated — (Use additional code to identify infection)
873.40	Open wound of face, unspecified site, without mention of complication
873.41	Open wound of cheek, without mention of complication
873.42	Open wound of forehead, without mention of complication
873.43	Open wound of lip, without mention of complication
873.44	Open wound of jaw, without mention of complication
873.49	Open wound of face, other and multiple sites, without mention of complication
873.50	Open wound of face, unspecified site, complicated — (Use additional code to identify infection)
873.51	Open wound of cheek, complicated — (Use additional code to identify infection)
873.52	Open wound of forehead, complicated — (Use additional code to identify infection)
873.53	Open wound of lip, complicated — (Use additional code to identify infection)
873.54	Open wound of jaw, complicated — (Use additional code to identify infection)
873.59	Open wound of face, other and multiple sites, complicated — (Use additional code to identify infection)
873.60	Open wound of mouth, unspecified site, without mention of complication
873.61	Open wound of buccal mucosa, without mention of complication
873.62	Open wound of gum (alveolar process), without mention of complication
873.63	Open wound of tooth (broken) (fractured) (due to trauma), without mention of complication
AHA: Q1, 2004, 17
873.64	Open wound of tongue and floor of mouth, without mention of complication
873.65	Open wound of palate, without mention of complication
873.69	Open wound of mouth, other and multiple sites, without mention of complication
873.70	Open wound of mouth, unspecified site, complicated — (Use additional code to identify infection)

Code	Description
873.71	Open wound of buccal mucosa, complicated — (Use additional code to identify infection)
873.72	Open wound of gum (alveolar process), complicated — (Use additional code to identify infection)
873.73	Open wound of tooth (broken) (fractured) (due to trauma), complicated — (Use additional code to identify infection) AHA: Q1, 2004, 17
873.74	Open wound of tongue and floor of mouth, complicated — (Use additional code to identify infection)
873.75	Open wound of palate, complicated — (Use additional code to identify infection)
873.79	Open wound of mouth, other and multiple sites, complicated — (Use additional code to identify infection)
873.8	Other and unspecified open wound of head without mention of complication
873.9	Other and unspecified open wound of head, complicated — (Use additional code to identify infection)

Coding Clarification

Cracked tooth unrelated to trauma is excluded from category 873 and is reported with code 521.81.

The term "complicated" describes wounds that have delayed healing, foreign body, infection, or wounds with delayed treatment.

874 Open wound of neck
AHA: Q4, 2001, 52

Code	Description
874.00	Open wound of larynx with trachea, without mention of complication
874.01	Open wound of larynx, without mention of complication
874.02	Open wound of trachea, without mention of complication
874.10	Open wound of larynx with trachea, complicated — (Use additional code to identify infection)
874.11	Open wound of larynx, complicated — (Use additional code to identify infection)
874.12	Open wound of trachea, complicated — (Use additional code to identify infection)
874.2	Open wound of thyroid gland, without mention of complication
874.3	Open wound of thyroid gland, complicated — (Use additional code to identify infection)
874.4	Open wound of pharynx, without mention of complication
874.5	Open wound of pharynx, complicated — (Use additional code to identify infection)
874.8	Open wound of other and unspecified parts of neck, without mention of complication
874.9	Open wound of other and unspecified parts of neck, complicated — (Use additional code to identify infection)

Coding Clarification

The term "complicated" describes wounds that have delayed healing, foreign body, infection, or wounds with delayed treatment.

875 Open wound of chest (wall)
AHA: Q3, 1993, 17; Q4, 2001, 52

Code	Description
875.0	Open wound of chest (wall), without mention of complication
875.1	Open wound of chest (wall), complicated — (Use additional code to identify infection)

Coding Clarification

The term "complicated" describes wounds that have delayed healing, foreign body, infection, or wounds with delayed treatment.

876 Open wound of back
AHA: Q4, 2001, 52

Code	Description
876.0	Open wound of back, without mention of complication
876.1	Open wound of back, complicated — (Use additional code to identify infection)

Coding Clarification

The term "complicated" describes wounds that have delayed healing, foreign body, infection, or wounds with delayed treatment.

877 Open wound of buttock
AHA: Q4, 2001, 52

Code	Description
877.0	Open wound of buttock, without mention of complication
877.1	Open wound of buttock, complicated — (Use additional code to identify infection)

Coding Clarification

The term "complicated" describes wounds that have delayed healing, foreign body, infection, or wounds with delayed treatment.

878 Open wound of genital organs (external), including traumatic amputation
AHA: Q4, 2001, 52

Code	Description
878.0	Open wound of penis, without mention of complication
878.1	Open wound of penis, complicated — (Use additional code to identify infection)
878.2	Open wound of scrotum and testes, without mention of complication
878.3	Open wound of scrotum and testes, complicated — (Use additional code to identify infection)
878.4	Open wound of vulva, without mention of complication
878.5	Open wound of vulva, complicated — (Use additional code to identify infection)
878.6	Open wound of vagina, without mention of complication
878.7	Open wound of vagina, complicated — (Use additional code to identify infection)
878.8	Open wound of other and unspecified parts of genital organs, without mention of complication
878.9	Open wound of other and unspecified parts of genital organs, complicated — (Use additional code to identify infection)

Injury and Poisoning

Coding Clarification
The term "complicated" describes wounds that have delayed healing, foreign body, infection, or wounds with delayed treatment.

879 Open wound of other and unspecified sites, except limbs
AHA: Q4, 2001, 52

Flank (879.4) can have two meanings: (1) the part of the body found between the ribs and the uppermost crest of the ilium; or (2) the lateral side of the hip, thigh, and buttock.

When using the term "complicated," described in the fourth-digit of codes 870-897, it includes wounds that have delayed healing, foreign body, infection, or wounds with delayed treatment.

879.0	Open wound of breast, without mention of complication
879.1	Open wound of breast, complicated — (Use additional code to identify infection)
879.2	Open wound of abdominal wall, anterior, without mention of complication
879.3	Open wound of abdominal wall, anterior, complicated — (Use additional code to identify infection)
879.4	Open wound of abdominal wall, lateral, without mention of complication
879.5	Open wound of abdominal wall, lateral, complicated — (Use additional code to identify infection)
879.6	Open wound of other and unspecified parts of trunk, without mention of complication
879.7	Open wound of other and unspecified parts of trunk, complicated — (Use additional code to identify infection)
879.8	Open wound(s) (multiple) of unspecified site(s), without mention of complication
879.9	Open wound(s) (multiple) of unspecified site(s), complicated — (Use additional code to identify infection)

Coding Clarification
The term "complicated" describes wounds that have delayed healing, foreign body, infection, or wounds with delayed treatment.

880 Open wound of shoulder and upper arm
AHA: Nov-Dec, 1985, 5; Q4, 2001, 52

The following fifth-digit subclassification is for use with category 880:
0 shoulder region
1 scapular region
2 axillary region
3 upper arm
9 multiple sites

880.0 ⌐sth	Open wound of shoulder and upper arm, without mention of complication
880.1 ⌐sth	Open wound of shoulder and upper arm, complicated — (Use additional code to identify infection)
	AHA: For code 880.13: Q2, 2006, 7
880.2 ⌐sth	Open wound of shoulder and upper arm, with tendon involvement

Coding Clarification
The term "complicated" describes wounds that have delayed healing, foreign body, infection, or wounds with delayed treatment.

881 Open wound of elbow, forearm, and wrist
AHA: Nov-Dec, 1985, 5; Q4, 2001, 52

The following fifth-digit subclassification is for use with category 881:
0 forearm
1 elbow
2 wrist

881.0 ⌐sth	Open wound of elbow, forearm, and wrist, without mention of complication
881.1 ⌐sth	Open wound of elbow, forearm, and wrist, complicated — (Use additional code to identify infection)
881.2 ⌐sth	Open wound of elbow, forearm, and wrist, with tendon involvement

882 Open wound of hand except finger(s) alone
AHA: Nov-Dec, 1985, 5; Q4, 2001, 52

882.0	Open wound of hand except finger(s) alone, without mention of complication
882.1	Open wound of hand except finger(s) alone, complicated — (Use additional code to identify infection)
882.2	Open wound of hand except finger(s) alone, with tendon involvement

Coding Clarification
The term "complicated" describes wounds that have delayed healing, foreign body, infection, or wounds with delayed treatment.

883 Open wound of finger(s)
AHA: Nov-Dec, 1985, 5; Q4, 2001, 52

883.0	Open wound of finger(s), without mention of complication
883.1	Open wound of finger(s), complicated — (Use additional code to identify infection)
883.2	Open wound of finger(s), with tendon involvement

Coding Clarification
The term "complicated" describes wounds that have delayed healing, foreign body, infection, or wounds with delayed treatment.

884 Multiple and unspecified open wound of upper limb
AHA: Nov-Dec, 1985, 5; Q4, 2001, 52

884.0	Multiple and unspecified open wound of upper limb, without mention of complication
884.1	Multiple and unspecified open wound of upper limb, complicated — (Use additional code to identify infection)
884.2	Multiple and unspecified open wound of upper limb, with tendon involvement

Coding Clarification
The term "complicated" describes wounds that have delayed healing, foreign body, infection, or wounds with delayed treatment.

885 Traumatic amputation of thumb (complete) (partial)
AHA: Nov-Dec, 1985, 5; Q4, 2001, 52

885.0	Traumatic amputation of thumb (complete) (partial), without mention of complication
885.1	Traumatic amputation of thumb (complete) (partial), complicated — (Use additional code to identify infection)

Coding Clarification
The term "complicated" describes wounds that have delayed healing, foreign body, infection, or wounds with delayed treatment.

886 Traumatic amputation of other finger(s) (complete) (partial)
AHA: Nov-Dec, 1985, 5; Q4, 2001, 52

886.0	Traumatic amputation of other finger(s) (complete) (partial), without mention of complication
886.1	Traumatic amputation of other finger(s) (complete) (partial), complicated — (Use additional code to identify infection)

Coding Clarification
The term "complicated" describes wounds that have delayed healing, foreign body, infection, or wounds with delayed treatment.

887 Traumatic amputation of arm and hand (complete) (partial)
AHA: Nov-Dec, 1985, 5; Q4, 2001, 52

887.0	Traumatic amputation of arm and hand (complete) (partial), unilateral, below elbow, without mention of complication
887.1	Traumatic amputation of arm and hand (complete) (partial), unilateral, below elbow, complicated — (Use additional code to identify infection)
887.2	Traumatic amputation of arm and hand (complete) (partial), unilateral, at or above elbow, without mention of complication
887.3	Traumatic amputation of arm and hand (complete) (partial), unilateral, at or above elbow, complicated — (Use additional code to identify infection)
887.4	Traumatic amputation of arm and hand (complete) (partial), unilateral, level not specified, without mention of complication
887.5	Traumatic amputation of arm and hand (complete) (partial), unilateral, level not specified, complicated — (Use additional code to identify infection)
887.6	Traumatic amputation of arm and hand (complete) (partial), bilateral (any level), without mention of complication
887.7	Traumatic amputation of arm and hand (complete) (partial), bilateral (any level), complicated — (Use additional code to identify infection)

Coding Clarification
The term "complicated" describes wounds that have delayed healing, foreign body, infection, or wounds with delayed treatment.

890–897 Open Wound of Lower Limb
Traumatic Amputations: Traumatic amputation injuries are capable of amelioration due to the ability to reattach the severed part. The severed part must be kept on ice to slow the process of decay and the patient must be brought to the operating room within a six- to eight-hour window. The nerves must regrow to the injured part and grow at a rate of about an inch a month.

When using the term "complicated," described in the fourth-digit of codes 870-897, it includes wounds that have delayed healing, a foreign body, infection, or wounds with delayed treatment.

890 Open wound of hip and thigh
AHA: Nov-Dec, 1985, 5; Q4, 2001, 52

890.0	Open wound of hip and thigh, without mention of complication
890.1	Open wound of hip and thigh, complicated — (Use additional code to identify infection)
890.2	Open wound of hip and thigh, with tendon involvement

Coding Clarification
The term "complicated" describes wounds that have delayed healing, foreign body, infection, or wounds with delayed treatment.

891 Open wound of knee, leg (except thigh), and ankle
AHA: Nov-Dec, 1985, 5; Q4, 2001, 52

891.0	Open wound of knee, leg (except thigh), and ankle, without mention of complication
891.1	Open wound of knee, leg (except thigh), and ankle, complicated — (Use additional code to identify infection)
891.2	Open wound of knee, leg (except thigh), and ankle, with tendon involvement

Coding Clarification
The term "complicated" describes wounds that have delayed healing, foreign body, infection, or wounds with delayed treatment.

892 Open wound of foot except toe(s) alone
AHA: Nov-Dec, 1985, 5; Q4, 2001, 52

892.0	Open wound of foot except toe(s) alone, without mention of complication
892.1	Open wound of foot except toe(s) alone, complicated — (Use additional code to identify infection)
892.2	Open wound of foot except toe(s) alone, with tendon involvement

893 Open wound of toe(s)
AHA: Nov-Dec, 1985, 5; Q4, 2001, 52

893.0	Open wound of toe(s), without mention of complication
893.1	Open wound of toe(s), complicated — (Use additional code to identify infection)
893.2	Open wound of toe(s), with tendon involvement

Coding Clarification
The term "complicated" describes wounds that have delayed healing, foreign body, infection, or wounds with delayed treatment.

894 Multiple and unspecified open wound of lower limb
AHA: Nov-Dec, 1985, 5; Q4, 2001, 52

894.0	Multiple and unspecified open wound of lower limb, without mention of complication
894.1	Multiple and unspecified open wound of lower limb, complicated — (Use additional code to identify infection)
894.2	Multiple and unspecified open wound of lower limb, with tendon involvement — (Use additional code to identify infection)

Coding Clarification
The term "complicated" describes wounds that have delayed healing, foreign body, infection, or wounds with delayed treatment.

895 Traumatic amputation of toe(s) (complete) (partial)
AHA: Nov-Dec, 1985, 5; Q4, 2001, 52

895.0	Traumatic amputation of toe(s) (complete) (partial), without mention of complication
895.1	Traumatic amputation of toe(s) (complete) (partial), complicated — (Use additional code to identify infection)

Coding Clarification
The term "complicated" describes wounds that have delayed healing, foreign body, infection, or wounds with delayed treatment.

896 Traumatic amputation of foot (complete) (partial)
AHA: Nov-Dec, 1985, 5; Q4, 2001, 52

896.0	Traumatic amputation of foot (complete) (partial), unilateral, without mention of complication
896.1	Traumatic amputation of foot (complete) (partial), unilateral, complicated — (Use additional code to identify infection)
896.2	Traumatic amputation of foot (complete) (partial), bilateral, without mention of complication
896.3	Traumatic amputation of foot (complete) (partial), bilateral, complicated — (Use additional code to identify infection)

Coding Clarification
The term "complicated" describes wounds that have delayed healing, foreign body, infection, or wounds with delayed treatment.

897 Traumatic amputation of leg(s) (complete) (partial)
AHA: Nov-Dec, 1985, 5; Q4, 2001, 52

897.0	Traumatic amputation of leg(s) (complete) (partial), unilateral, below knee, without mention of complication
897.1	Traumatic amputation of leg(s) (complete) (partial), unilateral, below knee, complicated — (Use additional code to identify infection)
897.2	Traumatic amputation of leg(s) (complete) (partial), unilateral, at or above knee, without mention of complication
897.3	Traumatic amputation of leg(s) (complete) (partial), unilateral, at or above knee, complicated — (Use additional code to identify infection)
897.4	Traumatic amputation of leg(s) (complete) (partial), unilateral, level not specified, without mention of complication
897.5	Traumatic amputation of leg(s) (complete) (partial), unilateral, level not specified, complicated — (Use additional code to identify infection)
897.6	Traumatic amputation of leg(s) (complete) (partial), bilateral (any level), without mention of complication
897.7	Traumatic amputation of leg(s) (complete) (partial), bilateral (any level), complicated — (Use additional code to identify infection)

Coding Clarification
The term "complicated" describes wounds that have delayed healing, foreign body, infection, or wounds with delayed treatment.

900–904 Injury to Blood Vessels
Vascular trauma results from penetrating and blunt injury. A traumatic aneurysm is a weakening in the arterial wall that bulges with the pumping of the blood, posing the threat of rupture. A traumatic

fistula is an abnormal communication between an artery and a vein. (These conditions also can arise from a disease process, and are classified elsewhere in ICD 9-CM.)

Not only must the physician accurately assess the extent of trauma, but must control any hemorrhage as soon as possible, as mortality risk is a function of the amount of blood loss. Arterial blood loss manifests as profuse and bright red, while venous loss is steady and dark. Injury to the great vessels that enter and leave the heart is an enormous threat, as are injuries to most arteries.

900 Injury to blood vessels of head and neck
AHA: Q3, 1990, 5

900.00	Injury to carotid artery, unspecified
900.01	Common carotid artery injury
900.02	External carotid artery injury
900.03	Internal carotid artery injury
900.1	Internal jugular vein injury
900.81	External jugular vein injury
900.82	Injury to multiple blood vessels of head and neck
900.89	Injury to other specified blood vessels of head and neck
900.9	Injury to unspecified blood vessel of head and neck

901 Injury to blood vessels of thorax
AHA: Q3, 1990, 5

901.0	Thoracic aorta injury
901.1	Innominate and subclavian artery injury
901.2	Superior vena cava injury
901.3	Innominate and subclavian vein injury
901.40	Injury to unspecified pulmonary vessel(s)
901.41	Pulmonary artery injury
901.42	Pulmonary vein injury
901.81	Intercostal artery or vein injury
901.82	Internal mammary artery or vein injury
901.83	Injury to multiple blood vessels of thorax
901.89	Injury to specified blood vessels of thorax, other
901.9	Injury to unspecified blood vessel of thorax

902 Injury to blood vessels of abdomen and pelvis
AHA: Q3, 1990, 5

902.0	Abdominal aorta injury
902.10	Unspecified inferior vena cava injury
902.11	Hepatic vein injury
902.19	Injury to specified branches of inferior vena cava, other
902.20	Unspecified celiac and mesenteric artery injury
902.21	Gastric artery injury
902.22	Hepatic artery injury
902.23	Splenic artery injury
902.24	Injury to specified branches of celiac axis, other
902.25	Superior mesenteric artery (trunk) injury
902.26	Injury to primary branches of superior mesenteric artery
902.27	Inferior mesenteric artery injury
902.29	Injury to celiac and mesenteric arteries, other
902.31	Injury to superior mesenteric vein and primary subdivisions
902.32	Inferior mesenteric vein injury
902.33	Portal vein injury
902.34	Splenic vein injury
902.39	Injury to portal and splenic veins, other
902.40	Renal vessel(s) injury, unspecified
902.41	Renal artery injury
902.42	Renal vein injury
902.49	Renal blood vessel injury, other
902.50	Unspecified iliac vessel(s) injury
902.51	Hypogastric artery injury
902.52	Hypogastric vein injury
902.53	Iliac artery injury
902.54	Iliac vein injury
902.55	Uterine artery injury
902.56	Uterine vein injury
902.59	Injury to iliac blood vessels, other
902.81	Ovarian artery injury
902.82	Ovarian vein injury
902.87	Injury to multiple blood vessels of abdomen and pelvis
902.89	Injury to specified blood vessels of abdomen and pelvis, other
902.9	Injury to blood vessel of abdomen and pelvis, unspecified

903 Injury to blood vessels of upper extremity
AHA: Q3, 1990, 5

903.00	Axillary vessel(s) injury, unspecified
903.01	Axillary artery injury
903.02	Axillary vein injury
903.1	Brachial blood vessels injury
903.2	Radial blood vessels injury
903.3	Ulnar blood vessels injury
903.4	Palmar artery injury
903.5	Digital blood vessels injury
903.8	Injury to specified blood vessels of upper extremity, other
903.9	Injury to unspecified blood vessel of upper extremity

904 Injury to blood vessels of lower extremity and unspecified sites
AHA: Q3, 1990, 5

904.0	Common femoral artery injury
904.1	Superficial femoral artery injury
904.2	Femoral vein injury
904.3	Saphenous vein injury
904.40	Unspecified popliteal vessel(s) injury
904.41	Popliteal artery injury
904.42	Popliteal vein injury
904.50	Unspecified tibial vessel(s) injury
904.51	Anterior tibial artery injury
904.52	Anterior tibial vein injury
904.53	Posterior tibial artery injury
904.54	Posterior tibial vein injury
904.6	Deep plantar blood vessels injury

904.7	Injury to specified blood vessels of lower extremity, other	905.7	Late effect of sprain and strain without mention of tendon injury
904.8	Injury to unspecified blood vessel of lower extremity	905.8	Late effect of tendon injury
904.9	Injury to blood vessels, unspecified site	905.9	Late effect of traumatic amputation

905–909 Late Effects of Injuries, Poisonings, Toxic Effects, and Other External Causes

After exiting the acute phase of a closed head injury, the victim faces problems that may be lifelong, including functional cognitive deficits involving working memory, behavioral, affective disorders requiring antipsychotics and antidepressants, and impaired visuospatial ability. Skull fracture injuries pose a higher degree of neuropsychological dysfunction than head trauma without skull fracture. Studies have shown that the ability to find employment is affected by the patient's physical, cognitive, and behavioral functioning from time of admission to discharge, and injury severity as reflected by the initial Glasgow Coma Scale, the highest Glasgow Coma Scale, and the duration of the coma.

Late effects of musculoskeletal injuries include bursitis, traumatic arthritis, joint instability, synovitis, and tenosynovitis.

Late effects of injury to peripheral nerves are quite common, and recovery is very unpredictable. Expert and technically perfect microsurgical repair of a damaged nerve does not predict a full recovery since sensation may not be regained.

Late effects of spinal cord injury include paralysis, loss of bowel and bladder control, muscular atrophy, and limb contracture.

Late effects of burns include scarring, joint immobility, nerve, and psychological damage.

Radiation can result in burns, paralysis, and tissue death.

905 Late effects of musculoskeletal and connective tissue injuries
AHA: Q2, 1994, 3; Q1, 1995, 10

905.0	Late effect of fracture of skull and face bones
905.1	Late effect of fracture of spine and trunk without mention of spinal cord lesion
905.2	Late effect of fracture of upper extremities
905.3	Late effect of fracture of neck of femur
905.4	Late effect of fracture of lower extremities
905.5	Late effect of fracture of multiple and unspecified bones
905.6	Late effect of dislocation

906 Late effects of injuries to skin and subcutaneous tissues

906.0	Late effect of open wound of head, neck, and trunk
906.1	Late effect of open wound of extremities without mention of tendon injury
906.2	Late effect of superficial injury
906.3	Late effect of contusion
906.4	Late effect of crushing
906.5	Late effect of burn of eye, face, head, and neck
	AHA: Q4, 2004, 76
906.6	Late effect of burn of wrist and hand
906.7	Late effect of burn of other extremities
906.8	Late effect of burns of other specified sites
906.9	Late effect of burn of unspecified site

907 Late effects of injuries to the nervous system

907.0	Late effect of intracranial injury without mention of skull fracture
907.1	Late effect of injury to cranial nerve
907.2	Late effect of spinal cord injury
907.3	Late effect of injury to nerve root(s), spinal plexus(es), and other nerves of trunk
907.4	Late effect of injury to peripheral nerve of shoulder girdle and upper limb
907.5	Late effect of injury to peripheral nerve of pelvic girdle and lower limb
907.9	Late effect of injury to other and unspecified nerve

908 Late effect of other and unspecified injury

908.0	Late effect of internal injury to chest
908.1	Late effect of internal injury to intra-abdominal organs
908.2	Late effect of internal injury to other internal organs
908.3	Late effect of injury to blood vessel of head, neck, and extremities
908.4	Late effect of injury to blood vessel of thorax, abdomen, and pelvis
908.5	Late effect of foreign body in orifice
908.6	Late effect of certain complications of trauma
908.9	Late effect of unspecified injury

909 Late effects of other and unspecified external causes

909.0	Late effect of poisoning due to drug, medicinal or biological substance
909.1	Late effect of toxic effects of nonmedical substances
909.2	Late effect of radiation
909.3	Late effect of complications of surgical and medical care
909.4	Late effect of certain other external causes
909.5	Late effect of adverse effect of drug, medical or biological substance

909.9	Late effect of other and unspecified external causes		912.5	Shoulder and upper arm, insect bite, nonvenomous, infected
910	**Superficial injury of face, neck, and scalp, except eye** AHA: Q2, 1989, 15		912.6	Shoulder and upper arm, superficial foreign body (splinter), without major open wound and without mention of infection
910.0	Face, neck, and scalp, except eye, abrasion or friction burn, without mention of infection		912.7	Shoulder and upper arm, superficial foreign body (splinter), without major open wound, infected
910.1	Face, neck, and scalp except eye, abrasion or friction burn, infected		912.8	Other and unspecified superficial injury of shoulder and upper arm, without mention of infection
910.2	Face, neck, and scalp except eye, blister, without mention of infection		912.9	Other and unspecified superficial injury of shoulder and upper arm, infected
910.2	Face, neck, and scalp except eye, blister, without mention of infection		**913**	**Superficial injury of elbow, forearm, and wrist** AHA: Q2, 1989, 15
910.3	Face, neck, and scalp except eye, blister, infected		913.0	Elbow, forearm, and wrist, abrasion or friction burn, without mention of infection
910.4	Face, neck, and scalp except eye, insect bite, nonvenomous, without mention of infection		913.1	Elbow, forearm, and wrist, abrasion or friction burn, infected
910.5	Face, neck, and scalp except eye, insect bite, nonvenomous, infected		913.2	Elbow, forearm, and wrist, blister, without mention of infection
910.6	Face, neck, and scalp, except eye, superficial foreign body (splinter), without major open wound or mention of infection		913.3	Elbow, forearm, and wrist, blister infected
			913.4	Elbow, forearm, and wrist, insect bite, nonvenomous, without mention of infection
910.7	Face, neck, and scalp except eye, superficial foreign body (splinter), without major open wound, infected		913.5	Elbow, forearm, and wrist, insect bite, nonvenomous, infected
910.8	Other and unspecified superficial injury of face, neck, and scalp, without mention of infection		913.6	Elbow, forearm, and wrist, superficial foreign body (splinter), without major open wound and without mention of infection
910.9	Other and unspecified superficial injury of face, neck, and scalp, infected		913.7	Elbow, forearm, and wrist, superficial foreign body (splinter), without major open wound, infected
911	**Superficial injury of trunk** AHA: Q2, 1989, 15		913.8	Other and unspecified superficial injury of elbow, forearm, and wrist, without mention of infection
911.0	Trunk abrasion or friction burn, without mention of infection		913.9	Other and unspecified superficial injury of elbow, forearm, and wrist, infected
911.1	Trunk abrasion or friction burn, infected		**914**	**Superficial injury of hand(s) except finger(s) alone** AHA: Q2, 1989, 15
911.2	Trunk blister, without mention of infection			
911.3	Trunk blister, infected		914.0	Hand(s) except finger(s) alone, abrasion or friction burn, without mention of infection
911.4	Trunk, insect bite, nonvenomous, without mention of infection		914.1	Hand(s) except finger(s) alone, abrasion or friction burn, infected
911.5	Trunk, insect bite, nonvenomous, infected		914.2	Hand(s) except finger(s) alone, blister, without mention of infection
911.6	Trunk, superficial foreign body (splinter), without major open wound and without mention of infection		914.3	Hand(s) except finger(s) alone, blister, infected
			914.4	Hand(s) except finger(s) alone, insect bite, nonvenomous, without mention of infection
911.7	Trunk, superficial foreign body (splinter), without major open wound, infected		914.5	Hand(s) except finger(s) alone, insect bite, nonvenomous, infected
911.8	Other and unspecified superficial injury of trunk, without mention of infection		914.6	Hand(s) except finger(s) alone, superficial foreign body (splinter), without major open wound and without mention of infection
911.9	Other and unspecified superficial injury of trunk, infected		914.7	Hand(s) except finger(s) alone, superficial foreign body (splinter) without major open wound, infected
912	**Superficial injury of shoulder and upper arm** AHA: Q2, 1989, 15			
912.0	Shoulder and upper arm, abrasion or friction burn, without mention of infection		914.8	Other and unspecified superficial injury of hand(s) except finger(s) alone, without mention of infection
912.1	Shoulder and upper arm, abrasion or friction burn, infected			
912.2	Shoulder and upper arm, blister, without mention of infection			
912.3	Shoulder and upper arm, blister, infected			
912.4	Shoulder and upper arm, insect bite, nonvenomous, without mention of infection			

Injury and Poisoning

| 914.9 | Other and unspecified superficial injury of hand(s) except finger(s) alone, infected |

915 Superficial injury of finger(s)
AHA: Q2, 1989, 15

915.0	Abrasion or friction burn of finger, without mention of infection
915.1	Finger, abrasion or friction burn, infected
915.2	Finger, blister, without mention of infection
915.3	Finger, blister, infected
915.4	Finger, insect bite, nonvenomous, without mention of infection
915.5	Finger, insect bite, nonvenomous, infected
915.6	Finger, superficial foreign body (splinter), without major open wound and without mention of infection
915.7	Finger, superficial foreign body (splinter), without major open wound, infected
915.8	Other and unspecified superficial injury of finger without mention of infection
915.9	Other and unspecified superficial injury of finger, infected

916 Superficial injury of hip, thigh, leg, and ankle
AHA: Q2, 1989, 15

916.0	Hip, thigh, leg, and ankle, abrasion or friction burn, without mention of infection
916.1	Hip, thigh, leg, and ankle, abrasion or friction burn, infected
916.2	Hip, thigh, leg, and ankle, blister, without mention of infection
916.3	Hip, thigh, leg, and ankle, blister, infected
916.4	Hip, thigh, leg, and ankle, insect bite, nonvenomous, without mention of infection
916.5	Hip, thigh, leg, and ankle, insect bite, nonvenomous, infected
916.6	Hip, thigh, leg, and ankle, superficial foreign body (splinter), without major open wound and without mention of infection
916.7	Hip, thigh, leg, and ankle, superficial foreign body (splinter), without major open wound, infected
916.8	Other and unspecified superficial injury of hip, thigh, leg, and ankle, without mention of infection
916.9	Other and unspecified superficial injury of hip, thigh, leg, and ankle, infected

917 Superficial injury of foot and toe(s)
AHA: Q2, 1989, 15

917.0	Abrasion or friction burn of foot and toe(s), without mention of infection
917.1	Foot and toe(s), abrasion or friction burn, infected
917.2	Foot and toe(s), blister, without mention of infection
917.3	Foot and toe(s), blister, infected
917.4	Foot and toe(s), insect bite, nonvenomous, without mention of infection
917.5	Foot and toe(s), insect bite, nonvenomous, infected
917.6	Foot and toe(s), superficial foreign body (splinter), without major open wound and without mention of infection
917.7	Foot and toe(s), superficial foreign body (splinter), without major open wound, infected
917.8	Other and unspecified superficial injury of foot and toes, without mention of infection
917.9	Other and unspecified superficial injury of foot and toes, infected

918 Superficial injury of eye and adnexa
AHA: Q2, 1989, 15

918.0	Superficial injury of eyelids and periocular area
918.1	Superficial injury of cornea
918.2	Superficial injury of conjunctiva
918.9	Other and unspecified superficial injuries of eye

919 Superficial injury of other, multiple, and unspecified sites
AHA: Q2, 1989, 15

919.0	Abrasion or friction burn of other, multiple, and unspecified sites, without mention of infection
919.1	Other, multiple, and unspecified sites, abrasion or friction burn, infected
919.2	Other, multiple, and unspecified sites, blister, without mention of infection
919.3	Other, multiple, and unspecified sites, blister, infected
919.4	Other, multiple, and unspecified sites, insect bite, nonvenomous, without mention of infection
919.5	Other, multiple, and unspecified sites, insect bite, nonvenomous, infected
919.6	Other, multiple, and unspecified sites, superficial foreign body (splinter), without major open wound and without mention of infection
919.7	Other, multiple, and unspecified sites, superficial foreign body (splinter), without major open wound, infected
919.8	Other and unspecified superficial injury of other, multiple, and unspecified sites, without mention of infection
919.9	Other and unspecified superficial injury of other, multiple, and unspecified sites, infected

920–924 Contusion with Intact Skin Surface

The skin of the face is vulnerable to severe contusions due to its proximity to unyielding bone. Any blunt trauma to the face may be noticed immediately due to swelling and discoloration.

A black eye can result in permanent vision loss, cataracts, and infection, though these complications are rare.

Gastrocnemius and the quadriceps femoris are the muscle groups most prone to contusions. If a muscle is repeatedly contused, it may become predisposed to developing myositis ossificans in the area of injury.

Hematomas, a large extravascular clot of blood, may require surgical evacuation, though most resorb naturally.

A contusion is a crushing of tissue that causes visible bruising due to trauma and blood leaking from microscopic vessels. A crushing injury occurs when the force deforms tissues beyond their failure limits; the injury may be internal, even though skin surface may be intact. A crushing injury can result in anatomical damage (i.e., fractures), physiologic damage (i.e., central nervous system injury), and death.

Bullets from gunshots injure first by crushing those structures that lie in the bullet path. The extent of injury depends on which structures are penetrated. A Type V fracture is a crushing injury to the end of a tubular bone, which can lead to injury to the vascular supply in the germinal cells of the plate and may not be initially apparent despite x-ray. Premature osseous fusion of the injured portion of the plate may occur. The agricultural industry has a high percentage of deaths due to crushing, as compared to other occupations. For example, an agricultural worker can easily become crushed between a tractor and the machinery being attached when the worker is standing between the tractor and the machine as the operator is backing up the tractor.

920 Contusion of face, scalp, and neck except eye(s)

921 Contusion of eye and adnexa
921.0	Black eye, not otherwise specified
921.1	Contusion of eyelids and periocular area
921.2	Contusion of orbital tissues
921.3	Contusion of eyeball
921.9	Unspecified contusion of eye

922 Contusion of trunk
922.0	Contusion of breast
922.1	Contusion of chest wall
922.2	Contusion of abdominal wall
922.31	Contusion of back
922.32	Contusion of buttock
922.33	Contusion of interscapular region
922.4	Contusion of genital organs
922.8	Contusion of multiple sites of trunk
922.9	Contusion of unspecified part of trunk

923 Contusion of upper limb
923.00	Contusion of shoulder region
923.01	Contusion of scapular region
923.02	Contusion of axillary region
923.03	Contusion of upper arm
923.09	Contusion of multiple sites of shoulder and upper arm
923.10	Contusion of forearm
923.11	Contusion of elbow
923.20	Contusion of hand(s)
923.21	Contusion of wrist
923.3	Contusion of finger
923.8	Contusion of multiple sites of upper limb
923.9	Contusion of unspecified part of upper limb

924 Contusion of lower limb and of other and unspecified sites
924.00	Contusion of thigh
924.01	Contusion of hip
924.10	Contusion of lower leg
924.11	Contusion of knee
924.20	Contusion of foot
924.21	Contusion of ankle
924.3	Contusion of toe
924.4	Contusion of multiple sites of lower limb
924.5	Contusion of unspecified part of lower limb
924.8	Contusion of multiple sites, not elsewhere classified
924.9	Contusion of unspecified site

925–929 Crushing Injury

This injury occurs when a body part is subjected to a high degree of force or pressure, typically after being pressed between two heavy or motionless objects. Damage related to crush injury can include lacerations, fractures, bleeding, bruising, and compartment syndrome.

Severe crush injuries cause extensive damage to skin, muscle, nerves, and bone. There may be bleeding, internally and/or externally, or blood supply to extremities may be cut off. Plasma may leak from the blood vessels into the damaged tissues, causing swelling and shock. When the crushed part is released, toxic chemicals produced by damaged muscles get into general circulation, leading to kidney failure in severe cases.

Use an additional code to identify any associated injuries, such as: fractures, 800-829; internal injuries, 860.0-869.1; or intracranial injury, 850.0-854.1.

925 Crushing injury of face, scalp, and neck
AHA: Q2, 1993, 7; Q4, 2003, 77
925.1	Crushing injury of face and scalp — (Use additional code to identify any associated injuries: 800-829, 850.0-854.1, 860.0-869.1)
925.2	Crushing injury of neck — (Use additional code to identify any associated injuries: 800-829, 850.0-854.1, 860.0-869.1)

926 Crushing injury of trunk
AHA: Q2, 1993, 7; Q4, 2003, 77

- **926.0** Crushing injury of external genitalia — (Use additional code to identify any associated injuries: 800-829, 850.0-854.1, 860.0-869.1)
- **926.11** Crushing injury of back — (Use additional code to identify any associated injuries: 800-829, 850.0-854.1, 860.0-869.1)
- **926.12** Crushing injury of buttock — (Use additional code to identify any associated injuries: 800-829, 850.0-854.1, 860.0-869.1)
- **926.19** Crushing injury of other specified sites of trunk — (Use additional code to identify any associated injuries: 800-829, 850.0-854.1, 860.0-869.1)
- **926.8** Crushing injury of multiple sites of trunk — (Use additional code to identify any associated injuries: 800-829, 850.0-854.1, 860.0-869.1)
- **926.9** Crushing injury of unspecified site of trunk — (Use additional code to identify any associated injuries: 800-829, 850.0-854.1, 860.0-869.1)

927 Crushing injury of upper limb
AHA: Q2, 1993, 7; Q4, 2003, 77

- **927.00** Crushing injury of shoulder region — (Use additional code to identify any associated injuries: 800-829, 850.0-854.1, 860.0-869.1)
- **927.01** Crushing injury of scapular region — (Use additional code to identify any associated injuries: 800-829, 850.0-854.1, 860.0-869.1)
- **927.02** Crushing injury of axillary region — (Use additional code to identify any associated injuries: 800-829, 850.0-854.1, 860.0-869.1)
- **927.03** Crushing injury of upper arm — (Use additional code to identify any associated injuries: 800-829, 850.0-854.1, 860.0-869.1)
- **927.09** Crushing injury of multiple sites of upper arm — (Use additional code to identify any associated injuries: 800-829, 850.0-854.1, 860.0-869.1)
- **927.10** Crushing injury of forearm — (Use additional code to identify any associated injuries: 800-829, 850.0-854.1, 860.0-869.1)
- **927.11** Crushing injury of elbow — (Use additional code to identify any associated injuries: 800-829, 850.0-854.1, 860.0-869.1)
- **927.20** Crushing injury of hand(s) — (Use additional code to identify any associated injuries: 800-829, 850.0-854.1, 860.0-869.1)
- **927.21** Crushing injury of wrist — (Use additional code to identify any associated injuries: 800-829, 850.0-854.1, 860.0-869.1)
- **927.3** Crushing injury of finger(s) — (Use additional code to identify any associated injuries: 800-829, 850.0-854.1, 860.0-869.1)
- **927.8** Crushing injury of multiple sites of upper limb — (Use additional code to identify any associated injuries: 800-829, 850.0-854.1, 860.0-869.1)
- **927.9** Crushing injury of unspecified site of upper limb — (Use additional code to identify any associated injuries: 800-829, 850.0-854.1, 860.0-869.1)

928 Crushing injury of lower limb
AHA: Q2, 1993, 7; Q4, 2003, 77

- **928.00** Crushing injury of thigh — (Use additional code to identify any associated injuries: 800-829, 850.0-854.1, 860.0-869.1)
- **928.01** Crushing injury of hip — (Use additional code to identify any associated injuries: 800-829, 850.0-854.1, 860.0-869.1)
- **928.10** Crushing injury of lower leg — (Use additional code to identify any associated injuries: 800-829, 850.0-854.1, 860.0-869.1)
- **928.11** Crushing injury of knee — (Use additional code to identify any associated injuries: 800-829, 850.0-854.1, 860.0-869.1)
- **928.20** Crushing injury of foot — (Use additional code to identify any associated injuries: 800-829, 850.0-854.1, 860.0-869.1)
- **928.21** Crushing injury of ankle — (Use additional code to identify any associated injuries: 800-829, 850.0-854.1, 860.0-869.1)
- **928.3** Crushing injury of toe(s) — (Use additional code to identify any associated injuries: 800-829, 850.0-854.1, 860.0-869.1)
- **928.8** Crushing injury of multiple sites of lower limb — (Use additional code to identify any associated injuries: 800-829, 850.0-854.1, 860.0-869.1)
- **928.9** Crushing injury of unspecified site of lower limb — (Use additional code to identify any associated injuries: 800-829, 850.0-854.1, 860.0-869.1)

929 Crushing injury of multiple and unspecified sites
AHA: Q2, 1993, 7; Q4, 2003, 77

- **929.0** Crushing injury of multiple sites, not elsewhere classified — (Use additional code to identify any associated injuries: 800-829, 850.0-854.1, 860.0-869.1)
- **929.9** Crushing injury of unspecified site — (Use additional code to identify any associated injuries: 800-829, 850.0-854.1, 860.0-869.1)

930–939 Effects of Foreign Body Entering Through Orifice

Instances of foreign bodies in orifices are one of the most common reasons for emergency department visits. Foreign bodies in the eye are particularly common and only a physician should remove a foreign body in the eye because of the danger of damaging the eye. If the foreign body is not removed, or is improperly removed, infection and permanent vision loss can result.

Children frequently aspirate foreign bodies into the right main bronchus. Often, the act is not observed, and the child may present with pneumonia or a lung abscess if the foreign body has been present for a long time. Hypoxia may result from objects obstructing breathing. Typically, the foreign body is located by use of the flexible bronchoscope and removed in the operating room with a rigid bronchoscope.

Ingested foreign bodies generally do not cause problems unless impacted. An impacted foreign body may erode through the walls of the organ and cause mediastinitis in the chest cavity or peritonitis in the abdominal cavity.

930   Foreign body on external eye
930.0   Foreign body in cornea
930.1   Foreign body in conjunctival sac
930.2   Foreign body in lacrimal punctum
930.8   Foreign body in other and combined sites on external eye
930.9   Foreign body in unspecified site on external eye

931   Foreign body in ear OK

932   Foreign body in nose OK

933   Foreign body in pharynx and larynx
933.0   Foreign body in pharynx
933.1   Foreign body in larynx

934   Foreign body in trachea, bronchus, and lung
934.0   Foreign body in trachea
934.1   Foreign body in main bronchus
934.8   Foreign body in other specified parts of trachea, bronchus, and lung
934.9   Foreign body in respiratory tree, unspecified

935   Foreign body in mouth, esophagus, and stomach
935.0   Foreign body in mouth
935.1   Foreign body in esophagus
935.2   Foreign body in stomach

936   Foreign body in intestine and colon OK

937   Foreign body in anus and rectum OK

938   Foreign body in digestive system, unspecified OK

939   Foreign body in genitourinary tract
939.0   Foreign body in bladder and urethra
939.1   Foreign body in uterus, any part
939.2   Foreign body in vulva and vagina
939.3   Foreign body in penis
939.9   Foreign body in unspecified site in genitourinary tract

940–949   Burns

Burns are classified by the degree of the burn (first degree through fourth degree) and the type of burn such as thermal, chemical, radiation, light, and electrical. The muscles, nerves, bones, blood vessels, respiratory system function, temperature regulation, joint function, fluid/electrolyte balance, physical appearance, and psychological functioning are all affected by a major burn injury.

The impact of burn injuries is magnified according to the amount of body surface burned. Children have much smaller thresholds for what is considered severe. Radiation burns are the most dangerous burns, though they may have a more benign appearance than a third degree thermal burn.

Category 948 classifies the extent of body surface affected by the burn and is useful as an adjunctive set of codes in assessing morbidity and mortality in burn centers. It may also be used when no further information is available, as in a patient who is briefly brought to an emergency department, stabilized, and transported to a specialty unit.

940   Burn confined to eye and adnexa
AHA: March-April, 1986, 9; Q4, 1988, 3; Q2, 1990, 7; Q4, 1994, 22
940.0   Chemical burn of eyelids and periocular area
940.1   Other burns of eyelids and periocular area
940.2   Alkaline chemical burn of cornea and conjunctival sac
940.3   Acid chemical burn of cornea and conjunctival sac
940.4   Other burn of cornea and conjunctival sac
940.5   Burn with resulting rupture and destruction of eyeball
940.9   Unspecified burn of eye and adnexa

Documentation Issues
For the correct ICD-9-CM code to be assigned, the medical record documentation must contain clear and concise information regarding the site of the burn, the degree of burn, if the burn is healed or nonhealed, any complications existing, and any late effect that may be present.

Coding Clarification
Abrasion Burn: Also indicated as "road rash," abrasion burns, if noted as deep, are not classified as burns, but as open wounds or abrasions. When the medical record documentation indicates that the patient is being treated for deep abrasion burns, indicate the appropriate open wound or abrasion code, not a burn code. If only superficial, code the abrasion burn as a superficial injury.

Infected Burn: When a patient is treated for infected burns, after the initial treatment of burns, two codes are necessary. Indicate the appropriate code for the burn (940-949) and the additional code 958.3 *Posttraumatic wound infection not elsewhere classified* to identify the complication of infection.

Late Effect of Burn: The treatment of current, unhealed burns is classified to categories 940-949.

The late effects of burns are coded to subcategories 906.5-906.9. The codes indicate healed burns resulting in sequelae, such as scarring. When coding the late effect of a burn, the appropriate code for describing the late effect itself is coded first, followed by the code identifying it as a late effect of another injury.

Because of the nature of burns, it is possible for a patient to have both healed and nonhealed burns during a single encounter. For this reason, it is appropriate to use a code for currently unhealed burns (940-949) and a code for late effects (906.5-906.9).

Multiple Burns: Patients are often treated with multiple burns. When coding multiple burns, assign separate codes for each burn site. Category 948 is used to classify burns according to the body surface involved. This code is used as an additional code for reporting purposes when there are third-degree burns involving 20 percent or more of the body surface or when further information is needed for evaluating burn mortality.

When there are burns of the same local site (identified by the three-digit category) but of varying degrees, use the fourth digit indicating the highest degree documented in the medical record.

Sequence first the code with the highest degree of burn in cases of multiple burns.

941 Burn of face, head, and neck
AHA: March-April, 1986, 9; Q4, 1988, 3; Q2, 1990, 7; Q4, 1994, 22

The following fifth-digit subclassification is for use with category 941:

0 face and head, unspecified site
1 ear [any part]
2 eye (with any other parts of face, head, and neck)
3 lip(s)
4 chin
5 nose (septum)
6 scalp [any part]
7 forehead and cheek
8 neck
9 multiple sites [except with eye] of face, head, and neck

941.0 Burn of face, head, and neck, unspecified degree
941.1 Erythema due to burn (first degree) of face, head, and neck
AHA: Q3, 2005, 10

941.2 Blisters with epidermal loss due to burn (second degree) of face, head, and neck
941.3 Full-thickness skin loss due to burn (third degree NOS) of face, head, and neck
941.4 Deep necrosis of underlying tissues due to burn (deep third degree) of face, head, and neck without mention of loss of a body part
941.5 Deep necrosis of underlying tissues due to burn (deep third degree) of face, head, and neck with loss of a body part

942 Burn of trunk
AHA: March-April, 1986, 9; Q4, 1988, 3; Q2, 1990, 7; Q4, 1994, 22

The following fifth-digit subclassification is for use with category 942:

0 trunk, unspecified site
1 breast
2 chest wall, excluding breast and nipple
3 abdominal wall
4 back [any part]
5 genitalia
9 other and multiple sites of trunk

942.0 Burn of trunk, unspecified degree
942.1 Erythema due to burn (first degree) of trunk
942.2 Blisters with epidermal loss due to burn (second degree) of trunk
942.3 Full-thickness skin loss due to burn (third degree NOS) of trunk
942.4 Deep necrosis of underlying tissues due to burn (deep third degree) of trunk without mention of loss of a body part
942.5 Deep necrosis of underlying tissues due to burn (deep third degree) of trunk with loss of a body part

943 Burn of upper limb, except wrist and hand
AHA: March-April, 1986, 9; Q4, 1988, 3; Q2, 1990, 7; Q4, 1994, 22

The following fifth-digit subclassification is for use with category 943:

0 upper limb, unspecified site
1 forearm
2 elbow
3 upper arm
4 axilla
5 shoulder
6 scapular region
9 multiple sites of upper limb, except wrist and hand

943.0 Burn of upper limb, except wrist and hand, unspecified degree
943.1 Erythema due to burn (first degree) of upper limb, except wrist and hand

Coders' Desk Reference for Diagnoses

- **943.2** ⌐sth Blisters with epidermal loss due to burn (second degree) of upper limb, except wrist and hand
- **943.3** ⌐sth Full-thickness skin loss due to burn (third degree NOS) of upper limb, except wrist and hand
- **943.4** ⌐sth Deep necrosis of underlying tissues due to burn (deep third degree) of upper limb, except wrist and hand, without mention of loss of a body part
- **943.5** ⌐sth Deep necrosis of underlying tissues due to burn (deep third degree) of upper limb, except wrist and hand, with loss of a body part

944 Burn of wrist(s) and hand(s)
AHA: March-April, 1986, 9; Q4, 1988, 3; Q2, 1990, 7; Q4, 1994, 22

The following fifth-digit subclassification is for use with category 944:

0 and, unspecified site
1 single digit [finger (nail)] other than the thumb
2 thumb (nail)
3 two or more digits, not including thumb
4 two or more digits including thumb
5 palm
6 back of hand
7 wrist
8 multiple sites of wrist(s) and hands

- **944.0** ⌐sth Burn of wrist(s) and hand(s), unspecified degree
- **944.1** ⌐sth Erythema due to burn (first degree) of wrist(s) and hand(s)
- **944.2** ⌐sth Blisters with epidermal loss due to burn (second degree) of wrist(s) and hand(s)
- **944.3** ⌐sth Full-thickness skin loss due to burn (third degree NOS) of wrist(s) and hand(s)
- **944.4** ⌐sth Deep necrosis of underlying tissues due to burn (deep third degree) of wrist(s) and hand(s), without mention of loss of a body part
- **944.5** ⌐sth Deep necrosis of underlying tissues due to burn (deep third degree) of wrist(s) and hand(s), with loss of a body part

945 Burn of lower limb(s)
AHA: March-April, 1986, 9; Q4, 1988, 3; Q2, 1990, 7; Q4, 1994, 22

The following fifth-digit subclassification is for use with category 945:

0 lower limb (leg), unspecified site
1 toe(s) (nail)
2 foot
3 ankle
4 lower leg
5 knee
6 thigh (any part)
9 multiple sites of lower limb(s)

- **945.0** ⌐sth Burn of lower limb(s), unspecified degree
- **945.1** ⌐sth Erythema due to burn (first degree) of lower limb(s)
- **945.2** ⌐sth Blisters with epidermal loss due to burn (second degree) of lower limb(s)
- **945.3** ⌐sth Full-thickness skin loss due to burn (third degree NOS) of lower limb(s)
- **945.4** ⌐sth Deep necrosis of underlying tissues due to burn (deep third degree) of lower limb(s) without mention of loss of a body part
- **945.5** ⌐sth Deep necrosis of underlying tissues due to burn (deep third degree) of lower limb(s) with loss of a body part

946 Burns of multiple specified sites
AHA: March-April, 1986, 9; Q4, 1988, 3; Q2, 1990, 7; Q4, 1994, 22

- **946.0** Burns of multiple specified sites, unspecified degree
- **946.1** Erythema due to burn (first degree) of multiple specified sites
- **946.2** Blisters with epidermal loss due to burn (second degree) of multiple specified sites
- **946.3** Full-thickness skin loss due to burn (third degree NOS) of multiple specified sites
- **946.4** Deep necrosis of underlying tissues due to burn (deep third degree) of multiple specified sites, without mention of loss of a body part
- **946.5** Deep necrosis of underlying tissues due to burn (deep third degree) of multiple specified sites, with loss of a body part

947 Burn of internal organs
AHA: March-April, 1986, 9; Q4, 1988, 3; Q2, 1990, 7; Q4, 1994, 22

- **947.0** Burn of mouth and pharynx
- **947.1** Burn of larynx, trachea, and lung
- **947.2** Burn of esophagus
- **947.3** Burn of gastrointestinal tract
- **947.4** Burn of vagina and uterus
- **947.8** Burn of other specified sites of internal organs
- **947.9** Burn of internal organs, unspecified site

948 Burns classified according to extent of body surface involved
AHA: Nov-Dec, 1984, 13; March-April, 1986, 9; Q4, 1988, 3; Q2, 1990, 7; Q4, 1994, 22

The rule of nines is a method for rapidly estimating the percent of total body surface area affected by a burn, which, in burn victims, is a strong predictor of the patient's prognosis. This metric helps emergency clinicians to decide whether a patient needs to be transferred to a regional burn center for specialized care and helps in estimating the amount of fluid replacement the patient will need to replace losses through the burned area. The rule of nines derives its name from the fact that an adult body may be divided into anatomic regions that have surface area percentages that are all multiples of 9 percent. According to this system, the head and each limb each account for 9 percent of the body surface area

Injury and Poisoning

for a total of 45 percent when added together (two legs, two arms, and the head). The genital area accounts for 1 percent, and the back and front of the torso each account for 18 percent of the body surface area.

The following fifth-digit subclassification is for use with category 948 to indicate the percent of body surface with third degree burn; valid digits are in [brackets] under each code:

0   less than 10 percent or unspecified
1   10-19%
2   20-29%
3   30-39%
4   40-49%
5   50-59%
6   60-69%
7   70-79%
8   80-89%
9   90% or more of body surface

948.0 [✓5th] Burn (any degree) involving less than 10% of body surface
948.1 [✓5th] Burn (any degree) involving 10-19% of body surface
948.2 [✓5th] Burn (any degree) involving 20-29% of body surface
948.3 [✓5th] Burn (any degree) involving 30-39% of body surface
948.4 [✓5th] Burn (any degree) involving 40-49% of body surface
948.5 [✓5th] Burn (any degree) involving 50-59% of body surface
948.6 [✓5th] Burn (any degree) involving 60-69% of body surface
948.7 [✓5th] Burn (any degree) involving 70-79% of body surface
948.8 [✓5th] Burn (any degree) involving 80-89% of body surface
948.9 [✓5th] Burn (any degree) involving 90% or more of body surface

949 Burn, unspecified site
AHA: March-April, 1986, 9; Q4, 1994, 22

949.0   Burn of unspecified site, unspecified degree
949.1   Erythema due to burn (first degree), unspecified site
949.2   Blisters with epidermal loss due to burn (second degree), unspecified site
949.3   Full-thickness skin loss due to burn (third degree NOS), unspecified site
949.4   Deep necrosis of underlying tissue due to burn (deep third degree), unspecified site without mention of loss of body part
949.5   Deep necrosis of underlying tissues due to burn (deep third degree, unspecified site with loss of body part

950–957   Injury to Nerves and Spinal Cord

The body's nerves report to the central nervous system (CNS), which is composed of the brain and the spinal cord. Twelve pairs of cranial nerves originate in the brain, and 31 pairs of spinal nerves emanate from the spinal cord, developing major branches and associated complexes known as peripheral nerves. Every nerve has two roots: sensory and motor. The anatomical arrangement of the spinal nerve roots places the motor root anteriorly and the sensory root posteriorly.

Cranial Nerves	Impairment by Injury to Motor Root
1st - Olfactory	Loss of smell
2nd - Optic	Traumatic blindness
3rd - Oculomotor	Ptosis of eyelid, double vision
4th - Trochlear	Unnatural rotation of eyeball, double vision
5th - Trigeminal	Eccentric jaw alignment, chewing
6th - Abducens	Unnatural rotation of eyeball (outwards); double vision
7th - Facial	Inability to move facial muscles of expression and animation
8th - Vestibulocochlear	Traumatic deafness; loss of balance
9th - Glossopharyngeal	Loss of taste; swallowing difficulty
10th - Vagus	Disturbance of innervation of heart, lungs, digestive organs
11th - Spinal accessory	Inability to rotate head
12th - Hypoglossopharyngeal	Loss of tongue mobility , thick speech or garbled speech

The table above lists impairments due to injury to specific cranial nerves.

If a nerve is transected, expert and expeditious microsurgery is no guarantee that full functioning will return. Regeneration can lead to appropriate motor and sensory impulses or an aberrant response may later be manifest, such as crying crocodile tears involuntarily when sensing the smell of food.

950 Injury to optic nerve and pathways
950.0	Optic nerve injury
950.1	Injury to optic chiasm
950.2	Injury to optic pathways
950.3	Injury to visual cortex
950.9	Injury to unspecified optic nerve and pathways

951 Injury to other cranial nerve(s)
951.0	Injury to oculomotor nerve
951.1	Injury to trochlear nerve
951.2	Injury to trigeminal nerve
951.3	Injury to abducens nerve
951.4	Injury to facial nerve
951.5	Injury to acoustic nerve
951.6	Injury to accessory nerve
951.7	Injury to hypoglossal nerve
951.8	Injury to other specified cranial nerves
951.9	Injury to unspecified cranial nerve

952 Spinal cord injury without evidence of spinal bone injury

Refer to category 806 for comprehensive descriptions.

952.00	C1-C4 level spinal cord injury, unspecified
952.01	C1-C4 level with complete lesion of spinal cord
952.02	C1-C4 level with anterior cord syndrome
952.03	C1-C4 level with central cord syndrome
952.04	C1-C4 level with other specified spinal cord injury
952.05	C5-C7 level spinal cord injury, unspecified
952.06	C5-C7 level with complete lesion of spinal cord
952.07	C5-C7 level with anterior cord syndrome
952.08	C5-C7 level with central cord syndrome
952.09	C5-C7 level with other specified spinal cord injury
952.10	T1-T6 level spinal cord injury, unspecified
952.11	T1-T6 level with complete lesion of spinal cord
952.12	T1-T6 level with anterior cord syndrome
952.13	T1-T6 level with central cord syndrome
952.14	T1-T6 level with other specified spinal cord injury
952.15	T7-T12 level spinal cord injury, unspecified
952.16	T7-T12 level with complete lesion of spinal cord
952.17	T7-T12 level with anterior cord syndrome
952.18	T7-T12 level with central cord syndrome
952.19	T7-T12 level with other specified spinal cord injury
952.2	Lumbar spinal cord injury without spinal bone injury
952.3	Sacral spinal cord injury without spinal bone injury
952.4	Cauda equina spinal cord injury without spinal bone injury
952.8	Multiple sites of spinal cord injury without spinal bone injury
952.9	Unspecified site of spinal cord injury without spinal bone injury

953–957 Injury to Nerve Roots, Peripheral, and Superficial Nerves

A plexus or ganglion is a bundle of nerves that serves a particular region of the body. A plexus lies relatively deep in the body as opposed to superficial nerves, which are close to the surface of the skin.

Sympathetic nerves are under the conscious control of the body, whereas parasympathetic nerves are considered to be involuntary, allowing the body to carry on without distraction by routine functions such as breathing, heart beating, digesting, and staying oriented in space. These parasympathetic activities are considered the duties of the autonomic nervous system.

953 Injury to nerve roots and spinal plexus
953.0	Injury to cervical nerve root
953.1	Injury to dorsal nerve root
953.2	Injury to lumbar nerve root
953.3	Injury to sacral nerve root
953.4	Injury to brachial plexus
953.5	Injury to lumbosacral plexus
953.8	Injury to multiple sites of nerve roots and spinal plexus
953.9	Injury to unspecified site of nerve roots and spinal plexus

954 Injury to other nerve(s) of trunk, excluding shoulder and pelvic girdles
954.0	Injury to cervical sympathetic nerve, excluding shoulder and pelvic girdles
954.1	Injury to other sympathetic nerve, excluding shoulder and pelvic girdles
954.8	Injury to other specified nerve(s) of trunk, excluding shoulder and pelvic girdles
954.9	Injury to unspecified nerve of trunk, excluding shoulder and pelvic girdles

955 Injury to peripheral nerve(s) of shoulder girdle and upper limb
955.0	Injury to axillary nerve
955.1	Injury to median nerve
955.2	Injury to ulnar nerve
955.3	Injury to radial nerve
955.4	Injury to musculocutaneous nerve
955.5	Injury to cutaneous sensory nerve, upper limb
955.6	Injury to digital nerve, upper limb
955.7	Injury to other specified nerve(s) of shoulder girdle and upper limb
955.8	Injury to multiple nerves of shoulder girdle and upper limb
955.9	Injury to unspecified nerve of shoulder girdle and upper limb

956 Injury to peripheral nerve(s) of pelvic girdle and lower limb

- 956.0 Injury to sciatic nerve
- 956.1 Injury to femoral nerve
- 956.2 Injury to posterior tibial nerve
- 956.3 Injury to peroneal nerve
- 956.4 Injury to cutaneous sensory nerve, lower limb
- 956.5 Injury to other specified nerve(s) of pelvic girdle and lower limb
- 956.8 Injury to multiple nerves of pelvic girdle and lower limb
- 956.9 Injury to unspecified nerve of pelvic girdle and lower limb

957 Injury to other and unspecified nerves

- 957.0 Injury to superficial nerves of head and neck
- 957.1 Injury to other specified nerve(s)
- 957.8 Injury to multiple nerves in several parts
- 957.9 Injury to nerves, unspecified site

958–959 Certain Traumatic Complications and Unspecified Injuries

A potentially fatal air embolism, whether arterial or venous, may result from a penetrating and blunt chest trauma or from blast injuries. Signs are sudden cardiovascular collapse, air bubbles in arterial blood samples, air bubbles in retinal and coronary arteries, and frothy blood coming from a chest wound. Treatment must commence immediately.

A fat embolism is typically associated with fracture of one of the long bones, especially the femur. Children are vulnerable to throwing multiple fat emboli if subjected to blunt trauma such as in child abuse situations.

Secondary hemorrhage is usually arterial and most often associated with sepsis arising from traumatized tissues that have been repaired. Slipping of a ligature on repaired vessels is the second most frequent cause for secondary hemorrhage.

Posttraumatic wound infection, NEC, includes injuries such as an infected, non-healing burn.

Traumatic shock sets in when the heart fails to deliver oxygenated blood and other nutrients to the body, usually because of a high rate of blood loss. The shock triggers other organ failure, with the kidney among the first affected. Blood volume must be restored as soon as possible to prevent the appearance of shock and its sequelae. Traumatic anuria runs a mortality rate of 60 percent.

Volkmann's ischemic contracture can appear in either the hand or the foot. In the hand, constriction of the radial artery produces the characteristic pronation and flexion. In the foot, a tibial fracture leading to an embolus or thrombus is more likely to be the causative agent.

Traumatic subcutaneous emphysema is tissue rupture that allows gas bubbles to form beneath the skin, a result of a high-pressure injury.

Compartment syndrome is an early complication of trauma, resulting from compression of nerves and tendons. Pain is extreme and is not easily relieved. Any compressive agent such as a cast or splint is immediately removed, though if removal is ineffective, the patient is surgically decompressed. Delayed diagnosis can result in permanent nerve injury and loss of muscle function; this can occur after 12 to 24 hours of compression. In the most severe cases, amputation may be required.

958 Certain early complications of trauma

- 958.0 Air embolism as an early complication of trauma
- 958.1 Fat embolism as an early complication of trauma
- 958.2 Secondary and recurrent hemorrhage as an early complication of trauma
- 958.3 Posttraumatic wound infection not elsewhere classified

Coding Clarification
Code 958.3 excludes infected open wounds that should be coded to complicated open wound of the site.

958 Certain early complications of trauma

- 958.4 Traumatic shock
- 958.5 Traumatic anuria
- 958.6 Volkmann's ischemic contracture
- 958.7 Traumatic subcutaneous emphysema
- 958.8 Other early complications of trauma
- 958.90 Compartment syndrome, unspecified
- 958.91 Traumatic compartment syndrome of upper extremity — *arm, forearm, shoulder, wrist, hand, fingers*
- 958.92 Traumatic compartment syndrome of lower extremity — *hip, buttock, thigh, leg, foot, toes*
- 958.93 Traumatic compartment syndrome of abdomen
- 958.99 Traumatic compartment syndrome of other sites

Coding Clarification
For nontraumatic compartment syndrome, see subcategory 729.7.

959 Injury, other and unspecified

- 959.01 Head injury, unspecified
- 959.09 Injury of face and neck, other and unspecified
- 959.11 Other injury of chest wall
- 959.12 Other injury of abdomen

959.13	Other injury, Fracture of corpus cavernosum penis — *a break in the spongy body of the penis; columns of erectile tissue forming the dorsum and the sides of the penis*	
959.14	Other injury of external genitals	
959.19	Other injury of other sites of trunk	
959.2	Injury, other and unspecified, shoulder and upper arm	
959.3	Injury, other and unspecified, elbow, forearm, and wrist	
959.4	Injury, other and unspecified, hand, except finger	
959.5	Injury, other and unspecified, finger	
959.6	Injury, other and unspecified, hip and thigh	
959.7	Injury, other and unspecified, knee, leg, ankle, and foot	
959.8	Injury, other and unspecified, other specified sites, including multiple	
959.9	Injury, other and unspecified, unspecified site	

960–979 Poisoning by Drugs, Medicinal and Biological Substances

Poisons are chemicals that cause illness, injury, or death when taken in very small quantities. The legal definition of a poison is a chemical that takes less than 50 mg per kilogram of body weight to kill 50 percent of the victims exposed (e.g., about 3/4 of a teaspoon for the average adult and about 1/8 of a teaspoon for a 2-year-old). Symptoms displayed and the systemic effect differ with the type of poison ingested.

Poisoning by drugs, medicinal, and biological substances is the major cause of childhood accidents in the home and can occur by many routes, including oral ingestion, inhalation, dermal absorption, and ocular instillation. Sources of poisoning for children and adults include:

- Acetaminophen overdose, which is rarely fatal. Symptoms are usually mild though prolonged abnormal liver function test results can occur.

- Ingestion of strong acids and alkalis (e.g.., drain and toilet bowl cleaners), which cause burns and damage tissues. Liquid preparations are often more dangerous since they are more often swallowed than the solid preparations and, thus, affect the entire esophagus and stomach. Pain is immediate in severe cases. Initially, the patient may drool, and there may be swelling at the burned areas. The airway may become obstructed. Respiration is shallow and shock is common. Patients who survive the initial poisoning may die of secondary infections, or the esophagus or stomach may perforate after a week or more.

- Exposure to methyl salicylate, which is found in liniments and in solutions used in hot vaporizers and is potentially lethal. The early symptoms are nausea and vomiting, tinnitus, hyperactivity, hyperthermia, and seizures. The central nervous system becomes depressed, followed by lethargy, respiratory failure, and collapse.

Hyperbaric oxygen (HBO) therapy is an accepted form of treatment for a number of serious illnesses including carbon monoxide poisoning. When carbon monoxide is inhaled, the CO combines with the hemoglobin to form carboxyhemoglobin or COHb. The CO displaces the oxygen on hemoglobin and the strong COHb bond makes it difficult for the body to eliminate CO buildups from the bloodstream. Carbon monoxide can poison slowly over a period of several hours, even in low concentrations. Sensitive organs such as the brain, heart, and lungs suffer the most from a lack of oxygen. In HBO therapy, a patient receives pure oxygen by mask, respiratory hood, tent, or endotracheal tube while in a hyperbaric chamber pressurized from two to three atmospheres absolute. HBO accelerates the process to halt carbon monoxide binding to hemoglobin; extra oxygen dissolved in plasma at high oxygen pressure may preserve tissue oxygenation even with lethal levels of carboxyhemoglobin and helps to minimize brain damage that at times accompanies or follows severe poisoning.

960   Poisoning by antibiotics
AHA: Q2, 1990, 11

960.0	Poisoning by penicillins — (Use additional code to specify the effects of the poisoning)
960.1	Poisoning by antifungal antibiotics — (Use additional code to specify the effects of the poisoning)
960.2	Poisoning by chloramphenicol group — (Use additional code to specify the effects of the poisoning)
960.3	Poisoning by erythromycin and other macrolides — (Use additional code to specify the effects of the poisoning)
960.4	Poisoning by tetracycline group — (Use additional code to specify the effects of the poisoning)
960.5	Poisoning of cephalosporin group — (Use additional code to specify the effects of the poisoning)
960.6	Poisoning of antimycobacterial antibiotics — (Use additional code to specify the effects of the poisoning)
960.7	Poisoning by antineoplastic antibiotics — (Use additional code to specify the effects of the poisoning)
960.8	Poisoning by other specified antibiotics — (Use additional code to specify the effects of the poisoning)

Injury and Poisoning

960.9	Poisoning by unspecified antibiotic — (Use additional code to specify the effects of the poisoning)	962.9	Poisoning by other and unspecified hormones and synthetic substitutes — (Use additional code to specify the effects of the poisoning)

961 Poisoning by other anti-infectives
AHA: Q2, 1990, 11

- **961.0** Poisoning by sulfonamides — (Use additional code to specify the effects of the poisoning)
- **961.1** Poisoning by arsenical anti-infectives — (Use additional code to specify the effects of the poisoning)
- **961.2** Poisoning by heavy metal anti-infectives — (Use additional code to specify the effects of the poisoning)
- **961.3** Poisoning by quinoline and hydroxyquinoline derivatives — (Use additional code to specify the effects of the poisoning)
- **961.4** Poisoning by antimalarials and drugs acting on other blood protozoa — (Use additional code to specify the effects of the poisoning)
- **961.5** Poisoning by other antiprotozoal drugs — (Use additional code to specify the effects of the poisoning)
- **961.6** Poisoning by anthelmintics — (Use additional code to specify the effects of the poisoning)
- **961.7** Poisoning by antiviral drugs — (Use additional code to specify the effects of the poisoning)
- **961.8** Poisoning by other antimycobacterial drugs — (Use additional code to specify the effects of the poisoning)
- **961.9** Poisoning by other and unspecified anti-infectives — (Use additional code to specify the effects of the poisoning)

962 Poisoning by hormones and synthetic substitutes
AHA: Q2, 1990, 11

- **962.0** Poisoning by adrenal cortical steroids — (Use additional code to specify the effects of the poisoning)
- **962.1** Poisoning by androgens and anabolic congeners — (Use additional code to specify the effects of the poisoning)
- **962.2** Poisoning by ovarian hormones and synthetic substitutes — (Use additional code to specify the effects of the poisoning)
- **962.3** Poisoning by insulins and antidiabetic agents — (Use additional code to specify the effects of the poisoning)
- **962.4** Poisoning by anterior pituitary hormones — (Use additional code to specify the effects of the poisoning)
- **962.5** Poisoning by posterior pituitary hormones — (Use additional code to specify the effects of the poisoning)
- **962.6** Poisoning by parathyroid and parathyroid derivatives — (Use additional code to specify the effects of the poisoning)
- **962.7** Poisoning by thyroid and thyroid derivatives — (Use additional code to specify the effects of the poisoning)
- **962.8** Poisoning by antithyroid agents — (Use additional code to specify the effects of the poisoning)

963 Poisoning by primarily systemic agents
AHA: Q2, 1990, 11

- **963.0** Poisoning by antiallergic and antiemetic drugs — (Use additional code to specify the effects of the poisoning)
- **963.1** Poisoning by antineoplastic and immunosuppressive drugs — (Use additional code to specify the effects of the poisoning)
- **963.2** Poisoning by acidifying agents — (Use additional code to specify the effects of the poisoning)
- **963.3** Poisoning by alkalizing agents — (Use additional code to specify the effects of the poisoning)
- **963.4** Poisoning by enzymes, not elsewhere classified — (Use additional code to specify the effects of the poisoning)
- **963.5** Poisoning by vitamins, not elsewhere classified — (Use additional code to specify the effects of the poisoning)
- **963.8** Poisoning by other specified systemic agents — (Use additional code to specify the effects of the poisoning)
- **963.9** Poisoning by unspecified systemic agent — (Use additional code to specify the effects of the poisoning)

964 Poisoning by agents primarily affecting blood constituents
AHA: Q2, 1990, 11

- **964.0** Poisoning by iron and its compounds — (Use additional code to specify the effects of the poisoning)
- **964.1** Poisoning by liver preparations and other antianemic agents — (Use additional code to specify the effects of the poisoning)
- **964.2** Poisoning by anticoagulants — (Use additional code to specify the effects of the poisoning)
- **964.3** Poisoning by vitamin K (phytonadione) — (Use additional code to specify the effects of the poisoning)
- **964.4** Poisoning by fibrinolysis-affecting drugs — (Use additional code to specify the effects of the poisoning)
- **964.5** Poisoning by anticoagulant antagonists and other coagulants — (Use additional code to specify the effects of the poisoning)
- **964.6** Poisoning by gamma globulin — (Use additional code to specify the effects of the poisoning)
- **964.7** Poisoning by natural blood and blood products — (Use additional code to specify the effects of the poisoning)
- **964.8** Poisoning by other specified agents affecting blood constituents — (Use additional code to specify the effects of the poisoning)
- **964.9** Poisoning by unspecified agent affecting blood constituents — (Use additional code to specify the effects of the poisoning)

965 Poisoning by analgesics, antipyretics, and antirheumatics
AHA: Q2, 1990, 11

- **965.00** Poisoning by opium (alkaloids), unspecified — (Use additional code to specify the effects of the poisoning)
- **965.01** Poisoning by heroin — (Use additional code to specify the effects of the poisoning)
- **965.02** Poisoning by methadone — (Use additional code to specify the effects of the poisoning)
- **965.09** Poisoning by opiates and related narcotics, other — (Use additional code to specify the effects of the poisoning)
- **965.1** Poisoning by salicylates — (Use additional code to specify the effects of the poisoning)
- **965.4** Poisoning by aromatic analgesics, not elsewhere classified — (Use additional code to specify the effects of the poisoning)
- **965.5** Poisoning by pyrazole derivatives — (Use additional code to specify the effects of the poisoning)
- **965.61** Poisoning by propionic acid derivatives — (Use additional code to specify the effects of the poisoning)
- **965.69** Poisoning by other antirheumatics — (Use additional code to specify the effects of the poisoning)
- **965.7** Poisoning by other non-narcotic analgesics — (Use additional code to specify the effects of the poisoning)
- **965.8** Poisoning by other specified analgesics and antipyretics — (Use additional code to specify the effects of the poisoning)
- **965.9** Poisoning by unspecified analgesic and antipyretic — (Use additional code to specify the effects of the poisoning)

966 Poisoning by anticonvulsants and anti-Parkinsonism drugs
AHA: Q2, 1990, 11

- **966.0** Poisoning by oxazolidine derivatives — (Use additional code to specify the effects of the poisoning)
- **966.1** Poisoning by hydantoin derivatives — (Use additional code to specify the effects of the poisoning)
- **966.2** Poisoning by succinimides — (Use additional code to specify the effects of the poisoning)
- **966.3** Poisoning by other and unspecified anticonvulsants — (Use additional code to specify the effects of the poisoning)
- **966.4** Poisoning by anti-Parkinsonism drugs — (Use additional code to specify the effects of the poisoning)

967 Poisoning by sedatives and hypnotics
AHA: Q2, 1990, 11

- **967.0** Poisoning by barbiturates — (Use additional code to specify the effects of the poisoning)
- **967.1** Poisoning by chloral hydrate group — (Use additional code to specify the effects of the poisoning)
- **967.2** Poisoning by paraldehyde — (Use additional code to specify the effects of the poisoning)
- **967.3** Poisoning by bromine compounds — (Use additional code to specify the effects of the poisoning)
- **967.4** Poisoning by methaqualone compounds — (Use additional code to specify the effects of the poisoning)
- **967.5** Poisoning by glutethimide group — (Use additional code to specify the effects of the poisoning)
- **967.6** Poisoning by mixed sedatives, not elsewhere classified — (Use additional code to specify the effects of the poisoning)
- **967.8** Poisoning by other sedatives and hypnotics — (Use additional code to specify the effects of the poisoning)
- **967.9** Poisoning by unspecified sedative or hypnotic — (Use additional code to specify the effects of the poisoning)

968 Poisoning by other central nervous system depressants and anesthetics
AHA: Q2, 1990, 11

- **968.0** Poisoning by central nervous system muscle-tone depressants — (Use additional code to specify the effects of the poisoning)
- **968.1** Poisoning by halothane — (Use additional code to specify the effects of the poisoning)
- **968.2** Poisoning by other gaseous anesthetics — (Use additional code to specify the effects of the poisoning)
- **968.3** Poisoning by intravenous anesthetics — (Use additional code to specify the effects of the poisoning)
- **968.4** Poisoning by other and unspecified general anesthetics — (Use additional code to specify the effects of the poisoning)
- **968.5** Poisoning by surface (topical) and infiltration anesthetics — (Use additional code to specify the effects of the poisoning)
- **968.6** Poisoning by peripheral nerve- and plexus-blocking anesthetics — (Use additional code to specify the effects of the poisoning)
- **968.7** Poisoning by spinal anesthetics — (Use additional code to specify the effects of the poisoning)
- **968.9** Poisoning by other and unspecified local anesthetics — (Use additional code to specify the effects of the poisoning)

969 Poisoning by psychotropic agents
AHA: Q2, 1990, 11

- **969.0** Poisoning by antidepressants — (Use additional code to specify the effects of the poisoning)
- **969.1** Poisoning by phenothiazine-based tranquilizers — (Use additional code to specify the effects of the poisoning)
- **969.2** Poisoning by butyrophenone-based tranquilizers — (Use additional code to specify the effects of the poisoning)
- **969.3** Poisoning by other antipsychotics, neuroleptics, and major tranquilizers — (Use additional code to specify the effects of the poisoning)

969.4	Poisoning by benzodiazepine-based tranquilizers — (Use additional code to specify the effects of the poisoning)			

969.4 Poisoning by benzodiazepine-based tranquilizers — (Use additional code to specify the effects of the poisoning)
969.5 Poisoning by other tranquilizers — (Use additional code to specify the effects of the poisoning)
969.6 Poisoning by psychodysleptics (hallucinogens) — (Use additional code to specify the effects of the poisoning)
969.7 Poisoning by psychostimulants — (Use additional code to specify the effects of the poisoning)
969.8 Poisoning by other specified psychotropic agents — (Use additional code to specify the effects of the poisoning)
969.9 Poisoning by unspecified psychotropic agent — (Use additional code to specify the effects of the poisoning)

Coding Scenario
A patient is seen in the emergency department after ingesting an unknown amount of antidepressants in a suicide attempt. She is in a comatose state.

Code assignment: 969.0 *Poisoning by psychotropic agents, antidepressants*, 780.01 *Alteration of consciousness, coma*, and E950.3 *Suicide and self-inflicted poisoning by solid or liquid substances, tranquilizers and other psychotropic agents*

A 3-year-old girl is seen in the emergency department after ingesting a single tablet of Amitriptyline found on the floor. She appears sleepy but in no distress and no physiological abnormal findings are noted. She will be observed for the next 24-hours to determine that there are no ill effects.

Code assignment: 969.0 *Poisoning by psychotropic agents, antidepressants*, 780.7 *Malaise and fatigue*, and E854.0 *Accidental poisoning by other psychotropic agents, antidepressants*

970 Poisoning by central nervous system stimulants
AHA: Q2, 1990, 11

970.0 Poisoning by analeptics — (Use additional code to specify the effects of the poisoning)
970.1 Poisoning by opiate antagonists — (Use additional code to specify the effects of the poisoning)
970.8 Poisoning by other specified central nervous system stimulants — (Use additional code to specify the effects of the poisoning)
AHA: Q1, 2005, 6
970.9 Poisoning by unspecified central nervous system stimulant — (Use additional code to specify the effects of the poisoning)

971 Poisoning by drugs primarily affecting the autonomic nervous system
AHA: Q2, 1990, 11

971.0 Poisoning by parasympathomimetics (cholinergics) — (Use additional code to specify the effects of the poisoning)
971.1 Poisoning by parasympatholytics (anticholinergics and antimuscarinics) and spasmolytics — (Use additional code to specify the effects of the poisoning)
971.2 Poisoning by sympathomimetics (adrenergics) — (Use additional code to specify the effects of the poisoning)
971.3 Poisoning by sympatholytics (antiadrenergics) — (Use additional code to specify the effects of the poisoning)
971.9 Poisoning by unspecified drug primarily affecting autonomic nervous system — (Use additional code to specify the effects of the poisoning)

972 Poisoning by agents primarily affecting the cardiovascular system
AHA: Q2, 1990, 11

972.0 Poisoning by cardiac rhythm regulators — (Use additional code to specify the effects of the poisoning)
972.1 Poisoning by cardiotonic glycosides and drugs of similar action — (Use additional code to specify the effects of the poisoning)
972.2 Poisoning by antilipemic and antiarteriosclerotic drugs — (Use additional code to specify the effects of the poisoning)
972.3 Poisoning by ganglion-blocking agents — (Use additional code to specify the effects of the poisoning)
972.4 Poisoning by coronary vasodilators — (Use additional code to specify the effects of the poisoning)
972.5 Poisoning by other vasodilators — (Use additional code to specify the effects of the poisoning)
972.6 Poisoning by other antihypertensive agents — (Use additional code to specify the effects of the poisoning)
972.7 Poisoning by antivaricose drugs, including sclerosing agents — (Use additional code to specify the effects of the poisoning)
972.8 Poisoning by capillary-active drugs — (Use additional code to specify the effects of the poisoning)
972.9 Poisoning by other and unspecified agents primarily affecting the cardiovascular system — (Use additional code to specify the effects of the poisoning)

973 Poisoning by agents primarily affecting the gastrointestinal system
AHA: Q2, 1990, 11

973.0 Poisoning by antacids and antigastric secretion drugs — (Use additional code to specify the effects of the poisoning)

Code	Description
973.1	Poisoning by irritant cathartics — (Use additional code to specify the effects of the poisoning)
973.2	Poisoning by emollient cathartics — (Use additional code to specify the effects of the poisoning)
973.3	Poisoning by other cathartics, including intestinal atonia drugs — (Use additional code to specify the effects of the poisoning)
973.4	Poisoning by digestants — (Use additional code to specify the effects of the poisoning)
973.5	Poisoning by antidiarrheal drugs — (Use additional code to specify the effects of the poisoning)
973.6	Poisoning by emetics — (Use additional code to specify the effects of the poisoning)
973.8	Poisoning by other specified agents primarily affecting the gastrointestinal system — (Use additional code to specify the effects of the poisoning)
973.9	Poisoning by unspecified agent primarily affecting the gastrointestinal system — (Use additional code to specify the effects of the poisoning)

974 Poisoning by water, mineral, and uric acid metabolism drugs
AHA: Q2, 1990, 11

Code	Description
974.0	Poisoning by mercurial diuretics — (Use additional code to specify the effects of the poisoning)
974.1	Poisoning by purine derivative diuretics — (Use additional code to specify the effects of the poisoning)
974.2	Poisoning by carbonic acid anhydrase inhibitors — (Use additional code to specify the effects of the poisoning)
974.3	Poisoning by saluretics — (Use additional code to specify the effects of the poisoning)
974.4	Poisoning by other diuretics — (Use additional code to specify the effects of the poisoning)
974.5	Poisoning by electrolytic, caloric, and water-balance agents — (Use additional code to specify the effects of the poisoning)
974.6	Poisoning by other mineral salts, not elsewhere classified — (Use additional code to specify the effects of the poisoning)
974.7	Poisoning by uric acid metabolism drugs — (Use additional code to specify the effects of the poisoning)

975 Poisoning by agents primarily acting on the smooth and skeletal muscles and respiratory system
AHA: Q2, 1990, 11

Code	Description
975.0	Poisoning by oxytocic agents — (Use additional code to specify the effects of the poisoning)
975.1	Poisoning by smooth muscle relaxants — (Use additional code to specify the effects of the poisoning)
975.2	Poisoning by skeletal muscle relaxants — (Use additional code to specify the effects of the poisoning)
975.3	Poisoning by other and unspecified drugs acting on muscles — (Use additional code to specify the effects of the poisoning)
975.4	Poisoning by antitussives — (Use additional code to specify the effects of the poisoning)
975.5	Poisoning by expectorants — (Use additional code to specify the effects of the poisoning)
975.6	Poisoning by anti-common cold drugs — (Use additional code to specify the effects of the poisoning)
975.7	Poisoning by antiasthmatics — (Use additional code to specify the effects of the poisoning)
975.8	Poisoning by other and unspecified respiratory drugs — (Use additional code to specify the effects of the poisoning)

976 Poisoning by agents primarily affecting skin and mucous membrane, ophthalmological, otorhinolaryngological, and dental drugs
AHA: Q2, 1990, 11

Code	Description
976.0	Poisoning by local anti-infectives and anti-inflammatory drugs — (Use additional code to specify the effects of the poisoning)
976.1	Poisoning by antipruritics — (Use additional code to specify the effects of the poisoning)
976.2	Poisoning by local astringents and local detergents — (Use additional code to specify the effects of the poisoning)
976.3	Poisoning by emollients, demulcents, and protectants — (Use additional code to specify the effects of the poisoning)
976.4	Poisoning by keratolytics, keratoplastics, other hair treatment drugs and preparations — (Use additional code to specify the effects of the poisoning)
976.5	Poisoning by eye anti-infectives and other eye drugs — (Use additional code to specify the effects of the poisoning)
976.6	Poisoning by anti-infectives and other drugs and preparations for ear, nose, and throat — (Use additional code to specify the effects of the poisoning)
976.7	Poisoning by dental drugs topically applied — (Use additional code to specify the effects of the poisoning)
976.8	Poisoning by other agents primarily affecting skin and mucous membrane — (Use additional code to specify the effects of the poisoning)
976.9	Poisoning by unspecified agent primarily affecting skin and mucous membrane — (Use additional code to specify the effects of the poisoning)

977 Poisoning by other and unspecified drugs and medicinal substances
AHA: Q2, 1990, 11

Code	Description
977.0	Poisoning by dietetics — (Use additional code to specify the effects of the poisoning)
977.1	Poisoning by lipotropic drugs — (Use additional code to specify the effects of the poisoning)
977.2	Poisoning by antidotes and chelating agents, not elsewhere classified — (Use additional code to specify the effects of the poisoning)

977.3	Poisoning by alcohol deterrents — (Use additional code to specify the effects of the poisoning)		979.7	Poisoning by mixed viral-rickettsial and bacterial vaccines, except combinations with pertussis component — (Use additional code to specify the effects of the poisoning)
977.4	Poisoning by pharmaceutical excipients — (Use additional code to specify the effects of the poisoning)		979.9	Poisoning by other and unspecified vaccines and biological substances — (Use additional code to specify the effects of the poisoning)
977.8	Poisoning by other specified drugs and medicinal substances — (Use additional code to specify the effects of the poisoning)			
977.9	Poisoning by unspecified drug or medicinal substance — (Use additional code to specify the effects of the poisoning)			

978 Poisoning by bacterial vaccines
AHA: Q2, 1990, 11

978.0	Poisoning by bcg vaccine — (Use additional code to specify the effects of the poisoning)
978.1	Poisoning by typhoid and paratyphoid vaccine — (Use additional code to specify the effects of the poisoning)
978.2	Poisoning by cholera vaccine — (Use additional code to specify the effects of the poisoning)
978.3	Poisoning by plague vaccine — (Use additional code to specify the effects of the poisoning)
978.4	Poisoning by tetanus vaccine — (Use additional code to specify the effects of the poisoning)
978.5	Poisoning by diphtheria vaccine — (Use additional code to specify the effects of the poisoning)
978.6	Poisoning by pertussis vaccine, including combinations with pertussis component — (Use additional code to specify the effects of the poisoning)
978.8	Poisoning by other and unspecified bacterial vaccines — (Use additional code to specify the effects of the poisoning)
978.9	Poisoning by mixed bacterial vaccines, except combinations with pertussis component — (Use additional code to specify the effects of the poisoning)

979 Poisoning by other vaccines and biological substances
AHA: Q2, 1990, 11

979.0	Poisoning by smallpox vaccine — (Use additional code to specify the effects of the poisoning)
979.1	Poisoning by rabies vaccine — (Use additional code to specify the effects of the poisoning)
979.2	Poisoning by typhus vaccine — (Use additional code to specify the effects of the poisoning)
979.3	Poisoning by yellow fever vaccine — (Use additional code to specify the effects of the poisoning)
979.4	Poisoning by measles vaccine — (Use additional code to specify the effects of the poisoning)
979.5	Poisoning by poliomyelitis vaccine — (Use additional code to specify the effects of the poisoning)
979.6	Poisoning by other and unspecified viral and rickettsial vaccines — (Use additional code to specify the effects of the poisoning)

980–989 Toxic Effects of Substances Chiefly Nonmedicinal as to Source

The toxicity of a substance is due to its ability to damage or disrupt metabolism. An acutely toxic substance can cause damage as the result of a single or short-duration exposure. A chronically toxic substance causes damage after repeated or long-duration exposure or becomes evident only after a long latency period. Toxicity varies with the route of exposure and the effectiveness at which the material is absorbed. A chemical that enters the body in large quantities but is not easily absorbed is a much lower risk than one that is easily absorbed into the bloodstream.

Skin contact is the most common route of exposure but often the best barrier since the skin guards against the entry of most chemicals. Once a chemical passes through the skin (i.e., through a wound), it enters the bloodstream and is carried to all parts of the body.

Inhalation is the most dangerous route of entry because the lungs are ineffective barriers. Chemicals that pass the lung membrane are absorbed into the bloodstream and carried to all parts of the body. Absorption can be extremely rapid. The rate of absorption depends on the concentration of the toxic substance, its solubility in water, the depth of respiration, and the rate of blood circulation.

Ingested materials are absorbed into the bloodstream anywhere along the gastrointestinal tract. If the material cannot be absorbed, it will be eliminated from the body.

Toxins are not due to absorption of purified or fermented foodstuffs, nor are they absorbed from the colon in conditions of constipation. A toxic reaction can be similar to an allergic reaction but more severe. If the liver is functioning normally, it may allow a small amount of the toxic material to enter the body, but eliminate the rest. If the liver is not functioning normally, the substance may enter the body and cause a toxic chemical overload that may result in blood poisoning and death. Toxemia is a poisoned condition of the blood caused by the presence of toxic materials, usually bacterial but occasionally chemical or hormonal in nature.

As a general rule, the more known about the poisoning agent, the better the treatment plan and outcome. Poison Control Centers have been invaluable in supplying the health care professional with the exact composition of the thousands of poisonous substances. If the information is unknown, treatment must revolve around general supportive measures.

Treatment includes the use of corticosteroids and mannitol drips to minimize cerebral edema, dialysis to combat renal failure, hasten the excretion of the poison, alkalinization or acidification of the urine, and remove lipid soluble substances from the blood, hemoperfusion, and chelating agents.

980 Toxic effect of alcohol
- **980.0** Toxic effect of ethyl alcohol — (Use additional code to identify any associated condition: 291.4, 303.0, 305.0)
- **980.1** Toxic effect of methyl alcohol — (Use additional code to specify the nature of the toxic effect)
- **980.2** Toxic effect of isopropyl alcohol — (Use additional code to specify the nature of the toxic effect)
- **980.3** Toxic effect of fusel oil — (Use additional code to specify the nature of the toxic effect)
- **980.8** Toxic effect of other specified alcohols — (Use additional code to specify the nature of the toxic effect)
- **980.9** Toxic effect of unspecified alcohol — (Use additional code to specify the nature of the toxic effect)

981 Toxic effect of petroleum products ✓

982 Toxic effect of solvents other than petroleum-based
- **982.0** Toxic effect of benzene and homologues — (Use additional code to specify the nature of the toxic effect)
- **982.1** Toxic effect of carbon tetrachloride — (Use additional code to specify the nature of the toxic effect)
- **982.2** Toxic effect of carbon disulfide — (Use additional code to specify the nature of the toxic effect)
- **982.3** Toxic effect of other chlorinated hydrocarbon solvents — (Use additional code to specify the nature of the toxic effect)
- **982.4** Toxic effect of nitroglycol — (Use additional code to specify the nature of the toxic effect)
- **982.8** Toxic effect of other nonpetroleum-based solvents — (Use additional code to specify the nature of the toxic effect)

983 Toxic effect of corrosive aromatics, acids, and caustic alkalis
- **983.0** Toxic effect of corrosive aromatics — (Use additional code to specify the nature of the toxic effect)
- **983.1** Toxic effect of acids — (Use additional code to specify the nature of the toxic effect)
- **983.2** Toxic effect of caustic alkalis — (Use additional code to specify the nature of the toxic effect)
- **983.9** Toxic effect of caustic, unspecified — (Use additional code to specify the nature of the toxic effect)

984 Toxic effect of lead and its compounds (including fumes)
- **984.0** Toxic effect of inorganic lead compounds — (Use additional code to specify the nature of the toxic effect)
- **984.1** Toxic effect of organic lead compounds — (Use additional code to specify the nature of the toxic effect)
- **984.8** Toxic effect of other lead compounds — (Use additional code to specify the nature of the toxic effect)
- **984.9** Toxic effect of unspecified lead compound — (Use additional code to specify the nature of the toxic effect)

985 Toxic effect of other metals
- **985.0** Toxic effect of mercury and its compounds — (Use additional code to specify the nature of the toxic effect)
- **985.1** Toxic effect of arsenic and its compounds — (Use additional code to specify the nature of the toxic effect)
- **985.2** Toxic effect of manganese and its compounds — (Use additional code to specify the nature of the toxic effect)
- **985.3** Toxic effect of beryllium and its compounds — (Use additional code to specify the nature of the toxic effect)
- **985.4** Toxic effect of antimony and its compounds — (Use additional code to specify the nature of the toxic effect)
- **985.5** Toxic effect of cadmium and its compounds — (Use additional code to specify the nature of the toxic effect)
- **985.6** Toxic effect of chromium — (Use additional code to specify the nature of the toxic effect)
- **985.8** Toxic effect of other specified metals — (Use additional code to specify the nature of the toxic effect)
- **985.9** Toxic effect of unspecified metal — (Use additional code to specify the nature of the toxic effect)

986 Toxic effect of carbon monoxide ✓

987 Toxic effect of other gases, fumes, or vapors
- **987.0** Toxic effect of liquefied petroleum gases — (Use additional code to specify the nature of the toxic effect)

987.1	Toxic effect of other hydrocarbon gas — (Use additional code to specify the nature of the toxic effect)		989.4	Toxic effect of other pesticides, not elsewhere classified — (Use additional code to specify the nature of the toxic effect)
987.2	Toxic effect of nitrogen oxides — (Use additional code to specify the nature of the toxic effect)		989.5	Toxic effect of venom — (Use additional code to specify the nature of the toxic effect)
987.3	Toxic effect of sulfur dioxide — (Use additional code to specify the nature of the toxic effect)			
987.4	Toxic effect of freon — (Use additional code to specify the nature of the toxic effect)			
987.5	Toxic effect of lacrimogenic gas — (Use additional code to specify the nature of the toxic effect)			
987.6	Toxic effect of chlorine gas — (Use additional code to specify the nature of the toxic effect)			
987.7	Toxic effect of hydrocyanic acid gas — (Use additional code to specify the nature of the toxic effect)			
987.8	Toxic effect of other specified gases, fumes, or vapors — (Use additional code to specify the nature of the toxic effect)			
987.9	Toxic effect of unspecified gas, fume, or vapor — (Use additional code to specify the nature of the toxic effect)			

AHA: Q3, 2005, 10

988 Toxic effect of noxious substances eaten as food

988.0	Toxic effect of fish and shellfish — (Use additional code to specify the nature of the toxic effect)
988.1	Toxic effect of mushrooms — (Use additional code to specify the nature of the toxic effect)
988.2	Toxic effect of berries and other plants — (Use additional code to specify the nature of the toxic effect)
988.8	Toxic effect of other specified noxious substances — (Use additional code to specify the nature of the toxic effect)
988.9	Toxic effect of unspecified noxious substance — (Use additional code to specify the nature of the toxic effect)

Coding Clarification
Category 988 excludes spoiled food that causes illness (food poisoning). The mistletoe berry is an example of poisonous flora belonging in this category.

989 Toxic effect of other substances, chiefly nonmedicinal as to source

989.0	Toxic effect of hydrocyanic acid and cyanides — (Use additional code to specify the nature of the toxic effect)
989.1	Toxic effect of strychnine and salts — (Use additional code to specify the nature of the toxic effect)
989.2	Toxic effect of chlorinated hydrocarbons — (Use additional code to specify the nature of the toxic effect)
989.3	Toxic effect of organophosphate and carbamate — (Use additional code to specify the nature of the toxic effect)

Each of the 48 contiguous states in the United States harbor at least one species of venomous snake. The pit vipers (copperhead, cottonmouth, and rattlesnakes) and coral snakes are two venomous families widely spread in the United States. Approximately 8,000 of the estimated 45,000 annual snakebites in this country are by poisonous snakes. Snake venoms are rated on a lethality index, with the Mojave rattlesnake having the highest index of any North American snake. Pit viper bites are associated with pain, swelling, and edema. Ecchymosis is common, ranging from moderate to severe. The patient may hemorrhage from the gums and develop hematemesis, melena, and hematuria. The coral snake bite generally produces nerve conduction damage and CNS damage. Annual fatalities are fewer than 15, most of which can be attributed to rattlesnake venom.

Survival often depends on the time it takes until medical help. If the patient is more than 40 minutes from a hospital, an incision over the bite may be made and suction applied. Envenomation must be assessed whenever a patient presents at the medical center with a snake bite since about 20 to 30 percent of all pit viper bites do not involve venom injection, and about 50 percent from the same class as coral snakes does not involve venom injection. Protocol calls for treating snakebites without envenomation as puncture wounds. If envenomation does occur, the patient presents a complex poisoning picture. Depending on the type of snake, the patient may weaken several hours after the bite, experience difficulty salivating or speaking, or experience respiratory distress and cardiovascular failure in fatal cases.

Antivenom is needed in only 60 percent of pit viper bites. The young or elderly require antivenom for copperhead bites. Coral snake envenomation is not typically associated with pain or swelling and three vials of antivenom are routinely administered once envenomation by coral snake bite is determined.

Two lizards, the Gila monster and the beaded lizard, are poisonous. Treatment protocols are similar to those for pit viper bites, though there is no antivenom for these bites.

There are numerous venomous spider species in the United States. Most bites require only local care, although in cases of severe envenomation the victim must be hospitalized for supportive measures. Fatalities are few, with the greatest risk for children and the elderly.

989.6	Toxic effect of soaps and detergents — (Use additional code to specify the nature of the toxic effect)
989.7	Toxic effect of aflatoxin and other mycotoxin (food contaminants) — (Use additional code to specify the nature of the toxic effect)
989.81	Toxic effect of asbestos — (Use additional code to specify the nature of the toxic effect)
989.82	Toxic effect of latex — (Use additional code to specify the nature of the toxic effect)
989.83	Toxic effect of silicone — (Use additional code to specify the nature of the toxic effect)
989.84	Toxic effect of tobacco — (Use additional code to specify the nature of the toxic effect)
989.89	Toxic effect of other substances — (Use additional code to specify the nature of the toxic effect)
989.9	Toxic effect of unspecified substance, chiefly nonmedicinal as to source — (Use additional code to specify the nature of the toxic effect)

990–995 Other and Unspecified Effects of External Causes

990 Effects of radiation, unspecified

A substance emitting ionizing radiation is capable of creating radiation sickness. Acute radiation sickness is classified as cerebral, gastrointestinal, or hematopoietic. The cerebral syndrome is fatal within a few hours of exposure to a dose in an amount greater than 30 Gy. The gastrointestinal syndrome involves a dose of at least 4 Gy, with death occurring within two or three weeks. The hematopoietic syndrome is also fatal, with neutropenia the contributing cause of death due to lowered immune resistance. The dose is 2 to 10 Gy.

Recovery from a radiation accident depends on the size of the dose, the rate at which the dose is received, and the distribution of the dose over the body. While a large dose all at once over the entire body is fatal, the same dose administered therapeutically to a small area for a brief period of time may be repeated over time without fear of fatality. Therapeutic doses may cause radiation sickness, involving nausea, vomiting, and diarrhea with malaise and tachycardia. These symptoms decline spontaneously, over time.

991 Effects of reduced temperature

Accidental hypothermia results from conduction, convection, and radiation. Examples of conduction hypothermia are wet clothing and skin freezing upon metal contact. Convection injuries are from wind chill. The body core temperature can drop as low as 79° Fahrenheit. The rule is to resuscitate until the patient is warm. The extremities are at great risk of hypothermia, as well as the nose. They should be warm and dry at all times. While dry, cold injury such as frostbite can result in gangrene, the gangrene is usually superficial, with a large reservoir of intact skin underneath the affected part. Wet, cold injury is more pernicious, leading to wet gangrene. As the patient recovers from frostbite, the skin may slough from the affected part. This skin is treated with burn protocols.

991.0	Frostbite of face
991.1	Frostbite of hand
991.2	Frostbite of foot
991.3	Frostbite of other and unspecified sites
991.4	Effects of immersion of foot
991.5	Effects of chilblains
991.6	Effects of hypothermia

Coding Clarification
This code excludes hypothermia not associated with environmental temperature (780.99).

991.8	Other specified effects of reduced temperature
991.9	Unspecified effect of reduced temperature

992 Effects of heat and light

Heat related illnesses are arranged in order from the most deadly to the mildest. Heat stroke has many names and is a major medical emergency, causing death in 10 percent of its victims.

Heat stroke is partitioned into two categories, equally dangerous — exertional and classic. Classic heat stroke victims typically are older, debilitated from chronic health problems, sedentary, and do not present with major systemic disorders. Exertional heat stroke, which may cause multiple systemic derangement, more often strikes younger, healthier individuals engaged in strenuous activity.

Both types of heat stroke must be treated immediately by immersing the patient in cold water. Water temperature must be monitored to prevent hypothermia. Stroke victims should be transported to the hospital, though prior to summoning help, the patient must be relieved from excessive temperature in the body core greater than 104.9° Fahrenheit.

Heat exhaustion is excessive body core temperature in the range of 100.4° to 104.9° Fahrenheit. The patient must be cooled and orally rehydrated, although there may be gastrointestinal distress necessitating intravenous administration of fluids. The patient generally recovers in two to three hours with appropriate support, though some cases are unresponsive and require hospitalization.

Heat syncope occurs from dehydration, lack of acclimatization to heat when undertaking exercise, and failure to undergo a cool-down period after exercise. Once the patient is prostrate, recovery is immediate.

Heat edema is the swelling of the extremities, typically the legs, in hot weather. Exercise and elevation of the affected parts lessens the swelling.

992.0	Heat stroke and sunstroke
992.1	Heat syncope
992.2	Heat cramps
992.3	Heat exhaustion, anhydrotic
992.4	Heat exhaustion due to salt depletion
992.5	Heat exhaustion, unspecified
992.6	Heat fatigue, transient
992.7	Heat edema
992.8	Other specified heat effects
992.9	Unspecified effects of heat and light

993 Effects of air pressure

993.0   Barotrauma, otitic

Otitic barotrauma can affect aviators, divers, or tunnel workers. Symptoms include pain, hearing loss, rupture of the tympanic membrane, vertigo, and disorientation, which is perhaps the most dangerous manifestation since it can interfere with the ability to move to safety.

993.1   Barotrauma, sinus

Congestion in the sinuses is likely to cause pain and possibly nosebleeds if diving or swift ascent occurs.

993.2   Other and unspecified effects of high altitude

The higher the altitude, the thinner the atmosphere and the greater reduction in oxygen content. The effect is magnified by the proximity of the peak to the earth's poles. At 18,000 feet above sea level, the oxygen content of the atmosphere is reduced by 50 percent and the body must produce a greater number of red blood cells to carry oxygen. Given time to spend at various levels of ascent, most individuals can successfully adapt to the thinner atmosphere.

There are three levels of acute mountain sickness: mild, moderate, and severe. If the moderate degree should manifest, the victim must descend 1,000 feet, rest, and adapt. Climbers must take precautions against the severe form of this life-threatening condition, which requires immediate descent of 2,000- to 4000-feet. The moderate to severe forms can alter mental status, change the degree of consciousness, and cause ataxia and shortness of breath with cyanosis, all of which can be fatal if the patient is not removed from the environment.

993.3   Caisson disease

Other common names for this disorder are the bends and decompression sickness. The term "the bends" refers to the pain associated with decompression sickness, though it has become synonymous for the sickness.

Nitrogen gas dissolved in the tissues forms potentially lethal bubbles in the blood. Women who have a higher proportion of fat are at higher risk of decompression sickness than men.

993.4	Effects of air pressure caused by explosion
993.8	Other specified effects of air pressure
993.9	Unspecified effect of air pressure

994 Effects of other external causes

994.0   Effects of lightning

There are an estimated 750 lightning strikes of humans per year, with an associated mortality rate of 3 to 10 percent. Lightning strikes the highest points, so standing in a meadow, standing under a big tree, or carrying an umbrella, increase the chances of a strike. Electrical energy travels along the earth's surface and can enter the human by the leg closest to the strike and exit through the other leg.

The nerves, muscles, and blood vessels are excellent electrical conductors. Once an individual is struck, the results are typically cardiac arrest, respiratory arrest, vascular spasm, neurological damage, and autonomic instability, rather than burns and renal failure.

994.1   Drowning and nonfatal submersion

The great mortality risk in near drowning is posed by respiratory insufficiency leading to hypoxia and respiratory acidosis. These conditions are always addressed first, and aspiration is managed secondarily. Aspiration of seawater is rarely life threatening, although such aspiration can cause mild elevations of sodium and chloride. Aspiration of large quantities of fresh water can cause massive increase of blood volume, life threatening electrolyte imbalance, and hemolysis leading to asphyxia and ventricular fibrillation.

The water temperature and duration of immersion are other factors when predicting survival from immersion. If an individual is exposed to cool water, over time hypothermia will set in, with its attendant problems. However, if the victim is suddenly tipped into cold water, the mammalian diving reflex reduces the body's oxygen need, thus increasing the chance of survival. The rule is to continue resuscitation efforts even if submerged for more than one hour.

994.2	Effects of hunger
994.3	Effects of thirst
994.4	Exhaustion due to exposure
994.5	Exhaustion due to excessive exertion
994.6	Motion sickness
994.7	Asphyxiation and strangulation
994.8	Electrocution and nonfatal effects of electric current

The extent of an injury by electric shock is a function of the amount of voltage delivered, current type, resistance to the current, and the length of contact to the current. If the skin is thick and dry, it will present greater resistance to the current, resulting in extensive burns, though only slight damage to internal organs. Of the two types of current, direct current is the least deadly since it throws the victim, cutting short the exposure to the current.

Alternating current is three times more dangerous than direct current since the chances of tetanic contractions multiply threefold. Tetany is likely to occur when the "let-go reflex" is depressed, increasing the victim's length of contact with the current.

994.9	Other effects of external causes

995 Certain adverse effects not elsewhere classified

995.0	Other anaphylactic shock not else where classified — (Use additional E code to identify external cause: E930-E949)

The key to understanding an allergy is to recognize that the previously sensitized individual has been re-exposed to the dose that begins the allergic reaction. Vasodilation and consequent loss of plasma into the tissues (productive of hives and angioedema) lead to hypovolemia. After receiving the "insult," the agitated system may present with reddened skin, pruritus, laryngeal edema, or bronchospasm. Shock can set in within a short time and, unless the process is arrested, the patient can die of vascular collapse.

995.1	Angioneurotic edema not elsewhere classified

Subcategory 995.2 reports other and unspecified adverse effects of drugs, medicinal, or biological substances. Various adverse effects or allergic reactions may be caused by local or general anesthesia, insulin, or other drugs or biological substances. Treatment options vary and are dependent upon the manifestation.

995.20	Unspecified adverse effect of unspecified drug, medicinal and biological substance
995.21	Arthus phenomenon — *Arthus reaction*

Arthus' phenomenon, also known as Arthus' reaction, refers to local inflammation seen in the skin some time after intradermal injection of an antigen, or substance that triggers an immune response. It is a type of hypersensitivity reaction in an individual who has been previously sensitized and has a high level of circulating antibody against that antigen. Thrombi destroy the small blood vessels, resulting in edema and a hemorrhagic reaction. In this reaction, immune complexes in the walls of blood vessels begin an inflammatory response; irritation and tissue damage can occur. It is not an acute, immediately overwhelming condition and most often develops over six to 12 hours if antibody levels are already high. Alternately, it may develop over a number of days as antibody levels increase and antigen persists. Localized Arthus' reactions are distinguished by pain, swelling, hardening of the soft tissues, and excessive fluid accumulation.

995.22	Unspecified adverse effect of anesthesia
995.23	Unspecified adverse effect of insulin
995.27	Other drug allergy — *allergy or hypersensitivity not otherwise specified*
995.29	Unspecified adverse effect of other drug, medicinal and biological substance
995.3	Allergy, unspecified not elsewhere classified
995.4	Shock due to anesthesia not elsewhere classified

Anesthetic drugs can cause vasodilation, which can lead to hypovolemic shock and vascular collapse. Patients are carefully monitored during anesthesia for any signs of inappropriate vasodilation.

995.50	Child abuse, unspecified
995.51	Child emotional/psychological abuse
995.52	Child neglect (nutritional)
995.53	Child sexual abuse
995.54	Child physical abuse
995.55	Shaken infant syndrome — (Use additional code(s) to identify any associated injuries)
995.59	Other child abuse and neglect
995.60	Anaphylactic shock due to unspecified food
995.61	Anaphylactic shock due to peanuts
995.62	Anaphylactic shock due to crustaceans
995.63	Anaphylactic shock due to fruits and vegetables
995.64	Anaphylactic shock due to tree nuts and seeds
995.65	Anaphylactic shock due to fish
995.66	Anaphylactic shock due to food additives
995.67	Anaphylactic shock due to milk products
995.68	Anaphylactic shock due to eggs
995.69	Anaphylactic shock due to other specified food
995.7	Other adverse food reactions, not elsewhere classified — (Use additional code to identify the type of reaction: 708.0, 786.07)
995.80	Adult maltreatment, unspecified — (Use additional code to identify any associated injury and perpetrator)
995.81	Adult physical abuse — (Use additional code to identify any associated injury, nature of abuse, and perpetrator)
995.82	Adult emotional/psychological abuse — (Use additional E code to identify perpetrator)

Injury and Poisoning

995.83	Adult sexual abuse — (Use additional code to identify any associated injury and perpetrator)
995.84	Adult neglect (nutritional) — (Use additional E code to identify intent of neglect and perpetrator)
995.85	Other adult abuse and neglect — (Use additional code to identify any associated injury, intent of neglect, nature of abuse, and perpetrator)
995.86	Malignant hyperthermia
995.89	Certain adverse effects, not elsewhere classified, other **AHA:** Q2, 2004, 18

Hyperthermia and hypothermia due to adverse reaction to anesthesia result from a combination of muscle relaxant and inhalation general anesthetic. When an adverse reaction occurs, the operation must be stopped and a reversal agent such as dantrolene must be administered. Family members should be tested for the same sensitivity.

995.9 ⌐5th	Systemic inflammatory response syndrome (SIRS)
995.90	Systemic inflammatory response syndrome, unspecified — (Code first underlying condition)
995.91	Sepsis — (Code first underlying infection) — systemic inflammatory response syndrome due to infectious process without acute organ dysfunction **AHA:** Q2, 2004, 16
995.92	Severe sepsis — (Code first underlying infection. Use additional code to specify acute organ dysfunction, such as 286.6, 348.31, 357.82, 359.81, 570, 518.81, 584.5-584.9) — systemic inflammatory response syndrome due to infectious process with acute organ dysfunction; sepsis with acute organ dysfunction; sepsis with multiple organ dysfunction (MOD) **AHA:** Q4, 2002, 71; Q4, 2003, 73, 79; Q2, 2004, 16; Q1, 2005, 7; Q2, 2005, 18, 19
995.93	Systemic inflammatory response syndrome due to non-infectious process without acute organ dysfunction — (Code first underlying condition, such as acute pancreatitis (577.0) or trauma)
995.94	Systemic inflammatory response syndrome due to noninfectious process with acute organ dysfunction — (Code first underlying condition, such as acute pancreatitis (577.0) or trauma. Use additional code to specify organ dysfunction, such as 286.6, 348.31, 357.82, 359.81, 570, 518.81, 584.5-584.9) **AHA:** Q4, 2002, 71; Q4, 2003, 79

Documentation Issues

The majority of these codes in rubric 995.20-995.29 should not be used in the inpatient setting; documentation in inpatient records should identify some sign or symptom of the adverse effect or reaction. As with other codes in this chapter, an additional E code may be assigned to identify the external cause.

Coding Clarification

Current official coding guidelines assume the terms "sepsis" and "severe sepsis" are associated with SIRS. Code the underlying condition first, then assign the code for sepsis (995.91) or severe sepsis (995.92). By contrast, the term "septicemia" prompts physician query regarding whether "sepsis" and therefore "SIRS" are also present. Sequencing for sepsis, septicemia, SIRS, and septic shock are determined by the circumstances of admission and instructional terms within the text.

996–999 Complications of Surgical and Medical Care, NEC

996 Complications peculiar to certain specified procedures
AHA: Q1, 1994, 3

Patients may experience idiosyncratic reactions to the materials used in prostheses, from lens implants to artificial skin. Prostheses can also cause problems when displaced from the site of original insertion.

Problems classified as mechanical, complications, infectious or inflammatory reactions, or "other" complications include associated pain, embolism, hemorrhage, organ transplant rejections, and complications of reattached extremities or body parts. When the reason for an admission is linked to complications of medical or surgical care, the complication code is listed as the principal diagnosis, with any explanatory codes following. For example, a patient may be readmitted with sepsis following a previous medical contact. In this case, determine if the sepsis is linked to the previous contact since it may be attributable to either an infected line or a postoperative infection.

996.00	Mechanical complication of unspecified cardiac device, implant, and graft
996.01	Mechanical complication due to cardiac pacemaker (electrode) **AHA:** Q2, 2006, 15
996.02	Mechanical complication due to heart valve prosthesis
996.03	Mechanical complication due to coronary bypass graft
996.04	Mechanical complication due to automatic implantable cardiac defibrillator **AHA:** Q2, 2005, 3
996.09	Mechanical complication of cardiac device, implant, and graft, other

Code	Description
996.1	Mechanical complication of other vascular device, implant, and graft AHA: Q2, 2005, 8; Q1, 2006, 10
996.2	Mechanical complication of nervous system device, implant, and graft
996.30	Mechanical complication of unspecified genitourinary device, implant, and graft
996.31	Mechanical complication due to urethral (indwelling) catheter
996.32	Mechanical complication due to intrauterine contraceptive device
996.39	Mechanical complication of genitourinary device, implant, and graft, other

Total joint replacement is one of the most commonly performed and successful orthopedic procedures. The occurrence of total joint replacement is expected to increase in the future with ever-advancing technologies that result in longer-lasting quality of life improvement. The codes in this subcategory help capture the different specific causes that a total joint replacement, most often hip or knee, has failed.

Code	Description
996.40	Unspecified mechanical complication of internal orthopedic device, implant, and graft — (Use additional code to identify prosthetic joint with mechanical complication, V43.60-V43.69) AHA: Q4, 2005, 91
996.41	Mechanical loosening of prosthetic joint— (Use additional code to identify prosthetic joint with mechanical complication, V43.60-V43.69) — aseptic loosening AHA: Q4, 2005, 91, 112

Mechanical loosening of a prosthetic joint is the most common cause of long-term failure in both hip and knee replacements. Loosening may occur regardless of fixation material employed.

Code	Description
996.42	Dislocation of prosthetic joint — (Use additional code to identify prosthetic joint with mechanical complication, V43.60-V43.69) — instability or subluxation of prosthetic joint AHA: Q4, 2005, 91

Dislocation of a joint replacement is most common with hip replacement procedures among the elderly, older than age 70, who have certain types of arthritic disease, although displacement can occur at any age and with any type of prosthetic joint. Factors such as surgical technique, mechanical device, and health and mobility of the patient play a part in potential subluxation of a prosthetic joint.

Code	Description
996.43	Prosthetic joint implant failure — (Use additional code to identify prosthetic joint with mechanical complication, V43.60-V43.69) — Breakage or fracture of prosthetic joint AHA: Q4, 2005, 91
996.44	Peri-prosthetic fracture around prosthetic joint — (Use additional code to identify prosthetic joint with mechanical complication, V43.60-V43.69) AHA: Q4, 2005, 91, 93

Implants performed on compromised bone can result in fracture of the bony tissue that is adjacent to the supporting prosthesis. Falls and external trauma can also result in a fracture of the bone around the implant.

Code	Description
996.45	Peri-prosthetic osteolysis — (Use additional code to identify major osseous defect, if applicable (731.3); use additional code to identify prosthetic joint with mechanical complication, V43.60-V43.69) AHA: Q4, 2005, 91

Wear on the prosthetic surface creates "dust" or debris that causes a biological response in the natural bone. The host bone begins to break down and results in bone resorption. This may occur in more active patients with total hip replacement, especially those with polyethylene plastics in the implant.

Code	Description
996.46	Articular bearing surface wear of prosthetic joint — (Use additional code to identify prosthetic joint with mechanical complication, V43.60-V43.69) AHA: Q4, 2005, 91

Wear of the articular bearing surface occurs over time, particularly dependent on the age and activity level of the patient.

Code	Description
996.47	Other mechanical complication of prosthetic joint implant — (Use additional code to identify prosthetic joint with mechanical complication, V43.60-V43.69) — prosthetic joint mechanical complication NOS AHA: Q4, 2005, 91
996.49	Other mechanical complication of other internal orthopedic device, implant, and graft — (Use additional code to identify prosthetic joint with mechanical complication, V43.60-V43.69) AHA: Q4, 2005, 91

Do not report 996.49 for mechanical complication of a prosthetic joint implant, which is coded to 996.41-996.47.

Code	Description
996.51	Mechanical complication due to corneal graft
996.52	Mechanical complication due to other tissue graft, not elsewhere classified
996.53	Mechanical complication due to ocular lens prosthesis
996.54	Mechanical complication due to breast prosthesis
996.55	Mechanical complications due to artificial skin graft and decellularized allodermis
996.56	Mechanical complications due to peritoneal dialysis catheter
996.57	Mechanical complication, Due to insulin pump
996.59	Mechanical complication due to other implant and internal device, not elsewhere classified
996.60	Infection and inflammatory reaction due to unspecified device, implant, and graft — (Use additional code to identify specified infections)

Injury and Poisoning

996.61 Infection and inflammatory reaction due to cardiac device, implant, and graft — (Use additional code to identify specified infections)

996.62 Infection and inflammatory reaction due to other vascular device, implant, and graft — (Use additional code to identify specified infections)
AHA: Q1, 2004, 5; Q2, 2004, 16

996.63 Infection and inflammatory reaction due to nervous system device, implant, and graft — (Use additional code to identify specified infections)

996.64 Infection and inflammatory reaction due to indwelling urinary catheter — (Use additional code to identify specified infections: 038.0-038.9, 595.0-595.9)

996.65 Infection and inflammatory reaction due to other genitourinary device, implant, and graft — (Use additional code to identify specified infections)

996.66 Infection and inflammatory reaction due to internal joint prosthesis — (Use additional code to identify specified infections) (Use additional code to identify infected prosthetic joint, V43.60-V43.69)
AHA: Q4, 2005, 91, 113

996.67 Infection and inflammatory reaction due to other internal orthopedic device, implant, and graft — (Use additional code to identify specified infections)

996.68 Infection and inflammatory reaction due to peritoneal dialysis catheter — (Use additional code to identify specified infections)

996.69 Infection and inflammatory reaction due to other internal prosthetic device, implant, and graft — (Use additional code to identify specified infections)

996.70 Other complications due to unspecified device, implant, and graft — (Use additional codes to identify complications, such as pain due to the presence of device, implant, or graft (338.18, 338.19, 338.28, 338.29)
AHA: Q4, 2005, 94

996.71 Other complications due to heart valve prosthesis — (Use additional codes to identify complications, such as pain due to the presence of device, implant, or graft (338.18, 338.19, 338.28, 338.29)
AHA: Q4, 2005, 94

996.72 Other complications due to other cardiac device, implant, and graft — (Use additional codes to identify complications, such as pain due to the presence of device, implant, or graft (338.18, 338.19, 338.28, 338.29)
AHA: Q4, 2005, 94

996.73 Other complications due to renal dialysis device, implant, and graft — (Use additional codes to identify complications, such as pain due to the presence of device, implant, or graft (338.18, 338.19, 338.28, 338.29)
AHA: Q4, 2005, 94

996.74 Other complications due to other vascular device, implant, and graft — (Use additional codes to identify complications, such as pain due to the presence of device, implant, or graft (338.18, 338.19, 338.28, 338.29)
AHA: Q4, 2005, 94

996.75 Other complications due to nervous system device, implant, and graft — (Use additional codes to identify complications, such as pain due to the presence of device, implant, or graft (338.18, 338.19, 338.28, 338.29)
AHA: Q4, 2005, 94

996.76 Other complications due to genitourinary device, implant, and graft — (Use additional codes to identify complications, such as pain due to the presence of device, implant, or graft (338.18, 338.19, 338.28, 338.29)
AHA: Q4, 2005, 94

996.77 Other complications due to internal joint prosthesis — (Use additional codes to identify complications, such as pain due to the presence of device, implant, or graft (338.18, 338.19, 338.28, 338.29)
AHA: Q4, 2005, 91, 94

996.78 Other complications due to other internal orthopedic device, implant, and graft — (Use additional codes to identify complications, such as pain due to the presence of device, implant, or graft (338.18, 338.19, 338.28, 338.29)
AHA: Q4, 2005, 94

996.79 Other complications due to other internal prosthetic device, implant, and graft — (Use additional codes to identify complications, such as pain due to the presence of device, implant, or graft (338.18, 338.19, 338.28, 338.29)
AHA: Q2, 2004, 7; Q4, 2005, 94

996.80 Complications of transplanted organ, unspecified site — (Use additional code to identify nature of complication, 078.5)

996.81 Complications of transplanted kidney — (Use additional code to identify nature of complication, 078.5)

996.82 Complications of transplanted liver — (Use additional code to identify nature of complication, 078.5)

996.83 Complications of transplanted heart — (Use additional code to identify nature of complication, 078.5)

996.84 Complications of transplanted lung — (Use additional code to identify nature of complication, 078.5)

996.85 Complications of bone marrow transplant — (Use additional code to identify nature of complication, 078.5)

996.86 Complications of transplanted pancreas — (Use additional code to identify nature of complication, 078.5)

996.87 Complications of transplanted organ, intestine — (Use additional code to identify nature of complication, 078.5)

996.89 Complications of other transplanted organ — (Use additional code to identify nature of complication, 078.5)

Code	Description
996.90	Complications of unspecified reattached extremity
996.91	Complications of reattached forearm
996.92	Complications of reattached hand
996.93	Complications of reattached finger(s)
996.94	Complications of reattached upper extremity, other and unspecified
996.95	Complications of reattached foot and toe(s)
996.96	Complications of reattached lower extremity, other and unspecified
996.99	Complications of other specified reattached body part

Coding Clarification

Acute Coronary Graft Closure: A common complication following coronary bypass surgery is occlusion of the graft. This condition is classified to ICD-9-CM code 996.03 *Mechanical complication of cardiac device, implant and graft, due to coronary bypass graft*.

As noted by the excludes note in the tabular list, this code is not used to indicate atherosclerosis of the graft. When the documentation indicates that this is the cause of the blockage, the appropriate code from 414.02-414.03 should be assigned.

Another common complication following coronary bypass graft is delayed closure of the graft. This is also reported with code 996.03.

Breast Implant Complications: Patients with augmentation mammoplasty may develop complications due to the implant. Such complications may include periprosthetic mammary capsular contracture, rupture, or infection.

When assigning a code to identify periprosthetic mammary capsular contracture, use code 996.79 *Other complications due to other internal prosthetic device, implant and graft*. Code 996.54 classifies the rupture of the implant. Infection or inflammatory reactions to the implant are identified by 996.69 *Infection and inflammatory reaction due to internal prosthetic device, implant, and graft, due to other internal prosthetic device, implant, and graft*.

Complications of Artificial Skin: Advances in the treatment of burns and other severe conditions affecting the skin have provided new technologies that are able to permanently regenerate or replace skin layers. These include artificial skin, decellularized allodermis, and cultured epithelial cells. As with any procedure, complications can occur, mainly infection and mechanical failure.

Complications such as dislodgment, displacement, non-adherence, poor incorporation, shearing or failure are assigned code 996.55. Infection and/or inflammatory reaction to the graft should be assigned code 996.69.

Mechanical Complication of Peritoneal Dialysis Catheter: It is not uncommon for patients with peritoneal dialysis catheters to experience complications associated with the catheter. Such complications include infection or leakage of the catheter. When a complication of a peritoneal dialysis catheter occurs, code 996.56.

Code 996.56 does not indicate a complication of an arteriovenous dialysis catheter. If the complication is of an A-V catheter, code 996.1 should be reported.

Coronary Artery Stent Stenosis: A complication of stent insertion procedures is the formation of scar tissue at the site of the stent. This is not considered to be a mechanical complication of the stent, as the stent is in working order. The scar tissue formation is the body's natural reaction to the introduction of the stent. The scar tissue formed at the stent should not be considered an infection and/or inflammatory reaction to the stent.

When assigning a code for stenosis of a stent, use a code from subcategory 996.7 *Other complications of internal (biological) (synthetic) prosthetic device, implant, and graft*. In the case of a coronary artery stent stenosis, the fifth-digit code assigned would be 996.72 *Due to other cardiac device, implant, and graft*.

When a patient develops sepsis due to an infection of a vascular catheter, the sepsis is a complication of the medical device. An appropriate 996-999 code is assigned. Code also the underlying condition, 038 series, and the appropriate code for the sepsis or SIRS, 995.91-995.92.

Coding Scenario

A patient is seen by the surgeon due to leakage of the peritoneal dialysis graft.

> Code assignment: 996.56 *Mechanical complication of other specified prosthetic device, implant or graft, due to peritoneal dialysis catheter*

A patient is seen four days post coronary artery bypass graft for blockage of the graft.

> Code assignment: 996.03 *Mechanical complication of cardiac device, implant, and graft, due to coronary bypass graft*

A patient is seen seven years post breast augmentation. She is complaining of pain. The physician documents periprosthetic mammary capsular contracture.

Code assignment: 996.79 *Other complications of internal (biological) (synthetic) prosthetic device, implant, and graft due to other internal prosthetic device, implant, and graft*

997 Complications affecting specified body systems, not elsewhere classified
AHA: Q1, 1993, 26; Q1, 1994, 4

Complications in the 997 category are organized according to body system. For example, urinary catheterization is an intervention or procedure and a urinary infection attributed to catheterization is coded with the 997.5 subcategory first and the appropriate urinary infection code secondarily. The more typical scenario with postoperative urinary tract infections is that following back, abdominal, or pelvic surgery, the patient is unable to void and, thus, catheterized. The extended period of catheterization leads to a postoperative urinary tract infection, and is coded as such. In all cases, the medical record must clearly link the complication to the procedure. If unclear, the coder should ask the physician to document the existing link in an addendum to the report.

Code	Description
997.00	Unspecified nervous system complication — (Use additional code to identify complications)
997.01	Central nervous system complication — (Use additional code to identify complications) **AHA:** Q1, 2006, 15
997.02	Iatrogenic cerebrovascular infarction or hemorrhage — (Use additional code to identify complications) **AHA:** Q2, 2004, 8
997.09	Other nervous system complications — (Use additional code to identify complications)
997.1	Cardiac complications — (Use additional code to identify complications)
997.2	Peripheral vascular complications — (Use additional code to identify complications)
997.3	Respiratory complications — (Use additional code to identify complications)

Coding Clarification
Transfusion-related acute lung injury (TRALI) is not reported with this code but with code 518.7.

Code	Description
997.4	Digestive system complication — (Use additional code to identify complications)
997.5	Urinary complications — (Use additional code to identify complications)
997.60	Late complications of amputation stump, unspecified — (Use additional code to identify complications)
997.61	Neuroma of amputation stump — (Use additional code to identify complications)
997.62	Infection (chronic) of amputation stump — (Use additional code to identify organism. Use additional code to identify complications) **AHA:** Q1, 2005, 14
997.69	Other late amputation stump complication — (Use additional code to identify complications) **AHA:** Q1, 2005, 15
997.71	Vascular complications of mesenteric artery — (Use additional code to identify complications)
997.72	Vascular complications of renal artery — (Use additional code to identify complications)
997.79	Vascular complications of other vessels — (Use additional code to identify complications)
997.91	Hypertension — (Use additional code to identify complications)
997.99	Other complications affecting other specified body systems, NEC — (Use additional code to identify complications)

Coding Clarification
Infection of Amputation Stump: Unless it is the original admission for treatment of a current traumatic amputation, a code from subcategory 997.6x should be identified for any type of amputation stump complication. Specifically, code 997.62 *Amputation stump complication, infection* should be identified in this scenario.

Complication of Amputation vs. Atherosclerotic Gangrene: Progressive atherosclerosis of the extremities with gangrene that necessitates successive amputations should be considered progression of the disease rather than complication of the previous amputation. Assign the code for the disease that necessitated the amputation and use additional codes to report any comorbidities and complications that affect treatment.

Postoperative Urinary Tract Infection: To indicate that a urinary tract infection is a postoperative complication, two codes are necessary. Assign code 997.5 *Urinary complications* first and code 599.0 *Urinary tract infection, site not specified* as a secondary diagnosis.

Postoperative urinary retention following surgery may lead to urinary tract infection. In this instance, one code, 997.5, is indicated on the claim. Likewise, secretion of a decreased amount of urine as opposed to fluid intake can cause a urinary tract infection and also is indicated by code 997.5.

Postoperative Pneumonia: When the physician documents that the patient is being treated for postoperative pneumonia, two codes are necessary. First assign code 997.3 *Complications affecting specified body systems, not elsewhere classified, respiratory complications* followed by the appropriate code from categories 480-487 or 507 for the pneumonia to specify the nature of the complication.

Cholangitis Following Percutaneous Transhepatic Cholangiogram: Cholangitis is an inflammation of the bile duct and can occur following a cholangiogram. Two codes are required to indicate that the condition occurred as a complication to a surgical procedure. First assign code 997.4 *Digestive system complications* to identify that the condition is due to the procedure followed by code 576.1 *Cholangitis* to further elucidate the condition.

Complications Following Bone Marrow Transplant: When complications arise following bone marrow transplant, report with code 996.85 *Complications of transplanted organ, bone marrow* followed by an additional code identifying the nature of the complication such as an infection.

Complications Following Coronary Artery Procedures: Complications resulting from coronary artery procedures generally occur intraoperatively or within the first 24 hours to one week after surgery. The types of complications include thrombus formation, myocardial infarction, graft closures, infection, pulmonary embolism, stroke, and renal failure.

- Thrombus formation: to identify this condition use code 997.2 *Peripheral vascular complication.* If the thrombus is due to an implant or catheter device, code 996.62 should be used.
- Myocardial infarction: When the documentation indicates that the myocardial infarction is a complication from a procedure, report code 997.1 *Cardiac complications,* followed by the appropriate code from category 410 *Acute myocardial infarction* to further identify the specific complication.
- Pulmonary embolism: To report this type of complication, assign codes 997.3 *Respiratory complication* and code 415.11 *Iatrogenic pulmonary embolism and infarction.*
- Stroke: Code 997.02 *Iatrogenic cerebrovascular infarction or hemorrhage* and a code from category 434, with a fifth digit of '1' (describing the cerebral infarction), should be assigned.
- Renal failure: When classifying renal failure following surgery, assign code 997.5 *Urinary complications* and the appropriate code from categories 584-586.

Postoperative Adhesions: Postoperative adhesions are adhesions of the gastrointestinal tract and are attributed to previous abdominal surgery. This condition causes abdominal pain and/or impaired bowel mobility. When the documentation indicates that the adhesions are postoperative, code 997.4 *Digestive system complications* is assigned.

Postoperative Hypertension and Hypotension: Code 997.91 is reported for postoperative hypertension. The physician must state that the hypertension was related to or was a complication of the procedure for this code to be accurately assigned. An additional code from the 401-405 series may be assigned to clarify the nature of the hypertension.

Postoperative Pain: Postoperative pain is assigned to the ICD-9-CM code that describes the pain of the specified site and not to a complication of procedures category.

Postoperative Urinary Retention: When a patient is documented as having postoperative urinary retention, code 997.5 *Urinary complications* and code 788.2x should be reported.

Subhepatic Fluid Accumulation Following Cholecystectomy: When the physician indicates that a subhepatic fluid accumulation resulted following a cholecystectomy, code 997.4 *Digestive system complications* should be assigned.

Complications of Esophagostomy: Report 530.86 for infection of esophagostomy and 530.87 for mechanical complication of esophagostomy.

Coding Scenario
Four days following a hysterectomy, a patient is complaining of urinary frequency and burning. The physician documents that she has a postoperative complication of a UTI and starts her on Bactrim DS, bid.

> Code assignment: 997.5 *Urinary complications* and 599.0 *Urinary tract infection, site unspecified*

Ten days following a below-the-knee amputation, the patient sees her physician. The physician notes that the amputation stump is not healing well and appears to be infected.

> Code assignment: 997.62 *Amputation stump complication, infection*

A 72-year-old female complaining of abdominal pain is seen by her family physician. She has a history of multiple abdominal surgeries including a hysterectomy, appendectomy, bowel resection, and cholecystectomy. The physician documents postoperative bowel adhesions.

> Code assignment: 997.4 *Digestive system complications*

998 Other complications of procedures, not elsewhere classified
AHA: Q1, 1994, 4

998.0	Postoperative shock, not elsewhere classified
998.11	Hemorrhage complicating a procedure

998.12	Hematoma complicating a procedure	
998.13	Seroma complicating a procedure	
998.2	Accidental puncture or laceration during procedure	
	AHA: Q1, 2006, 15	
998.31	Disruption of internal operation wound	
998.32	Disruption of external operation wound	
	AHA: Q1, 2005, 11; Q1, 2006, 8	
998.4	Foreign body accidentally left during procedure, not elsewhere classified	
998.51	Infected postoperative seroma — (Use additional code to identify organism)	
998.59	Other postoperative infection — (Use additional code to identify infection)	
	AHA: Q4, 2004, 76; Q2, 2006, 23	

Coding Clarification
Bleb-associated endophthalmitis is not reported with this, but with code 379.63.

998.6	Persistent postoperative fistula, not elsewhere classified	
998.7	Acute reaction to foreign substance accidentally left during procedure, not elsewhere classified	
998.81	Emphysema (subcutaneous) (surgical) resulting from a procedure	
998.82	Cataract fragments in eye following surgery	
998.83	Non-healing surgical wound	
998.89	Other specified complications	
	AHA: Q3, 2005, 16	
998.9	Unspecified complication of procedure, not elsewhere classified	

Coding Clarification
Other Postoperative Infections: When the infection is specified as a seroma, use code 998.51 *Infected postoperative seroma* followed by a code identifying the infectious organism if known.

For other postoperative infections such as stitch abscess, intraabdominal abscess, wound abscess, or septicemia use code 998.59 *Other postoperative infection*. In addition, identify the infectious organism if known.

Postoperative Peritonitis: This condition requires the assignment of two codes. First identify the postoperative infection using code 998.59 *Postoperative infection, other postoperative infection* followed by code 567.2 *Other suppurative peritonitis*.

Coding Scenario
Two days after a bowel resection a patient has a fever and abdominal pain. The physician indicates that the patient is suffering from postoperative peritonitis.

Code assignment: 998.59 *Other postoperative infection* and 567.2 *Other suppurative peritonitis*

999 Complications of medical care, not elsewhere classified

Transfusion reactions, a major complication of medical care, is found in this category. Reaction to dialysis is another common cause of admission to acute care that falls under 999.9. Postvaccinal encephalitis is excluded from this rubric and is reported with code 323.51.

999.0	Generalized vaccinia as complication of medical care, not elsewhere classified
999.1	Air embolism as complication of medical care, not elsewhere classified
999.2	Other vascular complications of medical care, not elsewhere classified
999.3	Other infection due to medical care, not elsewhere classified
999.4	Anaphylactic shock due to serum, not elsewhere classified
999.5	Other serum reaction, not elsewhere classified
999.6	Abo incompatibility reaction, not elsewhere classified
999.7	Rh incompatibility reaction, not elsewhere classified
999.8	Other transfusion reaction, not elsewhere classified

Coding Clarification
This code excludes transfusion-related acute lung injury, which is reported with code 518.7.

999.9	Other and unspecified complications of medical care, not elsewhere classified
	AHA: Q2, 2006, 25

V01–V86

Supplementary Classification of Factors Influencing Health Status and Contact with Health Services

The Supplementary Classification of Factors Influencing Health Status and Contact with Health Services (V Codes) describes occasions when circumstances other than a disease or an injury justify an encounter with the health care delivery system or influence the patient's current condition.

The V codes are sequenced depending on the circumstance or problem being coded. Some V codes are sequenced first to describe the reason for the encounter, while others are sequenced second because they identify a circumstance that affects the patient's health status but is not in itself a current illness.

The V codes immediately follow the injury and poisoning codes. Only in specific circumstances are these alphanumerical codes listed as the principal diagnosis for inpatient coding or primary diagnosis for outpatient coding based on coding guidelines.

The V codes are divided into three main classifications:

1. **Problem-oriented V Code:** this type of code identifies a circumstance that could affect the patient in the future but is neither a current illness or injury. Use a V code to describe an existing circumstance or problem that may influence future medical care or a patient's health status. Problem-oriented V codes are not usually listed first on the medical claim form because they represent supplemental information. An example of this use would be in the case of a patient with a personal history of cancer. Another example would be in the case of a patient with a family history of ischemic heart disease.

2. **Service-oriented V Code:** this type of code identifies or defines examinations, aftercare, ancillary services, or therapy. Use this type of V code to describe when a person with a known disease or injury, whether it is current or resolving, encounters the health care system for a specific treatment of that disease or injury. Review the outpatient coding guidelines to determine if this type of V code can be used as the primary diagnosis. Examples of when to use a service-oriented V code would be in the case of patient sterilization and in patient orthopaedic aftercare.

3. **Fact-oriented V Code:** this type of code does not describe a problem or a service; it simply states a fact. This type of code generally does not serve as an outpatient or inpatient principal diagnosis. Categories V30-V39 are applied to all live births (fourth and fifth digits) and are always the principal diagnosis if the birth occurred during admission. Categories V40-V49 classify conditions that may influence a patient's health status, such as the presence of a cardiac pacemaker or colostomy.

V01–V06 Persons with Potential Health Hazards Related to Communicable Diseases

This category identifies patients with potential health risks from communicable diseases or diseases that are transferable from one person to another. This includes contact with someone who has the disease, a person who is a carrier of an infectious disease (caused or transferred by infection), or someone in need of preventive immunizations.

Preventive immunizations are the introduction of an immunity and may be active or passive. Active immunizations stimulate the immune system to give protection against disease. Usually this is performed by the administration of a vaccine or toxoid. A passive immunization takes lymphoid cells or serum from immune individuals and administers them to nonimmune individuals to provide specific immune reactivity.

V01 Contact with or exposure to communicable diseases

A communicable disease is an infectious disease that can be transferred from one person to another. In most cases, the patient's immune system can successfully defeat the infective agent. In this instance, the patient may test positive for exposure to the disease but show no symptoms of the active disease. Factors that can influence a person's ability to resist an infection are age, underlying diseases, or some types of current medical treatments. The following codes are used for patients who have been exposed to an infectious disease but have not contracted the condition.

V01.0	Contact with or exposure to cholera — *spread though food, water contaminated with feces of infected person* AHA: Jan-Feb, 1987, 8
V01.1	Contact with or exposure to tuberculosis — *macrophages, immune cells that detect and destroy foreign matter, ingest the TB bacteria and transport them to the lymph nodes* AHA: Jan-Feb, 1987, 8
V01.2	Contact with or exposure to poliomyelitis — *polio enters the body through the digestive tract and spreads along nerve cells* AHA: Jan-Feb, 1987, 8
V01.3	Contact with or exposure to smallpox — *smallpox can be transmitted by infected blankets, linens and clothing* AHA: Jan-Feb, 1987, 8
V01.4	Contact with or exposure to rubella — *also called German measles* AHA: Jan-Feb, 1987, 8
V01.5	Contact with or exposure to rabies — *caused by neurotropic virus found in the saliva of rabid animals* AHA: Jan-Feb, 1987, 8
V01.6	Contact with or exposure to venereal diseases — *caused by sexual contact with infected person or can be transferred from mother to baby* AHA: Jan-Feb, 1987, 8
V01.71	Contact or exposure to varicella
V01.79	Contact or exposure to other viral diseases
V01.81	Contact with or exposure to anthrax — *can enter the body through a cut in the skin, inhalation, and/or gastrointestinally* AHA: Jan-Feb, 1987, 8; July-Aug, 1987, 24; Q4, 2002, 70, 78
V01.82	Exposure to SARS-associated coronavirus — *Severe Acute Respiratory Syndrome* AHA: Q4, 2003, 46-47
V01.83	Contact or exposure to Escherichia coli (E. coli)
V01.84	Contact or exposure to meningococcus
V01.89	Contact or exposure to other communicable diseases
V01.9	Contact with or exposure to unspecified communicable disease

Documentation Issues
Documentation should state that the person was exposed to the disease and does not have any acute symptoms at this time.

Coding Clarification
Category V01 codes may be used as the first listed or additional diagnosis.

These codes exclude V18.8 *Family history of infectious and parasitic diseases* and V12.0 *Personal history of infectious and parasitic diseases.*

Coding Scenario
A patient presents to the physician after traveling to Asia and was exposed to SARS. The patient does not have current symptoms of the disease.

> Code assignment: V01.82 *Exposure to SARS-associated coronavirus*

V02 Carrier or suspected carrier of infectious diseases

A carrier of infectious diseases has a specific disease even though he or she does not exhibit signs or symptoms of the disease. A suspected carrier is one who has been in contact with an individual who has an infectious disease, but does not have signs or symptoms. This person is capable of spreading the disease to others. Some of these diseases can be spread from an asymptomatic mother to an unborn child.

V02.0	Carrier or suspected carrier of cholera — *infection of the bowel caused by Vibrio cholerae* AHA: Jan-Feb, 1987, 8; Q3, 1994, 4; Q3, 1995, 18
V02.1	Carrier or suspected carrier of typhoid — *systemic bacterial disease caused by the human strain of Salmonella typhi* AHA: Jan-Feb, 1987, 8; Q3, 1994, 4; Q3, 1995, 18

Supplementary Classification of Factors Influencing Health Status and Contact with Health Services

V02.2 Carrier or suspected carrier of amebiasis — *amebiasis protozoa can live in the large intestine without causing symptoms.*
  AHA: Jan-Feb, 1987, 8; Q3, 1994, 4; Q3, 1995, 18

V02.3 Carrier or suspected carrier of other gastrointestinal pathogens

V02.4 Carrier or suspected carrier of diphtheria — *caused by Corynebacterium diphtheriae.*
  AHA: Jan-Feb, 1987, 8; Q3, 1994, 4; Q3, 1995, 18

V02.51 Carrier or suspected carrier of Group B streptococcus — *common pharyngeal infection*
  AHA: Jan-Feb, 1987, 8; Q3, 1994, 4; Q3, 1995, 18; Q4, 1998, 56; Q1, 2002, 14

V02.52 Carrier or suspected carrier of other streptococcus

V02.59 Carrier or suspected carrier of other specified bacterial diseases

V02.6 ⌐sth Carrier or suspected carrier of viral hepatitis — *can be transmitted through contaminated blood, fecal contamination, and raw shellfish*
  AHA: Jan-Feb, 1987, 8; Q3, 1994, 4; Q3, 1995, 18

V02.60 Unspecified viral hepatitis carrier

V02.61 Hepatitis B carrier — *limited to direct contact with blood or blood products or sexual contact*
  AHA: Jan-Feb, 1987, 8; Q3, 1994, 4; Q3, 1995, 18; Q4, 1997, 47

V02.62 Hepatitis C carrier — *eighty percent of cases result from blood transfusions*
  AHA: Jan-Feb, 1987, 8; Q3, 1994, 4; Q3, 1995, 18; Q4, 1997, 47

V02.69 Other viral hepatitis carrier

V02.7 Carrier or suspected carrier of gonorrhea — *an acute infection caused by Neisseria Gonorrhoeae, usually transmitted sexually*
  AHA: Jan-Feb, 1987, 8; Q3, 1994, 4; Q3, 1995, 18

V02.8 Carrier or suspected carrier of other venereal diseases

V02.9 Carrier or suspected carrier of other specified infectious organism

Documentation Issues
Documentation should include that the patient is a confirmed carrier or suspected carrier of the disease.

Coding Clarification
Category V02 codes may be used as the first listed or additional diagnosis.

Coding Scenario
A heath care worker is suspected of carrying group B streptococcus.

Code assignment: V02.51 *Carrier or suspected carrier of group B streptococcus*

V03 Need for prophylactic vaccination and inoculation against bacterial diseases
Vaccinations help the body fight off specific diseases. The vaccine contains weakened or dead bacteria, viruses, or toxins. Vaccines can be given orally, intramuscularly, or by subcutaneous injection. Once the immunization is given, the body creates antibodies against the vaccine, which provides immunity to the patient. Most immunizations are given during the early childhood years. However, some vaccinations such as for influenza and pneumonia are recommended for adults. Often more than one vaccine is included in one injection.

V03.0 Need for prophylactic vaccination and inoculation against cholera alone — *Vibrio cholerae*
  AHA: Jan-Feb, 1987, 8

V03.1 Need for prophylactic vaccination with typhoid-paratyphoid alone (TAB) — *systemic bacterial disease caused by the human strain of Salmonella typhi*
  AHA: Jan-Feb, 1987, 8

V03.2 Need for prophylactic vaccination with tuberculosis (BCG) vaccine — *Tuberculin bacillus*
  AHA: Jan-Feb, 1987, 8

V03.3 Need for prophylactic vaccination and inoculation against plague — *Yersinia pestis carried by rodents*
  AHA: Jan-Feb, 1987, 8

V03.4 Need for prophylactic vaccination and inoculation against tularemia — *Francisella tularensis*
  AHA: Jan-Feb, 1987, 8

V03.5 Need for prophylactic vaccination and inoculation against diphtheria alone — *Corynebacterium diphtheria*
  AHA: Jan-Feb, 1987, 8

V03.6 Need for prophylactic vaccination and inoculation against pertussis alone — *whooping cough*
  AHA: Jan-Feb, 1987, 8

V03.7 Need for prophylactic vaccination with tetanus toxoid alone — *caused by spore-forming bacillus Clostridium tetani, lock jaw*
  AHA: Jan-Feb, 1987, 8

V03.81 Need for prophylactic vaccination against Hemophilus influenza type B (Hib) — *can cause meningitis*
  AHA: Jan-Feb, 1987, 8

V03.82 Need for prophylactic vaccination against Streptococcus pneumoniae (pneumococcus) — *kills more people a year than any other disease that may be prevented by vaccination*
  AHA: Jan-Feb, 1987, 8

V03.89 Need for prophylactic vaccination against other specified vaccination

V03.9 Need for prophylactic vaccination and inoculation against unspecified single bacterial disease

Coding Clarification
If a contraindication for vaccination is evident in the patient, whether because of another condition or personal wishes, it should be coded within V64.00-V64.09 *Vaccination not carried out* Vaccinations against combinations of diseases should be coded with V06.0-V06.9.

If the disease is currently an active disease, codes 001.0-041.2 should be reported.

Coding Scenario
An elderly woman presents to the physician for her pneumococcal vaccination.

    Code assignment: V03.82 *Need for prophylactic vaccination against Streptococcus pneumoniae (pneumococcus)*

V04 Need for prophylactic vaccination and inoculation against certain viral diseases

V04.0 Need for prophylactic vaccination and inoculation against poliomyelitis — *polio lives in the throat and intestinal tract*
AHA: Jan-Feb, 1987, 8

V04.1 Need for prophylactic vaccination and inoculation against smallpox — *variolae major; variolae minor*
AHA: Jan-Feb, 1987, 8

V04.2 Need for prophylactic vaccination and inoculation against measles alone — *spreads very easily*
AHA: Jan-Feb, 1987, 8

V04.3 Need for prophylactic vaccination and inoculation against rubella alone — *can cause birth defects in unborn children*
AHA: Jan-Feb, 1987, 8

V04.4 Need for prophylactic vaccination and inoculation against yellow fever — *transmitted by mosquitos*
AHA: Jan-Feb, 1987, 8

V04.5 Need for prophylactic vaccination and inoculation against rabies — *causes acute encephalitis*
AHA: Jan-Feb, 1987, 8

V04.6 Need for prophylactic vaccination and inoculation against mumps alone — *spread through the air by coughing, sneezing, or talking*
AHA: Jan-Feb, 1987, 8

V04.7 Need for prophylactic vaccination and inoculation against common cold — *several hundreds of strains of the virus*
AHA: Jan-Feb, 1987, 8

V04.81 Need for prophylactic vaccination and inoculation, Influenza — *can be dangerous for elderly*

V04.82 Need for prophylactic vaccination and inoculation, Respiratory syncytial virus [RSV] — *most children are affected by a mild form of the virus*

V04.89 Need for prophylactic vaccination and inoculation, Other viral diseases

Coding Clarification
If a contraindication is evident in the patient, whether it is because of another condition or the patient's wishes, it should be coded with V64.0 *Vaccination not carried out because of contraindication*. Vaccinations against combinations of diseases should be coded with V06.0-V06.9.

Coding Scenario
A man traveling to South America presents for a yellow fever vaccination.

    Code assignment: V04.4 *Need for prophylactic vaccination and inoculation against yellow fever*

V05 Need for other prophylactic vaccination and inoculation against single diseases

V05.0 Need for prophylactic vaccination and inoculation against arthropod-borne viral encephalitis — *affects animals, wild birds, and transmitted by blood-sucking insects*
AHA: Jan-Feb, 1987, 8

V05.1 Need for prophylactic vaccination and inoculation against other arthropod-borne viral diseases

V05.2 Need for prophylactic vaccination and inoculation against Leishmaniasis — *causes lesions that look like leprosy*
AHA: Jan-Feb, 1987, 8

V05.3 Need for prophylactic vaccination and inoculation against viral hepatitis — *can be caused by IV drug use and unprotected sex*
AHA: Jan-Feb, 1987, 8

V05.4 Need for prophylactic vaccination and inoculation against varicella — *also called chicken pox*
AHA: Jan-Feb, 1987, 8

V05.8 Need for prophylactic vaccination and inoculation against other specified disease

V05.9 Need for prophylactic vaccination and inoculation against unspecified single disease

Coding Clarification
If a contraindication is evident in the patient, whether it is because of another condition or the patient's wishes, it should be coded with the appropriate code from subcategory V64.0 *Vaccination not carried out*. Vaccinations against combinations of diseases should be coded with V06.0-V06.9.

V06 Need for prophylactic vaccination and inoculation against combinations of diseases

AHA: Jan-Feb, 1987, 8

Code	Description
V06.0	Need for prophylactic vaccination against cholera with typhoid-paratyphoid (cholera + TAB) vaccine — (Use additional single vaccination codes from categories V03-V05 to identify any vaccinations not included in a combination code)
V06.1	Vaccination and inoculation need, prophylactic, combined diphtheria-tetanus-pertussis [DTP] [DTaP] — (Use additional single vaccination codes from categories V03-V05 to identify any vaccinations not included in a combination code)
V06.2	Need for prophylactic vaccination with diphtheria-tetanus-pertussis with typhoid-paratyphoid (DTP + TAB) vaccine
V06.3	Need for prophylactic vaccination with tetanus-pertussis with poliomyelitis (DTP + polio) vaccine — (Use additional single vaccination codes from categories V03-V05 to identify any vaccinations not included in a combination code)
V06.4	Need for prophylactic vaccination with measles-mumps-rubella (MMR) vaccine — (Use additional single vaccination codes from categories V03-V05 to identify any vaccinations not included in a combination code)
V06.5	Vaccination and inoculation need, prophylactic, tetanus-diphtheria [Td] [DT] — (Use additional single vaccination codes from categories V03-V05 to identify any vaccinations not included in a combination code)
V06.6	Need for prophylactic vaccination with Streptococcus pneumoniae (pneumococcus) and influenza — (Use additional single vaccination codes from categories V03-V05 to identify any vaccinations not included in a combination code)
V06.8	Need for prophylactic vaccination and inoculation against other combinations of diseases — (Use additional single vaccination codes from categories V03-V05 to identify any vaccinations not included in a combination code)
V06.9	Need for prophylactic vaccination with unspecified combined vaccine — (Use additional single vaccination codes from categories V03-V05 to identify any vaccinations not included in a combination code)

Documentation Issues

Combination vaccines should be clearly documented. Some vaccines are administered alone and some are combined into one injection.

Coding Clarification

If any additional vaccinations are given to the patient that are not included in the combination codes, they should be reported separately with V03-V05.

This category excludes V18.8 *Family history of infectious and parasitic diseases* and V12.0 *Personal history of infectious and parasitic diseases.*

Code V06.8 *Need for prophylactic vaccination and inoculation against other combinations of diseases* excludes multiple single-vaccination codes V03.0-V05.9.

Coding Scenario

A patient presents for routine Td administration.

> Code assignment: V06.5 *Vaccination and inoculation need, prophylactic, tetanus-diphtheria [Td] [DT]*

V07-V09 Persons with Need for Isolation, Other Potential Health Hazards and Prophylactic Measures

Isolation is provided to patients in cases where the patient has been exposed to a disease that could be transferred from one person to another or to protect a person from his or her surroundings.

Patients who have allergies to specific items (trees, plants, etc.) are typically given a series of shots over a period of time to improve their immunity or to desensitize their allergies.

Prophylactic measures include the administration of a substance for prevention of certain diseases or conditions, such as antivenin, RhoGAM, or tetanus administration in prophylactic immunotherapy.

V07 Need for isolation and other prophylactic measures

Isolation may be necessary to protect a patient from contamination or to protect other people from a patient who has been exposed to a highly transmissible disease. Isolation is designed to prevent the spread of a disease from one person to another. A person may contract an infectious disease by any of the following ways:

- Inhalation of air-borne evaporated or nonevaporated droplets or dust particles carrying microorganisms or spores, such as a sneeze from an infected patient
- Transmission from one host to another by a carrier of the disease, such as a mosquito
- Ingestion of a microorganism transmitted through water, such as when bathing

Some patients are more at risk of infection due to age, current state of health, and indwelling devices, such as catheters. Patients may be put in isolation while conditions are ruled out. Patients who are immunocompromised may be very susceptible to infections. Prophylactic isolation or other measures may be necessary to protect the patient.

V07.0	Need for isolation — *separating a patient from others* AHA: Jan-Feb, 1987, 8
V07.1	Need for desensitization to allergens — *gradual administration of allergens to prevent severe allergic reactions* AHA: Jan-Feb, 1987, 8
V07.2	Need for prophylactic immunotherapy — *therapeutic administration of serum containing antibodies to strengthen immune system* AHA: Jan-Feb, 1987, 8
V07.31	Need for prophylactic fluoride administration — *for the prevention of cavities* AHA: Jan-Feb, 1987, 8
V07.39	Need for other prophylactic chemotherapy — *may be given for hydatidiform mole* AHA: Jan-Feb, 1987, 8

This code excludes maintenance chemotherapy following disease, V58.11.

V07.4	Hormone replacement therapy (postmenopausal)
V07.8	Need for other specified prophylactic measure
V07.9	Need for unspecified prophylactic measure

Coding Clarification
If the patient is isolated as a result of terrorist acts, report V07.0 *Need for isolation.*

Use V07.2 *Need for prophylactic immunotherapy* for the administration of antivenin, immune sera (gamma globulin) RhoGAM, or tetanus antitoxin.

Coding Scenario
A woman presents to the OB/GYN clinic 48 hours after the birth of her baby for a postpartum injection of RhoGAM.

Code assignment: V07.2 *Need for prophylactic immunotherapy*

V08 Asymptomatic human immunodeficiency virus (HIV) infection status OK
AHA: Q2, 2004, 11

Human immunodeficiency virus (HIV) is a serious health concern. Two types of HIV are known to exist: HIV-1 and HIV-2. HIV-1 is widespread throughout the world and causes acquired immune deficiency syndrome (AIDS). HIV-2 is found primarily in West Africa and is seldom seen in the United States. Category V08 should be used during the first phase when the patient is asymptomatic. This usually occurs four weeks to six months after infected with HIV-1.

Documentation Issues
Documentation should clearly state that the patient is HIV positive but does not have and has never had any HIV-related illness.

Coding Clarification
Use this code when the patient presents with no HIV symptoms or conditions although the patient tests positive for HIV. If the patient has HIV symptoms or conditions, report 042. For exposure to HIV, use V01.7. For nonspecific serologic evidence of HIV, use 795.71.

Coding Scenario
An asymptomatic 23-year-old male presents for a follow-up of his HIV medication. The patient tested positive for HIV but reports that he has had no symptoms.

Code assignment: V08 *Asymptomatic human immunodeficiency virus (HIV) infection status*

V09 Infection with drug-resistant microorganisms
AHA: Jan-Feb, 1987, 8; Q4, 1993, 22; Q3, 1994, 4

Since the availability of penicillin and streptomycin, drug-resistance bacteria, parasites, viruses, and fungi have increasingly become a problem. Because of this, many common bacterial infections that were treated with antibiotics may become untreatable. Many of the new drugs used to treat drug-resistant diseases are expensive, which may limit the treatment of some patients. Drug resistance occurs as a result of overuse or underuse of antibiotic drugs, or from patients not completing treatment as prescribed. Health care professionals are more aware of drug resistance and are responding to this problem. New drugs are being developed to help fight these drug-resistant infections.

V09.0	Infection with microorganisms resistant to penicillins — (Use codes from this category as an additional code for infectious conditions classified elsewhere to indicate drug-resistance of the infectious organism) AHA: Jan-Feb, 1987, 8; Q4, 1993, 22; Q3, 1994, 4; Q4, 2003, 104, 106; Q2, 2006, 16
V09.1	Infection with microorganisms resistant to cephalosporins and other B-lactam antibiotics — (Use this code as an additional code for infectious conditions classified elsewhere to indicate drug-resistance of the infectious organism) AHA: Jan-Feb, 1987, 8; Q4, 1993, 22; Q3, 1994, 4
V09.2	Infection with microorganisms resistant to macrolides — (Use this code as an additional code for infectious conditions classified

Supplementary Classification of Factors Influencing Health Status and Contact with Health Services

Code	Description
	elsewhere to indicate drug-resistance of the infectious organism)
	AHA: Jan-Feb, 1987, 8; Q4, 1993, 22; Q3, 1994, 4
V09.3	Infection with microorganisms resistant to tetracyclines — (Use this code as an additional code for infectious conditions classified elsewhere to indicate drug-resistance of the infectious organism)
	AHA: Jan-Feb, 1987, 8; Q4, 1993, 22; Q3, 1994, 4
V09.4	Infection with microorganisms resistant to aminoglycosides — (Use this code as an additional code for infectious conditions classified elsewhere to indicate drug-resistance of the infectious organism)
	AHA: Jan-Feb, 1987, 8; Q4, 1993, 22; Q3, 1994, 4
V09.50	Infection with microorganisms resistant to quinolones and fluoroquinolones without mention of resistance to multiple quinolones and fluoroquinolones
V09.51	Infection with microorganisms resistant to quinolones and fluoroquinolones with resistance to multiple quinolones and fluoroquinolones
V09.6	Infection with microorganisms resistant to sulfonamides — (Use this code as an additional code for infectious conditions classified elsewhere to indicate drug-resistance of the infectious organism)
	AHA: Jan-Feb, 1987, 8; Q4, 1993, 22; Q3, 1994, 4
V09.70	Infection with microorganisms resistant to other specified antimycobacterial agents without mention of resistance to multiple antimycobacterial agents
V09.71	Infection with microorganisms resistant to other specified antimycobacterial agents with resistance to multiple antimycobacterial agents
V09.80	Infection with microorganisms resistant to other specified drugs without mention of resistance to multiple drugs
V09.81	Infection with microorganisms resistant to other specified drugs with resistance to multiple drugs — (Use this code as an additional code for infectious conditions classified elsewhere to indicate drug-resistance of the infectious organism)
V09.90	Infection with unspecified drug-resistant microorganisms, without mention of multiple drug resistance — (Use this code as an additional code for infectious conditions classified elsewhere to indicate drug-resistance of the infectious organism)
V09.91	Infection with unspecified drug-resistant microorganisms, with multiple drug resistance — (Use this code as an additional code for infectious conditions classified elsewhere to indicate drug-resistance of the infectious organism)

Coding Clarification
The infectious condition should be coded first; category V09 may be used only as a secondary diagnosis.

Code V09.4 *Infection with microorganisms resistant to aminoglycosides* includes amikacin, kanamycin, and streptomycin.

Coding Scenario
A patient is in for a follow-up of lobar pneumonia. A recent sputum culture identified *Streptococcus pneumoniae* as the infecting organism with resistance to penicillin.

Code assignment: 481 *Pneumococcal pneumonia (Streptococcus pneumoniae pneumonia)* and V09.0 *Infection with microorganisms resistant to penicillins*

V10–V19 Persons with Potential Health Hazards Related to Personal and Family History

Categories V10-V19 contain personal and family history codes. Personal history codes include a history of neoplasms, mental disorders, diseases, and allergies. Family history codes include a history of neoplasms and diseases. Personal history codes are often reported to indicate the need for adjunctive surgery and treatment; family history codes are often used to indicate the need for prophylactic surgery and treatment. Family history codes are frequently used with screening codes to justify a test or procedure. This range of codes should be used as secondary codes if the historical condition or family history has an impact on current care or influences treatment.

V10 Personal history of malignant neoplasm

In a malignancy, the neoplasm invades surrounding tissue or sheds cells that seed malignancy in other body sites. Codes in the V10 category describe a personal history of a malignant neoplasm. A personal history of malignant neoplasms identifies a malignancy that has been previously treated or removed but for which there is no current treatment for the condition and no evidence of the disease.

Code	Description
V10.0 ✓5th	Personal history of malignant neoplasm of gastrointestinal tract — *history of conditions reported by 140-159*
	AHA: May-June, 1985, 10; Jan-Feb, 1987, 1, 8; Q2, 1990, 9; Q3, 1992, 5; Q1, 1995, 4; Q4, 1998, 69; Q4, 2002, 80
V10.00	Personal history of malignant neoplasm of unspecified site in gastrointestinal tract

Code	Description
V10.01	Personal history of malignant neoplasm of tongue
V10.02	Personal history of malignant neoplasm of other and unspecified parts of oral cavity and pharynx
V10.03	Personal history of malignant neoplasm of esophagus
V10.04	Personal history of malignant neoplasm of stomach
V10.05	Personal history of malignant neoplasm of large intestine
V10.06	Personal history of malignant neoplasm of rectum, rectosigmoid junction, and anus
V10.07	Personal history of malignant neoplasm of liver
V10.09	Personal history of malignant neoplasm of other site in gastrointestinal tract
V10.1 ⌐sth	Personal history of malignant neoplasm of trachea, bronchus, and lung — *history of conditions reported by 162* **AHA:** May-June, 1985, 10; Jan-Feb, 1987, 1, 8; Q2, 1990, 9; Q3, 1992, 5; Q1, 1995, 4; Q4, 1998, 69; Q4, 2002, 80
V10.11	Personal history of malignant neoplasm of bronchus and lung
V10.12	Personal history of malignant neoplasm of trachea
V10.2 ⌐sth	Personal history of malignant neoplasm of other respiratory and intrathoracic organs — *history of conditions reported as 160, 161, 163-165* **AHA:** May-June, 1985, 10; Jan-Feb, 1987, 1, 8; Q2, 1990, 9; Q3, 1992, 5; Q1, 1995, 4; Q4, 1998, 69; Q4, 2002, 80
V10.20	Personal history of malignant neoplasm of unspecified respiratory organ
V10.21	Personal history of malignant neoplasm of larynx
V10.22	Personal history of malignant neoplasm of nasal cavities, middle ear, and accessory sinuses
V10.29	Personal history of malignant neoplasm of other respiratory and intrathoracic organs
V10.3	Personal history of malignant neoplasm of breast — *history of conditions reported by 174 and 175* **AHA:** May-June, 1985, 10; Jan-Feb, 1987, 1, 8; Q1, 1990, 21; Q2, 1990, 9; Q1, 1991, 16; Q3, 1992, 5; Q1, 1995, 4; Q4, 1997, 50; Q4, 1998, 65; Q4, 1998, 69; Q4, 2001, 66; Q4, 2002, 80; Q2, 2003, 5
V10.4 ⌐sth	Personal history of malignant neoplasm of genital organs — *history of conditions reported by 179-187* **AHA:** May-June, 1985, 10; Jan-Feb, 1987, 1, 8; Q2, 1990, 9; Q3, 1992, 5; Q1, 1995, 4; Q4, 1998, 69; Q4, 2002, 80
V10.40	Personal history of malignant neoplasm of unspecified female genital organ
V10.41	Personal history of malignant neoplasm of cervix uteri
V10.42	Personal history of malignant neoplasm of other parts of uterus
V10.43	Personal history of malignant neoplasm of ovary
V10.44	Personal history of malignant neoplasm of other female genital organs
V10.45	Personal history of malignant neoplasm of unspecified male genital organ
V10.46	Personal history of malignant neoplasm of prostate
V10.47	Personal history of malignant neoplasm of testis
V10.48	Personal history of malignant neoplasm of epididymis
V10.49	Personal history of malignant neoplasm of other male genital organs
V10.5 ⌐sth	Personal history of malignant neoplasm of urinary organs — *history of conditions reported by 188 and 189* **AHA:** May-June, 1985, 10; Jan-Feb, 1987, 1, 8; Q2, 1990, 9; Q3, 1992, 5; Q1, 1995, 4; Q4, 1998, 69; Q4, 2002, 80
V10.50	Personal history of malignant neoplasm of unspecified urinary organ
V10.51	Personal history of malignant neoplasm of bladder
V10.52	Personal history of malignant neoplasm of kidney **AHA:** Q2, 2004, 4
V10.53	Personal history of malignant neoplasm, renal pelvis
V10.59	Personal history of malignant neoplasm of other urinary organ
V10.6 ⌐sth	Personal history of leukemia — *history of conditions reported as 204-208* **AHA:** May-June, 1985, 10; Jan-Feb, 1987, 1, 8; Q2, 1990, 9; Q4, 1990, 3; Q4, 1991, 26; Q2, 1992, 13; Q3, 1992, 5; Q1, 1995, 4; Q4, 1998, 69; Q4, 2002, 80
V10.60	Personal history of unspecified leukemia
V10.61	Personal history of lymphoid leukemia
V10.62	Personal history of myeloid leukemia
V10.63	Personal history of monocytic leukemia
V10.69	Personal history of other leukemia
V10.7 ⌐sth	Personal history of other lymphatic and hematopoietic neoplasms — *history of conditions reported as 200-203* **AHA:** May-June, 1985, 10; May-June, 1985, 18; Jan-Feb, 1987, 1, 8; Q2, 1990, 9; Q3, 1992, 5; Q1, 1995, 4; Q4, 1998, 69; Q4, 2002, 80
V10.71	Personal history of lymphosarcoma and reticulosarcoma
V10.72	Personal history of Hodgkin's disease
V10.79	Personal history of other lymphatic and hematopoietic neoplasm
V10.8 ⌐sth	Personal history of malignant neoplasm of other sites — *history of conditions reported by 170-173, 190-195* **AHA:** May-June, 1985, 10; Jan-Feb, 1987, 1, 8; Q2, 1990, 9; Q3, 1992, 5; Q1, 1995, 4; Q4, 1998, 69; Q4, 2002, 80
V10.81	Personal history of malignant neoplasm of bone
V10.82	Personal history of malignant melanoma of skin
V10.83	Personal history of other malignant neoplasm of skin
V10.84	Personal history of malignant neoplasm of eye

Supplementary Classification of Factors Influencing Health Status and Contact with Health Services

Code	Description
V10.85	Personal history of malignant neoplasm of brain
V10.86	Personal history of malignant neoplasm of other parts of nervous system
V10.87	Personal history of malignant neoplasm of thyroid
V10.88	Personal history of malignant neoplasm of other endocrine glands and related structures
V10.89	Personal history of malignant neoplasm of other site
V10.9	Unspecified personal history of malignant neoplasm

Documentation Issues
Documentation should include that the malignancy has resolved and there is no further treatment directed at the site.

Coding Clarification
These codes should never be used if active disease is present. When a previously excised malignant neoplasm recurs at the same site, it is still considered a primary malignancy of that site and the history code should not be used. If the malignant neoplasm recurs at a different site, it is reported as a secondary malignant neoplasm and an additional code to identify a history of the malignancy site is reported using category V10.

Report V10.89 for a personal history of a malignant neoplasm of the peripheral, sympathetic, and parasympathetic nerves.

For leukemia in remission, report 204.xx-208.xx. For lymphatic and hematopoietic neoplasms in remission, report 200.xx-203.xx.

Observation of obstetric patients where the malignancy might affect the fetus should be reported with 655.0-655.9.

Coding Scenario
A 70-year-old female patient is admitted for a biopsy of a mass in the right breast. Ten years ago, the patient was treated with lumpectomy and chemotherapy for a malignancy in the left breast. The pathology report stated the right breast mass was benign.

> Code assignment: 217 *Benign neoplasms of the breast* and V10.3 *Personal history of malignant neoplasm of breast*

V11 Personal history of mental disorder
Mental illness covers a broad range of conditions. The causes of mental illness are not well understood. Some believe it is a functioning of the neurotransmitters in the brain; others believe that stress, drugs, and heredity may play a role in mental illness. Because heredity is believed to be a factor in mental illness, code the family history of mental illness when appropriate. Although prescription drugs may help, there is no known cure for these conditions.

Code	Description
V11.0	Personal history of schizophrenia — *withdraw into world of delusions* AHA: Jan-Feb, 1987, 1, 8
V11.1	Personal history of affective disorder — *pertaining to mood* AHA: Jan-Feb, 1987, 1, 8
V11.2	Personal history of neurosis — *anxiety, nervous disease* AHA: Jan-Feb, 1987, 1, 8
V11.3	Personal history of alcoholism — *alcohol addiction* AHA: Jan-Feb, 1987, 1, 8
V11.8	Personal history of other mental disorder
V11.9	Personal history of unspecified mental disorder

Documentation Issues
Documentation should include dates of illness, treatment, and that the illness is no longer present.

Coding Clarification
For patients who have a personal history of schizophrenia, but are in remission, report 295.0x-295.9x with a fifth digit of 5. For patients who have a personal history of manic-depressive psychosis, but are in remission, report 296.0x-296.6x with a fifth digit of 5 or 6.

Category V11 codes are so nonspecific, or potentially redundant with other codes in the classification, that there can be little justification for their use in the inpatient setting. Their use in the outpatient setting should be limited to those instances when there is no further documentation to permit more precise coding. Otherwise, any sign or symptom or any other reason for the visit that is captured in another code should be used.

Coding Scenario
A 75-year-old male presents from the nursing home with intermittent altered mental status. Past history includes alcoholism, although the patient went through a treatment program 10 years ago and has been clean and sober since. Blood alcohol is negative.

> Code assignment: 780.02 *Transient alteration of awareness* and V11.3 *Personal history of alcoholism*

V12 Personal history of certain other diseases
This category of codes is used to report that the patient had a particular disease but that the disease is no longer present and the patient is no longer receiving treatment for the illness.

Coders' Desk Reference for Diagnoses

V12.0 ⌐sth	Personal history of infectious and parasitic diseases — *disease capable of being transmitted from one person to another or disease caused by a parasite* **AHA:** Jan-Feb, 1987, 1, 8; Q3, 1992, 11		

This subcategory excludes personal history of infectious diseases specific to a body system.

V12.00	Personal history of unspecified infectious and parasitic disease
V12.01	Personal history of tuberculosis — *infection by Mycobacterium tuberculosis* **AHA:** Jan-Feb, 1987, 1, 8; Q3, 1992, 11
V12.02	Personal history of poliomyelitis — *polio enters the body through the digestive tract and spreads along nerve cells* **AHA:** Jan-Feb, 1987, 1, 8; Q3, 1992, 11
V12.03	Personal history of malaria — *caused by a parasite* **AHA:** Jan-Feb, 1987, 1, 8; Q3, 1992, 11
V12.09	Personal history of other infectious and parasitic disease
V12.1	Personal history of nutritional deficiency — *deprived of nutrition for an extended period of time* **AHA:** Jan-Feb, 1987, 1, 8; Q3, 1992, 11
V12.2	Personal history of endocrine, metabolic, and immunity disorders
V12.3	Personal history of diseases of blood and blood-forming organs
V12.4 ⌐sth	Personal history of disorders of nervous system and sense organs
V12.40	Personal history of unspecified disorder of nervous system and sense organs
V12.41	Personal history of benign neoplasm of the brain — *growth in the brain that is not malignant* **AHA:** Jan-Feb, 1987, 1, 8; Q3, 1992, 11; Q4, 1997, 48
V12.42	Personal history of infections of the central nervous system — *encephalitis, meningitis* **AHA:** Q4, 2005, 95
V12.49	Personal history of other disorders of nervous system and sense organs
V12.5 ⌐sth	Personal history of diseases of circulatory system — *related to blood flow throughout the body* **AHA:** Jan-Feb, 1987, 1, 8; Q3, 1992, 11; Q4, 1995, 61
V12.50	Unspecified circulatory disease
V12.51	Venous thrombosis and embolism — *use for pulmonary embolism* **AHA:** Jan-Feb, 1987, 1, 8; Q3, 1992, 11; Q4, 1995, 61; Q1, 2002, 15; Q4, 2003, 108
V12.52	Thrombophlebitis — *inflammation of the veins with clot* **AHA:** Jan-Feb, 1987, 1, 8; Q3, 1992, 11; Q4, 1995, 61
V12.59	Other diseases of circulatory system
V12.6 ⌐sth	Personal history of diseases of respiratory system

This subcategory excludes personal history of tuberculosis, V12.01.

V12.60	Personal history of unspecified disease of respiratory system
V12.61	Personal history of pneumonia (recurrent) **AHA:** Q4, 2005, 95
V12.69	Personal history of other diseases of respiratory system
V12.70	Personal history of unspecified digestive disease
V12.71	Personal history of peptic ulcer disease — *ulceration of the stomach* **AHA:** Jan-Feb, 1987, 1, 8; Q2, 1989, 16; Q3, 1992, 11; Q1, 1995, 3
V12.72	Personal history of colonic polyps — *benign growth in the colon* **AHA:** Jan-Feb, 1987, 1, 8; Q2, 1989, 16; Q3, 1992, 11; Q1, 1995, 3; Q3, 2002, 15
V12.79	Personal history of other diseases of digestive disease

Documentation Issues

Category V12 codes should be used when the presence of previous disease may affect the treatment or outcome of a current illness. The history of an illness should always be reported when documented.

Coding Clarification

Report V12.59 *Diseases of circulatory system* only when there are no lasting effects of the condition. If a patient has an old myocardial infarction, report 412; report 411.0 for postmyocardial infarction syndrome.

Coding Scenario

A patient presents to the emergency department with severe left lower abdominal pain. Past history is significant for colon polyps, which were removed a year ago.

> Code assignment: 789.04 *Pain left lower quadrant* and V12.72 *Personal history of colonic polyps*

V13 Personal history of other diseases

Personal history of other diseases codes are used to report that the patient had a particular disease but that the disease is no longer present. These codes also indicate that the patient is no longer receiving treatment for the illness.

V13.00	Personal history of unspecified urinary disorder
V13.01	Personal history of urinary calculi — *kidney stone* **AHA:** Jan-Feb, 1987, 1, 8
V13.02	Personal history of urinary (tract) infection **AHA:** Q4, 2005, 95

Code	Description
V13.03	Personal history of nephrotic syndrome AHA: Q4, 2005, 95
V13.09	Personal history of other disorder of urinary system
V13.1	Personal history of trophoblastic disease — *cell layer that erodes the uterine mucosa* AHA: Jan-Feb, 1987, 1, 8
V13.21	Personal history of pre-term labor — *22 to before 37 completed weeks of gestation* AHA: Jan-Feb, 1987, 1, 8; Q4, 2002, 78
V13.29	Personal history of other genital system and obstetric disorders
V13.3	Personal history of diseases of skin and subcutaneous tissue
V13.4	Personal history of arthritis — *inflammation of a joint* AHA: Jan-Feb, 1987, 1, 8
V13.5	Personal history of other musculoskeletal disorders
V13.61	Personal history of hypospadias — *urethra under the penis* AHA: Jan-Feb, 1987, 1, 8; Q4, 1998, 63
V13.69	Personal history of other congenital malformations\ AHA: Q1, 2004, 16
V13.7	Personal history of perinatal problems
V13.8	Personal history of other specified diseases
V13.9	Personal history of unspecified disease

Documentation Issues

Category V13 codes may be documented if the presence of a previous disease may affect the treatment or outcome of a current illness.

Coding Clarification

Category V13 codes may be listed as the primary or secondary diagnosis except for V13.4 *Personal history of arthritis* and V13.69 *Personal history of congenital malformations,* which are so nonspecific, or potentially redundant with other codes in the classification, that there can be little justification for their use in the inpatient setting. V13.61 *Personal history of hypospadias,* may only be used as a secondary diagnosis. Their use in the outpatient setting should be limited to those instances when there is no further documentation to permit more precise coding. Otherwise, any sign or symptom or any other reason for the visit that is captured in another code should be used.

Congenital malformations are typically lifelong problems and do not fall into the definition of "history." Congenital malformations such as hypospadias may be surgically repaired and would then qualify as a history as long as there are no residual or continued problems related to the malformation. Report V13.6x only if it directly affects the care of the patient.

Coding Scenario

A patient presents with right upper quadrant pain. Past medical history is significant for kidney stones, which were treated with lithotripsy.

Code assignment: 789.01 *Abdominal pain right upper quadrant* and V13.01 *Personal history of urinary calculi*

V14 Personal history of allergy to medicinal agents

Drug allergies should not be confused with normal side effects of the drug. Drug allergies can be life threatening. Symptoms of an allergy can be hives, skin rash, itching, wheezing, swelling of lips, tongue, or face, difficulty breathing, and rapid pulse. Allergic reactions are caused by an increased sensitivity of the immune system to the drug. An allergic reaction may not happen the first time the drug is taken, but as the body's immune system creates antibodies against the drug, the allergic reaction may appear in subsequent use of the drug. Treatment may include oral or topical antihistamines, nebulizer treatments, and epinephrine injections.

Code	Description
V14.0	Personal history of allergy to penicillin — *specific type of antibiotic* AHA: Jan-Feb, 1987, 1, 8
V14.1	Personal history of allergy to other antibiotic agent
V14.2	Personal history of allergy to sulfonamides — *specific type of antibiotic* AHA: Jan-Feb, 1987, 1, 8
V14.3	Personal history of allergy to other anti-infective agent
V14.4	Personal history of allergy to anesthetic agent — *usually local anesthetic* AHA: Jan-Feb, 1987, 1, 8
V14.5	Personal history of allergy to narcotic agent
V14.6	Personal history of allergy to analgesic agent — *a chemical that reduces pain* AHA: Jan-Feb, 1987, 1, 8
V14.7	Personal history of allergy to serum or vaccine
V14.8	Personal history of allergy to other specified medicinal agents
V14.9	Personal history of allergy to unspecified medicinal agent

Documentation Issues

Documentation should include the type and amount of the drug or agent taken and all symptoms the patient is experiencing as a result of the allergic reaction.

Coding Clarification

Codes from this category may only be reported as additional codes.

Coding Scenario
A 21-year-old female presents to the emergency department with a sore throat. A rapid strep test is given and results are positive. Past medical history is significant for allergy to penicillin.

>Code assignment: 034.0 *Streptococcal sore throat* and V14.0 *Personal history of allergy to penicillin*

V15 Other personal history presenting hazards to health

Food allergies are caused by the body's immune system building up antibodies to the food. Children whose parents both have allergies are more likely to have allergic reactions. The most common foods to cause an allergic reaction are peanuts, milk, eggs, and shellfish. Other reactions include allergies to insect bites, latex, and iodine found in some radiographic dye. Category V15 codes also include a personal history of surgery, abuse, psychological trauma, injury, tobacco use, and exposure to harmful substances that present hazards to the patient's health.

A personal history of extracorporeal membrane oxygenation (ECMO) is also included in category V15. ECMO gives respiratory support by circulating blood through an artificial lung, consisting of two compartments separated by a gas-permeable membrane, with blood on one side and the ventilating gas on the other. This is typically given to babies, but may be used in adults with acute respiratory distress.

Code	Description
V15.01	Personal history of allergy to peanuts
V15.02	Personal history of allergy to milk products
V15.03	Personal history of allergy to eggs
V15.04	Personal history of allergy to seafood — *octopus, squid ink, shellfish* **AHA:** Jan-Feb, 1987, 1, 8; Q4, 2000, 42, 49
V15.05	Personal history of allergy to other foods — *food additives, nuts (other than peanuts)* **AHA:** Jan-Feb, 1987, 1, 8; Q4, 2000, 42, 49
V15.06	Personal history of allergy to insects — *insect bites and stings* **AHA:** Jan-Feb, 1987, 1, 8; Q4, 2000, 42, 49
V15.07	Personal history of allergy to latex — *natural rubber latex allergy, type IV hypersensitivity reaction* **AHA:** Jan-Feb, 1987, 1, 8; Q4, 2000, 42, 49
V15.08	Personal history of allergy to radiographic dye — *contrast media used for diagnostic x-rays* **AHA:** Jan-Feb, 1987, 1, 8; Q4, 2000, 42, 49
V15.09	Personal history of other allergy, other than to medicinal agents
V15.1	Personal history of surgery to heart and great vessels, presenting hazards to health **AHA:** Q1, 2004, 16
V15.2	Personal history of surgery to other major organs, presenting hazards to health
V15.3	Personal history of irradiation, presenting hazards to health — *previous exposure to therapeutic or other ionizing radiation* **AHA:** Jan-Feb, 1987, 1, 8
V15.41	Personal history of physical abuse, presenting hazards to health — *rape, domestic violence* **AHA:** Jan-Feb, 1987, 1, 8; Q3, 1999, 15
V15.42	Personal history of emotional abuse, presenting hazards to health — *neglect* **AHA:** Jan-Feb, 1987, 1, 8; Q3, 1999, 15
V15.49	Other personal history of psychological trauma, presenting hazards to health
V15.5	Personal history of injury, presenting hazards to health
V15.6	Personal history of poisoning, presenting hazards to health
V15.7	Personal history of contraception, presenting hazards to health
V15.81	Personal history of noncompliance with medical treatment, presenting hazards to health
V15.82	Personal history of tobacco use, presenting hazards to health
V15.84	Personal history of exposure to asbestos, presenting hazards to health
V15.85	Personal history of exposure to potentially hazardous body fluids, presenting hazards to health
V15.86	Personal history of exposure to lead, presenting hazards to health
V15.87	History of extracorporeal membrane oxygenation [ECMO]
V15.88	Personal history of fall — *at risk for falling* **AHA:** Q4, 2005, 95
V15.89	Other specified personal history presenting hazards to health
V15.9	Unspecified personal history presenting hazards to health

Coding Clarification
A patient that has had a past allergic reaction to a substance should always be considered allergic to that agent.

This category of codes may only be reported as a secondary diagnosis, except V15.7 *Personal history of contraception*, which is so nonspecific, or potentially redundant with other codes in the classification, that there can be little justification for their use in the inpatient setting. V15.88 *Personal history of fall* may be used as a primary or secondary diagnosis. Their use in the outpatient setting should be limited to those instances when there is no further documentation to permit more precise coding. Otherwise, any sign or symptom or any other reason for the visit that is captured in another code should be used.

Report the medical condition in addition to V15.81 *Personal history of noncompliance with medical treatment, presenting hazards to health* if the condition is caused by noncompliance to medical instructions.

Coding Scenario
A patient presents with a productive cough, which has been present for the past three days. The past medical history is significant for a previous pack-a-day habit. The patient quit smoking one year ago.

    Code assignment: 786.2 *Cough* and V15.82 *Personal history of tobacco use, presenting hazards to health*

V16 Family history of malignant neoplasm
Many people with a family history of cancer have an increased risk of developing cancer. This is particularly true of the most common cancers of the breast, colon, ovary, and prostate. Family history codes are frequently used to indicate the need for prophylactic surgery and treatment.

V16.0	Family history of malignant neoplasm of gastrointestinal tract — *history of conditions reported by 140-159* AHA: Jan-Feb, 1987, 1, 8; Q1, 1999, 4
V16.1	Family history of malignant neoplasm of trachea, bronchus, and lung — *history of conditions reported by 162* AHA: Jan-Feb, 1987, 1, 8
V16.2	Family history of malignant neoplasm of other respiratory and intrathoracic organs — *history of conditions reported as 163-165* AHA: Jan-Feb, 1987, 1, 8
V16.3	Family history of malignant neoplasm of breast — *history of conditions reported by 174* AHA: Jan-Feb, 1987, 1, 8; Q1, 1992, 11; Q2, 2000, 8; Q2, 2003, 4; Q4, 2004, 107
V16.4 ⌐sth	Family history of malignant neoplasm of genital organs — *history of conditions reported by 179-187* AHA: Jan-Feb, 1987, 1, 8; Q4, 1997, 48
V16.40	Family history of malignant neoplasm, unspecified genital organ
V16.41	Family history of malignant neoplasm, ovary
V16.42	Family history of malignant neoplasm, prostate
V16.43	Family history of malignant neoplasm, testis
V16.49	Family history of other malignant neoplasm AHA: Q2, 2006, 3
V16.5 ⌐sth	Family history of malignant neoplasm of urinary organs — *history of conditions reported by 189* AHA: Jan-Feb, 1987, 1, 8
V16.51	Family history of malignant neoplasm of kidney
V16.59	Family history of malignant neoplasm of other urinary organs
V16.6	Family history of leukemia — *history of conditions reported by 204-208* AHA: Jan-Feb, 1987, 1, 8
V16.7	Family history of other lymphatic and hematopoietic neoplasms — *history of conditions reported by 200-203* AHA: Jan-Feb, 1987, 1, 8
V16.8	Family history of other specified malignant neoplasm — *history of conditions reported by 140-199* AHA: Jan-Feb, 1987, 1, 8
V16.9	Family history of unspecified malignant neoplasm

Documentation Issues
Documentation should include which family member had the cancer, at what age, and the outcome.

Coding Clarification
These codes are often used with screening codes, such as colonoscopy, to justify the test or procedure.

Coding Scenario
A 60-year-old female comes into the office for postmenopausal bleeding. She has a mother who died at the age of 61 of ovarian cancer.

    Code assignment: 627.1 *Postmenopausal bleeding* and V16.42 *Family history of malignant neoplasm, ovary*

V17 Family history of certain chronic disabling diseases
A family history of chronic disabling diseases includes psychiatric conditions, stroke, neurological diseases, ischemic heart disease, other cardiovascular diseases, asthma, other respiratory diseases, arthritis, and other musculoskeletal diseases. Many of these diseases are hereditary. Knowing the family history can help physicians order the appropriate screening or diagnostic tests, and diagnose and treat the patient's condition or symptoms.

V17.0	Family history of psychiatric condition — *history of conditions reported by 18.4* AHA: Jan-Feb, 1987, 1, 8
V17.1	Family history of stroke (cerebrovascular)
V17.2	Family history of other neurological diseases — *includes epilepsy and Huntington's chorea* AHA: Jan-Feb, 1987, 1, 8
V17.3	Family history of ischemic heart disease
V17.4	Family history of other cardiovascular diseases AHA: Q1, 2004, 6
V17.5	Family history of asthma
V17.6	Family history of other chronic respiratory conditions
V17.7	Family history of arthritis

V17.81	Family history of osteoporosis **AHA:** Q4, 2005, 95		V19.7	Family history of consanguinity — *blood-related kin* **AHA:** Jan-Feb, 1987, 1, 8
V17.89	Family history of other musculoskeletal diseases		V19.8	Family history of other condition

V18 Family history of certain other specific conditions

A family history of certain other specific conditions includes diabetes mellitus, other endocrine and metabolic diseases, anemia, other blood disorders, mental retardation, colon polyps or other digestive disorders, kidney diseases, other genitourinary diseases, and infectious and parasitic diseases. Knowing the family history can help physicians order the appropriate screening or diagnostic tests, and diagnose and treat the patient's condition or symptoms.

V18.0	Family history of diabetes mellitus **AHA:** Q1, 2004, 8
V18.1	Family history of other endocrine and metabolic diseases
V18.2	Family history of anemia
V18.3	Family history of other blood disorders
V18.4	Family history of mental retardation
V18.51	Family history, Colonic polyps

Coding Clarification
This code excludes family history of malignant neoplasm of gastrointestinal tract, which is reported with code V16.0.

V18.59	Family history, other digestive disorders
V18.61	Family history of polycystic kidney
V18.69	Family history of other kidney diseases
V18.7	Family history of other genitourinary diseases
V18.8	Family history of infectious and parasitic diseases
V18.9	Family history of genetic disease carrier **AHA:** Q4, 2005, 95

V19 Family history of other conditions

This category includes a family history of visual loss, other eye disorders, hearing loss, other ear disorders, skin conditions, congenital anomalies, allergic disorders, consanguinity, and other conditions. Knowing the family history can help physicians order the appropriate screening or diagnostic tests, and diagnose and treat the patient's condition or symptoms.

V19.0	Family history of blindness or visual loss
V19.1	Family history of other eye disorders
V19.2	Family history of deafness or hearing loss
V19.3	Family history of other ear disorders
V19.4	Family history of skin conditions
V19.5	Family history of congenital anomalies
V19.6	Family history of allergic disorders

V20–V28 Persons Encountering Health Services in Circumstances Related to Reproduction and Development

This section of codes is used to indicate the supervision of an uncomplicated pregnancy and perceived problems which, after evaluation, are determined to be normal states in development (e.g., onset of menses, teething). Codes used to report the outcome of a delivery on the mother's record (used in addition to codes from the obstetric section of ICD-9-CM) are also included.

V20 Health supervision of infant or child

Health supervision of an infant or a child involves medical or nursing care supervision of a healthy infant in cases of: physical or psychiatric maternal illness, adverse condition(s) at home, or too many children at home preventing normal care of the child. These codes include developmental testing of an infant or a child, immunizations appropriate for age, and routine vision and hearing testing.

V20.0	Health supervision of foundling
V20.1	Health supervision of other healthy infant or child receiving care
V20.2	Routine infant or child health check — (Use additional code(s) to identify special screening exams performed: V73.0-V82.9) — *initial/ subsequent routine newborn check* **AHA:** Q1, 2004, 15

Coding Clarification
Category V20 codes may only be reported as the primary diagnosis. Use additional codes to identify any special screening examinations performed.

Code V20.1 *Health supervision of other healthy infant or child receiving care* should not be reported on the baby's record after a routine C-section.

V21 Constitutional states in development

Constitutional states describe developmental conditions of a child during the growth period. This includes rapid growth, puberty, other development of adolescence, and low birth weight. Low birth weight status, which is 2,500 grams (5.59 pounds) or less, may affect the patient's health throughout life.

V21.0	Period of rapid growth in childhood

Supplementary Classification of Factors Influencing Health Status and Contact with Health Services

V21.1	Puberty — *sexual maturity*	
	AHA: Jan-Feb, 1987, 8	
V21.2	Other development of adolescence — *period beginning at puberty and ending at maturity*	
	AHA: Jan-Feb, 1987, 8	
V21.30	Low birth weight status, unspecified	
V21.31	Low birth weight status, less than 500 grams — *1.1 pounds or less*	
	AHA: Jan-Feb, 1987, 8; Q4, 2000, 51	
V21.32	Low birth weight status, 500-999 grams — *1.68-2.23 pounds*	
	AHA: Jan-Feb, 1987, 8; Q4, 2000, 51	
V21.33	Low birth weight status, 1000-1499 grams — *2.24-3.34 pounds*	
	AHA: Jan-Feb, 1987, 8; Q4, 2000, 51	
V21.34	Low birth weight status, 1500-1999 grams — *3.35-4.5 pounds*	
	AHA: Jan-Feb, 1987, 8; Q4, 2000, 51	
V21.35	Low birth weight status, 2000-2500 grams — *4.51-5.58 pounds*	
	AHA: Jan-Feb, 1987, 8; Q4, 2000, 51	
V21.8	Other specified constitutional states in development	
V21.9	Unspecified constitutional state in development	

Coding Clarification
Do not report status V codes for patients who have a condition that is classifiable to perinatal codes 760-779.

Report low birth weight status codes for patients who no longer have the condition but exhibit the consequences throughout life. Code V21.3 *Low birth weight status* excludes a history of perinatal problems.

Category V21 codes may be reported only as secondary/additional codes.

V22 Normal pregnancy
Normal pregnancies occur when there is no condition or problem that complicates the pregnancy. Complications may include ectopic and molar pregnancy, hydatidiform mole, spontaneous abortion, ectopic pregnancy, high blood pressure, and excessive vomiting.

Incidental pregnancy is when the patient comes in to see the provider for a reason other than the pregnancy, but the care of the patient may be affected by the pregnancy.

V22.0	Supervision of normal first pregnancy
V22.1	Supervision of other normal pregnancy
V22.2	Pregnant state, incidental

Coding Clarification
If a pregnant patient comes into the hospital for a non-stress test on the baby, V72.8 should be reported as the primary diagnosis with a secondary diagnosis code from category V22 or V23.

Codes V22.0 *Supervision of normal first pregnancy* and V22.1 *Supervision of other normal pregnancy* are generally used in outpatient settings. When a complication of the pregnancy is present, the code for that condition is assigned rather than a code from category V22. These codes are not used with any other pregnancy code.

Codes V22.0 *Supervision of normal first pregnancy* and V22.1 *Supervision of other normal pregnancy* are acceptable as first-listed only codes. Code V22.2 *Pregnancy state, incidental* may be used as an additional code only.

Coding Scenario
A patient presents to the office for a routine prenatal examination. The patient is 32 weeks along in her first pregnancy. Examination is normal and the patient has not experienced any complications with this pregnancy.

Code assignment: V22.0 *Supervision of normal first pregnancy*

V23 Supervision of high-risk pregnancy
Trophoblastic disease or hydatidiform mole is an abnormal product of conception in which the epithelial covering of the chorionic villi (the cellular, outmost membrane) disseminates and the avascular stroma of the villi proliferates and has cystic cavitation. The result is a mass of cells that resembles a bunch of grapes. This condition is also called cystic or vesicular mole.

V23.0	Pregnancy with history of infertility
V23.1	Pregnancy with history of trophoblastic disease — *includes hydatidiform mole and vesicular mole*
	AHA: Jan-Feb, 1987, 8; Q1, 1990, 10
V23.2	Pregnancy with history of abortion — *history of conditions reported with 634-638*
	AHA: Jan-Feb, 1987, 8; Q1, 1990, 10
V23.3	Pregnancy with grand multiparity
V23.4 ✔sth	Pregnancy with other poor obstetric history — *history of conditions reported by 630-676*
	AHA: Jan-Feb, 1987, 8; Q1, 1990, 10
V23.41	Supervision of pregnancy with history of pre-term labor
V23.49	Supervision of pregnancy with other poor obstetric history
V23.5	Pregnancy with other poor reproductive history — *history of stillbirth or neonatal death*
	AHA: Jan-Feb, 1987, 8; Q1, 1990, 10
V23.7	Insufficient prenatal care — *history of little or no prenatal care*
	AHA: Jan-Feb, 1987, 8; Q1, 1990, 10

V23.81	Supervision of high-risk pregnancy of elderly primigravida — *age 35 and older* **AHA:** Jan-Feb, 1987, 8; Q1, 1990, 10; Q4, 1998, 56,63	V24.1	Postpartum care and examination of lactating mother — *supervision of lactation* **AHA:** Jan-Feb, 1987, 8
V23.82	Supervision of high-risk pregnancy of elderly multigravida — *age 35 and older, 2nd or more pregnancies* **AHA:** Jan-Feb, 1987, 8; Q1, 1990, 10; Q4, 1998, 56,63	V24.2	Routine postpartum follow-up

V24.2 Routine postpartum follow-up

Coding Clarification
If the mother delivers outside of the hospital and is subsequently admitted for postpartum care, report V24.0 *Postpartum care and examination immediately after delivery*. Category V24 codes are normally used in the outpatient setting. If a postpartum complication is found, the appropriate pregnancy diagnosis codes should be assigned rather than a code from category V24.

Category V24 codes may be used only as the first listed diagnosis.

Coding Scenario
The patient presents for a routine postpartum visit. There are no complications present.

> Code assignment: V24.2 *Routine postpartum follow-up*

V23.83	Supervision of high-risk pregnancy of young primigravida — *less than 16 years of age* **AHA:** Jan-Feb, 1987, 8; Q1, 1990, 10; Q4, 1998, 56,63
V23.84	Supervision of high-risk pregnancy of young multigravida — *less than 16 years of age, 2nd or more pregnancies.* **AHA:** Jan-Feb, 1987, 8; Q1, 1990, 10; Q4, 1998, 56,63
V23.89	Supervision of other high-risk pregnancy
V23.9	Unspecified high-risk pregnancy

Documentation Issues
Documentation should include the risk factor of the patient and that there are no current complications of the pregnancy.

Health care providers must define "insufficient" prenatal care (V23.7) and consistently document this for the information to be useful.

Coding Clarification
Category V23 codes provide information on conditions that may add risk to a present pregnancy. A code from Chapter 11 in ICD-9-CM can be assigned with a code from category V23. The codes should be used when there is a history of a complication, but the pregnancy is progressing normally or when the patient's age could affect the pregnancy.

Coding Scenario
A 23-year-old female presents for her 36-week prenatal visit. A past medical history includes a spontaneous abortion at six weeks. This occurred one year ago. The current pregnancy is progressing normally.

> Code assignment: V23.2 *Pregnancy with history of abortion*

V24 Postpartum care and examination
The postpartum period (also called postnatal) of pregnancy begins at the birth of the child and continues for six weeks.

V24.0	Postpartum care and examination immediately after delivery — *care and observation in uncomplicated cases* **AHA:** Jan-Feb, 1987, 8

V25 Contraceptive management
Contraceptive management is used for patients who are trying to prevent pregnancy. There are many types of contraception, such as oral medication, that stops ovulation with the use of hormones, usually estrogen and/or progesterone; a barrier, such as a diaphragm, that is inserted into the uterus prior to coitus (intercourse), preventing the spermatozoa from entering the endometrial cavity and fallopian tubes; and an intrauterine device (IUD), which is typically a plastic or metal device fitted into the uterus.

Emergency contraceptive counseling is done postcoital (after intercourse), where a medication is prescribed within the first 72 hours after coitus to avoid pregnancy.

Another form of contraception is implantable medication that is inserted under the dermis. This medication is time released and usually lasts for a period of three months.

V25.01	General counseling for prescription of oral contraceptives
V25.02	General counseling for initiation of other contraceptive measures — *diaphragm fitting, prescription of foams, creams, or other agents* **AHA:** Jan-Feb, 1987, 8; Q4, 1992, 24; Q3, 1997, 7
V25.03	Encounter for emergency contraceptive counseling and prescription — *morning after pill* **AHA:** Q4, 2003, 84
V25.09	Other general counseling and advice for contraceptive management

Supplementary Classification of Factors Influencing Health Status and Contact with Health Services

Code	Description
V25.1	Insertion of intrauterine contraceptive device — IUD **AHA:** Jan-Feb, 1987, 8; Q4, 1992, 24
V25.2	Sterilization — *admission for tubal ligation or vasectomy* **AHA:** Jan-Feb, 1987, 8; Q4, 1992, 24
V25.3	Menstrual extraction — *menstrual regulation* **AHA:** Jan-Feb, 1987, 8; Q4, 1992, 24
V25.40	Unspecified contraceptive surveillance
V25.41	Surveillance of previously prescribed contraceptive pill
V25.42	Surveillance of previously prescribed intrauterine contraceptive device — *checking, reinsertion, or removal of IUD* **AHA:** Jan-Feb, 1987, 8; Q4, 1992, 24
V25.43	Surveillance of previously prescribed implantable subdermal contraceptive
V25.49	Surveillance of other previously prescribed contraceptive method
V25.5	Insertion of implantable subdermal contraceptive
V25.8	Other specified contraceptive management — *family planning advice* **AHA:** Jan-Feb, 1987, 8; Q4, 1992, 24; Q3, 1996, 9
V25.9	Unspecified contraceptive management

Coding Clarification
Report V45.5 if an intrauterine contraceptive device is already present.

Category V25 codes may be reported as either principal or secondary diagnoses.

Coding Scenario
An 18-year-old female presents for prescription of birth control pills.

> Code assignment: V25.01 *General counseling for prescription of oral contraceptives*

V26 Procreative management
Procreative management category codes describe health care services related to producing offspring. Services related to genetic testing and infertility services can be described with these codes. Health care encounters for reversal of a previous tubal ligation or vasectomy, artificial insemination, investigation and testing, and genetic counseling are included here.

Code	Description
V26.0	Tuboplasty or vasoplasty after previous sterilization
V26.1	Artificial insemination
V26.21	Fertility testing — *fallopian insufflation, sperm count for fertility testing* **AHA:** Jan-Feb, 1987, 8; Q4, 2000, 56

Code V26.21 excludes genetic counseling and testing, V26.31-V26.39.

Code	Description
V26.22	Aftercare following sterilization reversal — *fallopian insufflation following sterilization reversal, sperm count following sterilization reversal* **AHA:** Jan-Feb, 1987, 8; Q4, 2000, 56
V26.29	Other investigation and testing
V26.31	Testing of female for genetic disease carrier status **AHA:** Q4, 2005, 96
V26.32	Other genetic testing of female — (Use additional code to identify habitual aborter: 629.81, 646.3x) **AHA:** Q4, 2005, 96
V26.33	Genetic counseling **AHA:** Q4, 2005, 96
V26.34	Testing of male for genetic disease carrier status
V26.35	Encounter for testing of male partner of habitual aborter
V26.39	Other genetic testing of male
V26.4	General counseling and advice for procreative management
V26.51	Tubal ligation sterilization status
V26.52	Vasectomy sterilization status
V26.8	Other specified procreative management
V26.9	Unspecified procreative management

Coding Clarification
Codes used to describe a person's sterilization status are included here for both men and women. Code V25.2 *Sterilization* is often assigned as an additional diagnosis when a sterilization procedure is performed during the same admission as a delivery. It may also be assigned as a principal diagnosis when the admission is solely for sterilization.

If a failed tubal ligation results in pregnancy, code the pregnancy. If the visit is to evaluate tube patency, report V26.21 *Fertility testing*. Do not report V26.21 for genetic testing. Report 628.0-628.9 for infertility not due to previous tubal ligation.

The genetic counseling and testing codes allow for differentiating between patients who seek care to evaluate their genetic carrier status and those who have already tested positive as a carrier of genetic disease (V18.9). It is inappropriate to assign codes for genetic diseases not confirmed to be carried. Those who are carriers remain asymptomatic, but are capable of passing the disease on to offspring, who would be affected.

Category V26.3 excludes nonprocreative genetic screening, which is reported with code V82.71 or V82.72.

Coding Scenario
A 23-year-old female is admitted as an outpatient for fertility testing by fallopian insufflation.

Code assignment: V26.21 *Fertility testing*

V27 Outcome of delivery
AHA: Jan-Feb, 1987, 8; Q2, 1991, 16

Code	Description
V27.0	Outcome of delivery, single liveborn — (This code is intended for the coding of the outcome of delivery on the mother's record) AHA: Q4, 2005, 81
V27.1	Outcome of delivery, single stillborn — (This code is intended for the coding of the outcome of delivery on the mother's record)
V27.2	Outcome of delivery, twins, both liveborn — (This code is intended for the coding of the outcome of delivery on the mother's record)
V27.3	Outcome of delivery, twins, one liveborn and one stillborn — (This code is intended for the coding of the outcome of delivery on the mother's record)
V27.4	Outcome of delivery, twins, both stillborn — (This code is intended for the coding of the outcome of delivery on the mother's record)
V27.5	Outcome of delivery, other multiple birth, all liveborn — (This code is intended for the coding of the outcome of delivery on the mother's record)
V27.6	Outcome of delivery, other multiple birth, some liveborn — (This code is intended for the coding of the outcome of delivery on the mother's record)
V27.7	Outcome of delivery, other multiple birth, all stillborn — (This code is intended for the coding of the outcome of delivery on the mother's record)
V27.9	Outcome of delivery, unspecified — (This code is intended for the coding of the outcome of delivery on the mother's record) AHA: Jan-Feb, 1987, 8; Q2, 1991, 16

Documentation Issues
This category includes an unspecified code (V27.9); however, the health record should be reviewed again for more specific information.

Coding Clarification
Category V27 codes contain an optional code that may be assigned as an additional diagnosis on the mother's health record to indicate whether the outcome of delivery was single or multiple and liveborn or stillborn. These codes are intended for coding the outcome of delivery on the mother's record; the codes should not appear on the baby's record. These codes should also be used on all maternal delivery records. These codes should be reported for an attempted abortion that results in a live birth.

Category V27 codes are to be used as additional codes only.

Coding Scenario
A 25-year-old female is admitted for delivery of a full-term live infant.

Code assignment: 650 *Normal delivery* and V27.0 *Outcome of delivery, single liveborn*

V28 Encounter for antenatal screening of mother
AHA: Q1, 2004, 11

Antenatal screening is the testing of a baby before birth for a disease or disease precursors in seemingly well individuals so that early detection and treatment can be provided for those who test positive for the disease.

During amniocentesis, a needle is inserted into the womb and amniotic fluid is withdrawn. A number of tests can be performed on the fluid to confirm or rule out certain conditions.

Isoimmunization is the incompatibility of Rh and ABO between a mother and a fetus. The incompatibility is when an Rh-negative mother carries an Rh-positive fetus. Antibodies that are carried across the placenta into the fetus lead to hemolysis of the fetal blood. Symptoms that typically occur include edema, cardiomegaly, hepatomegaly, splenomegaly, pale skin, and severe generalized edema (hydrops fetalis).

Code	Description
V28.0	Screening for chromosomal anomalies by amniocentesis — *variation in the DNA strand that carries genetic information* AHA: Jan-Feb, 1987, 8
V28.1	Screening for raised alpha-fetoprotein levels in amniotic fluid — *abnormal levels may indicate, neural tube defects, anencephaly, omphalocele* AHA: Jan-Feb, 1987, 8
V28.2	Other antenatal screening based on amniocentesis
V28.3	Antenatal screening for malformation using ultrasonics — *abnormally formed fetus* AHA: Jan-Feb, 1987, 8
V28.4	Antenatal screening for fetal growth retardation using ultrasonics — *slow growth of the fetus* AHA: Jan-Feb, 1987, 8
V28.5	Antenatal screening for isoimmunization — *test for Rh factor* AHA: Jan-Feb, 1987, 8
V28.6	Screening of Streptococcus B
V28.8	Other specified antenatal screening
V28.9	Unspecified antenatal screening

Coding Clarification
Category V28 codes should only be used if no specific condition is found to exist during the screening process. Code the condition, not the screening, if one is discovered.

Supplementary Classification of Factors Influencing Health Status and Contact with Health Services

Coding Scenario
A 37-year-old female is admitted for an amniocentesis to rule out Down's syndrome.

> Code assignment: V28.0 *Antenatal screening for chromosomal anomalies by amniocentesis*

V29 Observation and evaluation of newborns and infants for suspected condition not found

Observation and evaluation of a newborn and infant are performed when a neonate (the first 28 days of life) is suspected of having a particular condition, resulting from exposure from the mother or birth process, which is ruled out after examination and observation.

V29.0	Observation and evaluation of newborns and infants for suspected infectious condition not found
V29.1	Observation and evaluation of newborns and infants for suspected neurological condition not found
V29.2	Observation and evaluation of newborns and infants for suspected respiratory condition not found
V29.3	Observation for suspected genetic or metabolic condition **AHA:** Q2, 2005, 21
V29.8	Observation and evaluation of newborns and infants for other specified suspected condition not found
V29.9	Observation and evaluation of newborns and infants for unspecified suspected condition not found

Coding Clarification
Category V29 codes may be reported only as primary diagnoses, unless they are documented with codes V30-V39. In this case, category V30-V39 codes will be listed as primary diagnoses and V29 codes will be listed as secondary diagnoses.

Coding Scenario
A five-day-old newborn is admitted to the hospital with suspected sepsis. Following blood cultures, the sepsis is ruled out.

> Code assignment: V29.0 *Observation and evaluation of newborns and infants for suspected infectious condition not found*

V30–V39 Liveborn Infants According to Type of Birth

Category V30-V39 codes are used for the primary diagnosis and describe the type of birth: single or multiple. These codes are used in the inpatient setting for most patients (fourth digit 0) but may be used for those born before admission (fourth digit 1) or not admitted to the hospital (fourth digit 2). The fifth digit identifies whether the delivery was vaginal or cesarean. A cesarean delivery is performed through an incision in the mother's abdomen. Most incisions are performed through a low horizontal incision but a vertical incision may be used in severe fetal distress.

V30 Single liveborn
AHA: Q1, 2004, 8, 16; Q4, 2005, 88

The following fourth-digit subdivisions are for use with categories V30-V39:

0 Born in hospital
1 Born before admission to hospital
2 Born outside hospital and not hospitalized

The following two fifth-digits are for use with the fourth-digit.0, Born in hospital:

0 delivered without mention of cesarean delivery
1 delivered by cesarean delivery

Cesarean delivery is performed through an incision into the mother's abdomen. Most incisions are performed through a low horizontal incision but a vertical incision may be used in severe fetal distress.

Coding Clarification
Category V30 codes may be used only as the first listed diagnosis and should only be used on the baby's record. If the baby is transferred to another hospital, the receiving hospital should not use this category of codes. The hospital that the baby is transferred to should report the condition of the baby that caused the need for transfer. These codes are intended for the coding of liveborn infants who are consuming health care (e.g., crib or bassinet occupancy).

Coding Scenario
A liveborn male infant is delivered in a hospital via a vaginal delivery.

> Code assignment: V30.00 *Single liveborn, born in hospital, delivered without mention of cesarean delivery*

V31 Twin birth, mate liveborn

Coding Clarification
Category V31 codes may be used only as the first listed diagnosis and should only be used on the baby's record. If the baby is transferred to another hospital, the receiving hospital should not use this category of codes. The hospital that the baby is transferred to should report the condition of the baby that caused the need for transfer. These codes are intended for the coding of liveborn infants who

are consuming health care (e.g., crib or bassinet occupancy).

Coding Scenario
Twin live males are born in the hospital by cesarean delivery.

> Code assignment: V31.01 *Twin birth, mate liveborn, born in hospital, delivered by cesarean delivery*

V32 Twin birth, mate stillborn
A stillborn is the delivery of a baby who is dead.

Coding Clarification
Category V32 codes may be used only as the first listed diagnosis and should only be used on the baby's record. If the baby is transferred to another hospital, the receiving hospital should not use this category of codes. The hospital that the baby is transferred to should report the condition of the baby that caused the need for transfer.

V33 Twin birth, unspecified whether mate liveborn or stillborn

Coding Clarification
Category V33 codes may be used only as the first listed diagnosis and should only be used on the baby's record. If the baby is transferred to another hospital, the receiving hospital should not use this category of codes. The hospital that the baby is transferred to should report the condition of the baby that caused the need for transfer. Category V33 codes are intended for the coding of liveborn infants who are consuming health care (e.g., crib or bassinet occupancy).

V34 Other multiple birth (three or more), mates all liveborn
Multiple births with more than three neonates may be a result of heredity or the use of a fertility drug. Typically, the neonates are delivered prematurely and have a low birth weight.

Coding Clarification
Category V34 codes may be used only as the first listed diagnosis and should only be used on the baby's record. If the baby is transferred to another hospital, the receiving hospital should not use these codes. The hospital that the baby is transferred to should report the condition of the baby that caused the need for transfer.

Coding Scenario
Triplets were born via low transverse cesarean section. All babies were liveborn and healthy.

> Code assignment: V34.01 *Other multiple birth, mates all liveborn, born in the hospital, delivered by cesarean delivery*

V35 Other multiple birth (three or more), mates all stillborn

Coding Clarification
Category V35 codes may be used only as the first listed diagnosis and should only be used on the baby's record. If the baby is transferred to another hospital, the receiving hospital should not use these codes. The hospital that the baby is transferred to should report the condition of the baby that caused the need for transfer. Category V35 codes are intended for the coding of liveborn infants who are consuming health care (e.g., crib or bassinet occupancy).

V36 Other multiple birth (three or more), mates liveborn and stillborn

Coding Clarification
Category V36 codes may be used only as the first listed diagnosis and should only be used on the baby's record. If the baby is transferred to another hospital, the receiving hospital should not use these codes. The hospital that the baby is transferred to should report the condition of the baby that caused the need for transfer. Category V36 codes are intended for the coding of liveborn infants who are consuming health care (e.g., crib or bassinet occupancy).

V37 Other multiple birth (three or more), unspecified whether mates liveborn or stillborn

Coding Clarification
Category V37 codes may be used only as the first listed diagnosis and should only be used on the baby's record. If the baby is transferred to another hospital, the receiving hospital should not use these codes. The hospital that the baby is transferred to should report the condition of the baby that caused the need for transfer. Category V37 codes are intended for the coding of liveborn infants who are consuming health care (e.g., crib or bassinet occupancy).

V39 Liveborn, unspecified whether single, twin, or multiple

Coding Clarification
Category V39 codes may be used only as the first listed diagnosis and should only be used on the baby's record. If the baby is transferred to another hospital, the receiving hospital should not use these

codes. The hospital that the baby is transferred to should report the condition of the baby that caused the need for transfer. Category V39 codes are intended for the coding of liveborn infants who are consuming health care (e.g., crib or bassinet occupancy).

V40–V49 Persons with a Condition Influencing Their Health Status

Category V40-V49 codes are used to describe circumstances other than a disease or an injury that influences a patient's health status. These codes describe the residual of a past disease or a condition that in some way affects the way the patient's treatment is carried out. The status codes are different from the history codes in that a history code indicates that the patient no longer has the disease. These codes should be used when the condition is documented as a diagnosis or problem.

V40 Mental and behavioral problems
AHA: Jan-Feb, 1987, 8

Mental problems include any conditions that affect the mood or behavior of a person. The conditions may include depression, dysphoria, personality disorder, and phobias. Mental problems may be caused by the malfunction of the brain's neurotransmitters, heredity, stress, or substance abuse.

Behavior problems affect the way people act. Problems include self-injury, aggressive behavior, hostility, and the inability to control actions.

V40.0	Problems with learning — (This code is intended for use when these conditions are recorded as diagnoses or problems) **AHA:** Jan-Feb, 1987, 8
V40.1	Problems with communication (including speech) — (This code is intended for use when these conditions are recorded as diagnoses or problems)
V40.2	Other mental problems — (This code is intended for use when these conditions are recorded as diagnoses or problems)
V40.3	Other behavioral problems — (This code is intended for use when these conditions are recorded as diagnoses or problems)
V40.9	Unspecified mental or behavioral problem — (This code is intended for use when these conditions are recorded as diagnoses or problems)

Coding Clarification
Category V40 codes are so nonspecific, or potentially redundant with other codes in the classification, that there can be little justification for their use in the inpatient setting. Their use in the outpatient setting should be limited to those instances when there is no further documentation to permit more precise coding. Otherwise, any sign or symptom or any other reason for the visit that is captured in another code should be used.

V41 Problems with special senses and other special functions
AHA: Jan-Feb, 1987, 8

V41.0	Problems with sight — (This code is intended for use when these conditions are recorded as diagnoses or problems)
V41.1	Other eye problems — (This code is intended for use when these conditions are recorded as diagnoses or problems)
V41.2	Problems with hearing — (This code is intended for use when these conditions are recorded as diagnoses or problems)
V41.3	Other ear problems — (This code is intended for use when these conditions are recorded as diagnoses or problems)
V41.4	Problems with voice production — (This code is intended for use when these conditions are recorded as diagnoses or problems)
V41.5	Problems with smell and taste — (This code is intended for use when these conditions are recorded as diagnoses or problems)
V41.6	Problems with swallowing and mastication — (This code is intended for use when these conditions are recorded as diagnoses or problems) **AHA:** Jan-Feb, 1987, 8
V41.7	Problems with sexual function — (This code is intended for use when these conditions are recorded as diagnoses or problems)
V41.8	Other problems with special functions — (This code is intended for use when these conditions are recorded as diagnoses or problems)
V41.9	Unspecified problem with special functions — (This code is intended for use when these conditions are recorded as diagnoses or problems)

Coding Clarification
This category of codes is generic. Check in the disease/condition section of ICD-9-CM to verify that no other code better describes the symptoms and/or disease/condition of the patient.

Category V41 codes are so nonspecific, or potentially redundant with other codes in the classification, that there can be little justification for their use in the inpatient setting. Their use in the outpatient setting should be limited to those instances when there is no further documentation to permit more precise coding. Otherwise, any sign or symptom or any other reason for the visit that is captured in another code should be used.

V42 Organ or tissue replaced by transplant
AHA: Jan-Feb, 1987, 8; Q3, 1998, 3, 4

Patients who require organ transplantation may have a variety or diseases and/or conditions. They may have end-stage renal disease (kidney) or mitral or aortic valve stenosis (heart valve).

Code	Description
V42.0	Kidney replaced by transplant — (This code is intended for use when these conditions are recorded as diagnoses or problems) **AHA:** Q1, 2003, 10
V42.1	Heart replaced by transplant — (This code is intended for use when these conditions are recorded as diagnoses or problems)
V42.2	Heart valve replaced by transplant — (This code is intended for use when these conditions are recorded as diagnoses or problems)
V42.3	Skin replaced by transplant — (This code is intended for use when these conditions are recorded as diagnoses or problems)
V42.4	Bone replaced by transplant — (This code is intended for use when these conditions are recorded as diagnoses or problems)
V42.5	Cornea replaced by transplant — (This code is intended for use when these conditions are recorded as diagnoses or problems)
V42.6	Lung replaced by transplant — (This code is intended for use when these conditions are recorded as diagnoses or problems)
V42.7	Liver replaced by transplant — (This code is intended for use when these conditions are recorded as diagnoses or problems)
V42.81	Bone marrow replaced by transplant — (This code is intended for use when these conditions are recorded as diagnoses or problems)
V42.82	Peripheral stem cells replaced by transplant — (This code is intended for use when these conditions are recorded as diagnoses or problems)
V42.83	Pancreas replaced by transplant — (This code is intended for use when these conditions are recorded as diagnoses or problems) **AHA:** Q1, 2003, 10
V42.84	Organ or tissue replaced by transplant, intestines — (This code is intended for use when these conditions are recorded as diagnoses or problems)
V42.89	Other organ or tissue replaced by transplant — (This code is intended for use when these conditions are recorded as diagnoses or problems)
V42.9	Unspecified organ or tissue replaced by transplant — (This code is intended for use when these conditions are recorded as diagnoses or problems)

Coding Clarification
Category V42 codes should be used for homologous or heterologous (animal) (human) transplant organ status. Transplant status codes indicate that a person has had an organ replaced but there are no current complications with the transplant. Do not report V42 category codes with 996.8 *Complications of a transplanted organ.*

Category V42 codes are to be used as additional codes only.

Coding Scenario
A patient presents to the clinic for an annual check of his transplanted kidney. Lab work and examination are normal.

> Code assignment: V42.0 *Kidney replaced by transplant*

V43 Organ or tissue replaced by other means
AHA: Jan-Feb, 1987, 8

"Other means" describes anatomical parts that have been replaced with an artificial or mechanical device or prosthesis rather than from another body part or another person.

Code	Description
V43.0	Eye globe replaced by other means — (This code is intended for use when these conditions are recorded as diagnoses or problems) **AHA:** Jan-Feb, 1987, 8
V43.1	Lens replaced by other means — (This code is intended for use when these conditions are recorded as diagnoses or problems) **AHA:** Jan-Feb, 1987, 8; Q4, 1998, 65
V43.21	Status, Organ or tissue replaced by other means, Heart assist device — (This code is intended for use when these conditions are recorded as diagnoses or problems)
V43.22	Status, Organ or tissue replaced by other means, Fully implantable artificial heart — (This code is intended for use when these conditions are recorded as diagnoses or problems)
V43.3	Heart valve replaced by other means — (This code is intended for use when these conditions are recorded as diagnoses or problems)
V43.4	Blood vessel replaced by other means — (This code is intended for use when these conditions are recorded as diagnoses or problems)
V43.5	Bladder replaced by other means — (This code is intended for use when these conditions are recorded as diagnoses or problems)
V43.60	Unspecified joint replacement by other means — (This code is intended for use when these conditions are recorded as diagnoses or problems) **AHA:** Q4, 2005, 91
V43.61	Shoulder joint replacement by other means — (This code is intended for use when these conditions are recorded as diagnoses or problems) **AHA:** Q4, 2005, 91
V43.62	Elbow joint replacement by other means — (This code is intended for use when these conditions are recorded as diagnoses or problems) **AHA:** Q4, 2005, 91

Supplementary Classification of Factors Influencing Health Status and Contact with Health Services

V43.63 Wrist joint replacement by other means — (This code is intended for use when these conditions are recorded as diagnoses or problems)
AHA: Q4, 2005, 91

V43.64 Hip joint replacement by other means — (This code is intended for use when these conditions are recorded as diagnoses or problems)
AHA: Jan-Feb, 1987, 8; Q2, 2004, 15; Q4, 2005, 91, 93, 112

V43.65 Knee joint replacement by other means — (This code is intended for use when these conditions are recorded as diagnoses or problems)
AHA: Q4, 2005, 91

V43.66 Ankle joint replacement by other means — (This code is intended for use when these conditions are recorded as diagnoses or problems)
AHA: Q4, 2005, 91

V43.69 Other joint replacement by other means — (This code is intended for use when these conditions are recorded as diagnoses or problems)
AHA: Q4, 2005, 91

V43.7 Limb replaced by other means — (This code is intended for use when these conditions are recorded as diagnoses or problems)

V43.81 Larynx replaced by other means — (This code is intended for use when these conditions are recorded as diagnoses or problems)
AHA: Jan-Feb, 1987, 8; Q4, 1995, 55

V43.82 Breast replaced by other means — (This code is intended for use when these conditions are recorded as diagnoses or problems)

V43.83 Organ or tissue replaced by artificial skin — (This code is intended for use when these conditions are recorded as diagnoses or problems)

V43.89 Other organ or tissue replaced by other means — (This code is intended for use when these conditions are recorded as diagnoses or problems)

Coding Clarification
Category V43 codes may be reported only as secondary diagnoses except for V43.22, which may be used as either the primary or secondary diagnosis.

Coding Scenario
A patient presents to the emergency department with a closed fracture of the right medial malleolus. A past medical history indicates that the patient had total hip placement on the right side five years ago.

Code assignment: 824.0 *Fracture of medial malleolus closed* and V43.64 *Hip joint replacement by other means*

V44 Artificial opening status
AHA: Jan-Feb, 1987, 8

A stoma is an artifical opening between the body cavities or organs and the body's surface.

V44.0 Tracheostomy status — (This code is intended for use when these conditions are recorded as diagnoses or problems)
AHA: Jan-Feb, 1987, 8; Q1, 2001, 6; Q4, 2003, 103, 107, 111

V44.1 Gastrostomy status — (This code is intended for use when these conditions are recorded as diagnoses or problems)
AHA: Jan-Feb, 1987, 8; Q1, 1993, 26; Q3, 1997, 12; Q1, 2001, 12; Q4, 2003, 103, 107-108, 110

V44.2 Ileostomy status — (This code is intended for use when these conditions are recorded as diagnoses or problems)
AHA: Jan-Feb, 1987, 8

V44.3 Colostomy status — (This code is intended for use when these conditions are recorded as diagnoses or problems)
AHA: Jan-Feb, 1987, 8; Q4, 2003, 110

V44.4 Status of other artificial opening of gastrointestinal tract — (This code is intended for use when these conditions are recorded as diagnoses or problems)

V44.5 Cystostomy status — (This subcategory is intended for use when these conditions are recorded as diagnoses or problems)
AHA: Jan-Feb, 1987, 8

V44.50 Unspecified cystostomy status — (This code is intended for use when these conditions are recorded as diagnoses or problems)

V44.51 Cutaneous-vesicostomy status — (This code is intended for use when these conditions are recorded as diagnoses or problems)
AHA: Jan-Feb, 1987, 8

V44.52 Appendico-vesicostomy status — (This code is intended for use when these conditions are recorded as diagnoses or problems)
AHA: Jan-Feb, 1987, 8

V44.59 Other cystostomy status — (This code is intended for use when these conditions are recorded as diagnoses or problems)

V44.6 Status of other artificial opening of urinary tract — (This code is intended for use when these conditions are recorded as diagnoses or problems)
AHA: Jan-Feb, 1987, 8

V44.7 Artificial vagina status — (This code is intended for use when these conditions are recorded as diagnoses or problems)

V44.8 Other artificial opening status — (This code is intended for use when these conditions are recorded as diagnoses or problems)

V44.9 Unspecified artificial opening status — (This code is intended for use when these conditions are recorded as diagnoses or problems)

Coding Clarification
Category V44 codes should be used when the reason for the visit is for attention or management of an artificial opening such as a tracheostomy, colostomy, or cystostomy and should only be reported as secondary diagnoses.

Category V44 codes are to be used as additional codes only.

V45 Other postsurgical states
AHA: Jan-Feb, 1987, 8; Q4, 2003, 85

Acquired absence of an organ indicates that an organ was removed surgically and not as a result of a congenital abnormality.

V45.00	Unspecified cardiac device in situ — (This code is intended for use when these conditions are recorded as diagnoses or problems)
V45.01	Cardiac pacemaker in situ — (This code is intended for use when these conditions are recorded as diagnoses or problems)— hemodialysis status, peritoneal dialysis status
V45.02	Automatic implantable cardiac defibrillator in situ — (This code is intended for use when these conditions are recorded as diagnoses or problems)
V45.09	Other specified cardiac device in situ — (This code is intended for use when these conditions are recorded as diagnoses or problems) AHA: Jan-Feb, 1987, 8
V45.1	Renal dialysis status — (This code is intended for use when these conditions are recorded as diagnoses or problems) AHA: Jan-Feb, 1987, 8; Q2, 2001, 12, 13; Q2, 2003, 7; Q1, 2004, 22-23; Q4, 2005, 96
V45.2	Presence of cerebrospinal fluid drainage device — (This code is intended for use when these conditions are recorded as diagnoses or problems) AHA: Jan-Feb, 1987, 8; Q4, 2003, 106
V45.3	Intestinal bypass or anastomosis status — (This code is intended for use when these conditions are recorded as diagnoses or problems)

Coding Clarification
Report bariatric surgery, gastric bypass, or obesity surgery status with code V45.86.

V45.4	Arthrodesis status — (This code is intended for use when these conditions are recorded as diagnoses or problems) AHA: Nov-Dec, 1984, 18; Jan-Feb, 1987, 8
V45.51	Presence of intrauterine contraceptive device — (This code is intended for use when these conditions are recorded as diagnoses or problems) AHA: Jan-Feb, 1987, 8
V45.52	Presence of subdermal contraceptive device — (This code is intended for use when these conditions are recorded as diagnoses or problems) AHA: Jan-Feb, 1987, 8
V45.59	Presence of other contraceptive device — (This code is intended for use when these conditions are recorded as diagnoses or problems)
V45.61	Cataract extraction status — (Use additional code for associated artificial lens status, V43.1)
V45.69	Other states following surgery of eye and adnexa — (This code is intended for use when these conditions are recorded as diagnoses or problems)
V45.71	Acquired absence of breast — (This code is intended for use when these conditions are recorded as diagnoses or problems)
V45.72	Acquired absence of intestine (large) (small) — (This code is intended for use when these conditions are recorded as diagnoses or problems)
V45.73	Acquired absence of kidney — (This code is intended for use when these conditions are recorded as diagnoses or problems)
V45.74	Acquired absence of organ, other parts of urinary tract — (This code is intended for use when these conditions are recorded as diagnoses or problems) AHA: Jan-Feb, 1987, 8; Q4, 1997, 50; Q4, 1998, 65; Q4, 2000, 51
V45.75	Acquired absence of organ, stomach — (This code is intended for use when these conditions are recorded as diagnoses or problems)
V45.76	Acquired absence of organ, lung — (This code is intended for use when these conditions are recorded as diagnoses or problems)
V45.77	Acquired absence of organ, genital organs — (This code is intended for use when these conditions are recorded as diagnoses or problems) AHA: Jan-Feb, 1987, 8; Q4, 1997, 50; Q4, 1998, 65; Q4, 2000, 51; Q1, 2003, 13-14
V45.78	Acquired absence of organ, eye — (This code is intended for use when these conditions are recorded as diagnoses or problems)
V45.79	Other acquired absence of organ — (This code is intended for use when these conditions are recorded as diagnoses or problems)
V45.81	Postsurgical aortocoronary bypass status — (This code is intended for use when these conditions are recorded as diagnoses or problems) AHA: Jan-Feb, 1987, 8; Q3, 1997, 16; Q3, 2001, 15; Q4, 2003, 105
V45.82	Postsurgical percutaneous transluminal coronary angioplasty status — (This code is intended for use when these conditions are recorded as diagnoses or problems) AHA: Jan-Feb, 1987, 8
V45.83	Breast implant removal status — (This code is intended for use when these conditions are recorded as diagnoses or problems)
V45.84	Dental restoration status — (This code is intended for use when these conditions are recorded as diagnoses or problems) AHA: Jan-Feb, 1987, 8; Q4, 2001, 54
V45.85	Insulin pump status — (This code is intended for use when these conditions are recorded as diagnoses or problems)
V45.86	Bariatric surgery status — *gastric banding, gastric bypass, obesity surgery status*

This code excludes bariatric surgery status complicating pregnancy, childbirth, and the puerperium, which is reported with a code from subcategory 649.2. Also excluded is intestinal bypass or anastomosis status (V45.3).

V45.89 Other postsurgical status — (This code is intended for use when these conditions are recorded as diagnoses or problems)
AHA: Jan-Feb, 1987, 8; Q1, 1995, 11

Coding Clarification

Category V45 codes may be reported only as secondary diagnoses except for codes in subcategory V45.7, which may be reported either as the primary or secondary diagnosis.

Female genital mutilation status is not reported with code V45.77, but with a code from range 629.20–629.29.

For the malfunction of a nervous system device, implant, or graft, report 996.2. For the complication of a contraceptive device, report 996.32.

V46 Other dependence on machines
AHA: Jan-Feb, 1987, 8

Patients who are dependent on machines typically have had a chronic illness in which the disease or condition has decreased their lung capacity or have suffered some form of significant trauma. Hyperbaric chambers reduce hypoxia and edema from injuries, which may include crush injuries and acute traumatic peripheral ischemias.

V46.0 Dependence on aspirator — (This code is intended for use when these conditions are recorded as diagnoses or problems)
V46.11 Dependence on respirator, status
AHA: Q4, 2004, 100; Q4, 2005, 96
V46.12 Encounter for respirator dependence during power failure
AHA: Q4, 2004, 100; Q4, 2005, 96
V46.13 Encounter for weaning from respirator [ventilator]
AHA: Q4, 2005, 96
V46.14 Mechanical complication of respirator [ventilator] — mechanical failure of respirator [ventilator]
V46.2 Dependence on machine for supplemental oxygen — (This code is intended for use when these conditions are recorded as diagnoses or problems)
AHA: Jan-Feb, 1987, 8; Q4, 2002, 79; Q4, 2003, 108
V46.8 Dependence on other enabling machine — (This code is intended for use when these conditions are recorded as diagnoses or problems)
AHA: Jan-Feb, 1987, 8

V46.9 Unspecified machine dependence — (This code is intended for use when these conditions are recorded as diagnoses or problems)

Coding Clarification

Category V46 codes may be used only as an additional diagnosis, except within subcategory V46.1, when the sole reason for the visit may be to sustain respiratory function needs due to power or mechanical failure of equipment, or to receive aid in breathing independently without the respirator [ventilator].

V47 Other problems with internal organs
AHA: Jan-Feb, 1987, 8

V47.0 Deficiencies of internal organs — (This code is intended for use when these conditions are recorded as diagnoses or problems)
V47.1 Mechanical and motor problems with internal organs — (This code is intended for use when these conditions are recorded as diagnoses or problems)
V47.2 Other cardiorespiratory problems — (This code is intended for use when these conditions are recorded as diagnoses or problems)
V47.3 Other digestive problems — (This code is intended for use when these conditions are recorded as diagnoses or problems)
V47.4 Other urinary problems — (This code is intended for use when these conditions are recorded as diagnoses or problems)
V47.5 Other genital problems — (This code is intended for use when these conditions are recorded as diagnoses or problems)
V47.9 Unspecified problems with internal organs — (This code is intended for use when these conditions are recorded as diagnoses or problems)

Coding Clarification

This category of codes is generic. Check in the disease/condition section of ICD-9-CM to verify that no other code better describes the symptoms and/or disease/condition of the patient.

Category V47 codes are so nonspecific, or potentially redundant with other codes in the classification, that there can be little justification for their use in the inpatient setting. Their use in the outpatient setting should be limited to those instances when there is no further documentation to permit more precise coding. Otherwise, any sign or symptom or any other reason for the visit that is captured in another code should be used.

Code V47.2 *Other cardiorespiratory problems* includes cardiovascular exercise intolerance with pain at rest, with less than ordinary activity, and with ordinary activity.

V48 Problems with head, neck, and trunk
AHA: Jan-Feb, 1987, 8

V48.0   Deficiencies of head — (This code is intended for use when these conditions are recorded as diagnoses or problems)

V48.1   Deficiencies of neck and trunk — (This code is intended for use when these conditions are recorded as diagnoses or problems)

V48.2   Mechanical and motor problems with head — (This code is intended for use when these conditions are recorded as diagnoses or problems)

V48.3   Mechanical and motor problems with neck and trunk — (This code is intended for use when these conditions are recorded as diagnoses or problems)

V48.4   Sensory problem with head — (This code is intended for use when these conditions are recorded as diagnoses or problems)

V48.5   Sensory problem with neck and trunk — (This code is intended for use when these conditions are recorded as diagnoses or problems)

V48.6   Disfigurements of head — (This code is intended for use when these conditions are recorded as diagnoses or problems)

V48.7   Disfigurements of neck and trunk — (This code is intended for use when these conditions are recorded as diagnoses or problems)

V48.8   Other problems with head, neck, and trunk — (This code is intended for use when these conditions are recorded as diagnoses or problems)

V48.9   Unspecified problem with head, neck, or trunk — (This code is intended for use when these conditions are recorded as diagnoses or problems)

Coding Clarification
This category of codes is generic. Check in the disease/condition section of ICD-9-CM to verify that no other code better describes the symptoms and/or disease/condition of the patient. Category V48 codes may be used only as an additional diagnosis.

Report V48.8 for deficiencies of the ears, eyelids, and nose.

V49 Problems with limbs and other problems
AHA: Jan-Feb, 1987, 8

V49.0   Deficiencies of limbs — (This code is intended for use when these conditions are recorded as diagnoses or problems)

V49.1   Mechanical problems with limbs — (This code is intended for use when these conditions are recorded as diagnoses or problems)

V49.2   Motor problems with limbs — (This code is intended for use when these conditions are recorded as diagnoses or problems)

V49.3   Sensory problems with limbs — (This code is intended for use when these conditions are recorded as diagnoses or problems)

V49.4   Disfigurements of limbs — (This code is intended for use when these conditions are recorded as diagnoses or problems)

V49.5   Other problems of limbs — (This code is intended for use when these conditions are recorded as diagnoses or problems)

V49.60   Upper limb amputation, unspecified level — (This code is intended for use when these conditions are recorded as diagnoses or problems)
AHA: Q4, 2005, 94

V49.61   Upper limb amputation, thumb — (This code is intended for use when these conditions are recorded as diagnoses or problems)
AHA: Q4, 2005, 94

V49.62   Upper limb amputation, other finger(s) — (This code is intended for use when these conditions are recorded as diagnoses or problems)
AHA: Q2, 2005, 7; Q4, 2005, 94

V49.63   Upper limb amputation, hand — (This code is intended for use when these conditions are recorded as diagnoses or problems)
AHA: Q4, 2005, 94

V49.64   Upper limb amputation, wrist — (This code is intended for use when these conditions are recorded as diagnoses or problems)
AHA: Jan-Feb, 1987, 8; Q4, 1994, 39; Q4, 1998, 42; Q4, 2005, 94

V49.65   Upper limb amputation, below elbow — (This code is intended for use when these conditions are recorded as diagnoses or problems)
AHA: Q4, 2005, 94

V49.66   Upper limb amputation, above elbow — (This code is intended for use when these conditions are recorded as diagnoses or problems)
AHA: Jan-Feb, 1987, 8; Q4, 1994, 39; Q4, 1998, 42; Q4, 2005, 94

V49.67   Upper limb amputation, shoulder — (This code is intended for use when these conditions are recorded as diagnoses or problems)
AHA: Jan-Feb, 1987, 8; Q4, 1994, 39; Q4, 1998, 42; Q4, 2005, 94

V49.70   Upper limb amputation, unspecified level — (This code is intended for use when these conditions are recorded as diagnoses or problems)
AHA: Q4, 2005, 94

V49.71   Upper limb amputation, great toe — (This code is intended for use when these conditions are recorded as diagnoses or problems)
AHA: Q4, 2005, 94

V49.72   Upper limb amputation, other toe(s) — (This code is intended for use when these conditions are recorded as diagnoses or problems)
AHA: Q4, 2005, 94

V49.73   Upper limb amputation, foot — (This code is intended for use when these conditions are recorded as diagnoses or problems)
AHA: Q4, 2005, 94

Code	Description
V49.74	Upper limb amputation, ankle — (This code is intended for use when these conditions are recorded as diagnoses or problems) AHA: Jan-Feb, 1987, 8; Q4, 1994, 39; Q4, 1998, 42; Q4, 2005, 94
V49.75	Lower limb amputation, below knee — (This code is intended for use when these conditions are recorded as diagnoses or problems) AHA: Q4, 2005, 94
V49.76	Lower limb amputation, above knee — (This code is intended for use when these conditions are recorded as diagnoses or problems) AHA: Jan-Feb, 1987, 8; Q4, 1994, 39; Q4, 1998, 42; Q2, 2005, 14; Q4, 2005, 94
V49.77	Upper limb amputation, hip — (This code is intended for use when these conditions are recorded as diagnoses or problems) AHA: Jan-Feb, 1987, 8; Q4, 1994, 39; Q4, 1998, 42; Q4, 2005, 94
V49.81	Asymptomatic postmenopausal status (age-related) (natural) — (This code is intended for use when these conditions are recorded as diagnoses or problems)
V49.82	Dental sealant status — (This code is intended for use when these conditions are recorded as diagnoses or problems)
V49.83	Awaiting organ transplant status
V49.84	Bed confinement status AHA: Q4, 2005, 96
V49.89	Other specified conditions influencing health status — (This code is intended for use when these conditions are recorded as diagnoses or problems) AHA: Q4, 2005, 94
V49.9	Unspecified problems with limbs and other problems — (This code is intended for use when these conditions are recorded as diagnoses or problems)

Coding Clarification

This category of codes is generic. Check in the disease/condition section of ICD-9-CM to verify that no other code better describes the symptoms and/or disease/condition of the patient. Code V49.84 provides a unique code for identifying those patients who cannot ambulate without assistance due to a disease or condition specified elsewhere. This provides a means of reporting the complexity and level of care required in caring for this particular population of patients.

Category V49 codes are nonspecific, except for V49.6x, V49.7x, and V49.81–V49.83, which can be reported as either the primary or secondary diagnosis. These codes are so nonspecific, or potentially redundant with other codes in the classification, that there can be little justification for their use in the inpatient setting. Their use in the outpatient setting should be limited to those instances when there is no further documentation to permit more precise coding. Otherwise, any sign or symptom or any other reason for the visit that is captured in another code should be used.

V50–V59 Persons Encountering Health Services for Specific Procedures and Aftercare

The codes in this section are used for patients who have already been treated for some disease or injury, but may need aftercare or adjunctive treatment to consolidate the treatment, deal with residual states, or prevent recurrence.

Encounters for plastic surgery are classified in two ways: procedures used for cosmetic surgery or for conditions of a healed injury or operation.

V50 Elective surgery for purposes other than remedying health states

Prophylactic gland, breast, or ovary removal may be performed on a patient with a family or personal history of cancer or another disease.

Code	Description
V50.0	Elective hair transplant for purposes other than remedying health states
V50.1	Other plastic surgery for unacceptable cosmetic appearance — *breast augmentation or reduction, face lift* AHA: Jan-Feb, 1987, 8
V50.2	Routine or ritual circumcision — *circumcision in the absence of significant medical indication* AHA: Jan-Feb, 1987, 8
V50.3	Ear piercing
V50.41	Prophylactic breast removal AHA: Q4, 2004, 107
V50.42	Prophylactic ovary removal
V50.49	Other prophylactic gland removal
V50.8	Other elective surgery for purposes other than remedying health states
V50.9	Unspecified elective surgery for purposes other than remedying health states

Coding Scenario

A patient presents to the plastic surgery clinic for an elective breast augmentation. Her present cup size is a small A. Following the surgery, the patient is a small C cup.

Code assignment: V50.1 *Other plastic surgery for unacceptable cosmetic appearance*

V51 Aftercare involving the use of plastic surgery

Plastic surgery may be performed on patients who have previously had surgery or had an injury heal in which another procedure is required to put the anatomical site back to its natural state.

Coding Clarification

Plastic surgery as treatment for current injury should be coded to the current condition. Plastic surgery on scar tissue should be coded to the scar, such as a keloid scar.

Code V51 codes are so nonspecific, or potentially redundant with other codes in the classification, that there can be little justification for their use in the inpatient setting. Their use in the outpatient setting should be limited to those instances when there is no further documentation to permit more precise coding. Otherwise, any sign or symptom or any other reason for the visit that is captured in another code should be used.

V52 Fitting and adjustment of prosthetic device and implant
AHA: Q4, 2005, 94

Fitting and adjustment of prosthetic devices are for devices that have been previously placed in or on the patient.

V52.0	Fitting and adjustment of artificial arm (complete) (partial)
V52.1	Fitting and adjustment of artificial leg (complete) (partial)
V52.2	Fitting and adjustment of artificial eye
V52.3	Fitting and adjustment of dental prosthetic device
V52.4	Fitting and adjustment of breast prosthesis and implant
V52.8	Fitting and adjustment of other specified prosthetic device
V52.9	Fitting and adjustment of unspecified prosthetic device

V53 Fitting and adjustment of other device

Communicating hydrocephalus occurs when there is a slight ventricular enlargement of the cerebrospinal fluid spaces outside of the brain. Shunts are the only treatment for this condition. The shunt has three major components. The first major component is a hollow tube with holes that is inserted through the skull and into the ventricular system where it is connected to the second component, which is a pressure valve that regulates the amount of cerebrospinous fluid that is released. The third component is a distal catheter, which is a long thin tube that attaches to the valve. This is placed under the skin and ends in a distal body cavity, usually in the peritoneum.

A neuropacemaker is an implanted device that is used to relieve nerve injury pain or to help movement disorders. Electrodes are implanted into the brain and attached to a pacemaker that is implanted in the basal ganglia. Electrical pulses are emitted and stimulate the brain.

V53.01	Fitting and adjustment of cerebral ventricular (communicating) shunt
V53.02	Neuropacemaker (brain) (peripheral nerve) (spinal cord)
V53.09	Fitting and adjustment of other devices related to nervous system and special senses — *auditory substitution device, visual substitution device*
	AHA: Jan-Feb, 1987, 8; Q4, 1997, 51; Q4, 1998, 66; Q2, 1999, 4
V53.1	Fitting and adjustment of spectacles and contact lenses
V53.2	Fitting and adjustment of hearing aid
V53.3 ⌐5th	Fitting and adjustment of cardiac device — *reprogramming*
	AHA: Nov-Dec, 1984, 18; May-June, 1987, 8; Jan-Feb, 1987, 8; Q1, 1990, 7; Q3, 1992, 3
V53.31	Fitting and adjustment of cardiac pacemaker
V53.32	Fitting and adjustment of automatic implantable cardiac defibrillator
	AHA: Q3, 2005, 8
V53.39	Fitting and adjustment of other cardiac device
V53.4	Fitting and adjustment of orthodontic devices
V53.5	Fitting and adjustment of other intestinal appliance
V53.6	Fitting and adjustment of urinary device — *urinary catheter*
	AHA: Jan-Feb, 1987, 8
V53.7	Fitting and adjustment of orthopedic device — *orthopedic brace, cast, corset shoes*
	AHA: Jan-Feb, 1987, 8
V53.8	Fitting and adjustment of wheelchair
V53.90	Fitting and adjustment, Unspecified device
V53.91	Fitting and adjustment of insulin pump — *insulin pump titration*
V53.99	Fitting and adjustment, Other device

Coding Clarification

For mechanical complications of a cardiac pacemaker, report 996.01.

V54 Other orthopedic aftercare

A fracture is a break or a rupture in a bone. A traumatic fracture is the result of an injury resulting from direct or indirect force against a bone. A pathologic fracture can occur from a weakening of the bone structure due to disease, such as osteoporosis. This category excludes malfunction of an internal orthopedic device, which is reported with 996.40-996.49.

V54.01	Encounter for removal of internal fixation device
V54.02	Encounter for lengthening/adjustment of growth rod
V54.09	Other aftercare involving internal fixation device
V54.10	Aftercare for healing traumatic fracture of arm, unspecified

Supplementary Classification of Factors Influencing Health Status and Contact with Health Services

Code	Description
V54.11	Aftercare for healing traumatic fracture of upper arm
V54.12	Aftercare for healing traumatic fracture of lower arm
V54.13	Aftercare for healing traumatic fracture of hip
V54.14	Aftercare for healing traumatic fracture of leg, unspecified
V54.15	Aftercare for healing traumatic fracture of upper leg
V54.16	Aftercare for healing traumatic fracture of lower leg
V54.17	Aftercare for healing traumatic fracture of vertebrae
V54.19	Aftercare for healing traumatic fracture of other bone **AHA:** Q1, 2005, 13
V54.20	Aftercare for healing pathologic fracture of arm, unspecified
V54.21	Aftercare for healing pathologic fracture of upper arm
V54.22	Aftercare for healing pathologic fracture of lower arm
V54.23	Aftercare for healing pathologic fracture of hip
V54.24	Aftercare for healing pathologic fracture of leg, unspecified
V54.25	Aftercare for healing pathologic fracture of upper leg
V54.26	Aftercare for healing pathologic fracture of lower leg
V54.27	Aftercare for healing pathologic fracture of vertebrae
V54.29	Aftercare for healing pathologic fracture of other bone
V54.81	Aftercare following joint replacement — (Use additional code to identify joint replacement site: V43.60-V43.69) **AHA:** Q2, 2004, 15
V54.89	Other orthopedic aftercare
V54.9	Unspecified orthopedic aftercare — *aftercare for healing fracture NOS* **AHA:** Jan-Feb, 1987, 8; Q3, 1995, 3

Coding Clarification
Use V54.81 and an additional code from V43.60-V43.69 to identify joint replacement. If there is a malfunction of an internal orthopedic device, report 996.40-996.49.

Coding Scenario
A patient presents to the orthopedic clinic for follow-up care of a fracture of the radius and ulna. X-rays are taken and show the fracture to be in alignment.

> Code assignment: V54.12 *Aftercare for healing traumatic fracture of lower arm*

V55 Attention to artificial openings
An ostomy refers to an opening that is created in an operation. An ostomy in the following refers to a surgically formed opening connecting the bowel, bladder, or trachea to outside the body.

These codes include the adjustment or repositioning of a catheter, closure, passage of sounds or bougies, reforming, or removal or replacement of a catheter.

Code	Description
V55.0	Attention to tracheostomy
V55.1	Attention to gastrostomy
V55.2	Attention to ileostomy
V55.3	Attention to colostomy **AHA:** Q2, 2005, 4
V55.4	Attention to other artificial opening of digestive tract **AHA:** Q2, 2005, 14
V55.5	Attention to cystostomy
V55.6	Attention to other artificial opening of urinary tract — *nephrostomy, urethrostomy, ureterostomy* **AHA:** Jan-Feb, 1987, 8
V55.7	Attention to artificial vagina
V55.8	Attention to other specified artificial opening
V55.9	Attention to unspecified artificial opening

Coding Clarification
For complications of an external stoma, report from codes 519.00-519.09, 569.60-569.69, 997.4 or 997.5.

V56 Encounter for dialysis and dialysis catheter care
AHA: Jan-Feb, 1987, 8; Q1, 1993, 29; Q4, 1998, 66

Hemodialysis is the removal of toxins in the blood through a semipermeable membrane. In peritoneal dialysis, the peritoneal lining in the peritoneum acts as the membrane. Fluid is infused into the peritoneum through a catheter and drained from the body after absorbing the toxins.

Code	Description
V56.0	Encounter for extracorporeal dialysis — (Use additional code to identify the associated condition) **AHA:** Jan-Feb, 1987, 8; Q1, 1993, 29; Q2, 1998, 20; Q3, 1998, 6; Q4, 1998, 66; Q4, 2000, 40; Q1, 2004, 23; Q4, 2005, 79
V56.1	Fitting and adjustment of extracorporeal dialysis catheter — (Use additional code for any concurrent extracorporeal dialysis, V56.0. Use additional code to identify the associated condition) **AHA:** Jan-Feb, 1987, 8; Q1, 1993, 29; Q2, 1998, 20; Q4, 1998, 66
V56.2	Fitting and adjustment of peritoneal dialysis catheter — (Use additional code for any concurrent peritoneal dialysis, V56.8. Use additional code to identify the associated condition)
V56.31	Encounter for adequacy testing for hemodialysis — (Use additional code to identify the associated condition)

Coders' Desk Reference for Diagnoses

V56.32	Encounter for adequacy testing for peritoneal dialysis — (Use additional code to identify the associated condition) AHA: Jan-Feb, 1987, 8; Q1, 1993, 29; Q4, 1998, 66; Q4, 2000, 55
V56.8	Encounter other dialysis — (Use additional code to identify the associated condition) AHA: Jan-Feb, 1987, 8; Q1, 1993, 29; Q4, 1998, 55; Q4, 1998, 66

Coding Clarification
Any concurrent extracorporeal or peritoneal dialysis should be reported in addition to category V56 codes.

Category V56 codes are to be used as additional codes only with the exception of V56.0 *Extracorporeal dialysis,* which is to be used as first-listed only.

V57 Care involving use of rehabilitation procedures
AHA: Sept-Oct, 1986, 3; Jan-Feb, 1987, 8; Q1, 1990, 6; Q3, 1997, 12; Q1, 2002, 19

Rehabilitation is typically needed for patients who after suffering an illness or injury need additional help to return to normal form and/or function or to an optimal functioning level.

In orthoptic training, exercises are performed to adjust the visual axes of one or both eyes. Orthoptic training is conducted in cases where the eyes are not properly coordinated to allow for good vision out of both eyes.

V57.0	Care involving breathing exercises — (Use additional code to identify underlying condition)
V57.1	Other physical therapy — (Use additional code to identify underlying condition) AHA: Sept-Oct, 1986, 3; Jan-Feb, 1987, 8; Q1, 1990, 6; Q3, 1997, 12; Q4, 1999, 5; Q1, 2002, 19; Q4, 2002, 56; Q2, 2004, 15
V57.21	Encounter for occupational therapy — (Use additional code to identify underlying condition)
V57.22	Encounter for vocational therapy — (Use additional code to identify underlying condition) AHA: Sept-Oct, 1986, 3; Jan-Feb, 1987, 8; Q1, 1990, 6; Q3, 1997, 12; Q1, 2002, 19
V57.3	Speech therapy — (Use additional code to identify underlying condition)
V57.4	Orthoptic training — (Use additional code to identify underlying condition)
V57.8 ⌐sth	Other specified rehabilitation procedure — (Use additional code to identify underlying condition) AHA: Sept-Oct, 1986, 3; Jan-Feb, 1987, 8; Q1, 1990, 6; Q3, 1997, 12; Q1, 2002, 19
V57.81	Orthotic training — (Use additional code to identify underlying condition) AHA: Sept-Oct, 1986, 3; Jan-Feb, 1987, 8; Q1, 1990, 6; Q3, 1997, 12; Q1, 2002, 19
V57.89	Other specified rehabilitation procedure — (Use additional code to identify underlying condition) AHA: Sept-Oct, 1986, 3; Sept-Oct, 1986, 4; Jan-Feb, 1987, 8; Q1, 1990, 6; Q3, 1997, 12; Q3, 1997, 11, 12; Q3, 2001, 21; Q1, 2002, 16; Q1, 2002, 19; Q2, 2003, 16; Q4, 2003, 105-106, 108
V57.9	Unspecified rehabilitation procedure — (Use additional code to identify underlying condition)

Coding Clarification
An additional diagnosis code should be reported indicating the condition requiring the rehabilitative services or therapy (V57.1, V57.2, V57.3, or V57.89).

Coding Scenario
A patient presents for physical therapy after fracturing a hip in a fall.

Code assignment: V57.1 *Care involving use of rehabilitation procedures, other physical therapy* and V54.13 *Aftercare for healing traumatic fracture of the hip*

V58 Encounter for other and unspecified procedure and aftercare
Drug monitoring is the measurement of the level of a specific drug in the body or of a specific function. Patients who take a specific drug on a long-term basis oftentimes need to be monitored to evaluate the continued effectiveness of the drug.

V58.0	Radiotherapy — *encounter or admission for radiotherapy* AHA: Jan-Feb, 1987, 8; Jan-Feb, 1987, 13; Q2, 1990, 7; Q3, 1992, 5

This subcategory excludes chemotherapy and immunotherapy that is administered for nonneoplastic conditions.

V58.1 ⌐sth	Encounter for antineoplastic chemotherapy and immunotherapy AHA: Sept-Oct, 1984, 5; Jan-Feb, 1987, 8; Q2, 1990, 7; Q2, 1991, 17; Q2, 1992, 6; Q3, 1993, 4; Q2, 2003, 16; Q1, 2004, 13
V58.11	Encounter for antineoplastic chemotherapy AHA: Q2, 2006, 20; 4Q, 2005, 98
V58.12	Encounter for antineoplastic immunotherapy AHA: Q4, 2005, 98
V58.2	Blood transfusion, without reported diagnosis

Subcategory V58.3 excludes attention to drains (V58.49) and planned postoperative wound closure (V58.41).

V58.30	Encounter for change or removal of nonsurgical wound dressing — *change or removal of wound dressing not otherwise specified* AHA: Jan-Feb, 1987, 8; Q2, 2005, 14

Supplementary Classification of Factors Influencing Health Status and Contact with Health Services

Code	Description
V58.31	Encounter for change or removal of surgical wound dressing **AHA:** Jan-Feb, 1987, 8; Q2, 2005, 14
V58.32	Encounter for removal of sutures — *removal of sutures or staples* **AHA:** Jan-Feb, 1987, 8; Q2, 2005, 14
V58.41	Planned postoperative wound closure — (This code should be used in conjunction with other aftercare codes to fully identify the reason for the aftercare encounter)
V58.42	Aftercare following surgery for neoplasm — (This code should be used in conjunction with other aftercare codes to fully identify the reason for the aftercare encounter) **AHA:** Jan-Feb, 1987, 8; Nov-Dec, 1987, 9; Q4, 1999, 9; Q4, 2002, 80
V58.43	Aftercare following surgery for injury and trauma — (This code should be used in conjunction with other aftercare codes to fully identify the reason for the aftercare encounter) **AHA:** Jan-Feb, 1987, 8; Nov-Dec, 1987, 9; Q4, 1999, 9; Q4, 2002, 80
V58.44	Aftercare following organ transplant **AHA:** Q4, 2004, 101
V58.49	Other specified aftercare following surgery — (This code should be used in conjunction with other aftercare codes to fully identify the reason for the aftercare encounter)
V58.5	Orthodontics aftercare
V58.61	Encounter for long-term (current) use of anticoagulants **AHA:** Q3, 2004, 7
V58.62	Encounter for aftercare for long-term (current) use of antibiotics
V58.63	Long-term (current) use of antiplatelet/antithrombotic
V58.64	Long-term (current) use of nonsteroidal anti-inflammatories
V58.65	Long-term (current) use of steroids
V58.66	Long-term (current) use of aspirin **AHA:** Q4, 2004, 102
V58.67	Long-term (current) use of insulin **AHA:** Q4, 2004, 55-56, 103
V58.69	Encounter for long-term (current) use of other medications — *high risk medications* **AHA:** Jan-Feb, 1987, 8; Q4, 1995, 61; Q2, 1996, 7; Q1, 1997, 12; Q2, 1999, 17; Q3, 1999, 13; Q2, 2000, 8; Q3, 2002, 15; Q4, 2002, 84; Q1, 2003, 11; Q1, 2004, 13; Q2, 2004, 10
V58.71	Aftercare following surgery of the sense organs, NEC — (This code should be used in conjunction with other aftercare codes to fully identify the reason for the aftercare encounter) **AHA:** Jan-Feb, 1987, 8; Q4, 2002, 80
V58.72	Aftercare following surgery of the nervous system, NEC — (This code should be used in conjunction with other aftercare codes to fully identify the reason for the aftercare encounter) **AHA:** Jan-Feb, 1987, 8; Q4, 2002, 80
V58.73	Aftercare following surgery of the circulatory system, NEC — (This code should be used in conjunction with other aftercare codes to fully identify the reason for the aftercare encounter) **AHA:** Jan-Feb, 1987, 8; Q4, 2002, 80; Q4, 2003, 105
V58.74	Aftercare following surgery of the respiratory system, NEC — (This code should be used in conjunction with other aftercare codes to fully identify the reason for the aftercare encounter) **AHA:** Jan-Feb, 1987, 8; Q4, 2002, 80
V58.75	Aftercare following surgery of the teeth, oral cavity, and digestive system, NEC — (This code should be used in conjunction with other aftercare codes to fully identify the reason for the aftercare encounter) **AHA:** Jan-Feb, 1987, 8; Q4, 2002, 80; Q2, 2005, 14
V58.76	Aftercare following surgery of the genitourinary system, NEC — (This code should be used in conjunction with other aftercare codes to fully identify the reason for the aftercare encounter) **AHA:** Jan-Feb, 1987, 8; Q4, 2002, 80; Q1, 2005, 11-12
V58.77	Aftercare following surgery of the skin and subcutaneous tissue, NEC — (This code should be used in conjunction with other aftercare codes to fully identify the reason for the aftercare encounter) **AHA:** Jan-Feb, 1987, 8; Q4, 2002, 80
V58.78	Aftercare following surgery of the musculoskeletal system, NEC — (This code should be used in conjunction with other aftercare codes to fully identify the reason for the aftercare encounter) **AHA:** Jan-Feb, 1987, 8; Q4, 2002, 80
V58.81	Fitting and adjustment of vascular catheter — *removal or replacement of catheter, toilet or cleaning* **AHA:** Jan-Feb, 1987, 8; Q2, 1994, 8; Q4, 1994, 45
V58.82	Encounter for fitting and adjustment of non-vascular catheter NEC — *removal or replacement of catheter, toilet or cleansing* **AHA:** Jan-Feb, 1987, 8; Q2, 1994, 8; Q4, 1994, 45
V58.83	Encounter for therapeutic drug monitoring — (Use additional code for any associated long-term current drug use: V58.61-V58.69) **AHA:** Q1, 2004, 13; Q2, 2004, 10
V58.9	Unspecified aftercare

Coding Clarification

When a patient is admitted for radiotherapy, chemotherapy, or immunotherapy report V58.0, V58.11 or V58.12 as the primary diagnosis and the cancer, disease, or condition as a secondary diagnosis. When procedures V58.0 and V58.11 or V58.12 are performed simultaneously, both may be reported on the same record, with either one sequenced first.

Immunotherapy, also called biologic therapy, is not classified as chemotherapy. Immunotherapy stimulates the body's own immune defense system to fight infection and disease. Whereas traditional cytotoxic chemotherapies attack the cancer cells themselves, biologic therapy lends support to the body's defenses by mimicking naturally occurring substances that activate the immune system. This stimulates cancer-killing cells activity to treat malignancies. Reporting an encounter for chemotherapy is not suitable for patients admitted to have immunotherapy.

Codes V58.2, V58.5, and V58.9 may be reported only as secondary diagnoses.

Codes for long-term (current) drug use can be used for medication that a patient is currently taking that was either prescribed by a physician to treat a medical condition or self-administered of a patient's own initiative for palliative effect or preventative measures.

Code V58.67 should be assigned with Type 2 and gestational diabetes to indicate insulin usage. Code assignment is optional with Type 1 diabetes, since insulin is an inherent part of treatment of the disease.

V59 Donors

This category of codes is used when the sole purpose of the admission of a patient to a hospital is to donate an organ.

Code	Description
V59.01	Whole blood donor
V59.02	Stem cell donor
V59.09	Blood donor, other
V59.1	Skin donor
V59.2	Bone donor
V59.3	Bone marrow donor
V59.4	Kidney donor
V59.5	Cornea donor
V59.6	Liver donor
V59.70	Egg (oocyte) (ovum) donor, unspecified AHA: Q4, 2005, 99
V59.71	Egg (oocyte) (ovum) donor, under age 35, anonymous recipient AHA: Q4, 2005, 99
V59.72	Egg (oocyte) (ovum) donor, under age 35, designated recipient AHA: Q4, 2005, 99
V59.73	Egg (oocyte) (ovum) donor, age 35 and over, anonymous recipient AHA: Q4, 2005, 99
V59.74	Egg (oocyte) (ovum) donor, age 35 and over, designated recipient AHA: Q4, 2005, 99
V59.8	Donor of other specified organ or tissue
V59.9	Donor of unspecified organ or tissue

Documentation Issues
Donor information must be documented in the patient's chart to verify cross-matching of donor parts.

Coding Clarification
Category V59 codes may only be reported as primary diagnoses and must report the donor of the tissue only.

For self-donation of an organ or tissue, report the condition.

V60–V68 Persons Encountering Health Services in Other Circumstances

Category V60-V68 codes contain additional information that must be included in the medical record regarding family, household, administrative, follow up, and psychosocial circumstances. Included in this section is category V64 *Persons encountering health services for specific procedures, not carried out.* Code sequencing is dependent upon the reason the procedure was not performed.

V60 Housing, household, and economic circumstances

Housing may pose a problem for a patient. The patient may have no place of residence, or inadequate resources to maintain a household, or be unable to care for self, or may need to be housed in an institution.

Holiday relief care is reported when a patient who normally receives care at home is provided health care in another facility to enable a relative or caretaker to take a vacation.

Code	Description
V60.0	Lack of housing — *hobos, social migrants, tramps, transients, vagabonds* AHA: Jan-Feb, 1987, 8
V60.1	Inadequate housing — *lack of heating, restricted space, technical defects in home, preventing adequate care* AHA: Jan-Feb, 1987, 8
V60.2	Inadequate material resources — *economic problem, poverty NOS* AHA: Jan-Feb, 1987, 8
V60.3	Person living alone
V60.4	No other household member able to render care — *person requiring care (has) (is): family*

Supplementary Classification of Factors Influencing Health Status and Contact with Health Services

member too handicapped, ill, or otherwise unsuited to render care
AHA: Jan-Feb, 1987, 8

V60.5 Holiday relief care
V60.6 Person living in residential institution — boarding school resident
AHA: Jan-Feb, 1987, 8
V60.8 Other specified housing or economic circumstances
V60.9 Unspecified housing or economic circumstance

Coding Clarification
Category V60 codes may be reported only as secondary diagnoses.

V61 Other family circumstances
Category V61 codes are used to report circumstances for seeking or receiving medical advice or care.

V61.0 Family disruption — divorce, estrangement
AHA: Jan-Feb, 1987, 8; Q1, 1990, 9
V61.10 Counseling for marital and partner problems, unspecified — marital conflict, partner conflict
AHA: Jan-Feb, 1987, 8; Q1, 1990, 9
V61.11 Counseling for victim of spousal and partner abuse
V61.12 Counseling for perpetrator of spousal and partner abuse
V61.20 Counseling for parent-child problem, unspecified — parent-child conflict or relationship problem
AHA: Jan-Feb, 1987, 8; Q1, 1990, 9
V61.21 Counseling for victim of child abuse — child battering, child neglect
AHA: Jan-Feb, 1987, 8; Q1, 1990, 9
V61.22 ☐ Counseling for perpetrator of parental child abuse
V61.29 Counseling for perpetrator of parental child abuse — problem concerning adopted or foster child
AHA: Jan-Feb, 1987, 8; Q1, 1990, 9; Q3, 1999, 16
V61.3 Problems with aged parents or in-laws
V61.41 Alcoholism in family
V61.49 Other health problem within the family — care of or presence of sick or handicapped person in family or household
AHA: Jan-Feb, 1987, 8; Q1, 1990, 9
V61.5 Multiparity — many children
AHA: Jan-Feb, 1987, 8; Q1, 1990, 9
V61.6 Illegitimacy or illegitimate pregnancy — pregnancy without two married parents
AHA: Jan-Feb, 1987, 8; Q1, 1990, 9
V61.7 Other unwanted pregnancy
V61.8 Other specified family circumstances — sibling relationship problem, problem with family members NEC
AHA: Jan-Feb, 1987, 8; Q1, 1990, 9
V61.9 Unspecified family circumstance

Coding Clarification
If the abuse causes injuries, report all current injuries with codes from 995.50-995.59.

Coding Scenario
A married couple presents for a weekly counseling session.

Code assignment: V61.10 Counseling for marital and partner problems, unspecified.

V62 Other psychosocial circumstances
These codes are used to report circumstances for seeking or receiving medical advice or care.

V62.0 Unemployment
V62.1 Adverse effects of work environment
V62.2 Other occupational circumstance or maladjustment — career choice problem, dissatisfaction with employment, occupational problem
AHA: Jan-Feb, 1987, 8
V62.3 Educational circumstance — dissatisfaction with school, educational handicap, academic problem
AHA: Jan-Feb, 1987, 8
V62.4 Social maladjustment — culture deprivation, political, religious, or sex discrimination, social isolation, persecution, acculturation problem
AHA: Jan-Feb, 1987, 8
V62.5 Legal circumstance — imprisonment, legal investigation, litigation, prosecution
AHA: Jan-Feb, 1987, 8
V62.6 Refusal of treatment for reasons of religion or conscience
V62.81 Interpersonal problem, not elsewhere classified—relationship problem NOS
V62.82 Bereavement, uncomplicated
V62.83 Counseling for perpetrator of physical/sexual abuse
V62.84 Suicidal ideation
AHA: Q4, 2005, 99

This code excludes suicidal tendencies, reported with 300.9.

V62.89 Other psychological or physical stress, not elsewhere classified — life circumstance problems, phase of life problem, borderline intellectual functioning, religious or spiritual problems
AHA: Jan-Feb, 1987, 8

Coding Clarification
Category V62 codes may be reported only as secondary diagnoses.

For circumstances where the main problem is economic inadequacy or poverty, report V60.2.

For bereavement as an adjustment reaction, report 309.0.

For suicidal tendencies, report 300.9. Suicidal ideation is the term used for thoughts of committing suicide. These are problematic thoughts in people who may not have been diagnosed with a mental or behavioral disorder. Some patients may follow through with attempts to commit suicide after the ideation has been expressed, creating the need for such a code reporting the necessity of further evaluation and follow-up. Suicidal ideation is reported for thoughts of suicide, whether the patient actually formulates a plan for committing suicide or not.

V63 Unavailability of other medical facilities for care

Medical facilities may not be accessible to patients for a variety of reasons, such as a patient's resident is too far removed from a health care facility or medical services are not available to a patient at a patient's home. Another reason is a patient is suffering from a disease or condition that requires a specific type of treatment that was unavailable at the time of admission and is awaiting admission to an adequate facility elsewhere.

V63.0	Residence remote from hospital or other health care facility
V63.1	Medical services in home not available
V63.2	Person awaiting admission to adequate facility elsewhere
V63.8	Other specified reason for unavailability of medical facilities — *person on waiting list undergoing social agency investigation* **AHA:** Jan-Feb, 1987, 8; Q1, 1991, 21
V63.9	Unspecified reason for unavailability of medical facilities

V64 Persons encountering health services for specific procedures, not carried out

Services and/or procedures may not be carried out due to a condition that renders the patient untreatable (e.g., reaction to anesthesia, extremely high blood pressure) or because the patient refuses treatment.

In certain instances, procedures performed by scopes are converted into open procedures due to the inability to perform the procedure with the scope (e.g., extensive adhesions) or because the procedure is more extensive than originally anticipated.

V64.00	Vaccination not carried out, unspecified reason **AHA:** Q4, 2005, 99
V64.01	Vaccination not carried out because of acute illness **AHA:** Q4, 2005, 99
V64.02	Vaccination not carried out because of chronic illness or condition **AHA:** Q4, 2005, 99
V64.03	Vaccination not carried out because of chronic illness or condition **AHA:** Q4, 2005, 99
V64.04	Vaccination not carried out because of allergy to vaccine or component **AHA:** Q4, 2005, 99
V64.05	Vaccination not carried out because of caregiver refusal **AHA:** Q4, 2005, 99
V64.06	Vaccination not carried out because of patient refusal **AHA:** Q4, 2005, 99
V64.07	Vaccination not carried out for religious reasons **AHA:** Q4, 2005, 99
V64.08	Vaccination not carried out because patient had disease being vaccinated against **AHA:** Q4, 2005, 99
V64.09	Vaccination not carried out for other reason **AHA:** Q4, 2005, 99
V64.1	Surgical or other procedure not carried out because of contraindication
V64.2	Surgical or other procedure not carried out because of patient's decision
V64.3	Procedure not carried out for other reasons
V64.41	Laparoscopic surgical procedure converted to open procedure
V64.42	Thoracoscopic surgical procedure converted to open procedure
V64.43	Arthroscopic surgical procedure converted to open procedure

Documentation Issues
The medical necessity of the conversion from a scope procedure to an open procedure should be well documented in the patient's health record.

Coding Clarification
Category V64 codes may be reported only as secondary diagnoses.

Coding Scenario
A patient is admitted to the ambulatory surgery center for a laparoscopic right inguinal hernia repair. Due to the patient's anatomy, the physician was not able to perform the repair through the scope. The patient was redraped and the hernia repair was performed through an open incision.

> Code assignment: 550.90 *Unilateral inguinal hernia repair unspecified* and V64.41 *Laparoscopic surgical procedure converted to open procedure*

V65 Other persons seeking consultation without complaint or sickness

Insulin pump training is provided to patients who require insulin for diabetes. It is an alternative to daily shots, in which insulin is supplied by a pump worn externally through a tube into the subcutaneous tissue. A large amount of insulin is supplied to the patient prior to mealtime and a continuous amount of insulin is maintained throughout the day.

V65.0	Healthy person accompanying sick person — boarder
	AHA: Jan-Feb, 1987, 8
V65.11	Pediatric pre-birth visit for expectant mother
V65.19	Other person consulting on behalf of another person
V65.2	Person feigning illness — *malingerer, peregrinating patient*
	AHA: Jan-Feb, 1987, 8; Q3, 1999, 20
V65.3	Dietary surveillance and counseling — (Use additional code to identify body mass index (BMI) if known: V85.0-V85.54) — *colitis, diabetes, allergies, gastritis, high cholesterol, hypoglycemia, obesity*
	AHA: Jan-Feb, 1987, 8; Q4, 2005, 96
V65.4 ✎5th	Other counseling, not elsewhere classified — *health advice, education, instruction*
	AHA: Jan-Feb, 1987, 8
V65.40	Counseling NOS
V65.41	Excercise counseling — *cardiovascular disease, obesity*
	AHA: Jan-Feb, 1987, 8
V65.42	Counseling on substance use and abuse
V65.43	Counseling on injury prevention
V65.44	Human immunodeficiency virus (HIV) counseling
V65.45	Counseling on other sexually transmitted diseases — *herpes simplex, syphilis, gonorrhea, viral hepatitis B*
	AHA: Jan-Feb, 1987, 8
V65.46	Encounter for insulin pump training — *diabetes*
V65.49	Other specified counseling
V65.5	Person with feared complaint in whom no diagnosis was made — *feared condition not demonstrated, problem was normal stated, "worried well"*
	AHA: Jan-Feb, 1987, 8
V65.8	Other reasons for seeking consultation
V65.9	Unspecified reason for consultation

Coding Clarification
For consultations conducted on behalf of another person, report with codes V65.11-V65.19.

V66 Convalescence and palliative care
Palliative care is given at the end of a person's life, including hospice and terminal care. Palliative care is given to patients whose illness is terminal and the treatment is aimed toward making the patient comfortable rather than treating the illness. It may be used when a patient is admitted for treatment, but during the process of the treatment it is determined that the illness is terminal.

V66.0	Convalescence following surgery
V66.1	Convalescence following radiotherapy
V66.2	Convalescence following chemotherapy
V66.3	Convalescence following psychotherapy and other treatment for mental disorder
V66.4	Convalescence following treatment of fracture
V66.5	Convalescence following other treatment
V66.6	Convalescence following combined treatment
V66.7	Encounter for palliative care — (Code first underlying disease)
	AHA: Jan-Feb, 1987, 8; Q4, 1996, 47, 48; Q1, 1998, 11; Q4, 2003, 107; Q2, 2005, 9
V66.9	Unspecified convalescence

Documentation Issues
The physician must document that admission is for palliative care. Terms meaning the same as palliative care may be hospice, end-of-life, or comfort care. Terms synonymous with palliative care must be well documented in the medical record.

Coding Clarification
Category V66 codes may only be as primary diagnoses except for V66.7, which should be reported as a secondary diagnosis. Report the underlying condition before V66.7.

V67 Follow-up examination
Follow-up treatment may be necessary to check on a patient following surgery, after different types of therapy, or after a fracture has healed to verify the success of treatment.

V67.00	Follow-up examination, following unspecified surgery
V67.01	Following surgery follow-up vaginal pap smear — (Use additional code to identify condition: V10.40-V10.44, V45.77)
	AHA: Jan-Feb, 1987, 8; Q3, 1992, 11; Q4, 1994, 48; Q1, 1995, 4; Q2, 1995, 8; Q4, 1997, 50; Q4, 1998, 69; Q4, 2000, 56
V67.09	Follow-up examination, following other surgery
V67.1	Radiotherapy follow-up examination
V67.2	Chemotherapy follow-up examination — *cancer chemotherapy follow-up*
	AHA: Jan-Feb, 1987, 8; Q4, 1994, 48
V67.3	Psychotherapy and other treatment for mental disorder follow-up examination
V67.4	Treatment of healed fracture follow-up examination
V67.51	Follow-up examination following completed treatment with high-risk medications, not elsewhere classified
V67.59	Other follow-up examination
V67.6	Combined treatment follow-up examination
V67.9	Unspecified follow-up examination

Coding Clarification
Report the acquired absence of uterus (V15.77) and personal history of malignant neoplasm (V10.40-10.44) in addition to V67.01.

Diagnostic exams performed as a follow-up to surgery to determine if there is evidence of recurrence or metastasis are reported using the appropriate follow-up exam V code. If the exam reveals malignancy, then the appropriate malignancy code is reported, not the follow-up exam V code.

Routine follow-up encounters for heart transplant that involve cardiac cath or biopsy are assigned the V code for the follow-up exam (following other surgery) as the first-listed code. Code also the V code for transplant status. However, if there is evidence of rejection upon exam, assign the complication of transplanted heart code as the first-listed code.

Coding Scenario
A 57-year-old female presents to the OB/GYN clinic for a follow-up Pap smear following a total abdominal hysterectomy one year ago with a diagnosis of a malignancy of the cervix. Treatment ended about six months ago and there has been no further sign of the disease.

> Code assignment: V67.01 *Following surgery follow-up vaginal Pap smear;* V10.41 *Personal history of malignant neoplasm, cervix uteri;* and V45.77 *Acquired absence of uterus*

V68 Encounters for administrative purposes
Medical certificates include death certificates, disability papers, and fitness verification. Repeat prescriptions include appliances, orthotics, glasses, and medication.

A request for expert evidence includes medical testimony and depositions.

V68.0	Issue of medical certificates — *cause of death, fitness, incapacity*
	AHA: Jan-Feb, 1987, 8
V68.1	Issue of repeat prescriptions
V68.2	Request for expert evidence
V68.81	Referral of patient without examination or treatment
V68.89	Encounters for other specified administrative purpose
V68.9	Encounters for unspecified administrative purpose

Coding Clarification
Category V68 codes may only be reported as primary diagnoses.

V69 Problems related to lifestyle
Some experts agree that lack of exercise can be as damaging as smoking a pack of cigarettes every day. Lack of exercise may contribute to heart disease and increase the risk for diabetes and high blood pressure. Inappropriate diet may also contribute to health related problems.

High-risk sexual behaviors include homosexuality and promiscuity. This behavior puts the patient at risk for sexually transmitted diseases.

V69.0	Problems related to lack of physical excercise — *sedentary*
	AHA: Jan-Feb, 1987, 8; Q4, 1994, 48
V69.1	Problems related to inappropriate diet and eating habits — *malnutrition*
	AHA: Jan-Feb, 1987, 8; Q4, 1994, 48
V69.2	Problems related to high-risk sexual behavior — *sexually-transmitted diseases*
	AHA: Jan-Feb, 1987, 8; Q4, 1994, 48
V69.3	Problems related to gambling and betting — *financial issues*
	AHA: Jan-Feb, 1987, 8; Q4, 1994, 48
V69.4	Lack of adequate sleep
V69.5	Behavioral insomnia of childhood
	AHA: Q4, 2005, 99

Sleep problems in a child can result from a variety of causes, including teething, disruptions in routine, family stress, illness, dietary intake of sugar or other stimulants, and inadequate enforcement of bedtime by a caregiver. These changes can negatively affect a child's sleep schedule, sometimes leading to behavioral issues of stalling or refusing to go to bed, and the effect can result in childhood insomnia.

V69.8	Other problems related to lifestyle — *self-damaging behavior*
	AHA: Jan-Feb, 1987, 8; Q4, 1994, 48
V69.9	Unspecified problems related to lifestyle

Documentation Issues
The health care provider must document that the patient has a risk factor related to lifestyle.

Coding Clarification
Report from codes 260-269.9 for malnutrition and other nutritional deficiencies; 307.1 for anorexia nervosa; and 783.6 for bulimia.

V70–V82 Persons Without Reported Diagnosis Encountered During Examination and Investigation of Individuals and Populations

Category V70-V85 codes represent encounters with health services for general physical and mental examinations, routine tests on specific body systems, and screenings. The special screening codes are used only when screening procedures are done on defined population groups, such as armed forces personnel or pre-employment physicals.

Observation for suspected condition codes should be reported when a patient presents with a suspected condition but after further examination it is ruled out. This category may be used for administrative or legal observations.

Special investigations and screening codes should be reported for examination of a specific body system or screening for a specific disease that, after examination, is not found to exist. This includes routine eye examination and diabetes screening. If a diagnosis is found or confirmed, assign the code for the disease or illness rather than a V code.

V70 General medical examination
AHA: Jan-Feb, 1987, 8

This section of codes may include a yearly physical, examination for admission to school or camp, receipt of a driver's license, insurance certification, blood alcohol levels, and examination to participate in clinical research or trials. These services may be requested by the patient or could come from another administrative source, such as the military, employer, or legal authority. This also includes special screening studies for potential organ or tissue donors.

V70.0	Routine general medical examination at health care facility — (Use additional code(s) to identify any special screening examination(s) performed: V73.0-V82.9) AHA: Jan-Feb, 1987, 8
V70.1	General psychiatric examination requested by the authority — (Use additional code(s) to identify any special screening examination(s) performed: V73.0-V82.9)
V70.2	Other and unspecified general psychiatric examination — (Use additional code(s) to identify any special screening examination(s) performed: V73.0-V82.9)
V70.3	Other general medical examination for administrative purposes — (Use additional code(s) to identify any special screening examination(s) performed: V73.0-V82.9) AHA: Jan-Feb, 1987, 8; Q1, 1990, 6
V70.4	Examination for medicolegal reason — (Use additional code(s) to identify any special screening examination(s) performed: V73.0-V82.9) AHA: Jan-Feb, 1987, 8
V70.5	Health examination of defined subpopulation — (Use additional code(s) to identify any special screening examination(s) performed: V73.0-V82.9)
V70.6	Health examination in population survey — (Use additional code(s) to identify any special screening examination(s) performed: V73.0-V82.9) AHA: Jan-Feb, 1987, 8
V70.7	Examination of participant in clinical trial — (Use additional code(s) to identify any special screening examination(s) performed: V73.0-V82.9) AHA: Jan-Feb, 1987, 8; Q4, 2001, 55; Q2, 2006, 5
V70.8	Other specified general medical examination — (Use additional code(s) to identify any special screening examination(s) performed: V73.0-V82.9) AHA: Jan-Feb, 1987, 8
V70.9	Unspecified general medical examination — (Use additional code(s) to identify any special screening examination(s) performed: V73.0-V82.9)

Coding Clarification
Category V70 codes may only be reported as primary diagnoses except for V70.7, which may be reported as either the primary or secondary diagnosis.

Use codes from V73.0-V82.9 in addition to category V70 codes to identify any special screening examinations.

Code V70.0 excludes a general physical examination done as a pre-procedural measure, coded to V72.83.

V71 Observation and evaluation for suspected conditions not found

These codes are used when a patient presents with a suspected condition, that is ruled out after further examination; no further treatment or follow-up is required for the suspected condition. This category may be used for legal and administrative observation.

Antisocial behavior is behavior that is negative and outside what is perceived as normal. This may include irresponsibility, lack of concern for the feelings of others, inability to maintain relationships, easy frustration and aggression, and the inability to learn from experience.

Tuberculosis (TB) is a bacterial infection that usually attacks the lungs, but which may also affect other organs. The disease is caused by *Mycobacterium tuberculosis*. TB is transmitted by inhaling air droplets exhaled by an infected person or, sometimes, the infection is absorbed by the skin.

Observation for suspected abuse and neglect should be reported for adults or children who are examined for abuse but it is ruled out.

With increased threat of terrorism, a code for suspected exposure to anthrax was developed.

Anthrax is a potentially deadly bacterial infection that can be transmitted through contact with the skin, inhalation, and eating undercooked meat from infected animals.

V71.0 ⌐sth	Observation for suspected mental condition — *without manifest psychiatric disorder* **AHA:** March-April, 1987, 1; Jan-Feb, 1987, 8; Q2, 1990, 5; Q4, 1994, 47
V71.01	Observation of adult antisocial behavior — *gang activity in child or adolescent* **AHA:** March-April, 1987, 1; Jan-Feb, 1987, 8; Q2, 1990, 5; Q4, 1994, 47
V71.02	Observation of childhood or adolescent antisocial behavior
V71.09	Observation of other suspected mental condition
V71.1	Observation for suspected malignant neoplasm
V71.2	Observation for suspected tuberculosis — *can be spread by close contact to someone who has the disease* **AHA:** March-April, 1987, 1; Jan-Feb, 1987, 8; Q2, 1990, 5; Q4, 1994, 47
V71.3	Observation following accident at work
V71.4	Observation following other accident — *includes motor vehicle accident* **AHA:** March-April, 1987, 1; Jan-Feb, 1987, 8; Q2, 1990, 5; Q4, 1994, 47; Q1, 2006, 9
V71.5	Observation following alleged rape or seduction
V71.6	Observation following other inflicted injury
V71.7	Observation for suspected cardiovascular disease **AHA:** Q1, 2004, 6
V71.81	Observation for suspected abuse and neglect
V71.82	*Observation and evaluation for suspected exposure to anthrax*
V71.83	Observation and evaluation for suspected exposure to other biological agent
V71.89	Observation for other specified suspected conditions
V71.9	Observation for unspecified suspected condition

Coding Clarification

Category V71 codes may only be reported as primary diagnoses. Conditions that coexist at the time of observation for a suspected condition may be reported and sequenced after the V71 category codes.

Observation codes for alleged rape or seduction or following an injury may be used for the victim or the suspect.

Report from codes 995.80-995.85 for adult abuse and neglect and 995.50-995.59 for child abuse and neglect.

Code V71.81 should not be reported on an inpatient following outpatient surgery if a symptom or condition exists that can be coded, such as nausea and vomiting.

Report V29.9 for a baby less than 29 days old observed for a suspected condition that is ruled out.

Coding Scenario

A patient is admitted to the emergency department following a motor vehicle accident for observation of suspected head and internal injuries. After a thorough check, all injuries are ruled out.

Code assignment: V71.4 *Observation following other accident*

V72–V82 Screening Exams

Reason for Exam; Whenever a screening examination is performed, official coding guidelines require the screening code to be first-listed if the reason for the visit is specifically the screening exam. This guideline must be followed regardless of whether the exam reveals a reportable condition. The condition is reported as an additional diagnosis.

Additional Code: Screening codes may be listed as an additional code only when the reason for the encounter was for other health problems.

With Routine Exam: A screening code is not necessary if the screening is one as part of a routine exam.

Screening vs. Diagnostic: Testing to confirm or rule out suspected diagnoses due to the presence of a sign or symptom is a diagnostic exam, not a screening exam. The sign or symptom is used to explain the reason for the test.

V72 Special investigations and examinations
AHA: Jan-Feb, 1987, 8

Preoperative clearance exams are performed prior to surgery to ensure the patient is healthy enough to undergo anesthesia and surgical procedures. This category includes routine examinations or exams performed in the absence of symptoms.

V72.0	Examination of eyes and vision — (Use additional code(s) to identify any special screening examination(s) performed: V73.0-V82.9) **AHA:** Q1, 2004, 15
V72.11	Encounter for hearing examination following failed hearing screening **AHA:** Q1, 2004, 15
V72.19	Other examination of ears and hearing **AHA:** Q1, 2004, 15
V72.2	Dental examination — (Use additional code(s) to identify any special screening examination(s) performed: V73.0-V82.9)

Supplementary Classification of Factors Influencing Health Status and Contact with Health Services

Code	Description
V72.3 ✓5th	Gynecological examination — (Use additional code to identify routine vaginal pap smear, V76.47.) **AHA:** Jan-Feb, 1987, 8
V72.31	Routine gynecological examination **AHA:** Q4, 2005, 98; Q2, 2006, 3
V72.32	Encounter for Papanicolaou cervical smear to confirm findings of recent normal smear following initial abnormal smear **AHA:** Q2, 2006, 4
V72.4 ✓5th	Pregnancy examination or test, pregnancy unconfirmed — (Use additional code(s) to identify any special screening examination(s) performed: V73.0-V82.9) **AHA:** Jan-Feb, 1987, 8; Q4, 2005, 98
V72.40	Pregnancy examination or test, pregnancy unconfirmed
V72.41	Pregnancy examination or test, negative result
V72.42	Pregnancy examination or test, positive result
V72.5	Radiological examination, not elsewhere classified — (Use additional code(s) to identify any special screening examination(s) performed: V73.0-V82.9) **AHA:** Jan-Feb, 1987, 8; Q1, 1990, 19
V72.6	Laboratory examination — (Use additional code(s) to identify any special screening examination(s) performed: V73.0-V82.9) **AHA:** Q2, 2006, 4
V72.7	Diagnostic skin and sensitization tests — (Use additional code(s) to identify any special screening examination(s) performed: V73.0-V82.9) **AHA:** Jan-Feb, 1987, 8
V72.81	Pre-operative cardiovascular examination — (Use additional code(s) to identify any special screening examination(s) performed: V73.0-V82.9)— pre-procedural cardiovascular exam
V72.82	Pre-operative respiratory examination — (Use additional code(s) to identify any special screening examination(s) performed: V73.0-V82.9)— pre-procedural respiratory exam
V72.83	Other specified pre-operative examination — (Use additional code(s) to identify any special screening examination(s) performed: V73.0-V82.9)— pre-procedural general physical exam
V72.84	Unspecified pre-operative examination — (Use additional code(s) to identify any special screening examination(s) performed: V73.0-V82.9)— pre-procedural exam NOS
V72.85	Other specified examination — (Use additional code(s) to identify any special screening examination(s) performed: V73.0-V82.9) **AHA:** Q1, 2004, 12; Q4, 2005, 96
V72.86	Encounter for blood typing

This code is used to code heath care encounters specifically for the purpose of testing Rh status and other blood typing purposes when a specific condition is not the reason for an encounter.

Code	Description
V72.9	Unspecified examination — (Use additional code(s) to identify any special screening examination(s) performed: V73.0-V82.9)

Coding Clarification

Category V72 codes may only be reported as primary diagnoses. Codes V72.5 and V72.6 are not to be used if any sign, symptom, or reason for a test is documented.

V73 Special screening examination for viral and chlamydial diseases
AHA: Q1, 2004, 11

Viruses are pathogens that can attach to the cell membrane and take over cell functions. They can only grow and reproduce after infecting a host. There are more than 400 types of viruses that cause a variety of diseases ranging from the common cold to hemorrhagic fever. Viruses may immediately cause a disease or remain dormant for several years.

Chlamydial infections are classified as bacterial. They only grow inside a cell and are responsible for causing a variety of diseases including pneumonia and genital infections in men and women.

Poliomyelitis is an infectious viral disease of the central nervous system that sometimes results in paralysis. The World Health Organization (WHO) declared the Western Hemisphere polio-free in 1994. Today polio is most prevalent in areas of Africa, the Middle East and South Asia.

Smallpox is a highly contagious human disease caused by the virus variolae, of which there are two strains: variolae major, which has severe symptoms and a mortality rate of 20 to 40 percent; and variolae minor, which has less severe symptoms and a 1 percent mortality rate. The disease can be spread from person to person and through infected blankets, linens, and clothing.

Measles is an acute infection caused by paramyxovirus and presents with a hacking cough, rash, and fever.

Rubella or German measles is a highly contagious virus, but the symptoms are mild and short-lived in most people. Symptoms include malaise, arthralgia, rash, headache, and fever. Rubella during pregnancy can result in abortion, stillbirth, or congenital defects.

Yellow fever is transmitted from mosquito to man. In cities, the bite of an Aedes aegypti mosquito causes the infection; in the jungle, Haemagogus and other forest canopy mosquitoes acquire the virus from jungle primates and transmit the virus to man. In the United States, cases of yellow fever are usually limited to people who have been abroad.

Trachoma is caused by infection with the organism *Chlamydia trachomatis*. It begins slowly as a mild conjunctivitis that develops into a severe onset infection.

V73.0   Screening examination for poliomyelitis — *viral disease of the central nervous system*
AHA: Jan-Feb, 1987, 8

V73.1   Screening examination for smallpox — *caused by virus variolae*
AHA: Jan-Feb, 1987, 8

V73.2   Screening examination for measles — *caused by paramyxovirus*
AHA: Jan-Feb, 1987, 8

V73.3   Screening examination for rubella — *German measles*
AHA: Jan-Feb, 1987, 8

V73.4   Screening examination for yellow fever — *transmitted from mosquito to man*
AHA: Jan-Feb, 1987, 8

V73.5   Screening examination for other arthropod-borne viral diseases — *dengue fever, viral encephalitis, hemorrhagic fever*
AHA: Jan-Feb, 1987, 8

V73.6   Screening examination for trachoma — *caused by chlamydia trachomatis*
AHA: Jan-Feb, 1987, 8

V73.88   Special screening examination for other specified chlamydial diseases

V73.89   Special screening examination for other specified viral diseases

V73.98   Special screening examination for unspecified chlamydial disease

V73.99   Special screening examination for unspecified viral disease

Coding Clarification
Category V73 codes may be reported as primary or secondary diagnoses.

V74   Special screening examination for bacterial and spirochetal diseases
AHA: Q1, 2004, 11

Bacterial and spirochetal diseases include diagnostic skin tests for the diseases. Bacteria are one-cell organisms that cause a wide variety of diseases. A bacterium is capable of undergoing mutations, which makes fighting diseases caused by bacteria an ongoing battle.

A spiral shaped bacterium causes a spirochetal infection. It is responsible for diseases such as syphilis and Lyme disease.

V74.0   Screening examination for cholera — *infectious disease of the bowel*
AHA: Jan-Feb, 1987, 8

V74.1   Screening examination for pulmonary tuberculosis — *caused by Mycobacterium tuberculosis*
AHA: Jan-Feb, 1987, 8

V74.2   Screening examination for leprosy (Hansen's disease) — *highest incidence in India and Brazil*
AHA: Jan-Feb, 1987, 8

V74.3   Screening examination for diphtheria — *caused by Corynebacterium diphtheriae*
AHA: Jan-Feb, 1987, 8

V74.4   Screening examination for bacterial conjunctivitis — *pink eye*
AHA: Jan-Feb, 1987, 8

V74.5   Screening examination for venereal disease — *sexually transmitted diseases*
AHA: Jan-Feb, 1987, 8

V74.6   Screening examination for yaws — *infectious nonvenereal disease*
AHA: Jan-Feb, 1987, 8

V74.8   Screening examination for other specified bacterial and spirochetal diseases

V74.9   Screening examination for unspecified bacterial and spirochetal diseases

Coding Clarification
Category V74 codes may be reported as primary or secondary diagnoses.

Coding Scenario
A patient presents to the clinic for a routine TB test. The test is read as negative.

    Code assignment: V74.1 *Screening examination for pulmonary tuberculosis*

V75   Special screening examination for other infectious diseases
AHA: Q1, 2004, 11

An infectious disease is caused by a microorganism that can be transmitted with or without contact. A parasite is an organism that attacks a host but does not contribute to the survival of a host.

Rickettsial diseases include Rocky Mountain spotted fever, catscratch disease, Q fever, louse-born typhus, and rickettsial pox and are caused by the microorganism rickettsiae. The organism is somewhere between a virus and a bacterium. The diseases can be serious and various organs and tissues can be affected.

Malaria is a parasite that is transmitted by an infected mosquito. It is a potentially deadly disease that affects 300-500 million people. There are about 1,200 cases each year, mostly contracted by immigrants and people who have traveled to malaria-risk areas.

Leishmaniasis is a disease caused by a parasite. It is transmitted by the bite of infected sand flies. It occurs most often in developing countries and found more in rural than urban areas.

A fungus causes mycotic infections. It can affect a variety of body systems including the skin.

Schistosomiasis, also know as bilharzia or blood fluke, is a water-borne parasitic disease carried by water snails. The disease is caused by infested water. The eggs of the schistomosomes in the excreta of an infected host open on contact with water and release a parasite, the miracidium, which seeks a fresh water snail. Once it has found its snail host, the miracidium produces thousands of new parasites. The snail excretes the parasites into the surrounding water.

Filarial infections are roundworms that are transmitted through the bites of arthropods. The larvae travel through the body to sites such as lymphatic vessels, lymph nodes, subcutaneous tissue, and body cavities and surrounding tissue.

Helminthiases are parasitic worms that can be found in the gastrointestinal tract or under the skin.

Code	Description
V75.0	Screening examination for rickettsial diseases — most common is Rocky Mountain spotted fever AHA: Jan-Feb, 1987, 8
V75.1	Screening examination for malaria — less than 1000 are diagnosed in the United States each year AHA: Jan-Feb, 1987, 8
V75.2	Screening examination for leishmaniasis — seen most in developing nations AHA: Jan-Feb, 1987, 8
V75.3	Screening examination for trypanosomiasis — disease can affect the central nervous system and major organs and can be fatal AHA: Jan-Feb, 1987, 8
V75.4	Screening examination for mycotic infections — condition that is caused by a fungus AHA: Jan-Feb, 1987, 8
V75.5	Screening examination for schistosomiasis — caused by a parasite AHA: Jan-Feb, 1987, 8
V75.6	Screening examination for filariasis — caused by filarial parasites AHA: Jan-Feb, 1987, 8
V75.7	Screening examination for intestinal helminthiasis
V75.8	Screening examination for other specified parasitic infections
V75.9	Screening examination for unspecified infectious disease

Coding Clarification
Category V75 codes may be reported as primary or secondary diagnoses.

V76 Special screening for malignant neoplasms
AHA: Q1, 2004, 11

This category is broken down by body site, such as breast, bladder, skin, and cervix. It is used for routine screenings or for patients who present without any signs, symptoms, or history of the disease.

Code	Description
V76.0	Special screening for malignant neoplasm of the respiratory organs
V76.10	Unspecified breast screening — *manual breast exam* AHA: Jan-Feb, 1987, 8; Q4, 1998, 67
V76.11	Screening mammogram for high-risk patient
V76.12	Other screening mammogram AHA: Q2, 2006, 10
V76.19	Other screening breast examination
V76.2	Screening for malignant neoplasm of the cervix — *routine cervical Pap smear; excludes that as part of general gynecological exam* AHA: Jan-Feb, 1987, 8
V76.3	Screening for malignant neoplasm of the bladder
V76.41	Screening for malignant neoplasm of the rectum
V76.42	Screening for malignant neoplasm of the oral cavity
V76.43	Screening for malignant neoplasm of the skin
V76.44	Special screening for malignant neoplasm of prostate
V76.45	Special screening for malignant neoplasm of testis
V76.46	Special screening for malignant neoplasms, ovary
V76.47	Special screening for malignant neoplasms, vagina — (Use additional code to identify acquired absence of uterus, V45.77)
V76.49	Special screening for malignant neoplasms, other sites
V76.50	Special screening for malignant neoplasms, intestine, unspecified
V76.51	Special screening for malignant neoplasms, colon
V76.52	Special screening for malignant neoplasms, small intestine
V76.81	Special screening for malignant neoplasms, nervous system
V76.89	Special screening for other malignant neoplasm
V76.9	Screening for unspecified malignant neoplasm

Coding Clarification
V76 Screening exams are used to report malignancy screen exams for patients, regardless of the risk factors involved. Use an additional code to indicate the risk factor, such as personal or family history. In either case, should a condition be discovered during the screening, then code the condition as an additional diagnosis to the screening exam.

Diagnostic mammograms are reported using the diagnosis, sign, symptom, or other problem as the first-listed diagnosis. Do not report diagnostic mammograms using the screening mammogram V codes.

Coding Scenario

A screening cervical Pap smear specimen is sent to the pathologist for reading. The specimen is normal.

> Code assignment: V76.2 *Screening for malignant neoplasm of the cervix*

V77 Special screening for endocrine, nutritional, metabolic, and immunity disorders
AHA: Q1, 2004, 11

Endocrine glands are ductless glands, such as the thyroid and pancreas, that secrete directly into the blood system. Nutritional deficiencies include deficiencies in vitamins, minerals, and protein-calorie malnutrition. Metabolic disorders are when the body is not able to break down or utilize certain nutrients. This includes problems with amino-acid transport, carbohydrate transport, lipid metabolism, and gout.

The thyroid is an organ located in the front of the neck that excretes hormones into the blood stream. The main hormones released are thyroxine (T4) and triiodothyronine (T3). Symptoms of thyroid disorders can include nervousness, irritability, feeling hot or cold, weight loss or gain, and loss of energy.

Diabetes mellitus is a condition in which the body does not produce enough insulin or does not correctly use the insulin it does produce. The body needs insulin to convert sugars and starches into energy.

Malnutrition results from inadequate intake or malabsorption of nutrients. Infants and children are at the highest risk for malnutrition, since there is a high demand for nutrients during the growth years. Pregnancy and old age also pose other significant risks for malnutrition.

Phenylketonuria (PKU) is an inherited error of metabolism affecting phenylalanine. This condition is a failure to break down amino acids found in many foods. This can cause mental retardation and hyperphenylalaninemia.

Galactosemia is a congenital condition marked by the body's inability to break down galactose. This is due to an absence of enzymes needed to convert galactose to glucose.

Gout is caused by deposits of monosodium urate or monohydrate crystals. The most common site for these deposits is around the joints, especially around the big toe.

Cystic fibrosis is caused by a defect in the manufacture of cystic fibrosis transmembrane conductance regulator (CFTR). Normally, CFTR forms a channel through which chloride ions transverse the cells lining in the lungs, pancreas, sweat glands, and small intestine. Cystic fibrosis causes a thick, sticky mucus that blocks the airway and can interfere with enzyme production in the pancreas.

Obesity is defined as a condition in which the body weight of the patient is at least 30 percent above the ideal weight as seen on standardized weight charts.

Lipoid disorders are disorders of lipoproteins. There are three types of lipoproteins that carry cholesterol through the bloodstream including high-density lipoproteins (HDL), also known as good cholesterol; low-density lipoproteins (LDL), also know as bad cholesterol; and very low-density lipoproteins (VLDL), also known as very bad cholesterol.

V77.0	Screening for thyroid disorder — *hypothyroid, hyperthyroid* **AHA:** Jan-Feb, 1987, 8
V77.1	Screening for diabetes mellitus — *body does not produce enough insulin* **AHA:** Jan-Feb, 1987, 8
V77.2	Screening for malnutrition
V77.3	Screening for phenylketonuria (PKU) — *failure to break down an amino acid found in many food products* **AHA:** Jan-Feb, 1987, 8
V77.4	Screening for galactosemia — *failure to break down galactose* **AHA:** Jan-Feb, 1987, 8
V77.5	Screening for gout — *monosodium crystals in the joint* **AHA:** Jan-Feb, 1987, 8
V77.6	Screening for cystic fibrosis — *mucoviscidosis* **AHA:** Jan-Feb, 1987, 8
V77.7	Screening for other inborn errors of metabolism — *defective proteins, metabolism, cholesterol, lipoprotein, amino acids, fatty acids, and nucleotide* **AHA:** Jan-Feb, 1987, 8
V77.8	Screening for obesity
V77.91	Screening for lipoid disorders — *cholesterol level, hypercholesterolemia, hyperlipidemia* **AHA:** Jan-Feb, 1987, 8; Q4, 2000, 53
V77.99	Other and unspecified endocrine, nutritional, metabolic, and immunity disorders

V78 Special screening for disorders of blood and blood-forming organs
AHA: Q1, 2004, 11

The term anemia refers to a lower than normal erythrocyte count or level of hemoglobin in the circulating blood. Iron deficiency anemia is almost always caused by blood loss in adults.

Sickle-cell anemia is a severe, chronic, and incurable form of anemia occurring in patients who inherit hemoglobin S genes from both parents. Less severe variations of the disease occur when the patient inherits one hemoglobin S gene from one parent and one hemoglobin C, D, or E gene from the other.

V78.0	Screening for iron deficiency anemia
V78.1	Screening for other and unspecified deficiency anemia
V78.2	Screening for sickle-cell disease or trait — highest among African-Americans, native African, and Mediterranean cultures **AHA:** Jan-Feb, 1987, 8
V78.3	Screening for other hemoglobinopathies
V78.8	Screening for other disorders of blood and blood-forming organs
V78.9	Screening for unspecified disorder of blood and blood-forming organs

Coding Clarification
Category V78 codes may be reported as primary or secondary diagnoses.

V79 Special screening for mental disorders and developmental handicaps
AHA: Q1, 2004, 11

Depression is marked by a loss of interest in activities and feeling sad for long periods of time. There are several kinds of depression that affects more than 20 million people in the United States.

Alcoholism is both a mental and physical condition, resulting from excessive alcohol consumption. It is characterized by behavioral and other responses that always include a compulsion to take alcohol on a continuous or periodic basis in order to experience its psychic effects and sometimes to avoid the discomfort of its absence; tolerance may or may not be present.

Mental retardation is defined as general intellectual functioning at least two standard deviations below the norm as measured in a standardized intelligence test. It must be accompanied by significant limitation in communication, self care, home living, interpersonal skills, self-direction, work, leisure, health, or safety. This onset must occur before adulthood.

A developmental delay is the failure to obtain developmental milestones that are related to a specific age. This may include sitting, crawling, and walking.

V79.0	Screening for depression
V79.1	Screening for alcoholism
V79.2	Screening for mental retardation
V79.3	Screening for developmental handicaps in early childhood
V79.8	Screening for other specified mental disorders and developmental handicaps
V79.9	Screening for unspecified mental disorder and developmental handicap

Coding Clarification
Category V79 codes may be reported as primary or secondary diagnoses.

Coding Scenario
A mother of a one-year-old male presents to the pediatric clinic with concerns that the child is not walking. After examination and testing it is determined that there is no problem with the child.

Code assignment: V79.3 *Screening for developmental handicaps in early childhood*

V80 Special screening for neurological, eye, and ear diseases
AHA: Q1, 2004, 11

Neurological conditions are those that affect the central nervous system. This can include epilepsy, dementia, migraines, and neuromuscular diseases.

Glaucoma is an increase in intraocular pressure due to an abnormal aqueous humor outflow from the anterior chamber or, rarely, from an above normal rate of aqueous humor production by the ciliary body. If untreated, glaucoma ultimately leads to optic nerve damage and loss of vision.

V80.0	Screening for neurological conditions
V80.1	Screening for glaucoma
V80.2	Screening for other eye conditions — *cataract, senile macular lesions* **AHA:** Jan-Feb, 1987, 8
V80.3	Screening for ear diseases

Coding Clarification
Category V80 codes may be reported as primary or secondary diagnoses.

V81 Special screening for cardiovascular, respiratory, and genitourinary diseases
AHA: Q1, 2004, 11

Ischemic heart disease is an inadequate flow of blood through the coronary arteries to the tissue of the heart. The predominant etiology of the ischemia is arteriosclerosis. Partially obstructed coronary artery blood flow can manifest in angina pectoris; complete obstruction results in an infarction of the myocardium.

Hypertension is a condition in which the diastolic pressure exceeds 100 mm Hg in persons 60 years of age and older or 90 mm Hg in persons younger than 60 years of age. WHO defines hypertension as pressures exceeding 160/90 mm Hg, but studies have shown that increased morbidity and mortality are associated with diastolic pressures of just 85 mm Hg. It is generally asymptomatic until complications develop. Complications may include retinal changes, loud aortic sounds, and early systolic ejection click heard on auscultation, headache, tinnitus, and palpations.

Bronchitis is defined as a persistent cough with sputum production occurring on most days for at least three months of the year for at least two years.

Emphysema refers to any condition in which air is present in a small area of an organ or tissue. This causes over inflation of the lungs. The most common cause of emphysema is smoking; however, environmental factors may have an influence.

Nephropathy refers to diseases of the kidney. Included in this are nephritis and sclerotic lesions of the kidney.

V81.0	Screening for ischemic heart disease
V81.1	Screening for hypertension
V81.2	Screening for other and unspecified cardiovascular conditions
V81.3	Screening for chronic bronchitis and emphysema
V81.4	Screening for other and unspecified respiratory condition
V81.5	Screening for nephropathy — *asymptomatic bacteriuria*
	AHA: Jan-Feb, 1987, 8
V81.6	Screening for other and unspecified genitourinary condition

Coding Clarification
Category V81 codes may be reported as primary or secondary diagnoses.

Coding Scenario
A 65-year-old male presents to the family practice clinic for a routine blood pressure check. The patient has no history of hypertension.

> Code assignment: V81.1 *Screening for hypertension*

V82 Special screening for other condition
AHA: Q1, 2004, 11

Rheumatoid arthritis is a chronic, systemic inflammatory disease of unknown etiology, characterized by a variable but prolonged course with swelling. In early stages, the disease attacks the joints of the hands and feet. As the disease progresses, more joints become involved. Also known as primary progressive arthritis and proliferative arthritis, the disease often leads to progressive deformities, which may develop rapidly and cause permanent disability.

Congenital dislocation of the hip is caused by failure of the hip joint to form correctly. This is characterized by a hip click that can be heard when the leg is moved.

Chromosomal anomalies are either lack of genetic material or extra genetic material. Mothers can pass genetic anomalies to their children without having the specific disease. Genetic anomalies can also occur at conception when genetic material from the mother and father are joined.

Multiphasic screening refers to multiple tests that are used to identify illness or disease.

Osteoporosis is generalized bone disease characterized by decreased osteoblastic formation of matrix combined with increased osteoclastic resorption of bone, resulting in a marked decrease in bone mass.

V82.0	Screening for skin condition
V82.1	Screening for rheumatoid arthritis
V82.2	Screening for other rheumatic disorder
V82.3	Screening for congenital dislocation of hip
V82.4	Maternal postnatal screening of chromosomal anomalies
V82.5	Screening for chemical poisoning and other contamination
V82.6	Multiphasic screening
V82.71	Screening for genetic disease carrier status
V82.79	Other genetic testing

Coding Clarification
Report genetic testing for procreative management with codes V26.31 and V26.32.

V82.81	Special screening for osteoporosis — (Use additional code to identify postmenopausal status: V07.4, V49.81)
V82.89	Special screening for other specified conditions
V82.9	Screening for unspecified condition

Coding Clarification
Category V82 codes may reported as primary or secondary diagnoses.

Report V07.4 for postmenopausal hormone replacement therapy status or V49.81 for postmenopausal (age-related) (natural) status in addition to V82.81.

V83–V84 Genetics

V83 Genetic carrier status

Category V83 codes are used to report genetic carrier status. The codes are mainly used for women who are pregnant or are considering pregnancy and are known carriers of a disease. The codes listed are for asymptomatic carriers except for V83.02, which is for carriers of hemophilia A, who have trouble with blood coagulation.

Hemophilia A is abnormal coagulation characterized by subcutaneous and intramuscular hemorrhage and caused by a mutant gene on the X chromosome.

Cystic fibrosis is caused by a defect in the manufacture of cystic fibrosis transmembrane conductance regulator (CFTR). Normally, CFTR forms a channel through which chloride ions transverse the cells lining in the lungs, pancreas, sweat glands, and small intestine. Cystic fibrosis causes a thick, sticky mucus that blocks the airway and can interfere with enzyme production in the pancreas.

V83.01	Asymptomatic hemophilia A carrier
V83.02	Symptomatic hemophilia A carrier
V83.81	Cystic fibrosis gene carrier
V83.89	Other genetic carrier status

V84 Genetic susceptibility to diseases
AHA: Q4, 2004, 106

Having a genetic susceptibility to a disease, in particular a malignancy, is not the same as being a carrier of a disease, that may be passed on to offspring. Those people who are genetically susceptibility is a red flag a person is at higher risk and has a greater chance of getting a disease or malignant growth because of their inborn predisposition. These patients sometimes request to have the particular organ at risk removed prophylactically in the hope that taking such a step will prevent the disease from occurring. Most of these requests are for prophylactic breast or ovary removal.

V84.01	Genetic susceptibility to malignant neoplasm of breast **AHA:** Q4, 2004, 107
V84.02	Genetic susceptibility to malignant neoplasm of ovary
V84.03	Genetic susceptibility to malignant neoplasm of prostate
V84.04	Genetic susceptibility to malignant neoplasm of endometrium
V84.09	Genetic susceptibility to other malignant neoplasm
V84.8	Genetic susceptibility to other disease

V85 Body Mass Index [BMI]

V85 Body mass index [BMI]
AHA: Q4, 2005, 97; Q2, 2006, 5

BMI is measured in kilograms per meters squared. The calculation is based on height and weight determined by dividing a person's weight in kilograms by height in meters squared. The index score can also be calculated by multiplying a patient's weight in kilograms by 704.5, and dividing the result by the patient's height in inches twice. BMI measurements are a guideline for categorizing weight in a more specific manner than relying solely on "overweight" or "obese" terminology.

By definition, an adult is generally considered overweight if he or she has a BMI between 25 and 29.9 kg/m2. Obesity is defined as a BMI of 30 or higher. Individual variances such as the presence or absence of muscle mass and the distribution of body fat also need to be taken into consideration. For example, a body builder with an excess of healthy muscle mass may be considered "overweight." Also, persons with fat distributed primarily in the upper body are at a higher risk for diseases such as hypertension and cardiovascular disease than those patients with fat mainly distributed in the lower body, below the waist.

The CDC provides four weight classifications for children:

- "Underweight" refers to a weight that is under the fifth percentile for the child's age.
- "Healthy" refers to a weight between the fifth and 85th percentile.
- "At risk" refers to a weight between the 85th and 95th percentile for the child's age. This corresponds to a BMI of 25, which is considered overweight for an adult.
- "Overweight" refers to a weight ranking above the 95th percentile for the child's age. This is the most severe level of childhood obesity, corresponding to a BMI of at least 30. This is the same indicator used to classify adult obesity.

A differentiation is made between the terms "overweight" and "obese." The difference is severity of condition and potential outcomes. Treatment for these conditions and the associated health risks differ in relationship to its progression and severity. These codes have been created to distinguish overweight patients from obese patients and to provide a mechanism of severity measurement based on Body Mass Indices.

V85.0	Body Mass Index less than 19, adult
V85.1	Body Mass Index between 19-24, adult
V85.21	Body Mass Index 25.0-25.9, adult
V85.22	Body Mass Index 26.0-26.9, adult
V85.23	Body Mass Index 27.0-27.9, adult
V85.24	Body Mass Index 28.0-28.9, adult
V85.25	Body Mass Index 29.0-29.9, adult
V85.30	Body Mass Index 30.0-30.9, adult
V85.31	Body Mass Index 31.0-31.9, adult
V85.32	Body Mass Index 32.0-32.9, adult
V85.33	Body Mass Index 33.0-33.9, adult
V85.34	Body Mass Index 34.0-34.9, adult
V85.35	Body Mass Index 35.0-35.9, adult
V85.36	Body Mass Index 36.0-36.9, adult
V85.37	Body Mass Index 37.0-37.9, adult
V85.38	Body Mass Index 38.0-38.9, adult
V85.39	Body Mass Index 39.0-39.9, adult
V85.4	Body Mass Index 40 and over, adult

Category V85 codes are to be used as additional codes only.

V85.51	Body Mass Index, pediatric, less than 5th percentile for age
V85.52	Body Mass Index, pediatric, 5th percentile to less than 85th percentile for age
V85.53	Body Mass Index, pediatric, 85th percentile to less than 95th percentile for age
V85.54	Body Mass Index, pediatric, greater than or equal to 95th percentile for age

Coding Clarification

BMI pediatric codes are to be used for persons aged 2 to 20 years only. The percentiles specified above are based on growth charts published by the Centers for Disease Control and Prevention (CDC).

V86   Estrogen Receptor Status

V86   Estrogen receptor status

In breast cancer, the hormone receptor status of the cells is a useful tool for determining treatment and prognosis. Cancers in which the cells express estrogen receptor (ER) in their nuclei generally have a better prognosis, since these cells are better differentiated and can respond to hormonal manipulation. According to the National Cancer Institute, seven out of 10 breast cancer patients have ER-positive tumors.

V86.0	Estrogen receptor positive status [ER+] — (Code first the malignant neoplasm of the breast)
V86.1	Estrogen receptor negative status [ER-] — (Code first the malignant neoplasm of the breast)

E800–E999

Supplementary Classification of External Causes

E codes are used to indicate how an accident occurred, what caused an injury, whether a drug overdose was accidental, an adverse drug reaction, or the location of an injury. This information can be used by payers to determine if another insurance company (e.g., automobile insurance) should be billed, but the primary intent is to gather information for injury research and prevention. These codes are used as an additional diagnosis and should never be listed first; the most serious condition or injury should be coded as the primary diagnosis.

When accidents involve more than one motor vehicle, the following order should be used:

- Aircraft and spacecraft (E840-E845)
- Watercraft (E830-E838)
- Motor vehicle (E810-E825)
- Railway (E800-E807)
- Other road vehicles (E826-E829)
- If injuries are sustained from more than one cause, report as many E codes as necessary. The codes should be listed in the following order:
- E codes for abuse
- E codes for terrorism
- E codes for catastrophe or natural disaster
- E codes for transport accidents
- Assign the code for the most serious injuries in each category first.

Transport accidents (E800-E848) involve a vehicle that is primarily used to transport people or products. Agriculture and construction vehicle accidents are considered transport accidents if the machinery is under its own power on a highway.

E800–E807 Railway Accidents

Railway accidents involve vehicles that travel on rails and transport people or products. Use this category whether or not the train is moving. A train is defined as an electric car or a street car that is operated on its own right-of-way and is not open to other traffic, a railway train, a car on a flexible cable either monorail or two rail, a subway or elevated train and any other vehicle designed to run on a railway track. Excluded from this category are interurban electric cars (streetcars) specified to be operating on a street that forms part of the public street or highway.

According to ICD-9-CM guidelines, a railway or railroad is a right-of-way designed for traffic on rails, which is used by carriages or wagons transporting passengers or freight, and by other rolling stock, and which is not open to other public vehicular traffic.

A passenger on the train is any authorized person traveling on the train. Use fourth digit .8 *Other specified person,* for passengers waiting to get on the train or unauthorized riders.

The following fourth-digit subdivisions are for use with categories E800-E807 to identify the injured person:

0 Railway employee
1 Passenger on railway
2 Pedestrian
3 Pedal cyclist
8 Other specified person
9 Unspecified person

E800 ⌐sth Railway accident involving collision with rolling stock

Rolling stock is any kind of car or vehicle that travels on a track. Included in this code category is any kind of collision that involves a railway train or railway vehicle, a collision not otherwise specified (NOS) on railway, or a derailment with preceding collision with rolling stock.

A railway accident is one that involves a train and another vehicle that travels on rails.

An antecedent collision with derailment means the engine collides with an object causing the train to derail.

Coding Clarification
Category E800 codes may only be reported as a secondary diagnosis.

E code reporting varies from state to state and hospital to hospital. Check with payers and hospital policies to determine if E codes should be reported.

Use an additional code from category E849 to identify the place of occurrence.

E801 ✓5th   Railway accident involving collision with other object
Included in this code category is the collision of a railway train with buffers, which includes fallen trees or rocks on the railway, a gate, a platform, a streetcar, a bicycle, or any other object that is not a motorized vehicle.

Coding Clarification
Category E801 codes may only be reported as a secondary diagnosis.

Use an additional code from category E849 to identify the place of occurrence.

Coding Scenario
A train engineer presented to the emergency department with a left radial and ulnar shaft fracture after the train he was driving hit a tree that had fallen on to the track.

> Code assignment: 813.2 *Closed fracture of shaft of the radius and ulna*, E800.0 *Railway accident involving collision with other object, railroad employee*, E849.8 *Place of occurrence, other specified place.*

E802 ✓5th   Railway accident involving derailment without antecedent collision
Railway accidents involving derailment without antecedent collision means a train derailment that is not caused by the engine hitting an object.

Coding Clarification
Category E802 codes may only be reported as a secondary diagnosis.

Use an additional code from category E849 to identify the place of occurrence.

E803 ✓5th   Railway accident involving explosion, fire, or burning
A railway accident that is caused by or involves a type of fire or explosion may be a mechanical issue related to the train's engine, a fire in a commuter train caused by an individual or cooking vessel, or other flammable items.

Coding Clarification
Category E803 codes may only be reported as a secondary diagnosis.

Report the code for the injury sustained in the accident before the E code.

Use an additional code from category E849 to identify the place of occurrence.

E804 ✓5th   Fall in, on, or from railway train
Category E804 codes are used to report a fall in, on, or from the railway train, which includes a fall while getting on or off the train. Report the ICD-9-CM code for the injury before the E code.

Coding Clarification
Category E804 codes may only be reported as a secondary diagnosis.

Use an additional code from category E849 to identify the place of occurrence.

Coding Scenario
A 54-year-old female presents to the emergency department with pain in the right ankle. She fell while stepping off the train at the station. X-rays show no fracture. The final diagnosis is a sprained right ankle.

> Code assignment: 845.00 *Unspecified site of ankle sprain and strain*, E804.1 *Fall in, on, or from railway train, passenger on railway*, E849.8 *Place of occurrence, other specified place*

E805 ✓5th   Hit by rolling stock
Category E805 codes are used to describe railway accidents caused by a hit to rolling stock. Rolling stock is defined as anything that travels on the track. These kinds of accidents include persons being crushed, injured, killed, knocked down, or run over stock by a railway train or part.

Coding Clarification
Category E805 codes may only be reported as a secondary diagnosis.

Use an additional code from category E849 to identify the place of occurrence.

E806 ⚐sth Other specified railway accident
Category E806 codes are used to describe any other specified railway accident. This code category includes an object falling on and hitting a pedestrian in the railway train, pedestrian injuries caused by a door or window on a railway train, an object set in motion by a railway train hitting a non-motor-road vehicle or pedestrian, or falling earth NOS, a rock, a tree, or other object hitting a railway train.

Coding Clarification
Category E806 codes may only be reported as a secondary diagnosis.

Use an additional code from category E849 to identify the place of occurrence.

Coding Scenario
A 48-year-old male was found on a railroad track with a severe laceration to the thigh. He could not provide any details of the accident.

> Code assignment: 890.0 *Open wound of the thigh without mention of complication* and E806.9 *Railway accident of unspecified nature, unspecified person*

E807 ⚐sth Railway accident of unspecified nature
Category E807 codes are used to report an unspecified railway accident. Included in these types of accidents are a person found dead or injured on the railway right-of-way and a railway accident NOS.

Coding Clarification
Category E807 codes may only be reported as a secondary diagnosis.

Use an additional code from category E849 to identify the place of occurrence.

E810–E819 Motor Vehicle Traffic Accidents

According to ICD-9-CM guidelines, a motor vehicle accident is a transport accident involving a vehicle that is motorized. A motor vehicle accident is an accident that occurs on the highway and is assumed to have occurred on the highway unless otherwise specified. An accident that involves an off-road vehicle, such as an ATV or a snowmobile, is considered a nontraffic accident unless otherwise specified. All codes require fourth digits.

A motor vehicle is defined as a self-powered device intended to move people or objects. Motor vehicles travel on the highway and not on rails. Included in this category are automobiles, buses, construction machinery, farm and industrial machinery, steam rollers, tractors, army tanks, highway graders or similar vehicles on wheels or treads while in transport under its own power, fire engines, motorcycles, motorized bicycles, mopeds, scooters, trolley buses (not operating on rails), trucks, and vans.

A driver is considered the occupant of a car who is operating the vehicle. All other occupants are considered passengers.

A pedal cycle is any vehicle operated solely by pedal power. A pedal cyclist includes any person riding on a pedal cycle, including a passenger.

A pedestrian is defined as a person not riding in a vehicle, on a motorcycle, or on an animal. A pedestrian can be a person changing a tire, operating a pedestrian conveyance, fixing a vehicle, or traveling on foot.

The following fourth-digit subdivisions are for use with categories E810-E819 to identify the injured person:
0 Driver of motor vehicle other than motorcycle
1 Passenger in motor vehicle other than motorcycle
2 Motorcyclist
3 Passenger on motorcycle
4 Occupant of streetcar
5 Rider of animal; occupant of animal-driven vehicle
6 Pedal cyclist
7 Pedestrian
8 Other specified person
9 Unspecified person

E810 ⚐sth Motor vehicle traffic accident involving collision with train
Category E810 codes are used to report an accident involving a motor vehicle and a train.

Coding Clarification
Category E810 codes may only be reported as a secondary diagnosis.

Use an additional code from category E849 to identify the place of occurrence.

E811 ⚐sth Motor vehicle traffic accident involving re-entrant collision with another motor vehicle
Category E811 is used to report a motor vehicle traffic accident involving a re-entrant collision with another motor vehicle. A re-entry accident includes the collision between two motor vehicles caused by one motor vehicle accidentally leaving the roadway and then re-entering the same roadway or a motor vehicle that crosses over to the opposite roadway or a divided highway.

Coding Clarification

Category E811 codes may only be reported as a secondary diagnosis.

Use an additional code from category E849 to identify the place of occurrence.

E812 ✓5th Other motor vehicle collision with unmoving motor vehicle

Category E812 codes are used to report a motor vehicle accident involving a collision with another motor vehicle. This code category includes the collision of one motor vehicle with another motor vehicle that is parked, stopped, stalled, disabled, or abandoned on the highway and a motor vehicle collision NOS.

Coding Clarification

Category E812 codes may only be reported as a secondary diagnosis.

Use an additional code from category E849 to identify the place of occurrence.

E813 ✓5th Motor vehicle collision with nonmotor transport vehicle

Category E813 codes are used to report a motor vehicle collision with another vehicle. This includes a collision between a motor vehicle of any kind and other road (non-motor-transport) vehicles, such as an animal carrying a person, an animal-drawn vehicle, a pedal cycle, or a streetcar.

Coding Clarification

Category E813 codes may only be reported as a secondary diagnosis.

Use an additional code from category E849 to identify the place of occurrence.

Coding Scenario

A 21-year-old female was brought into the emergency department following a car vs. bicycle accident. The patient was riding her bike in the street and was hit by a car from behind. The patient complains of pain in her right wrist. X-rays were negative for a fracture. The final diagnosis is sprain of the right wrist.

> Code assignment: 842.00 *Sprain and strain of unspecified part of the wrist*, E813.3 *Motor vehicle traffic accident involving collision with other vehicle, Pedal cyclist*, and E849.5 *Place of occurrence street and highway*

E814 ✓5th Motor vehicle collision with pedestrian

Category E14 codes identify a motor vehicle collision with a pedestrian. This code category includes all kinds of motor vehicles. A pedestrian dragged, hit, or run over by a motor vehicle is included in this category.

Coding Clarification

Category E814 codes may only be reported as a secondary diagnosis.

Use an additional code from category E849 to identify the place of occurrence.

E815 ✓5th Other motor vehicle collision with object on the highway

Category E815 codes are used to report other motor vehicle collisions on the highway. This code category includes a collision due to loss of control on the highway between a motor vehicle and an abutment (a structure that receives force or pressure), a bridge, an overpass, an animal, fallen stone, a traffic sign, a tree, a utility pole, a guard rail, a fence, a highway divider, a landslide (not moving), an object set in motion by a railway train or road vehicles, fixed, moveable, or moving object thrown in front of motor vehicle safety island, a temporary traffic signs or markers, or walls.

Coding Clarification

Category E815 codes may only be reported as a secondary diagnosis.

Report E816.0-E816.9 for collision with any object that normally would have been off the highway and is not stated as having been on it.

Use an additional code from category E849 to identify the place of occurrence.

E816 ✓5th Motor vehicle traffic accident due to loss of control, without collision on the highway

Category E816 codes are used to report traffic accidents due to loss of control of a motor vehicle without collision on the highway. This code category includes a motor vehicle that fails to make a curve, a motor vehicle going out of control due to a tire blowout, the driver falling asleep, the driver not paying attention, excessive speeding, or the failure of mechanical parts. This type of accident also includes an out-of-control vehicle colliding with an object off the highway, overturning the car, and stopping abruptly off the highway.

Coding Clarification

Category E816 codes may only be reported as a secondary diagnosis.

Use an additional code from category E849 to identify the place of occurrence.

Coding Scenario

A 16-year-old male is brought into the emergency department following a one-car rollover accident. He went out of control after overcorrecting on a turn. He complains of left elbow pain. There are no other injures. The final diagnosis is a fracture of the distal humerus.

> Code assignment: 812.4 *Fracture lower end of humerus*, E816.0 *Motor vehicle traffic accident due to loss of control without collision on the highway, driver*, E849.5 *Place of occurrence, street and highway*
>
> **E817** ✓5th Noncollision motor vehicle traffic accident while boarding or alighting

Category E817 codes are used to report non-collision, motor-vehicle-traffic accidents while boarding or alighting (getting out of the car). This code category includes a fall while getting on or off a bus, a fall getting in or out of a car, an injury by a moving part of a vehicle, or a passenger trapped by the door of a bus.

Coding Clarification

Category E817 codes may only be reported as a secondary diagnosis.

Use an additional code from category E849 to identify the place of occurrence.

> **E818** ✓5th Other noncollision motor vehicle traffic accident

Category E818 codes are used to report other noncollision motor vehicle traffic accidents. This code category includes most accidents that are not caused by one vehicle colliding with another vehicle. Examples of this are accidental poisoning from exhaust gas; falling, jumping, or being accidentally pushed from a moving car; a fire starting in a moving car; and an injury from being hit by an object thrown into or on a moving vehicle.

A traffic accident is one that occurs on a public highway. A motor vehicle accident is assumed to have occurred on the highway unless otherwise specified.

Coding Clarification

Category E818 codes may only be reported as a secondary diagnosis.

Use an additional code from category E849 to identify the place of occurrence.

> **E819** ✓5th Motor vehicle traffic accident of unspecified nature

Category E819 codes are used to report motor vehicle accidents of an unspecified nature. This code category includes motor vehicle traffic accidents NOS and traffic accidents NOS.

A traffic accident is one that occurs on a public highway. A motor vehicle accident is assumed to have occurred on the highway unless otherwise specified.

A motor vehicle is one that is mechanically or electrically powered and primarily used on a highway. Any object being towed by the motor vehicle is considered a part of the vehicle.

Coding Clarification

Category E819 codes may only be reported as a secondary diagnosis.

Use an additional code from category E849 to identify the place of occurrence.

Coding Scenario

An 18-year-old male is brought into the emergency department following a motor vehicle accident with another car at an intersection. He is the restrained driver. The patient has a small laceration on his forehead. No other injuries were found.

> Code assignment: 873.42 *Open wound, forehead, without complication*, E819.0 *Motor vehicle traffic accident of unspecified nature, driver of motor vehicle other than motorcycle*, and E849.5 *Place of occurrence, street and highway*

E820–E825 Motor Vehicle Nontraffic Accidents

Category E820-E825 codes are used to report nontraffic accidents. Nontraffic accidents are defined as those that occur in a place other than a public highway. This code category includes snowmobile accidents, off-road vehicle accidents, and collisions with stationary objects. Also included in this category is an accident while boarding and alighting a vehicle not on a public highway. Accidents that involve off-road vehicles, such as all-terrain vehicles (ATVs) and snowmobiles, are assumed to be nontraffic accidents unless otherwise specified. Fourth digits are required for all of the codes.

A driver is considered the occupant of a car who is operating the vehicle. All other occupants are considered passengers.

A pedal cycle is any vehicle operated solely by pedal power. A pedal cyclist includes any person riding on a pedal cycle, including a passenger.

A pedestrian is defined as a person not riding in a vehicle, on a motorcycle, or on an animal. A pedestrian can be a person changing a tire, operating a pedestrian conveyance, fixing a motor vehicle, or traveling on foot.

A pedestrian conveyance is defined as a device powered by a human to transport a person other than by walking. This includes a baby carriage, coaster wagon, ice skates, perambulator, pushcart, pushchair, roller skates, scooter, skateboard, skis, sled, or wheelchair. For coding purposes, a person in or on a pedestrian conveyance is considered a pedestrian.

A streetcar is a vehicle that normally runs on rails but is subject to traffic signals and forms part of the traffic way. A trailer being towed by a streetcar is considered part of the streetcar.

Accidents involving off-road vehicles are assumed to be nontraffic accidents unless otherwise specified.

The following fourth-digit subdivisions are for use with categories E820-E825 to identify the injured person:
0   Driver of motor vehicle other than motorcycle
1   Passenger in motor vehicle other than motorcycle
2   Motorcyclist
3   Passenger on motorcycle
4   Occupant of streetcar
5   Rider of animal; occupant of animal-drawn vehicle
6   Pedal cyclist
7   Pedestrian
8   Other specified person
9   Unspecified person

E820 ⌐5th⌐   Nontraffic accident involving motor-driven snow vehicle

Category E820 codes are used to report nontraffic accidents involving motor-driven snow vehicles. This code category is used to report an injury from falling off of or being dragged by a snowmobile. Also included in this code category is any injury caused by a rough landing of the snow vehicle.

Alcohol and excessive speed contribute to the majority of snowmobile injuries and death.

Nontraffic accidents are those that occur any place other than a public highway. Off-road vehicle accidents are considered nontraffic accidents unless otherwise specified.

Coding Clarification
Category E820 codes may only be reported as a secondary diagnosis.

Use an additional code from category E849 to identify the place of occurrence.

E821 ⌐5th⌐   Nontraffic accident involving other off-road motor vehicle

Category E821 codes are used to report nontraffic accidents involving other off-road motor vehicles. An off-road motor vehicle is one specially designed to negotiate rough or soft terrain (e.g., vehicles that are

high in construction, have special wheels and tires, or are driven by treads). A non-motor-vehicle accident is one that occurs any place other than a public highway. Off-road vehicle accidents are considered nontraffic accidents unless otherwise specified.

Coding Clarification
Category E821 codes may only be reported as a secondary diagnosis.

Use an additional code from category E849 to identify the place of occurrence.

Coding Scenario
A 45-year-old male is brought into the emergency department with an abrasion to the right hip after falling off the ATV he was driving. X-rays are negative for a fracture. The final diagnosis is an abrasion the right hip.

> Code assignment: 916.0 *Hip, thigh, and ankle abrasion or friction burn without mention of infection*, E821.0 *Nontraffic accident involving other off-road motor vehicle, driver*

E822 ⌐5th⌐   Other motor vehicle nontraffic accident involving collision with moving object

Category E822 codes are used to report other motor vehicle accidents involving collision with a moving object. This code category includes collision between a motor vehicle and an animal, a non-motor-vehicle, another motor vehicle, a pedestrian, a train, or another moving object. A non-motor-vehicle accident is one that occurs any place other than a public highway. Do not use this code for off-road motor vehicles.

Coding Clarification
Category E822 codes may only be reported as a secondary diagnosis.

Use an additional code from category E849 to identify the place of occurrence.

E823 ⌐5th⌐   Other motor vehicle nontraffic accident involving collision with stationary object

Category E823 codes are used to report a nontraffic collision between a motor vehicle and any other object that is not moving. This type of accident includes collisions with objects that are fixed or moveable. Nontraffic accidents are those that occur any place other than a public highway. Do not use this code for off-road motor vehicles. A motor vehicle is one that is mechanically or electrically powered and primarily used on a highway. Any object being towed by the motor vehicle is considered a part of the vehicle.

Coding Clarification
Category E823 codes may only be reported as a secondary diagnosis.

Use an additional code from category E849 to identify the place of occurrence.

Coding Scenario
A 17-year-old female is admitted to the emergency department with a suspected head injury after the ATV she was driving hit a rock and flipped her out. All x-rays and tests are negative for a head injury and she is sent home.

> Code assignment: V71.4 *Observation following other accident* and E823.0 *Other motor vehicle nontraffic accident involving collision with stationary object, driver of motor vehicle other than motorcycle*

E824 [✓5th] Other motor vehicle nontraffic accident while boarding and alighting

Category E824 codes are used to report injuries while getting in or out of a motor vehicle or on or off a motorcycle. This code category also includes injury from any moving part of the vehicle or being trapped by the door of the vehicle. Codes in this category are used to report an injury that occurs when the vehicle is not moving. Do not use this code for off-road motor vehicles. An off-road motor vehicle is one specifically designed to negotiate rough or soft terrain (e.g., vehicles that are high in construction, have special wheels and tires, or driven by treads). A motor vehicle is one that is mechanically or electrically powered and primarily used on a highway. Any object being towed by the motor vehicle is considered a part of the vehicle.

Coding Clarification
Category E824 codes may only be reported as a secondary diagnosis.

Use an additional code from category E849 to identify the place of occurrence.

E825 [✓5th] Other motor vehicle nontraffic accident of other and unspecified nature

Category E825 codes are used to report other and unspecified injuries sustained as a result of a nontraffic accident. A nontraffic accident is one that occurs any place other than on a public highway. Unspecified injuries include injury from accidental carbon monoxide poisoning and injury from a part of a moving vehicle. Also included is injury that occurs when from falling, jumping, or being accidentally pushed from a moving vehicle. This category also includes an injury sustained from an object thrown into a moving vehicle.

Coding Clarification
Category E825 codes may only be reported as a secondary diagnosis.

Use an additional code from category E849 to identify the place of occurrence.

E826–E829 Other Road Vehicle Accidents

Other road vehicle accidents are those that involve any device other than motor vehicles. This type of accident includes those that occur while a person is riding on an animal, and any accident that involves an animal-drawn carriage, a bicycle, a tricycle, or a streetcar.

A pedestrian is defined as a person not riding in a vehicle, on a motorcycle, or on an animal. A pedestrian can be a person changing a tire, operating a pedestrian conveyance, fixing a motor vehicle, or traveling on foot.

A streetcar is a vehicle that normally runs on rails but is subject to traffic signals and forms part of the traffic way. A trailer being towed by a streetcar is considered part of the streetcar.

> The following fourth-digit subdivisions are for use with categories E826-E829 to identify the injured person:
> 0 Pedestrian
> 1 Pedal cyclist
> 2 Rider of animal
> 3 Occupant of animal-drawn vehicle
> 4 Occupant of streetcar
> 8 Other specified person
> 9 Unspecified person

E826 [✓5th] Pedal cycle accident

Category E826 codes are used to report an accident involving a pedal cycle. A pedal cycle is defined as any vehicle that is run solely by pedal power. A pedal cyclist is any person riding a pedal cycle or riding in a sidecar. This code category includes most injuries caused by parts of the cycle or by a person becoming entangled in a part. Also included in this code category is injury sustained from a fall off of the cycle or from an object thrown at the cycle.

Coding Clarification
Category E826 codes may only be reported as a secondary diagnosis.

Use an additional code from category E849 to identify the place of occurrence.

Coding Scenario
A 34-year-old male, riding in the street, fell off his bicycle and sustained a laceration to his right hand.

> Code assignment: 882.0 *Open wound to hand alone*, E826.1 *Pedal cycle accident, pedal cyclist*, and E849.5 *Place of occurrence, street and highway*

E827 ⌐sth   Animal-drawn vehicle accident — *carriage, sled*
Animal-drawn-vehicle accidents include those caused by a breakage of any part of the vehicle. Included in this category are injuries sustained from a collision with an animal-drawn vehicle and an animal, a nonmotor vehicle, a pedestrian, or a pedestrian conveyance. Also included in this category is an injury sustained by falling off of or being thrown from an animal-drawn vehicle. This does not include an accident between an animal-drawn-vehicle and a pedal cycle. A non-motor-vehicle accident is one that occurs any place other than on a public highway.

A pedestrian is defined as a person not riding in a vehicle, on a motorcycle, or on an animal. A pedestrian can be a person changing a tire, operating a pedestrian conveyance, fixing a vehicle, or traveling on foot. A pedestrian conveyance is defined as a device powered by a human to transport a person other than by walking, which includes a baby carriage, a coaster wagon, ice skates, a perambulator, a pushcart, a pushchair, roller skates, a scooter, a skateboard, skis, a sled, or a wheelchair. For coding purposes, a person in or on a pedestrian conveyance is considered a pedestrian.

Coding Clarification
Category E827 codes may only be reported as a secondary diagnosis.

Use an additional code from category E849 to identify the place of occurrence.

Only fourth digits 0, 2-4, 8, and 9 may be used with category E827.

Coding Scenario
A 10-year-old female is admitted to the emergency department with a left arm injury. The girl was ice skating on a frozen lake and was hit and knocked down by a horse-drawn sleigh. The final diagnosis is a sprain of the left wrist.

> Code assignment: 842.00 *Sprain and strain of unspecified site of wrist*, E 827.0 *Animal-drawn vehicle accident, pedestrian*, and E849.4 *Place of occurrence, place for recreation and sport*

E828 ⌐sth   Accident involving animal being ridden

Category E828 codes are used to report accidents that involve an animal being ridden. This type of accident includes a collision with another animal, a nonmotor vehicle except pedal cycle, an animal-drawn vehicle, a pedestrian, or a pedestrian conveyance. Also included in this category are injuries caused by a fall from, being knocked down by, being thrown from, or being trampled by an animal.

A non-motor-vehicle accident is one that occurs any place other than a public highway. A pedestrian is defined as a person not riding in a vehicle, on a motorcycle, or on an animal. A pedestrian can be a person changing a tire, operating a pedestrian conveyance, fixing a motor vehicle, or traveling on foot. A pedestrian conveyance is defined as a device powered by a human to transport a person other than by walking, which includes a baby carriage, a coaster wagon, ice skates, a perambulator, a pushcart, a pushchair, roller skates, a scooter, a skateboard, skis, a sled, or a wheelchair. For coding purposes, a person in or on a pedestrian conveyance is considered a pedestrian.

Coding Clarification
Category E828 codes may only be reported as a secondary diagnosis.

Use an additional code from category E849 to identify the place of occurrence.

Only fourth digits 1, 2, 4, 8, and 9 may be used with category E828.

E829 ⌐sth   Other road vehicle accidents
Category E828 codes are used to report accidents that involve an animal being ridden. This type of accident includes a collision with another animal, a nonmotor vehicle except pedal cycle, an animal-drawn vehicle, a pedestrian, or a pedestrian conveyance. Also included in this category are injuries caused by a fall from, being knocked down by, being thrown from, or being trampled by an animal.

A non-motor-vehicle accident is one that occurs any place other than a public highway. A pedestrian is defined as a person not riding in a vehicle, on a motorcycle, or on an animal. A pedestrian can be a person changing a tire, operating a pedestrian conveyance, fixing a motor vehicle, or traveling on foot. A pedestrian conveyance is defined as a device powered by a human to transport a person other than by walking, which includes a baby carriage, a coaster wagon, ice skates, a perambulator, a pushcart, a pushchair, roller skates, a scooter, a skateboard, skis, a sled, or a wheelchair. For coding purposes, a person in or on a pedestrian conveyance is considered a pedestrian.

Coding Clarification
Category E829 codes may only be reported as a secondary diagnosis.

Use an additional code from category E849 to identify the place of occurrence.

Only fourth digits 0, 4, 8, and 9 may be used with category E829.

Coding Scenario
A 65-year-old woman presents to the emergency room after getting her hand caught in the door of a streetcar. The diagnosis is a fracture at the base of the third metacarpal.

> Code assignment: 815.02 *Closed fracture base of other metacarpal*, E829.4 *Other road vehicle accidents, occupant of streetcar*, and E849.5 *Place of occurrence, street and highway*

E830–E838 Water Transport Accidents

Water transport accidents involve vehicles that travel in the water and are used for transporting people or products. This definition includes recreational boating.

A small boat is defined as a boat propelled by paddles, oars, or a small engine that carries fewer than 10 people. Small boats can be canoes, cobles, dinghies, punts, rafts, rowboats, rowing shells, sculls, skiffs, and small motorboats. Excluded from this definition are barges, lifeboats, rafts (anchored), and yachts.

The crew of a watercraft is defined as people who are working on a boat or ship, which includes ship operators, people providing passenger services, entertainment personnel, and shop operators.

Dockers and stevedores are longshoreman employed on the dock and work loading and unloading a ship.

The following fourth-digit subdivisions are for use with categories E830-E838 to identify the injured person:
0 Occupant of small boat, unpowered
1 Occupant of small boat, powered
2 Occupant of other watercraft - crew
3 Occupant of other watercraft - other than crew
4 Water skier
5 Swimmer
6 Dockers, stevedores
8 Other specified person
9 Unspecified person

E830 ✓sth Accident to watercraft causing submersion
Category E830 codes are used to report injuries sustained from an overturned or sinking watercraft, which include submerging and drowning, falling or jumping from a boat that is on fire, or falling or jumping from a crushed watercraft.

Drowning is death from suffocation after submersion that occurs within 24 hours of injury. At first a person holds his or her breath and carbon dioxide levels increase and hypoxia progresses. There are then two types of drowning: wet drowning, when water is taken into the lungs and dry drowning, when the patient experiences a laryngospasm. Near drowning is now more commonly referred to as a submersion accident.

A watercraft is a device traveling on the water that transports goods or people.

Coding Clarification
Category E830 codes may only be reported as a secondary diagnosis.

Use an additional code from category E849 to identify the place of occurrence.

E831 ✓sth Accident to watercraft causing other injury
Category E831 codes are used to report any injury, except sinking and drowning, that involves a watercraft. Use these codes to report burns sustained from a ship fire, and injuries from being crushed between ships during a collision, or by a lifeboat after abandoning ship. Also included are injuries sustained from a colliding watercrafts, falling objects during a watercraft accident, and falling or jumping from a damaged boat and being struck by another boat or part of a boat.

A watercraft is a device traveling on the water that transports goods or people.

Coding Clarification
Category E831 codes may only be reported as a secondary diagnosis.

Use an additional code from category E849 to identify the place of occurrence.

E832 ✓sth Other accidental submersion or drowning in water transport accident
Category E832 codes are used to report accidental submerging or drowning in a watercraft accident other than from the boat sinking, which includes injuries sustained from falling from the boat, falling overboard, or falling from the gangplank. Also

included are injuries from being thrown overboard by the motion of the boat or being washed overboard.

Drowning is death from suffocation after submersion that occurs within 24 hours of injury. At first a person holds his or her breath and carbon dioxide levels increase and hypoxia progresses. There are then two types of drowning: wet drowning, when water is taken into the lungs and dry drowning, when the patient experiences a laryngospasm. Near drowning is now more commonly referred to as a submersion accident.

Coding Clarification
Category E832 codes may only be reported as a secondary diagnosis.

Use an additional code from category E849 to identify the place of occurrence.

E833 ✓5th Fall on stairs or ladders in water transport
Category E833 codes are used to report a fall on stairs or a ladder of a boat or ship. This includes slipping, tripping, and falling. Excluded from this section are falls due to an accident of the watercraft.

Coding Clarification
Category E833 codes may only be reported as a secondary diagnosis.

Use an additional code from category E849 to identify the place of occurrence.

Coding Scenario
A 38-year-old male is admitted to the emergency department with a 4.0 cm laceration to his right knee. The patient was climbing up the ladder in his motorboat and slipped and hit his leg on the ladder.

> Code assignment: 891.1 *Open wound knee, without mention of complication*, E833.1 *Fall on stairs or ladders in water transport, occupant of small boat, powered*, and E849.8 *Place of occurrence, other specified place*

E834 ✓5th Other fall from one level to another in water transport
Category E834 codes are used to report injury from a fall from one level to another in a watercraft, such as falling from the deck to the lower cabin. Excluded from this code category is a fall that is the result of a watercraft accident.

A watercraft is a device traveling on the water that transports goods or people.

Coding Clarification
Category E834 codes may only be reported as a secondary diagnosis.

Use an additional code from category E849 to identify the place of occurrence.

E835 ✓5th Other and unspecified fall in water transport
Category E835 codes are used to report other and unspecified falls in water transport. Excluded from this code is a fall caused by an accident in a watercraft.

A watercraft is a device traveling on the water that transports goods or people.

Coding Clarification
Category E835 codes may only be reported as a secondary diagnosis.

Use an additional code from category E849 to identify the place of occurrence.

Coding Scenario
An 8-year-old boy is admitted to the emergency department with an injured wrist. He was at the lake on a scout activity and slipped and fell in the canoe. The diagnosis is a sprained right wrist.

> Code assignment: 842.00 *Sprain or strain unspecified part of wrist*, E835.0 *Other and unspecified fall in water transport, occupant of a small boat, unpowered*, and E849.8 *Place of occurrence, other specified place*

E836 ✓5th Machinery accident in water transport
Category E836 codes are used to report machinery accidents in water transport. This includes injuries caused by machinery on the deck, machinery in the engine room, galley, or laundry room, and loading machinery onto the ship.

Coding Clarification
Category E836 codes may only be reported as a secondary diagnosis.

Use an additional code from category E849 to identify the place of occurrence.

E837 ✓5th Explosion, fire, or burning in watercraft
Category E837 codes are used to report the explosion, fire, or burning of a watercraft, which includes localized fire on a watercraft and explosion of a boiler. Excluded from this category are fires caused by collision or explosion that results in sinking, submerging, or other injury. Near drowning is now more commonly referred to as a submersion accident.

A watercraft is a device traveling on the water that transports goods or people.

Coding Clarification
Category E837 codes may only be reported as a secondary diagnosis.

Use an additional code from category E849 to identify the place of occurrence.

Coding Scenario
A 39-year-old female chef on a cruise ship suffered second degree burns to her right hand when a small fire started on the stove.

> Code assignment: 944.20 *Second degree burn, unspecified part of hand*, E837.2 *Explosion, fire, or burning in watercraft, occupant of watercraft, crew*, and E849.8 *Place of occurrence, other specified place*

E838 ✓sth Other and unspecified water transport accident
Category E838 codes are used to report other and unspecified water transport accidents. This category includes a person crushed between the dock and the watercraft, a person crushed by a falling object while loading or unloading the ship, or a person hit by a boat while water-skiing. Also included in this category are injuries caused by being struck by boat or part of a boat, accidental poisoning by gas or fumes, or atomic power plant malfunction on the ship. Note that fourth category.4 identifies a water skier. Transport accidents are those involving a vehicle being used primarily for transporting people or goods from one place or another.

Coding Clarification
Category E838 codes may only be reported as a secondary diagnosis.

Use an additional code from category E849 to identify the place of occurrence.

E840–E845 Air and Space Transport Accidents

The chances of being in an airline-related accident while traveling on one of the top 25 airlines are one in 3.72 million. Rubrics E840-E845 describe air- and space-transport accidents. An aircraft is a vehicle that transports products or people by air. This includes commercial or noncommercial flights. Categories E840-E845 include accidents during take off and landing, accidents to unpowered aircraft, falls in, on, or from an aircraft, and accidents involving spacecraft.

> The following fourth-digit subdivisions are for use with categories E840-E845 to identify the injured person. Valid fourth digits are in [brackets] under codes E842-E845.
> 0   Occupant of spacecraft
> 1   Occupant of military aircraft, any
> 2   Crew of commercial aircraft (powered) in surface to surface transport

> 3   Other occupant of commercial aircraft (powered) in surface to surface transport
> 4   Occupant of commercial aircraft (powered) in surface to air transport
> 5   Occupant of other powered aircraft
> 6   Occupant of unpowered aircraft, except parachutist
> 7   Parachutist (military) (other)
> 8   Ground crew, airline employee
> 9   Other person

E840 ✓sth Accident to powered aircraft at takeoff or landing
Category E840 codes are used to report aircraft accidents during takeoff or landing, which includes the collision of a plane with any object, a crash, an explosion, a fire, or a forced landing.

An aircraft is a device traveling in the air that transports goods or people.

Coding Clarification
Category E840 codes may only be reported as a secondary diagnosis.

Use an additional code from category E849 to identify the place of occurrence.

Coding Scenario
A patient is admitted to the emergency room following a plane crash while the plane was taking off. The patient has an open femur fracture.

> Code assignment: 821.1 *Open fracture, unspecified part of femur*, E840.3 *Accident to powered aircraft at takeoff or landing, other occupant of commercial aircraft (powered) in surface to surface transport*, and E849.8 *Place of occurrence, other specified places*

E841 ✓sth Accident to powered aircraft, other and unspecified
Category E841 codes are used to report accidents to powered aircraft. Included in this category are aircraft accidents NOS, an aircraft crash or wreck NOS, collisions with other aircraft or another object, aircraft explosions while traveling, or a fire on the aircraft. Use this category for an accident when it is not specified that the accident took place during take off, landing, or in transit.

An aircraft is a device traveling in the air that transports goods or people.

Coding Clarification
Category E841 codes may only be reported as a secondary diagnosis.

Use an additional code from category E849 to identify the place of occurrence.

E842 ✎5th Accident to unpowered aircraft

Category E842 codes are used to report accidents to unpowered aircraft except for collision with a powered aircraft. Unpowered aircraft include hot air balloons, gliders, hang gliders, or a kite carrying a person.

Coding Clarification
Category E842 codes may only be reported as a secondary diagnosis.

Use an additional code from category E849 to identify the place of occurrence.

Only fourth digits 6-9 may be used with category E842.

E843 ✎5th Fall in, on, or from aircraft

Category E843 codes describe falls in, on, or from an aircraft. This code category includes falls that occur when people are getting on or off an aircraft, and falling in, on, or from an aircraft while traveling, taking off, or landing, except as a result of an aircraft accident.

An aircraft is a device traveling in the air that transports goods or people.

Coding Clarification
Category E843 codes may only be reported as a secondary diagnosis.

Use an additional code from category E849 to identify the place of occurrence.

E844 ✎5th Other specified air transport accidents

Category E844 codes describe other specified air transport accidents. This code category includes injuries sustained from a wide variety of causes such as an injury from an object that falls from the aircraft, an injury from machinery on the aircraft, an injury from a rotating propeller, or an injury involving a voluntary parachute descent. Also included in this category is poisoning by carbon monoxide while traveling on an aircraft. All of the previously mentioned causes are without accident to the aircraft. Excluded from this category is airsickness, effects of high altitude or pressure change, and injury to a parachutist due to an accident to the aircraft.

An aircraft is a device traveling in the air that transports goods or people. Transport accidents are those involving a vehicle being used primarily for transporting people or goods from one place or another.

Coding Clarification
Category E844 codes may only be reported as a secondary diagnosis.

Use an additional code from category E849 to identify the place of occurrence.

E845 ✎5th Accident involving spacecraft

Category E845 codes include accidents involving spacecraft. Excluded from this category is the effect of weightlessness in a spacecraft.

Coding Clarification
Category E845 codes may only be reported as a secondary diagnosis.

Use an additional code from category E849 to identify the place of occurrence.

Only fourth digits 0, 8, and 9 may be used with category E845.

E846–E848 Vehicle Accidents Not Elsewhere Classifiable

Codes in this rubric are assigned for vehicle accidents that are not well described by other categories. This code category includes accidents that involve vehicles used exclusively in commercial buildings or premises, accidents that involve cable cars not on rails, and accidents that involve other types of vehicles such as yachts.

E846 Accidents involving powered vehicles used solely within the buildings and premises of industrial or commercial establishment

Code E846 is used to report accidents that involve vehicles used solely within the building or premises of an industrial or a commercial establishment. Included in E846 are accidents involving battery powered airport passenger vehicles, battery powered trucks, coal cars, or trams, trucks or tubs used in a mine or quarry. This may involve a collision with a pedestrian or another vehicle. This code category also includes explosion of, fall from, overturning of, or being struck by an industrial or commercial powered vehicle. Excluded from E846 is accidental poisoning by exhaust gas and injury by a crane, forklift, or an elevator.

A pedestrian is defined as a person who is not riding in a vehicle, on a motorcycle, or on an animal. A pedestrian can be a person changing a tire, operating a pedestrian conveyance, fixing a motor vehicle, or traveling on foot.

Coding Clarification
Code E846 may only be reported as a secondary diagnosis.

Use an additional code from category E849 to identify the place of occurrence.

E847 Accidents involving cable cars not running on rails

Code E847 is used to report accidents involving cable cars not running on rails, ski chair lifts, ski lifts with gondolas, or teleferique (means transfer on the ground). This code also is used to report accidents caused by a broken cable.

Coding Clarification
Code E847 may only be reported as a secondary diagnosis.

Use an additional code from category E849 to identify the place of occurrence.

Coding Scenario
A 25-year-old male presents to the emergency department with left knee pain. The patient says that he jumped off a ski lift after missing the exit. He fell a distance of about six feet. He is diagnosed with a tear of the medial meniscus on the left knee.

> Code assignment: 836.0 *Tear of medial cartilage of the knee, current injury*, E847 *Accident involving cable cars not running on rails*, and E849.4 *Place of occurrence, places for recreation and sport*

E848 Accidents involving other vehicles, not elsewhere classifiable

Code E848 is used to report accidents involving other vehicles, not elsewhere classified. This code category includes accidents involving yachts that have the capacity to carry more than 10 people and vehicles not otherwise specified.

A watercraft is a device traveling on the water that transports goods or people.

Coding Clarification
Use an additional code from category E849 to identify the place of occurrence.

E849 Place of occurrence
Category E849 codes are used to identify where the injury or poisoning occurred. The place of occurrence should describe where the accident happened and not what the patient was doing at the time of the accident.

A home is defined as an apartment, a boarding house, a farmhouse, a noninstitutional place of residence, a private driveway, a private garage, a garden home, or a yard. Report a home under construction but not yet occupied with E849.3. Report an institutional place of residence with E849.7.

A farm includes farm buildings and land under cultivation.

A quarry and mine include gravel pits, sand pits, and any tunnel under construction.

An industrial place includes a building under construction, a dockyard, a dry dock, a factory, an industrial yard, a shop, a warehouse, and a loading platform.

A place for recreation and sports includes an amusement park, a baseball field, a basketball court, a football field, a golf course, a gymnasium, a hockey field, a skating rink, a resort, a playground, a public park, a stadium, and a tennis court.

A public building includes an airport, a bank, a cafe, a casino, a church, a hotel, a store, a theater, a nightclub, a office building, a post office, and a school.

A residential institution includes a children's home, a dormitory, a hospital, a jail, a retirement home, an orphanage, a prison, and a reform school.

Other specified places include a beach, desert, dock, forest, harbor, hill, lake, mountain, parking lot, pond, river, sea, stream, swamp, and trailer court.

Code	Description
E849.0	Place of occurrence, home
E849.1	Place of occurrence, farm
E849.2	Place of occurrence, mine and quarry
E849.3	Place of occurrence, industrial places and premises
E849.4	Place of occurrence, place for recreation and sport
E849.5	Place of occurrence, street and highway
E849.6	Place of occurrence, public building
E849.7	Place of occurrence, residential institution
E849.8	Other specified place of occurrence
E849.9	Unspecified place of occurrence

Coding Clarification
According to ICD-9-CM guidelines, code E849.9 should not be used if the place of occurrence is not stated.

Guidelines pertaining to place of occurrence codes may vary by payer and hospital policy. Check with payers to determine if E849 codes are required.

Coding Scenario
A patient presents with a sprained right ankle after falling at home.

> Code assignment: 845.00 *Sprain, unspecified part of ankle*, E888.9 *Unspecified fall*, and E849.0 *Place of occurrence, home*

E850–E858 Accidental Poisoning by Drugs, Medicinal Substances, and Biologicals

Poisoning by drugs, medicinal, and biological substances is the major cause of childhood accidents in the home and can occur by many routes, including oral ingestion, inhalation, dermal absorption, and ocular instillation.

Accidental poisoning codes identify accidental overdose of a drug, a wrong substance given or taken, a drug taken inadvertently, and accidents in the use of drugs and biologicals in medical and surgical procedures. The alphabetical index of ICD-9-CM can give a more complete list of specific drugs classified under a fourth-digit category; however, codes should not be assigned directly from the table of drugs and chemicals. Always consult the tabular section of ICD-9-CM before assigning the accidental poisoning codes. Many of the common medications can be found in the pharmacological listings found in the back of ICD-9-CM.

As a general rule, the more known about the poisoning agent, the better the treatment plan and outcome. Poison control centers have been invaluable in supplying the health care professional with the exact composition of the thousands of poisonous substances. If the information is unknown, treatment must revolve around general supportive measures.

E850 Accidental poisoning by analgesics, antipyretics, and antirheumatics

Category E850 codes are used to report accidental poisoning by analgesics, antipyretics and antirheumatics. An analgesic medication is one that provides pain relief or reduces pain. An antipyretic is a medication that is used to eliminate or reduce a fever. An antirheumatic is an anti-inflammatory medication.

Heroin is a highly addictive drug. It can be injected, snorted or smoked. Accidental overdoses can occur as a result of varying strength of the street drug. Drug users are not always sure of the purity of the drug. Heroin is usually mixed with other substances. Drug users may experience an accidental overdose using the same amount of heroin because of the purity.

Methadone is a synthetic form of heroin. It blocks the effects of heroin which results in a reduced craving. Methadone overdose is a serious medical condition that usually affects people who are using the drug illegally. Symptoms of methadone overdose include muscle spasm, difficulty breathing, pin point pupils and death.

Opiates are drugs derived from a Papaver somniferum plant. Common names are opium, codeine, morphine, Dilaudid, Percodan, Vicodin, Demerol, and fentanyl. Symptoms of overdose include decreased respiration, clammy skin, coma and possible death.

Salicylates are found in many commonly used drugs. Aspirin is the most common salicylate. Because aspirin is found in many common drugs, accidental overdose can occur from taking more than one medication that includes salicylates.

Aromatic analgesics include acetaminophen, acetanilid and acetophenetidin. Tylenol is a common form of aromatic analgesic.

Pyrazole is a non-narcotic pain reliever and fever reducer that includes aminophenazone and phenylbutazone.

Antirheumatics include gold salts and indomethacin. Excluded in this section are salicylates and steroids. Symptoms of overdose may include ringing in ears, blurred vision, nausea and vomiting.

E850.0	Accidental poisoning by heroin
E850.1	Accidental poisoning by methadone
E850.2	Accidental poisoning by other opiates and related narcotics
E850.3	Accidental poisoning by salicylates
E850.4	Accidental poisoning by aromatic analgesics, not elsewhere classified
E850.5	Accidental poisoning by pyrazole derivatives
E850.6	Accidental poisoning by antirheumatics (antiphlogistics)
E850.7	Accidental poisoning by other non-narcotic analgesics
E850.8	Accidental poisoning by other specified analgesics and antipyretics
E850.9	Accidental poisoning by unspecified analgesic or antipyretic

Coding Clarification

If a reaction is the result of medicine and alcohol, assign a code for each drug and/or the alcohol.

Apply each E code only once even if the agent is responsible for more than one adverse reaction.

When coding accidental poisoning use as many codes as necessary to completely describe the drug, medicinal, or biological poisoning. Sequence poisoning first, manifestation second, and the E code third. Assign an additional code for drug dependency, if applicable.

When assigning codes for the late effect of a poisoning, code the nature of the late effect first, the cause of the late effect second, and then the applicable E code describing the cause of the poisoning.

Use a secondary E code from category E849 to identify the place of occurrence.

E851   Accidental poisoning by barbiturates ☑

Barbiturates are depressant type drugs used for sleep and relaxation. Most barbiturate overdoses are combinations such as barbiturates and alcohol. For combination overdoses, use as many E codes as necessary to describe the overdose. There are no antidotes to barbiturate overdoses. Maintenance of airway and drugs to make the urine less acidic can be used to treat barbiturate overdose.

Coding Clarification
Code E851 codes may only be reported as a secondary diagnosis.

Use a secondary E code from category E849 to identify the place of occurrence.

E852   Accidental poisoning by other sedatives and hypnotics

Sedatives are agents used to calm and quiet the body. Several types and compounds of sedatives are available for use today. Accidental overdose can occur when a patient forgets that he or she has taken a dose or accidentally takes too much medication.

Chloral hydrate is the oldest sleep medication. It may still be used for children prior to dental or medical procedures. Mixed with alcohol, it produces the infamous knockout drops, or Mickey. Symptoms of an overdose include gastrointestinal (GI) irritation, vomiting, GI bleed, and a pear like odor of the breath.

Paraldehyde is used to treat certain convulsive disorders. It may also be used in the treatment of alcoholism and used to calm or relax patients. The medication should be taken with a metal spoon because paraldehyde tends to react with plastic. The medication will cause the patient to have bad breath. Signs of overdose are confusion, muscle tremors, nausea, vomiting, stomach cramps, weakness, depressed breathing, and slow heartbeat. This medication has generally been replaced by safer and more effective drugs.

Bromine compounds are central nervous center depressants and are mixed with other drugs to form compound drugs. They have a tranquilizing effect on the body.

E852.0	Accidental poisoning by chloral hydrate group
E852.1	Accidental poisoning by paraldehyde
E852.2	Accidental poisoning by bromine compounds
E852.3	Accidental poisoning by methaqualone compounds
E852.4	Accidental poisoning by glutethimide group
E852.5	Accidental poisoning by mixed sedatives, not elsewhere classified
E852.8	Accidental poisoning by other specified sedative and hypnotic
E852.9	Accidental poisoning by unspecified sedative or hypnotic

Coding Clarification
Category E852 codes may only be reported as a secondary diagnosis.

Use a secondary E code from category E849 to identify the place of occurrence.

Coding Scenario
A 75-year-old male is brought into the emergency department following an accidental overdose of Ambien. The patient misunderstood the dosage and took additional medication. The patient is experiencing nausea and vomiting.

Code assignment: 967.8 *Poisoning by other sedatives and hypnotics*, 787.01 *Nausea and vomiting*, and E852.8 *Accidental poisoning by other specified sedative or hypnotic*

E853   Accidental poisoning by tranquilizers

Tranquilizers are antianxiety medications used to calm a patient. Phenothiazine-based tranquilizers include chlorpromazine, fluphenazine, prochlorperazine and promazine. Butyrophenone-based tranquilizers include haloperidol, spiperone, and trifluperidol. Other specified tranquilizers include hydroxyzine and meprobamate.

E853.0	Accidental poisoning by phenothiazine-based tranquilizers
E853.1	Accidental poisoning by butyrophenone-based tranquilizers
E853.2	Accidental poisoning by benzodiazepine-based tranquilizers
E853.8	Accidental poisoning by other specified tranquilizers
E853.9	Accidental poisoning by unspecified tranquilizer

Coding Clarification
Category E853 codes may only be reported as a secondary diagnosis.

Use a secondary E code from category E849 to identify the place of occurrence.

E854 Accidental poisoning by other psychotropic agents

Category E854 codes describe accidental poisoning by antidepressants, psychodysleptics, psychostimulants, and central nervous system stimulants.

Antidepressants are used to treat mood disorders. Symptoms of mood disorders include sadness, loss of appetite, sleep problems, hopelessness, helplessness, guilt, loss of energy, agitation, and lack of pleasure. Overdoses of antidepressants can cause central nervous symptom problems, cardiovascular symptoms, and parasympathetic nervous system symptoms.

Psychodysleptics are hallucinogenic drugs that include cannabis derivatives, LSD, marihuana derivatives, mescaline, psilocin, and psilocybin.

Psychostimulants include amphetamine and caffeine. Psychostimulants are often used to treat children with attention deficit hyperactivity disorder (ADHD).

Central nervous system stimulants include analeptics and opiate antagonists. Central nervous system stimulants speed up the mental and physical processes. They are used to treat children with ADHD and other people with attention span disorders. Opiate antagonists reduce the affects of opiates.

Code	Description
E854.0	Accidental poisoning by antidepressants
E854.1	Accidental poisoning by psychodysleptics (hallucinogens)
E854.2	Accidental poisoning by psychostimulants
E854.3	Accidental poisoning by central nervous system stimulants
E854.8	Accidental poisoning by other psychotropic agents

Coding Clarification

Category E854 codes may only be reported as a secondary diagnosis.

Use a secondary E code from category E849 to identify the place of occurrence.

E855 Accidental poisoning by other drugs acting on central and autonomic nervous system

Category E855 codes are used to report accidental poisoning by other drugs acting on the central nervous system, which includes anti-Parkinsonism drugs, central nervous system depressants, anesthetics, parasympatholytics, sympathomimetics, and sympatholytics.

Parkinson's disease is a progressive neurologic disease that affects walking, talking, and movement. Symptoms of the disease include tremors, stiffness, and slow movement. The cause of Parkinson's disease is not known. The disease causes a degeneration of nerves in the brain that produce a chemical called dopamine. There is no treatment for the disease; however, medications are used to decrease the symptoms.

Anesthetics can be used to produce a loss of consciousness or a local pain blocking effect. Overdose can cause reduced cardiac output and arrhythmias.

Parasympathomimetics are drugs that produce the effects of parasympathetic nerve stimulation. Therapeutic use of the drugs includes stimulation and motility of the GI tract and bladder following surgery, glaucoma, diagnosis of myasthenia gravis, and treatment of delayed gastric emptying time.

Parasympatholytics relax smooth muscles. Drugs in this category include atropine, homatropine, hyoscine, and quaternary ammonium derivatives.

Sympathomimetic agents are used to increase myocardial contractility, increase blood pressure, maintain blood pressure, treat bronchospasm, reduce systemic local anesthetic absorption, and manage severe allergic reactions. Drugs in this category include epinephrine and levarterenol.

Sympatholytics stimulate smooth muscles. This category of drugs is used to treat hypertension, angina, glaucoma, and to prevent migraines. Medications include phenoxybenzamine and tolazoline hydrochloride.

Code	Description
E855.0	Accidental poisoning by anticonvulsant and anti-Parkinsonism drugs
E855.1	Accidental poisoning by other central nervous system depressants
E855.2	Accidental poisoning by local anesthetics
E855.3	Accidental poisoning by parasympathomimetics (cholinergics)
E855.4	Accidental poisoning by parasympatholytics (anticholinergics and antimuscarinics) and spasmolytics
E855.5	Accidental poisoning by sympathomimetics (adrenergics)
E855.6	Accidental poisoning by sympatholytics (antiadrenergics)
E855.8	Accidental poisoning by other specified drugs acting on central and autonomic nervous systems
E855.9	Accidental poisoning by unspecified drug acting on central and autonomic nervous systems

Supplementary Classification of External Causes

Coding Clarification
Category E855 codes may only be reported as a secondary diagnosis.

Use a secondary E code from category E849 to identify the place of occurrence.

Coding Scenario
A 10-year-old female presents to the emergency department with an accidental overdose of Dilantin. The young girl suffers from a seizure disorder. The patient's mother forgot when the medication was given and administered two extra doses to the child. The child has nystagmus on examination.

> Code assignment: 966.1 *Poisoning by hydantoin derivatives*, 379.50 *Unspecified nystagmus*, 780.39 *Other convulsions*, and E855.0 *Accidental poisoning by anticonvulsant and anti-Parkinsonism drugs*

E856 Accidental poisoning by antibiotics OK

Antibiotics are used to fight infections including pneumonia, cystitis, strep infections, and ear infections. They can be administered topically, intravenously (IV), intramuscularly (IM), and orally. Overuse of antibiotics has lead to a decrease in their effectiveness. Symptoms of an overdose can include decreased respiration, tightness in the chest, low blood pressure, and unconsciousness.

Coding Clarification
Code E856 codes may only be reported as a secondary diagnosis.

Use a secondary E code from category E849 to identify the place of occurrence.

Coding Scenario
A 2-year-old female presents to the emergency department with diaphoresis after getting into the ampicillin prescribed for her brother. The diagnosis is diaphoresis and ampicillin poisoning.

> Code assignment: 960.0 *Poisoning by penicillins*, 780.8 *Hyperhidrosis*, and E856 *Accidental poisoning by antibiotics*

E857 Accidental poisoning by other anti-infectives OK

Anti-infectives include medications such as sulfonamides, arsenical anti-infectives, heavy metal anti-infectives, hydroxyquinoline derivatives, antimalarials, antiprotozoal drugs, anthelmintics, antiviral drugs, and drugs acting on other blood forming protozoa.

Coding Clarification
Code E857 codes may only be reported as a secondary diagnosis.

Use a secondary E code from category E849 to identify the place of occurrence.

E858 Accidental poisoning by other drugs

Category E858 codes are used to report accidental poisoning by the following kinds of drugs: hormones, synthetic substitutes, and systemic agents. Also included are drugs that affect the following systems: blood constituents, cardiovascular system, gastrointestinal system, uric acid metabolism, smooth and skeletal muscles, and respiratory system. Additionally, agents that affect skin, mucous membranes, eyes, ears, nose, throat and mouth are included in this category.

Poisoning by hormones and synthetic substitutes include adrenal cortical steroids, androgens and anabolic congeners, ovarian hormones, insulin and antidiabetic agents, anterior pituitary hormones, posterior pituitary hormones, parathyroid and parathyroid derivatives, thyroid and thyroid derivatives, and antithyroid agents.

E858.0	Accidental poisoning by hormones and synthetic substitutes
E858.1	Accidental poisoning by primarily systemic agents
E858.2	Accidental poisoning by agents primarily affecting blood constituents
E858.3	Accidental poisoning by agents primarily affecting cardiovascular system
E858.4	Accidental poisoning by agents primarily affecting gastrointestinal system
E858.5	Accidental poisoning by water, mineral, and uric acid metabolism drugs
E858.6	Accidental poisoning by agents primarily acting on the smooth and skeletal muscles and respiratory system
E858.7	Accidental poisoning by agents primarily affecting skin and mucous membrane, ophthalmological, otorhinolaryngological, and dental drugs
E858.8	Accidental poisoning by other specified drugs — central appetite depressants
E858.9	Accidental poisoning by unspecified drug

Coding Clarification
Category E858 codes may only be reported as a secondary diagnosis.

Use a secondary E code from category E849 to identify the place of occurrence.

E860–E869 Accidental Poisoning by Other Solid and Liquid Substances, Gases, and Vapors

The toxicity of a substance is due to its ability to damage or disrupt the metabolism. An acutely toxic substance can cause damage as the result of a single- or short-duration exposure. A chronically toxic substance causes damage after repeated or long-duration exposure or becomes evident only after a long latency period. Toxicity varies with the route of exposure and the effectiveness at which the material is absorbed. A chemical that enters the body in large quantities, but is not easily absorbed, is a much lower risk than one that is easily absorbed into the bloodstream.

Ingested materials are absorbed into the bloodstream anywhere along the gastrointestinal tract. If the material cannot be absorbed, it will be eliminated from the body.

A toxic reaction can be similar to an allergic reaction, but more severe. If the liver is functioning normally, it may allow a small amount of the toxic material to be absorbed into the body, but eliminate the rest. If the liver is not functioning normally, the substance may be absorbed and cause a toxic chemical overload that may result in blood poisoning and death. Toxemia is a poisoned condition of the blood caused by the presence of toxic materials, usually bacterial but occasionally chemical or hormonal in nature.

Skin contact can be a common route of exposure but the skin acts as a barrier against the entry of most chemicals. Once a chemical passes through the skin (i.e., through a wound), it enters the bloodstream and is carried to all parts of the body.

Inhalation can be the most dangerous route of entry because the lungs are ineffective barriers. Chemicals that pass the lung membrane are absorbed into the bloodstream and carried to all parts of the body. Absorption can be extremely rapid. The rate of absorption depends on the concentration of the toxic substance, its solubility in water, the depth of respiration, and the rate of blood circulation.

Treatment includes the use of corticosteroids and mannitol drips to minimize cerebral edema dialysis to combat renal failure and hasten the excretion of the poison, and removal of lipoid soluble substances from the blood by hemoperfusion and chelating agents.

Categories E860-E869 are primarily used to indicate the cause of poisoning (980-989), however, they may also be used to indicate the cause of a localized reaction (001-799).

E860 Accidental poisoning by alcohol, not elsewhere classified

Alcohol poisoning occurs from consuming too much alcohol. Factors that affect alcohol poisoning are the strength or concentration of alcohol in a drink, how fast it is consumed, and the amount of food in the system. Combining certain drugs, such as sedatives, tranquilizers, pain medication, and certain anti-seizure medication, can be harmful if consumed in addition to alcohol. The signs and symptoms of alcohol intoxication include giddiness, slurred speech, uninhibited behavior, and coordination problems. Signs and symptoms of alcohol poisoning or ethanol overdose are mental confusion, vomiting, seizures, slow or irregular breathing, paleness, bluish skin, and unconsciousness. If a reaction is the result of medicine and alcohol, assign the codes for both.

Wood alcohol and methanol is a common substance found in paint thinner and antifreeze. Methanol poisoning can cause serious kidney damage and blindness. This can be absorbed by skin contact or inhalation but is far more serious when ingested. Symptoms include headache, nausea, vomiting, ringing in the ears, diarrhea, constipation, lethargy, central nervous system depression, stupor, cerebral edema, coma, and profound metabolic acidosis.

Rubbing alcohol consists mainly of isopropyl alcohol. Poisoning from this substance can occur from skin contact, inhalation, and ingestion. Symptoms include headache, dizziness, mental depression, nausea, vomiting, and coma.

Fuel oil is irritating to the mucous membranes. Symptoms of overdose include headache, dizziness, pungent taste, nausea, vomiting, diarrhea, delirium, and central nervous center depression.

E860.0	Accidental poisoning by alcoholic beverages
E860.1	Accidental poisoning by other and unspecified ethyl alcohol and its products
E860.2	Accidental poisoning by methyl alcohol
E860.3	Accidental poisoning by isopropyl alcohol
E860.4	Accidental poisoning by Fuel oil
E860.8	Accidental poisoning by other specified alcohols
E860.9	Accidental poisoning by unspecified alcohol

Coding Clarification
When coding accidental poisoning use as many codes as necessary to completely describe the drug, medicinal, or biological poisoning.

Coding Scenario
A 21-year-old male college student is brought to the emergency department by his friends for nausea and vomiting and confusion. This patient has been

drinking vodka for the last eight hours. The diagnosis is acute alcohol toxicity, intoxication, and confusion.

> Code assignment: 980.0 *Toxic effects of alcohol*, 305.0 *Alcohol intoxication*, 787.01 *Nausea and vomiting*, 298.2 *Reactive confusion*, and E860.0 *Accidental poisoning by alcoholic beverages*

E861 Accidental poisoning by cleansing and polishing agents, disinfectants, paints, and varnishes

Poisoning continues to be one of the leading causes of pediatric admission. Although the numbers have declined, this is still a significant threat. The second most common cause of poisoning is from cleaning supplies. Keeping cleaning supplies out of children's reach is the most effective way of preventing poisoning. Treatment for poisoning includes ipecac syrup, gastric lavage, medication to increase GI motility, and administration of activated charcoal.

Lead is a highly toxic metal that was used for many years in paint and other products found around the home. Lead poisoning has steadily decreased over the years. In 1978 there were three to four million children with lead in their blood. In the 1990s the number has dropped to 434,000. Lead poisoning usually happens slowly and most children show no symptoms. Children between the ages of one to two, when they are crawling, learning to walk, and putting things in their mouth, are most likely to get lead poisoning. Many older homes were painted with lead-based paint. These paint chips and dust can poison a child. Acute lead poisoning is rare but it can cause abdominal pain, vomiting, diarrhea, weakness in the extremities, behavioral problems, seizures, coma, and death. This would only occur if a person ingested a large amount of lead at once. If the lead level in a child is high, a treatment called chelation can be used to bind the lead and help the body pass it through the urine. Report E866.4 for poisoning from lead and its compounds and fumes other than paint.

E861.0	Accidental poisoning by synthetic detergents and shampoos
E861.1	Accidental poisoning by soap products
E861.2	Accidental poisoning by polishes
E861.3	Accidental poisoning by other cleansing and polishing agents
E861.4	Accidental poisoning by disinfectants — excludes carbolic acid or phenol
E861.5	Accidental poisoning by lead paints
E861.6	Accidental poisoning by other paints and varnishes
E861.9	Accidental poisonings by unspecified cleansing and polishing agents, disinfectants, paints, and varnishes

Coding Clarification
Category E861 codes may only be reported as a secondary diagnosis.

Use a secondary E code from category E849 to identify the place of occurrence.

E862 Accidental poisoning by petroleum products, other solvents and their vapors, not elsewhere classified

Petroleum products include solvents, fuels, cleaners, oils, and wax. Symptoms of poisoning are anal seepage and irritation, lipid granuloma, lipid pneumonia, eczematous dermatitis, and melanosis. Vomiting is generally not recommended for petroleum product ingestion as vomiting causes an increased risk of pneumonia.

E862.0	Accidental poisoning by petroleum solvents
E862.1	Accidental poisoning by petroleum fuels and cleaners
E862.2	Accidental poisoning by lubricating oils
E862.3	Accidental poisoning by petroleum solids
E862.4	Accidental poisoning by other specified solvents
E862.9	Accidental poisoning by unspecified solvent

Coding Clarification
Category E862 codes may only be reported as a secondary diagnosis.

Use a secondary E code from category E849 to identify the place of occurrence.

E863 Accidental poisoning by agricultural and horticultural chemical and pharmaceutical preparations other than plant foods and fertilizers

Pesticides can readily be absorbed through the skin or cause harm from ingestion or inhalation. Death from insecticide poisoning can occur between five minutes and 24 hours after ingestion. The most common cause of death is respiratory failure. Symptoms include headache, nausea, pupil dilation, excessive sweating, salivation, respiratory distress, and death.

Rodenticides are one of the most toxic substances found in the home. Until 20 years ago, arsenic was the main ingredient. Most rodenticides today contain an anticoagulant. They are toxic to almost every organ system in the body. Most accidental poisoning by rodenticides affects children. Adults who ingest this substance are usually attempting suicide. Symptoms include abdominal pain, shortness of breath, nausea, vomiting, abdominal pain, dizziness, hair loss, muscle pain or twitching, facial grimace, pulmonary edema, and a garlic taste in the mouth. Patients may require dialysis or blood transfusions. Activated charcoal is usually given to inhibit additional absorption of the toxin.

E863.0	Accidental poisoning by insecticides of organochlorine compounds
E863.1	Accidental poisoning by insecticides of organophosphorus compounds
E863.2	Accidental poisoning by carbamates
E863.3	Accidental poisoning by mixtures of insecticides
E863.4	Accidental poisoning by other and unspecified insecticides
E863.5	Accidental poisoning by herbicides
E863.6	Accidental poisoning by fungicides
E863.7	Accidental poisoning by rodenticides
E863.8	Accidental poisoning by fumigants
E863.9	Accidental poisoning by other and unspecified agricultural and horticultural chemical and pharmaceutical preparations other than plant foods and fertilizers

Coding Clarification
Category E863 codes may only be reported as a secondary diagnosis.

Use a secondary E code from category E849 to identify the place of occurrence.

E864 Accidental poisoning by corrosives and caustics, not elsewhere classified

A corrosive is a substance that destroys living tissue. The most common types of corrosives are hydrochloric acid, sulfuric acid, nitric acid, acetic acid, phosphoric acid, oxalic acid, chronic acid, formic acid, and boric acid. These corrosives are commonly found in metal cleaners, toilet and drain cleaners, batteries, and antirust compounds. Symptoms of ingestion include a severe burning pain in the mouth, throat, and abdomen; dysphagia; vomiting; diarrhea; and cold, clammy skin. Symptoms will usually begin immediately after swallowing. Symptoms of inhalation include cough, dyspnea, pleuritic chest pain, pulmonary edema, and frothy sputum. These symptoms could be delayed several hours. Eye exposure can cause burning, irritation and swelling eyes, photophobia, corneal erosion, and perforation of the conjunctiva and cornea.

E864.0	Accidental poisoning by corrosive aromatics not elsewhere classified
E864.1	Accidental poisoning by acids not elsewhere classified
E864.2	Accidental poisoning by caustic alkalis not elsewhere classified
E864.3	Accidental poisoning by other specified corrosives and caustics not elsewhere classified
E864.4	Accidental poisoning by unspecified corrosives and caustics not elsewhere classified

Coding Clarification
Category E864 codes may only be reported as a secondary diagnosis.

Use a secondary E code from category E849 to identify the place of occurrence.

E865 Accidental poisoning from poisonous foodstuffs and poisonous plants

Category E865 codes identify poisoning from food and plants. This type of poisoning does not include bacterial food poisoning or toxic reactions to venomous plants. This category does include poisoning from food or plants that should not be eaten, such as a child ingesting plants or berries that are poisonous to humans.

The four main types of toxic shellfish poisoning are paralytic, amnesic, neurotoxic, and diarrhetic. Paralytic shellfish poisoning differs in effect based on the species of shellfish and the species of algae producing the toxin. Symptoms of amnesic poisoning are neurological in nature and usually begin within 24 to 48 hours. Neurotoxic shellfish toxins affect the nervous system. Symptoms, which will appear within 24 hours, include difficulty swallowing, double vision, tremor, nausea, diarrhea, vomiting, numbness, and tingling in the mouth, lips, and extremities. Diarrhetic shellfish poisoning cause GI problems such as nausea, vomiting, diarrhea, and abdominal pain.

Relatively few plants are fit for human consumption. Many have toxins that are designed to deter predators from eating them. Many of these forms of toxic plants are houseplants or plants that are commonly found in people's flower gardens. Some plants, such as herbs, spices, and condiments are safe to eat in small quantities. Polluted water may add to the toxicity of plants. Examples of toxic plants are hyacinth, daffodil, oleander, larkspur, iris, bleeding heart, rhubarb leaf blades, daphne berries, jasmine berries, mistletoe berries, and jimson weed. Toadstools that are commonly found outside are also toxic. Some types of poisoning cause mild GI symptoms and some can be fatal.

E865.0	Accidental poisoning by meat
E865.1	Accidental poisoning by shellfish
E865.2	Accidental poisoning from other fish
E865.3	Accidental poisoning from berries and seeds
E865.4	Accidental poisoning from other specified plants
E865.5	Accidental poisoning from mushrooms and other fungi
E865.8	Accidental poisoning from other specified foods
E865.9	Accidental poisoning from unspecified foodstuff or poisonous plant

Supplementary Classification of External Causes

Coding Clarification
Category E865 codes may only be reported as a secondary diagnosis.

Use a secondary E code from category E849 to identify the place of occurrence.

E866 Accidental poisoning by other and unspecified solid and liquid substances

Category E866 codes are used to report poisoning by other and unspecified solid or liquid substances. Excluded from this section are substances as components of medicines, paints, pesticides, petroleum fuels, lead paint, and fertilizers mixed with herbicides.

E866.0	Accidental poisoning by lead and its compounds and fumes
E866.1	Accidental poisoning by mercury and its compounds and fumes
E866.2	Accidental poisoning by antimony and its compounds and fumes
E866.3	Accidental poisoning by arsenic and its compounds and fumes
E866.4	Accidental poisoning by other metals and their compounds and fumes
E866.5	Accidental poisoning by plant foods and fertilizers
E866.6	Accidental poisoning by glues and adhesives
E866.7	Accidental poisoning by cosmetics
E866.8	Accidental poisoning by other specified solid or liquid substances
E866.9	Accidental poisoning by unspecified solid or liquid substance

Coding Clarification
Category E866 codes may only be reported as a secondary diagnosis.

Use a secondary E code from category E849 to identify the place of occurrence.

E867 Accidental poisoning by gas distributed by pipeline OK

The most common poisoning by gas distributed by pipeline is from carbon monoxide poisoning. Carbon monoxide is produced whenever pipeline gas is burned. The amount produced is usually not hazardous. Improper ventilation and malfunctioning equipment can result in a deadly amount of carbon monoxide emitted into the air. Although the lead in gas has decreased over the years, gasoline fumes can also cause short- or long-term health problems.

Coding Clarification
Code E867 codes may only be reported as a secondary diagnosis.

Use a secondary E code from category E849 to identify the place of occurrence.

E868 Accidental poisoning by other utility gas and other carbon monoxide

Carbon monoxide poisoning can be deadly. There is no smell and it can't been seen, but it can kill in just a matter of minutes. If appliances that burn fuel are not properly working, toxic levels of carbon monoxide can be produced. Accidental carbon monoxide poisoning kills hundreds of people each year. Symptoms of carbon monoxide poisoning include severe headache, dizziness, mental confusion, nausea, and fainting. Since the symptoms are similar to many other causes, carbon monoxide poisoning has been hard to diagnose. Use of carbon monoxide alarms has greatly reduced the mortality rate from carbon monoxide poisoning.

E868.0	Accidental poisoning by liquefied petroleum gas distributed in mobile containers
E868.1	Accidental poisoning by other and unspecified utility gas
E868.2	Accidental poisoning by motor vehicle exhaust gas
E868.3	Accidental poisoning by carbon monoxide from incomplete combustion of other domestic fuels
E868.8	Accidental poisoning by carbon monoxide from other sources
E868.9	Accidental poisoning by unspecified carbon monoxide

Coding Clarification
Category E868 codes may only be reported as a secondary diagnosis.

Use a secondary E code from category E849 to identify the place of occurrence.

Coding Scenario
A 57-year-old male presents to the emergency department with a severe headache. It is found that the man was in his barn working on his tractor engine with all doors and windows closed. The tractor had been running for several minutes. The diagnosis is carbon monoxide poisoning.

> Code assignment: 986 *Toxic effect of carbon monoxide,* E868.2 *Accidental poisoning by motor vehicle exhaust gas,* and E849.1 *Place of occurrence, farm*

E869 Accidental poisoning by other gases and vapors

Symptoms from exposure to gas and vapors can range from mild to severe. These include headache, nausea, vomiting, eye irritation, pulmonary edema, confusion, drowsiness, loss of consciousness, shortness of breath, cough, and bronchospasm. Life-threatening symptoms may appear as late as several weeks after exposure to some gases.

E869.0	Accidental poisoning by nitrogen oxides

E869.1	Accidental poisoning by sulfur dioxide
E869.2	Accidental poisoning by freon
E869.3	Accidental poisoning by lacrimogenic gas (tear gas)
E869.4	Accidental poisoning by second-hand tobacco smoke
E869.8	Accidental poisoning by other specified gases and vapors
E869.9	Accidental poisoning by unspecified gases and vapors

Coding Clarification
Category E869 codes may only be reported as a secondary diagnosis.

Use a secondary E code from category E849 to identify the place of occurrence.

E870–E876 Misadventures to Patients During Surgical and Medical Care

Many people are incapacitated as a result of medical errors. As many people as 98,000 Americans die each year as a result of medical errors, approximately the eighth leading cause of death. These errors increase health care costs significantly. The following kinds of errors unfortunately are often made: prescribing the wrong medication, administering an anesthetic improperly, operating a mechanical device incorrectly, causing an infection by improper wound treatment, contaminating blood or other pathological tests, completing a surgical procedure incorrectly.

E870 Accidental cut, puncture, perforation, or hemorrhage during medical care

Category E870 codes are used to report accidental puncture, perforation, or hemorrhage during medical care. Procedures where these accidents might take place are surgery, infusion or transfusion, dialysis, perfusion, injection or vaccination, endoscopic exam, aspiration of fluid or tissue, puncture, catheterization, heart catheterization, and administration of an enema. One study indicates that 3.29 out of 1,000 discharges and 31.17 per 100,000 people experience a complication from an accidental puncture, perforation, or hemorrhage.

Hemodialysis is the use of an artificial kidney to clear waste products from the blood when the patient's own kidneys are not functioning. Risk of accidental perforation could happen when connecting the dialysis machine to the catheter implanted in the patient.

Accidental laceration, when performing an endoscopy, was the second highest complication reported by ambulatory surgery centers in 1999. During the endoscopy, the physician's field is closed and the physician's view is limited to what is in the camera's line of site. Most physicians are proficient in performing endoscopic procedures; however, the closed surgical field increases the chance of puncturing a structure.

Accidental dural puncture during an epidural is one of the most common complications of that procedure. Symptoms may include a severe headache. An epidural blood patch may be necessary to treat the dural puncture.

During a cardiac catheterization a puncture is made in a blood vessel in the groin and a catheter is fed through this to the heart. Different vessels of the heart are imaged and often a repair can be made at the same time as the diagnosis. One risk of the procedure is an inadvertent puncture of an artery.

Enemas are performed to evacuate the bowel or in some instances to instill radio opaque dye to image the bowel. There is a slight risk that the bowel may be punctured during the process.

E870.0	Accidental cut, puncture, perforation, or hemorrhage during surgical operation
E870.1	Accidental cut, puncture, perforation, or hemorrhage during infusion or transfusion
E870.2	Accidental cut, puncture, perforation, or hemorrhage during kidney dialysis or other perfusion
E870.3	Accidental cut, puncture, perforation, or hemorrhage during injection or vaccination
E870.4	Accidental cut, puncture, perforation, or hemorrhage during endoscopic examination
E870.5	Accidental cut, puncture, perforation, or hemorrhage during aspiration of fluid or tissue, puncture, and catheterization
E870.6	Accidental cut, puncture, perforation, or hemorrhage during heart catheterization
E870.7	Accidental cut, puncture, perforation, or hemorrhage during administration of enema
E870.8	Accidental cut, puncture, perforation, or hemorrhage during other specified medical care
E870.9	Accidental cut, puncture, perforation, or hemorrhage during unspecified medical care

Documentation Issues
The physician should document clearly that a misadventure occurred and the nature of the complication.

Rubrics E870-E876 must be assigned if documented by the physician. Office or hospital policies cannot state that these codes never be used.

Supplementary Classification of External Causes

Coding Clarification
Category E870 codes may only be reported as a secondary diagnosis.

Do not assign traumatic injury codes (800-959) in addition to 998.2 *Accidental puncture or laceration during a procedure.*

Report a code from the E878-E879 rubric for an abnormal reaction or later complication of a procedure that the physician does not document as a misadventure. Codes E870-E876 should be assigned if the physician documents the misadventure.

Coding Scenario
A 23-year-old female suffers a puncture into the dura during an epidural injection.

> Code assignment: 998.2 *Accidental puncture or laceration during a procedure* and E870.5 *Accidental cut, puncture, perforation, or hemorrhage during aspiration of fluid or tissue, puncture, and catheterization*

E871 Foreign object left in body during procedure

Category E871 codes are used to report foreign objects left in the body during surgery. This set of codes should not be used if the foreign body was left in intentionally. Foreign bodies include sponges, needles, catheters, instruments, and any other object not intended to remain in the patient.

Code	Description
E871.0	Foreign object left in body during surgical operation
E871.1	Foreign object left in body during infusion or transfusion
E871.2	Foreign object left in body during kidney dialysis or other perfusion
E871.3	Foreign object left in body during injection or vaccination
E871.4	Foreign object left in body during endoscopic examination
E871.5	Foreign object left in body during aspiration of fluid or tissue, puncture, and catheterization
E871.6	Foreign object left in body during heart catheterization
E871.7	Foreign object left in body during removal of catheter or packing
E871.8	Foreign object left in body during other specified procedure
E871.9	Foreign object left in body during unspecified procedure

Documentation Issues
The physician should document clearly that a misadventure occurred and the nature of the complication.

Coding Clarification
Category E871 codes may only be reported as a secondary diagnosis.

Codes E870-E876 should be assigned if the physician documents the misadventure.

Report a code from the E878-E879 rubric for an abnormal reaction or later complication of a procedure that the physician does not document as a misadventure.

E872 Failure of sterile precautions during procedure

Category E872 codes are used to report failure of sterile precautions during a procedure. Sterile technique is the process of keeping the operating area free from all germs. This involves ensuring that anything that will be used during the procedure is sterile. This is primarily done by autoclaving the instruments.

An autoclave is a machine that heats instruments to a high enough temperature to kill bacteria. Color change indicators wrapped with the instruments show operating room personnel that the sterilization process was successful.

All surgeons and scrub personnel are responsible for maintaining a sterile field. This is accomplished by wearing sterile gowns and gloves and by the use of sterile drapes and instruments. These should be carefully inspected to ensure that there are no cuts or holes in the attire or in the packages in which the instruments are wrapped. Even the smallest hole will breach the integrity of the sterile field.

The surgical site should only be touched by items that are sterile. Each member of the surgical team has the responsibility to ensure that there is not a break in the sterile technique. A break in sterile technique may go unnoticed, but it is the responsibility of all operating room personnel to report any problem with sterile technique so it can be quickly corrected.

Code	Description
E872.0	Failure of sterile precautions during surgical operation
E872.1	Failure of sterile precautions during infusion or transfusion
E872.2	Failure of sterile precautions during kidney dialysis and other perfusion
E872.3	Failure of sterile precautions during injection or vaccination
E872.4	Failure of sterile precautions during endoscopic examination
E872.5	Failure of sterile precautions during aspiration of fluid or tissue, puncture, and catheterization
E872.6	Failure of sterile precautions during heart catheterization

Coders' Desk Reference for Diagnoses

E872.8	Failure of sterile precautions during other specified procedure
E872.9	Failure of sterile precautions during unspecified procedure

Coding Clarification

Category E872 codes may only be reported as a secondary diagnosis.

Codes E870-E876 should be assigned if the physician documents the misadventure.

Report a code from the E878-E879 rubric for an abnormal reaction or later complication of a procedure that the physician does not document as a misadventure.

E873 Failure in dosage

Category E873 codes are used to report failure in dosage. This could mean excessive fluid or blood administration, which can cause heart failure or electrolyte imbalance in the patient or an excess amount of iron in the blood in the case of excessive blood transfusion.

Excess radiation can cause short-term effects such as burns on the skin to long-term effects such as cancer and birth defects. Radiation is commonly used to treat certain types of cancer.

Drug administration errors can include giving the patient too much medication, not enough medication, or failing to give an ordered drug.

E873.0	Excessive amount of blood or other fluid during transfusion or infusion
E873.1	Incorrect dilution of fluid during infusion
E873.2	Overdose of radiation in therapy
E873.3	Inadvertent exposure of patient to radiation during medical care
E873.4	Failure in dosage in electroshock or insulin-shock therapy
E873.5	Inappropriate (too hot or too cold) temperature in local application and packing
E873.6	Nonadministration of necessary drug or medicinal substance
E873.8	Other specified failure in dosage
E873.9	Unspecified failure in dosage

Coding Clarification

Category E873 codes may only be reported as a secondary diagnosis.

Codes E870-E876 should be assigned if the physician documents the misadventure.

Report a code from the E878-E879 rubric for an abnormal reaction or later complication of a procedure that the physician does not document as a misadventure.

E874 Mechanical failure of instrument or apparatus during procedure

Category E874 codes are used to report the mechanical failure of an instrument or apparatus during a procedure, which includes the malfunction of instruments or equipment used during a surgical procedure. Procedures during which equipment malfunctions might occur include infusion, transfusion, dialysis, perfusion, endoscopy, aspiration, puncture, catheterization, heart catheterization, and other procedures. The practice of testing equipment and instrumentation will help eliminate problems in this area.

E874.0	Mechanical failure of instrument or apparatus during surgical operation
E874.1	Mechanical failure of instrument or apparatus during infusion and transfusion
E874.2	Mechanical failure of instrument or apparatus during kidney dialysis and other perfusion
E874.3	Mechanical failure of instrument or apparatus during endoscopic examination
E874.4	Mechanical failure of instrument or apparatus during aspiration of fluid or tissue, puncture, and catheterization
E874.5	Mechanical failure of instrument or apparatus during heart catheterization
E874.8	Mechanical failure of instrument or apparatus during other specified procedure
E874.9	Mechanical failure of instrument or apparatus during unspecified procedure

Coding Clarification

Category E874 codes may only be reported as a secondary diagnosis.

Codes E870-E876 should be assigned if the physician documents the misadventure.

Report a code from the E878-E879 rubric for an abnormal reaction or later complication of a procedure that the physician does not document as a misadventure.

E875 Contaminated or infected blood, other fluid, drug, or biological substance

Blood can be transfused as whole blood, red blood cells, plasma, cryoprecipitated AHF, platelets, white blood cells, and plasma derivatives. Blood can be stored from five days to 10 years depending on the component of the blood being stored. Currently blood is tested for Hepatitis B surface antigen, Hepatitis B core antibody, Hepatitis C virus antibody, HIV-1 antibody, HIV 2 antibody, HTLV-I antibody, HTLV-II antibody, syphilis, and nucleic acid amplification. Nucleic acid amplification testing, which detects the genetic material of viruses, is also performed. These tests are all considered screening tests. The tests are sensitive and may result in false positives. Confirmatory tests can be done to confirm a positive result. The Food and Drug Administration (FDA) allows investigational tests for the West Nile virus, which can be transmitted through a blood transfusion.

E875.0	Contaminated substance transfused or infused
E875.1	Contaminated substance injected or used for vaccination
E875.2	Contaminated drug or biological substance administered by other means
E875.8	Other contamination of patient during medical care
E875.9	Unspecified contamination of patient during medical care

Coding Clarification
Category E875 codes may only be reported as a secondary diagnosis.

Codes E870-E876 should be assigned if the physician documents the misadventure.

Report a code from the E878-E879 rubric for an abnormal reaction or later complication of a procedure that the physician does not document as a misadventure.

E876 Other and unspecified misadventures during medical care

A patient given the incorrect blood type can suffer clotting problems, kidney failure, and death. A blood type is the presence or absence of certain proteins on the red blood cells. If the wrong blood type is given, the body's immune system would try to fight off the unfamiliar virus.

An endotracheal tube (ET) is placed into a patient's trachea to provide ventilation. Often the patient is paralyzed before the procedure so the patient is completely dependent on the ET tube to provide oxygen to the body. If this tube is incorrectly placed into the esophagus, the patient can die from lack of oxygen.

The Joint Commission on Accreditation of Healthcare Organizations (JCAHO) states that since 1996 more than 150 cases of wrong-site surgery has occurred. This means the physician operated on the wrong side or wrong body part. There are also incidences where surgery was performed on the wrong patient.

E876.0	Mismatched blood in transfusion
E876.1	Wrong fluid in infusion
E876.2	Failure in suture and ligature during surgical operation
E876.3	Endotracheal tube wrongly placed during anesthetic procedure
E876.4	Failure to introduce or to remove other tube or instrument
E876.5	Performance of inappropriate operation
E876.8	Other specified misadventure during medical care
E876.9	Unspecified misadventure during medical care

Coding Clarification
Category E876 codes may only be reported as a secondary diagnosis.

Codes E870-E876 should be assigned if the physician documents the misadventure.

Report a code from the E878-E879 rubric for an abnormal reaction or later complication of a procedure that the physician does not document as a misadventure.

E878–E879 Surgical and Medical Procedures as the Cause of Abnormal Reaction of Patient or Later Complication, Without Mention of Misadventure at the Time of Procedure

Rubric E878-E879 codes are used to report abnormal reactions that patients have following surgical and medical procedures. These codes can also be used to report a later complication of a misadventure that occurred at the time of a procedure. Examples of these kinds of procedures are those that cause an abnormal reaction such as displacement or malfunction of a prosthetic device, liver or renal failure, malfunction of an external stoma, postoperative intestinal obstruction, or rejection of a transplanted organ. Excluded from this category are anesthetic management properly carried out as the cause of an adverse effect and infusion and transfusion without mention of misadventure in the technique. These codes should be used when a physician documents that an abnormal reaction or later complication is a result of a medical or surgical procedure, but does not mention any misadventure at the time of the procedure.

E878 Surgical operation and other surgical procedures as the cause of abnormal reaction of patient, or of later complication, without mention of misadventure at the time of operation

Transplanted organs are rejected because the body's immune system sees the transplanted organ as a potentially harmful foreign body. Although tissue typing is performed prior to the transplant, no two people (except identical twins) have the same tissue antigens. Other than with corneal transplants, patients have to be on immunosuppressive drugs all of their lives. Symptoms of organ rejection include the following:

- Organ does not function properly
- General feeling of uneasiness or illness
- Fever and pain or swelling at the organ site

A stoma is an artificial opening from an internal organ to outside the body. A gastrostomy is an opening from the stomach to the skin. This allows feeding directly into the stomach. A jejunostomy is an opening from the first portion of the bowel to outside the body, which also can be used for feeding. An ileostomy is an opening from the small bowel to outside the body, which allows feces to leave the body without passing through the large intestine. A colostomy is an opening from the large bowel to outside the body, which allows feces to be eliminated from the body bypassing the anus. A urostomy is a connection between the urinary system and the abdominal wall. This procedure also may be referred to as a urinary conduit. Some stomas may be temporary and will require another surgery to close them.

Also included in this category are surgical procedures to remove a limb or organ, such as an amputated limb and a cholecystectomy.

E878.0	Surgical operation with transplant of whole organ causing abnormal patient reaction, or later complication, without mention of misadventure at time of operation
E878.1	Surgical operation with implant of artificial internal device causing abnormal patient reaction, or later complication, without mention of misadventure at time of operation
E878.2	Surgical operation with anastomosis, bypass, or graft, with natural or artificial tissues used as implant causing abnormal patient reaction, or later complication, without mention of misadventure at time of operation
E878.3	Surgical operation with formation of external stoma causing abnormal patient reaction, or later complication, without mention of misadventure at time of operation
E878.4	Other restorative surgery causing abnormal patient reaction, or later complication, without mention of misadventure at time of operation
E878.5	Amputation of limb(s) causing abnormal patient reaction, or later complication, without mention of misadventure at time of operation
E878.6	Removal of other organ (partial) (total) causing abnormal patient reaction, or later complication, without mention of misadventure at time of operation
E878.8	Other specified surgical operation and procedure causing abnormal patient reaction, or later complication, without mention of misadventure at time of operation
E878.9	Unspecified surgical operation and procedure causing abnormal patient reaction, or later complication, without mention of misadventure at time of operation

Coding Clarification

Category E878 codes may only be reported as a secondary diagnosis.

Report a code from the E878-E879 rubric for an abnormal reaction or later complication of a procedure that the physician does not document as a misadventure.

For misadventures during a surgical or medical procedure, report E870-E876.

Coding Scenario

A patient who has undergone appendectomy experiences a dehiscence of the skin wound. The patient is taken back to the operating room and the wound is repaired. There is no sign of infection.

> Code assignment: 998.32 *Dehiscence of external wound*, and E878.6 *Removal of other organ (partial) (total) causing abnormal patient reaction, or later complication, without mention of misadventure at time of operation*

E879 Other procedures, without mention of misadventure at the time of procedure, as the cause of abnormal reaction of patient, or of later complication

During a cardiac catheterization a puncture is made into a blood vessel in the groin and a catheter is fed through this to the heart. Different vessels of the heart are imaged and often a repair can be made at the same time as the diagnosis.

Hemodialysis is the use of an artificial kidney to clear waste products from the blood when the patient's own kidneys are not functioning.

Between 100,000 to 150,000 patients are given electroconvulsive therapy (shock therapy) every year to treat schizophrenia and depression. Anesthetic and muscle relaxants are given to the patient prior to the administration of the therapy.

E879.0	Cardiac catheterization as the cause of abnormal reaction of patient, or of later complication, without mention of misadventure at time of procedure
E879.1	Kidney dialysis as the cause of abnormal reaction of patient, or of later complication, without mention of misadventure at time of procedure
E879.2	Radiological procedure and radiotherapy as the cause of abnormal reaction of patient, or of later complication, without mention of misadventure at time of procedure

E879.3	Shock therapy as the cause of abnormal reaction of patient, or of later complication, without mention of misadventure at time of procedure	
E879.4	Aspiration of fluid as the cause of abnormal reaction of patient, or of later complication, without mention of misadventure at time of procedure	
E879.5	Insertion of gastric or duodenal sound as the cause of abnormal reaction of patient, or of later complication, without mention of misadventure of time of procedure	
E879.6	Urinary catheterization as the cause of abnormal reaction of patient, or of later complication, without mention of misadventure at time of procedure	
E879.7	Blood sampling as the cause of abnormal reaction of patient, or of later complication, without mention of misadventure at time of procedure	
E879.8	Other specified procedure as the cause of abnormal reaction of patient, or of later complication, without mention of misadventure at time of procedure	
E879.9	Unspecified procedure as the cause of abnormal reaction of patient, or of later complication, without mention of misadventure at time of procedure	

Coding Clarification
Category E879 codes may only be reported as a secondary diagnosis.

Report a code from the E878-E879 rubric for an abnormal reaction or later complication of a procedure that the physician does not document as a misadventure.

E880–E888 Accidental Falls

Accidental fall codes are one of the most frequently assigned series of E codes. A fall is the most common cause of fatal injury in the elderly and a common cause of injury in children.

Accidental falls are broken down into specific types depending on whether the fall was from a bed, a chair, a ladder, the toilet, or the sidewalk curb. Also included in this category is a fall that results in the person striking against an object.

Excluded from this rubric is a fall in or from a burning building; into a fire; into water with submerging and drowning; in or from operating machinery; on an edged, painted, or sharp object; and in or from a transport or other vehicle.

E880 Accidental fall on or from stairs or steps
Category E880 codes describe falls from an escalator, a sidewalk curb, stairs, or steps. An escalator is defined as mechanically moving stairs or steps. This category does not include moving sidewalks.

E880.0	Accidental fall on or from escalator
E880.1	Accidental fall on or from sidewalk curb
E880.9	Accidental fall on or from other stairs or steps

Coding Clarification
Category E880 codes may only be reported as a secondary diagnosis.

Use a secondary E code from category E849 to identify the place of occurrence.

E881 Accidental fall on or from ladders or scaffolding
Category E881 codes are used to report falls from a ladder or scaffolding. A scaffolding is a temporary platform used to stand on when performing tasks above the ground.

E881.0	Accidental fall from ladder
E881.1	Accidental fall from scaffolding

Coding Clarification
Category E881 codes may only be reported as a secondary diagnosis.

Use a secondary E code from category E849 to identify the place of occurrence.

E882 Accidental fall from or out of building or other structure
Code E882 is used to report falls from out of a building or other structure. Included in this category is a fall from a turret, viaduct, wall, window, balcony, bridge, building, flagpole, tower, and a fall through the roof. Excluded from this category is a fall or jump from a burning building or a fall due to a collapse of a building.

Coding Clarification
Code E882 codes may only be reported as a secondary diagnosis.

Use a secondary E code from category E849 to identify the place of occurrence.

E883 Accidental fall into hole or other opening in surface
Category E883 codes are used to report a fall into a hole or opening in the surface. This includes a hole, pit quarry, shaft, and tank. There are specific codes for accidents caused by diving or jumping into water, falling into a well, and falling into a storm drain or manhole.

E883.0	Accident from diving or jumping into water (swimming pool)
E883.1	Accidental fall into well
E883.2	Accidental fall into storm drain or manhole

E883.9   Accidental fall into other hole or other opening in surface

Coding Clarification
Category E883 codes may only be reported as a secondary diagnosis.

Use a secondary E code from category E849 to identify the place of occurrence.

Coding Scenario
A 29-year-old male presents to the emergency department with a neck injury. The patient was diving into a pool in his back yard and hit his head on the bottom. The diagnosis is a strained neck.

> Code assignment: 847.0 *Neck strain or sprain*, E883.0 *Accident from diving or jumping into water*, and E849.0 *Place of occurrence, home*

E884   Other accidental fall from one level to another
Category E884 codes are used to report any fall from one level to another. Specific codes are available to report a fall from playground equipment, a cliff, chair, wheelchair, bed, other furniture, and a commode.

Many playground accidents involve falls from playground equipment onto hard surfaces. This is one of the major types of falls for children ages 5 to 14.

Code	Description
E884.0	Accidental fall from playground equipment
E884.1	Accidental fall from cliff
E884.2	Accidental fall from chair
E884.3	Accidental fall from wheelchair
E884.4	Accidental fall from bed
E884.5	Accidental fall from other furniture
E884.6	Accidental fall from commode
E884.9	Other accidental fall from one level to another

Coding Clarification
Category E884 codes may only be reported as a secondary diagnosis.

Use a secondary E code from category E849 to identify the place of occurrence.

E885   Accidental fall on same level from slipping, tripping, or stumbling
Category E885 codes are used to describe falls on the same level. This code category includes falls from scooters, roller skates, skateboards, skis, snowboards, or from slipping, tripping, and stumbling.

Code	Description
E885.0	Fall on same level from (nonmotorized) scooter
E885.1	Fall from roller skates
E885.2	Fall from skateboard
E885.3	Fall from skis
E885.4	Fall from snowboard
E885.9	Fall from other slipping, tripping, or stumbling

Coding Clarification
Category E885 codes may only be reported as a secondary diagnosis.

Use a secondary E code from category E849 to identify the place of occurrence.

E886   Accidental fall on same level from collision, pushing, or shoving, by or with other person
Category E886 codes are used to describe falls from the same level due to a collision, push, or shove, by or with another person. Code E886.0 is used to report colliding, pushing, or shoving injuries that occur in sports. Code 886.9 includes a fall from or a collision with a pedestrian conveyance. A pedestrian conveyance is a device that is human powered and used to move a pedestrian, which includes a baby carriage, coaster wagon, ice skates, pushcart, and pushchair.

Code	Description
E886.0	Accidental fall on same level from collision, pushing, or shoving, by or with other person in sports
E886.9	Other and unspecified accidental falls on same level from collision, pushing, or shoving, by or with other person

Coding Clarification
Category E886 codes may only be reported as a secondary diagnosis.

Use a secondary E code from category E849 to identify the place of occurrence.

Coding Scenario
A 17-year-old male presents to the emergency department with a dislocated right shoulder. The patient was playing in a high school football game and was tackled landing on his right shoulder. The diagnosis is a closed dislocation of the right shoulder.

> Code assignment: 831.0 *Closed dislocation of shoulder*, E886.0 *Accidental fall on same level from collision, pushing, or shoving, by or with other person in sports*, and E849.4 *Place of occurrence, place for recreation and sport*

E887   Fracture in accidental fall, cause unspecified
Code E887 is used to report a fracture caused by a fall when the cause of the fall is not specified. This code should only be used if the information cannot be obtained from the patient or the physician.

Coding Clarification
Code E887 codes may only be reported as a secondary diagnosis.

Use a secondary E code from category E849 to identify the place of occurrence.

E888 Other and unspecified accidental fall
Category E888 codes are used to report other and unspecified falls. Specific codes in this category are for falls that result in striking against a sharp object and falls that result in striking against other objects.

E888.0	Fall resulting in striking against sharp object
E888.1	Fall resulting in striking against other object
E888.8	Other fall
E888.9	Unspecified fall

Coding Clarification
Category E888 codes may only be reported as a secondary diagnosis.

Use an additional E code from category E920 to identify the sharp object.

Use a secondary E code from category E849 to identify the place of occurrence.

E890–E899 Accidents Caused by Fire and Flames
Rubrics E890-E899 are used to describe accidents caused by fire and flames. This code category includes asphyxia or poisoning due to fire. Asphyxia is suffocation or lack of oxygen intake, which can occur in a very short amount of time. In the United States, fires are the third leading cause of accidental death, with the number one cause being smoke inhalation. Smoke contents are heated particles and gases. The exact composition of smoke and the toxicity are dependent on the material that is on fire.

E890 Conflagration in private dwelling
Category E890 codes are used to report conflagration in a private dwelling. A private dwelling is defined as an apartment, a boarding house, camping place, farmhouse, house, mobile home, or private garage. Conflagration is a widespread, general burning. One of the harmful gases that can be generated in a fire is polyvinylchloride (PVC). PVC is a flame and water-resistant plastic material that can be found in communication and building cables.

E890.0	Explosion caused by conflagration in private dwelling
E890.1	Fumes from combustion of polyvinylchloride (PVC) and similar material in conflagration in private dwelling
E890.2	Other smoke and fumes from conflagration in private dwelling
E890.3	Burning caused by conflagration in private dwelling
E890.8	Other accident resulting from conflagration in private dwelling
E890.9	Unspecified accident resulting from conflagration in private dwelling

Coding Clarification
Category E890 codes may only be reported as a secondary diagnosis.

Use a secondary E code from category E849 to identify the place of occurrence.

E891 Conflagration in other and unspecified building or structure
Category E891 codes are used to report conflagration in a structure other than a private dwelling. A nonprivate dwelling is defined as a barn, church, retirement home, factory, hospital, hotel, school, store, or theater. Conflagration is a widespread, general burning. One of the harmful gases that can be generated in a fire is PVC. PVC is a flame- and water-resistant plastic material that can be found in communication and building cables.

E891.0	Explosion caused by conflagration in other and unspecified building or structure
E891.1	Fumes from combustion of polyvinylchloride (PVC) and similar material in conflagration in other and unspecified building or structure
E891.2	Other smoke and fumes from conflagration in other and unspecified building or structure
E891.3	Burning caused by conflagration in other and unspecified building or structure
E891.8	Other accident resulting from conflagration in other and unspecified building or structure
E891.9	Unspecified accident resulting from conflagration of other and unspecified building or structure

Coding Clarification
Category E891 codes may only be reported as a secondary diagnosis.

Use a secondary E code from category E849 to identify the place of occurrence.

E892 Conflagration not in building or structure
Code E892 is used to report conflagration not in a building or structure, which includes forest, grass, and lumber fires. This code category also includes fire in a transport vehicle when the vehicle is not moving. Conflagration is a widespread, general burning.

Coding Clarification
Code E892 codes may only be reported as a secondary diagnosis.

Use a secondary E code from category E849 to identify the place of occurrence.

E893 Accident caused by ignition of clothing

Category E893 codes are used to describe accidents caused by ignition of clothing. The United States government issued regulations to restrict the use of flammable materials in children's clothing.

Legislation classifies clothing into the following three different categories:

- Class one is normal flammability. These are textiles without raised fiber in which flames spread in four seconds or more.
- Class two is intermediate flammability. These are textiles having raised fiber in which flames spread between four and seven seconds.
- Class three is rapid and intense burning. These are textiles without raised fiber in which flames spread in less than four seconds.

E893.0	Accident caused by ignition of clothing from controlled fire in private dwelling
E893.1	Accident caused by ignition of clothing from controlled fire in other building or structure
E893.2	Accident caused by ignition of clothing from controlled fire not in building or structure
E893.8	Accident caused by ignition of clothing from other specified sources
E893.9	Accident caused by ignition of clothing by unspecified source

Coding Clarification
Category E893 codes may only be reported as a secondary diagnosis.

Use a secondary E code from category E849 to identify the place of occurrence.

Coding Scenario
A 40-year-old male is admitted to the emergency department with second-degree burns of his upper arm. The patient was using a torch at work and his shirt was ignited.

> Code assignment: 942.23 *Second degree burn of upper arm*, E893.8 *Accident caused by ignition of clothing from other specified source*, and E849.3 *Place of occurrence, industrial place and premises*

E894 Ignition of highly inflammable material

Code E894 is used to report ignition of clothing by highly inflammable material. These are materials such as gasoline, fat, kerosene, paraffin, and benzine. Excluded from this category is ignition of highly inflammable materials with conflagration or explosion. Conflagration is a widespread burning.

Coding Clarification
Code E894 codes may only be reported as a secondary diagnosis.

Use a secondary E code from category E849 to identify the place of occurrence.

E895 Accident caused by controlled fire in private dwelling

Code E895 is used to describe accidents caused by a controlled fire in a private dwelling. The definition of a private dwelling is an apartment, a boarding house, camping place, caravan, farmhouse, house, lodging house, mobile home, private garage, rooming house, and tenement. Examples of controlled burns are those in a brazier, fireplace, furnace, and stove. A brazier is a device that holds coal or charcoal and is used to heat food.

Coding Clarification
Code E895 codes may only be reported as a secondary diagnosis.

Use a secondary E code from category E849 to identify the place of occurrence.

E896 Accident caused by controlled fire in other and unspecified building or structure

Code E896 is used to report accidents caused by a controlled fire in other and unspecified buildings or structures. The following are kinds of buildings or structures: a barn, church, convalescent home, residential home, dormitory, factory, any type of farm outbuilding, hospital, hotel, school, store, and theater. Examples of controlled burns are those in a brazier, fireplace, furnace, and stove. A brazier is a device that holds coal or charcoal and is used to heat food.

Coding Clarification
Code E896 codes may only be reported as a secondary diagnosis.

Use a secondary E code from category E849 to identify the place of occurrence.

E897 Accident caused by controlled fire not in building or structure

Code E897 is used to report accidents caused by a controlled fire not in a building or structure. Examples of this type of controlled fire include a bonfire, brazier fire, trash fire, and campfire. A brazier is a device that holds coal or charcoal and is used to heat food.

Coding Clarification
Code E897 codes may only be reported as a secondary diagnosis.

Use a secondary E code from category E849 to identify the place of occurrence.

Supplementary Classification of External Causes

E898   Accident caused by other specified fire and flames

Burning bedclothes can be the cause of flashover. Flashover is a temperature that is so intense it causes everything in the room to burst into flames. This happens at a heat-release rate of about 1,000 kilowatts. King-size bedclothes can contribute to more than 400 kilowatts and a mattress and box spring can contribute to more than 500 kilowatts.

| E898.0 | Accident caused by burning bedclothes |
| E898.1 | Accident caused by other burning materials |

Coding Clarification
Category E898 codes may only be reported as a secondary diagnosis.

Use a secondary E code from category E849 to identify the place of occurrence.

E899   Accident caused by unspecified fire OK

Code E899 is used to describe fires of an unspecified nature. This should only be used if more specific information cannot be obtained from the physician or patient.

Coding Clarification
Code E899 codes may only be reported as a secondary diagnosis.

Use a secondary E code from category E849 to identify the place of occurrence.

E900–E909 Accidents due to Natural and Environmental Factors

E900   Accident caused by excessive heat

Sunstroke is a rise in temperature caused by exposure to the sun, hot climates, overcrowding, and poor ventilation. It may also be called siriasis. Symptoms of heatstroke include heat syncope, sudden seizure, flushed face, quick pulse, gasping or sighing respiration, headache, vomiting, nausea, and thermic fever, which is a body temperature of 110 degrees or more.

E900.0	Accident due to excessive heat weather conditions
E900.1	Accident due to excessive heat, man-made origin
E900.9	Accident due to excessive heat, unspecified origin

Coding Clarification
Category E900 codes may only be reported as a secondary diagnosis.

Use a secondary E code from category E849 to identify the place of occurrence.

E901   Accident due to excessive cold

Chilblains are painful, small, itchy, red areas of the skin that appear on the skin after exposure to cold temperature. They are more common in cold, humid climates. Chilblains are most common on the toes but can appear on the fingers, nose, and ears also. The skin breaks down and ulcers and infection can occur. Chilblains are more common in females and can be recurrent for the rest of the patient's life or last only a few years.

Immersion foot occurs when the feet have been submerged or subjected to wet conditions for long periods of time. It is less serious than frost bite but can cause gangrene and necrosis.

E901.0	Accident due to excessive cold, weather conditions
E901.1	Accident due to excessive cold, man-made origin
E901.8	Accident due to excessive cold, other specified origin
E901.9	Accident due to excessive cold, unspecified origin

Coding Clarification
Category E901 codes may only be reported as a secondary diagnosis.

Use a secondary E code from category E849 to identify the place of occurrence.

E902   Accident due to high and low air pressure and changes in air pressure

Altitude sickness can occur when people are above 6,000 to 8,000 feet. Susceptibility to altitude sickness does not seem to be affected by training or the physical condition of the patient. The three types of altitude sickness are:

- Acute mountain sickness (AMS). This is the most common type. It can occur in altitudes as low as 4,000 to 6,000 feet but most often occurs in rapid ascents to greater than 9,000 feet. Symptoms include headache, fatigue, loss of appetite, nausea, and vomiting. Symptoms can occur between six and 24 hours after ascent.

- High-altitude cerebral edema (HACE). This is a severe progression of AMS. The patient may have the symptoms of AMS plus profound confusion and ataxia during a tandem gait test. A tandem gait test is walking heel to toe in a straight line. A person who fails the tandem gait test has HACE and should descend immediately.

- High-altitude pulmonary edema (HAPE). This can occur by itself or in conjunction with high-altitude cerebral edema. Symptoms include increased breathlessness with exertion and eventually increased loss of breath at rest. If the increased loss of breath continues after several minutes at rest, the patient should descend immediately.

The bends or diver's sickness is caused by nitrogen bubble formation in the blood and tissues. This is usually caused by a diver ascending to the surface too fast. The symptoms include headache, vertigo, disturbed sensation, paralysis, and death.

E902.0	Accident due to residence or prolonged visit at high altitude
E902.1	Accident due to changes in airpressure in aircraft
E902.2	Accident due to changes in air pressure due to diving
E902.8	Accident due to changes in air pressure due to other specified cause
E902.9	Accident due to changes in air pressure from unspecified cause

Coding Clarification
Category E902 codes may only be reported as a secondary diagnosis.

Use a secondary E code from category E849 to identify the place of occurrence.

E903 Accident due to travel and motion OK

Motion sickness is caused by a disturbance in the balance center in the middle ear. Many people will experience motion sickness when there is increased turbulence. Symptoms include dizziness, nausea, and vomiting.

Coding Clarification
Code E903 codes may only be reported as a secondary diagnosis.

Use a secondary E code from category E849 to identify the place of occurrence.

Coding Scenario
A 42-year-old female traveling by air from Salt Lake City to Cincinnati experiences nausea and vomiting. She presents to the emergency department for treatment. The diagnosis is nausea and vomiting due to motion sickness.

Code assignment: 787.01 *Nausea and vomiting*, E903 *Accidents due to travel and motion*, and E849.8 *Place of occurrence, other specified place*

E904 Accident due to hunger, thirst, exposure, and neglect

Malnutrition results from inadequate intake of nutrients. Infants and children are at the highest risk for malnutrition, since there is a high demand for nutrients during the growth years. Pregnancy and old age also pose other significant risks for malnutrition. Malnutrition as the result of abandonment and neglect should be reported with E904.0. When neglect is determined to be due to abandonment or neglect, E904.0 should be the first listed E code.

E904.0	Accident due to abandonment or neglect of infant and helpless person
E904.1	Accident due to lack of food
E904.2	Accident due to lack of water
E904.3	Accident due to exposure (to weather conditions), not elsewhere classifiable
E904.9	Accident due to unqualified privation

Coding Clarification
Category E904 codes may only be reported as a secondary diagnosis. Code E904.2 excludes dehydration due to acute fluid loss, which is reported with 276.51.

Use a secondary E code from category E849 to identify the place of occurrence.

E905 Venomous animals and plants as the cause of poisoning and toxic reactions

Each of the 48 contiguous states in the United States harbors at least one species of venomous snake. The pit vipers (copperhead, cottonmouth, and rattlesnakes) and coral snakes are two venomous families widely spread throughout the United States. Approximately 8,000 of the estimated 45,000 annual snakebites in this country are by poisonous snakes. Snake venoms are rated on a lethality index, with the Mojave rattlesnake having the highest index of any North American snake. Pit viper bites are associated with pain, swelling, and edema. Ecchymosis is common, ranging from moderate to severe. The patient may hemorrhage from the gums and develop hematemesis, melena, and hematuria. The coral snake bite generally produces conduction damage and central nervous system (CNS) damage. Annual fatalities are fewer than 15, most of which can be attributed to rattlesnake venom.

Two lizards, the Gila monster and the bearded lizard, are poisonous. There is currently no antivenom for these bites.

There are numerous venomous spider species in the United States. Most bites require only local care, although in cases of severe envenomation, the victim must be hospitalized for supportive measures. Fatalities are few, with the greatest risks for children and elderly.

As many as 85 percent of all people will develop a reaction if exposed to poison ivy, poison oak, or poison sumac. It may take several exposures to develop a sensitivity or the effects may appear with the initial contact. Although the toxin is only found in the sap of the plant, they are fragile and are often damaged causing the sap to come to the surface.

E905.0	Venomous snakes and lizards as the cause of poisoning and toxic reactions
E905.1	Venomous spiders as the cause of poisoning and toxic reactions
E905.2	Scorpion sting as the cause of poisoning and toxic reactions
E905.3	Sting of hornets, wasps, and bees as the cause of poisoning and toxic reactions
E905.4	Centipede and venomous millipede (tropical) bite as the cause of poisoning and toxic reactions
E905.5	Other venomous arthropods as the cause of poisoning and toxic reactions
E905.6	Venomous marine animals and plants as the cause of poisoning and toxic reactions
E905.7	Poisoning and toxic reactions caused by other plants
E905.8	Poisoning and toxic reactions caused by other specified animals and plants
E905.9	Poisoning and toxic reactions caused by unspecified animals and plants

Coding Clarification
Category E905 codes may only be reported as a secondary diagnosis.

Use a secondary E code from category E849 to identify the place of occurrence.

E906 Other injury caused by animals
There are an estimated 4.7 million people bitten by dogs each year. Injuries can range from minor and superficial to vicious, harmful attacks. There are steps people can take to avoid being bitten, such as staying away from unfamiliar dogs, not running from dogs, slowly backing away from a dog once it loses interest, and, if knocked down by a dog, rolling into a ball and staying motionless.

Although instances of rat bites are on the decline, children in poverty stricken areas are still at risk. There is a high probability of transmission of disease with wild rat bites. Diseases include streptobacillary rat-bite fever and spirillary rat-bite fever.

There are approximately 94 out of 120 snakes found in the United States that are not venomous. Bites from nonvenomous snakes are more common than venomous types. Nonvenomous snakebites are treated much like any other puncture wound.

E906.0	Dog bite
E906.1	Rat bite
E906.2	Bite of nonvenomous snakes and lizards
E906.3	Bite of other animal except arthropod
E906.4	Bite of nonvenomous arthropod
E906.5	Bite by unspecified animal
E906.8	Other specified injury caused by animal
E906.9	Unspecified injury caused by animal

Coding Clarification
Category E906 codes may only be reported as a secondary diagnosis.

Use a secondary E code from category E849 to identify the place of occurrence.

E907 Accident due to lightning OK
Lightning strikes can cause a wide variety of injuries. Many people struck by lightning suffer temporary paralysis that is distinctive to a lightning strike. Cardiac injuries such as cardiac arrest, arrhythmias, and infarction, as well as superficial burns and neurologic injuries, can occur as a result of lightning strikes. The eardrum is commonly ruptured causing hearing loss and pain.

Coding Clarification
Code E907 codes may only be reported as a secondary diagnosis.

Use a secondary E code from category E849 to identify the place of occurrence.

E908 Accident due to cataclysmic storms, and floods resulting from storms
A cataclysmic event is one that is caused by the force of nature. Hurricanes, tornadoes, floods, blizzards, and dust storms are considered cataclysmic events.

Hurricanes are storms containing two parts, an eye or calm portion in the middle and a wall of clouds that surround the eye. Hurricanes can be several hundred feet in diameter. A hurricane can maintain winds of 74 miles per hour or higher.

There are approximately 1,200 tornadoes each year causing more than 1,500 injuries and 80 deaths. A tornado is a violent storm that consists of a column of air that rotates violently. Tornadoes can range in speed from 30 to 70 miles per hour.

E908.0	Accident due to hurricane
E908.1	Accident due to tornado
E908.2	Accident due to floods
E908.3	Accident due to blizzard (snow) (ice)
E908.4	Accident due to dust storm
E908.8	Accident due to other cataclysmic storms
E908.9	Accident due to unspecified cataclysmic storms and floods resulting from storms

Coding Clarification
Category E908 codes may only be reported as a secondary diagnosis.

Use a secondary E code from category E849 to identify the place of occurrence.

E codes for cataclysmic events take priority over all other E codes except child and adult abuse and terrorism.

E909 Accident due to cataclysmic earth surface movements and eruptions

A cataclysmic event is one that is caused by the force of nature. Category E909 codes include earthquakes, volcanic eruptions, avalanches, landslides or mudslides, collapse of dams or man-made structures, and tidal waves caused by earthquakes.

Earthquakes are caused by shifting of the earth because of faults or a pre-existing weakness in the earth. Earthquakes are measured on a Richter scale. If the earthquake registers at less than a 3.5 on the scale, the earthquake is generally not felt, 3.5 to 5.4 and the earthquake can be felt but generally does not cause damage, 5.5 to 6.0 may cause damage to poorly constructed buildings, 6.1 to 6.9 can cause damage, 7.0 to 7.9 is a major earthquake and can cause major damage over large areas, and 8.0 is a great earthquake that can cause damage to areas more than 100 kilometers.

Volcanic eruptions do both harm and good. An eruption can destroy hundreds of acres of land but is key in forming land masses, such as the islands of Hawaii. Geologists are still unsure of exactly how volcanoes work but continue to study them. By learning how they work, scientists may better learn how to predict their eruption.

E909.0	Earthquakes
E909.1	Volcanic eruptions
E909.2	Avalanche, landslide, or mudslide
E909.3	Collapse of dam or man-made structure
E909.4	Tidalwave caused by earthquake
E909.8	Other cataclysmic earth surface movements and eruptions
E909.9	Unspecified cataclysmic earth surface movements and eruptions

Coding Clarification
Category E909 codes may only be reported as a secondary diagnosis.

Use a secondary E code from category E849 to identify the place of occurrence.

E codes for cataclysmic events take priority over all other E codes except child and adult abuse and terrorism.

E910–E915 Accidents Caused by Submersion, Suffocation, and Foreign Bodies

Rubric E910-E915 is used to report accidents caused by submersion, suffocation, and foreign bodies. The great mortality risk in near drowning is posed by respiratory insufficiency leading to hypoxia and respiratory acidosis. Aspiration of large quantities of fresh water can cause massive increase of blood volume, life-threatening electrolyte imbalance, and hemolysis leading to asphyxia and ventricular fibrillation. Near drowning is now more commonly referred to as a submersion accident.

The water temperature and duration of immersion are factors when predicting survival from immersion. If an individual is exposed to cool water, over time hypothermia will set in, with its attendant problems.

E910 Accidental drowning and submersion

Drowning can cause serious long-term effects such as brain damage or death. Alcohol and drugs contribute to drowning and near drowning, now more commonly referred to as a submersion accident. Nearly three-fourths of boating-related deaths are a result of drowning. More than one-third of adults are unable to swim.

Drowning is the third leading cause of death in children younger than five years of age. Children can drown in only a few inches of water and in a short period of time. Children should never be left unattended in the bathtub for any reason.

E910.0	Accidental drowning and submersion while water-skiing
E910.1	Accidental drowning and submersion while engaged in other sport or recreational activity with diving equipment
E910.2	Accidental drowning and submersion while engaged in other sport or recreational activity without diving equipment
E910.3	Accidental drowning and submersion while swimming or diving for purposes other than recreation or sport
E910.4	Accidental drowning and submersion in bathtub
E910.8	Other accidental drowning or submersion
E910.9	Unspecified accidental drowning or submersion

Coding Clarification
Category E910 codes may only be reported as a secondary diagnosis.

Use a secondary E code from category E849 to identify the place of occurrence.

E911 Inhalation and ingestion of food causing obstruction of respiratory tract or suffocation [OK]

Inhalation of food or a foreign object can cause obstruction of the airway. This can be caused by talking and eating at the same time, drinking alcohol and talking, and in older people due to dentures. Dentures do not have the chewing power of natural teeth, which can cause the patient to try to swallow larger pieces of food that get lodged in the airway.

People who are choking usually have a look of panic on their face. Their face may turn red or purple. The universal signal for someone choking is putting their hands to their throat. Using the Heimlich maneuver will help to dislodge an item blocking the airway by using the air already in the lungs to push the foreign body out.

Coding Clarification
Code E911 codes may only be reported as a secondary diagnosis.

Use a secondary E code from category E849 to identify the place of occurrence.

E912 Inhalation and ingestion of other object causing obstruction of respiratory tract or suffocation [OK]

In 2001, there were more than 17,000 visits to the emergency department due to choking in children 0 to 14 years of age. The highest incidence is for children younger than age one because they tend to put everything in their mouths. This includes small toys and coins. Of the children treated in 2001 for choking incidences, 10.5 percent were admitted or transferred to another facility.

Coding Clarification
Coded E912 codes may only be reported as a secondary diagnosis.

Use a secondary E code from category E849 to identify the place of occurrence.

E913 Accidental mechanical suffocation

Accidental mechanical suffocation codes are used for suffocation on items other than food. Specific codes exist for suffocation in a bed or cradle, by a plastic bag, due to lack of air in a closed in place, such as a refrigerator, and by falling earth or other substance.

Shopping bags, dry cleaning bags, and even mattress bags can cause instances of suffocation in children. All items that could cause airway obstruction in children should be kept out of their reach.

E913.0 Accidental mechanical suffocation in bed or cradle
E913.1 Accidental mechanical suffocation by plastic bag
E913.2 Accidental mechanical suffocation due to lack of air (in closed place)
E913.3 Accidental mechanical suffocation by falling earth or other substance
E913.8 Accidental mechanical suffocation by other specified means
E913.9 Accidental mechanical suffocation by unspecified means

Coding Clarification
Category E913 codes may only be reported as a secondary diagnosis.

Use a secondary E code from category E849 to identify the place of occurrence.

E914 Foreign body accidentally entering eye and adnexa [OK]

A foreign body in the eye can cause anything from a minor irritation to a serious penetrating eye trauma. The eye's natural tears remove many foreign bodies. Those that aren't removed require medical treatment. Most foreign bodies can be removed using a slit lamp for vision and sometimes a special instrument. Symptoms of a foreign body in the eye include, irritation, pain, redness, tearing, decreased vision, itching, and sensitivity to light.

Coding Clarification
Code E914 codes may only be reported as a secondary diagnosis.

Use a secondary E code from category E849 to identify the place of occurrence.

E915 Foreign body accidentally entering other orifice [OK]

Foreign bodies accidentally entering another orifice include a foreign body in the ear, genitourinary tract, or the gastrointestinal tract. Children may put things like toys, food, or other small objects in their ear. Adults can have things such as a hearing aid battery, insect, or even a lost button in their ear. Symptoms include pain, decreased hearing, and strange sounds. Many people do not know they have a foreign body in their ear until they have a foul-smelling discharge from the ear.

Coding Clarification
Code E915 codes may only be reported as a secondary diagnosis.

Use a secondary E code from category E849 to identify the place of occurrence.

E916–E928 Other Accidents

Rubric E916-E928 identifies other accidents. Accidents in this code category include being struck accidentally by a falling object, striking against an object or a person, and being caught accidentally in or between objects. Also included are accidents caused by machinery, cutting instruments, explosion of a pressure vessel (i.e., a boiler), guns, explosives, corrosive materials, electricity, and radiation. Environmental accidents, vibration, human bite, and constriction caused by hair are also types of accidents in this code category.

E916 Struck accidentally by falling object [OK]

Code E916 is used to report injuries caused by a falling object. Injuries from cataclysmic events take priority over other E codes except for terrorism and adult and child abuse. For example, if a piece of a building falls and injures a person during a hurricane, the code for the hurricane would be used rather than E916.

Coding Clarification
Code E916 codes may only be reported as a secondary diagnosis.

Use a secondary E code from category E849 to identify the place of occurrence.

E917 Striking against or struck accidentally by objects or persons

Category E917 codes are used to describe accidents caused by striking against an object or person without a subsequent fall. The appropriate code from the fall category (E888) should be used if the collision with an object or person causes a subsequent fall or if the fall is from an object.

E917.0	Striking against or struck accidentally by objects or persons in sports
E917.1	Striking against or struck accidentally by crowd, by collective fear or panic
E917.2	Striking against or struck accidentally in running water
E917.3	Strike against or struck accidentally by furniture without subsequent fall
E917.4	Strike against or struck accidentally by other stationary object without subsequent fall
E917.5	Strike against or struck accidentally by other object in sports with subsequent fall
E917.6	Strike against or struck accidentally by crowd, by collective fear or panic with subsequent fall
E917.7	Strike against or struck accidentally by furniture with subsequent fall
E917.8	Strike against or struck accidentally by other stationary object with subsequent fall
E917.9	Other accident caused by striking against or being struck accidentally by objects or persons

Coding Clarification
Category E917 codes may only be reported as a secondary diagnosis.

Use a secondary E code from category E849 to identify the place of occurrence.

Coding Scenario
A 16-year-old female injured her right ankle playing soccer for the school team. Another girl stepped on her and her right ankle twisted. She felt pain immediately. The diagnosis is a sprained deltoid ligament of the right ankle.

> Code assignment: 845.01 *Sprain or strain of the deltoid ligament ankle,* E917.0 *Striking against or struck accidentally by objects or person in sports, without subsequent fall,* and E849.4 *Place of occurrence, place for recreation and sport*

E918 Caught accidentally in or between objects [OK]

Code E918 is used to report a mishap caused by a person accidentally caught in an object or between objects, which includes moving objects such as an escalator, folding doors, and sliding doors. Pinching injuries often happen to the hands and fingers but can occur anywhere on the body.

Coding Clarification
Code E918 codes may only be reported as a secondary diagnosis.

Use a secondary E code from category E849 to identify the place of occurrence.

E919 Accident caused by machinery

Category E919 codes are used to report accidents caused by machinery. Accidents caused by machinery under their own power on a highway are classified as transport accidents. Transport accidents are those involving a vehicle being used primarily for transporting people or goods from one place to another.

Pinching injuries are when body parts or clothing are caught between two pieces of machinery, at least one of them moving. Wrapping injuries are caused by machinery parts that are rotating. Body parts or clothing can be caught and wrapped around the rotating part. Cutting injuries are caused by sharp parts of machinery, such as blades. These pieces can cut or even sever limbs. Crushing injuries are caused by machinery rolling or falling on a person or body part. Also included in this category are injuries by an object being thrown from machinery, such as a rock.

Supplementary Classification of External Causes

E919.0	Accident caused by agricultural machines
E919.1	Accident caused by mining and earth-drilling machinery
E919.2	Accident caused by lifting machines and appliances
E919.3	Accident caused by metalworking machines
E919.4	Accident caused by woodworking and forming machines
E919.5	Accident caused by prime movers, except electrical motors
E919.6	Accident caused by transmission machinery
E919.7	Accident caused by earth moving, scraping, and other excavating machines
E919.8	Accident caused by other specified machinery
E919.9	Accident caused by unspecified machinery

Coding Clarification
Category E919 codes may only be reported as a secondary diagnosis.

Use a secondary E code from category E849 to identify the place of occurrence.

E920 Accident caused by cutting and piercing instruments or objects

Lawn mowers are considered one of the most dangerous pieces of equipment around the home. They can cause minor cuts, broken bones, and severed fingers and toes. Many of these injuries can be prevented by simple precautions: wear heavy duty shoes when mowing and make sure the engine is off, the spark plug is removed, and the blades have stopped completely before removing debris.

Needle stick injuries are one of the most common injuries in the health care field. Injuries by hypodermic needle punctures can increase the risk of disease as well as HIV. In 1991, OSHA issued standards regulating the exposure to blood-borne pathogens, which has greatly reduced the risk of workers contracting a blood-borne disease while working.

E920.0	Accident caused by powered lawn mower
E920.1	Accident caused by other powered hand tools
E920.2	Accident caused by powered household appliances and implements
E920.3	Accident caused by knives, swords, and daggers
E920.4	Accident caused by other hand tools and implements
E920.5	Accident caused by hypodermic needle
E920.8	Accident caused by other specified cutting and piercing instruments or objects
E920.9	Accident caused by unspecified cutting and piercing instrument or object

Coding Clarification
Category E920 codes may only be reported as a secondary diagnosis.

Use a secondary E code from category E849 to identify the place of occurrence.

E921 Accident caused by explosion of pressure vessel

Category E921 codes are used to report injuries as a result of accidents caused by the explosion of a pressure vessel, which includes boilers and gas cylinders, such as air tanks, aerosol cans, and pressure cookers.

E921.0	Accident caused by explosion of boilers
E921.1	Accident caused by explosion of gas cylinders
E921.8	Accident caused by explosion of other specified pressure vessels
E921.9	Accident caused by explosion of unspecified pressure vessel

Coding Clarification
Category E921 codes may only be reported as a secondary diagnosis.

Use a secondary E code from category E849 to identify the place of occurrence.

E922 Accident caused by firearm, and air gun missiles

Paintball gun injuries have increased over the past several years. Paintballs can travel up to 300 feet per second. Eye injuries are the most serious cause of injury from a paintball and can cause permanent damage. These most often occur when people do not wear protective eye gear when using the paintball guns.

Although most injuries are unintentional, as many as 30,00 people are injured each year by BB guns and pellet guns.

E922.0	Accident caused by handgun
E922.1	Accident caused by shotgun (automatic)
E922.2	Accident caused by hunting rifle
E922.3	Accident caused by military firearms
E922.4	Accident caused by air gun
E922.5	Accident caused by paintball gun
E922.8	Accident caused by other specified firearm missile
E922.9	Accident caused by unspecified firearm missile

Coding Clarification
Category E922 codes may only be reported as a secondary diagnosis.

Use a secondary E code from category E849 to identify the place of occurrence.

E923 Accident caused by explosive material

Many fireworks can be used with relative safety. However, all fireworks are potentially hazardous and can cause injury. Some states allow all types of fireworks, some limit fireworks, and some do not allow any type of consumer fireworks. The following safety precautions should be observed when lighting any kind of fireworks: have a bucket of water handy; all children should be supervised by an adult; make sure the area is free from debris, such as dry leaves or grass; if a firework does not light, do not try to relight it; and make sure everyone is clear before lighting.

E923.0	Accident caused by fireworks
E923.1	Accident caused by blasting materials
E923.2	Accident caused by explosive gases
E923.8	Accident caused by other explosive materials
E923.9	Accident caused by unspecified explosive material

Coding Clarification
Category E923 codes may only be reported as a secondary diagnosis.

Use a secondary E code from category E849 to identify the place of occurrence.

E924 Accident caused by hot substance or object, caustic or corrosive material, and steam

Skin exposed to 140-degree water for three seconds or less may be seriously burned. Children and the elderly have skin that is more sensitive to burns. Steps can be taken to reduce the risk of scalding burns. Turn the temperature down on the water heater, install faucets with scald prevention technology, always check the water temperature before entering the bath or shower or putting a child in the tub, keep hot liquids away from a counter edge and table, keep pan handles out of a child's reach, and remove lids from hot foods carefully to avoid steam burns.

E924.0	Accident caused by hot liquids and vapors, including steam
E924.1	Accident caused by caustic and corrosive substances
E924.2	Accident caused by hot (boiling) tap water
E924.8	Accident caused by other hot substance or object
E924.9	Accident caused by unspecified hot substance or object

Coding Clarification
Category E924 codes may only be reported as a secondary diagnosis.

Use a secondary E code from category E849 to identify the place of occurrence.

Coding Scenario
An 11-year-old female is admitted to the emergency department with third-degree burns on her left knee. The young girl was home carrying a pan of bacon from the stove to the table and the pan slipped spilling hot grease onto her leg. The diagnosis is a third-degree burn to the left knee.

Code assignment: 945.35 *Third degree burn, left knee*, E924.0 *Accident caused by liquids and vapors, including steam*, and E849.0 *Place of occurrence, home*

E925 Accident caused by electric current

Faulty wiring, malfunctioning appliances, or loose connectors can cause electric injuries. Approximately one person a day dies from electrocution at work. This is the fourth leading cause of death from work accidents. Because the body is made mostly of water, it is susceptible to injuries from electrical currents. Electrical injuries may result in burns and respiratory or heart failure.

E925.0	Electrical accident caused by domestic wiring and appliances
E925.1	Electrical accident caused by electric current in electric power generating plants, distribution stations, transmission lines
E925.2	Electrical accident caused by industrial wiring, appliances, and electrical machinery
E925.8	Accident caused by other electric current
E925.9	Accident caused by unspecified electric current

Coding Clarification
Category E925 codes may only be reported as a secondary diagnosis.

Use a secondary E code from category E849 to identify the place of occurrence.

E926 Exposure to radiation

The sun is the primary source of ultra violet radiation. About 10 percent of ultra violet radiation from the sun reaches the earth. However, artificial sources such as tanning beds, sun lamps, welders, and lasers also produce ultra violet radiation. A sunburn is a reaction to overexposure of this radiation. The effects of a sunburn may not be felt until eight to 10 hours after exposure. The intensity of ultra violet radiation from the sun can vary based on time of day, time of year, cloud cover, and proximity to the equator. Symptoms of sunburn are redness, blisters, swelling, pain, fever, chills, and weakness. Sunburned skin may peel several days after the burn.

E926.0	Exposure to radiofrequency radiation
E926.1	Exposure to infrared radiation from heaters and lamps
E926.2	Exposure to visible and ultraviolet light sources
E926.3	Exposure to x-rays and other electromagnetic ionizing radiation
E926.4	Exposure to lasers
E926.5	Exposure to radioactive isotopes

Supplementary Classification of External Causes

E926.8	Exposure to other specified radiation
E926.9	Exposure to unspecified radiation

Coding Clarification
Category E926 codes may only be reported as a secondary diagnosis.

Use a secondary E code from category E849 to identify the place of occurrence.

Assign E926.2 for welder's flash burns.

E927 Overexertion and strenuous movements ✓

Overexertion and strenuous movements may cause small tears in the muscle, which are referred to as muscle strain. This occurs when the muscle is suddenly stretched beyond its limit. Muscle strains are graded according to their severity. Muscle strains can heal rapidly in the cases of mild strain or take months to heal for more severe strains. Standard treatment for muscle strains is rest, ice, compression, and elevation. Properly warming up, using correct body mechanics, strengthening muscles, and regular exercise can prevent muscle strains.

Coding Clarification
Code E927 codes may only be reported as a secondary diagnosis.

Use a secondary E code from category E849 to identify the place of occurrence.

Coding Scenario
A 45-year-old male presents to the emergency department with back pain. The patient was helping his son move over the weekend and slowly developed back pain. The diagnosis is back strain due to heavy lifting.

> Code assignment: 847.9 *Strains and sprains of unspecified part of back*, E927 *Overexertion and strenuous movements*, and E849.0 *Place of occurrence, home*

E928 Other and unspecified environmental and accidental causes

Loss of hearing due to noise can be the result of one loud exposure. However, the most common cause is an accumulation of noise over a period of time. Loss of hearing is caused by damage to the nerve cells in the ear and progresses with exposure. Hearing loss onset is often subtle. It is recommended that workers exposed to noise levels higher than 85 decibels wear ear protection.

E928.0	Prolonged stay in weightless environment
E928.1	Exposure to noise
E928.2	Accident caused by vibration
E928.3	Accidental human bite
E928.4	External constriction caused by hair
E928.5	External constriction caused by other object
E928.8	Other accident
E928.9	Unspecified accident

Coding Clarification
Category E928 codes may only be reported as a secondary diagnosis.

Use a secondary E code from category E849 to identify the place of occurrence.

E929 Late Effects of Accidental Injury

A late effect is the residual effect that remains after the acute phase of an illness or injury has terminated. Terminology that may be found in diagnostic statements that indicate a late effect include residuals of, old, sequela of, late, and due to or following previous illness or injury. There are late-effect E codes for injuries and poisonings. There are no late-effect E codes for the adverse effects of drugs, misadventures, and surgical complications.

Late effects of accidents are used for the presence of a residual condition caused by the accident. Examples of this category are scars, nonunion of fractures, functional and cognitive deficits, behavioral disorders, bursitis, traumatic arthritis, joint instability, paralysis, muscular atrophy, contracture, nerve damage, and psychological damage. Category E929 codes should be used to report the cause of the accident that resulted in late effects.

E929.0	Late effects of motor vehicle accident
E929.1	Late effects of other transport accident
E929.2	Late effects of accidental poisoning
E929.3	Late effects of accidental fall
E929.4	Late effects of accident caused by fire
E929.5	Late effects of accident due to natural and environmental factors
E929.8	Late effects of other accidents
E929.9	Late effects of unspecified accident

Coding Clarification
Do not use a late effect E code with a related current injury code.

Coding Scenario
A patient has a scar on the hand secondary to a laceration sustained in an automobile accident.

> Code assignment: 709.2 *Scar conditions and fibrosis of skin*, 906.1 *Late effect of open wound of extremities, without mention of tendon injuries*, E929.0 *Late effects of motor vehicle accident*, and E849.5 *Place of occurrence, street and highway*

E930–E949 Drugs, Medicinal and Biological Substances Causing Adverse Effects in Therapeutic Use

Rubric E930-E949 is used to report adverse reactions causing adverse reaction in therapeutic dose. This category is not used to report overdoses but rather allergic reaction or hypersensitivity. Symptoms can range from hives or skin rash to anaphylactic shock. Anaphylaxis is a severe allergic reaction and, in some cases, can produce bronchospasm and laryngeal edema, which can be deadly.

E930 Antibiotics causing adverse effects in therapeutic use

An adverse effect in antibiotics is any unintentional, unwanted reaction that is caused when the drug is taken at the appropriate dose. Because antibiotic allergic reactions can be the same as those of the disease being treated, such as rash, some patients may be labeled as having an allergic reaction where none exists.

Code	Description
E930.0	Penicillins causing adverse effect in therapeutic use
E930.1	Antifungal antibiotics causing adverse effect in therapeutic use
E930.2	Chloramphenicol group causing adverse effect in therapeutic use
E930.3	Erythromycin and other macrolides causing adverse effect in therapeutic use
E930.4	Tetracycline group causing adverse effect in therapeutic use
E930.5	Cephalosporin group causing adverse effect in therapeutic use
E930.6	Antimycobacterial antibiotics causing adverse effect in therapeutic use
E930.7	Antineoplastic antibiotics causing adverse effect in therapeutic use
E930.8	Other specified antibiotics causing adverse effect in therapeutic use
E930.9	Unspecified antibiotic causing adverse effect in therapeutic use

Coding Clarification
Category E930 codes may only be reported as a secondary diagnosis.

E931 Other anti-infectives causing adverse effect in therapeutic use

Anti-infectives cover medications such as sulfonamides, arsenical anti-infectives, heavy metal anti-infectives, quinoline and hydroxyquinoline derivatives, antimalarials and drugs acting on other blood forming protozoa, antiprotozoal drugs, anthelmintics, and antiviral drugs. Therapeutic use is taking the drug as prescribed to treat a disease.

Code	Description
E931.0	Sulfonamides causing adverse effect in therapeutic use
E931.1	Arsenical anti-infectives causing adverse effect in therapeutic use
E931.2	Heavy metal anti-infectives causing adverse effect in therapeutic use
E931.3	Quinoline and hydroxyquinoline derivatives causing adverse effect in therapeutic use
E931.4	Antimalarials and drugs acting on other blood protozoa causing adverse effect in therapeutic use
E931.5	Other antiprotozoal drugs causing adverse effect in therapeutic use
E931.6	Anthelmintics causing adverse effect in therapeutic use
E931.7	Antiviral drugs causing adverse effect in therapeutic use
E931.8	Other antimycobacterial drugs causing adverse effect in therapeutic use
E931.9	Other and unspecified anti-infectives causing adverse effect in therapeutic use

Coding Clarification
Category E931 codes may only be reported as a secondary diagnosis.

E932 Hormones and synthetic substitutes causing adverse effect in therapeutic use

A hormone is a substance in a gland or organ that, when released, stimulates a part of the body to decrease or increase function. Examples of this include growth hormones, hormones that stimulate the beginning of puberty, digestive hormones, and pancreatic hormones.

Code	Description
E932.0	Adrenal cortical steroids causing adverse effect in therapeutic use
E932.1	Androgens and anabolic congeners causing adverse effect in therapeutic use
E932.2	Ovarian hormones and synthetic substitutes causing adverse effect in therapeutic use
E932.3	Insulins and antidiabetic agents causing adverse effect in therapeutic use
E932.4	Anterior pituitary hormones causing adverse effect in therapeutic use
E932.5	Posterior pituitary hormones causing adverse effect in therapeutic use
E932.6	Parathyroid and parathyroid derivatives causing adverse effect in therapeutic use
E932.7	Thyroid and thyroid derivatives causing adverse effect in therapeutic use
E932.8	Antithyroid agents causing adverse effect in therapeutic use
E932.9	Other and unspecified hormones and synthetic substitutes causing adverse effect in therapeutic use

Supplementary Classification of External Causes

Coding Clarification
Category E932 codes may only be reported as a secondary diagnosis.

E933 Primarily systemic agents causing adverse effect in therapeutic use

Antineoplastic drugs are those that fight cancer. They can have many side effects such as nausea, vomiting, and hair loss. Antineoplastic drugs can also weaken the immune system as they are destroying the cancer cells. Cancer cells and hair cells are both fast growing. Many antineoplastic drugs attack fast growing cells, which is why many people lose their hair when on chemotherapy. Gastrointestinal (GI) squamous cells and bone marrow cells are also fast growing and may be affected by chemotherapy.

E933.0	Antiallergic and antiemetic drugs causing adverse effect in therapeutic use
E933.1	Antineoplastic and immunosuppressive drugs causing adverse effect in therapeutic use
E933.2	Acidifying agents causing adverse effect in therapeutic use
E933.3	Alkalizing agents causing adverse effect in therapeutic use
E933.4	Enzymes, not elsewhere classified, causing adverse effect in therapeutic use
E933.5	Vitamins, not elsewhere classified, causing adverse effect in therapeutic use
E933.8	Other systemic agents, not elsewhere classified, causing adverse effect in therapeutic use
E933.9	Unspecified systemic agent causing adverse effect in therapeutic use

Coding Clarification
Category E933 codes may only be reported as a secondary diagnosis.

E934 Agents primarily affecting blood constituents causing adverse effect in therapeutic use

Anticoagulants are used to prevent blood clots from forming or reduce blood clots that are already present. One of the biggest problems with anticoagulants is regulating the dosages. Patients have to be monitored regularly to ensure that the levels are high enough to be effective but not high enough to cause bleeding.

E934.0	Iron and its compounds causing adverse effect in therapeutic use
E934.1	Liver preparations and other antianemic agents causing adverse effect in therapeutic use
E934.2	Anticoagulants causing adverse effect in therapeutic use
E934.3	Vitamin K (phytonadione) causing adverse effect in therapeutic use
E934.4	Fibrinolysis-affecting drugs causing adverse effect in therapeutic use
E934.5	Anticoagulant antagonists and other coagulants causing adverse effect in therapeutic use
E934.6	Gamma globulin causing adverse effect in therapeutic use
E934.7	Natural blood and blood products causing adverse effect in therapeutic use
E934.8	Other agents affecting blood constituents causing adverse effect in therapeutic use
E934.9	Unspecified agent affecting blood constituents causing adverse effect in therapeutic use

Coding Clarification
Category E934 codes may only be reported as a secondary diagnosis.

E935 Analgesics, antipyretics, and antirheumatics causing adverse effect in therapeutic use

An analgesic medication is one that provides pain relief or reduces pain. An antipyretic is a medication that is used to eliminate or reduce a fever. An antirheumatic is an anti-inflammatory medication.

Methadone is a synthetic form of heroin. It blocks the effects of heroin, which results in a reduced craving.

Opiates are drugs derived from a Papaver somniferum plant. Common names are opium, codeine, morphine, Dilaudid, Percodan, Vicodin, Demerol, and fentanyl.

Salicylates are found in many commonly used drugs. Aspirin is the most common salicylate.

Aromatic analgesics include acetaminophen, acetanilid, and acetophenetidin. Tylenol is a common form of aromatic analgesic.

Pyrazole is a non-narcotic pain reliever and fever reducer, which includes aminophenazone and phenylbutazone.

E935.0	Heroin causing adverse effect in therapeutic use
E935.1	Methadone causing adverse effect in therapeutic use
E935.2	Other opiates and related narcotics causing adverse effect in therapeutic use
E935.3	Salicylates causing adverse effect in therapeutic use
E935.4	Aromatic analgesics, not elsewhere classified, causing adverse effect in therapeutic use
E935.5	Pyrazole derivatives causing adverse effect in therapeutic use
E935.6	Antirheumatics (antiphlogistics) causing adverse effect in therapeutic use
E935.7	Other non-narcotic analgesics causing adverse effect in therapeutic use
E935.8	Other specified analgesics and antipyretics causing adverse effect in therapeutic use
E935.9	Unspecified analgesic and antipyretic causing adverse effect in therapeutic use

Coding Clarification
Category E935 codes may only be reported as a secondary diagnosis.

E936 Anticonvulsants and anti-Parkinsonism drugs causing adverse effect in therapeutic use
Parkinson's disease is a progressive neurologic disease that affects walking, talking, and moving. Symptoms of the disease include tremors, stiffness, and slow movement. The cause of Parkinson's disease is not known. The disease causes a degeneration of nerves in the brain that produces a chemical called dopamine. There is no treatment for the disease; however, medications are used to decrease the symptoms.

E936.0	Oxazolidine derivatives causing adverse effect in therapeutic use
E936.1	Hydantoin derivatives causing adverse effect in therapeutic use
E936.2	Succinimides causing adverse effect in therapeutic use
E936.3	Other and unspecified anticonvulsants causing adverse effect in therapeutic use
E936.4	Anti-Parkinsonism drugs causing adverse effect in therapeutic use

Coding Clarification
Category E936 codes may only be reported as a secondary diagnosis.

E937 Sedatives and hypnotics causing adverse effect in therapeutic use
Sedatives are agents used to calm and quiet the body. Several types and compounds of sedatives are available for use today.

Chloral hydrate is the oldest sleep medication. It may still be used for children prior to dental or medical procedures. Mixed with alcohol, it produces the infamous knockout drops, also called a Mickey.

Paraldehyde is used to treat certain convulsive disorders. It may also be used in the treatment of alcoholism and used to calm or relax patients. The medication should be taken with a metal spoon because paraldehyde tends to react with the plastic. The medication will cause the patient to have bad breath.

Bromine compounds are central nervous center depressants and are mixed with other drugs to form compound drugs. They have a tranquilizing effect on the body.

E937.0	Barbiturates causing adverse effect in therapeutic use
E937.1	Chloral hydrate group causing adverse effect in therapeutic use
E937.2	Paraldehyde causing adverse effect in therapeutic use
E937.3	Bromine compounds causing adverse effect in therapeutic use
E937.4	Methaqualone compounds causing adverse effect in therapeutic use
E937.5	Glutethimide group causing adverse effect in therapeutic use
E937.6	Mixed sedatives, not elsewhere classified, causing adverse effect in therapeutic use
E937.8	Other sedatives and hypnotics causing adverse effect in therapeutic use
E937.9	Unspecified sedatives and hypnotics causing adverse effect in therapeutic use

Coding Clarification
Category E937 codes may only be reported as a secondary diagnosis.

E938 Other central nervous system depressants and anesthetics causing adverse effect in therapeutic use
Anesthetics can be used to produce a loss of consciousness or a local pain blocking effect. Side effects of anesthesia drugs include nausea, vomiting, urinary retention, myalgia, pruritus, alteration of mental status, and vasodilation. Vasodilatation can lead to hypovolemic shock and vascular collapse. Patients are carefully monitored during anesthesia for any signs of inappropriate vasodilation.

E938.0	Central nervous system muscle-tone depressants causing adverse effect in therapeutic use
E938.1	Halothane causing adverse effect in therapeutic use
E938.2	Other gaseous anesthetics causing adverse effect in therapeutic use
E938.3	Intravenous anesthetics causing adverse effect in therapeutic use
E938.4	Other and unspecified general anesthetics causing adverse effect in therapeutic use
E938.5	Surface and infiltration anesthetics causing adverse effect in therapeutic use
E938.6	Peripheral nerve- and plexus-blocking anesthetics causing adverse effect in therapeutic use
E938.7	Spinal anesthetics causing adverse effect in therapeutic use
E938.9	Other and unspecified local anesthetics causing adverse effect in therapeutic use

Coding Clarification
Category E938 codes may only be reported as a secondary diagnosis.

E939 Psychotropic agents causing adverse effect in therapeutic use
Tranquilizers are antianxiety medications used to calm a patient. Phenothiazine-based tranquilizers include chlorpromazine, fluphenazine, prochlorperazine, and promazine. Butyrophenone-

based tranquilizers include haloperidol, spiperone, and trifluperidol. Benzodiazepine-based tranquilizers include haloperidol, spiperone, and trifluperidol. Other specified tranquilizers include hydroxyzine and meprobamate.

E939.0	Antidepressants causing adverse effect in therapeutic use
E939.1	Phenothiazine-based tranquilizers causing adverse effect in therapeutic use
E939.2	Butyrophenone-based tranquilizers causing adverse effect in therapeutic use
E939.3	Other antipsychotics, neuroleptics, and major tranquilizers causing adverse effect in therapeutic use
E939.4	Benzodiazepine-based tranquilizers causing adverse effect in therapeutic use
E939.5	Other tranquilizers causing adverse effect in therapeutic use
E939.6	Psychodysleptics (hallucinogens) causing adverse effect in therapeutic use
E939.7	Psychostimulants causing adverse effect in therapeutic use
E939.8	Other psychotropic agents causing adverse effect in therapeutic use
E939.9	Unspecified psychotropic agent causing adverse effect in therapeutic use

Coding Clarification
Category E939 codes may only be reported as a secondary diagnosis.

E940 Central nervous system stimulants causing adverse effect in therapeutic use

An analeptic is a drug that stimulates the central nervous system. One of the uses is for ventilatory failure in patients who have chronic obstructive airway disease. Some side effects may include epilepsy and liver impairment. This type of drug is given only with strict supervision.

E940.0	Analeptics causing adverse effect in therapeutic use
E940.1	Opiate antagonists causing adverse effect in therapeutic use
E940.8	Other specified central nervous system stimulants causing adverse effect in therapeutic use
E940.9	Unspecified central nervous system stimulant causing adverse effect in therapeutic use

Coding Clarification
Category E940 codes may only be reported as a secondary diagnosis.

E941 Drugs primarily affecting the autonomic nervous system causing adverse effect in therapeutic use

Parasympathomimetics are drugs that produce the affects of parasympathetic nerve stimulation. Therapeutic use of the drugs includes stimulation and motility of the GI tract and bladder following surgery, glaucoma, diagnosis of myasthenia gravis, and treatment of delayed gastric emptying syndrome.

Parasympatholytics relax smooth muscles. Drugs in this category include atropine, homatropine, hyoscine, and quaternary ammonium derivatives.

Sympathomimetic agents are used to increase myocardial contractility, increase blood pressure, maintain blood pressure, treat bronchospasm, reduce systemic local anesthetic absorption, and manage severe allergic reactions. Drugs in this category include epinephrine and levarterenol.

Sympatholytics stimulate smooth muscles. This category of drugs is used to treat hypertension, angina, glaucoma, and to prevent migraines. Medications include phenoxybenzamine, and tolazoline hydrochloride.

E941.0	Parasympathomimetics (cholinergics) causing adverse effect in therapeutic use
E941.1	Parasympatholytics (anticholinergics and antimuscarinics) and spasmolytics causing adverse effect in therapeutic use
E941.2	Sympathomimetics (adrenergics) causing adverse effect in therapeutic use
E941.3	Sympatholytics (antiadrenergics) causing adverse effect in therapeutic use
E941.9	Unspecified drug primarily affecting the autonomic nervous system causing adverse effect in therapeutic use

Coding Clarification
Category E941 codes may only be reported as a secondary diagnosis.

E942 Agents primarily affecting the cardiovascular system causing adverse effect in therapeutic use

Vasodilators are medications that widen the blood vessels. They allow blood to flow through the blood vessels more easily and are used to treat high blood pressure. Untreated blood pressure increases the risk of heart disease, stroke, and heart failure. Side effects of these medications include headaches and dizziness.

E942.0	Cardiac rhythm regulators causing adverse effect in therapeutic use
E942.1	Cardiotonic glycosides and drugs of similar action causing adverse effect in therapeutic use
E942.2	Antilipemic and antiarteriosclerotic drugs causing adverse effect in therapeutic use
E942.3	Ganglion-blocking agents causing adverse effect in therapeutic use
E942.4	Coronary vasodilators causing adverse effect in therapeutic use

Coders' Desk Reference for Diagnoses

E942.5	Other vasodilators causing adverse effect in therapeutic use
E942.6	Other antihypertensive agents causing adverse effect in therapeutic use
E942.7	Antivaricose drugs, including sclerosing agents, causing adverse effect in therapeutic use
E942.8	Capillary-active drugs causing adverse effect in therapeutic use
E942.9	Other and unspecified agents primarily affecting the cardiovascular system causing adverse effect in therapeutic use

Coding Clarification
Category E942 codes may only be reported as a secondary diagnosis.

E943 Agents primarily affecting gastrointestinal system causing adverse effect in therapeutic use

An ulcer is a sore in the lining of the stomach that is usually caused by the bacteria *Helicobacter pylori* and can be treated in a couple of weeks with antibiotics. Some ulcers can be due to the use of anti-inflammatory medications. In all of these cases, bacteria, medication, or cancer weaken the mucous lining of the stomach and the stomach acid irritates the lining and causes an ulcer. One symptom of an ulcer is dull, gnawing ache. It may come and go for several weeks. It usually occurs a couple of hours after a meal and it is worse at night or when the stomach is empty. Other symptoms may include weight loss, poor appetite, bloating, burping, nausea, and vomiting.

E943.0	Antacids and antigastric secretion drugs causing adverse effect in therapeutic use
E943.1	Irritant cathartics causing adverse effect in therapeutic use
E943.2	Emollient cathartics causing adverse effect in therapeutic use
E943.3	Other cathartics, including intestinal atonia drugs, causing adverse effect in therapeutic use
E943.4	Digestants causing adverse effect in therapeutic use
E943.5	Antidiarrheal drugs causing adverse effect in therapeutic use
E943.6	Emetics causing adverse effect in therapeutic use
E943.8	Other specified agents primarily affecting the gastrointestinal system causing adverse effect in therapeutic use
E943.9	Unspecified agent primarily affecting the gastrointestinal system causing adverse effect in therapeutic use

Coding Clarification
Category E943 codes may only be reported as a secondary diagnosis.

E944 Water, mineral, and uric acid metabolism drugs causing adverse effect in therapeutic use

Diuretics stimulate the kidney to produce more urine. Diuretics also reduce the amount of minerals, such as sodium, in the body. Diuretics are used to treat high blood pressure, congestive heart failure, and edema. Side effects of the drug may include numbness, tingling, or burning in the hands, feet, fingers, and toes, potassium deficiency, and increased blood sugar in diabetics.

E944.0	Mercurial diuretics causing adverse effect in therapeutic use
E944.1	Purine derivative diuretics causing adverse effect in therapeutic use
E944.2	Carbonic acid anhydrase inhibitors causing adverse effect in therapeutic use
E944.3	Saluretics causing adverse effect in therapeutic use
E944.4	Other diuretics causing adverse effect in therapeutic use
E944.5	Electrolytic, caloric, and water-balance agents causing adverse effect in therapeutic use
E944.6	Other mineral salts, not elsewhere classified, causing adverse effect in therapeutic use
E944.7	Uric acid metabolism drugs causing adverse effect in therapeutic use

Coding Clarification
Category E944 codes may only be reported as a secondary diagnosis.

E945 Agents primarily acting on the smooth and skeletal muscles and respiratory system causing adverse effect in therapeutic use

Muscle relaxants are medications that relax certain muscles in the body. They are used to treat muscle strain and muscle spasms. They do not cure the muscle injury but help reduce the pain by reducing the muscle spasms. Side effects may include drowsiness, confusion, and light-headedness.

E945.0	Oxytocic agents causing adverse effect in therapeutic use
E945.1	Smooth muscle relaxants causing adverse effect in therapeutic use
E945.2	Skeletal muscle relaxants causing adverse effect in therapeutic use
E945.3	Other and unspecified drugs acting on muscles causing adverse effect in therapeutic use
E945.4	Antitussives causing adverse effect in therapeutic use
E945.5	Expectorants causing adverse effect in therapeutic use
E945.6	Anti-common cold drugs causing adverse effect in therapeutic use
E945.7	Antiasthmatics causing adverse effect in therapeutic use

Supplementary Classification of External Causes

E945.8 Other and unspecified respiratory drugs causing adverse effect in therapeutic use

Coding Clarification
Category E945 codes may only be reported as a secondary diagnosis.

E946 Agents primarily affecting skin and mucous membrane, ophthalmological, otorhinolaryngological, and dental drugs causing adverse effect in therapeutic use

Keratolytics are medications that loosen and soften the tough outer layer of the skin. These are topical solutions applied directly to the skin. They are normally used for about six weeks. Adverse reactions may include discoloration of the treated area, peeling, blistering, swelling, and skin irritation.

E946.0 Local anti-infectives and anti-inflammatory drugs causing adverse effect in therapeutic use
E946.1 Antipruritics causing adverse effect in therapeutic use
E946.2 Local astringents and local detergents causing adverse effect in therapeutic use
E946.3 Emollients, demulcents, and protectants causing adverse effect in therapeutic use
E946.4 Keratolytics, keratoplastics, other hair treatment drugs and preparations causing adverse effect in therapeutic use
E946.5 Eye anti-infectives and other eye drugs causing adverse effect in therapeutic use
E946.6 Anti-infectives and other drugs and preparations for ear, nose, and throat causing adverse effect in therapeutic use
E946.7 Dental drugs topically applied causing adverse effect in therapeutic use
E946.8 Other agents primarily affecting skin and mucous membrane causing adverse effect in therapeutic use
E946.9 Unspecified agent primarily affecting skin and mucous membrane causing adverse effect in therapeutic use

Coding Clarification
Category E946 codes may only be reported as a secondary diagnosis.

E947 Other and unspecified drugs and medicinal substances causing adverse effect in therapeutic use

Lipotropics prevent abnormal accumulation of fat in the liver. They help keep cholesterol more soluble and reduce the build up in the blood stream.

E947.0 Dietetics causing adverse effect in therapeutic use
E947.1 Lipotropic drugs causing adverse effect in therapeutic use
E947.2 Antidotes and chelating agents, not elsewhere classified, causing adverse effect in therapeutic use
E947.3 Alcohol deterrents causing adverse effect in therapeutic use
E947.4 Pharmaceutical excipients causing adverse effect in therapeutic use
E947.8 Other drugs and medicinal substances causing adverse effect in therapeutic use
E947.9 Unspecified drug or medicinal substance causing adverse effect in therapeutic use

Coding Clarification
Category E947 codes may only be reported as a secondary diagnosis.

E948 Bacterial vaccines causing adverse effect in therapeutic use

Tuberculosis (TB) is a bacterial infection that usually attacks the lungs, but which may also affect other organs. The disease is caused by *Mycobacterium tuberculosis*. TB is transmitted by inhaling air droplets exhaled by an infected person or, sometimes, the infection is absorbed through the skin.

Vaccinations prevent a patient from getting a disease. Although there are small risks with every vaccine, the benefits far outweigh the risks.

E948.0 BCG vaccine causing adverse effect in therapeutic use
E948.1 Typhoid and paratyphoid vaccines causing adverse effect in therapeutic use
E948.2 Cholera vaccine causing adverse effect in therapeutic use
E948.3 Plague vaccine causing adverse effect in therapeutic use
E948.4 Tetanus vaccine causing adverse effect in therapeutic use
E948.5 Diphtheria vaccine causing adverse effect in therapeutic use
E948.6 Pertussis vaccine, including combinations with pertussis component, causing adverse effect in therapeutic use
E948.8 Other and unspecified bacterial vaccines causing adverse effect in therapeutic use
E948.9 Mixed bacterial vaccines, except combinations with pertussis component, causing adverse effect in therapeutic use

Coding Clarification
Category E948 codes may only be reported as a secondary diagnosis.

E949 Other vaccines and biological substances causing adverse effect in therapeutic use

Measles is an acute infection caused by paramyxovirus and presents with a hacking cough, rash, and fevers. Measles are usually transmitted from person to person via airborne respiratory droplets. Pharyngitis is common. Koplik's spots are white, grainy spots that can occur in the buccal mucosa and are an early symptom of measles. In the United States, measles outbreaks have been greatly reduced by government immunization programs. Measles has a low mortality rate in healthy individuals.

Vaccinations prevent a patient from getting a disease. Although there are small risks with every vaccine, the benefits far outweigh the risks.

E949.0	Smallpox vaccine causing adverse effect in therapeutic use
E949.1	Rabies vaccine causing adverse effect in therapeutic use
E949.2	Typhus vaccine causing adverse effect in therapeutic use
E949.3	Yellow fever vaccine causing adverse effect in therapeutic use
E949.4	Measles vaccine causing adverse effect in therapeutic use
E949.5	Poliomyelitis vaccine causing adverse effect in therapeutic use
E949.6	Other and unspecified viral and rickettsial vaccines causing adverse effect in therapeutic use
E949.7	Mixed viral-rickettsial and bacterial vaccines, except combinations with pertussis component, causing adverse effect in therapeutic use
E949.9	Other and unspecified vaccines and biological substances causing adverse effect in therapeutic use

Coding Clarification
Category E949 codes may only be reported as a secondary diagnosis.

E950–E959 Suicide and Self–Inflicted Injury

Rubric E950-E959 is used to report suicide and self-inflicted injury, which includes injury and suicide by self-inflicted poisoning, hanging, strangulating, suffocating, shooting, submerging and drowning, and cutting or piercing. Near drowning is now more commonly referred to as a submersion accident.

If the intent is not specified, is unknown, or documented as questionable, probable, or suspected, assign the E code for cause undetermined.

Suicide is the third leading cause of death among people ages 15 to 24 and is the 11th leading cause of death for all Americans.

The following signs may be observed in a person thinking about suicide:

- Talks about or has tried suicide before
- Experiences disturbances in sleeping and eating
- Exhibits a drastic behavior change
- Withdraws from life
- Loses interest in hobbies, work, school
- Writes a will or makes final arrangements
- Seems preoccupied with death and dying
- Increases use of alcohol and drugs
- Loses interest in personal appearance

E950 Suicide and self-inflicted poisoning by solid or liquid substances

Attempted suicides are classified as one third of all drug abuse incidences. Females are more likely to attempt suicide by overdose than males. Alcohol consumption is commonly used in suicides and suicide attempts.

E950.0	Suicide and self-inflicted poisoning by analgesics, antipyretics, and antirheumatics
E950.1	Suicide and self-inflicted poisoning by barbiturates
E950.2	Suicide and self-inflicted poisoning by other sedatives and hypnotics
E950.3	Suicide and self-inflicted poisoning by tranquilizers and other psychotropic agents
E950.4	Suicide and self-inflicted poisoning by other specified drugs and medicinal substances
E950.5	Suicide and self-inflicted poisoning by unspecified drug or medicinal substance
E950.6	Suicide and self-inflicted poisoning by agricultural and horticultural chemical and pharmaceutical preparations other than plant foods and fertilizers
E950.7	Suicide and self-inflicted poisoning by corrosive and caustic substances
E950.8	Suicide and self-inflicted poisoning by arsenic and its compounds
E950.9	Suicide and self-inflicted poisoning by other and unspecified solid and liquid substances

Coding Clarification
Category E950 codes may only be reported as a secondary diagnosis.

E951 Suicide and self-inflicted poisoning by gases in domestic use

Symptoms of inhaling natural gas are dizziness and vomiting. Natural gas does have an odor and this type of suicide may be interrupted before it is completed.

E951.0	Suicide and self-inflicted poisoning by gas distributed by pipeline
E951.1	Suicide and self-inflicted poisoning by liquefied petroleum gas distributed in mobile containers
E951.8	Suicide and self-inflicted poisoning by other utility gas

Coding Clarification
Category E951 codes may only be reported as a secondary diagnosis.

Supplementary Classification of External Causes

E952 Suicide and self-inflicted poisoning by other gases and vapors

Carbon monoxide poisoning can be deadly. There is no smell and it cannot be seen but it can kill in just a matter of minutes. Symptoms of carbon monoxide poisoning include severe headache, dizziness, mental confusion, nausea, and fainting. Since the symptoms are similar to many other causes, carbon monoxide poisoning has been hard to diagnose.

E952.0	Suicide and self-inflicted poisoning by motor vehicle exhaust gas
E952.1	Suicide and self-inflicted poisoning by other carbon monoxide
E952.8	Suicide and self-inflicted poisoning by other specified gases and vapors
E952.9	Suicide and self-inflicted poisoning by unspecified gases and vapors

Coding Clarification
Category E952 codes may only be reported as a secondary diagnosis.

E953 Suicide and self-inflicted injury by hanging, strangulation, and suffocation

Suicide by hanging is on the increase. Men are more likely than women to commit suicide by hanging. Hangings can be categorized as complete where the body is totally suspended and does not touch the floor, or incomplete where some part of the body is touching the floor. The human neck is susceptible to injury due to the location of the spinal cord, airway, and major blood vessels.

Suffocation deprives the body of oxygen and can quickly cause death. Symptoms include venous obstruction, arterial and airway obstruction, low cerebral blood flow, and collapse.

E953.0	Suicide and self-inflicted injury by hanging
E953.1	Suicide and self-inflicted injury by suffocation by plastic bag
E953.8	Suicide and self-inflicted injury by other specified means
E953.9	Suicide and self-inflicted injury by unspecified means

Coding Clarification
Category E953 codes may only be reported as a secondary diagnosis.

E954 Suicide and self-inflicted injury by submersion (drowning)

Drowning is death from suffocation after submersion that occurs within 24 hours of injury. At first the person holds his or her breath and carbon dioxide levels increase and hypoxia progresses. There are then two types of drowning: wet drowning when water is taken into the lungs and dry drowning when the patient experiences a laryngospasm. Near drowning is now more commonly referred to as a submersion accident.

Coding Clarification
Code E954 codes may only be reported as a secondary diagnosis.

E955 Suicide and self-inflicted injury by firearms, air guns and explosives

It is estimated that in 2001, 55 percent of all suicides were committed with guns. Suicide is the leading cause of death from firearms. Unlike other forms of suicide, most suicide attempts with guns are successful. Suicide from handguns is usually to the head. Suicides by more than one shot are uncommon. However, the victim may test fire the gun before the suicide.

E955.0	Suicide and self-inflicted injury by handgun
E955.1	Suicide and self-inflicted injury by shotgun
E955.2	Suicide and self-inflicted injury by hunting rifle
E955.3	Suicide and self-inflicted injury by military firearms
E955.4	Suicide and self-inflicted injury by other and unspecified firearm
E955.5	Suicide and self-inflicted injury by explosives
E955.6	Suicide and self-inflicted injury by air gun
E955.7	Suicide and self-inflicted injury by paintball gun
E955.9	Suicide and self-inflicted injury by firearms and explosives, unspecified

Coding Clarification
Category E955 codes may only be reported as a secondary diagnosis.

E956 Suicide and self-inflicted injury by cutting and piercing instrument

This category includes suicide and self-inflicted injury by cutting and piercing with sharp instruments. This includes self-mutilation. Self-mutilation is cutting the skin enough to damage the tissue, which is done in an attempt to change the mood or state. It is not considered self-harming if it is done to fit in with a crowd, as a part of tattooing or piercing, for sexual gratification, or as a ritual.

Coding Clarification
Code E956 codes may only be reported as a secondary diagnosis.

Coding Scenario
A 17-year-old female is brought to the emergency department for lacerations of the left forearm. The patient has a history of depression and gets a sense of relief from cutting herself with a razor blade. The diagnosis is a laceration of the left forearm and depression.

Code assignment: 881 *Laceration of wrist, forearm, elbow without mention of complication,* 311 *Depressive disorder NOS,* and E956 *Suicide and self inflicted injury by cutting and piercing instrument*

E957 Suicide and self-inflicted injuries by jumping from high place

Category E957 codes are used to describe suicide or self-inflicted injuries by jumping from high places. This includes residential premises, other man-made structures such as bridges or commercial buildings, or natural structures.

E957.0	Suicide and self-inflicted injuries by jumping from residential premises
E957.1	Suicide and self-inflicted injuries by jumping from other man-made structures
E957.2	Suicide and self-inflicted injuries by jumping from natural sites
E957.9	Suicide and self-inflicted injuries by jumping from unspecified site

Coding Clarification
Category E957 codes may only be reported as a secondary diagnosis.

E958 Suicide and self-inflicted injury by other and unspecified means

Category E958 codes describe other suicide and self-inflicted injuries. This includes jumping or lying before a moving object, burning, scalding, freezing, electrocuting, crashing a motor vehicle, crashing an aircraft, or injury caused by caustic substance, except poisoning.

E958.0	Suicide and self-inflicted injury by jumping or lying before moving object
E958.1	Suicide and self-inflicted injury by burns, fire
E958.2	Suicide and self-inflicted injury by scald
E958.3	Suicide and self-inflicted injury by extremes of cold
E958.4	Suicide and self-inflicted injury by electrocution
E958.5	Suicide and self-inflicted injury by crashing of motor vehicle
E958.6	Suicide and self-inflicted injury by crashing of aircraft
E958.7	Suicide and self-inflicted injury by caustic substances, except poisoning
E958.8	Suicide and self-inflicted injury by other specified means
E958.9	Suicide and self-inflicted injury by unspecified means

Coding Clarification
Category E958 codes may only be reported as a secondary diagnosis.

E959 Late effects of self-inflicted injury

Code E959 is used to describe a late effect of a self-inflicted injury. A late effect is the residual effect that remains after the acute phase of an illness or injury has terminated. A residual is the temporary or permanent health care problem that follows the acute phase of an illness or injury. Terminology that may be found in diagnostic statements that indicate a late effect include residuals of, old, sequela of, late, due to, or following previous illness or injury. The late-effect E codes should be used with any report of a late effect. Do not use a late-effect E code with a related current injury code.

Coding Clarification
Code E959 codes may only be reported as a secondary diagnosis.

E960–E969 Homicide and Injury Purposely Inflicted by Other Persons

This section includes fights, rape, assault by corrosive substance, assault by poisoning, and assault by firearm. Also included in this section are codes to describe the perpetrator of child and adult abuse.

E codes for child and adult abuse take priority over all other E codes. An E code for the type of abuse should be listed first, followed by the code for perpetrator. Report an accidental neglect code first if the intent is an accidental abandonment of an adult or a child.

If the intent is not specified, unknown, or documented as questionable, probable, or suspected, assign the E code for cause undetermined.

E960 Fight, brawl, rape

Rape is sexual contact without consent. Rape is usually an act of power and is not related to sexual desire. Many sexual assault victims report that the attack occurred in their own home, home of a friend, or home of a neighbor. Some rapes happen because the victim is under the influence of alcohol or drugs. However, it is still a crime and should be reported as such. A sexual assault should be reported with E968.8.

E960.0	Unarmed fight or brawl
E960.1	Rape

Coding Clarification
Category E960 codes may only be reported as a secondary diagnosis.

E961 Assault by corrosive or caustic substance, except poisoning

Code E961 is used to report assault by corrosive or caustic substances, except poisoning, which includes acid, corrosive substance, and vitriol. Burns from hot liquids and chemical burns from swallowing a corrosive substance are excluded from this code.

Coding Clarification
Code E961 codes may only be reported as a secondary diagnosis.

E962 Assault by poisoning
Poisons are chemicals that cause illness, injury, or death when taken in very small quantities. The legal definition of a poison is a chemical that takes less than 50 mg per kilogram of body weight to kill 50 percent of the victims exposed (e.g., about three-fourths of a teaspoon for the average adult and about one-eighth of a teaspoon for a two-year-old child). Symptoms displayed and the systemic effect differs with the type of poison ingested.

E962.0	Assault by drugs and medicinal substances
E962.1	Assault by other solid and liquid substances
E962.2	Assault by other gases and vapors
E962.9	Assault by unspecified poisoning

Coding Clarification
Category E962 codes may only be reported as a secondary diagnosis.

E963 Assault by hanging and strangulation OK
Hangings can be categorized as complete where the body is totally suspended and does not touch the floor, or incomplete where some part of the body is touching the floor. The human neck is susceptible to injury due to the location of the spinal cord, airway, and major blood vessels.

Coding Clarification
Code E963 codes may only be reported as a secondary diagnosis.

E964 Assault by submersion (drowning) OK
Drowning is death from suffocation after submersion that occurs within 24 hours of injury. At first a person holds his or her breath and carbon dioxide levels increase and hypoxia progresses. There are then two types of drowning: wet drowning when water is taken into the lungs and dry drowning when the patient experiences a laryngospasm. Near drowning is now more commonly referred to as a submersion accident.

Coding Clarification
Code E964 codes may only be reported as a secondary diagnosis.

E965 Assault by firearms and explosives
There are a wide variety of firearms such as, handguns, single shot pistols, Derringers, revolvers, rifles, shotguns, submachine guns, and machine guns. As the primer strikes the primer compound, a fire is ignited, which starts the gunpowder burning, and changes it into a gas. This causes pressure to build up in the cartridge and forces the bullet down the barrel. The bullet explodes out of the gun.

E965.0	Assault by handgun
E965.1	Assault by shotgun
E965.2	Assault by hunting rifle
E965.3	Assault by military firearms
E965.4	Assault by other and unspecified firearm
E965.5	Assault by antipersonnel bomb
E965.6	Assault by gasoline bomb
E965.7	Assault by letter bomb
E965.8	Assault by other specified explosive
E965.9	Assault by unspecified explosive

Coding Clarification
Category E965 codes may only be reported as a secondary diagnosis.

E966 Assault by cutting and piercing instrument OK
The following sharp objects are used as weapons in an assault: glass, sword, razor, switchblade, butterfly knife, automatic knife, kitchen knife, military knife, survival knife, stiletto, tonto knife, and pair of scissors. There are different types of wounds that can be caused by these various devices. An incised wound is a sharp cutting injury, usually made with a knife or broken glass, etc. In a slash wound, the length is greater than the depth. In a stab wound, the depth is greater than the length. The seriousness of the wound can range from a scratch to deep, life threatening wounds.

Coding Clarification
Code E966 codes may only be reported as a secondary diagnosis.

E967 Child and adult battering and other maltreatment
Category E967 codes are used to report the perpetrator of child or adult abuse. This code selection should be based on the relationship of the perpetrator and the victim. If the intent of the assault is not known, code the intent with the undetermined cause E codes. Codes E960-E968 should be the first listed E codes, followed by a code from category E967. Codes for child and adult abuse take priority over all other E codes.

E967.0	Child and adult battering and other maltreatment by father or stepfather

E967.1	Child and adult battering and other maltreatment by other specified person
E967.2	Child and adult battering and other maltreatment by mother or stepmother
E967.3	Child and adult battering and other maltreatment by spouse or partner
E967.4	Child and adult battering and other maltreatment by child
E967.5	Child and adult battering and other maltreatment by sibling
E967.6	Child and adult battering and other maltreatment by grandparent
E967.7	Child and adult battering and other maltreatment by other relative
E967.8	Child and adult battering and other maltreatment by non-related caregiver
E967.9	Child and adult battering and other maltreatment by unspecified person

Coding Clarification
Category E967 codes may only be reported as a secondary diagnosis.

Coding Scenario
A 1-year-old child is brought into the emergency department with burns on both feet. The mother plunged the baby into a hot bath when the baby wouldn't stop crying. The diagnosis is a second-degree burn on both feet caused by child abuse by mother.

Code assignment: 945.22 *Blister with epidermal loss due to burns, feet*, 995.54 *Child maltreatment syndrome, child physical abuse*, E978.3 *Assault by hot liquid*, and E967.2 *Child and adult battering and other maltreatment by mother or stepmother*

E968 Assault by other and unspecified means
Category E968 codes are used to identify assault by other and unspecified means. This category includes injuries sustained from the following malicious acts: being burned by an intentionally set fire or with a hot liquid, being pushed from a high place, and being struck by blunt or thrown object. Also included is criminal neglect, which includes abandonment of child, infant, or other helpless person with intent to injure or kill. Also included in this category is assault by an air gun, a human bite, and a transport vehicle.

E968.0	Assault by fire
E968.1	Assault by pushing from high place
E968.2	Assault by striking by blunt or thrown object
E968.3	Assault by hot liquid
E968.4	Criminal neglect
E968.5	Assault by transport vehicle
E968.6	Assault by air gun
E968.7	Assault by human bite
E968.8	Assault by other specified means
E968.9	Assault by unspecified means

Coding Clarification
Category E968 codes may only be reported as a secondary diagnosis.

E969 Late effects of injury purposely inflicted by other person OK
Code E969 is used to describe a late effect of an injury purposely inflicted by another person. A late effect is the residual effect that remains after the acute phase of an illness or injury has terminated. A residual is the temporary or permanent health care problem that follows the acute phase of an illness or injury. Terminology indicating a late effect that may be found in diagnostic statements includes residuals of, old, sequela of, late, due to, or following previous illness or injury. The late-effect E codes should be used with any report of a late effect. Do not use a late-effect E code with a related current injury code.

Coding Clarification
Code E969 codes may only be reported as a secondary diagnosis.

E970–E978 Legal Intervention
Rubric E970-E978 is used to report legal intervention injuries. These are injuries inflicted by police, law enforcement, or military police officers while arresting criminals or suspected criminals, suppressing disturbances, maintaining order, or during other legal action.

E970 Injury due to legal intervention by firearms OK
There are a wide variety of firearms such as, handguns, Derringers, revolvers, rifles, lever action, bolt action, pump action, auto-loading, shotguns, submachine guns, and machine guns. As the primer strikes the primer compound, a fire is ignited, which starts the gunpowder burning and changes it into a gas. This causes pressure to build up in the cartridge and forces the bullet down the barrel. The bullet explodes out of the gun.

Coding Clarification
Code E970 codes may only be reported as a secondary diagnosis.

E971 Injury due to legal intervention by explosives OK
Code E971 is used to report legal intervention by explosives. This includes injury by dynamite, explosive shell, grenade, and mortar bomb. Injuries sustained by civilians during a war should be reported by E990-E999.

Coding Clarification
Code E971 codes may only be reported as a secondary diagnosis.

E972 Injury due to legal intervention by gas ⦿

When used correctly, there are no lasting effects of tear gas. It is used by legal authorities to control civilian crowds and subdue criminals. The two most widely used forms of tear gas are chlorobenzylidenemalononitrile and chloroacetophenone. Although tear gas causes only temporary disability, injuries from a tear bomb explosion have been reported.

Coding Clarification
Code E972 codes may only be reported as a secondary diagnosis.

E973 Injury due to legal intervention by blunt object ⦿

A nightstick is a short, club like instrument used by police in close combat to subdue a suspect.

Coding Clarification
Code E973 codes may only be reported as a secondary diagnosis.

E974 Injury due to legal intervention by cutting and piercing instrument ⦿

The following sharp objects are used as weapons during a legal intervention: glass, sword, razor, switchblade, butterfly knife, automatic knife, kitchen knife, military knife, survival knife, stiletto, tonto knife, and pair of scissors. There are different types of wounds that can be caused by these various devices. An incised wound is a sharp cutting injury, usually made with a knife or broken glass, etc. In a slash wound, the length is greater than the depth. In a stab wound, the depth is greater than the length. The seriousness of the wound can range from a scratch to deep, life threatening wounds.

Coding Clarification
Code E974 codes may only be reported as a secondary diagnosis.

E975 Injury due to legal intervention by other specified means ⦿

Code E975 is used to report an injury due to legal intervention by other specified means. Use this code if the other legal intervention codes do not apply. This includes injuries by a blow or by manhandling.

Coding Clarification
Code E975 codes may only be reported as a secondary diagnosis.

E976 Injury due to legal intervention by unspecified means ⦿

Use this code as a last resort if the method of injury is not documented or cannot be obtained.

Coding Clarification
Code E976 codes may only be reported as a secondary diagnosis.

E977 Late effects of injuries due to legal intervention ⦿

A late effect is the residual effect that remains after the acute phase of an illness or injury has terminated. A residual is the temporary or permanent health care problem that follows the acute phase of an illness or injury. Terminology that may be found in diagnostic statements that indicate a late effect include residuals of, old, sequela of, late, due to, or following previous illness or injury. The late effect E codes should be used with any report of a late effect. Do not use a late effect E code with a related current injury code. This code should be used to indicate circumstances classifiable to E970-E976.

Coding Clarification
Code E977 codes may only be reported as a secondary diagnosis.

E978 Legal execution ⦿

A legal execution is one that is performed at the direction of the judiciary or ruling authority. Methods can include asphyxiating by gas, decapitating, electrocuting, hanging, shooting, administering lethal injection, or other specified means.

Many states use a three-drug cocktail to perform lethal injections. First a drug that renders the prisoner unconscious is administered, followed by a muscle relaxant that paralyzes the diaphragm and lungs. Finally, a drug is administered that causes cardiac arrest.

Coding Clarification
Code E978 codes may only be reported as a secondary diagnosis.

E979 Terrorism

Due to the events of September 11, 2001, new codes were developed to track injuries as a result of terrorism. The cause of the injury attributed to terrorism must by identified by the FBI as terrorism. Terrorism is defined as injuries resulting from the unlawful use of force or violence against persons or property to intimidate or coerce a government, the civilian population, or any segment, in furtherance of political or social objective.

If terrorism is suspected, category E979 codes should not be used. Assign an E code based on the documentation and the facts that are known. Terrorism codes take priority over all other E codes except child and adult abuse.

E979.0	Terrorism involving explosion of marine weapons
E979.1	Terrorism involving destruction of aircraft
E979.2	Terrorism involving other explosions and fragments
E979.3	Terrorism involving fires, conflagration and hot substances
E979.4	Terrorism involving firearms
E979.5	Terrorism involving nuclear weapons
E979.6	Terrorism involving biological weapons
E979.7	Terrorism involving chemical weapons
E979.8	Terrorism involving other means
E979.9	Terrorism, secondary effects

Coding Clarification
Category E979 codes may only be reported as a secondary diagnosis.

E980–E989 Injury Undetermined Whether Accidentally or Purposely Inflicted

If the intent of an injury, a suicide, or an assault is undetermined or unspecified, use rubric E980-E989.

E980   Poisoning by solid or liquid substances, undetermined whether accidentally or purposely inflicted

An analgesic medication is one that provides pain relief or reduces pain. An antipyretic is a medication that is used to eliminate or reduce a fever. An antirheumatic is an anti-inflammatory medication.

Barbiturates are drugs used to treat convulsions, anxiety, and aid in sleep.

Sedatives are agents used to calm and quiet the body. Several types and compounds of sedatives are available for use today.

A tranquilizer helps reduce tension and anxiety. Tranquilizers may cause dependence or addiction.

A corrosive is a substance that destroys living tissue. The most common types of corrosives are hydrochloric acid, sulfuric acid, nitric acid, acetic acid, phosphoric acid, oxalic acid, chronic acid, formic acid, and boric acid. These corrosives are commonly found in metal cleaners, toilet and drain cleaners, batteries, and antirust compounds.

Symptoms of ingestion include severe burning pain in the mouth, throat, and abdomen; dysphagia; vomiting; diarrhea; and cold, clammy skin. Symptoms will usually begin immediately after swallowing. Symptoms of inhalation include cough, dyspnea, pleuritic chest pain, pulmonary edema, and frothy sputum. These symptoms could be delayed several hours. Eye exposure can cause burning, irritation, and swelling eyes; photophobia; corneal erosion; and perforation of the conjunctiva and cornea.

E980.0	Poisoning by analgesics, antipyretics, and antirheumatics, undetermined whether accidentally or purposely inflicted
E980.1	Poisoning by barbiturates, undetermined whether accidentally or purposely inflicted
E980.2	Poisoning by other sedatives and hypnotics, undetermined whether accidentally or purposely inflicted
E980.3	Poisoning by tranquilizers and other psychotropic agents, undetermined whether accidentally or purposely inflicted
E980.4	Poisoning by other specified drugs and medicinal substances, undetermined whether accidentally or purposely inflicted
E980.5	Poisoning by unspecified drug or medicinal substance, undetermined whether accidentally or purposely inflicted
E980.6	Poisoning by corrosive and caustic substances, undetermined whether accidentally or purposely inflicted
E980.7	Poisoning by agricultural and horticultural chemical and pharmaceutical preparations other than plant foods and fertilizers, undetermined whether accidentally or purposely inflicted
E980.8	Poisoning by arsenic and its compounds, undetermined whether accidentally or purposely inflicted
E980.9	Poisoning by other and unspecified solid and liquid substances, undetermined whether accidentally or purposely inflicted

Coding Clarification
Category E980 codes may only be reported as a secondary diagnosis.

E981   Poisoning by gases in domestic use, undetermined whether accidentally or purposely inflicted

The most common poisoning by gas distributed by pipeline is from carbon monoxide poisoning. Carbon monoxide is produced whenever pipeline gas is burned. The amount produced is usually not hazardous. Improper ventilation and malfunctioning equipment can result in a deadly amount of carbon monoxide emitted into the air. Although the lead in gas has decreased over the years, gasoline fumes can also cause short- or long-term health problems.

Supplementary Classification of External Causes

E981.0	Poisoning by gas distributed by pipeline, undetermined whether accidentally or purposely inflicted
E981.1	Poisoning by liquefied petroleum gas distributed in mobile containers, undetermined whether accidentally or purposely inflicted
E981.8	Poisoning by other utility gas, undetermined whether accidentally or purposely inflicted

Coding Clarification
Category E981 codes may only be reported as a secondary diagnosis.

E982   Poisoning by other gases, undetermined whether accidentally or purposely inflicted

Carbon monoxide poisoning can be deadly. It cannot be seen or smelled, but it can kill in just a matter of minutes. If appliances that burn fuel are not properly working, toxic levels of carbon monoxide can be produced. Accidental carbon monoxide poisoning kills hundreds of people each year. Symptoms of carbon monoxide poisoning include severe headache, dizziness, mental confusion, nausea, and fainting. Since the symptoms are similar to many other causes, carbon monoxide poisoning has been hard to diagnose. Use of carbon monoxide alarms has greatly reduced the mortality from carbon monoxide poisoning.

E982.0	Poisoning by motor vehicle exhaust gas, undetermined whether accidentally or purposely inflicted
E982.1	Poisoning by other carbon monoxide, undetermined whether accidentally or purposely inflicted
E982.8	Poisoning by other specified gases and vapors, undetermined whether accidentally or purposely inflicted
E982.9	Poisoning by unspecified gases and vapors, undetermined whether accidentally or purposely inflicted

Coding Clarification
Category E982 codes may only be reported as a secondary diagnosis.

E983   Hanging, strangulation, or suffocation, undetermined whether accidentally or purposely inflicted

Hangings can be categorized as complete where the body is totally suspended and does not touch the floor, or incomplete where some part of the body is touching the floor. The human neck is susceptible to injury due to the location of the spinal cord, airway, and major blood vessels.

E983.0	Hanging, undetermined whether accidentally or purposely inflicted
E983.1	Suffocation by plastic bag, undetermined whether accidentally or purposely inflicted
E983.8	Strangulation or suffocation by other specified means, undetermined whether accidentally or purposely inflicted
E983.9	Strangulation or suffocation by unspecified means, undetermined whether accidentally or purposely inflicted

Coding Clarification
Category E983 codes may only be reported as a secondary diagnosis.

E984   Submersion (drowning), undetermined whether accidentally or purposely inflicted

Drowning is death from suffocation after submersion that occurs within 24 hours of injury. At first a person holds his or her breath and carbon dioxide levels increase and hypoxia progresses. There are then two types of drowning: wet drowning when water is taken into the lungs and dry drowning when the patient experiences a laryngospasm. Near drowning is now more commonly referred to as a submersion accident.

Coding Clarification
Code E984 codes may only be reported as a secondary diagnosis.

E985   Injury by firearms, air guns and explosives, undetermined whether accidentally or purposely inflicted

There are a wide variety of firearms such as handguns, Derringers, revolvers, rifles, shotguns, submachine guns, and machine guns. As the primer strikes the primer compound, a fire is ignited that starts the gunpowder burning and changes it into a gas. This causes pressure to build up in the cartridge and forces the bullet down the barrel. The bullet explodes out of the gun.

Paintballs can travel up to 300 feet per second. The increased used of paintball guns over the past few years has increased the incidence of injuries. Eye injuries are the most serious and can cause permanent damage.

E985.0	Injury by handgun, undetermined whether accidentally or purposely inflicted
E985.1	Injury by shotgun, undetermined whether accidentally or purposely inflicted
E985.2	Injury by hunting rifle, undetermined whether accidentally or purposely inflicted
E985.3	Injury by military firearms, undetermined whether accidentally or purposely inflicted
E985.4	Injury by other and unspecified firearm, undetermined whether accidentally or purposely inflicted
E985.5	Injury by explosives, undetermined whether accidentally or purposely inflicted

E985.6   Injury by air gun, undetermined whether accidental,or purposefully inflicted

E985.7   Injury by paintball gun, undetermined whether accidentally or purposefully inflicted

Coding Clarification
Category E985 codes may only be reported as a secondary diagnosis.

E986   Injury by cutting and piercing instruments, undetermined whether accidentally or purposely inflicted OK

The following sharp objects can cause either accidental or purposeful injury: glass, sword, razor, switchblade, butterfly knife, automatic knife, kitchen knife, military knife, survival knife, stiletto, tonto knife, and pair of scissors. There are different types of wounds that can be caused by these various devices. An incised wound is a sharp cutting injury, usually made with a knife or broken glass, etc. In a slash wound, the length is greater than the depth. In a stab wound, the depth is greater than the length. The seriousness of the wound can range from a scratch to deep, life threatening wounds.

Coding Clarification
Code E986 codes may only be reported as a secondary diagnosis.

E987   Falling from high place, undetermined whether accidentally or purposely inflicted

Category E987 codes are used to describe falling from high places, when the cause is undetermined to be accidental or purposely inflicted. This includes falls from residential premises, other man made structures, natural sites, or an unspecified site.

E987.0   Falling from high place on residential premises, undetermined whether accidentally or purposely inflicted

E987.1   Falling from high place on other man-made structures, undetermined whether accidentally or purposely inflicted

E987.2   Falling from high place on natural sites, undetermined whether accidentally or purposely inflicted

E987.9   Falling from unspecified high place, undetermined whether accidentally or purposely inflicted

Coding Clarification
Category E987 codes may only be reported as a secondary diagnosis.

E988   Injury by other and unspecified means, undetermined whether accidentally or purposely inflicted

Chilblains are painful, small, itchy, red areas of the skin that appear on the skin after exposure to cold temperature. They are more common in cold, humid climates. Chilblains are most common on the toes but can also appear on the fingers, nose, and ears. The skin breaks down and ulcers and infection can occur. Chilblains are more common in females and can be recurrent for the rest of the patient's life or last only a few years.

Skin exposed to 140-degree water for three seconds or less may be seriously burned. Children and the elderly have skin that is more sensitive to burns.

Electrocution can cause burns and the heart to stop. High voltage contact can cause death instantly.

E988.0   Injury by jumping or lying before moving object, undetermined whether accidentally or purposely inflicted

E988.1   Injury by burns or fire, undetermined whether accidentally or purposely inflicted

E988.2   Injury by scald, undetermined whether accidentally or purposely inflicted

E988.3   Injury by extremes of cold, undetermined whether accidentally or purposely inflicted

E988.4   Injury by electrocution, undetermined whether accidentally or purposely inflicted

E988.5   Injury by crashing of motor vehicle, undetermined whether accidentally or purposely inflicted

E988.6   Injury by crashing of aircraft, undetermined whether accidentally or purposely inflicted

E988.7   Injury by caustic substances, except poisoning, undetermined whether accidentally or purposely inflicted

E988.8   Injury by other specified means, undetermined whether accidentally or purposely inflicted

E988.9   Injury by unspecified means, undetermined whether accidentally or purposely inflicted

Coding Clarification
Category E988 codes may only be reported as a secondary diagnosis.

E989   Late effects of injury, undetermined whether accidentally or purposely inflicted OK

A late effect is the residual effect that remains after the acute phase of an illness or injury has terminated. A residual is the temporary or permanent health care problem that follows the acute phase of an illness or injury. Terminology that may be found in diagnostic statements indicating a late effect include residuals of, old, sequela of, late, due to, or following previous illness or injury. There are late-effect E codes for injuries and poisonings. There are not late effect E codes for the adverse effects of drugs, misadventures, and surgical complications. The late-effect E codes should be used with any report of a late effect. Do not use a late-effect E code with a related current injury code.

This code should be used to indicate circumstances classifiable to E980-E988.

Coding Clarification
Code E989 codes may only be reported as a secondary diagnosis.

E990–E999 Injury Resulting from Operations of War

Rubric E990-E999 is used to report injury resulting from operations of war. Operations of war are injuries to military personnel and civilians caused by war and civil revolt and occurring during the time of war. Excluded from this rubric are accidents during training of military personnel, manufacture of war material, and transport, unless attributable to enemy action.

E990 Injury due to war operations by fires and conflagrations
Category E990 codes are used to report fires and conflagration due to war. Conflagration is a widespread, general burning. This includes asphyxia, burns, or other injury originating from fire caused by a fire-producing device or indirectly by any conventional weapon.

E990.0	Injury due to war operations from gasoline bomb
E990.9	Injury due to war operations from other and unspecified source

Coding Clarification
Category E990 codes may only be reported as a secondary diagnosis.

E991 Injury due to war operations by bullets and fragments
Category E991 codes are used to report injuries due to war operations by bullets and fragments. Bullets and fragments are defined as rubber bullets, pellets, machine gun bullets, pistol bullets, rifle bullets, shotgun bullets, antipersonnel bomb fragments, fragments from artillery shells, bombs, grenades, guided missiles, land mines, rockets, shells, and shrapnel.

E991.0	Injury due to war operations from rubber bullets (rifle)
E991.1	Injury due to war operations from pellets (rifle)
E991.2	Injury due to war operations from other bullets
E991.3	Injury due to war operations from antipersonnel bomb (fragments)
E991.9	Injury due to war operations from other and unspecified fragments

Coding Clarification
Category E991 codes may only be reported as a secondary diagnosis.

E992 Injury due to war operations by explosion of marine weapons OK
Code E992 is used to report an injury due to war operations by explosion of marine weapons. This includes depth charge, mine explosions at sea or in a harbor, sea-based artillery shell, torpedo, and underwater blasts.

Coding Clarification
Code E992 codes may only be reported as a secondary diagnosis.

E993 Injury due to war operations by other explosion OK
Code E993 is used to report an injury due to war operations by other explosions. This includes accidental explosion of munitions being used in war, accidental explosion of weapons, air blast, explosion of artillery shell, breechblock, cannon block, mortar bomb, and weapon burst.

Coding Clarification
Code E993 codes may only be reported as a secondary diagnosis.

E994 Injury due to war operations by destruction of aircraft OK
Code E994 is used to report an injury due to war operations by destruction of aircraft. This includes the burning or exploding of an airplane, an airplane being shot down, and being crushed by a falling airplane.

Coding Clarification
Code E994 codes may only be reported as a secondary diagnosis.

E995 Injury due to war operations by other and unspecified forms of conventional warfare OK
Code E995 is used to report an injury due to war operations by other and unspecified forms of conventional warfare. This includes battle wounds, bayonet injuries, and drowning in war operations.

Coding Clarification
Code E995 codes may only be reported as a secondary diagnosis.

E996 Injury due to war operations by nuclear weapons OK
Code E996 is used to report an injury due to war operations by nuclear weapons. Nuclear weapons have four major destructive effects: blast, thermal radiation, initial nuclear radiation, and fallout. Blasts cause an energy explosion that creates great pressure. The pressure can be equal to several thousand pounds per square inch. It crushes and

destroys objects, including the human lungs. Thermal radiation includes light and heat. There is a huge amount of light emitted from a nuclear explosion. It is bright enough to blind people many miles away and burn skin. Initial nuclear radiation contains gamma rays and neutrons. These can enter the body directly and cause radiation exposure. This will kill a person within about six to seven weeks. Fallout consists of particles from objects that become irradiated by the explosion and can lodge in different parts of the body.

Coding Clarification
Code E996 codes may only be reported as a secondary diagnosis.

E997 Injury due to war operations by other forms of unconventional warfare

A laser is an acronym for light amplification by stimulated emission of radiation. It emits intense heat and power but is only effective at close range.

Biologic warfare is intentionally using viruses, bacteria, fungi, or toxins to kill or harm people, animals, or plants.

E997.0	Injury due to war operations by lasers
E997.1	Injury due to war operations by biological warfare
E997.2	Injury due to war operations by gases, fumes, and chemicals
E997.8	Injury due to other specified forms of unconventional warfare
E997.9	Injury due to unspecified form of unconventional warfare

Coding Clarification
Category E997 codes may only be reported as a secondary diagnosis.

E998 Injury due to war operations but occurring after cessation of hostilities

Code E998 is used to report injuries due to war operations but occurring after cessation of hostilities. This includes injuries by explosion of bombs or mines placed in the course of operations of war, if the explosion occurred after the hostilities cease.

Coding Clarification
Code E998 codes may only be reported as a secondary diagnosis.

E999 Late effect of injury due to war operations and terrorism

A late effect is the residual effect that remains after the acute phase of an illness or injury has terminated. A residual is the temporary or permanent health care problem that follows the acute phase of an illness or injury. Terminology found in diagnostic statements that indicate a late effect include residuals of, old, sequela of, late, due to, or following previous illness or injury. The late-effect E codes should be used with any report of a late effect. Do not use a late-effect E code with a related current injury code. This code should be used to indicate circumstances classifiable to E979 and E990-E998.

E999.0	Late effect of injury due to war operations
E999.1	Late effect of injury due to terrorism

Coding Clarification
Category E999 codes may only be reported as a secondary diagnosis.